# Brain–Computer Interfaces Handbook

## Technological and Theoretical Advances

# Brain–Computer Interfaces Handbook

## Technological and Theoretical Advances

Edited by
Chang S. Nam
Anton Nijholt
Fabien Lotte

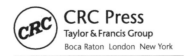

CRC Press
Taylor & Francis Group
Boca Raton London New York

CRC Press is an imprint of the
Taylor & Francis Group, an informa business

CRC Press
Taylor & Francis Group
6000 Broken Sound Parkway NW, Suite 300
Boca Raton, FL 33487-2742

First issued in paperback 2019

© 2018 by Taylor & Francis Group, LLC
CRC Press is an imprint of Taylor & Francis Group, an Informa business

No claim to original U.S. Government works

ISBN-13: 978-1-4987-7343-0 (hbk)
ISBN-13: 978-0-367-37545-4 (pbk)

**Library of Congress Cataloging-in-Publication Data**

Names: Nam, Chang S., editor. | Nijholt, Anton, 1946- editor. | Lotte, Fabien, editor.
Title: Brain-computer interfaces handbook : technological and theoretical advances / edited by Chang S. Nam, Anton Nijholt, Fabien Lotte.
Description: Boca Raton : Taylor & Francis, CRC Press, 2018. | Includes bibliographical references and index.
Identifiers: LCCN 2017035052 | ISBN 9781498773430 (hardback : alk. paper)
Subjects: LCSH: Neuroergonomics. | Brain-computer interfaces. | Self-help devices for people with disabilities. | Brain--Research. | Computer games--Equipment and supplies. | Augmented reality. | Human-machine systems.
Classification: LCC QP360.7 .B7345 2018 | DDC 612.80285--dc23
LC record available at https://lccn.loc.gov/2017035052

**Visit the Taylor & Francis Web site at
http://www.taylorandfrancis.com**

**and the CRC Press Web site at
http://www.crcpress.com**

# Contents

Foreword .................................................................................................................. xi
Preface.................................................................................................................... xiii
Handbook Website .................................................................................................. xv
Editors.................................................................................................................... xvii
Contributors .......................................................................................................... xix
Reviewers .............................................................................................................. xxv

**Introduction: Evolution of Brain–Computer Interfaces**............................................. 1
    *Fabien Lotte, Chang S. Nam, and Anton Nijholt*

## PART I    Brain–Computer Interface Applications

## SECTION A    Brain–Computer Interfaces Introduction

**Chapter 1**    Brain–Computer Interface: An Emerging Interaction Technology ........................... 11

              *Chang S. Nam, Inchul Choi, Amy Wadeson, and Mincheol Whang*

**Chapter 2**    Facilitating the Integration of Modern Neuroscience into Noninvasive BCIs........... 53

              *Mark Wronkiewicz, Eric Larson, and Adrian K.C. Lee*

**Chapter 3**    Passive Brain–Computer Interfaces: A Perspective on Increased Interactivity......... 69

              *Laurens R. Krol, Lena M. Andreessen, and Thorsten O. Zander*

## SECTION B    Therapeutic Applications

**Chapter 4**    Brain–Computer Interfaces for Motor Rehabilitation, Assessment
              of Consciousness, and Communication ...............................................................89

              *Christoph Guger, Rossella Spataro, Jitka Annen, Rupert Ortner, Danut Irimia,*
              *Brendan Allison, Vincenzo La Bella, Woosang Cho, Günter Edlinger,*
              *and Steven Laureys*

**Chapter 5**    Therapeutic Applications of BCI Technologies ...................................................... 101

              *Dennis J. McFarland*

**Chapter 6**    Advances in Neuroprosthetics: Past, Present, and Future........................................ 113

              *Stuart Mason Dambrot*

**Chapter 7**  Design and Customization of SSVEP-Based BCI Applications Aimed
              for Elderly People .............................................................................. 133

              *Piotr Stawicki, Felix Gembler, and Ivan Volosyak*

## SECTION C  *Affective and Artistic Brain–Computer Interfaces*

**Chapter 8**  Affective Brain–Computer Interfacing and Methods for Affective State
              Detection .......................................................................................... 147

              *Ian Daly*

**Chapter 9**  Toward Practical BCI Solutions for Entertainment and Art Performance ............... 165

              *Paruthi Pradhapan, Ulf Großekathöfer, Giuseppina Schiavone,*
              *Bernard Grundlehner, and Vojkan Mihajlović*

**Chapter 10**  BCI for Music Making: Then, Now, and Next .......................................... 193

              *Duncan A.H. Williams and Eduardo R. Miranda*

## SECTION D  *BCI Control of Entertainment and Multimedia*

**Chapter 11**  BCI and Games: Playful, Experience-Oriented Learning by Vivid Feedback? ...... 209

              *Silvia E. Kober, Manuel Ninaus, Elisabeth V.C. Friedrich, and Reinhold Scherer*

**Chapter 12**  Brain–Computer Interfaces for Mediating Interaction in Virtual
              and Augmented Reality ..................................................................... 235

              *Josef Faller, Neil Weiss, Nicholas Waytowich, and Paul Sajda*

**Chapter 13**  Brain–Computer Interfaces and Haptics: A Literature Review .............................. 253

              *Jan B.F. van Erp*

## PART II  *Signal Acquisition and Open Source Platform in BCI*

**Chapter 14**  Utilizing Subdermal Electrodes as a Noninvasive Alternative
              for Motor-Based BCIs ....................................................................... 269

              *Melissa M. Smith, Jared D. Olson, Felix Darvas, and Rajesh P.N. Rao*

**Chapter 15**  Validation of Neurotrophic Electrode Long-Term Recordings in Human Cortex .... 279

              *Philip R. Kennedy, Dinal S. Andreasen, Jess Bartels, Princewill Ehirim,*
              *Edward Joe Wright, Steven Seibert, and Andre Joel Cervantes*

**Chapter 16**  ECoG-Based BCIs ............................................................................... 297

Aysegul Gunduz and Gerwin Schalk

**Chapter 17**  BCI Software .................................................................................... 323

Peter Brunner and Gerwin Schalk

## PART III    Signal Processing, Feature Extraction, and Classification in BCI

**Chapter 18**  Gentle Introduction to Signal Processing and Classification for Single-Trial
EEG Analysis ................................................................................... 343

Benjamin Blankertz

**Chapter 19**  Riemannian Classification for SSVEP-Based BCI: Offline versus Online
Implementations ............................................................................... 371

Sylvain Chevallier, Emmanuel K. Kalunga, Quentin Barthélemy,
and Florian Yger

**Chapter 20**  The Fundamentals of Signal Processing for Evoked Potential BCIs:
A Guided Tutorial .............................................................................. 397

Garett D. Johnson and Dean J. Krusienski

**Chapter 21**  Bayesian Learning for EEG Analysis ................................................ 407

Yu Zhang

**Chapter 22**  Transfer Learning for BCIs ............................................................... 425

Vinay Jayaram, Karl-Heinz Fiebig, Jan Peters, and Moritz Grosse-Wentrup

## PART IV    Brain–Computer Interface Paradigms

**Chapter 23**  A Step-by-Step Tutorial for a Motor Imagery–Based BCI ..................... 445

Hohyun Cho, Minkyu Ahn, Moonyoung Kwon, and Sung Chan Jun

**Chapter 24**  Eye Gaze Collaboration with Brain–Computer Interfaces: Using Both
Modalities for More Robust Interaction ................................................ 461

Gaye Lightbody, Chris P. Brennan, Paul J. McCullagh, and Leo Galway

**Chapter 25** Designing a BCI Stimulus Presentation Paradigm Using a Performance-Based
Approach ...................................................................................................................487

Boyla O. Mainsah, Leslie M. Collins, and Chandra S. Throckmorton

**Chapter 26** Issues and Challenges in Designing P300 and SSVEP Paradigms...........................501

Ali Haider and Reza Fazel-Rezai

**Chapter 27** Hybrid Brain–Computer Interfaces and Their Applications ....................................525

Jiahui Pan and Yuanqing Li

**Chapter 28** Augmenting Attention with Brain–Computer Interfaces.........................................549

Mehdi Ordikhani-Seyedlar and Mikhail A. Lebedev

## PART V   Human Factors, Design, and Evaluation in BCI

**Chapter 29** Toward Usability Evaluation for Brain–Computer Interfaces ..................................563

Ilsun Rhiu, Yushin Lee, Inchul Choi, Myung Hwan Yun, and Chang S. Nam

**Chapter 30** Why User-Centered Design Is Relevant for Brain–Computer Interfacing
and How It Can Be Implemented in Study Protocols ...............................................585

Sonja C. Kleih and Andrea Kübler

**Chapter 31** A Generic Framework for Adaptive EEG-Based BCI Training and Operation ......595

Jelena Mladenović, Jérémie Mattout, and Fabien Lotte

**Chapter 32** Mind the Traps! Design Guidelines for Rigorous BCI Experiments ......................613

Camille Jeunet, Stefan Debener, Fabien Lotte, Jérémie Mattout,
Reinhold Scherer, and Catharina Zich

**Chapter 33** Evaluation and Performance Assessment of the Brain–Computer
Interface System ......................................................................................................635

Md Rakibul Mowla, Jane E. Huggins, and David E. Thompson

## PART VI   Emerging Issues and Future BCIs

**Chapter 34** Privacy and Ethics in Brain–Computer Interface Research ...................................653

Eran Klein and Alan Rubel

**Chapter 35** Associative Plasticity Induced by a Brain–Computer Interface Based on Movement-Related Cortical Potentials ................................................................ 669

*Natalie Mrachacz-Kersting, Ning Jiang, Kim Dremstrup, and Dario Farina*

**Chapter 36** Past and Future of Multi-Mind Brain–Computer Interfaces .................................... 685

*Davide Valeriani and Ana Matran-Fernandez*

**Chapter 37** Bidirectional Neural Interfaces .............................................................................. 701

*Mikhail A. Lebedev and Alexei Ossadtchi*

**Chapter 38** Perspectives on Brain–Computer Interfaces ........................................................... 721

*Gerwin Schalk*

**Conclusion: Moving Forward in Brain–Computer Interfaces** ................................................. 725
*Chang S. Nam, Fabien Lotte, and Anton Nijholt*

**Author Index** ............................................................................................................................ 727

**Subject Index** .......................................................................................................................... 761

# Foreword

This rich and varied volume is a significant milestone in the continuing emergence of brain–computer interface (BCI) research and development as a new field with major scientific, clinical, and societal ramifications. Over the past 15 years, many BCI review articles have appeared, and several BCI textbooks have been published. Nevertheless, this handbook recognizes and confirms the new field in a further way as a unique new region of scientific and technical endeavor. Its sections are replete with detailed information about the nature of BCI technologies; about their essential principles, major goals, and most difficult challenges; and about both established and newly developing research endeavors. Together, they describe, essentially in the nature of a travel guide, what might be termed the Country of BCI. The handbook moves beyond theory and principles and prototypical examples—that is, beyond the standard substance of review articles and textbooks—to demarcate and populate the principal regions of the country and describe the kinds and centers of activity in this new territory, both the well-established hubs and the emerging settlements.

The handbook pays ample attention to the traditional BCI focus on restoring communication and control and also features the newer and very exciting focus on BCI-based rehabilitation for stroke and other disorders. For several reasons, this application may well prove to be the most important BCI use over the next several decades. BCIs that enhance recovery of function could help the many millions of people disabled by strokes, traumatic brain and spinal cord injuries, and other chronic neuromuscular disorders. Furthermore, unlike BCIs intended for important communication and control purposes—which need to be perfect or nearly perfect—BCIs intended for rehabilitation need only to enhance the results achieved with other rehabilitation methodology. Thus, the threshold for their effectiveness and widespread adoption is likely to be more readily achieved. The handbook also features important emerging areas, some overtly therapeutic, and some not. Thus, chapters discuss the new category of affective BCIs, and others describe BCIs for composing music or playing computer games. In chapters devoted to BCI methods and research practices, and also in the chapters addressing specific BCI applications, the handbook emphasizes and illustrates fundamental principles and critical caveats that distinguish serious BCI research and are essential for its success. The importance of appropriate signal processing, of recognizing and avoiding the impact of artifacts, of adequate online testing, and of focusing on the capacities and needs of the individual user is explicated and illustrated. In addition, the ethical issues involved in BCI research, both therapeutic and nontherapeutic, are considered.

The aggregate impact of the profuse and varied information provided by the handbook conveys to the reader what is unique and fundamental about this new field and what is most important for operating effectively in this new territory. In doing so, it demarcates the field very clearly and thereby separates and protects it from contamination by endeavors or technologies that do not adhere to the key principles and caveats it brings out. This is particularly important in view of the prominence of commercial devices that simply record electrical activity of some undefined kind from the head and purport to be BCIs, without incorporating the fundamental principles that define BCIs—systems that provide the CNS with new, non-muscular output channels through which to act on the world. By setting out the size, complexity, and standards of this new field, this handbook effectively charts the scientific and technological environment of BCI research and development. It constitutes a distinctive contribution that advances and recognizes the remarkably rapid maturation of this exciting new field.

**Jonathan R. Wolpaw, M.D.**
*National Center for Adaptive Neurotechnologies*
*Wadsworth Center*
*New York State Department of Health*
*120 New Scotland Avenue*
*Albany, New York 12208*
*Voice: 518-473-3631*
*Fax: 518-486-4910*
*Email: jonathan.wolpaw@health.ny.gov*

# Preface

Brain–computer interface (BCI) uses devices that enable their users to interact with computers and machines by using only their brain activity, which is measured and processed by the system. This handbook provides researchers, students, and practitioners, including those with no formal training in BCI research and development, with a synopsis of key findings, and theoretical and technical advances from BCI-related fields that have direct bearing on human brain–computer interfacing. Many BCI applications currently exist, allowing users to perform tasks such as writing sentences by selecting letters, moving a cursor on a computer screen, playing an electronic ping-pong game, and controlling an orthosis that provides a graspable hand. BCIs are also used to study the human brain in relation to performance at work, transportation, and other everyday settings, which can provide important guidelines and constraints for theories of information presentation and task design. These research approaches also aim at applications that are not necessarily in the clinical field and for impaired users. It is making BCI use possible for new potential user groups such as gamers and for applications in the domestic domain, human–computer interaction, robotics, and team performance.

This handbook is organized into an introductory chapter with an emphasis on BCI technology trend and historical events that paved the way for flourishing BCI technology, six main parts, and a conclusion chapter. Part I opens with various BCI applications and consists of four sections in which BCI introductory (Section A), therapeutic application (Section B), affective and artistic application (Section C), and BCI control of entertainment and multimedia application (Section D) chapters are presented. Part II focuses on the different ways to acquire brain signals and a summary of BCI software. Part III deals with various methods to process acquired brain signals, extract features, and classify the user's intention. Part IV is devoted to various BCI paradigms including guided tutorial chapters. Part V presents five chapters that discuss various issues associated with human factors, design, and evaluation of BCI systems. Part VI, consisting of four chapters, presents emerging issues and future BCI research directions. This book wraps up with final thoughts on what is on the horizon for BCI research and development and a variety of strategies and tasks that BCI researchers must take into account.

It is our hope that our readers will find something new and/or valuable in this handbook. We notably hope that, thanks to this book, readers would better understand the underlying neural bases of human brains, possess new insights into interfacing human brains with computing systems, and subsequently appreciate the opportunities afforded by BCI research and development.

We thank the contributing authors for their commitment to the success of this handbook, and we are honored to have worked with each one of contributors. We would also like to thank the many reviewers who contributed their time and expertise reviewing this handbook's chapters, thus improving the overall book quality. The production of the handbook was made possible with the very valuable assistance of Cindy Carelli (Taylor & Francis Acquiring Editor), Renee Nakash (Taylor & Francis Editorial Assistant), and Jonathan Achorn (MTC Project Manager), who so effectively coordinated the management of contributions.

**Chang S. Nam**
**Anton Nijholt**
**Fabien Lotte**

MATLAB® is a registered trademark of The MathWorks, Inc. For product information, please contact:

The MathWorks, Inc.
3 Apple Hill Drive
Natick, MA 01760-2098 USA
Tel: (508) 647-7000
Fax: (508) 647-7001
E-mail: info@mathworks.com
Web: www.mathworks.com

# Handbook Website

Additional material related to this handbook can be found at https://www.ise.ncsu.edu/bci/bci-handbook/, including

- Electronic versions of all figures, including high-quality color images where appropriate
- An expended index with additional keywords
- Other supplementary material

# Editors

**Chang S. Nam** is an associate professor of Edward P. Fitts Industrial and Systems Engineering at North Carolina State University, USA. He is also an associate professor of the UNC/NCSU Joint Department of Biomedical Engineering as well as the Department of Psychology. He received a PhD from the Grado Department of Industrial and Systems Engineering at Virginia Tech in 2003. Dr. Nam is the author or coauthor of more than 100 research publications including journal articles, books, book chapters, and conference proceedings. Dr. Nam's research interests center on brain–computer interface and rehabilitation, wearable sensor-based remote healthcare, neuroergonomics, neuroadaptive automation in large-scale unmanned aerial vehicles, and haptic–user interaction. His research has been supported by federal agencies including the National Science Foundation (NSF), the Air Force Research Laboratory, and the National Security Agency. Dr. Nam has received the NSF CAREER Award, Outstanding Researcher Award, and Best Teacher Award. Currently, Dr. Nam serves as the editor-in-chief of the journal *Brain–Computer Interfaces*.

**Anton Nijholt** is professor emeritus of the University of Twente, the Netherlands, and research fellow at the Imagineering Institute in Iskandar, Malaysia. He studied mathematics at Delft University of Technology and received a PhD in computer science from the Vrije Universiteit, Amsterdam. He held positions at McMaster University, Canada, University of Twente, Nijmegen University, and Vrije Universiteit Brussels, before becoming full professor at the University of Twente, where he established the Human Media Interaction research group. He supervised more than 50 PhD students in natural language processing, human–computer interaction, multi-party interaction, and brain–computer interfacing. His research has been supported by regional, national, and EU research agencies. Nijholt is the author of hundreds of research papers and he is the editor of books on brain–computer interfaces, entertainment computing, playful interfaces, and playable cities. Nijholt was research fellow at the Netherlands Institute for Advanced Study in the Humanities and Social Sciences, and for several years, he acted as an adviser for Philips Research. Nijholt also acted as general or program chair of all main international conferences on entertainment computing, virtual agents, affective computing and multimodal interaction. Currently, he is the editor of the Springer book series on Gaming Media and Social Effects, the specialty chief editor of the Human–Media Interaction section of the journal *Frontiers in Psychology*, and a member of editorial boards of various other journals.

**Fabien Lotte** has been a research scientist (with tenure) at Inria Bordeaux Sud-Ouest, France, since 2011. He obtained an MSc, a MEng, and a PhD degree in computer science, all from the National Institute of Applied Sciences, Rennes, France, in 2005 (MSc, MEng) and 2008 (PhD). In 2009 and 2010, he was a research fellow at the Institute for Infocomm Research in Singapore, working in the Brain–Computer Interface Laboratory. His research interests include brain–computer interfaces (BCI), human–computer interaction, pattern recognition, and brain signal processing. He is the author or coauthor of about 100 publications, several of which published in the best journals (e.g., *Journal of Neural Engineering, IEEE Transactions on Biomedical Engineering, Proceedings of the IEEE, IEEE Transactions on Signal Processing*, etc.) and conferences (ICASSP, UIST, CHI, etc.) in these fields. His PhD thesis received both the PhD Thesis award 2009 from AFRIF (French Association for Pattern Recognition) and the PhD Thesis award 2009 accessit (2nd prize) from ASTI (French Association for Information Sciences and Technologies). His research is supported, among others, by Inria, the French National Research Agency (ANR) and the European Research Council (ERC). He is part of the editorial boards of the journals *Brain–Computer Interfaces* and *Journal of Neural Engineering*.

# Contributors

**Minkyu Ahn**
School of Computer Science and Electrical
  Engineering
Handong Global University
Pohang, South Korea

**Brendan Allison**
g.tec medical engineering GmbH
Schiedlberg, Austria

**Dinal S. Andreasen**
Georgia Research Institute
Atlanta, Georgia

**Lena M. Andreessen**
Biological Psychology and Neuroergonomics
Technische Universität Berlin
Berlin, Germany

**Jitka Annen**
University Hospital of Liége
Liége, Belgium

**Jess Bartels**
Neural Signals Inc.
Duluth, Georgia

**Quentin Barthélemy**
Mensia Technologies S.A.
Paris, France

**Vincenzo La Bella**
University of Palermo
Palermo, Italy

**Benjamin Blankertz**
Neurotechnology Group
Technische Universität Berlin
Berlin, Germany

**Chris P. Brennan**
Smart Environments Research Group
Ulster University
Coleraine, United Kingdom

**Peter Brunner**
Department of Neurology
Albany Medical College
Albany, New York

**Andre Joel Cervantes**
Neurosurgical and Spinal Services Associates
Belize City, Belize

**Sylvain Chevallier**
LISV
Université de Versailles St Quentin
Versailles, France

**Hohyun Cho**
School of Electrical Engineering and Computer
  Science
Gwangju Institute of Science and Technology
Gwangju, South Korea

**Woosang Cho**
g.tec medical engineering GmbH
Schiedlberg, Austria

**Inchul Choi**
Department of Industrial and Systems
  Engineering
North Carolina State University
Raleigh, North Carolina

**Leslie M. Collins**
Department of Electrical and Computer
  Engineering
Duke University
Durham, North Carolina

**Ian Daly**
Brain–Computer Interfacing and Neural
  Engineering Laboratory
University of Essex
Colchester, United Kingdom

**Stuart Mason Dambrot**
Brain–Machine Interface Consortium
New York

**Felix Darvas**
Department of Neurosurgery
University of Washington
Seattle, Washington

**Stefan Debener**
Neuropsychology Lab/Cluster of Excellence/
    Research Center Neurosensory Systems
University of Oldenburg
Oldenburg, Germany

**Kim Dremstrup**
Department of Health Science and Technology
Aalborg University
Aalborg, Denmark

**Günter Edlinger**
g.tec medical engineering GmbH
Schiedlberg, Austria

**Princewill Ehirim**
Department of Neurosurgery
Gwinnett Medical Center
Lawrenceville, Georgia

**Josef Faller**
Department of Biomedical Engineering
Columbia University
New York

**Dario Farina**
Department of Bioengineering
Imperial College London
London, United Kingdom

**Reza Fazel-Rezai**
Department of Electrical Engineering
University of North Dakota
Grand Forks, North Dakota

**Karl-Heinz Fiebig**
Department of Computer Science
Technische Universität Darmstadt
Darmstadt, Germany

**Elisabeth V.C. Friedrich**
Department of Psychology
Ludwig-Maximilians-University Munich
Munich, Germany

**Leo Galway**
Smart Environments Research Group
Ulster University
Coleraine, United Kingdom

**Felix Gembler**
Rhine-Waal University of Applied Sciences
Kleve, Germany

**Ulf Großekathöfer**
Holst Centre/imec
Eindhoven, The Netherlands

**Moritz Grosse-Wentrup**
Institute of Statistics
Ludwig-Maximilian-Universität München
Munich, Germany

and

Department Empirical Inference
Max Planck Institute for Intelligent Systems
Tübingen, Germany

**Bernard Grundlehner**
Holst Centre/imec
Eindhoven, The Netherlands

**Christoph Guger**
Guger Technologies OG
g.tec medical engineering GmbH
Schiedlberg, Austria

**Aysegul Gunduz**
J. Crayton Pruitt Family Department
    of Biomedical Engineering
University of Florida
Gainesville, Florida

**Ali Haider**
Department of Electrical Engineering
University of North Dakota
Grand Forks, North Dakota

**Jane E. Huggins**
Department of Physical Medicine
    and Rehabilitation
University of Michigan
Ann Arbor, Michigan

**Danut Irimia**
g.tec medical engineering GmbH
Schiedlberg, Austria

**Vinay Jayaram**
Department of Empirical Inference
Max Planck Institute for Intelligent Systems
Tübingen, Germany

**Camille Jeunet**
Inria
Rennes, France

and

École Polytechnique Fédérale de Lausanne
Lausanne, Switzerland

**Ning Jiang**
Department of Systems Design Engineering
University of Waterloo
Waterloo, Ontario, Canada

**Garett D. Johnson**
Biomedical Engineering
Old Dominion University
Norfolk, Virginia

**Sung Chan Jun**
School of Electrical Engineering and Computer
  Science
Gwangju Institute of Science and Technology
Gwangju, South Korea

**Emmanuel K. Kalunga**
LISV
Université de Versailles St Quentin
Versailles, France

**Philip R. Kennedy**
Neural Signals Inc.
Duluth, Georgia

**Sonja C. Kleih**
Department of Psychology I
University of Würzburg
Würzburg, Germany

**Eran Klein**
Department of Neurology
Oregon Health and Science University
Portland, Oregon

**Silvia E. Kober**
Department of Psychology
University of Graz
Graz, Austria

**Laurens R. Krol**
Biological Psychology and Neuroergonomics
Technische Universität Berlin
Berlin, Germany

**Dean J. Krusienski**
Department of Electrical and Computer
  Engineering/Biomedical Engineering
Old Dominion University
Norfolk, Virginia

**Andrea Kübler**
Department of Psychology I
University of Würzburg
Würzburg, Germany

**Moonyoung Kwon**
School of Electrical Engineering and Computer
  Science
Gwangju Institute of Science and Technology
Gwangju, South Korea

**Eric Larson**
Institute for Learning & Brain Sciences
  (I-LABS)
University of Washington
Seattle, Washington

**Steven Laureys**
University Hospital of Liége
Liége, Belgium

**Mikhail A. Lebedev**
Department of Neurobiology
Duke University
Durham, North Carolina

**Adrian K.C. Lee**
Department of Speech and Hearing Sciences
University of Washington
Seattle, Washington

**Yushin Lee**
Department of Industrial Engineering
Seoul National University
Seoul, South Korea

**Yuanqing Li**
School of Automation Science and Engineering
South China University of Technology
and
Guangzhou Key Laboratory of Brain Computer
    Interface and Applications
Guangzhou, China

**Gaye Lightbody**
Smart Environments Research Group
Ulster University
Coleraine, United Kingdom

**Fabien Lotte**
Inria Bordeaux Sud-Ouest/LaBRI, team Potioc
Rennes, France

**Boyla O. Mainsah**
Department of Electrical and Computer
    Engineering
Duke University
Durham, North Carolina

**Ana Matran-Fernandez**
School of Computer Science and Electronic
    Engineering
University of Essex
Colchester, United Kingdom

**Jérémie Mattout**
Brain Dynamics and Cognition
Inserm Lyon
Lyon, France

**Paul J. McCullagh**
Smart Environments Research Group
Ulster University
Coleraine, United Kingdom

**Dennis J. McFarland**
National Center for Adaptive
    Neurotechnologies
Wadsworth Center
New York State Department of Health
Albany, New York

**Vojkan Mihajlović**
Holst Centre/imec
Eindhoven, The Netherlands

**Eduardo R. Miranda**
Interdisciplinary Center for Computer Music
    Research
Plymouth University
Plymouth, United Kingdom

**Jelena Mladenović**
Computer Science
Inria Bordeaux and Inserm Lyon
Lyon, France

**Md Rakibul Mowla**
Department of Electrical and Computer
    Engineering
Kansas State University
Manhattan, Kansas

**Natalie Mrachacz-Kersting**
Department of Health Science and Technology
Aalborg University
Aalborg, Denmark

**Chang S. Nam**
Department of Industrial and Systems
    Engineering
North Carolina State University
Raleigh, North Carolina

**Anton Nijholt**
Faculty Electrical Engineering, Mathematics
    and Computer Science
University of Twente
Enschede, The Netherlands

**Manuel Ninaus**
Leibniz-Institut für Wissensmedien
Tuebingen, Germany

**Jared D. Olson**
Department of Rehabilitation Medicine
University of Washington
Seattle, Washington

**Mehdi Ordikhani-Seyedlar**
Laboratory for Investigative Neurophysiology
Department of Radiology and Department
  of Clinical Neurosciences
The University Hospital Center and University
  of Lausanne
Lausanne, Switzerland

**Rupert Ortner**
g.tec medical engineering GmbH
Schiedlbcrg, Austria

**Alexei Ossadtchi**
Centre for Cognition and Decision Making
and
Faculty of Computer Science
National Research University Higher School
  of Economics
Moscow, Russian Federation

**Jiahui Pan**
School of Software
South China Normal University
and
School of Automation Science and Engineering
South China University of Technology
Guangzhou, China

**Jan Peters**
Department of Computer Science
Technische Universität Darmstadt
Darmstadt, Germany

**Paruthi Pradhapan**
Holst Centre/imec
Eindhoven, The Netherlands

**Rajesh P.N. Rao**
Department of Computer Science and
  Engineering
University of Washington
Seattle, Washington

**Ilsun Rhiu**
Division of Global Management Engineering
Hoseo University
Asan, South Korea

**Alan Rubel**
Information School
Center for Law, Justice, & Society
University of Wisconsin–Madison
Madison, Wisconsin

**Paul Sajda**
Department of Biomedical Engineering
Columbia University
New York

**Gerwin Schalk**
National Center for Adaptive Neurotechnologies
Wadsworth Center, New York State
  Department of Health
Albany, New York

**Reinhold Scherer**
Institute for Neural Engineering
Graz University of Technology
Graz, Austria

**Giuseppina Schiavone**
Holst Centre/imec
Eindhoven, The Netherlands

**Steven Seibert**
Neural Signals Inc.
Duluth, Georgia

**Melissa M. Smith**
Department of Computer Science and
  Engineering
University of Washington
Seattle, Washington

**Rossella Spataro**
University of Palermo
Palermo, Italy

**Piotr Stawicki**
Rhine-Waal University of Applied Sciences
Kleve, Germany

**David E. Thompson**
Department of Electrical and Computer
   Engineering
Kansas State University
Manhattan, Kansas

**Chandra S. Throckmorton**
Department of Electrical and Computer
   Engineering
Duke University
Durham, North Carolina

**Davide Valeriani**
School of Computer Science and Electronic
   Engineering
University of Essex
Colchester, United Kingdom

**Jan B.F. van Erp**
Department Human Media Interaction
University of Twente
Enschede, The Netherlands

**Ivan Volosyak**
Rhine-Waal University of Applied Sciences
Kleve, Germany

**Amy Wadeson**
Department of Industrial and Systems
   Engineering
North Carolina State University
Raleigh, North Carolina

**Nicholas Waytowich**
Department of Biomedical Engineering
Columbia University
New York

and

Human Research and Engineering Directorate
US Army Research Laboratory
Aberdeen Proving Ground, Maryland

**Neil Weiss**
Department of Biomedical Engineering
Columbia University
New York

**Mincheol Whang**
Department of Digital Media Engineering
Sangmyung University
Seoul, South Korea

**Duncan A.H. Williams**
Digital Creativity Labs
University of York
York, United Kingdom

**Edward Joe Wright**
Neural Signals Inc.
Duluth, Georgia

**Mark Wronkiewicz**
Graduate Program in Neuroscience
University of Washington
Seattle, Washington

**Florian Yger**
LAMSADE, CNRS
Université Paris-Dauphine, PSL Research
   University
Paris, France

**Myung Hwan Yun**
Department of Industrial Engineering
Seoul National University
Seoul, South Korea

**Thorsten O. Zander**
Biological Psychology and Neuroergonomics
Technische Universität Berlin
Berlin, Germany

**Yu Zhang**
East China University of Science and
   Technology
Shanghai, China

**Catharina Zich**
Neuropsychology Lab
University of Oldenburg
Oldenburg, Germany

and

Department of Experimental Psychology
University of Oxford
Oxford, United Kingdom

# Reviewers

To ensure the high-quality content of this book, in addition to being reviewed by the editors, all submitted chapters were reviewed by other scientists from the field as well. Most of these reviewers were also contributors to this book, but we also got reviews from external experts who did not contribute a chapter to the book. We would like to thank all of them here for their help and hard work, which certainly contributed to improving the quality of this handbook. Please find below a list of all the reviewers who contributed to this handbook of BCI, in alphabetical order:

| | |
|---|---|
| Brendan Allison | Boyla Mainsah |
| Marvin Andujar | Jérémie Mattout |
| Saugat Bhattacharya | Dennis McFarland |
| Benjamin Blankertz | Vojkan Mihajlović |
| Peter Brunner | Jelena Mladenovic |
| Sylvain Chevallier | Md Rakibul Mowla |
| Ian Daly | Natalie Mrachacz-Kersting |
| Stuart M. Dambrot | Ilsun Rhiu |
| Reza Fazel-Rezai | Paul Sajda |
| Christoph Guger | Reinhold Scherer |
| Keum-Shik Hong | Melissa Smith |
| Camille Jeunet | Piotr Stawicki |
| Philip Kennedy | Davide Valeriani |
| Pieter-Jan Kindermans | Jan van Erp |
| Sonja Kleih | Aleksandra Vuckovic |
| Eran Klein | Duncan Williams |
| Laurens R. Krol | Ellen Wittenberg |
| Mikhail Lebedev | Mark Wronkiewicz |
| Yuanqing Li | HaiHong Zhang |
| Gaye Lightbody | Yu Zhang |

# Introduction: Evolution of Brain–Computer Interfaces

*Fabien Lotte, Chang S. Nam, and Anton Nijholt*

Brain–computer interfaces (BCIs) are systems that translate a measure of a user's brain activity into messages or commands for an interactive application. A typical example of a BCI is a system that enables a user to move a ball on a computer screen toward the left or toward the right, by imagining left- or right-hand movement, respectively. The very term BCI was coined in the 1970s, and since then, interest and research efforts in BCIs have grown tremendously, with possibly hundreds of laboratories around the world studying this topic. This has resulted in a very large number of paradigms, methods, concepts, and applications of such technology. This handbook thus aims at providing an overview and tutorials of the multiple and rich facets of BCIs.

As an introduction to this vast endeavor, we a short and brief history of BCIs, in order to explain where they come from. Figure I.1 illustrates BCI technology trends and historical events. Since we are no historians of science, such a historical introduction is likely to be incomplete and biased, according to our background, views, and (conscious or not) preferences. Nonetheless, we hope this will enable the readers to get a quick overview of the development in BCIs these last 30 or 40 years and will motivate them to learn more about BCI concepts, which this handbook should make easier.

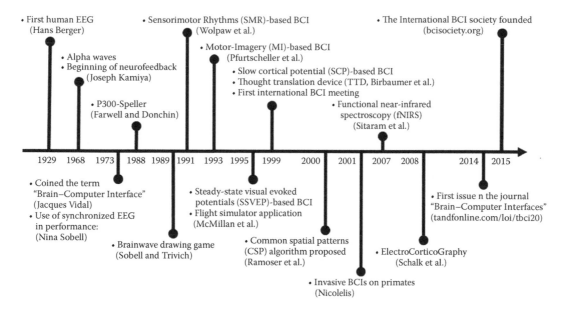

**FIGURE I.1**    BCI technology and historical events

1

## THE ORIGINS

In the 1920s, a German scientist named Hans Berger was the first to show that the human brain was producing electrical currents. Such currents reflected brain activity and could be measured on the scalp using electrodes: the concept of electroencephalography (EEG) was born (Berger 1929). EEG proved a key tool in neuroscience, notably to study cognitive functions and their neural correlates, for understanding or diagnosing neuropathologies. With the development of EEG, the idea that brain activity could be used as a communication channel or carrier of information also rapidly emerged. Kamiya, in 1968, has notably showed that features of EEG activity—in his studies he considered alpha waves—could purposely be controlled by a human subject after some training (Kamiya 1968). This was the beginning of neurofeedback, a field interested in training users to self-regulate their brain activity thanks to real-time feedback about this activity. This led artists to consider using EEG in their performances. For instance, in the early 1970s, artist Nina Sobell provided participants with a visualization of their synchronized brain activity, to encourage them to get synchronized EEG features (Sobell 2002) (see also Nijholt 2016 for more history on BCI and arts). Then, in 1973, a seminal paper by Jacques J. Vidal, a Belgium researcher working at the University of California in Los Angeles, coined the term "Brain–Computer Interface" (Vidal 1973). In particular, Vidal describe BCIs as "utilizing the brain signals in a man–computer dialogue" and "as a mean of control over external processes such as computers or prosthetic devices." Only the concepts were proposed at that time—implementations were ongoing—but the vision and several ideas proposed at that time are still explored and followed today.

While the field stayed kind of dormant in the 1970s and early 1980s, the end of the 1980s and the beginning of the 1990s saw a handful of researchers from the United States and Europe pioneering the BCI field, by proposing the first real-time and working BCI implementations, which defined several of the major paradigms used today.

## THE PIONEERS

In 1988, Farwell and Donchin published another seminal paper, which proposed the now very famous and widely used BCI paradigm known as the "P300 speller" (Farwell & Donchin 1988). More specifically, they proposed a BCI for spelling letters based on event-related potentials (ERP), which are EEG deflections in response to a specific event or stimulus. In the P300 speller, a $6 \times 6$ grid of letters and digits is displayed on a computer screen. The rows and columns of this grid are randomly flashing, and the user is asked to count the number of times the letter he wants to spell is flashed. This way, each time the target letter is flashed, this triggers an ERP known as the P300 in the user's EEG signals, which can be detected. After several flash repetitions, it thus becomes possible to detect which row and which column contains the letter the user wants to spell and thus to select this letter. Although this system was tested on healthy users only at that time, this showed that BCIs could potentially be used to enable severely paralyzed users to communicate and interact with their environment. In fact, the main driving force behind BCI research at that time, and still a major motivation today, was to use them as a new assistive technology for motor-impaired users and notably for those that may not have access to any alternative one.

Not long after, both in the United States and in Europe, researchers developed BCIs based on sensorimotor rhythms (SMR), that is, based on the oscillatory EEG activity and notably the mu rhythm (~7–13 Hz) over the sensorimotor part of the cortex. In the United States, Jonathan Wolpaw and his colleagues developed a BCI for 1D cursor control based on operant conditioning (Wolpaw et al. 1991). With this approach, users were trained to voluntarily self-regulate the amplitude of their SMR activity in order to move a ball up or down. This was made possible by using neurofeedback, that is, by displaying to users their SMR activity in real time, so that they can learn to modulate it. At about the same time in Europe, in Austria, Gert Pfurtscheller and his team were developing another SMR-based BCI, in which users had to explicitly imagine left- or right-hand movements that were translated into a command for the computer by using machine learning (Pfurtscheller et al. 1993). This defined the so-called motor imagery–based BCIs.

Still in Europe, and during the same period, Niels Birbaumer and his colleagues were working on a third type of BCI paradigm: BCIs based on slow cortical potential (SCP). SCPs are low-frequency variations of EEG signal amplitude, whose amplitude can be voluntarily increased or decreased using training and neurofeedback. This principle was used to design the "Thought Translation Device" (TTD), which enables a user to select one group of commands or another by respectively increasing or decreasing the SCP amplitude. The TTD was notably used by paralyzed users to spell letters (Birbaumer et al. 1999). The idea was to use the SCP-BCI to select between two groups of letters. The selected letter group was then divided into two subgroups and the process was repeated until only one letter remains in each group, so that they can be selected, enabling the user to communicate by brain activity alone. While SCP-BCIs are not really used anymore, owing to generally inferior performances, the TTD showed that BCIs were promising tools for severely paralyzed users.

While it did not get as much visibility at that time and even after, Jose Principe and his colleagues also developed an ERP-based BCI at that time in the United States. They developed the so-called cortical mouse, which enables a user to select one command among two based on the N400 response to a congruent or incongruent stimulus sentence (Childers et al. 1989; Konger et al. 1990; Principe 2013).

These pioneering groups essentially defined the BCI field and are all prominent figures in BCI research nowadays. Their work sparked the rapid increase in BCI research that follows the years after.

## THE BLOOM OF A RESEARCH FIELD

The end of the last century and the beginning of the new one saw BCI research becoming a research field on its own, with many new research groups joining the efforts and making the field evolve rapidly. New BCI paradigms were proposed, such as BCIs based on steady-state visual evoked potentials (SSVEPs). SSVEPs are oscillatory EEG activity whose frequency is synchronized to that of a flickering visual stimulus, to which the user pays attention. By using several stimuli, each with a specific flickering frequency, the specific SSVEP response to each of them can be associated to a specific BCI command. Such an SSVEP BCI was notably used to control the left and right movement of a plane in a flight simulator, using two different flickering lights situated on the left and right of the cockpit (McMillan et al. 1995).

While machine learning was already used for BCIs, more advanced and BCI-specific machine learning tools were proposed by different groups at that time to classify EEG signals in a more robust way, using, for example, support vector machines or neural classifiers (Anderson et al. 1996; Blankertz et al. 2002; Millan et al. 2002). The famous common spatial pattern (CSP) spatial filtering algorithm, which is still kind of a gold standard today, was also proposed back then (Ramoser et al. 2000).

At the same time, research in invasive BCIs on primates was starting. We can notably cite the work of the Nicolelis group, which showed that first rats and then monkeys could control a robotic arm using neural signals recorded directly from their motor cortex neurons, that is, with electrodes implanted in their brains (Chapin et al. 1999; Nicolelis 2001).

BCI research groups started at that time to organize themselves as a full research community, with notably the first International BCI meeting that took place in the United States in 1999 (Wolpaw et al. 2000). About 50 participants from 22 research groups participated. At that time, BCIs were defined as "a communication system in which messages or commands that an individual sends to the external world do not pass through the brain's normal output pathways of peripheral nerves and muscles" (Wolpaw et al. 2002).*

## MODERN HISTORY

From that time to about now (i.e., 2017), the BCI research field expanded drastically both in size and in scope (Brunner et al. 2015). In terms of size, the 6th (and most recent) International BCI meeting in 2016 gathered about 400 participants, from 188 research groups and organizations (Huggins et al. 2017). The journal *Brain–Computer Interfaces* was created in 2013 and published its first issue in 2014 (www.tandfonline.com/loi/tbci20). The international BCI society was also created in 2015, in order to "to foster research and development leading to technologies that enable people to interact with the world through brain signals" (bcisociety.org).

Research developments continue to propose many new results, such as new BCI paradigms including new visual or auditory evoked potential–based BCIs (Gao et al. 2014) or hybrid BCIs that combine one BCI with another interface or another BCI (Muller-Putz et al. 2015; Pfurtscheller et al. 2010). Invasive BCIs became much more efficient (Lebedev & Nicolelis 2006), including now on humans (Collinger et al. 2013; Hochberg et al. 2006). New brain recording technologies are being explored such as functional near-infrared spectroscopy (Girouard et al. 2010; Sitaram et al. 2007) or electrocorticography (Schalk et al. 2008). On the practical side, consumer-grade EEG sensors and BCI systems are now available on the market (see, e.g., openbci.com), while BCI software is available for free and open-source (Brunner et al. 2012). EEG signal processing algorithms improved (Makeig et al. 2012), as well as our understanding of the user side of BCIs, that is, the user experience, psychology, and training (Jeunet et al. 2016; Kübler et al. 2014; Lotte et al. 2013; Neuper et al. 2010).

The scope of BCIs also expanded, and many new BCI applications are now explored, including, among others, stroke rehabilitation (Ang et al. 2015), gaming (Lécuyer et al. 2008; Nijholt et al. 2009), many new uses of BCI as assistive technologies (Kübler et al. 2013; Millan et al. 2010), mobile BCI, that is, real-time EEG decoding with a moving user (Kranczioch et al. 2014; Lotte et al. 2009), or artistic applications (Andujar et al. 2015). Passive BCIs were also proposed as a new concept of BCI, which are not used for directly sending voluntary commands to an application, but for monitoring the users' mental states (e.g., attention or workload), to then adapt the target application according to this state (Zander et al. 2011). Subcategories of passive BCIs notably include affective BCIs, which monitor affective states (e.g., anger or joy) to design applications reacting to these states (Mühl et al. 2014).

This in turn led to increased interest for BCI technologies outside the BCI field, notably in the human–computer interaction field, where BCI proved useful for multimodal interaction, intelligent systems, or (neuro)ergonomics, among others (see, e.g., Frey et al. 2017 and Tan & Nijholt 2010). BCI technologies were also shown to be useful as a new tool for scientific research (Sanchez et al. 2014). To reflect and include such new usages of BCIs, the current definition of BCIs has expanded. A BCI is currently defined as "a system that measures central nervous system (CNS) activity and converts it into artificial output that replaces, restores, enhances, supplements, or improves natural CNS output and thereby changes the ongoing interactions between the CNS and its external or internal environment" (Wolpaw & Wolpaw 2012).

## THIS BOOK

As this brief historical—but incomplete and partial—chapter showed, the BCI research field is thus now a mature, very rich, and highly multidisciplinary research field. As such, starting to work on or

---

* This paper by Wolpaw and colleagues is a seminal one in BCI research and quite possibly the most cited BCI paper ever. It is a must read for anyone starting with BCIs, as this paper presents most of the concepts, paradigms, and challenges of BCI research.

with BCIs is a difficult endeavor, which requires learning and mastering multiple disciplines, tools, and concepts. In order to make that task easier, and contribute to spreading the use of BCIs and their potential benefits, we have put up together this handbook of BCI, with the help of many renowned scientists from the field. It is our hope that this book would enable any newcomer to the BCI field, or even anyone already working on the field but wanting to deepen their BCI knowledge, to find an overview of BCI developments, methods, results, and open challenges. We hope that this book will provide our readers with the necessary tools and knowledge to conduct new, rigorous, and relevant BCI studies as well as to design and build innovative and useful BCI applications and products.

This book is divided into six parts, dedicated respectively to BCI applications, brain signals acquisition and software, brain signal processing, BCI paradigms, design and evaluation of BCI experiments, and the future of BCI research.

More precisely, Part I, dedicated to BCI applications, first starts with an introduction to BCIs (Part I.A), with a general overview of BCI systems, how neuroscience and BCIs interact, and a presentation of passive BCIs. Then, Part I.B presents various therapeutic applications of BCI, including using BCI for motor rehabilitation, troubles of consciousness, cognitive rehabilitation, neuroprosthesis, or communication, including elderly users. Part I.C deals with affective and artistic applications of BCIs, for affect detection, art applications, and music. Applications of BCI for entertainment and multimedia are covered in Part I.D, with chapters dedicated to BCI games, BCIs for virtual and augmented realities, and BCI for haptics.

Part II gathers chapters dealing with brain signal acquisition, notably invasive ones, and BCI software. Notably, it contains chapters focused on subdermal electrodes (minimally invasive), electrocorticography (semi-invasive), and neurotrophic electrodes (fully invasive). This parts ends with a chapter dedicated to the different kinds of software that are available to acquire and process in real time various brain signals such as those above, in order to design a BCI.

Part III is dedicated to the next step in the BCI processing pipeline, namely, processing the acquired brain signals. As such, this part starts with a chapter providing a gentle introduction to EEG signal processing in BCIs, before presenting more advanced material in the subsequent chapters. In particular, the next chapters cover EEG signal classification based on Riemannian geometry, more advanced methods for ERP classification and Bayesian learning for BCIs, and transfer learning approaches for BCIs. Many of these methods aim at dealing with the variability of BCI performance over time and users, which is a critical problem in brain signal processing for BCIs.

Part IV explores in more detail the various types of BCI paradigms that are available. It indeed gathers chapters dedicated to the most common BCI paradigms, namely, motor imagery BCIs, P300, and SSVEP BCIs. It also presents more recent and complex BCI designs, namely, attention-based BCIs, BCIs with specific stimulus design, as well as hybrid BCIs. Two chapters are actually dedicated to hybrid BCIs, with an overview of such paradigms and a specific focus on hybrid BCIs combining SSVEP with eye tracking.

Part V focuses mostly on the last—but no less crucial—element of the brain–computer interaction loop: the user. As such, it focuses on human factors, design, and evaluation of BCI systems, by considering this key element that the human user is. In particular, this part contains chapters dedicated to usability evaluation in BCI, user-centred design, and adaptive BCI design to improve user training and experience. It also provides BCI experimenters and researchers with tools to successfully design and evaluate actual BCI studies on real users. A chapter is indeed dedicated to the design of rigorous BCI experiments, providing guidelines to avoid typical flaws and biases, while another chapter is dedicated to the many ways to evaluate BCI performances, both machine and user ones.

Finally, Part VI is dedicated to the future of BCIs and emerging research directions. It notably addresses important ethical issues associated with BCI research and applications, the impact of BCI use on brain plasticity, the emergence of multi-brain BCI systems—that is, BCI applications using as input brain signals from multiple users—as well as bidirectional BCIs, that is, systems that both directly measure from and stimulate the brain. The book concludes with a chapter offering perspectives for the whole BCI field.

Now, we invite our readers to dive into this book, to learn and get inspired from it, in order for the BCI community to continue to be a dynamic and innovative community, and to ensure that BCI technologies can benefit, in practice, those who need them!

## ACKNOWLEDGMENTS

F. Lotte was supported in part by the French National Research Agency with the REBEL project (grant ANR-15-CE23-0013-01). Chang S. Nam was supported in part by the National Science Foundation under grants IIS-1421948 and BCS-1551688. Any opinions, findings, and conclusions or recommendations expressed in this material are those of the authors and do not necessarily reflect the views of the NSF and the French National Research Agency.

## REFERENCES

Anderson, C. W., & Sijercic, Z. Classification of EEG signals from four subjects during five mental tasks. In *Solving Engineering Problems with Neural Networks: Proceedings of the Conference on Engineering Applications in Neural Networks (EANN'96)* (pp. 407–414). Turkey. 1996

Andujar, M., Crawford, C. S., Nijholt, A., Jackson, F., & Gilbert, J. E. Artistic brain–computer interfaces: The expression and stimulation of the user's affective state. *Brain–Computer Interfaces*, 2015, 2(2–3), 60–69.

Ang, K. K., & Guan, C. Brain–computer interface for neurorehabilitation of upper limb after stroke. *Proceedings of the IEEE*, 2015, 103, 944–953.

Berger, H. Ueber das Elektroenkephalogramm des Menschen. *Archiv für Psychiatrie und Nervenkrankheiten*, 1929, 87, 527–570.

Birbaumer, N., Ghanayim, N., Hinterberger, T., Iversen, I., Kotchoubey, B., Kübler, A., Perelmouter, J., Taub, E., & Flor, H. A spelling device for the paralysed. *Nature*, 1999, 398, 297–298.

Blankertz, B., Curio, G., & Müller, K. R. Classifying single trial EEG: Towards brain computer interfacing. *Advances in Neural Information Processing Systems (NIPS 01)*, 2002, 14, 157–164.

Brunner, C., Birbaumer, N., Blankertz, B., Guger, C., Kübler, A., Mattia, D., Millán, J. d. R., Miralles, F., Nijholt, A., Opisso, E., & others. BNCI Horizon 2020: Towards a roadmap for the BCI community. *Brain–Computer Interfaces*, 2015, 1–10.

Brunner, C., Andreoni, G., Bianchi, L., Blankertz, B., Breitwieser, C., Kanoh, S., Kothe, C. A., Lécuyer, A., Makeig, S., Mellinger, J., Perego, P., Renard, Y., Schalk, G., Susila, I. P., Venthur, B., & G. R. Muller-Putz. BCI software platforms. In *Towards Practical Brain–Computer Interfaces*, (2012), (pp. 303–331). Springer Berlin Heidelberg.

Chapin, J. K., Moxon, K. A., Markowitz, R. S., & Nicolelis, M. A. Real-time control of a robot arm using simultaneously recorded neurons in the motor cortex. *Nature Neuroscience*, 1999, 2(7), 664–670.

Childers, D., Principe, J. C., & Arroyo A. Rome Air Development Center Tech. Rep. F30602-88-D-0027, 1989.

Collinger, J. L., Wodlinger, B., Downey, J. E., Wang, W., Tyler-Kabara, E. C., Weber, D. J., ..., & Schwartz, A. B. High-performance neuroprosthetic control by an individual with tetraplegia. *The Lancet*, 2013, 381(9866), 557–564.

Farwell, L., & Donchin, E. Talking off the top of your head: Toward a mental prosthesis utilizing event-related brain potentials. *Electroencephalography and Clinical Neurophysiology*, 1988, 70, 510–523.

Frey, J., Hachet, M., & Lotte, F. EEG-based neuroergonomics for 3D user interfaces: Opportunities and challenges. *Le Travail Humain*, 2017, 80(1), 73–92.

Gao, S., Wang, Y., Gao, X., & Hong, B. Visual and auditory brain–computer interfaces. *IEEE Transactions on Biomedical Engineering*, 2014, 61(5), 1436–1447.

Girouard, A., Solovey, E. T., Hirshfield, L. M., Peck, E. M., Chauncey, K., Sassaroli, A., Fantini, S., & Jacob R. J. From brain signals to adaptive interfaces: Using fNIRS in HCI. *Brain–Computer Interfaces*, 2010, 221–237.

Hochberg, L., Serruya, M., Friehs, G., Mukand, J., Saleh, M., Caplan, A., Branner, A., Chen, D., Penn, R., & Donoghue, J. Neuronal ensemble control of prosthetic devices by a human with tetraplegia. *Nature*, 2006, 442, 164–171.

Huggins, J. E., Guger, C., Ziat, M., Zander, T. O., Taylor, D., Tangermann, M., ..., & Ruffini, G. Workshops of the Sixth International Brain–Computer Interface Meeting: Brain–computer interfaces past, present, and future. *Brain–Computer Interfaces*, 2017, 1–34.

Jeunet, C., N'Kaoua, B., & Lotte, F. Advances in user-training for mental-imagery-based BCI control: Psychological and cognitive factors and their neural correlates. *Progress in Brain Research*, 2016.

Kamiya, J. Conscious control of brain waves. *Psychology Today*, 1968, 1(11), 56–60.

Konger, C., Principe, J. C., & Taner, M. Neural network classification of event related potentials for the design of a new computer interface. In *Proc. Int. Joint Conf. Neural Networks*, 1990, vol. 1, pp. 367–372.

Kranczioch, C., Zich, C., Schierholz, I., & Sterr, A. Mobile EEG and its potential to promote the theory and application of imagery-based motor rehabilitation. *International Journal of Psychophysiology*, 2014, 91, 10–15.

Kübler, A., Holz, E. M., Riccio, A., Zickler, C., Kaufmann, T., Kleih, S. C., Staiger-Sälzer, P., Desideri, L., Hoogerwerf, E.-J., & Mattia, D. The user-centered design as novel perspective for evaluating the usability of BCI-controlled applications. *PLoS One*, 2014, 9, e112392.

Kübler, A., Mattia, D., Rupp, R., & Tangermann, M. Facing the challenge: Bringing brain–computer interfaces to end-users. *Artificial Intelligence in Medicine*, 2013, 59, 55–60.

Lebedev, M., & Nicolelis, M. Brain–machine interfaces: Past, present and future. *Trends in Neurosciences*, 2006, 29, 536–546.

Lécuyer, A., Lotte, F., Reilly, R. B., Leeb, R., Hirose, M., & Slater, M. Brain–computer interfaces, virtual reality, and videogames. *Computer*, 2008, 41(10).

Lotte, F., Fujisawa, J., Touyama, H., Ito, R., Hirose, M., & Lécuyer, A. Towards ambulatory brain-computer interfaces: A pilot study with P300 signals. In *5th Advances in Computer Entertainment Technology Conference (ACE)*, 2009, 336–339.

Lotte, F., Larrue, F., & Mühl, C. Flaws in current human training protocols for spontaneous Brain–Computer Interfaces: Lessons learned from instructional design. *Frontiers in Human Neuroscience*, 2013, 7.

Makeig, S., Kothe, C., Mullen, T., Bigdely-Shamlo, N., Zhang, Z., & Kreutz-Delgado, K. Evolving signal processing for brain–computer interfaces. *Proceedings of the IEEE*, 2012, 100, 1567–1584.

McMillan, G., Calhoun, G., Middendorf, M., Schuner, J., Ingle, D., & Nashman, V. Direct brain interface utilizing self-regulation of steady-state visual evoked response. *Proceedings of RESNA*, 1995, 693–695.

Millan, J., Franzé, M., Cincotti, F., Varsta, M., Heikkonen, J., & Babiloni, F. A local neural classifier for the recognition of EEG patterns associated to mental tasks. *IEEE Transactions on Neural Networks*, 2002, 13, 678–686.

Millan, J. D. R., Rupp, R., Mueller-Putz, G., Murray-Smith, R., Giugliemma, C., Tangermann, M., ..., & Neuper, C. Combining brain–computer interfaces and assistive technologies: State-of-the-art and challenges. *Frontiers in Neuroscience*, 2010, 4, 161.

Mühl, C., Allison, B., Nijholt, A., & Chanel, G. A survey of affective brain computer interfaces: Principles, state-of-the-art, and challenges. *Brain–Computer Interfaces*, 2014, 1(2), 66–84.

Muller-Putz, G., Leeb, R., Tangermann, M., Hohne, J., Kubler, A., Cincotti, F., Mattia, D., Rupp, R., Muller, K.-R., & Millan, J. D. R. Towards non-invasive hybrid brain–computer interfaces: Framework, practice, clinical application, and beyond. *Proceedings of the IEEE*, 2015, 103, 926–943.

Neuper, C., & Pfurtscheller, G. Brain–computer interfaces neurofeedback training for BCI control. *The Frontiers Collection*, 2010, 65–78.

Nicolelis, M. Actions from thoughts. *Nature*, 2001, 409, 403–407.

Nijholt, A. The future of brain–computer interfacing (keynote paper). In *5th International Conference on Informatics, Electronics and Vision (ICIEV)*, 2016 (pp. 156–161). IEEE, 2016.

Nijholt, A., Bos, D. P. O., & Reuderink, B. Turning shortcomings into challenges: Brain–computer interfaces for games. *Entertainment Computing*, 2009, 1(2), 85–94.

Pfurtscheller, G., Allison, B. Z., Bauernfeind, G., Brunner, C., Solis Escalante, T., Scherer, R., Zander, T. O., Mueller-Putz, G., Neuper, C., & Birbaumer, N. The hybrid BCI. *Frontiers in Neuroscience, Frontiers*, 2010, 4, 3.

Pfurtscheller, G., Flotzinger, D., & Kalcher, J. Brain–computer interface—A new communication device for handicapped persons. *Journal of Microcomputer Application*, 1993, 16, 293–299.

Principe, J. C. The cortical mouse: A piece of forgotten history in noninvasive brain–computer interfaces. *IEEE Pulse*, 2013, 4(4), 26–29.

Ramoser, H., Muller-Gerking, J., & Pfurtscheller, G. Optimal spatial filtering of single trial EEG during imagined hand movement. *IEEE Transactions on Rehabilitation Engineering*, 2000, 8, 441–446.

Sanchez, G., Daunizeau, J., Maby, E., Bertrand, O., Bompas, A., & Mattout, J. Toward a new application of real-time electrophysiology: Online optimization of cognitive neurosciences hypothesis testing. *Brain Sciences*, 2014, 4, 49–72.

Schalk, G., Miller, K., Anderson, N., Wilson, J., Smyth, M., Ojemann, J., Moran, D., Wolpaw, J., & Leuthardt, E. Two-dimensional movement control using electrocorticographic signals in humans. *Journal of Neural Engineering*, 2008, 5, 75–84.

Sitaram, R., Zhang, H., Guan, C., Thulasidas, M., Hoshi, Y., Ishikawa, A., Shimizu, K., & Birbaumer, N. Temporal classification of multi-channel near infrared spectroscopy signals of motor imagery for developing a brain–computer interface. *NeuroImage*, 2007, 34, 1416–1427.

Sobell, N. Streaming the brain. *IEEE Multimedia*, 2002, 9(3), 4–8.

Tan, D., & Nijholt, A. (Eds.). *Brain–Computer Interaction: Applying our Minds to Human–Computer Interaction*. Springer-Verlag: London, 2010.

Vidal, J. J. Toward direct brain–computer communication. *Annual Review of Biophysics and Bioengineering*, 1973, 2, 157–180.

Wolpaw, J. R., Birbaumer, N., Heetderks, W. J., McFarland, D. J., Peckham, P. H., Schalk, G., Donchin, E., Quatrano, L. A., Robinson, C. J., & Vaughan, T. M. Brain–computer interface technology: A review of the first international meeting. *IEEE Transaction on Rehabilitation Engineering*, 2000, 8, 164–173.

Wolpaw, J., Birbaumer, N., McFarland, D., Pfurtscheller, G., & Vaughan, T. Brain–computer interfaces for communication and control. *Clinical Neurophysiology*, 2002, 113, 767–791.

Wolpaw, J. R., McFarland, D. J., Neat, G. W., & Forneris, C. A. An EEG-based brain–computer interface for cursor control. *Electroencephalography and Clinical Neurophysiology*, 1991, 78, 252–259.

Wolpaw, J., & Wolpaw, E. *Brain–Computer Interfaces: Principles and Practice*. Oxford University Press, 2012.

Zander, T., & Kothe, C. Towards passive brain–computer interfaces: Applying brain–computer interface technology to human–machine systems in general. *Journal of Neural Engineering*, 2011, 8.

# Part I

---

## Brain–Computer Interface Applications

### Section A. Brain–Computer Interfaces Introduction

# 1 Brain–Computer Interface
## *An Emerging Interaction Technology*

Chang S. Nam, Inchul Choi, Amy Wadeson,
and Mincheol Whang

## CONTENTS

1.1 Introduction ........................................................................................................ 12
    1.1.1 How Does a BCI Work? .......................................................................... 13
    1.1.2 How Can BCIs Be Categorized? ............................................................ 13
1.2 Signal Acquisition Methods ................................................................................ 15
    1.2.1 Noninvasive Recording Methods ............................................................ 16
        1.2.1.1 Electroencephalography ............................................................. 16
        1.2.1.2 Magnetoencephalography .......................................................... 19
        1.2.1.3 Functional Magnetic Resonance Imaging ................................. 20
        1.2.1.4 Functional Near-Infrared Spectroscopy .................................... 20
        1.2.1.5 Positron Emission Tomography ................................................. 21
    1.2.2 Invasive Recording Methods ................................................................... 21
        1.2.2.1 Electrocorticography .................................................................. 21
        1.2.2.2 Intracortical Neuron Recording ................................................. 22
    1.2.3 Brain Signal Patterns for BCI Operation ................................................ 22
        1.2.3.1 P300 ERPs .................................................................................. 22
        1.2.3.2 Steady-State Evoked Potentials ................................................. 22
        1.2.3.3 Sensorimotor Rhythms .............................................................. 24
        1.2.3.4 Slow Cortical Potentials ............................................................ 25
1.3 Improving Signal Quality and Feature Extraction Methods ............................... 25
    1.3.1 Removing Noisy Signals and Artifacts ................................................... 25
    1.3.2 Spatial Filtering ...................................................................................... 26
        1.3.2.1 Referencing Methods ................................................................. 26
        1.3.2.2 Data-Dependent Spatial Filtering .............................................. 28
    1.3.3 Feature Extraction: SSVEPs ................................................................... 30
1.4 Feature Classification Methods .......................................................................... 30
    1.4.1 Linear Classifiers .................................................................................... 30
        1.4.1.1 Linear Discriminant Analysis .................................................... 31
        1.4.1.2 Support Vector Machine ............................................................ 31
    1.4.2 Artificial Neural Network Classifiers ..................................................... 32
        1.4.2.1 Multilayer Perceptron ................................................................ 32
        1.4.2.2 Other ANN Architectures .......................................................... 33
    1.4.3 Hidden Markov Model Classifiers .......................................................... 33
1.5 Example BCI Applications .................................................................................. 34
    1.5.1 P300-Based BCIs .................................................................................... 34
        1.5.1.1 Communication Applications ..................................................... 34
        1.5.1.2 Control Applications .................................................................. 36

      1.5.2   SSVEP-Based BCIs ........................................................................................36
            1.5.2.1   Communication .............................................................................36
            1.5.2.2   Control .........................................................................................36
      1.5.3   ERD/ERS-Based BCIs ..................................................................................38
            1.5.3.1   Communication .............................................................................38
            1.5.3.2   Control .........................................................................................38
1.6   Summary ....................................................................................................................39
Acknowledgments ..................................................................................................................39
References ...............................................................................................................................39

**Abstract**

During the last decades, a new capability has emerged by which the human brain can directly communicate with the environment, called a brain–computer interface (BCI), brain–machine interface (BMI), direct neural interface, or mind–machine interface (MMI). The BCI community has witnessed a substantial amount of work done on BCI technologies and many successful BCI applications. However, continuing effort is still needed to further optimize the capabilities, robustness, and usability of BCI systems for human use, including those who suffer from muscular disabilities such as amyotrophic lateral sclerosis, brainstem stroke, and severe cerebral palsy. This chapter reviews the state of the art of BCI as an emerging human–computer interaction technology. We first introduce a BCI classification scheme, along with different types of the signal recording methods and brain signal patterns for BCI operation. Next, the most commonly used signal processing techniques and feature extraction techniques are explained, in addition to classification methods used for identifying the user's intentions. Finally, we present and discuss various types of BCI applications with an emphasis on the future of BCI research and development through inter- and multidisciplinary collaborations and ongoing communication among neuroscientists, engineers, psychologists, human factors professionals, clinicians, and rehabilitation specialists.

## 1.1   INTRODUCTION

Individuals with healthy motor functions may take for granted the complicated biological, chemical, and electrical processes that occur within their body in order for them to easily communicate and interact with the outside world. Although the processes are complex, healthy individuals are able to complete them without much thought or effort. However, when certain neuron pathways are severed or degeneration brought on by an injury or a disease occurs, what once were simple tasks may become impossible or very cumbersome to complete.

During the last decades, a new capability has emerged by which the human brain can directly communicate with the environment, called a *brain–computer interface (BCI)*, *brain–machine interface (BMI)*, *direct neural interface*, or *mind–machine interface (MMI)*. BCI is defined as "a communication system in which messages or commands that an individual (Nam 2012) sends to the external world do not pass through the brain's normal output pathways of peripheral nerves and muscles" (Wolpaw et al. 2002, p. 769). That is, BCIs offer a way of bypassing typical nerve pathways by providing novel output pathways in order to interact with a variety of applications that replace, improve, enhance, restore, and supplement the human user's central nervous system output (Klein & Nam 2016; Nijholt & Nam 2015; Wolpaw & Wolpaw 2012). This is especially important for individuals with compromised neural tracts. For example, there are nearly 2 million people in the United States alone and many more worldwide who suffer from severe motor disabilities (Ficke 1992). Moreover, nearly 500,000 people suffer from locked-in syndrome worldwide (Moore & Kennedy 2000). Though research into brain–computer interfacing technology is still in early phases on these benefits, many significant developments have been made. BCI applications now enable individuals, in particular those with severe motor impairments but cognitively intact, to write sentences (Birbaumer et al. 2000; Li et al. 2010, 2014), control an unmanned aerial vehicle control (Shi et al. 2015) and a prosthetic (Tyler-Kabara et al. 2015), play video games (Beveridge et al. 2015), perform a collaborative work (Li & Nam 2015, 2016; Nam et al. 2013), and create arts (Mullen et al. 2015), all through brain signal acquisition, signal processing, and interpretation.

BCI systems consist of several sequential steps, which can be divided into four categories: brain activity pattern generation, signal acquisition, feature extraction, and classification. First, brain activity can be represented by electrical activity, magnetic fields created by electrical activity, and blood oxygenation, and it differs in spatial and temporal characteristics depending on stimulus type, stimulus intensity, mental effort, and mental status. Second, brain activity can be measured through various brain imaging techniques in the signal acquisition phase. The appropriate technique should be chosen according to the type of brain activity to be measured and the purpose of the measurement, largely divided into invasive and noninvasive methods. Third, in the feature extraction step, only the important and interesting brain activities are extracted from the measured brain signals. Finally, the extracted brain features are analyzed through various algorithms to classify the user's current intention and status.

In addition, BCI systems can be categorized as either active, reactive, or passive depending on the user's attention and efforts (Brouwer et al. 2013; Mühl et al. 2014; Zander et al. 2010). While active/reactive BCI systems use brain activity that occurs with external stimuli (reactive BCI) or modulated mental efforts (active BCI) to directly control the application, passive BCI systems use spontaneously generated brain activity such as users' cognitive state to utilize an additional signal to support and compensate ongoing human–computer interaction (Choi et al. 2017; Garcia–Molina et al. 2013; Khan & Hong 2015; Kim et al. 2017; Lim et al. 2012). In this chapter, only active and reactive BCIs will be introduced.

The goal of this chapter is to provide an overview of the state of the art of BCI as an emerging human–computer interaction technology. The outline of the chapter is as follows. This section features an example of illustrating how a typical BCI works, along with a classification scheme with which to catalog BCI systems. Section 1.2 discusses two main types of recording methods and six different brain signal patterns for BCI operation. Section 1.3 describes the most commonly used signal processing techniques that deal with artifacts and some of the feature extraction techniques that have become increasingly popular in BCIs. Section 1.4 covers different classification methods used for identifying the user's intentions. Section 1.5 introduces various types of BCI applications. Finally, the conclusions are drawn in Section 1.6.

### 1.1.1 How Does a BCI Work?

Imagine being completely unable to move. You want to communicate, but cannot speak or even move your eyeballs. You cannot even use general assistive technologies such as an eye tracker and speech recognition system, because they still require some degree of motor control such as eyeball control and vocal-cord vibration. BCIs can offer an effective communication alternative purely through the use of human brain signals. Take a look at an anecdotal story illustrating how a person with severe motor disability can write an e-mail to his daughter, Samantha, using a P300-based BCI, along with a BCI system framework in Figure 1.1.

### 1.1.2 How Can BCIs Be Categorized?

In general, BCI systems can be categorized by *brain signal pattern*, *stimulus modality*, *mode of operation*, *operation strategy*, and *recording method*. Figure 1.2 illustrates how BCI systems compare against each other based on these criteria.

There are many kinds of brain signal patterns that can be used to communicate with a BCI (Bryant et al. 2016; Wadeson et al. 2015). A brain signal is a set of electrical impulses that flows on groups of active neurons (for more details, see Section 1.3). BCIs that are categorized by brain

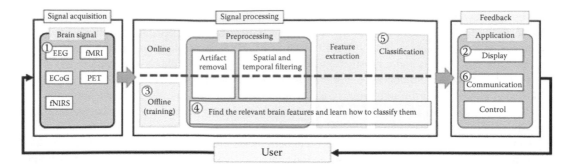

**FIGURE 1.1** Overview of a general BCI system framework. Tom, who is paralyzed but is cognitively intact, visits a BCI lab, and sits in front of the computer screen in his wheelchair, while the lab assistant places an EEG cap (1) on his head. On the computer screen, the letters and numbers are displayed in matrix form (2). Before he can type a letter to his daughter, he needs to train the system to properly record and respond to his brain signals (3). Rows and columns of the alphanumeric matrix flash randomly, and Tom is mentally counting how many times the character he wants to type flashes. The BCI system then processes his EEG signals, which include distinct brain patterns elicited by mental counting with respect to the desired characters, to extract the important brain features by filtering out irrelevant signals. From the extracted brain signal, the BCI system learns how to distinguish what letters he intends to select, so that future attempts to type will be more readily discernable (4). After a few letters, the training is complete and he is able to start typing his message. Again, he focuses on the letters that he wants to type, and the BCI system applies the classifier that was built through the training exercise to detect Tom's intention (5). One by one, the letters appear on the computer screen: D E A R   S A M A N T H A (6). He is well on his way to writing his letter, using only his brainwaves.

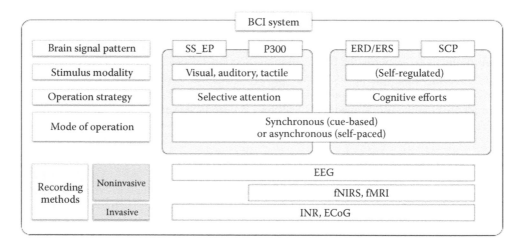

**FIGURE 1.2** Classification of BCI systems.

signals rely on different arrangements of impulses to communicate with the specific application. An example of a brain signal is **P300 event-related potentials (ERPs)** that reach a maximum positive peak in voltage about 300 ms after a stimulus onset (e.g., through the so-called oddball paradigm). Compared with other brain signals, P300 ERPs require little initial training—a huge advantage as compared to other brain signal types (Li et al. 2010; Powers et al. 2015). P300 can be evoked by visual, auditory, tactile, and even olfactory or gustatory paradigms (Linden 2011). Another widely used brain signal type is **steady-state evoked potentials (SSEPs)**, which are the electrical activity of the brain in response to stimulation of specific sensory nerve pathways, as distinct from spontaneous potentials. There are three kinds of SSEPs: **steady-state auditory evoked** potentials (SS**A**EPs), usually recorded from the scalp but originating at the brainstem level (Hill et al. 2012); **steady-state visually evoked potentials (SS**V**EPs)** found within the occipital lobe of the brain caused by focusing on a steady pattern of visual stimuli, such as a regularly flashing light (Nam et al. 2015); and **steady-state somatosensory evoked potentials (SS**S**EPs)**, a sinusoidal electrophysiological brain response elicited from mechanical vibrotactile stimulation delivered to the glabrous skin (e.g., fingertip), which is modulated by selective spatial attention (Giabbiconi et al. 2004). Among many SSEPs, SSVEP-based BCIs that utilize flickering light sources with different frequencies from either LED or LCD displays are well studied, because they could provide the quickest and most reliable path to communication (Volosyak 2011; Wang et al. 2008; Zhu et al. 2010). For example, when the user concentrates on a target stimulus with a certain frequency, that same frequency is synchronized to a certain area according to the modality (e.g., visual cortex for visual stimuli), and the amplitude at the frequency of the target stimulus is higher than those of the nontarget stimuli. The BCI system uses these distinct brain patterns to perform different actions (e.g., directions, on/off, and typing) according to the user's selective attention (Müller-Putz & Pfurtscheller 2008; Muller et al. 2011; Wang et al. 2011a). A lesser used brain signal method is **slow cortical potentials (SCPs)**, which are shifts in the cortical electrical activity lasting from several hundred milliseconds to several seconds (Gevensleben et al. 2014). Finally, there is **sensorimotor rhythm** (SMR), involving event-related desynchronization/synchronization (ERD/ERS), brain activity associated with imagining motor behavior.

There are two recording methods for use in BCIs (for more details, see Section 1.2). The safest and most prevalent of these methods is **noninvasive** (Han et al. 2015). This method requires equipment that either touches the scalp such as electroencephalogram (EEG) or near-infrared spectroscopy (fNIRS) or is otherwise outside of the cranium such as functional magnetic resonance imaging (fMRI), magnetoencephalography (MEG), or positron emission tomography (PET). Although there is controversy in categorizing PET as a noninvasive brain imaging method because of the radiotracer injection process, they were classified as noninvasive methods in this chapter because they did not require surgical intervention (Coyle et al. 2007; Krepki et al. 2003; Vallabhaneni et al. 2005). Unlike noninvasive methods, **invasive** techniques require surgery in order to place signal receptors within the brain (Birbaumer 2006). Examples of invasive recording methods are intracortical neuronal recording and electrocochleography (ECoG).

Another way to categorize BCIs is through their **Operation Strategy**. This is the way in which a BCI elicits brain signals during use. A BCI that utilizes **Selective Attention** presents users with auditory, visual, or tactile stimulation that can elicit brain signal responses (e.g., Allison et al. 2008; Zhang et al. 2010). **Cognitive Efforts**, another operation strategy, rely on biofeedback to train users to maintain a desirable level of brainwave frequency amplitude (e.g., Kamiya 1971). Some BCIs employ the unique operation strategy of **Motor Imagery**, which allows the user to imagine muscle movements, in order to cause a spike in neuronal activity in the motor cortex (e.g., Pfurtscheller & Neuper 2006).

The **Mode of Operation** for a BCI is the underlying way in which brain signals are elicited. They are either synchronous or asynchronous. **Synchronous** BCIs are cue based; information is presented to the user in order to elicit certain brain signal responses (e.g., Hazrati & Erfanian 2010). **Asynchronous** BCIs, on the other hand, are self-paced; they are controlled through user intention in the user's desired timing (e.g., Leeb et al. 2007).

Finally, BCIs can be categorized by their **Stimulus Modality**, or the form in which stimulus is presented to the user: **visual** (e.g., Sellers & Donchin 2006), **auditory** (e.g., Nijboer et al. 2008), **tactile** (e.g., Brouwer & van Erp 2010), or **hybrid**, which combines multiple BCIs such as imagined movement and visual attention, or P300 and SSVEP (Pfurtscheller et al. 2010a; Yin et al. 2013).

## 1.2  SIGNAL ACQUISITION METHODS

BCIs require a neuroimaging or neurophysiological device to acquire and transmit the brain signals from brain to computer. In general, neuroimaging methods are categorized by *invasiveness* of

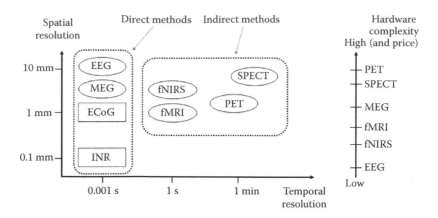

**FIGURE 1.3** A comparison of noninvasive (oval) and invasive (rectangular) recording methods for use in BCIs based on temporal resolution (x axis) and spatial resolution (y axis); The x-axis and y-axis scales are not evenly distributed. ECoG, electrocorticography; EEG, electroencephalography; fMRI, functional magnetic resonance imaging; fNIRS, functional near infrared spectroscopy; INR, intracortical neuron recordings; MEG, magnetoencephalography; PET, positron emission tomography.

the recording methods, but can be further classified by *spatial/temporal resolution, direct/indirect measurement*, and *complexity/price*. Each recording technique has strengths, weaknesses, and specific uses that help researchers decide which device is relevant to their study. Figure 1.3 visually compares different recording methods discussed in more detail in the following sections.

### 1.2.1 NONINVASIVE RECORDING METHODS

A noninvasive recording technique uses sensors placed on the skin, such as the scalp, or machinery that surrounds the cranium in whole. Two types of noninvasive recording methods discussed in this section include (1) *direct measures* that detect electrical (e.g., EEG) or magnetic activity (e.g., MEG) of the brain, and (2) *indirect measures* of brain function reflecting brain metabolism or hemodynamics of the brain (e.g., fMRI, fNIRS, and PET) that do not directly characterize the neuronal activity. Unlike invasive recording methods, these noninvasive techniques do not require surgery, internal chemical or machine implantation, or needle insertion in order to receive and record neural activity (Bhattacharyya et al. 2015).

#### 1.2.1.1 Electroencephalography

One of the most popular noninvasive neurophysiological recording techniques is electroencephalography, or EEG. This method measures electrical activity in the brain through the use of surface electrodes placed on the scalp (Niedermeyer & da Silva 2005). The first human EEG was recorded by Hans Berger, a German psychiatrist, in 1924.

The neurophysiological origin of EEG signals is the pyramidal neurons of the cortex (Cantor & Evans 2013). An electrical impulse is sent down the axon and into the synapse every time neurons are fired during excitation. Since electrical signals are not able to cross neuronal boundaries, a chemical reaction is created between neurons. This chemical reaction is triggered by the electrical impulse and causes an action potential. An action potential is the process of neuron depolarization, followed by repolarization. Chemical information can begin flowing through the synaptic cleft when a neuron is at its resting polarization level. The flow causes the depolarization, and repolarization is necessary before more chemical information can flow through the synapse again (Nunez 1995). EEG measures the electrical current, which Teplan explained as "that flow during synaptic excitations of the dendrites of many pyramidal neurons in the cerebral cortex" (Teplan

2002, p. 1). Because of the distance and impedance of bone and skin between the electrodes and the cerebral cortex, the EEG cannot accurately detect single neuron excitations. Instead, the EEG picks up local current flows on groups of active neurons within the cerebral cortex (Teplan 2002; Tonet et al. 2006).

Neural oscillations that are observed in EEG signals are popularly called "brainwaves," reflecting different aspects when they occur in different locations in the brain (Table 1.1). These brainwaves are identified by frequency (in hertz or cycles per second) and amplitude in the range of microvolts (μV or 1/1,000,000 of a volt). Each brainwave has its own set of characteristics representing a specific level of brain activity and mental states (Mühl et al. 2014). For example, Delta brainwaves reflect slow, loud, and functional mental states that prevail during the late sleep (Steriade et al. 1993), while the power decrease at the alpha band correlates to the presence of mental imagery (Pfurtscheller & Lopes da Silva 1999).

In order to record EEG signals, a head set consisting of an EEG cap with at least three electrodes (i.e., a ground, a reference, and a recording electrode) is needed (Figure 1.4b). In addition, an amplifier, an A/D converter, and a computing device (such as a computer) are necessary (Nicolas-Alonso & Gomez-Gil 2012). Electrodes are typically made of silver, silver chloride, or gold and can be considered wet, which requires conductive gel to be placed between electrode and scalp, or dry, where the electrode is placed directly onto the skin (Peng et al. 2015, 2016). Measurements from all electrodes are referred to one common electrode, called "reference" electrode (Schalk & Mellinger 2010). The active and reference electrodes serve as the signal receptors for potential difference comparisons. The ground electrode serves as the baseline of brainwave signals that helps weed out irrelevant data from the active and reference signals.

Correct EEG electrode placement is important to ensure proper location of electrodes in relation to cortical areas so that they can be reliably and precisely maintained from individual to individual. The international 10/20 system has been an internationally recognized standard system for electrode positioning with 21 electrodes for half a century (Homan et al. 1987; Jasper 1958). Under the 10/20 system, the skull is divided into six areas from nasion to inion with interval rates of 10%, 20%, 20%, 20%, 20%, and 10% (Fp: frontopolar, F: frontal, C: central, P: parietal, and O: occipital, respectively), and also divided into the same ratios from left to right preauricular points (T3: temporal, C3: central, Cz, C4, and T5, respectively) (Klem et al. 1958). With the advent of multichannel EEG acquisition systems and the concurrent development of topographic and tomographic signal

**TABLE 1.1**

**Five Categories of Brainwave Patterns**

| Brainwave | Sample Pattern | Frequency (Hz) | Amplitude (μV) |
|---|---|---|---|
| Delta | | 0.5–4 | 100–200 |
| Theta | | 4–8 | 5–10 |
| Alpha | | 8–12 | 20–80 |
| SMR | | 12–15 | |
| Beta | | 15–25 | 1–5 |
| Gamma | | 25–60 | 0.5–2 |

source localization methods, however, the international 10/20 system has been extended to higher-density electrode settings such as the 10/10 and 10/5 systems, allowing more than 500 electrode positions (for the effectiveness of 10/20-derived systems, see Jurcak et al. 2007). Figure 1.4a and b demonstrate the 10/20 international system of electrode placement and an example montage based on the 10/10 system, respectively. To accurately identify the location of scalp electrodes, anatomical landmarks should be determined for the essential positioning of the electrodes: (1) the nasion, which is the point between the forehead and the nose; (2) the inion, which is the lowest point of the skull from the back of the head and is normally indicated by a prominent bump; (3) the pre-auricular points anterior to the ear. The numbers "10" and "20" refer to the fact that the distances between adjacent electrodes are either 10% or 20% of the total front–back or right–left distance of the skull. Each site has a letter to identify the lobe (i.e., F, T, C, P, and O stand for Frontal, Temporal, Central, Parietal, and Occipital, respectively), the Z(ero) to refer to an electrode placed on the midline, and

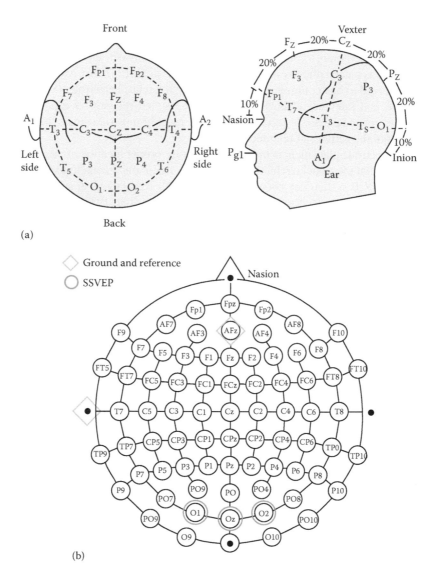

(a)

(b)

**FIGURE 1.4** (a) The 10/20 international system of electrode placement. (b) An example montage based on the 10/10 system, which measures O1 and O2 with Oz bipolar method to elicit SSVEPs.

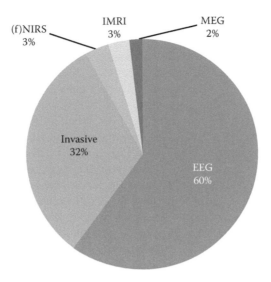

**FIGURE 1.5** BCI research articles published in 2007–2011 from Hwang et al. (2013).

a number to identify the hemisphere location (i.e., odd and even numbers referring to the left and right hemispheres, respectively). Also note that the smaller the number, the closer the position is to the midline. In Figure 1.4b, for example, electrode O1 identifies the left occipital, C4 identifies the right central, P3 identifies the left parietal, and A1 identifies the left ear reference.

Currently, EEGs are among the most popular techniques for brain–computer interfacing technology, making up 68% of BCI research articles published in 2007–2011 as shown in Figure 1.5 (Hwang et al. 2013). It is noninvasive, inexpensive, and portable, making it a popular device in current research. It does not, however, provide high spatial quality information on the location of brain signal activation. In addition, it is mathematically difficult to accurately compute the distribution of currents within the brain that generated these signals. This is referred to as the "inverse problem" (Castaño-Candamil et al. 2015).

### 1.2.1.2 Magnetoencephalography

MEG is another recording technique for noninvasively measuring the magnetic fields generated by neuronal activity of the brain. When active neurons generate electric currents, a miniscule magnetic field is created (Hämäläinen et al. 1993). This magnetic field is impossible to detect from the activation of a single neuron, but when many neurons fire together, a larger and more easily detectable magnetic field is created. MEG combines functional information from the magnetic field recordings with structural information from other anatomical images, such as magnetic resonance imaging (MRI).

The hardware required includes the MEG scanner that is equipped with a superconducting quantum interference device or SQUID that was invented in the 1960s as a sensor of magnetic field changes. The principle features of MEG are as follows: (1) a direct measure of brain function, (2) a very high temporal resolution on the order of milliseconds, (3) an excellent spatial resolution with millimeter precision, and (4) a noninvasive method that does not require the injection of isotopes or exposure to x-rays or magnetic fields (Uhlhaas 2015).

Despite MEGs having better spatial resolution and very similar temporal resolution to EEG, they are used less in BCI research—accounting for only 2% of relevant literature (Figure 1.5). This is likely due to the nonportability and high cost. In addition, MEG requires highly sensitive instrumentation and sophisticated methods, such as a magnetically shielded room for eliminating environmental magnetic interference (Tonet et al. 2006).

### 1.2.1.3 Functional Magnetic Resonance Imaging

Functional magnetic resonance imaging or functional MRI (fMRI) is a noninvasive, functional neuroimaging method that indirectly measures neuronal activity of the brain by identifying the hemodynamic response, known as the blood oxygen level–dependent (BOLD) contrast.

The fMRI principle is based on the so-called neurovascular coupling in which neuronal activation and metabolism with regional cerebral blood flow (rCBF) and regional cerebral blood oxygenation (rCBO) are tightly coupled (Lindauer et al. 2010). When neurons fire, the surrounding blood of the firing neurons experiences a decrease in oxygenated blood, and then a rapid increase in rCBF and oxygen metabolism (cerebral metabolic rate of oxygen, $CMRO_2$) as more oxygenated blood and glucose flow to the area for use in energy consumption (Dunn et al. 2005). The increased oxygen metabolism then converts the oxyhemoglobin in the blood (oxy-Hb) to the deoxygenated blood (deoxy-Hb). On the other hand, a disproportionately large increase in rCBF leads to a washout of deoxy-Hb from the activation area, resulting in a decrease of deoxy-Hb and an increase of oxy-Hb (Lindauer et al. 2001). It has long been suggested that rCBF increases exceed $CMRO_2$ increases by a factor of 2–10 (Lin et al. 2008). Deoxygenated blood transmits greater magnetic fields, interfering with the MRI's magnetic field. However, oxygenated blood creates less intense magnetic fields and therefore interferes with the MRI less, allowing activated neuron areas to be viewable owing to an increase in oxygenated blood flow (Weiskopf et al. 2004).

fMRI data imagery is shown very close to the blood flow, within approximately 1 mm of accuracy and within approximately 1 s of oxygenated blood flow increase (Nicolas-Alonso & Gomez-Gil 2012). That is, fMRIs offer highly accurate spatial information that could be very useful for detailed BCI tasks, but their temporal resolution is quite slow compared to techniques such as EEG or MEG. In addition, fMRI does not measure neural activity directly, but allows for inference of neural activity from measured blood volume and blood flow. Other downfalls include size, and expense of use, making them ineffective and impractical for everyday purposes. Research articles discussing fMRI-BCIs accounted for only 2% of the literature (Figure 1.5).

### 1.2.1.4 Functional Near-Infrared Spectroscopy

Similar to fMRI, functional near-infrared spectroscopy (fNIRS) relies on the changes in oxygenated and deoxygenated blood in the cerebral cortex. Oxygenated and deoxygenated blood absorb light at different rates. For example, deoxygenated blood absorbs more light below 800 nm light, while oxygenated blood does above 800 nm (Giardini et al. 2000; Wilcox et al. 2008). fNIRS takes advantage of the differences in light absorption to detect neuronal activity.

The hardware required for fNIRS includes an infrared light source, a light detector, signal processing devices, and a computing device such as a computer (Nicolas-Alonso & Gomez-Gil 2012). Through the use of an infrared light placed on the scalp and a light detection device placed nearby, levels of neuronal activation can be detected. The infrared light penetrates the scalp and bone and the upper level of the cerebral cortex and, depending on the amount of oxygenated or deoxygenated blood in the area, a certain amount of light is allowed to pass through, and some light is reflected back out of the scalp (Tonet et al. 2006). This penetrating light is identified by the light detector. As discussed in Section 1.2.1.3, neuron firings cause oxygenated blood to rush to the surrounding area, bringing glucose for energy. This shift in blood oxygen levels causes the light to act differently, providing a change in the signal sent to the light detector, which is then processed and recorded.

fNIRS BCIs are not nearly as popular as EEG systems. Research articles focused on fNIRS BCIs accounted for just 3% of the relevant published material (Figure 1.5). Coyle and colleagues (2007) found that fNIRS BCIs can be accurately and simply commanded through motor imagery and proper light and detector placement. Because of the latent nature of the blood flow response to neuron activated sites in the cerebral cortex, the temporal resolution is slower in fNIRS than in EEG or invasive methods that we will discuss in Section 1.2.2. In addition, fNIRS signals are vulnerable to motion and pulse artifacts caused by physical motions and heartbeats during the measurement, respectively (Matthews et al. 2008). Thus, fNIRS should be preprocessed with elaborate artifact removal methods, such as ICA and wavelet, to improve the signal-to-noise ratio (SNR) before feature extraction. fNIRS is also limited to detecting changes in the surface areas of the brain, as the infrared light can only penetrate so far. It is, however, a portable and inexpensive option, making it a decent candidate for home settings (Castermans et al. 2014).

### 1.2.1.5 Positron Emission Tomography

PET is a noninvasive, three-dimensional (3D) radiation or nuclear medicine imaging technique that is used to measure the functional processes within the human body, including neural activity (Stollfuss et al. 2015). The PET principle is based on the phenomenon of positron annihilation. That is, when a positron passes through matter, two photons are simultaneously emitted in almost exactly opposite directions. This method relies on a positron-emitting tracer atom that is introduced into the bloodstream in a biologically active molecule, such as fludeoxyglucose, which acts similarly to glucose in the body. Fludeoxyglucose will concentrate in areas with higher metabolic needs. Over time, this tracer molecule emits positrons, which are detected by a sensor. The spatial location of the tracer molecule in the brain can be determined based on the emitted positrons. This allows researchers to construct a 3D image of the areas of the brain that have the highest metabolic needs, typically those that are most active (Townsend 2008).

In general, the arrangement of a PET machine consists of coincidence detectors, scintillating crystals, and block detectors. However, most BCI research utilizing PET is limited to clinical studies because of its disadvantages, including its high cost and lower half-life of the radionuclide (Bhattacharyya et al. 2015; Boecker et al. 2002; Grafton et al. 1996; Winstein et al. 1997).

### 1.2.2 Invasive Recording Methods

Invasive recording methods are neuroimaging techniques in which the electrodes make direct contact with brain tissue. These methods can provide more accurate spatial and temporal information, but come at a greater risk to the individual. Two types of invasive recording methods—electrocorticography (ECoG) and intracortical neuron recording (INR)—are discussed in this section.

### 1.2.2.1 Electrocorticography

ECoG is also referred to as intracranial EEG, a method of recording electrical impulses with electrodes that are placed on the brain in order to bypass impeding material such as the scalp and skull. The physiology behind ECoG is the same as that for EEG, but sensitivity in ECoG is greater because of the close nature of the electrodes to the neurons. In order for the electrodes to be placed on the surface of the cortex, surgery involving removing part of the skull is required. A group of electrodes spaced about 1 cm apart from each other are placed lightly on either the epidural or subdural layer of the brain. The spacing and grouping of the electrodes are kept consistent through the use of clear, flexible grid structure. Electrodes can be placed temporarily and patients can complete tasks while cognizant during the surgical procedure or they can be placed permanently for use outside of the operating room.

ECoG offers higher temporal (Henle et al. 2013) and spatial resolution than EEG (e.g., tenths of millimeters vs. centimeters) (Freeman et al. 2003), broader bandwidth (e.g., 0–500 Hz vs. 0–50 Hz) (Staba et al. 2002), higher characteristic amplitude (i.e., 50–100 μV vs. 10–20 μV) (Schalk & Mellinger 2010), and far less vulnerability to artifacts such as EMG (Ball et al. 2009) or ambient noise (Schalk & Mellinger 2010). Leuthardt and colleagues found that users of ECoG BCIs had a quicker training rate than those who used EEG BCIs (Leuthardt et al. 2004). Invasive techniques accounted for 32% of the literature over the 2007–2011 period (Figure 1.5). Even still, the invasive nature of ECoG poses obvious risks, including the chance that electrodes can unintentionally move from their initial placement. In addition, patients are also at risk of postoperative infection and tissue reaction (Castermans et al. 2014; Daly & Wolpaw 2008; Mestais et al. 2015). Furthermore, the long-term stability of ECoG signals has not been well researched.

### 1.2.2.2 Intracortical Neuron Recording

INR is a technique that allows for neuronal activity in the gray matter of the brain to be recorded. Just like the EEG and ECoG, this technique relies on the electrical impulses of the brain. Through the use of a penetrating electrode made of glass, platinum or tungsten, placed near or within a neuron cell body, electrical currents are able to be observed. This technique can be so precise it detects one single neuron, known as single unit activity (SUA). Or it can be used to detect multiple neuronal impulses, known as multi-unit activity (MUA). Or more generally, INR can identify local field potentials (LFPs), which are the electrical impulses in the surrounding area of the electrode placement (Homer et al. 2013).

Research into INR began with animal subjects and has since been applied to humans—especially those with severe motor disorders. Coupled with ECoG, research into BCIs using these methods accounted for 32% of the literature (Figure 1.5). The spatial resolution of INR is very detailed and surpasses all other types of invasive and noninvasive neuroimaging techniques, whether recording SUA, MUA, or LFPs. The temporal resolution is similar to that of ECoG. This method has associated risks, including the diminishing of signal acquisition through the electrode over time, tissue damage, foreign body rejection, or electrode movement within the brain (Gunasekera et al. 2015).

### 1.2.3 Brain Signal Patterns for BCI Operation

Every BCI is created to respond to a certain type of brain signal. Figure 1.6 illustrates the most popular types of brain signals used for operating BCIs. What follows is an overarching review of the brain signal patterns in terms of their physiological bases, initial training requirement for use, and the rate at which information is transferred from brain to application. However, only neuroelectric signals, such as EEG, are discussed in the following sections, because it not only can cover most of brain patterns (P300, SSEP, and ERD/ERS) as shown in Figure 1.2 but also is the most studied BCI system because of its simplicity in application (Niedermeyer & da Silva 2005).

### 1.2.3.1 P300 ERPs

The P300 wave is an ERP component of the EEG that reaches a maximum positive peak in voltage about 300 ms after a stimulus onset (Figure 1.6). It is most commonly elicited in an "oddball" paradigm when a subject responds to target stimuli that occur infrequently and irregularly within a series of standard stimuli that occur frequently and regularly (Huettel & McCarthy 2004). The amplitude of the P300 wave is maximal at central and parietal scalp regions (e.g., Pz), varying with the improbability of the targets. Its latency is proportional to the difficulty of discriminating the target stimulus from the standard stimuli (Picton 1992). The stimulus can be visual (Bledowski et al. 2004), auditory (Musiek et al. 2005), or even tactile (Brouwer & van Erp 2010).

Since the P300 response to external stimuli is automatic, initial training is not required to teach users to control their brain signals. A short training may be necessary for certain applications using the P300 wave owing to complicated interfaces or for the sake of the classification algorithm (discussed in Section 1.4). Guger et al. (2009) found that healthy individuals were able to achieve high accuracy levels with very little training time. The high levels of accuracy coupled with the low-cost, easy-to-use EEGs used to measure this response make the P300 wave a useful and popular tool for BCIs. P300 BCIs can also provide the user with a large amount of options to choose.

### 1.2.3.2 Steady-State Evoked Potentials

When presented with steady-state (i.e., vibratory in nature) stimuli, the rhythmic brain activity in the associated cortical area will be generated, mimicking the frequency of the stimuli (Figure 1.6).

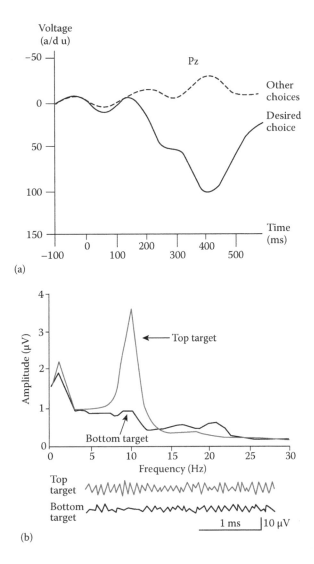

**FIGURE 1.6** Brain signal patterns for BCI operation. (a) P300 ERP. (From Wolpaw, J. R., Birbaumer, N., McFarland, D. J., Pfurtscheller, G., & Vaughan, T. M. (2002). Brain–computer interfaces for communication and control. *Clinical Neurophysiology, 113*(6), 767–791. http://doi.org/10.1016/S1388-2457(02)00057-3) (b) Sensorimotor rhythm. (From Wolpaw, J. R., Birbaumer, N., McFarland, D. J., Pfurtscheller, G., & Vaughan, T. M. (2002). Brain–computer interfaces for communication and control. *Clinical Neurophysiology, 113*(6), 767–791. http://doi.org/10.1016/S1388-2457(02)00057-3) *(Continued)*

The stimulus can be visual, auditory, or even tactile. For example, SSVEPs are currently the most popular choice for brain signals in BCI operations. SSSEPs to be elicited by vibrotactile stimuli (Severens et al. 2010) and SSAEPs to be elicited by auditory stimuli (Hill et al. 2012) have also been used in BCI research.

BCIs that use SSVEPs as their control signal usually have lights or other stimuli that flash at differing frequencies. Each light or pattern is linked with a control option (e.g., direction, on/off, etc.) for the BCI application. For example, a 9-Hz flickering light-emitting diode (LED) is for turning on TV, while an 11-Hz LED is for turning off TV. Selections are made through users focusing on whichever stimulus is associated with the action they want to perform. The neuroimaging device records the frequency of the brain signals and interprets the selection. SSVEP BCIs do not require

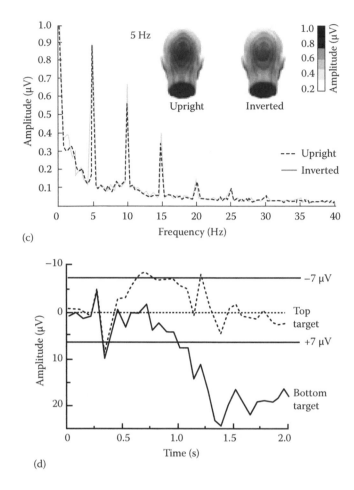

**FIGURE 1.6 (CONTINUED)** Brain signal patterns for BCI operation. (c) Steady-state visual evoked potential. (From Gruss, L. F., Wieser, M. J., Schweinberger, S. R., & Keil, A. (2012). Face-evoked steady-state visual potentials: Effects of presentation rate and face inversion. *Frontiers in Human Neuroscience, 6*.) (d) Slow cortical potential. (From Wolpaw, J. R., Birbaumer, N., McFarland, D. J., Pfurtscheller, G., & Vaughan, T. M. (2002). Brain–computer interfaces for communication and control. *Clinical Neurophysiology, 113*(6), 767–791. http://doi.org/10.1016/S1388-2457(02)00057-3)

training and provide the quickest and most reliable communication in EEG BCIs (Volosyak 2011; Wang et al. 2008; Zhu et al. 2010). However, as SSVEP BCIs required eye gaze and focus, they may not be suitable for users with severe motor disabilities and those who are visually impaired (Nicolas-Alonso & Gomez-Gil 2012). Moreover, staring for long periods of time at flashing lights or stimulus may also induce fatigue.

### 1.2.3.3 Sensorimotor Rhythms

SMRs are brainwave patterns recorded in the somatosensory and the motor cortices (Figure 1.6). These patterns can change due to either movement or imagined movement. There are two rhythms relevant to SMRs: the Mu band (7–13 Hz, alpha band present in the somatosensory and motor cortices) and the Beta band (14–30 Hz). Real and imagined movement creates what are known as event-related desynchronization (ERD) and event-related synchronization (ERS).

ERD is the decrease in frequency band amplitude in the sensorimotor areas of the brain related to movements or imagined movement. ERS is the increase in frequency band amplitude in the sensorimotor areas immediately after movement or imagined movement (Graimann et al. 2010). Mu band ERD starts right before movement onset, reaches the maximal ERD shortly after movement onset, and recovers its original level within a few seconds. In contrast, the beta band shows a short ERD during the initiation of movement, followed by ERS that reaches the maximum after movement execution. This ERS occurs when the Mu rhythm is still attenuated (Nicolas-Alonso & Gomez-Gil 2012). In order for the signal emitting from these movements or imagined movements to be strong enough, the area of usage in the brain needs to be large enough. The hands, feet, and tongue are represented over large areas of the somatosensory and motor cortices owing to the complex and regular motion they produce. BCIs using SMRs often use the imagined movement of feet, hands, or tongue for the purposes of control (Graimann et al. 2010). Since outside stimulation is not required for this BCI type, and the brainwaves and interactions with the BCI are controlled by thought processes, training—sometimes extensive training—is required, employing techniques such as operant conditioning.

### 1.2.3.4 Slow Cortical Potentials

Generalized changes in the polarization levels of superficial cortical neurons are known as slow cortical potentials (SCPs) (Strehl et al. 2014). A change in the direction of negative polarity is associated with increased cortical activity or movement, while a change in the direction of positive polarity is associated with decreased cortical activity and calm (Figure 1.6). SCPs are generally analyzed through the Thought Translation Device. Extensive and intensive training is required, using individualized cognitive and behavioral strategies (Studer et al. 2014). SCPs take anywhere from 1 s to several seconds to develop, and therefore the information transfer rate is quite slow compared to SSVEP and visual P300, which does not allow for much efficiency in use. Similar to SMR BCIs, SCP BCIs do not rely on external stimulus such as visual stimuli of SSVEP in order to elicit brainwave patterns to use to influence the interface. Instead, users control their thought processes in order to interact with the BCI.

## 1.3 IMPROVING SIGNAL QUALITY AND FEATURE EXTRACTION METHODS

In this section, we briefly discuss some methods to improve signal quality and extract important features (e.g., Nicolas-Alonso & Gomez-Gil 2012). First, a discussion of the different artifacts, their primary causes, and the main methods used to remove them is presented. Next, spatial filtering techniques used to enhance the quality of brain signals are discussed. Finally, an example illustrating how artifact removal methods and spatial and temporal filtering techniques are implemented in an SSVEP-based BCI system is presented, along with a summary of the feature extraction techniques widely used for BCI applications.

### 1.3.1 REMOVING NOISY SIGNALS AND ARTIFACTS

The raw signals recorded from the brain during the signal acquisition stage often contain other information that reduces signal quality (Wittenberg et al. 2017). This extra information is collectively known as "noisy signals" or "artifact" and is added by environmental and physiological sources (Wolpaw & Wolpaw 2012). The initial step in feature extraction is to remove the artifacts and excess noise because their presence hinders BCI performance. Figure 1.7 gives an overview of the different artifacts and their primary causes.

Since eye blinking, heart rate, and movement are all uncontrollable body functions that unavoidably intrude on the desired brain signal output necessary for controlling a BCI, preventative measures need to be taken. The signals caused by physiological sources are counteracted by recording electrical output at, or near, the site of the source so that those signals can be temporally compared to the overall brain signal recording. When a shift in the brain signal correlates to the signal recorded by the EKG, EOG, or EMG, that signal is no longer considered for controlling the BCI.

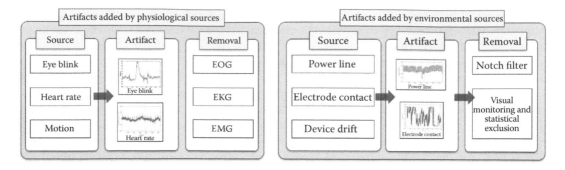

**FIGURE 1.7** Artifacts and noise sources, causal factors, and removal methods. EKG/ECG, electrocardiography; EMG, electromyography; EOG: electrooculography.

Other unavoidable electrical signals that interfere with brain signal data stem from power lines, incorrect electrode contact, and electrode drift. The electrode drift indicates abnormal peaks and trends in EEG signals, and it can be caused by eye-related artifacts, electrode cable movements, and unstable electrode contacts. A notch filter is applied at 60 Hz (main frequency in the United States) or 50 Hz (main frequency in Europe) to remove power line data from the incoming signal, while statistical analysis and visual monitoring are used to overcome irrelevant signals from issues with the EEG cap.

### 1.3.2 Spatial Filtering

The purpose of a spatial filter is to enhance sensitivity to particular brain sources, improve source localization, and suppress certain artifacts (Krusienski et al. 2012). Two main types of spatial filtering methods have been commonly used for BCIs: referencing and data-dependent spatial filters.

#### 1.3.2.1 Referencing Methods

Electric potentials are only defined with respect to a reference electrode that needs to be placed on a presumably "inactive" zone such as the mastoid, earlobe, nose, or base of the neck. Since no position on the scalp can have zero potentials, however, several methods have been used to eliminate task-unrelated background noise from the electrodes (Lee et al. 2017). Example methods include the common average reference (CAR), surface (small or large) Laplacian, and bipolar reference (Figure 1.8).

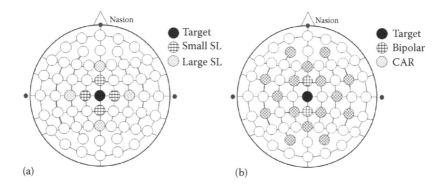

**FIGURE 1.8** The example of referencing methods. (a) Small and larger surface Laplacian method: inner four grid circles are used for the small surface Laplacian method while outer four checkers are used for the large surface Laplacian method. (b) Bipolar and CAR method: grid circles are used for the bipolar method while checkers are used for CAR method.

The choice of the EEG reference is a critical issue, because it can improve the SNR of the electrical activities at target and reference sites (Vatta et al. 2005) and may produce topographic distortion if not appropriately selected (Alhaddad et al. 2012).

### 1.3.2.1.1 Bipolar Reference

The simplest referencing method is bipolar reference, which is performed by measuring a potential difference between two electrodes placed anteriorly and posteriorly or to the left and right of the target position, or with bipolar chains. A bipolar reference is calculated by subtracting the secondary electrode $j$ from the recording electrode $i$:

$$V_{\text{bipolar}(i,j)} = V_{(i)} - V_{(j)}.$$

One advantage of bipolar reference is that it is easy to remove artifacts with relatively less electrodes, which occur at the same temporal, on the same position, and with the same amplitude such as eye blinking and jaw clenching. Moreover, it can easily detect spatial differences over a larger area by chain bipolar reference (Evans & Abarbanel 1999). For these reasons, bipolar reference has been commonly used for BCI applications, including motor imagery BCIs (e.g., Ramoser et al. 2000) and SSVEP-based BCIs (e.g., Wang et al. 2004). The disadvantages, however, are that measuring a specific position is not possible because of indirect measurement and that the information from the electrode could be cancelled out when the brain activities at two positions are temporally and spatially similar to each other (Arciniegas et al. 2013). An example of the bipolar method is shown in Figure 1.8a with grid circles while the gray circle is the target electrode.

### 1.3.2.1.2 Surface Laplacian Reference

The surface Laplacian reference methods can enhance EEG spatial resolution by filtering out spatially broad features among nearest-neighbor or next–nearest-neighbor electrodes. The procedure can be expressed in the following formula:

$$V_{\text{LAP}(i)} = V_{(i)} - \sum_{j \in S(i)} w_{i,j} V_{(j)}$$

$$\text{where } w_{i,j} = \frac{\dfrac{1}{d_{i,j}}}{\displaystyle\sum_{j \in S(i)} \dfrac{1}{d_{i,j}}},$$

where $S_{(i)}$ is the subset of the four adjacent electrodes surrounding the target electrode $i$ (i.e., anterior, posterior, left and right). If the distance from the target electrode $i$ to an adjacent electrode $j$, $d_{i,j}$, is identical for all $j$'s, then $w_{i,j}$ is just a reciprocal of the number of adjacent electrodes, 0.25. Note that the electrodes are not weighted according to their distance (Schalk & Mellinger 2010).

The advantages of the surface Laplacian reference method are that it can be used as a spatial filter to eliminate spatial noise (McFarland et al. 1997) and that it is a reference-independent approach (Tenke & Kayser 2005). However, it is limited in its ability to detect widely distributed brain activity on both the target and adjacent electrodes. An example of small (large) surface Laplacian methods is shown in Figure 1.8b where grid (checkerboard) circles are for adjacent electrode, while the gray circle is the target electrode.

### 1.3.2.1.3   Common Average Reference

The CAR is one of the common referencing methods where the potential is averaged over all electrodes (including the recording electrode) and is subtracted from the recording electrode. The procedure can be expressed in the following formula:

$$V_{\text{CAR}(i)} = V_{(i)} - \frac{1}{N} \sum_{j=1}^{N} V_{(j)},$$

where $N$ is the total number of electrodes used for the recording and $V_{(j)}$ is the potential between the recording electrode $i$ and the reference electrode $j$.

The CAR works well if small signal sources need to be identified in very noisy recordings (Cooper et al. 2003) or when 30 or more electrodes are used (Schmidt & Segalowitz 2007). The advantage of the CAR method is that it can measure spatially broad activities that cannot be measured by bipolar or surface Laplacian reference methods (Carmeli et al. 2012). An example of the CAR method is shown in Figure 1.8a with checkerboard circles while the gray circle is the target electrode.

## 1.3.2.2   Data-Dependent Spatial Filtering

It is often hard to know the exact characteristics of relevant brain activity. In this case, a spatial filter can be derived directly from each BCI user's data. Three common methods for deriving data-dependent spatial filters are introduced: principal component analysis (PCA), independent component analysis (ICA), and common spatial patterns (CSP).

### 1.3.2.2.1   Principal Component Analysis

PCA is a nonparametric statistical data analysis method for significant feature extraction and data reduction, which is accomplished by re-expressing a data set (Shlens 2014). In PCA, EEG data can be explained as a linear combination of principal component coefficients and associated weights by finding the eigenvectors of a covariance matrix (Kayser & Tenke 2003). The principal components of the signals can be derived by the singular value decomposition method (Wall et al. 2003). The EEG signal matrix with $n$ rows of temporal data (sampled data) and $m$ columns of spatial data (channels) can be decomposed into three components such as $\mathbf{U}$, $\mathbf{S}$, and $\mathbf{V}$ matrices as

$$\mathbf{X} = \mathbf{USV}^{T},$$

where $\mathbf{U}$ is an $n \times m$ matrix with $U^{T}U = I$, $\mathbf{S}$ is an $m \times m$ diagonal matrix, and $\mathbf{V}$ is an $m \times m$ orthonormal matrix with $V'V = VV' = I$. Then, the covariance matrix as is written as

$$\mathbf{C} = \frac{1}{n-1} XX^{T} = \frac{1}{n-1} US^{2}U^{T},$$

The eigenvectors and corresponding eigenvalues of $XX^{T}$ are calculated, and then select $m$ eigenvectors have the largest $m$ eigenvalues for the new basis because higher eigenvalues present more data characteristics than lower eigenvalues.

PCA has been proven especially effective at reconstructing the signals with fewer artifactual components in EEG signals (e.g., Boye et al. 2008) and reducing feature space dimensionality (e.g., McFarland et al. 2006).

### 1.3.2.2.2 Independent Component Analysis

The biological signals are measured by a set of electrodes, where each electrode receives an unknown combination of the source signals. ICA is a useful technique to separate unobserved and independent signals from the mixed signal containing artifacts such as facial EMG and blinks with the assumption that these signals are mutually independent (McMenamin et al. 2010). In the simple ICA, it is assumed that there are $n$ random $x_i$ arranged into a vector $x = (x_1, x_2, ..., x_m)^T$, which are linear combinations of $n$ unknown independent variables $s_i$ arranged into $(s_1, s_2, ..., s_n)^T$ (Mozaffar & Petr 2002). Thus, the linear combination form of the model is presented as

$$\mathbf{X} = \mathbf{AS},$$

where $\mathbf{X}$ consists of the $N$ observed signals, $\mathbf{A}$ is an unknown $m \times n$ "mixing matrix" that contains mixing coefficients, and $\mathbf{S}$ is a matrix consisting of coefficients $s_i$.

Then, the goal of ICA tries to find a best possible estimation of unmixing or separation matrix $W$, $W \approx A^{-1}$, such that

$$\mathbf{Y} = \mathbf{WX} = \mathbf{W(AS)} = \mathbf{S'} \approx \mathbf{S}.$$

While any ICA algorithm can be used to estimate the one-dimensional ICA components, large computational savings can be held by using an algorithm that makes use of pre-whitening such as FastICA.

Because of the main advantage of ICA of not requiring a priori knowledge or hypotheses, it has been commonly used as a preprocessing tool (e.g., Gao et al. 2010) or a classifier (Chiappa & Barber 2006). The shortcoming of the basic ICA estimation is, however, that the high computational cost comes about as a result of using high dimensions (Hyvärinen & Oja 2000).

### 1.3.2.2.3 Common Spatial Patterns

CSP is a data-driven supervised decomposition technique that transforms the multichannel EEG signal into a variance matrix to discriminate between two different classes (for a detailed theoretical description of CSP, see Wang et al. 2005). CSP helps to discriminate vague spatial information such as ERD/ERS effects among EEGs by maximizing the variance for one class while minimizing variance for the other classes (Blankertz et al. 2008; Lemm et al. 2005). CSP and its improved versions (e.g., wavelet common spatial pattern, WCSP; common spatio-spectral pattern, CSSP; common sparse spectral spatial pattern, CSSSP) have provided good results for synchronous BCIs, but less effective for asynchronous BCIs (Nicolas-Alonso & Gomez-Gil 2012) because of the nonstationary EEG properties (Galán et al. 2008).

Assuming a single-trial EEG data matrix, $X_{N \times S}$, consisting of $N$ channels and $S$ samples per channel, the normalized covariance matrix is

$$C_{C1} = \frac{X_{C1}X_{C1}^T}{\text{trace}\left(X_{C1}X_{C1}^T\right)}, \; C_{C2} = \frac{X_{C2}X_{C2}^T}{\text{trace}\left(X_{C2}X_{C2}^T\right)}, \; C_c = C_{C1} + C_{C2},$$

where $\text{trace}(XX^T)$ is the sum of diagonal elements of $XX^T$. The composite spatial covariance, $C_c$, and the factored composite spatial covariance are given as

$$C_c = C_{C1} + C_{C2} = U_c \lambda U_C^T,$$

where $U_C$ is a matrix of normalized eigenvectors with corresponding diagonal matrix of eigenvalues $\lambda$. The whitening transformation matrix is given as

$$P = \sqrt{\lambda} U_C^T.$$

Finally, the CSP projection matrix will be $W = U^T P$.

### 1.3.3 Feature Extraction: SSVEPs

In this section, we describe a feature extraction procedure with an EEG-based SSVEP BCI example. Assume that there is a robot that can move four directions in a grid cell environment. A user can control the robot by gazing at one of four flashing LED stimuli (i.e., flickering at 7, 13, 17, and 23 Hz) that correspond to directional commands (up, down, left, and right, respectively). A starting position of the robot is randomly set and the user moves the robot via a BCI system to hit a target position. The robot moves one cell from its current location when the classification of BCI detects one of the four SSVEP features. The classification is made only if the amplitude of one of the frequencies exceeds a certain threshold within the most recent 5 s of EEG data. Otherwise, the robot will not move and will stay at its current position.

EEG data record at a sampling rate of 512 Hz on the occipital area (O1 and O2). The recorded EEG data are first filtered by a 5-Hz high-pass filter, a 75-Hz low-pass filter, and a 60-Hz notch filter. The filtered EEG data are refined by the artifacts removal procedure, and subtract O1 channel to O2 channel by using the bipolar reference method. Then, the EEG data are transformed into the frequency domain by fast Fourier transform (FFT). The time window for FFT is 5 s and a 1-s (512 data points) sliding time window is used, so one decision can be made every second. For each time window, the power values of the fundamental, second, and third harmonics for each frequency are summed up. For example, the power value of 23, 46, and 69 Hz will be summed up for the stimulus of 23 Hz. If the maximum power sum value among four values is two times bigger than the average of the others, then the robot will move one cell from its current location to the corresponding direction of the maximum power frequency. Otherwise, the robot stays in its current position. This procedure will continue until the robot arrives at the target position.

## 1.4 FEATURE CLASSIFICATION METHODS

One important element in BCI operations is a data classifier, or a classification algorithm, that aims at automatically determining a user's intention by classifying extracted brain features. Comprehensive reviews on the classification techniques used for BCIs have been given elsewhere (e.g., Bashashati et al. 2007; Lotte et al. 2007; Nicolas-Alonso & Gomez-Gil 2012). Thus, this section is restricted to present three types of the commonly employed classifiers to design EEG-based BCI systems and highlights their most important properties for BCI applications: linear classifiers, artificial neural network classifiers, and hidden Markov model classifiers.

### 1.4.1 Linear Classifiers

Linear classifiers are discriminant algorithms that use a linear function to classify the data into mutually exclusive and exhaustive classes, assuming that the data come from a Gaussian mixture model. Because of their structural simplicity, competitive accuracy, and very fast training and testing, linear classifiers are one of the most popular algorithms used to design BCI applications. Two main kinds of linear classifier are described: linear discriminant analysis (LDA) and support vector machine (SVM).

### 1.4.1.1  Linear Discriminant Analysis

The aim of LDA is to separate the classes using a line (the number of dimensions $D = 2$), a plane ($D = 3$), or a hyperplane ($D > 3$) that maximizes the distance between the means of the classes (encoded in the between-class scatter matrix $S_B$) and minimize the intraclass variances (encoded in the within-class scatter matrix $S_W$). LDA works well under parametric assumptions (i.e., of the classes with equal class covariances) and linearity assumption (Duda et al. 2012).

To solve a two-class problem ($\omega_i$, $i = 1, 2$), for example, LDA seeks a good projection vector $w^*$ that maximizes the criterion function:

$$J(w) = \frac{\left|\tilde{\mu}_1 - \tilde{\mu}_2\right|^2}{\tilde{S}_1^2 + \tilde{S}_2^2} = \frac{\left|\tilde{S}_B\right|}{\left|\tilde{S}_W\right|} = \frac{w^T S_B w}{w^T S_W w},$$

where $\tilde{\mu}_i$ is the projected mean vector of each class $\omega_i$ in $x$ and $y$ feature space, and $\tilde{S}_i^2$ measures the variability within class $\omega_i$ after projecting it on the $y$ space. The matrix $S_B$ ($S_W$) is called the between-class (within-class) scatter of the original feature vectors, while $\tilde{S}_B(\tilde{S}_W)$ is the between-class (within-class) scatter of the projected samples $y$. Solving the generalized eigenvalue problem

$$S_W^{-1} S_B w = \lambda w, \text{ where } \lambda = J(w) = \text{Scalar}$$

yields

$$w^* = \begin{array}{c} \arg\max J(w) \\ w \end{array} = \begin{array}{c} \arg\max \\ w \end{array} \left( \frac{w^T S_B w}{w^T S_W w} \right) = S_W^{-1}(\mu_1 - \mu_2).$$

The LDA technique has several advantages that make it suitable for determining a BCI user's intention: low computational requirement and simple to use. In addition, LDA has given good results for motor imagery–based BCIs (e.g., Pfurtscheller 1999), P300 speller (e.g., Bostanov 2004), and asynchronous BCIs (e.g., Scherer et al. 2004). LDA has also been applied to multiclass BCI problems (e.g., Garrett et al. 2003), mainly using the "one-versus-the-rest" (OVR) strategy. The OVR method first constructs a set of binary classifiers, each one trained to separate class $C_i$ from all other classes, and then uses the outputs of each binary classifier to predict one of the C classes (Ramage et al. 2009). However, some limitations of LDA should also be noted when considering this approach for BCI applications. For example, parametric assumptions (multivariate normality and equality of covariance matrices) and linearity assumption are particularly restrictive and can provide poor results on complex nonlinear EEG data (Garcia et al. 2003). LDA is sensitive to the presence of outliers (Duda et al. 2012) and often fails when the discriminatory information is not in the mean but rather in the variance of the data (Bostanov 2004).

### 1.4.1.2  Support Vector Machine

SVM is similar to LDA in that it is a binary classification algorithm that uses a discriminant hyperplane to distinguish two classes, but it is also different from LDA in that the selected best hyperplane for an SVM means the one with the largest margin (i.e., largest "gap" or "distance") between the classes. The data points that are closest to or on the separating hyperplane (a linear decision surface) are called support vectors. SVMs have several advantages because of theoretical reasons such as good generalization properties (Bennett & Campbell 2000) and relative insensitive to overtraining (Jain et al. 2000) and the curse of dimensionality (Burges 1998). The disadvantages of SVMs include a poor performance if the number of features is much greater than the number of samples, an expensive $n$-fold cross-validation to calculate probability estimates, and a lower speed of execution (Bennett & Campbell 2000).

In addition to performing linear classification, SVMs can efficiently classify nonlinearly separable data using what is called the kernel trick. This method uses a kernel function $K(x,y)$ to implicitly map the data into another high-dimensional feature spaces. The radial basis function (RBF) or Gaussian kernel is the most widely used kernel function in BCI research:

$$K(x, y) = \exp\left(\frac{-\|x - y\|^2}{2\sigma^2}\right).$$

These RBF-based SVMs have been successfully applied to various BCI applications (e.g., Garrett et al. 2003). In addition, SVMs have provided good empirical results for synchronous BCI problems (e.g., Garrett et al. 2003), motor imagery–based BCIs (Lee & Choi 2003; Thomas et al. 2012), P3 speller (e.g., Krusienski et al. 2006; Rakotomamonjy & Guigue 2008; Salvaris & Sepulveda 2009), and multiclass BCI problems using the OVR strategy (Schlögl et al. 2005).

### 1.4.2 Artificial Neural Network Classifiers

One of the most successful for classification tasks in BCI applications is the so-called artificial neural networks or ANNs, a family of models inspired by biological neural networks (e.g., the structure of the human brain) (Wu et al. 2010). The key element of this paradigm is a large number of highly interconnected neurons or perceptrons, in which each neuron takes many input data, then, based on an internal weighting scheme, produces a single output that is often sent as input to another neuron. This section first describes the multilayer perceptron (MLP), the most widely used ANN for BCI applications, and then briefly presents other architectures of neural network used for BCIs.

#### 1.4.2.1 Multilayer Perceptron

The perhaps most widely used of all kinds of ANNs is the MLP, first proposed by Rumelhart et al. (1986). The MLP consists of a number of highly interconnected neurons or perceptrons organized into different layers. It has an input layer, an output layer, and in between one or more hidden layers. The MLP computes a single output from a set of (many) real-valued inputs ($x$) by forming a linear combination according to weighted connections between the inputs ($w$) and then possibly putting the output through some nonlinear activation function ($\varphi$). With the bias $b$, mathematically this can be written as

$$y = \varphi\left(\sum_{i=1}^{n} w_i x_i + b\right) = \varphi(w^T x + b).$$

There are important properties common to most ANNs and thus MLP (Forslund 2003):

1. *Learnability:* The ability to learn from examples to produce a certain output when presented with a certain input
2. *Generalizability:* The capability to produce good outputs even for inputs not encountered during training
3. *Nonlinearity:* Nonlinear information processing in each neuron, and hence a nonlinear mapping from an input space to an output space
4. *Fault tolerance:* Neural network systems that keep on functioning even if parts of them stop working

Because of these advantages, the MLP has been applied to many BCI problems such as binary (Palaniappan 2005), multiclass (Singha et al. 2007), synchronous (Haselsteiner & Pfurtscheller 2000), or motor imagery (Aguilar et al. 2015) BCIs.

### 1.4.2.2 Other ANN Architectures

The main advantage of the ANNs and thus MLP is that they are universal estimators (Hornik 1994). This means that a neural network can approximate any continuous function to an arbitrary degree of accuracy as the number of hidden layer neurons increases. However, it should also be noted that the universal approximation capability can make these ANN classifiers sensitive to overtraining, especially with noisy and nonstationary EEG data (Balakrishnan & Puthusserypady 2005). Thus, careful attention is required to select ANN architectures for BCI applications.

One of the most commonly used ANN architectures in the field of BCI is the Gaussian classifier, which has been successfully applied to motor imagery (Leeb et al. 2014) and asynchronous (Cincotti et al. 2003) BCIs. According to Lotte et al. (2007), several other ANN architectures have been used for BCI applications. Because of space limitations, we do not discuss these architectures. Interested readers can consult the corresponding references.

- Learning vector quantization (LVQ) neural network (e.g., Bascil et al. 2015)
- Fuzzy ARTMAP neural network (e.g., Palaniappan et al. 2002)
- RBF neural network (e.g., Hoya et al. 2003)
- Bayesian logistic regression neural network (BLRNN) (e.g., Penny et al. 2000)
- Adaptive logic network (ALN) (e.g., Kostov & Polak 2000)
- Probability estimating guarded neural classifier (PeGNC) (e.g., Felzer & Freisleben 2003)
- Finite impulse response neural network (FIRNN) (e.g., Haselsteiner & Pfurtscheller 2000)
- Gamma dynamic neural network (GDNN) (e.g., Barreto et al. 1996)

### 1.4.3 Hidden Markov Model Classifiers

A hidden Markov model (HMM) can be thought of as a bivariate stochastic process in which the most likely hidden state sequence that produces a given sequence of observations can be found using, for example, the well-known Viterbi algorithm (Hernando et al. 2005). Under an HMM, there are two basic assumptions:

1. The *first-order Markov hypothesis*: the current state is dependent only on the previous state.
2. The *output independence hypothesis*: the output observation at time *t* is dependent only on the current state.

HMMs have been used in many other areas of speech recognition, computational biology, and fault detection, but they have also proven to be promising classifiers for EEG-based BCIs (e.g., Cincotti et al. 2003) and ECoG-based BCIs (e.g., Zhao et al. 2014). Table 1.2 summarizes different types of HMMs that have been used to analyze time series data such as EEG and ECoG as well as for BCI applications. HMMs have been applied to classify EEG signals on a motor imagery task. For example, Souza et al. (2012) compared the HMM and ANN classifiers for the spontaneous EEG, EEG of two-class MI, and EEG of real movement. The HMM was also used to classify single-trial EEG data during imagination of a left or right hand movement (Obermaier et al. 2001) and four-class single-trial motor imagery EEG data (Argunşah & Çetin 2010). Zhong and Ghosh (2002) compared the performance of several HMM and CHMM models for a multichannel EEG data classification. Chiappa and Bengio (2003) compared two Markovian models, HMMs and IOHMMs, on three mental tasks for an asynchronous BCI. Suk and Lee (2010) constructed a two-layer HMM for the classification of motor imagery EEG signals in a multiclass BCI paradigm. Recently, ECoG

**TABLE 1.2**
**HMMs Used for EEG Signal Analyses and BCI Applications**

| HMM Classifier | Task | Brain Signal | BCI Study |
|---|---|---|---|
| HMM | Four-class single-trial motor imagery | EEG | Argunşah & Çetin 2010 |
| | Motor imagery | EEG | Souza et al. 2012 |
| | Two-class single-trial motor imagery | EEG | Obermaier et al. 2001 |
| Coupled HMM (CHMM) | Signal analysis | EEG | Zhong & Ghosh 2002 |
| | Hand motion | ECoG | Zhao et al. 2014 |
| Input–output HMM (IOHMM) | Signal analysis | EEG | Chiappa & Bengio 2003 |
| HMM + SVM | Finger movement | ECoG | Onaran et al. 2011 |
| Two-layer HMM | Motor imagery | EEG | Suk & Lee 2010 |

signals have been used for more sophisticated motor task classification such as finger (Onaran et al. 2011) and hand movement (Zhao et al. 2014). For example, Onaran et al. (2011) applied a hybrid approach combining SVM and HMM to classify ECoG signals during finger movements. On the other hand, Zhong and Ghosh (2002) employed the CHMM on multichannel ECoG signals to classify brain signals during a multidirection hand movement task.

## 1.5   EXAMPLE BCI APPLICATIONS

Relying on different neuroimaging and neurophysiological techniques, control signals, feature extractions, and classifications, many interesting BCI systems have been developed for a wide variety of applications. This section serves to highlight the importance of BCI applications based on each control signal type and their implications for future research and development.

### 1.5.1   P300-Based BCIs

One of the more common control signal types is the P300 ERP (as discussed in Section 1.2.3.1). Its most prevalent usage has been the P300 Speller (Farwell & Donchin 1988), which paved the way for many other communication and control applications to be developed using and expanding on their work (Li et al. 2012; Nam et al. 2008). Table 1.3 gives an overview of many different P300-based BCI application resources, comparing control mechanisms and application objectives.

#### 1.5.1.1   Communication Applications

The P300 Speller is not only the most popular spelling application, but it was also the first of its kind (Nam et al. 2009, 2010, 2012). Since then, many researchers have expanded on Farwell and Donchin's (1988) work to create more reliable, faster, and more accurate communication systems. To use the P300 Speller, the user gazes at the target letter while the system randomly flashes rows and columns. The user counts the number of flashes on the target letter and the BCI system then selects the letter with the highest probability with respect to rows and columns as described in the anecdotal story in Section 1.1.1 (Sellers & Donchin 2006). Much of the research has focused on changing the look of the interface in order to elicit either quicker or more intense ERPs. Furthermore, their research has been instrumental in the development of P300-based BCIs for human–machine interaction, entertainment, and art (see Table 1.3).

P300 ERPs that use visual stimulation may not be practical for users with decreased eyesight or eye movement ability. To overcome this limitation, P300-based BCIs relying on auditory and tactile stimulation have been researched. While visual, or a mixture of visual and auditory, stimulation

**TABLE 1.3**

**Example P300-Based BCI Applications**

| Application Type | | Stimulus Modality | | |
| --- | --- | --- | --- | --- |
| | | Visual | Auditory | Tactile |
| Communication | | • Farwell & Donchin 1988<br>• Krusienski et al. 2008<br>• Hex-o-Spell type: Treder & Blankertz 2010<br>• Checkerboard type: Townsend et al. 2010 | • Furdea et al. 2009<br>• Sellers et al. 2006<br>• Furdea et al. 2009<br>• 2D: Höhne et al. 2010<br>• Multi-class: Schreuder et al. 2010<br>• Fast: Schreuder et al. 2011 | • Circle: Brouwer & van Erp 2010<br>• Braille: van der Waal et al. 2012 |
| Control | Human–machine interaction (HMI) | • Robot: Bell et al. 2008<br>• Home devices: Corralejo & Nicolás-Alonso 2014<br>• Browser: Mugler et al. 2010<br>• Virtual smart home: Holzner et al. 2009 | • Robot: Hinic 2009 | • Robot: Mori et al. 2013<br>• Joystick: Kono & Rutkowski 2014 |
| | Rehabilitation | • Wheelchair: Iturrate et al. 2009<br>• Prosthesis: Pfurtscheller et al. 2008<br>• Internet browser: Mugler et al. 2008 | • Locked-in patients: Kübler et al. 2009<br>• ALS patients: Sellers & Donchin 2006 | • Wheelchair: Kaufmann et al. 2014<br>• Locked-in patients: Lugo et al. 2014 |
| | Entertainment | • 3D game: Finke et al. 2009<br>• Game: Congedo et al. 2011<br>• Virtual driving: Bayliss & Ballard 2000<br>• Chess: Kaplan et al. 2013 | • Game: Robinson et al. 2010 | • Game: Thurlings et al. 2013 |
| | Art | • Painting: Holz et al. 2015; Münßinger et al. 2010<br>• Composing: Grierson 2008 | • Music: Vamvakousis & Ramirez 2014 | |

has proven more effective than auditory stimulation alone (Sellers et al. 2006), BCIs using auditory stimuli are still viable for communication purposes (Furdea et al. 2009). Tactile stimulation has also proved effective (van der Waal et al. 2012), especially for users with the visual impairments discussed above.

### 1.5.1.2 Control Applications

P300-based BCI controls have many different uses such as human–machine interaction, entertainment and games, as well as art. Human–machine interaction encompasses robot control, wheelchair control, and many other human–device interactions. These types of applications are useful for individuals with physical disabilities, providing them with more independence and control over their environment. Certain devices are created to increase mobility, while others focus on control of in-home devices such as a TV or DVD player (Corralejo & Nicolás-Alonso 2014), and still others on robotic control to help with carrying tasks (Bell et al. 2008) and other odd jobs.

Although P300 ERPs are a popular control signal for many other BCIs, they are less popular in the entertainment area. This is perhaps due to the time it takes the computer to analyze the P300 data before making a decision and the nature of the task required by the user for P300 elicitation, which may not be well suited to game play (Kaplan et al. 2013). Even though they are not used regularly in BCI games, they are a prevalent choice in artistic BCIs. There are different types of artistic BCIs, ranging from musical applications that allow users to create music by visually selecting notes presented in a P300 Speller–type matrix (Miranda & Soucaret 2008) to a toolbox-style painting program that allows users to make creative choices with the options at their disposal (Münßinger et al. 2010). In-home artistic BCI usage (Holz et al. 2015) reignited the creative processes of two individuals presenting with amyotrophic lateral sclerosis (ALS), which increased their overall quality of life. Visual, auditory, and tactile stimulation applications have all been researched, although visual still appears to be the most popular for control purposes.

### 1.5.2 SSVEP-Based BCIs

Table 1.4 gives an overview of many different SSVEP-based BCI application resources, comparing control mechanisms and application objectives.

### 1.5.2.1 Communication

Most BCIs have developed from a need to make life easier for those who are physically disabled or suffering from a debilitating disease. Recent developments into SSVEP BCIs have geared toward making communication BCIs mobile friendly (Chi et al. 2012; Lin et al. 2013).

Other researchers (Wang et al. 2011b) have explored the development of an online chatting system using SSVEP BCIs, again seeking more independent and communally connected experiences for those with physical disabilities. SSVEP speller applications are becoming more present in the literature. One of the benefits of the SSVEP speller applications is that they require little to no training compared to P300 Spellers, are often quicker, and produce results with higher accuracies. Typically, in SSVEP systems, fewer options are presented at a time, but research into a QWERTY-style keyboard interface (Hwang et al. 2012) proved that increased speed and accuracies could still be accomplished with a large variety of choices. Communication applications using auditory steady-state responses (ASSRs) and SSSEPs have not shown to be as feasible or effective as those using SSVEPs, but research is still being conducted to attempt to implement these types of systems (Hill & Schölkopf 2012; Muller-Putz et al. 2006).

### 1.5.2.2 Control

SSVEP systems can provide users with a relatively simple and reliable means of interacting with their surroundings. Human–machine interaction, rehabilitation, and entertainment are all important

**TABLE 1.4**

**Example SSEP-Based BCI Applications**

| Application Type | | Stimulus Modality | | |
| --- | --- | --- | --- | --- |
| | | Visual | Auditory | Tactile |
| Communication | | • Mobile—LCD (Wang et al. 2011) <br> • Hierarchical design—LCD (Cecotti 2010) <br> • Online chatting—LCD (Wang et al. 2011) <br> • Qwerty keyboard—LED (Hwang et al. 2012) | • Binary choice task (Hill & Schölkopf 2012; Kim et al. 2011) | • Printer head (Muller-Putz et al. 2006) <br> • Braille (Severens et al. 2010) <br> • Solenoid stimulator (Choi et al. 2015) |
| Control | HMI | • Flight simulator—computer display (Müller-Putz et al. 2005) <br> • Remote control car (Gonzalez-Mendoza et al. 2015) <br> • Robot (Nam et al. 2015) | • GUI (Middleton et al. 2006) | • Wheelchair (Kim & Lee 2014) |
| | Regain functionality | • Prosthesis—LED (Muller-Putz & Pfurtscheller 2008) <br> • FES—LCD (Yao et al. 2012) <br> • Exoskeleton—LED (McDaid et al. 2013) | • Schizophrenia (Hong et al. 2004) | • (Colon et al. 2012; Muller-Putz et al. 2006; Severens et al. 2013) |
| | Entertainment | • Two-class—checker (Lalor et al. 2005) <br> • Four-direction—maze (Chumerin et al. 2012) <br> • Three-direction—VR (Faller et al. 2010) <br> • Two-class—eye-closed (Lim et al. 2013) | • Attention—Tetris (Roth et al. 2013) | |
| | Art | • Sketch (Todd et al. 2012) | | |

focuses of SSVEP-based BCIs. Research has been promising for SSVEP, SSAEP, and SSSEP systems for human–machine interactions.

In the field of rehabilitation, SSVEP BCIs have led to greater patient involvement in their therapeutic exercises (e.g., McDaid et al. 2013; Yao et al. 2012). Not only does patient involvement lead to more attentive participation, but it also helps the patient feel more in control of the process. Games developed using SSVEP-based BCI technology have also been used for rehabilitation purposes to keep the patient engaged in the process. From an entertainment perspective, SSVEP-based BCI applications are quite popular, with navigation games currently cornering the research market (e.g., spacecraft control, maze, etc.). Even able-bodied users can appreciate a BCI-driven game environment because of its novelty and uniqueness.

### 1.5.3    ERD/ERS-Based BCIs

Table 1.5 gives an overview of many different ERD/ERS-based BCI application resources; comparing control mechanisms and the application objectives.

#### 1.5.3.1    Communication

Seeking to overcome the time-related decline in P300 potentials and reduce visual fatigue caused by staring at high-contrast, blinking stimuli for too long, Yue et al. (2011) among others (e.g., Perdikis et al. 2014) have developed motor imagery–based BCI speller applications. Motor imagery communication BCIs could also be useful for individuals with reduced eye movement ability and decreased vision, as prolonged eye gaze or movement is not required to control the application.

#### 1.5.3.2    Control

BCI for control of machines using motor imagery has led researchers to test the controlled movements of a humanoid robot (Prataksita et al. 2014), a driving simulator (Bi et al. 2014), and a mouse within a web browser (Yu et al. 2012). All of these laying the bases for future research into more complex systems that continue to provide disabled users with more independence and autonomy

---

**TABLE 1.5**

**Example ERD/ERS-Based BCI Applications**

| | | |
|---|---|---|
| Communication | • SMR-Speller (Yue et al. 2011) | |
| | • BrainTree (Perdikis et al. 2014) | |
| | • NLP (D'albis et al. 2012) | |
| | • Communication board (Scherer et al. 2015) | |
| Control | HMI | • Robot (Prataksita et al. 2014) |
| | | • Simulated vehicle (Bi et al. 2014) |
| | | • 2-D cursor with target selection (Long et al. 2012) |
| | | • BCI mouse (Yu et al. 2012) |
| | Rehabilitation | • Virtual hand (Cincotti et al. 2012; Morone et al. 2015; Pichiorri et al. 2015) |
| | | • FES (Mukaino et al. 2014) |
| | | • Robot arm (Onose et al. 2012) |
| | | • Orthosis (Pfurtscheller et al. 2010b) |
| | | • Wheelchair (Choi & Cichocki 2008) |
| | Entertainment | • Maze (Bordoloi et al. 2012) |
| | | • Virtual helicopter (Doud et al. 2011) |
| | | • Co-BCI video game (Bonnet et al. 2013) |
| | | • Quadcopter (LaFleur et al. 2013) |
| | | • Continuous control (Coyle et al. 2011) |

(Jeon et al. 2011; Nam et al. 2011). Neurorehabilitation after a stroke often requires training undamaged part of the brain to perform the tasks that were previously performed by the affected area (Cincotti et al. 2012). Many stroke victims have impaired motor movements and using motor imagery therapies could potentially help rehabilitate motor function (Cincotti et al. 2012; Triponyuwasin & Wongsawat 2014). Certain motor imagery therapeutic techniques found that brainwave intensity, or "spectral power," increases over a short period of time. This is indicative of rebuilding damaged brain cells, training other brain cells to do different work, and greater ability to interact with a motor imagery BCI.

Research into games using motor imagery BCI can give insight into future techniques to improve other systems focused on rehabilitation or control. For example, Bonnet et al. (2013), through creating a collaborative football game, found that users preferred multiuser conditions as they improved fun and motivation. Incorporating those methods or game-like environments into rehabilitation could have a positive effect on patient outcomes.

## 1.6   SUMMARY

This chapter reviewed the state of the art of BCI as an emerging human–computer interaction technology, including a BCI classification scheme (Section 1.1), different types of the signal recording methods and brain signal patterns for BCI operation (Section 1.2), the most commonly used signal processing techniques and feature extraction techniques (Section 1.3), classification methods used for identifying the user's intentions (Section 1.4), and various types of BCI applications (Section 1.5).

In the last two decades, the BCI community has witnessed a substantial amount of work done on BCI technologies and many successful BCI applications. However, continuing effort is still needed to further optimize the capabilities, robustness, and usability of BCI systems for human use, including those who suffer from muscular disabilities such as ALS, brainstem stroke, and severe cerebral palsy. That is, more research and development is required to advance BCI technology in the areas of (1) invasive and noninvasive methods to monitor and obtain brain signals, (2) effective signal processing methods that extract signal features (e.g., spatial and temporal filters), (3) innovative algorithms that translate these features into device commands (e.g., linear and nonlinear classifiers), and (4) the development and evaluation of potential applications to enhance the value of brain–computer interfacing technology. Additionally, most BCI technology has strictly focused on supporting individuals with disabilities, and while those efforts continue to be necessary, applications outside of clinical settings, including passive BCI systems, could prove useful and beneficial as well (Zander & Kothe 2011). Finally, the future of BCI research and development, including readily available BCI applications, also depends on close inter- and multidisciplinary collaborations and ongoing communication among neuroscientists, engineers, psychologists, human factors professionals, clinicians, and rehabilitation specialists (Kothe & Makeig 2013; Nam et al. 2015; Schalk et al. 2004).

## ACKNOWLEDGMENTS

This work was supported in part by the National Science Foundation (NSF) under grants numbers IIS-1421948 and BCS-1551688. Any opinions, findings, and conclusions or recommendations expressed in this material are those of the authors and do not necessarily reflect the views of the NSF.

## REFERENCES

Aguilar, J. M., Castillo, J., & Elias, D. (2015). EEG signals processing based on fractal dimension features and classified by neural network and support vector machine in motor imagery for a BCI. In A. Braidot & A. Hadad (Eds.), *VI Latin American Congress on Biomedical Engineering CLAIB 2014, Paraná, Argentina 29, 30 & 31 October 2014 SE - 157* (Vol. 49, pp. 615–618). Springer International Publishing. http://doi.org/10.1007/978-3-319-13117-7_157

Alhaddad, M. J., Kamel, M., Malibary, H., Thabit, K., Dahlwi, F., & Hadi, A. (2012). P300 Speller efficiency with common average reference. In *Proceedings of the Third International Conference on
Autonomous and Intelligent Systems* (pp. 234–241). Berlin, Heidelberg: Springer-Verlag. http://doi
.org/10.1007/978-3-642-31368-4_28

Allison, B. Z., McFarland, D. J., Schalk, G., Zheng, S. D., Jackson, M. M., & Wolpaw, J. R. (2008). Towards
an independent brain–computer interface using steady state visual evoked potentials. *Clinical
Neurophysiology: Official Journal of the International Federation of Clinical Neurophysiology, 119*,
399–408. http://doi.org/10.1016/j.clinph.2007.09.121

Arciniegas, D. B., Anderson, C. A., & Filley, C. M. (Eds.). (2013). *Behavioral Neurology & Neuropsychiatry.*
Cambridge University Press.

Argunşah, A. Ö., & Çetin, M. (2010). AR-PCA-HMM approach for sensorimotor task classification in EEG-
based brain–computer interfaces. *Proceedings—International Conference on Pattern Recognition,*
113–116. http://doi.org/10.1109/ICPR.2010.36

Balakrishnan, D., & Puthusserypady, S. (2005). Multilayer perceptrons for the classification of brain computer
interface data. *Proceedings of the IEEE 31st Annual Northeast Bioengineering Conference, 2005*, 5–6.
http://doi.org/10.1109/NEBC.2005.1431953

Ball, T., Kern, M., Mutschler, I., Aertsen, A., & Schulze-Bonhage, A. (2009). Signal quality of simultaneously
recorded invasive and non-invasive EEG. *Neuroimage, 46*(3), 708–716.

Barreto, A. B., Taberner, A. M., & Vicente, L. M. (1996). Classification of spatio-temporal EEG readiness
potentials towards the development of a brain–computer interface. *Proceedings of SOUTHEASTCON
'96.* http://doi.org/10.1109/SECON.1996.510035

Bascil, M. S., Tesneli, A. Y., Temurtas, F., Pca, Á., & Mlnn, Á. L. V. Q. Á. (2015). Multi-channel EEG signal
feature extraction and pattern recognition on horizontal mental imagination task of 1-D cursor movement for brain computer interface. *Australasian Physical & Engineering Sciences in Medicine.* http://
doi.org/10.1007/s13246-015-0345-6

Bashashati, A., Fatourechi, M., Ward, R. K., & Birch, G. E. (2007). A survey of signal processing algorithms
in brain–computer interfaces based on electrical brain signals. *Journal of Neural Engineering, 4*(2), R32.

Bayliss, J. D., & Ballard, D. H. (2000). A virtual reality testbed for brain–computer interface research.
*Rehabilitation Engineering, IEEE Transactions on, 8*(2), 188–190.

Bell, C. J., Shenoy, P., Chalodhorn, R., & Rao, R. P. N. (2008). Control of a humanoid robot by a noninvasive brain–computer interface in humans. *Journal of Neural Engineering, 5*(2), 214–220. http://doi
.org/10.1088/1741-2560/5/2/012

Bennett, K. P., & Campbell, C. (2000). Support vector machines: Hype or hallelujah? *ACMSIGKDD
Explorations Newsletter, 2*(2), 1–13.

Beveridge, R., Marshall, D., Wilson, S., & Coyle, D. (2015). 3D game graphic complexity effects on motion-
onset visual evoked potentials. In *International Conference on Computer Games, Multimedia & Allied
Technology (CGAT)* (p. 139). Global Science and Technology Forum.

Bhattacharyya, S., Khasnobish, A., Ghosh, P., Mazumder, A., & Tibarewala, D. N. (2015). A review on brain
imaging techniques for BCI applications. *Biomedical Image Analysis and Mining Techniques for
Improved Health Outcomes, 39*.

Bi, L., He, T., & Fan, X. (2014). A driver-vehicle interface based on ERD/ERS potentials and alpha rhythm.
*Systems, Man and Cybernetics (SMC), 2014 IEEE International Conference on.* http://doi.org/10.1109
/SMC.2014.6974053

Birbaumer, N. (2006). Breaking the silence: Brain–computer interfaces (BCI) for communication and motor
control. *Psychophysiology, 43*(6), 517–532.

Birbaumer, N., Kubler, A., Ghanayim, N., Hinterberger, T., Perelmouter, J., Kaiser, J., … Flor, H. (2000).
The thought translation device (TTD) for completely paralyzed patients. *IEEE Transactions on
Rehabilitation Engineering, 8*(2), 190–193. http://doi.org/10.1109/86.847812

Blankertz, B., Tomioka, R., Lemm, S., Kawanabe, M., & Müller, K. R. (2008). Optimizing spatial filters for
robust EEG single-trial analysis. *IEEE Signal Processing Magazine, 25*(1), 41–56. http://doi.org/10.1109
/MSP.2008.4408441

Bledowski, C., Prvulovic, D., Hoechstetter, K., Scherg, M., Wibral, M., Goebel, R., & Linden, D. E. J. (2004).
Localizing P300 generators in visual target and distractor processing: A combined event-related potential and functional magnetic resonance imaging study. *The Journal of Neuroscience, 24*(42), 9353–9360.
http://doi.org/10.1523/JNEUROSCI.1897-04.2004

Boecker, H., Ceballos-Baumann, A. O., Bartenstein, P., Dagher, A., Forster, K., Haslinger, B., … Conrad, B.
(2002). AH 2 15 O positron emission tomography study on mental imagery of movement sequences—
The effect of modulating sequence length and direction. *NeuroImage, 17*(2), 999–1009.

Bonnet, L., Lotte, F., & Lécuyer, A. (2013). Two brains, one game: Design and evaluation of a multiuser BCI video game based on motor imagery. *Computational Intelligence and AI in Games, IEEE Transactions on*, *5*(2), 185–198.

Bordoloi, S., Sharmah, U., & Hazarika, S. M. (2012). Motor imagery based BCI for a maze game. In *Intelligent Human Computer Interaction (IHCI), 2012 4th International Conference on* (pp. 1–6).

Bostanov, V. (2004). BCI competition 2003-data sets Ib and IIb: feature extraction from event-related brain potentials with the continuous wavelet transform and the t-value scalogram. *Biomedical Engineering*, *51*(6), 1057–1061.

Boye, A. T., Kristiansen, U. Q., Billinger, M., do Nascimento, O. F., & Farina, D. (2008). Identification of movement-related cortical potentials with optimized spatial filtering and principal component analysis. *Biomedical Signal Processing and Control*, *3*(4), 300–304.

Brouwer, A. M., & Van Erp, J. B. (2010). A tactile P300 brain–computer interface. *Frontiers in Neuroscience*, *4*(19), 19. http://doi.org/10.3389/fnins.2010.00019

Brouwer, A. M., Van Erp, J., Heylen, D., Jensen, O., & Poel, M. (2013). Effortless passive BCIs for healthy users. *Lecture Notes in Computer Science (Including Subseries Lecture Notes in Artificial Intelligence and Lecture Notes in Bioinformatics)*, *8009 LNCS*(PART 1), 615–622. http://doi.org/10.1007/978-3-642-39188-0-66

Bryant, D., Wang, F., Deardeuff, K., Zoccoli, E., & Nam, C. S. (2016). The neural correlates of moral thinking: A meta-analysis. *International Journal of Computational & Neural Engineering*, *3*(2), 28–39.

Burges, C. J. (1998). A tutorial on support vector machines for pattern recognition. *Data Mining and Knowledge Discovery*, *2*(2), 121–167.

Cantor, D. S., & Evans, J. R. (2013). *Clinical Neurotherapy: Application of Techniques for Treatment*. Academic Press.

Carmeli, C., Knyazeva, M. G., Cuénod, M., & Do, K. Q. (2012). Glutathione precursor $N$-acetyl-cysteine modulates EEG synchronization in schizophrenia patients: A double-blind, randomized, placebo-controlled trial. *PloS One*, *7*(2), e29341. http://doi.org/10.1371/journal.pone.0029341

Castaño-Candamil, S., Höhne, J., Martinez-Vargas, J.-D., An, X.-W., Castellanos-Dominguez, G., & Haufe, S. (2015). Solving the EEG inverse problem based on space-time-frequency structured sparsity constraints. *NeuroImage*. http://doi.org/10.1016/j.neuroimage.2015.05.052

Castermans, T., Duvinage, M., Cheron, G., & Dutoit, T. (2014). Towards effective non-invasive brain–computer interfaces dedicated to gait rehabilitation systems. *Brain Sciences*, *4*, 1–48.

Cecotti, H. (2010). A self-paced and calibration-less SSVEP-based brain–computer interface speller. *IEEE Transactions on Neural Systems and Rehabilitation Engineering*, *18*(2), 127–133. http://doi.org/10.1109/TNSRE.2009.2039594

Chi, Y. M., Wang, Y.-T., Wang, Y., Maier, C., Jung, T.-P., & Cauwenberghs, G. (2012). Dry and noncontact EEG sensors for mobile brain–computer interfaces. *IEEE Transactions on Neural Systems and Rehabilitation Engineering*, *20*(2), 228–235.

Chiappa, S., & Barber, D. (2006). EEG classification using generative independent component analysis. *Neurocomputing*, *69*(7–9 SPEC. ISS.), 769–777. http://doi.org/10.1016/j.neucom.2005.12.028

Chiappa, S., & Bengio, S. (2003). *HMM and IOHMM Modeling of EEG Rhythms for Asynchronous BCI Systems*.

Choi, I., Bond, K., Krusienski, D., & Nam, C. (2015). Comparison of stimulation patterns to elicit steady-state somatosensory evoked potentials (SSSEPs): Implications for hybrid and SSSEP-based BCIs. In *IEEE International Conference on Systems, Man, and Cybernetics* (pp. 3122–3127). http://doi.org/10.1109/SMC.2015.542

Choi, I., Rhiu, I., Lee, Y., Yun, M. H., & Nam, C. S. (2017). A systematic review of hybrid brain-computer interfaces: Taxonomy and usability perspectives. *PloS One*, *12*(4), e0176674.

Choi, K., & Cichocki, A. (2008). Control of a wheelchair by motor imagery in real time. In *Intelligent Data Engineering and Automated Learning—IDEAL 2008* (pp. 330–337). Springer.

Chumerin, N., Manyakov, N. V. N. V., Combaz, A., Robben, A., van Vliet, M., & Van Hulle, M. M. (2012). Steady state visual evoked potential based computer gaming—The maze. *IEEE Transactions on Computational Intelligence and AI in Games*, *PP*(99), 28–37. http://doi.org/10.1109/TCIAIG.2012.2225623

Cincotti, F., Pichiorri, F., Aricò, P., Aloise, F., Leotta, F., de Vico Fallani, F., … Mattia, D. (2012). EEG-based brain–computer interface to support post-stroke motor rehabilitation of the upper limb. In *Engineering in Medicine and Biology Society (EMBC), 2012 Annual International Conference of the IEEE* (pp. 4112–4115).

Cincotti, F., Scipione, A., Timperi, A., Mattia, D., Marciani, A. G., Millan, J., & Bablioni, F. (2003). Comparison of different feature classifiers for brain computer interfaces. *First International IEEE EMBS Conference on Neural Engineering, 2003. Conference Proceedings*, 645–647. http://doi.org/10.1109/CNE.2003.1196911

Colon, E., Legrain, V., & Mouraux, A. (2012). Steady-state evoked potentials to study the processing of tactile and nociceptive somatosensory input in the human brain. *Neurophysiologie Clinique/Clinical Neurophysiology*, *42*(5), 315–323.

Congedo, M., Goyat, M., Tarrin, N., Ionescu, G., Varnet, L., Rivet, B., … Jutten, C. (2011). "Brain Invaders": A prototype of an open-source P300-based video game working with the OpenViBE platform. In *5th International Brain–Computer Interface Conference 2011 (BCI 2011)* (pp. 280–283). Graz, Austria.

Corralejo, R., & Nicolás-Alonso, L. (2014). A P300-based brain–computer interface aimed at operating electronic devices at home for severely disabled people. *Medical & Biological Engineering & Computing*, *52*(10), 861–872. http://doi.org/10.1007/s11517-014-1191-5

Coyle, D., Garcia, J., Satti, A. R., & McGinnity, T. M. (2011). EEG-based continuous control of a game using a 3 channel motor imagery BCI: BCI game. In *Computational Intelligence, Cognitive Algorithms, Mind, and Brain (CCMB), 2011 IEEE Symposium on* (pp. 1–7). http://doi.org/10.1109/CCMB.2011.5952128

Coyle, S. M., Ward, T. E. T. E., & Markham, C. M. (2007). Brain–computer interface using a simplified functional near-infrared spectroscopy system. *Journal of Neural Engineering*, *4*(3), 219–226. http://doi.org/10.1088/1741-2560/4/3/007

D'albis, T., Blatt, R., Tedesco, R., Sbattella, L., & Matteucci, M. (2012). A predictive speller controlled by a brain–computer interface based on motor imagery. *ACM Transactions on Computer-Human Interaction (TOCHI)*, *19*(3), 20.

Daly, J. J., & Wolpaw, J. R. (2008). Brain–computer interfaces in neurological rehabilitation. *The Lancet Neurology*, *7*(11), 1032–1043. http://doi.org/10.1016/S1474-4422(08)70223-0

Doud, A. J., Lucas, J. P., Pisansky, M. T., & He, B. (2011). Continuous three-dimensional control of a virtual helicopter using a motor imagery based brain–computer interface. *PloS One*, *6*(10), e26322.

Duda, R. O., Hart, P. E., & Stork, D. G. (2012). *Pattern Classification*. John Wiley & Sons.

Dunn, A. K., Devor, A., Dale, A. M., and Boas, D. A. (2005). Spatial extent of oxygen metabolism and hemodynamic changes during functional activation of the rat somatosensory cortex. *Neuroimage*, *27*, 279–290.

Evans, J. R., & Abarbanel, A. (1999). *Introduction to Quantitative EEG and Neurofeedback. Search* (Vol. 158). http://doi.org/10.1176/appi.ajp.158.5.827

Faller, J., Muller-Putz, G., Schmalstieg, D., & Pfurtscheller, G. (2010). An application framework for controlling an avatar in a desktop-based virtual environment via a software SSVEP brain–computer interface. *Presence*. http://doi.org/10.1162/pres.19.1.25

Farwell, L. A., & Donchin, E. (1988). Talking off the top of your head: Toward a mental prosthesis utilizing event-related brain potentials. *Electroencephalography and Clinical Neurophysiology*, *70*(6), 510–523.

Felzer, T., & Freisleben, B. (2003). Analyzing EEG signals using the probability estimating guarded neural classifier. *IEEE Transactions on Neural Systems and Rehabilitation Engineering: A Publication of the IEEE Engineering in Medicine and Biology Society*, *11*(4), 361–371. http://doi.org/10.1109/TNSRE.2003.819785

Ficke, R. (1992). *Digest of Data on Persons with Disabilities*. Washington, DC.

Finke, A., Lenhardt, A., & Ritter, H. (2009). The MindGame: A P300-based brain–computer interface game. *Neural Networks*, *22*(9), 1329–1333.

Forslund, P. (2003). A neural network based brain–computer interface for classification of movement related EEG.

Freeman, W. J., Holmes, M. D., Burke, B. C., & Vanhatalo, S., Freeman, W. J., Holmes, M. D., Burke, B. C., & Vanhatalo, S. (2003). Spatial spectra of scalp EEG and EMG from awake humans. *Clinical Neurophysiology*, *114*(6), 1053–1068.

Furdea, A., Halder, S., Krusienski, D. J., Bross, D., Nijboer, F., Birbaumer, N., & Kübler, A. (2009). An auditory oddball (P300) spelling system for brain–computer interfaces. *Psychophysiology*, *46*(3), 617–625. http://doi.org/10.1111/j.1469-8986.2008.00783.x

Galán, F., Nuttin, M., Lew, E., Ferrez, P. W., Vanacker, G., Philips, J., & Millan, J. del R. (2008). A brain-actuated wheelchair: Asynchronous and non-invasive brain–computer interfaces for continuous control of robots. *Clinical Neurophysiology*, *119*(9), 2159–2169. http://doi.org/10.1016/j.clinph.2008.06.001

Gao, J., Zheng, C., & Wang, P. (2010). Real-time removal of ocular artifacts from EEG signals using ICA and manifold algorithm. *Scandinavian Journal of Work, Environment & Health*, *36*(3), 113–118.

Garcia, G., Ebrahimi, T., & Vesin, J. (2003). Support vector EEG classification in the Fourier and time-frequency correlation. In *IEEE-EMBS First International Conference on Neural Engineering* (pp. 591–594).

Garcia–Molina, G., Tsoneva, T., & Nijholt, A. (2013). Emotional brain–computer interfaces. *International Journal of Autonomous and Adaptive Communications Systems*, *6*(1), 9–25.

Garrett, D., Peterson, D., Anderson, C. W., & Thaut, M. H. (2003). Comparison of linear, nonlinear, and feature selection methods for EEG signal classification. *Neural Systems and Rehabilitation Engineering, IEEE Transactions on, 11*(2), 141–144.

Gevensleben, H., Albrecht, B., Lütcke, H., Auer, T., Dewiputri, W. I., Schweizer, R., … Rothenberger, A. (2014). Neurofeedback of slow cortical potentials: Neural mechanisms and feasibility of a placebo-controlled design in healthy adults. *Frontiers in Human Neuroscience, 8*, 990. http://doi.org/10.3389/fnhum.2014.00990

Giabbiconi, C. M., Dancer, C., Zopf, R., Gruber, T., & Muller, M. M. (2004). Selective spatial attention to left or right hand flutter sensation modulates the steady-state somatosensory evoked potential. *Cognitive Brain Research, 20*, 58–66. http://doi.org/10.1016/j.cogbrainres.2004.01.004

Giardini, M. E., Lago, M. C. P., Gemetti, A., & Chimica, D. (2000). Portable microcontroller-based instrument for near infrared spectroscopy, *SPIE, 3911*, 250–255.

Gonzalez-Mendoza, A., Perez-Benitez, J. L., Perez-Benitez, J. A., & Espina-Hernandez, J. H. (2015). Brain computer interface based on SSVEP for controlling a remote control car. *Electronics, Communications and Computers (CONIELECOMP), 2015 International Conference on.* http://doi.org/10.1109/CONIELECOMP.2015.7086931

Grafton, S. T., Arbib, M. A., Fadiga, L., & Rizzolatti, G. (1996). Localization of grasp representations in humans by positron emission tomography. *Experimental Brain Research, 112*(1), 103–111.

Graimann, B., Allison, B., & Pfurtscheller, G. (2010). Brain–computer interfaces: A gentle introduction. *Brain–Computer Interfaces.*

Grierson, M. (2008). Composing with brainwaves: Minimal trial P300b recognition as an indication of subjective preference for the control of a musical instrument. In *Proceedings of the ICMC.*

Gruss, L. F., Wieser, M. J., Schweinberger, S. R., & Keil, A. (2012). Face-evoked steady-state visual potentials: Effects of presentation rate and face inversion. *Frontiers in Human Neuroscience, 6.*

Guger, C., Daban, S., Sellers, E., Holzner, C., Krausz, G., Carabalona, R., … Edlinger, G. (2009). How many people are able to control a P300-based brain–computer interface (BCI)? *Neuroscience Letters, 462*, 94–98. http://doi.org/10.1016/j.neulet.2009.06.045

Gunasekera, B., Saxena, T., Bellamkonda, R., & Karumbaiah, L. (2015). Intracortical recording interfaces: Current challenges to chronic recording function. *ACS Chemical Neuroscience, 6*(1), 68–83. http://doi.org/10.1021/cn5002864

Hämäläinen, M., Hari, R., Ilmoniemi, R. J., Knuutila, J., & Lounasmaa, O. V. (1993). Magnetoencephalography—Theory, instrumentation, and applications to noninvasive studies of the working human brain. *Reviews of Modern Physics, 65*(2), 413.

Han, J. H., Ji, S., Shi, C., Yu, S. B., & Shin, J., Han, J.-H., Ji, S., Shi, C., Yu, S.-B., & Shin, J. (2015). Recent progress of non-invasive optical modality to brain computer interface: A review study. In *The 3rd International Winter Conference on Brain–Computer Interface* (pp. 1–2). http://doi.org/10.1109/IWW-BCI.2015.7073037

Haselsteiner, E., & Pfurtscheller, G. (2000). Using time-dependent neural networks for EEG classification. *IEEE Transactions on Rehabilitation Engineering: A Publication of the IEEE Engineering in Medicine and Biology Society, 8*(4), 457–463. http://doi.org/10.1109/86.895948

Hazrati, M. K., & Erfanian, A. (2010). An online EEG-based brain–computer interface for controlling hand grasp using an adaptive probabilistic neural network. *Medical Engineering & Physics, 32*(7), 730–739. http://doi.org/10.1016/j.medengphy.2010.04.016

Henle, C., Schuettler, M., Rickert, J., & Stieglitz, T. (2013). Towards electrocorticographic electrodes for chronic use in BCI applications. In B. Z. Allison, S. Dunne, R. Leeb, J. Del R. Millán, & A. Nijholt (Eds.), *Towards Practical Brain–Computer Interfaces SE - 5* (pp. 85–103). Springer Berlin Heidelberg. http://doi.org/10.1007/978-3-642-29746-5_5

Hernando, D., Crespi, V., & Cybenko, G. (2005). Efficient computation of the hidden Markov model entropy for a given observation sequence. *Information Theory, IEEE Transactions on, 51*(7), 2681–2685.

Hill, N. J., Moinuddin, A., Häuser, A.-K., Kienzle, S., Schalk, G., & Hill, N. J., Moinuddin, A., Häuser, A. K., Kienzle, S., & Schalk, G. (2012). Communication and control by listening: Toward optimal design of a two-class auditory streaming brain–computer interface. *Frontiers in Neuroscience, 6*, 181. http://doi.org/10.3389/fnins.2012.00181

Hill, N. J., & Schölkopf, B. (2012). An online brain–computer interface based on shifting attention to concurrent streams of auditory stimuli. *Journal of Neural Engineering, 9*(2), 26011.

Hinic, V. (2009). Brain computer interface system for communication and robot control based on auditory evoked event-related potentials. ProQuest Dissertations and Theses.

Höhne, J., Schreuder, M., Blankertz, B., & Tangermann, M. (2010). Two-dimensional auditory p300 speller with predictive text system. In *Engineering in Medicine and Biology Society (EMBC), 2010 Annual International Conference of the IEEE* (pp. 4185–4188).

Holz, E. M., Botrel, L., & Kübler, A. (2015). Independent home use of Brain Painting improves quality of life of two artists in the locked-in state diagnosed with amyotrophic lateral sclerosis. *Brain–Computer Interfaces*, *2*(2–3), 117–134.

Holzner, C., Guger, C., Edlinger, G., Grönegress, C., & Slater, M. (2009). Virtual smart home controlled by thoughts. *Proceedings of the Workshop on Enabling Technologies: Infrastructure for Collaborative Enterprises, WETICE*, 236–239. http://doi.org/10.1109/WETICE.2009.41

Homan, R. W., Herman, J., & Purdy, P. (1987). Cerebral location of international 10–20 system electrode placement. *Electroencephalography and Clinical Neurophysiology*, *66*(4), 376–382.

Homer, M. L., Nurmikko, A. V., Donoghue, J. P., & Hochberg, L. R. (2013). Implants and decoding for intracortical brain computer interfaces. *Annual Review of Biomedical Engineering*, *15*, 383–405. http://doi.org/10.1146/annurev-bioeng-071910-124640

Hong, L. E., Summerfelt, A., McMahon, R., Adami, H., Francis, G., Elliott, A., … Thaker, G. K. (2004). Evoked gamma band synchronization and the liability for schizophrenia. *Schizophrenia Research*, *70*(2), 293–302.

Hornik, K. (1994). Neural networks: More than "Statistics for Amateurs"? In R. Dutter & W. Grossmann (Eds.), *Compstat SE - 25* (pp. 223–235). Physica-Verlag HD. http://doi.org/10.1007/978-3-642-52463-9_25

Hoya, T., Hori, G., Bakardjian, H., Nishimura, T., Suzuki, T., Miyawaki, Y., … Cao, J. (2003). Classification of single trial EEG signals by a combined principal + independent component analysis and probabilistic neural network approach. In *In International Symposium on Independent Component Analysis and Blind Signal Separation.* http://doi.org/10.1.1.6.9249

Huettel, S. A., & McCarthy, G. (2004). What is odd in the oddball task? *Neuropsychologia*, *42*(3), 379–386. http://doi.org/10.1016/j.neuropsychologia.2003.07.009

Hwang, H.-J., Kim, S., Choi, S., & Im, C.-H. (2013). EEG-based brain–computer interfaces: A thorough literature survey. *International Journal of Human–Computer Interaction*, *29*(12), 814–826. http://doi.org/10.1080/10447318.2013.780869

Hwang, H.-J., Lim, J.-H. H., Jung, Y.-J. J., Choi, H., Lee, S. W., & Im, C.-H. H. (2012). Development of an SSVEP-based BCI spelling system adopting a QWERTY-style LED keyboard. *Journal of Neuroscience Methods*, *208*(1), 59–65. http://doi.org/10.1016/j.jneumeth.2012.04.011

Hyvärinen, A., & Oja, E. (2000). Independent component analysis: Algorithms and applications. *Neural Networks: The Official Journal of the International Neural Network Society*, *13*(4–5), 411–430. http://doi.org/10.1016/S0893-6080(00)00026-5

Iturrate, I., Antelis, J., Kubler, A., & Minguez, J. (2009). A noninvasive brain-actuated wheelchair based on a p300 neurophysiological protocol and automated navigation. *IEEE Transactions on Robotics*, *25*(3), 1–14. http://doi.org/10.1109/TRO.2009.2020347

Jain, A. K., Duin, R. P., & Mao, J. (2000). Statistical pattern recognition: A review. *Pattern Analysis and Machine Intelligence, IEEE Transactions on*, *22*(1), 4–37.

Jasper, H. H. (1958). The 10/20 international electrode system. *EEG and Clinical Neurophysiology*, *10*, 371–375.

Jeon, Y., Nam, C. S., Kim, Y.-J., & Whang, M. (2011). Event-related (De) synchronization (ERD/ERS) during motor imagery tasks: Implications for brain–computer interfaces. *International Journal of Industrial Ergonomics*, *41*(5), 428–436.

Jurcak, V., Tsuzuki, D., Dan, I., & Jurcak, V., Tsuzuki, D., & Dan, I. (2007). 10/20, 10/10, and 10/5 systems revisited: Their validity as relative head-surface-based positioning systems. *NeuroImage*, *34*(4), 1600–1611. http://doi.org/10.1016/j.neuroimage.2006.09.024

Kamiya, J. (1971). *Biofeedback and Self-Control: An Aldine Reader on the Regulation of Bodily Processes and Consciousness*. Chicago: Aldine.

Kaplan, A., Shishkin, S., Ganin, I., Basyul, I., & Zhigalov, A. (2013). Adapting the P300-based brain–computer interface for gaming: A review. *IEEE Transactions on Computational Intelligence and AI in Games*, *5*(2), 141–149. http://doi.org/10.1109/TCIAIG.2012.2237517

Kaufmann, T., Herweg, A., & Kübler, A. (2014). Toward brain–computer interface based wheelchair control utilizing tactually-evoked event-related potentials. *Journal of Neuroengineering and Rehabilitation*, *11*(7), 1–17. http://doi.org/10.1186/1743-0003-11-7

Kayser, J., & Tenke, C. E. (2003). Optimizing PCA methodology for ERP component identification and measurement: Theoretical rationale and empirical evaluation. *Clinical Neurophysiology*, *114*(12), 2307–2325. http://doi.org/10.1016/S1388-2457(03)00241-4

Khan, M. J., & Hong, K.-S. (2015). Passive BCI based on drowsiness detection: An fNIRS study. *Biomedical Optics Express, 6*(10), 4063–4078. http://doi.org/10.1364/BOE.6.004063

Kim, D.-W., Cho, J.-H., Hwang, H.-J., Lim, J.-H., & Im, C.-H. (2011). A vision-free brain–computer interface (BCI) paradigm based on auditory selective attention. In *Engineering in Medicine and Biology Society, EMBC, 2011 Annual International Conference of the IEEE* (pp. 3684–3687).

Kim, K.-T., & Lee, S.-W. (2014). Steady-state somatosensory evoked potentials for brain-controlled wheelchair. In *Brain–Computer Interface (BCI), 2014 International Winter Workshop on* (pp. 1–2).

Kim, N. Y., Wittenberg, E., & Nam, C. S. (2017). Behavioral and neural correlates of executive function: Interplay between inhibition and updating processes. *Frontiers in Neuroscience, 11*, 378.

Klein, E., & Nam, C. S. (2016). Neuroethics and brain–computer interfaces (BCIs). *Brain-Computer Interfaces, 3*(3), 123–125.

Klem, G., Luders, H., Jasper, H., & Elger, C. (1958). The ten-twenty electrode system of the International Federation. *Electroencephalography and Clinical Neurophysiology, 10*(2), 371–375. http://doi.org/10.1016/0013-4694(58)90053-1

Kono, S., & Rutkowski, T. M. (2014). Tactile-force brain–computer interface paradigm. *Multimedia Tools and Applications,* 1–13.

Kostov, A., & Polak, M. (2000). Parallel man–machine training in development of EEG-based cursor control. *IEEE Transactions on Rehabilitation Engineering, 8*(2), 203–205. http://doi.org/10.1109/86.847816

Kothe, C. A., & Makeig, S. (2013). BCILAB: A platform for brain–computer interface development. *Journal of Neural Engineering, 10*(5), 56014. http://doi.org/10.1088/1741-2560/10/5/056014

Krepki, R., Blankertz, B., Curio, G., & Müller, K.-R. (2003). The Berlin Brain–Computer Interface (BBCI). *IEEE Transactions on Automatic Control, 23*(4), 538–544.

Krusienski, D. J., McFarland, D. J., & Wolpaw, J. R. (2012). Value of amplitude, phase, and coherence features for a sensorimotor rhythm-based brain–computer interface. *Brain Research Bulletin, 87*, 130–134. http://doi.org/10.1016/j.brainresbull.2011.09.019

Krusienski, D. J., Sellers, E. W., Cabestaing, F., Bayoudh, S., McFarland, D. J., Vaughan, T. M., … Krusienski, D. J., Sellers, E. W., Cabestaing, F., Bayoudh, S., McFarland, D. J., Vaughan, T. M., & Wolpaw, J. R. (2006). A comparison of classification techniques for the P300 Speller. *Journal of Neural Engineering, 3*(4), 299. http://doi.org/10.1088/1741-2560/3/4/007

Krusienski, D. J., Sellers, E. W., McFarland, D. J., Vaughan, T. M., & Wolpaw, J. R. (2008). Toward enhanced P300 speller performance. *Journal of Neuroscience Methods, 167*, 15–21. http://doi.org/10.1016/j.jneumeth.2007.07.017

Kübler, A., Furdea, A., Halder, S., Hammer, E. M., Nijboer, F., & Kotchoubey, B. (2009). A brain–computer interface controlled auditory event-related potential (p300) spelling system for locked-in patients. *Annals of the New York Academy of Sciences, 1157*, 90–100. http://doi.org/10.1111/j.1749-6632.2008.04122.x

LaFleur, K., Cassady, K., Doud, A., Shades, K., Rogin, E., & He, B. (2013). Quadcopter control in three-dimensional space using a noninvasive motor imagery-based brain–computer interface. *Journal of Neural Engineering, 10*(4), 46003.

Lalor, E. E. C., Kelly, S. P. S., Finucane, C., Burke, R., Smith, R., Reilly, R. B., & Mcdarby, G. (2005). Steady-state VEP-based brain–computer interface control in an immersive 3D gaming environment. *EURASIP Journal on Applied Signal Processing, 2005*, 3156–3164.

Lee, H., & Choi, S. (2003). PCA+HMM+SVM for EEG pattern classification. *Seventh International Symposium on Signal Processing and Its Applications, 2003. Proceedings, 1*(2), 1–4. http://doi.org/10.1109/ISSPA.2003.1224760

Lee, J.-Y., Lindquist, K. A., & Nam, C. S. (2017). Emotional granularity effects on event-related brain potentials during affective picture processing. *Frontiers in Human Neuroscience, 11*, 133.

Leeb, R., Friedman, D., Müller-Putz, G. R., Scherer, R., Slater, M., & Pfurtscheller, G. (2007). Self-paced (asynchronous) BCI control of a wheelchair in virtual environments: A case study with a tetraplegic. *Computational Intelligence and Neuroscience, 2007*, 8 pages. http://doi.org/10.1155/2007/79642

Leeb, R., Gwak, K., Kim, D.-S., & Millán, J. del R. (2014). Platform for analyzing multi-tasking capabilities during BCI operation. In *6th International Brain–Computer Interface Conference 2014*. http://doi.org/10.3217/978-3-85125-378-8-67

Lemm, S., Blankertz, B., Curio, G., & Müller, K. R. (2005). Spatio-spectral filters for improving the classification of single trial EEG. *IEEE Transactions on Biomedical Engineering, 52*(9), 1541–1548. http://doi.org/10.1109/TBME.2005.851521

Leuthardt, E. C., Schalk, G., Wolpaw, J. R., Ojemann, J. G., & Moran, D. W. (2004). A brain–computer interface using electrocorticographic signals in humans. *Journal of Neural Engineering, 1*(2), 63–71. http://doi.org/S1741-2560(04)76526-X [pii]\n10.1088/1741-2560/1/2/001

Li, Y., & Nam, C. S. (2015). A collaborative brain-computer interface (BCI) for ALS patients. In *Proceedings of the Human Factors and Ergonomics Society Annual Meeting* (Vol. 59, pp. 716–720). Sage CA: Los Angeles, CA: SAGE Publications.

Li, Y., & Nam, C. S. (2016). Collaborative brain–computer interface for people with motor disabilities. *IEEE Computational Intelligence Magazine*.

Li, Y., Bahn, S., Nam, C. S., & Lee, J. (2014). Effects of luminosity contrast and stimulus duration on user performance and preference in a P300-based brain–computer interface (BCI). *International Journal of Human–Computer Interaction*, *30*(2), 151–163.

Li, Y., Nam, C. S., Shadden, B. B., & Johnson, S. L. (2010). A P300-based brain–computer interface: effects of interface type and screen size. *International Journal of Human–Computer Interaction*, *27*(1), 52–68.

Li, Y., Woo, J., & Nam, C. S. (2012). A preliminary research on P300-based BCI application for people with motor disabilities. *Proceedings of the Human Factors and Ergonomics Society's 56th Annual Meeting* (pp. 1049–1053). New York: Human Factors and Ergonomics Society.

Lim, J.-H., Hwang, H.-J., Han, C., Jung, K.-Y., & Im, C.-H. (2013). Classification of binary intentions for individuals with impaired oculomotor function: "eyes-closed" SSVEP-based brain–computer interface (BCI). *Journal of Neural Engineering*, *10*(2), 26021. http://doi.org/10.1088/1741-2560/10/2/026021

Lim, S., Bahn, S., Woo, J., & Nam, C. S. (2012). The effects of Individual's mood state and personality trait on the cognitive processing of emotional stimuli. *Proceedings of the Human Factors and Ergonomics Society's 56th Annual Meeting* (pp. 1059–1063). New York: Human Factors and Ergonomics Society.

Lin, A.-L., Fox, P. T., Yang, Y., Lu, H., Tan, L.-H., and Gao, J.-H. (2008). No evaluation of MRI models in the measurement of CMRO2 and its relationship with CBF. *Magnetic Resonance in Medicine*, *60*(2), 380–389.

Lin, Y.-P., Wang, Y., & Jung, T.-P. (2013). A mobile SSVEP-based brain–computer interface for freely moving humans: The robustness of canonical correlation analysis to motion artifacts. In *Engineering in Medicine and Biology Society (EMBC), 2013 35th Annual International Conference of the IEEE* (pp. 1350–1353).

Lindauer, U., Dirnagl, U., Füchtemeier, M., Böttiger, C., Offenhauser, N., Leithner, C., & Royl, G. (2010). Pathophysiological interference with neurovascular coupling—When imaging based on hemoglobin might go blind. *Frontiers in Neuroenergetics*, *2*.

Lindauer, U., Royl, G., Leithner, C., Kühl, M., Gold, L., Gethmann, J., Kohl-Bareis, M., Villringer, A., and Dirnagl, U. (2001). No evidence for early decrease in blood oxygenation in rat whisker cortex in response to functional activation. *Neuroimage*, *13*, 988–1001.

Linden, D. (2011). *The Biology of Psychological Disorders*. Palgrave Macmillan.

Long, J., Li, Y., Yu, T., & Gu, Z. (2012). Target selection with hybrid feature for BCI-based 2-D cursor control. *Biomedical Engineering, IEEE Transactions on*, *59*(1), 132–140.

Lotte, F., Congedo, M., Lécuyer, A., Lamarche, F., & Arnaldi, B. (2007). A review of classification algorithms for EEG-based brain–computer interfaces. *Journal of Neural Engineering*, *4*(2), R1–R13. http://doi.org/10.1088/1741-2560/4/2/R01

Lugo, Z. R., Rodriguez, J., Lechner, A., Ortner, R., Gantner, I. S., Laureys, S., … Guger, C. (2014). A vibrotactile p300-based brain–computer interface for consciousness detection and communication. *Clinical EEG and Neuroscience*, *45*, 14–21. http://doi.org/10.1177/1550059413505533

Matthews, F., Pearlmutter, B. A., Ward, T. E., Soraghan, C., & Markham, C. (2008). Hemodynamics for brain–computer interfaces. *IEEE Signal Processing Magazine*, *25*(1), 87–94. http://doi.org/10.1109/MSP.2008.4408445

McDaid, A. J., Xing, S., & Xie, S. Q. (2013). Brain controlled robotic exoskeleton for neurorehabilitation. *2013 IEEE/ASME International Conference on Advanced Intelligent Mechatronics: Mechatronics for Human Wellbeing, AIM 2013*, 1039–1044. http://doi.org/10.1109/AIM.2013.6584231

McFarland, D. J., Anderson, C. W., Muller, K.-R., Schlogl, A., & Krusienski, D. J. (2006). BCI meeting 2005-workshop on BCI signal processing: Feature extraction and translation. *Neural Systems and Rehabilitation Engineering, IEEE Transactions on*, *14*(2), 135–138.

McFarland, D. J., McCane, L. M., David, S. V., & Wolpaw, J. R. (1997). Spatial filter selection for EEG-based communication. *Electroencephalography and Clinical Neurophysiology*, *103*, 386–394. http://doi.org/10.1016/S0013-4694(97)00022-2

McMenamin, B. W., Shackman, A. J., Maxwell, J. S., Bachhuber, D. R. W., Koppenhaver, A. M., Greischar, L. L., & Davidson, R. J. (2010). Validation of ICA-based myogenic artifact correction for scalp and source-localized EEG. *NeuroImage*, *49*(3), 2416–2432. http://doi.org/10.1016/j.neuroimage.2009.10.010

Mestais, C. S., Charvet, G., Sauter-Starace, F., Foerster, M., Ratel, D., & Benabid, A. L. (2015). WIMAGINE: Wireless 64-channel ECoG recording implant for long term clinical applications. *IEEE Transactions on Neural Systems and Rehabilitation Engineering, 23*(1), 10–21. http://doi.org/10.1109/TNSRE.2014.2333541

Middleton, S., Goli, A., & Ziarani, A. K. (2006). A software module for the adaptive estimation of steady state auditory evoked potentials. In *Engineering in Medicine and Biology Society, 2006. EMBS'06. 28th Annual International Conference of the IEEE* (pp. 3700–3703).

Miranda, E. R., & Soucaret, V. (2008). Mix-it-yourself with a brain–computer music interface. *7th ICDVRAT with ArtAbilitation, Maia/Porto, Portugal.*

Moore, M. M., & Kennedy, P. R. (2000). Human factors issues in the neural signals direct brain–computer interfaces. In *Proceedings of the Fourth International ACM Conference on Assistive Technologies* (pp. 114–120). New York, NY, USA: ACM. http://doi.org/10.1145/354324.354351

Mori, H., Makino, S., & Rutkowski, T. M. (2013). Multi-command chest tactile brain computer interface for small vehicle robot navigation. In *Brain and Health Informatics* (pp. 469–478). Springer.

Morone, G., Pisotta, I., Pichiorri, F., Kleih, S., Paolucci, S., Molinari, M., … Mattia, D. (2015). Proof of principle of a brain–computer interface approach to support poststroke arm rehabilitation in hospitalized patients: Design, acceptability, and usability. *Archives of Physical Medicine and Rehabilitation, 96*(3), S71–S78. http://doi.org/10.1016/j.apmr.2014.05.026

Mozaffar, S., & Petr, D. (2002). Artifact extraction from EEG data using independent component analysis. *Information Telecommunication and Technology Center, University of Kansas, Lawrence, KS, Tech. Rep. ITTC-FY2003-TR-03050-02.*

Mugler, E., Benschc, M., Haldera, S., Rosenstielc, W., Bogdancd, M., Birbaumerae, N., & Kübleraf, A. (2008). Control of an internet browser using the P300 event-related potential. *IJBEM, 10,* 56–63.

Mugler, E. M., Ruf, C. A., Halder, S., Bensch, M., & Kubler, A. (2010). Design and implementation of a P300-based brain–computer interface for controlling an internet browser. *IEEE Transactions on Neural Systems and Rehabilitation Engineering: A Publication of the IEEE Engineering in Medicine and Biology Society, 18*(6), 599–609. http://doi.org/10.1109/TNSRE.2010.2068059

Mühl, C., Allison, B., Nijholt, A., & Chanel, G. (2014). A survey of affective brain computer interfaces: Principles, state-of-the-art, and challenges. *Brain–Computer Interfaces, 1*(2), 66–84. http://doi.org/10.1080/2326263X.2014.912881

Mukaino, M., Ono, T., Shindo, K., Fujiwara, T., Ota, T., Kimura, A., … Ushiba, J. (2014). Efficacy of brain–computer interface-driven neuromuscular electrical stimulation for chronic paresis after stroke. *Journal of Rehabilitation Medicine, 46*(4), 378–382.

Mullen, T., Khalil, A., Ward, T., Iversen, J., Leslie, G., Warp, R., … Ojeda, A. (2015). MindMusic: Playful and social installations at the interface between music and the brain. In *More Playful User Interfaces* (pp. 197–229). Springer Singapore.

Muller, S. M. T. S., Bastos-Filho, T. F., & Sarcinelli-Filho, M. (2011). Using a SSVEP-BCI to command a robotic wheelchair. *2011 IEEE International Symposium on Industrial Electronics,* 957–962. http://doi.org/10.1109/ISIE.2011.5984288

Müller-Putz, G. R., & Pfurtscheller, G. (2008). Control of an electrical prosthesis with an SSVEP-based BCI. *IEEE Transactions on Biomedical Engineering, 55*(1), 361–364. http://doi.org/10.1109/TBME.2007.897815

Müller-Putz, G. R., Scherer, R., Brauneis, C., & Pfurtscheller, G. (2005). Steady-state visual evoked potential (SSVEP)-based communication: Impact of harmonic frequency components. *Journal of Neural Engineering, 2*(4), 123. http://doi.org/10.1088/1741-2560/2/4/008

Muller-Putz, G. R., Scherer, R. R., Neuper, C., & Pfurtscheller, G. (2006). Steady-state somatosensory evoked potentials: Suitable brain signals for brain–computer interfaces? *IEEE Transactions on Neural Systems and Rehabilitation Engineering, 14*(1), 30–37. http://doi.org/10.1109/TNSRE.2005.863842

Münßinger, J. I., Halder, S., Kleih, S. C., Furdea, A., Raco, V., Hösle, A., & Kübler, A. (2010). Brain painting: First evaluation of a new brain–computer interface application with ALS-patients and healthy volunteers. *Frontiers in Neuroscience, 4,* 182. http://doi.org/10.3389/fnins.2010.00182

Musiek, F. E., Froke, R., & Weihing, J. (2005). The auditory P300 at or near threshold. *Journal of the American Academy of Audiology, 16*(9), 698–707. Retrieved from http://www.ncbi.nlm.nih.gov/pubmed/16515141

Nam, C. S. (2012). Brain-computer interface (BCI) and ergonomics. *Ergonomics, 55*(5), 513–515.

Nam, C. S., Jeon, Y., Kim, Y.-J., Lee, I., & Park, K. (2011). Movement imagery-related lateralization of event-related (De)synchronization (ERD/ERS): Motor-imagery duration effects. *Clinical Neurophysiology, 122*(3), 567–577.

Nam, C. S., Jeon, Y., Li, Y., Kim, Y.-J., & Yoon, H. (2009). Usability of the P300 speller: Towards a more sustainable brain-computer interface. *eMinds: International Journal on Human–Computer Interaction, 1*(5), 111–125.

Nam, C. S., Johnson, S., & Li, Y., (2008). Environmental noise and P300-based brain-computer interface (BCI). *Proceedings of the Human Factors and Ergonomics Society's 52nd Annual Meeting* (pp. 803–807). New York: Human Factors and Ergonomics Society.

Nam, C. S., Lee, J., & Bahn, S. (2013). Brain-computer interface supported collaborative work: Implications for rehabilitation. In *Engineering in Medicine and Biology Society (EMBC), 2013 35th Annual International Conference of the IEEE* (pp. 269–272).

Nam, C. S., Li, Y., & Johnson, S. (2010). Evaluation of P300-based brain-computer interface (BCI) in real-world contexts. *International Journal of Human–Computer Interaction, 26*(6), 621–637.

Nam, C. S., Moore, M., Choi, I., & Li, Y. (2015). Designing better, cost-effective brain–computer interfaces. *Ergonomics in Design: The Quarterly of Human Factors Applications, 23*(4), 13–19.

Nam, C. S., Woo, J., & Bahn, S. (2012). Severe motor disability affects functional cortical differentiation in the context of BCI use. *Ergonomics, 55*(5), 581–591.

Nicolas-Alonso, L., & Gomez-Gil, J. (2012). Brain computer interfaces, a review. *Sensors.*

Niedermeyer, E., & da Silva, F. L. (2005). *Electroencephalography: Basic Principles, Clinical Applications, and Related Fields* (F. L. Niedermeyer, E., & da Silva, Eds.) (Vol. 1), Lippincott Williams & Wilkins. Retrieved from http://books.google.com/books?hl=en&lr=&id=tndqYGPHQdEC&oi=fnd&pg=PR11&dq=Niederm eyer+%26+da+Silva,+2005&ots=GN5p-139py&sig=-BRONsGjhkvpIvDY9cHAuG_i2UY

Nijboer, F., Furdea, A., Gunst, I., Mellinger, J., McFarland, D. J., Birbaumer, N., & Kübler, A. (2008). An auditory brain–computer interface (BCI). *Journal of Neuroscience Methods, 167*(1), 43–50.

Nijholt, A., & Nam, C. S. (2015). Arts and brain-computer interface. *Brain–Computer Interfaces, 2*(2–3), 57–59.

Nunez, P. L. (1995). *Neocortical Dynamics and Human EEG Rhythm.* New York: Oxford University Press.

Obermaier, B., Guger, C., Neuper, C., & Pfurtscheller, G. (2001). Hidden Markov models for online classification of single trial EEG data. *Pattern Recognition Letters, 22*(12), 1299–1309. http://doi.org/10.1016/S0167-8655(01)00075-7

Onaran, I., Ince, N. F., Cetin, A. E., & Abosch, A. (2011). A hybrid SVM/HMM based system for the state detection of individual finger movements from multichannel ECoG signals. *International IEEE/EMBS Conference on Neural Engineering,* 457–460. http://doi.org/10.1109/NER.2011.5910585

Onose, G., Grozea, C., Anghelescu, A., Daia, C., Sinescu, C. J., Ciurea, A. V., ... Popescu, F. (2012). On the feasibility of using motor imagery EEG-based brain—Computer interface in chronic tetraplegics for assistive robotic arm control: A clinical test and long-term post-trial follow-up. *Spinal Cord, 50*(8), 599–608.

Palaniappan, R. (2005). Brain computer interface design using band powers extracted during mental tasks. *2nd International IEEE EMBS Conference on Neural Engineering, 2005,* 321–324. http://doi.org/10.1109/CNE.2005.1419622

Palaniappan, R., Paramesran, R., Nishida, S., & Saiwaki, N. (2002). A new brain–computer interface design using fuzzy ARTMAP. *IEEE Transactions on Neural Systems and Rehabilitation Engineering: A Publication of the IEEE Engineering in Medicine and Biology Society, 10*(3), 140–148. http://doi.org/10.1109/TNSRE.2002.802854

Peng, H.-L., Liu, J.-Q., Tian, H.-C., Dong, Y.-Z., Yang, B., Chen, X., & Yang, C.-S. (2016). A novel passive electrode based on porous Ti for EEG recording. *Sensors and Actuators B: Chemical, 226,* 349–356.

Peng, H.-L., Liu, J.-Q., Tian, H.-C., Xu, B., Dong, Y.-Z., Yang, B., ... Yang, C.-S. (2015). Flexible dry electrode based on carbon nanotube/polymer hybrid micropillars for biopotential recording. *Sensors and Actuators A: Physical, 235,* 48–56. http://doi.org/10.1016/j.sna.2015.09.024

Penny, W. D., Roberts, S. J., Curran, E. A., & Stokes, M. J. (2000). EEG-based communication: A pattern recognition approach. *IEEE Transactions on Rehabilitation Engineering, 8*(2), 214–215. http://doi.org/10.1109/86.847820

Perdikis, S., Leeb, R., Williamson, J., Ramsay, A., Tavella, M., Desideri, L., ... d R Millán, J. (2014). Clinical evaluation of BrainTree, a motor imagery hybrid BCI speller. *Journal of Neural Engineering, 11*(3), 36003.

Pfurtscheller, G. (1999). Quantification of ERD and ERS in the time domain. In G. Pfurtscheller & F. H. Lopes da Silva (Eds.), *Handbook of Electroencephalography and Clinical Neuropsychology, Event-Related Desynchronization* (Vol. 6, pp. 89–105). Amsterdam: Elsevier.

Pfurtscheller, G., Allison, B. Z., Brunner, C., Bauernfeind, G., Solis-Escalante, T., Scherer, R., … Birbaumer, N. (2010a). The hybrid BCI. *Frontiers in Neuroscience, 4*(April), 30. http://doi.org/10.3389/fnpro.2010.00003

Pfurtscheller, G., & Lopes da Silva, F. H. (1999). Event-related EEG/MEG synchronization and desynchronization: Basic principles. *Clinical Neurophysiology, 110*(11), 1842–1857. http://doi.org/10.1016/S1388-2457(99)00141-8

Pfurtscheller, G., Muller-Putz, G. R., Scherer, R., & Neuper, C. (2008). Rehabilitation with brain–computer interface systems. *Computer, 41*(10), 58–65. http://doi.org/10.1109/MC.2008.432

Pfurtscheller, G., & Neuper, C. (2006). Future prospects of ERD/ERS in the context of brain–computer interface (BCI) developments. *Progress in Brain Research, 159*(159), 433–437.

Pfurtscheller, G., Solis-Escalante, T., Ortner, R., Linortner, P., Müller-Putz, G. R., & Muller-Putz, G. R. (2010b). Self-paced operation of an SSVEP-based orthosis with and without an imagery-based "brain switch": A feasibility study towards a hybrid BCI. *IEEE Transactions on Neural Systems and Rehabilitation Engineering, 18*(4), 409–414. http://doi.org/10.1109/TNSRE.2010.2040837

Pichiorri, F., Morone, G., Petti, M., Toppi, J., Pisotta, I., Molinari, M., … Mattia, D. (2015). Brain–computer interface boosts motor imagery practice during stroke recovery. *Annals of Neurology, 77*(5), 851–865. http://doi.org/10.1002/ana.24390

Picton, T. W. (1992). The P300 wave of the human event-related potential. *Journal of Clinical Neurophysiology: Official Publication of the American Electroencephalographic Society, 9*(4), 456–479. http://doi.org/10.1097/00004691-199210000-00002

Powers, J., Bieliaieva, K., Wu, S., & Nam, C. S. (2015). The human factors and ergonomics of P300-based brain–computer interfaces. *Brain Sciences, 5*, 318–356.

Prataksita, N., Lin, Y.-T., Chou, H.-C., & Kuo, C.-H. (2014). Brain-robot control interface: Development and application. *IEEE International Symposium on Bioelectronics and Bioinformatics (ISBB)*.

Rakotomamonjy, A., & Guigue, V. (2008). BCI competition III: Dataset II—Ensemble of SVMs for BCI P300 speller. *IEEE Transactions on Biomedical Engineering, 55*(3), 1147–1154. http://doi.org/10.1109/TBME.2008.915728

Ramage, D., Hall, D., Nallapati, R., & Manning, C. D. (2009). Labeled LDA: A supervised topic model for credit attribution in multi-labeled corpora. *Conference on Empirical Methods in Natural Language Processing*, (August), 248–256. http://doi.org/10.3115/1699510.1699543

Ramoser, H., Müller-Gerking, J., & Pfurtscheller, G. (2000). Optimal spatial filtering of single trial EEG during imagined hand movement. *IEEE Transactions on Rehabilitation Engineering, 8*(4), 441–446. http://doi.org/10.1109/86.895946

Robinson, C. W., Ahmar, N., & Sloutsky, V. M. (2010). Evidence for auditory dominance in a passive oddball task. In *Proceedings of the 32nd Annual Conference of the Cognitive Science Society* (pp. 2644–2649).

Roth, C., Gupta, C. N., Plis, S. M., Damaraju, E., Khullar, S., Calhoun, V. D., & Bridwell, D. A. (2013). The influence of visuospatial attention on unattended auditory 40 Hz responses. *Frontiers in Human Neuroscience, 7*.

Rumelhart, D. E., McClelland, J. L., & the Pop Research Group. (1986). *Parallel Distributed Processing, Vols 1 and 2*. Cambridge, MA: The MIT Press.

Salvaris, M., & Sepulveda, F. (2009). Visual modifications on the P300 speller BCI paradigm. *Journal of Neural Engineering, 6*(4), 46011. http://doi.org/10.1088/1741-2560/6/4/046011

Schalk, G., & Mellinger, J. (2010). *A Practical Guide to Brain–Computer Interfacing with BCI2000: General-Purpose Software for Brain–Computer Interface Research, Data Acquisition, Stimulus Presentation, and Brain Monitoring*. Springer Science & Business Media.

Schalk, G., McFarland, D. J., Hinterberger, T., Birbaumer, N., & Wolpaw, J. R. (2004). BCI2000: A general-purpose brain–computer interface (BCI) system. *IEEE Transactions on Biomedical Engineering, 51*, 1034–1043. http://doi.org/10.1109/TBME.2004.827072

Scherer, R., Billinger, M., Wagner, J., Schwarz, A., Hettich, D. T., Bolinger, E., … Müller-Putz, G. (2015). Thought-based row-column scanning communication board for individuals with cerebral palsy. *Annals of Physical and Rehabilitation Medicine, 58*(1), 14–22. http://doi.org/10.1016/j.rehab.2014.11.005

Scherer, R., Müller, G. R., Neuper, C., Graimann, B., & Pfurtscheller, G. (2004). An asynchronously controlled EEG-based virtual keyboard: Improvement of the spelling rate. *Biomedical Engineering, IEEE Transactions on, 51*(6), 979–984.

Schlögl, A., Lee, F., Bischof, H., & Pfurtscheller, G. (2005). Characterization of four-class motor imagery EEG data for the BCI-competition 2005. *Journal of Neural Engineering, 2*(4), L14.

Schmidt, L. A., & Segalowitz, S. J. (2007). *Developmental Psychophysiology: Theory, Systems, and Methods*. Cambridge University Press.

Schreuder, M., Blankertz, B., & Tangermann, M. (2010). A new auditory multi-class brain–computer interface paradigm: Spatial hearing as an informative cue. *PLoS ONE, 5*. http://doi.org/10.1371/journal.pone.0009813

Schreuder, M., Rost, T., & Tangermann, M. (2011). Listen, you are writing! Speeding up online spelling with a dynamic auditory BCI. *Frontiers in Neuroscience, 5*(112). http://doi.org/10.3389/fnins.2011.00112

Sellers, E. W., & Donchin, E. (2006). A P300-based brain–computer interface: Initial tests by ALS patients. *Clinical Neurophysiology, 117*(3), 538–548.

Sellers, E. W., Kübler, A., & Donchin, E. (2006). Brain–computer interface research at the University of South Florida cognitive psychophysiology laboratory: The P300 speller. *IEEE Transactions on Neural Systems and Rehabilitation Engineering, 14*, 221–224. http://doi.org/10.1109/TNSRE.2006.875580

Severens, M., Farquhar, J., Desain, P., Duysens, J., & Gielen, C. (2010). Transient and steady-state responses to mechanical stimulation of different fingers reveal interactions based on lateral inhibition. *Clinical Neurophysiology: Official Journal of the International Federation of Clinical Neurophysiology, 121*(12), 2090–6. http://doi.org/10.1016/j.clinph.2010.05.016

Severens, M., Farquhar, J., Duysens, J., & Desain, P. (2013). A multi-signature brain–computer interface: Use of transient and steady-state responses. *Journal of Neural Engineering, 10*(2), 26005. http://doi.org/10.1088/1741-2560/10/2/026005

Shi, T., Wang, H., & Zhang, C. (2015). Brain computer interface system based on indoor semi-autonomous navigation and motor imagery for unmanned aerial vehicle control. *Expert Systems with Applications, 42*(9), 4196–4206. http://doi.org/10.1016/j.eswa.2015.01.031

Shlens, J. (2014). A tutorial on principal component analysis. *arXiv Preprint arXiv:1404.1100.*

Singha, H., Lia, X., Hines, E. L., & Stocks, N. G. (2007). Classification and feature extraction strategies for multi channel multi trial BCI data. *International Journal of Bioelectromagnetism, 9*(4), 233–236.

Souza, A. P., Filho, S. A. S., Felix, L. B., Maia, C. A., & Tierra-Criollo, C. J. (2012). Classification of imaginary movements using the magnitude-squared coherence feature extractor. In *2012 ISSNIP Biosignals and Biorobotics Conference: Biosignals and Robotics for Better and Safer Living (BRC)* (pp. 1–6). IEEE. http://doi.org/10.1109/BRC.2012.6222181

Staba, R. J., Wilson, C. L., Bragin, A., Fried, I., & Engel, J. (2002). Quantitative analysis of high frequency oscillations (80–500 Hz) recorded in human epileptic hippocampus and entorhinal cortex. *Journal of Neurophysiology, 88*(4), 1743–1752.

Steriade, M., McCormick, D. A., & Sejnowski, T. J. (1993). Thalamocortical oscillations in the sleeping and aroused brain. *Science, 262*, 679.

Stollfuss, J., Landvogt, N., Abenstein, M., Ziegler, S., Schwaiger, M., Senekowitsch-Schmidtke, R., & Wieder, H. (2015). Non-invasive imaging of implanted peritoneal carcinomatosis in mice using PET and bioluminescence imaging. *EJNMMI Research, 5*(1), 1–8.

Strehl, U., Birkle, S. M., Wörz, S., & Kotchoubey, B. (2014). Sustained reduction of seizures in patients with intractable epilepsy after self-regulation training of slow cortical potentials—10 years after. *Frontiers in Human Neuroscience, 8*(604), 1–7. http://doi.org/10.3389/fnhum.2014.00604

Studer, P., Kratz, O., Gevensleben, H., Rothenberger, A., Moll, G. H., Hautzinger, M., & Heinrich, H. (2014). Slow cortical potential and theta/beta neurofeedback training in adults: Effects on attentional processes and motor system excitability. *Frontiers in Human Neuroscience, 8*(July), 555. http://doi.org/10.3389/fnhum.2014.00555

Suk, H.-I., & Lee, S.-W. (2010). Two-layer hidden Markov models for multi-class motor imagery classification. *2010 First Workshop on Brain Decoding: Pattern Recognition Challenges in Neuroimaging*, 5–8. http://doi.org/10.1109/WBD.2010.16

Tenke, C. E., & Kayser, J. (2005). Reference-free quantification of EEG spectra: Combining current source density (CSD) and frequency principal components analysis (fPCA). *Clinical Neurophysiology, 116*(12), 2826–2846. http://doi.org/10.1016/j.clinph.2005.08.007

Teplan, M. (2002). Fundamentals of EEG measurement. *Measurement Science Review, 2*(2).

Thomas, E., Fruitet, J., & Clerc, M. (2012). Investigating brief motor imagery for an ERD/ERS based BCI. *Conference Proceedings: Annual International Conference of the IEEE Engineering in Medicine and Biology Society. IEEE Engineering in Medicine and Biology Society. Annual Conference, 2012*, 2929–32. http://doi.org/10.1109/EMBC.2012.6346577

Thurlings, M. E., Van Erp, J. B. F., Brouwer, A.-M., & Werkhoven, P. (2013). Controlling a tactile ERP–BCI in a dual task. *IEEE Transactions on Computational Intelligence and AI in Games, 5*(2), 129–140. http://doi.org/10.1109/TCIAIG.2013.2239294

Todd, D. A., McCullagh, P. J., Mulvenna, M. D., & Lightbody, G. (2012). Investigating the use of brain–computer interaction to facilitate creativity. In *Proceedings of the 3rd Augmented Human International Conference* (p. 19).

Tonet, O., Tecchio, F., Sepulveda, F., Citi, L., Tombini, M., Marinelli, M., Focacci, F., Laschi, C., & Dario, P. (2006). Critical review and future perspectives of non-invasive brain–machine interfaces. *Journal of Neuroscience Methods*, *31*(0).

Townsend, D. W. (2008). Dual-modality imaging: Combining anatomy and function. *Journal of Nuclear Medicine*, *49*(6), 938–955.

Townsend, G., LaPallo, B. K., Boulay, C. B., Krusienski, D. J., Frye, G. E., Hauser, C. K., … Sellers, E. W. (2010). A novel P300-based brain–computer interface stimulus presentation paradigm: Moving beyond rows and columns. *Clinical Neurophysiology: Official Journal of the International Federation of Clinical Neurophysiology*, *121*(7), 1109–20. http://doi.org/10.1016/j.clinph.2010.01.030

Treder, M. S., & Blankertz, B. (2010). (C)overt attention and visual speller design in an ERP-based brain–computer interface. *Behavioral & Brain Functions*, *6*.

Triponyuwasin, P., & Wongsawat, Y. (2014). Brain–computer interface based stroke rehabilitation for hemiplegia. In *Biomedical Engineering International Conference (BMEiCON), 2014 7th* (pp. 1–4). http://doi.org/10.1109/BMEiCON.2014.7017402

Tyler-Kabara, E. C., Collinger, J., Wodlinger, B., Weber, D., Schwartz, A., Boninger, M., & Gaunt, R. (2015). Brain computer interface (BCI) controlled prosthetic arm movement is possible in the absence of visual input with proprioceptive feedback. *Journal of Neurosurgery*, *122*(6), A1560–A1561.

Uhlhaas, P. (2015). Magnetoencephalogrphy as a tool in cognitive neuroscience: A translational perspective. *Schizophrenia Bulletin*, *41*, S98–S99.

Vallabhaneni, A., Wang, T., & He, B. (2005). Brain–computer interface. *Neural Engineering*, 85–121. http://doi.org/10.1007/0-306-48610-5_3

Vamvakousis, Z., & Ramirez, R. (2014). P300 harmonies: A brain–computer musical interface. *ICMC| SMC| 2014*.

van der Waal, M., Severens, M., Geuze, J., & Desain, P. (2012). Introducing the tactile speller: An ERP-based brain–computer interface for communication. *Journal of Neural Engineering*, *9*(4), 45002. http://doi.org/10.1088/1741-2560/9/4/045002

Vatta, F., Bruno, P., Mininel, S., & Inchingolo, P. (2005). EEG simulation accuracy: Reference choice and head models extension. *Rdm*, *1*(2), 1.

Volosyak, I. (2011). SSVEP-based Bremen-BCI interface—Boosting information transfer rates. *Journal of Neural Engineering*, *8*(3), 36020. http://doi.org/10.1088/1741-2560/8/3/036020

Wadeson, A., Nijholt, A., & Nam, C. S. (2015). Artistic brain-computer interfaces: State-of-the-art control mechanisms. *Brain-Computer Interfaces*, *2*(2–3), 60–69.

Wall, M., Rechtsteiner, A., & Rocha, L. (2003). Singular value decomposition and principal component analysis. *A Practical Approach to Microarray Data Analysis*, 91–109. http://doi.org/10.1007/0-306-47815-3_5

Wang, X., Cao, T., Wang, B., Wan, F., Mak, P. U., Mak, P. I., … Li, C. (2011a). An online SSVEP-based chatting system. *Proceedings 2011 International Conference on System Science and Engineering, ICSSE 2011*, (June), 536–539. http://doi.org/10.1109/ICSSE.2011.5961961

Wang, Y.-T., Wang, Y., & Jung, T.-P. (2011b). A cell-phone-based brain–computer interface for communication in daily life. *Journal of Neural Engineering*, *8*(2), 25018.

Wang, Y., Gao, S., & Gao, X. (2005). Common spatial pattern method for channel selelction in motor imagery based brain–computer interface. In *27th Annual International Conference of the Engineering in Medicine and Biology Society (IEEE-EMBS)* (pp. 5392–5395). http://doi.org/10.1109/IEMBS.2005.1615701

Wang, Y., Gao, X., Hong, B., Jia, C., & Gao, S. (2008). Brain–computer interfaces based on visual evoked potentials: Feasibility of practical system designs. *IEEE Engineering in Medicine and Biology Magazine: The Quarterly Magazine of the Engineering in Medicine & Biology Society*, *27*(5), 64–71. http://doi.org/10.1109/MEMB.2008.923958

Wang, Y., Zhang, Z., Gao, X., & Gao, S. (2004). Lead selection for SSVEP-based brain–computer interface. *Conference Proceedings: Annual International Conference of the IEEE Engineering in Medicine and Biology Society. IEEE Engineering in Medicine and Biology Society. Conference*, *6*, 4507–10. http://doi.org/10.1109/IEMBS.2004.1404252

Weiskopf, N., Mathiak, K., Bock, S. W., Scharnowski, F., Veit, R., Grodd, W., & Birbaumer, N. (2004). Principles of a brain–computer interface (BCI) based on real-time functional magnetic resonance imaging (fMRI). *Biomedical Engineering, IEEE Transactions on*, *51*(6), 966–970.

Wilcox, T., Bortfeld, H., Woods, R., Wruck, E., & Boas, D. A. (2008). Hemodynamic response to featural changes in the occipital and inferior temporal cortex in infants: A preliminary methodological exploration: Paper. *Developmental Science*, *11*(3), 361–370. http://doi.org/10.1111/j.1467-7687.2008.00681.x

Winstein, C. J., Grafton, S. T., & Pohl, P. S. (1997). Motor task difficulty and brain activity: Investigation of goal-directed reciprocal aiming using positron emission tomography. *Journal of Neurophysiology*, *77*(3), 1581–1594.

Wittenberg, E., Thompson, J., Nam, C. S., & Franz, J. R. (2017). Neuroimaging of human balance control: A systematic review. *Frontiers in Human Neuroscience*, *11*, 170.

Wolpaw, J., & Wolpaw, E. W. (2012). *Brain–Computer Interfaces: Principles and Practice*. Oxford University Press.

Wolpaw, J. R., Birbaumer, N., McFarland, D. J., Pfurtscheller, G., & Vaughan, T. M. (2002). Brain–computer interfaces for communication and control. *Clinical Neurophysiology*, *113*(6), 767–791. http://doi.org/10.1016/S1388-2457(02)00057-3

Wu, T., Yang, B., & Sun, H. (2010). EEG classification based on artificial neural network in brain computer interface. *Life System Modeling and Intelligent Computing*.

Yao, L., Zhang, D., & Zhu, X. (2012). SSVEP based brain–computer interface controlled functional electrical stimulation system for knee joint movement. In C.-Y. Su, S. Rakheja, & H. Liu (Eds.), *Intelligent Robotics and Applications SE - 53* (Vol. 7506, pp. 526–535). Springer Berlin Heidelberg. http://doi.org/10.1007/978-3-642-33509-9_53

Yin, E., Zhou, Z., Jiang, J., Chen, F., Liu, Y., & Hu, D. (2013). A speedy hybrid BCI spelling approach combining P300 and SSVEP. *IEEE Transactions on Bio-Medical Engineering*, *61*(2), 473–483. http://doi.org/10.1109/TBME.2013.2281976

Yu, T., Li, Y., Long, J., & Gu, Z. (2012). Surfing the internet with a BCI mouse. *Journal of Neural Engineering*, *9*(3), 36012.

Yue, J., Jiang, J., Zhou, Z., & Hu, D. (2011). SMR-speller: A novel brain–computer interface spell paradigm. In *ICCRD2011 - 2011 3rd International Conference on Computer Research and Development* (Vol. 3, pp. 187–190). http://doi.org/10.1109/ICCRD.2011.5764276

Zander, T. O., & Kothe, C. (2011). Towards passive brain–computer interfaces: Applying brain–computer interface technology to human–machine systems in general. *Journal of Neural Engineering*, *8*(2), 25005. http://doi.org/10.1088/1741-2560/8/2/025005

Zander, T. O., Kothe, C., Jatzev, S., Gaertner, M., & Co-investigator, N. (2010). Enhancing human–computer interaction with input from active and passive brain–computer interfaces. In *Brain–Computer Interfaces* (Vol. 53, pp. 181–199). Springer. http://doi.org/10.1017/CBO9781107415324.004

Zhang, D., Maye, A., Gao, X., Hong, B., Engel, A. K., Gao, S., & Zhang, D., Maye, A., Gao, X., Hong, B., Engel, A. K., & Gao, S. (2010). An independent brain–computer interface using covert non-spatial visual selective attention. *Journal of Neural Engineering*, *7*(1), 16010. http://doi.org/10.1088/1741-2560/7/1/016010

Zhao, R., Schalk, G., & Ji, Q. (2014). Coupled hidden Markov model for electrocorticographic signal classification. In *Pattern Recognition (ICPR), 2014 22nd International Conference on* (pp. 1858–1862). http://doi.org/10.1109/ICPR.2014.325

Zhong, S., & Ghosh, J. (2002). HMMs and coupled HMMs for multi-channel EEG classification. *Proceedings of the 2002 International Joint Conference on Neural Networks. IJCNN'02 (Cat. No.02CH37290)*, 1154–1159. http://doi.org/10.1109/IJCNN.2002.1007657

Zhu, D., Bieger, J., Garcia Molina, G., & Aarts, R. M. (2010). A survey of stimulation methods used in SSVEP-based BCIs. *Computational Intelligence and Neuroscience*, *2010*. http://doi.org/10.1155/2010/702357

# 2 Facilitating the Integration of Modern Neuroscience into Noninvasive BCIs

*Mark Wronkiewicz, Eric Larson, and Adrian K.C. Lee*

## CONTENTS

2.1 Introduction..................................................................................................53
2.2 Mapping Noninvasive Signals to the Brain.................................................56
2.3 Application: Applying Neuroscience to Improve Classification Accuracy...........59
2.4 Application: Transfer Learning....................................................................61
2.5 Conclusions and Future Directions..............................................................63
Acknowledgments....................................................................................................64
References.................................................................................................................64

**Abstract**

There are still many obstacles that must be solved before brain–computer interfaces (BCIs) can advance out of controlled research settings and into real-world scenarios. Some of these obstacles arise because of a growing separation between neuroscience and neuroengineering. Much of modern neuroscience research operates at the cortical level, so it is difficult to leverage this basic science research in BCIs that use noninvasive recordings (e.g., electroencephalography or magnetoencephalography) because those BCI data are recorded from outside the head. A neuroimaging technique called "source imaging" may offer a way to alleviate this disconnect as it allows the estimation cortical activity (on the surface of the brain) from noninvasive data (recorded on or above the surface of the scalp). We start by explaining the fundamentals of source imaging and then explore research using this technique to address two issues in BCI research. First, targeting brain activity from the most relevant cortical region can improve classification accuracy compared to the traditional approach. Second, source imaging was shown to improve transfer learning—an area of research aimed at reducing the 20- to 30-min calibration period required for most noninvasive BCIs. Overall, this chapter illustrates how tools and research findings from neuroscience can serve as a principled way to advance BCI methodology.

## 2.1 INTRODUCTION

The notion of using brain–computer interfaces (BCIs) to liberate the mind from the physical constraints of the body is a captivating technological idea—an idea that, despite being over three-quarters of a century old (Wolpaw & Wolpaw 2012), continues to shape both science fiction stories and many scientists' careers. Regardless of their long-standing promise, however, the transition from fiction to reality has been sluggish; BCIs have yet to make a meaningful impact on clinical or commercial fields. Compared to other grand scientific accomplishments like mapping the human genome or establishing an international space station, it is puzzling as to why BCIs have not found success outside controlled laboratory settings.

Three conventional BCI paradigms—all published over a quarter-century ago—continue to comprise a large majority of noninvasive BCI research. Systems based on sensorimotor rhythms (SMRs) related to movement, for instance, were first reported in 1991 (Wolpaw et al. 1991). Other BCIs like those relying on the P300 event-related potential or steady-state visually evoked responses (SSVEPs) were published even earlier in 1988 and 1977, respectively (Farwell & Donchin 1988; Vidal 1977). The literature first reporting the underlying neurophysiology of the signals behind these BCIs is even older; SMRs related to motor activity were reported as reliably detectable in 1979 (Pfurtscheller & Aranibar 1979), the P300 ERP was characterized in a pair of papers from 1964 and 1965 (Chapman & Bragdon 1964; Sutton et al. 1965), and visually evoked potentials were first discussed in 1973 (Vidal 1973).

These three pillars of human BCI work were all established by the time the field of cortical mapping (using both MRI and electromagnetic methods) was about to begin its crescendo. Even the original SMR-based BCI—representing the youngest of the main paradigms—was published the same year as the first human functional magnetic resonance imaging (fMRI) experiment (Belliveau et al. 1991). This is important because, over 25 years later, those same three paradigms still dominate today's BCI research, and they continue to rely on the same neuroscience foundation that existed at the time of the original publications. Given that researchers are still working today to build a solid footing for real-world BCI applications, it is a fair question whether continued iterative research on these conventional paradigms represents the most encouraging path forward. With decades of neuroscience research since the original BCI publications, perhaps it is worth striving to incorporate novel neuroscience findings to expand the BCI field.

In this chapter, we start by dissecting some of the limitations that continue to hinder the advancement of BCIs. We then cover some effective methodologies that could accelerate the transition of BCIs into commercial and clinical spaces. Here, we focus on noninvasive EEG-based methods because they make up the majority of BCI applications, are portable, and are currently suitable for healthy users. In Section 2.2, we focus on neuroimaging tools that allow estimation of cortical activity from recordings made outside the head. We then discuss how infusing both knowledge (Section 2.3) and techniques (Section 2.4) from neuroimaging into BCIs addresses many of the obstacles covered later in this section. Finally, we speculate on additional opportunities worth exploring at the intersection of neuroimaging and BCIs (Section 2.5).

Machine learning is a vital component of modern BCIs used to predict a user's intended action from brain activity. Classifying segments of brain recordings, however, is more challenging than traditional machine learning problems for a few reasons. The task (in a machine-learning sense) is not predefined, time constraints rarely allow the collection of enough labeled data, and recorded EEG activity is difficult to interpret directly. To illustrate this point, consider instead the classical (supervised) machine learning problem of classifying handwritten digits. The canonical Mixed National Institute of Standards and Technology (MNIST) digits data set is composed of tens of thousands of images of handwritten digits. When analyzing this data set, the machine learning task is clear: categorize yet-to-be-seen images into 1 of the 10 possible classes of digits as accurately as possible. Comparatively, this problem setting is desirable for three reasons: (1) the class labels (i.e., "0" thru "9") are clearly defined, (2) there are thousands of exemplars for each class, and (3) researchers can view and quickly agree on the proper class label for practically every data sample.

BCIs face more convoluted circumstances. First, although the overarching goal of generating artificial output based solely on brain activity is clear, actual BCI experiments require researchers to select a specific paradigm of interest (e.g., P300 or motor imagery). Therefore, experimenters must implicitly choose the data class labels even though there is not always a principled basis for selecting any one of the many behaviors humans can accomplish (Schalk et al. 2008). Second, the collection of electrophysiological brain data is time consuming and known to exhibit high variability due to issues like nonstationarity, fatigue, and changes in mental strategy. Combined, this means that there are typically only a few dozen exemplars per class and the probability distributions of each class are often not sampled adequately. This poses a challenge when training a classifier that should generalize to new data. Third, it is difficult to fully verify that the subject actually performed the appropriate task, so ground truth concerning the data labels is usually not accessible. Moreover, relating these noninvasive data to the broader neuroscience literature is challenging, especially for nontraditional BCI paradigms where there is no empirical understanding of how brain activity is connected with the task at hand. Consider what it would mean if the MNIST data set were compromised in the same manner: perhaps discrete classes were difficult to define because some letters were mislabeled as numbers, only 50 exemplars were obtained for each digit class, or all the images were taken from the first week of an elementary school penmanship class. Connecting back to BCIs, it is therefore worth exploring any method that informs the choice in behavioral task (and, thus, the data classes), better accounts for sources of data variability, or increases interpretability by, for example, connecting the recorded data with basic neuroscience.

Basic functional neuroimaging research may alleviate some of these issues. As will be explored more in Section 2.3, this research can provide *a priori* information characterizing where and how brain activity is modulated during certain tasks. Therefore, this research may allow researchers to make more informed decisions when choosing BCI paradigms, focus resources only on the most relevant activity, and better relate the observed brain activity to basic science research. One of the central limitations facing BCI research, however, is the difficulty of incorporating these advances in neuroscience into new BCI systems. For example, recent insights into resting state networks or the functional brain areas involved in modulating attention are two examples of important neuroimaging findings not fully explored in noninvasive neuroengineering. A core reason for this divide is that noninvasive BCIs most often record electric potentials using EEG electrodes on the scalp; more formally, this domain is often referred to as the *sensor space* because it is where the EEG sensors reside (Figure 2.1, top row). However, recordings made in the sensor space are only an external proxy to the cortical activity that is truly of interest for much of the neuroscience community. This creates an unfortunate division between BCI and neuroscience research.

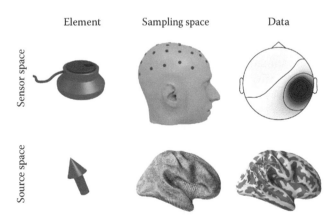

        Element        Sampling space        Data

**FIGURE 2.1** Comparison of sensor space and source space. Top row: The sensor space is traditionally where noninvasive EEG recordings are processed and visualized. Electric potentials are recorded at tens of electrodes (left) positioned against the scalp (middle) and data are analyzed at the scalp surface (right). Bottom row: In source imaging, the source space provides an alternative reference frame to process EEG data that better align with modern human neuroscience. Data are projected from the sensor space to the source space (here using source imaging) to estimate activity at model current dipoles (left). Several thousand dipoles are modeled at the gray/white matter boundary of each hemisphere (middle), and data are analyzed on the cortical surface (right).

Modern human neuroscience uses a number of different methods to acquire brain signals and map them to the brain. Therefore, it is challenging to develop new BCI paradigms or signal processing strategies from these advancements because they must be translated into an EEG context. For example, fMRI, electrocorticography, and single-unit recordings all represent major subdivisions of neuroscience research that produce data fundamentally different from EEG recordings. More specifically, a key difference with these techniques is that they operate in a cortical domain instead of the sensor space. Therefore, any methods that can port EEG data in this cortical reference frame can tighten the connection between noninvasive data and most modern neuroscience findings.

A neuroimaging tool called "source estimation" offers one solution to this issue. Source estimation attempts to calculate the sources of brain activity in the *source space* from recordings made in the sensor space using EEG or other methods. In contrast to the sensor space, the source space refers to the domain where brain activity originates. Throughout this chapter, we discuss a popular form of source estimation called "source imaging"—the topic of Section 2.2. The underlying goal of source imaging is to estimate cortical sources of activity at several thousand discrete points distributed across the entire cortex. In other words, it estimates whole-brain cortical activity from recorded EEG data (Figure 2.1, bottom row).

In certain situations, working with data in the source space carries important advantages over the sensor space, as the field of human neuroimaging also operates primarily in the source space. Therefore, collections of knowledge and techniques from neuroimaging become useful for improving BCIs after converting the sensor-based EEG data into a source space representation. This chapter focuses on two cases that leverage this rationale. First, functional imaging literature has localized numerous cortical regions where activity is modulated during certain behavioral tasks. With source imaging, we can focus on processing EEG activity originating only a specific cortical region of interest (ROI) and avoid expending resources on less relevant data. Second, neuroimaging often involves normalizing brain data across subjects for group-level statistics and visualizing data on a template brain. These same algorithms are useful for tackling noteworthy goals in BCIs like transfer learning, where the aim is to recycle training data across subjects to expedite BCI calibration. We will formally review the source imaging technique in Section 2.2 before detailing these two specific opportunities that the source space offers BCIs.

## 2.2 MAPPING NONINVASIVE SIGNALS TO THE BRAIN

Source estimation is the area of study concerned with bridging the sensor and source spaces. Specifically, it is used to estimate the sources of neural activity that gave rise to signals observed outside the head with noninvasive measurements like EEG. In this section, we specifically describe source imaging—a form of source estimation—and provide a mathematical overview of this procedure.

EEG largely reflects the summed activity from large populations of pyramidal neurons (Hämäläinen et al. 1993), which are the largest and most common excitatory neurons in the cortex. Pyramidal neurons are generally oriented with the "trunk" of their large dendritic tree (called the apical dendrite) oriented normal to the cortical surface. Therefore, when pyramidal neurons are influenced by excitatory or inhibitory postsynaptic potentials (PSPs), charged ions flow within the neuron primarily along an axis aligned with the apical dendrite. This charge flow is often referred to as the "primary current." Since charge cannot accumulate in the brain, "secondary" (or volume) current loops also flow extracellularly throughout the head to compensate for the primary current (Lopes da Silva & Van Rotterdam 2011). Therefore, an activation pattern resembling a source-sink configuration arises that mimics the characteristics of a current dipole—a fact that simplifies source imaging (Dale & Sereno 1993; Hämäläinen et al. 1993; Lopes da Silva & Van Rotterdam 2011) as discussed later. These PSP activations (lasting tens to hundreds of milliseconds) are much slower than action potentials (lasting ~1 ms), so the PSP activations of a population of neurons are more likely to temporally overlap (Lopes da Silva 2010). Combined with the aligned arrangement of these neurons, the field potentials of simultaneously active neurons add constructively in space and time to become detectible outside the head (Lopes da Silva & Van Rotterdam 2011).

The link between neural activity and EEG recordings can be difficult to establish because this activity is undesirably transformed before reaching the EEG sensors. One transformation arises because EEG electrodes are separated from the cortex by a few centimeters of tissue. This separation forces researchers to contend with the effects of volume conduction; activity from any given neural source is detected by a number of EEG electrodes, or equivalently, the voltage trace for any single EEG electrode is the sum of many separate sources of activity. A second transformation results because the tissues in the head all have different conductivity profiles (e.g., the skull is much less conductive than the scalp). These inhomogeneities between tissue layers cause further distortion as electromagnetic activity propagates to the EEG electrodes (Lopes da Silva 2010). At the group level, a related issue results from the substantial geometrical differences in the shape of head and brain tissues between subjects. Since these anatomical differences influence the spatial profile of brain activity on the scalp, even activations of hypothetically identical brain regions will appear different in the EEG recordings of different subjects because of geometric anatomical variability. In a similar problem, the specific location of each EEG sensor, including small deviations from the ideal placement, affects the profile of recorded activity. All of these components act to obscure the relationship between source space activity and recordings in the sensor space on a unique subject-by-subject basis.

Source estimation is a modeling approach that attempts to account for these transformations when estimating the active neural sources. As EEG does not allow us to directly observe the sources of cortical brain activity, we can view this problem as a member of a broader class of physics and mathematics questions often referred to as "inverse problems." To solve this particular inverse problem, we first construct a forward model to capture how neural signals are distorted by these transformations before reaching the EEG electrodes. We then generate an inverse solution that attempts to account for (or "undo") this collective transformation. In the end, solving this inverse problem provides a means to estimate unobservable cortical activity from observed EEG data.

There exist several major methods of carrying out source estimation, and each is based on different assumptions. As mentioned previously, this chapter is specifically focused on source imaging, which is a technique for estimating neural activity across the entire cortex simultaneously. This approach entails creating a cortical model of several thousand model current dipoles distributed evenly across the cortical surface. These dipoles are oriented orthogonal to and outward from the cortical surface to reflect the biophysical properties of the cortex, and each dipole can be thought to represent the primary current due to one cortical macrocolumn of pyramidal neurons. The goal in source imaging is to estimate the activity of many distributed elements that sample the entire cortical space (analogous to estimating the intensity of pixels in a digital image).

Putting these principles into practice, we must first quantitatively characterize how neural activity propagates to the EEG sensors by computing a forward model. This model is made up of two main components. First, a source space model describes the location and orientation of each simulated current dipole. As this consists of a set of 3D locations and normal vectors that define the dipoles' geometry, it can often be conveniently expressed as a 3D mesh or volumetric grid. Typically, this requires either a brain reconstruction segmented from a structural MRI scan or a generic brain model (like FreeSurfer's "fsaverage"; Fischl 2012). Second, a head conductivity model characterizes how neural activity is transformed when traversing the different head layers (like the skull and scalp) since the changes in conductivity at each layer boundary act to spatially smear the signals of interest. While a handful of different head models exist, two are used most commonly: spherical head models, which are mathematically efficient but simplistically approximate the head as a sphere, and boundary element models (BEMs), which are MRI-reconstructed anatomically accurate representations of the head layers (Ermer et al. 2001). Before an experiment, cardinal landmarks and the 3D location of each EEG electrode are also recorded to coregister their positions with this head model. For further review of the forward model, see Hämäläinen et al. (1993) or Baillet (2010).

Given the forward model, we can estimate the influence of each cortical dipole on each EEG sensor. The weight for each dipole–electrode pair serves as an entry in the forward (or "gain") matrix **A**. We can describe a pattern of cortical activity (i.e., the current at all dipoles) using the vector **j** and relate this cortical activity to the vector of sensor measurements **x** (i.e., the electric potential at all electrodes) as

$$\mathbf{x} = \mathbf{A}\mathbf{j} + \mathbf{n}. \tag{2.1}$$

Here, **n** is assumed to be additive white Gaussian noise. See Figure 2.2 for an illustration of the forward modeling problem.

Source imaging is aimed at estimating cortical activity from noninvasive measurements, that is, the reciprocal to the forward problem. This challenge is one example of an "ill-posed" problem, which are a class of problems that satisfy one of the following properties: there are infinite solutions, there is no solution, or the solution is noncontinuous such that a small amount of noise in the observation can lead to drastic changes in the estimated model parameters—here, the model parameters represent the activity of the modeled current dipoles. To transform an ill-posed problem into a well-posed one, we require regularization, which introduces additional assumptions to reduce the model's variance. There are a number of different regularization methods, all of which share the overarching goal of ensuring a unique and stable solution.

The commonly used minimum-norm estimate (MNE) approach to source imaging (Gramfort et al. 2014) attempts to minimize the $\ell_2$ (or Euclidean) norm using Tikhonov regularization (Baillet et al. 2001; Hämäläinen & Ilmoniemi 1984; Tikhonov & Arsenin 1977). A solution with these properties is obtained by calculating the pseudoinverse matrix **M** of the forward matrix. Given the inverse solution, we can then estimate the cortical activity $\hat{\mathbf{j}}$ from the sensor recordings as

$$\hat{\mathbf{j}} = \mathbf{M}\mathbf{x}. \tag{2.2}$$

This particular source imaging approach is equivalent to the Bayesian maximum *a posteriori* estimate of the measurements given the sensor and source covariance matrices and assuming that the

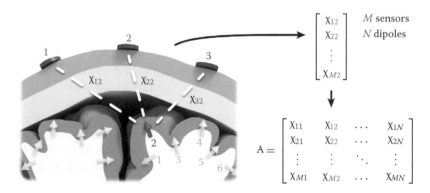

**FIGURE 2.2** Illustration of the EEG forward modeling process. Left: The relationship between an exemplar dipole (red) and the EEG electrodes (black) is calculated (white dashed lines) by solving for the electric potential of the propagating electromagnetic activity at the interface of each pair of conducting layers. These weights are compiled into a vector that quantifies how electrical current at one dipole in the source space influences the electric potential at each electrode in the sensor space. The weight vectors are computed for all dipoles and concatenated as columns to form the forward (or "gain") matrix A, which allows calculation of the electric potential x at all *M* electrodes given the activity j at all *N* dipoles. Head layers depicted here include the scalp (gray), skull (off-white), gray matter (pinkish gray), and white matter (white).

source amplitudes are normally distributed (Hämäläinen et al. 2010). The sensor noise covariance is often estimated from baseline activity, and the source covariance is typically assumed to be the identity matrix. Alternative source imaging methods to MNE include the minimum current estimate (Matsuura & Okabe 1995; Uutela et al. 1999), which uses a different regularization scheme (specifically, the $\ell_1$ norm) resulting in more focal source estimates, and beamforming, which attempts to estimate a spatial filter for each dipoles or region individually (Jensen & Hesse 2010; van Veen et al. 1997). For full mathematical derivations, see Baillet et al. (2001) or Hämäläinen et al. (2010).

Source imaging does come with some drawbacks that are worth reviewing. For example, the regularization scheme underlying the MNE approach is known to produce spatially diffuse cortical estimates even if the true brain activity is focal. There is also little biological evidence supporting any particular regularization technique as the brain is not known to minimize any norm of the total cortical current. Often, regularizers are chosen because they are intuitive, yield some desired activity distribution, and have a linear solution that makes the calculation computationally convenient (Baillet 2010). Ideally, the regularizer should also reflect what is known in neuroscience literature (e.g., with fMRI or invasive work) about the brain activation of interest (e.g., focal or diffuse) and the end goal (e.g., estimation of whole-brain activity or a single region) in order to develop a reasonable approach and solution. Note, however, that theoretical work suggests that the sensor noise covariance matrix has a more significant impact on results than the chosen regularization scheme (Mosher et al. 2003). Additionally, the researcher must choose a number of parameters associated with the forward and inverse models. Reasonable values exist for head layer conductivities and thicknesses, template brains are available for generic head models, and other parameters such as the regularizer parameter (often denoted as λ) can be estimated from the SNR of the data (Lin et al. 2004). Finally, we often assume time invariance in regard to the sensor and source covariance matrices, which are an important component in source imaging used to normalize the spatial coactivation patterns in EEG sensors and current dipoles, respectively. This assumption is not supported in theoretical (Friston 1997) or empirical studies (Brookes et al. 2014; de Pasquale et al. 2010) though recent work has proposed source imaging methods that are amenable to nonstationary brain signals (Castaño-Candamil et al. 2015; Gramfort et al. 2013; Woolrich et al. 2013).

Source imaging aside, a common task throughout many types of neuroimaging is to spatially normalize neural activity estimates across brains for statistical analysis and visualization. As mentioned previously, this is needed to account for the substantial intersubject anatomical variability. Often, researchers employ brain morphing, which uses either a surface- or volume-based algorithm to normalize spatial variability across different brains. Surface-based methods more accurately morph cortical regions (Fischl et al. 1999a), making them appropriate for transferring cortical source estimates. The spherical morphing procedure is one such example of surface-based morphing. This procedure starts by first transferring data onto a high-resolution version of the cortical surface mesh and smoothing it using an isotropic diffusion process (Gramfort et al. 2014). The mesh is then mapped onto a sphere using a procedure described in Fischl et al. (1999b). The convexity of sulcal/gyral regions, defined using a curvature threshold, is maximally aligned to a second spherical brain from a different subject. This alignment is crucial as cortical folding varies considerably between subjects, causing variation in how electromagnetic signals propagate to the sensor space (even for identical ROIs; Wronkiewicz et al. 2016). The cortical activations themselves are then transferred, the target brain is deflated, and finally the data are smoothed onto a standard resolution mesh. The entire process is often compiled into one morphing matrix, to allow data morphing with a single matrix multiplication. In BCIs, we can extend this tool to facilitate transfer learning—a method of recycling training data across subjects described in Section 2.4.

## 2.3 APPLICATION: APPLYING NEUROSCIENCE TO IMPROVE CLASSIFICATION ACCURACY

When comparing sensor- and source-based BCIs, the source domain carries with it a few theoretical advantages over the conventional sensor space approach. The sensor-based approach very often uses spatial filtering algorithms like independent component analysis (ICA) or the common spatial pattern (CSP) algorithm to spatially filter the brain activity into an algorithmically optimal data space. This strategy has proven useful empirically but has some limiting drawbacks. First, these spatial filtering algorithms, which linearly recombine EEG signals, are difficult to interpret neuroscientifically; by projecting data into an algorithmic space, they further complicate the (already loose) spatial relationship between scalp electrodes and the cortex. Second, it is difficult to directly compare these spatial projections (e.g., EEG activity projected onto subject-specific CSP components) across subjects (Devlaminck et al. 2011; Lotte 2015; Samek et al. 2013). These filters are typically recomputed for each recording session such that the projected data from one session will not share an easily identifiable common reference frame with the next (i.e., the projected recordings do not share a common vector space). This contributes to the challenges with sensor-based transfer learning as discussed in Section 2.4. Finally, many BCI signal processing algorithms require that useful signal features are punctate in space and/or time. While this is an appropriate assumption in event-related paradigms (e.g., P300 or SSVEP), this approach has limited generalizability. As a few groups have suggested (Vansteensel et al. 2010) that future BCIs may instead work better with distributed cognitive activity or some form of network synchronization—two topics currently at the center of the neuroimaging community's attention.

Source imaging projects brain activity directly to the cortex, thereby mitigating some important shortcomings associated with the sensor space. Most importantly, it allows a tighter link with modern neuroscience research since most modern human neuroscience experiments collect data in the source domain. The practical implication for BCI research is that novel neuroscience findings are more applicable in the source space. In functional neuroimaging experiments, for example, the goal is often to precisely determine the cortical region(s) involved in some task (e.g., as a discrete set of dipoles on a template brain). Therefore, these discoveries are readily translated into source-based BCIs by targeting brain activity only from relevant cortical regions. This targeted source approach is also more likely to generalize because the ROI originates from a separate study that has often statistically confirmed its spatial extent across a cohort of subjects. This represents a more scientifically informed and repeatable signal processing approach; it does not rely on either hand-picking electrodes or recomputed spatial filters for every recording session. This also largely sidesteps any trial-and-error process to find the optimal electrode(s) or signal processing technique for a given task-related activation. Additionally, in algorithms where spatial projections are difficult to rank in order of importance (like in ICA), this avoids the need for an expert to subjectively choose which projection(s) to use for later processing stages. Overall, the source space remains a principled way to inject insights from neuroscience research into the BCI development process.

In experimental work, source imaging has been used in about a dozen published BCI studies to date, and most have focused on classifying SMR activity. Some source-based BCI research used conventional sensor space features for SMR activity classification but then validated *post hoc* that the event-related synchronization/desynchronization signals originated from the SMR cortex (Yuan et al. 2008). Others classified motor imagery depending on whether source activity of a few ICA components was greater in the left or right hemisphere during hand-selected time periods of a motor task (Kamousi et al. 2005, 2007; Qin et al. 2004). More recent research has directly compared sensor- and source-based BCI strategies on motor tasks and found that the latter gave a moderate performance improvement (Ahn et al. 2012; Cincotti et al. 2008; Grosse-Wentrup et al. 2009). Others focused on using the source space to identify the most useful cortical regions and their frequency bands for individuals (Lotte et al. 2009). However, the overall notion that the most relevant signals for a motor task originate in the SMR cortex is not surprising. The functional map of the motor and somatosensory cortices has been well established since Penfield's work on the central sulcus over 65 years ago (Penfield & Rasmussen 1950).

The source space, however, is not limited to validating or improving the established BCI paradigms (discussed in Section 2.1)—it may also guide development of new BCIs. Recently, a few studies have used source estimation to focus on cortical regions previously unexplored in BCIs. Because source imaging brings data into the same reference frame as modern neuroimaging data, neuroimaging insights can then act to supply *a priori* information to directly target cortical ROIs in novel BCI paradigms. For example, some have demonstrated classification of nonmotor BCI tasks (e.g., mental calculation, visuospatial navigation) using features-based synchronization between cortical regions (Besserve et al. 2011)—currently, a burgeoning area of neuroimaging. Another recent work selectively targeted the superior parietal cortex in a task where subjects self-regulated gamma power through focused attention (Grosse-Wentrup & Schölkopf 2014). In addition, our laboratory has targeted the right temporoparietal junction to detect when a subject voluntarily switched auditory attention while listening to multiple talkers (Wronkiewicz et al. 2016). These studies demonstrate how recently published neuroimaging literature can act as a prior to focus on the most relevant cortical ROI (thereby selecting the most informative brain activity). Therefore, the source space can serve as a principled pathway to leverage new neuroscience discoveries for BCI advancement.

Of course, there are some disadvantages to using source imaging in a BCI context. A one-time 20- to 30-min structural MRI scan is needed to construct the anatomically accurate BEM, although multiple studies have suggested that accurate head-shape digitization can provide sufficient information to deform a surrogate MRI instead with minimal accuracy loss (Ermer et al. 2001; Fuchs et al. 2002; van't Ent et al. 2001). The experimenter also needs to choose one of the numerous regularization methods and its associated parameters and also record electrode positions before each recording session (as discussed in Section 2.2). Like most BCI signal processing pipelines, source imaging also does not account for nonstationarities in the underlying brain signal. See Section 2.2 for recent work addressing this challenge, as well as Wronkiewicz et al. (2016) for further discussion on the benefits and drawbacks of using source imaging in BCIs.

## 2.4 APPLICATION: TRANSFER LEARNING

Unlike early "operant-conditioning" BCIs where the processing pipeline was static, modern BCI systems now use machine learning classifiers to rapidly adapt to the statistics of a user's brain activity. This transition was a critical advancement in BCI methodology as it shortened BCI training periods from several weeks to 20–30 min (Guger et al. 2003; Krauledat et al. 2007) for some paradigms. However, a further reduction in calibration time is vital in order for BCIs to gain acceptance outside laboratories, and methods to do so are an active area of research (see Lotte 2015 for a review). In healthcare, any therapy that requires a half-hour of system calibration before each treatment session is financially prohibitive. For healthy users, this lengthy calibration period is a serious marketing and usability concern. As an analogy, imagine attempting to commercialize a car that required a 20- to 30-min start-up period to calibrate the steering wheel and pedals before *every single trip*.

There are some promising paths toward reducing this time-consuming training phase, but it remains an active research area (Kindermans et al. 2014; Krauledat et al. 2008; Lotte 2015; Lotte & Guan 2010). Most BCI laboratories have EEG data stored from many subjects who have completed the same task. A natural question to ask is whether these existing data from other subjects (or previous sessions from the same subject) can be recycled to speed up calibration for an upcoming BCI session. While conceptually straightforward, this is challenging in practice because EEG signals are affected by many sources of intersubject (and intersession) variability. A few examples of this variation include changes in electrode number or positioning, head anatomy, cortical folding, fatigue, and mental strategy. Thus, the reuse of training data across subjects or sessions is significantly constrained; these inconsistencies violate the implicit assumption of standard machine learning algorithms that the training and test data share an identical feature space and probability distribution. This hurdle forces most BCI systems to obey a subject-specific scheme and be recalibrated from scratch for every recording session (Figure 2.3a).

Within machine learning research, the field of "transfer learning" aims to address this problem of reusing training data even when the features or their distributions differ (Pan & Yang 2010).

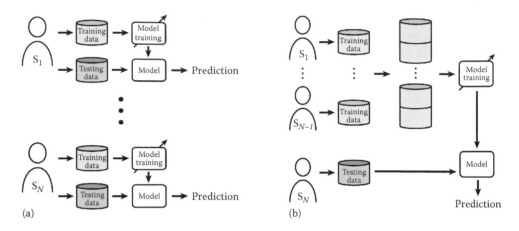

**FIGURE 2.3** Comparison of standard subject-specific training (a) with subject-independent training (b). (a) In most BCIs, a machine learning algorithm is trained and tested separately for every BCI recording session because the data's underlying statistics are highly subject and session dependent. Therefore, each classification model is typically only effective for one recording session. (b) Subject-independent BCIs attempt to account for intersubject variability with transfer learning techniques. In this way, pre-recorded data from $N - 1$ subjects are used to train a model that can quickly begin to make predictions on testing data from the $N$th subject. Here, the transfer of training data is depicted, but an equally valid approach is to transfer knowledge from a set of classifiers (each trained on one subject) into an aggregate classifier.

In BCIs specifically, an attractive application of this idea is to pool prerecorded EEG data from $N - 1$ subjects to train the upcoming ($N$th) subject's classifier (Figure 2.3b). A system that requires no training data for a new subject is referred to as a subject-independent BCI (Fazli et al. 2009). A few studies proposed similar methods that involve aggregating multiple spatial filters and/or classifiers (trained on different recordings) into a single ensemble classifier (Fazli et al. 2009, 2011). Formally, these are examples of "transductive transfer learning" because the classification task is the same while the data sets differ between subjects (Pan & Yang 2010). A number of studies have carried out transfer learning in the sensor space (see Lotte 2015 for a review), but directly transferring EEG activity neglects several sources of substantial variability related to the electrode positioning, head anatomy, and brain anatomy (as discussed in Section 2.2).

Source imaging represents a useful technique for normalizing many forms of intersubject variability. Specifically, source imaging includes an inverse model that incorporates variation in cortical folding as well as head and skull morphology. It also directly accounts for electrode positions as part of the forward model, thereby normalizing for deviations in their locations that otherwise lower the accuracy of sensor-based BCIs (Ramoser et al. 2000). This includes electrodes that must be excluded because of noise—a situation that changes the feature space in sensor-based BCIs. Once the EEG data are projected to the cortical surface, well-established neuroimaging tools exist to then morph data across subjects in a manner that optimally preserves the cortical sulcal/gyral alignment (see the end of Section 2.2). This is a critical normalization step because differences in cortical geometry will cause even identical ROI activity to manifest very differently in the sensor space (Wronkiewicz et al. 2016).

An empirical study of a source-based subject-independent BCI (using no training data from the subject being tested) supported these theoretical advantages (Wronkiewicz et al. 2015). We found that in both simulated and real data, this approach often surpassed the accuracy of a conventional subject-specific BCI even when trained only on data morphed from a few other subjects (i.e., in a subject-independent manner). While some sensor-based transfer learning approaches have also proven effective, all sustained small accuracy decreases compared to the traditional subject-specific approach. Thus, when compared to conventional subject-specific approaches, porting established neuroimaging tools into BCIs may shorten or eliminate the training period while also improving classification accuracy.

## 2.5 CONCLUSIONS AND FUTURE DIRECTIONS

Given that many of the ideal BCI applications have yet to be realized, the field still has a great deal of room to expand. Our brains engage in an almost innumerable number of behaviors and processes every day. Unexplored cortical activations may soon prove useful for integrating BCIs with technologies like virtual reality, alternative smartphone interfaces, or even scalable and effective stroke rehabilitation techniques. At present, however, the BCI community has continued its focus on only a handful of mainstream BCI paradigms. Moreover, some conventional paradigms like the P300- and SSVEP-based BCIs require stimuli like flashing letters and lights to elicit useful brain signals. In these cases, the relevant signal feature is not generated with pure volition, but rather as a reaction to presented stimuli. Ideally, the next generation of BCI signals should be under complete volitional control and not be encumbered by the need for additional stimulus-producing hardware. Coupled with burdensome calibration periods, these and other limitations continue to stifle the advancement and adoption of BCIs. Toward addressing these challenges, we reviewed how source imaging provides a way to incorporate new neuroimaging findings into BCIs and reduce calibration periods by recycling training data in a controlled manner. Even so, the source space still offers a number of other opportunities that are worth investigating in future work.

In this chapter, we focused on methods to improve BCIs using knowledge and tools borrowed from neuroscience. The relationship between neuroscience and BCIs, however, need not be unidirectional—it should be symbiotic. Put simply, BCI research could play a stronger role in guiding future neuroscience experiments. This is a unique opportunity for the technology because BCIs can modulate the user's experience in real time and in response to brain activity. For example, some have suggested investigating how brain processing changes during interaction with a continuously adapting agent (like the computer; Mattout 2012) or detecting neural correlates of an upcoming lapse in attention (O'Connell et al. 2009). Another area of research is focused on bidirectional BCIs where there are many addressable questions related to sensory coding and neural plasticity (Wander & Rao 2014) and methods to more flexibly probe the neural mechanisms behind SMR control (Golub et al. 2016). Source imaging in particular can provide a whole-brain perspective at an excellent temporal resolution (but lower spatial resolution) compared to other signal acquisition methods like fMRI, electrocorticography, or single-unit recordings. Answers to these neuroscience questions are likely to inspire new BCI paradigms and improve existing ones.

Another question related to source imaging arises because the conductivity component of the forward model can be defined in multiple ways. As discussed in Section 2.2, the head layers are usually modeled either generically using concentric spherical shells or by reconstructing an anatomically accurate BEM from an MRI scan. The source space model typically corresponds to this choice; spatially averaged template brains are often used with the generic conductivity model, and anatomically accurate cortical reconstructions usually accompany a BEM. While BEMs generally give more accurate source estimates (Darvas et al. 2006; Ermer et al. 2001; Vatta et al. 2010), this relative advantage has received little investigation in a BCI context (Wronkiewicz et al. 2016). The structural MRI scan required for a BEM is costly and time-consuming, so more examination is needed to determine which BCI paradigms benefit substantially enough to justify their use.

Source imaging may also facilitate the investigation of optimized electrode positioning. During the 1950s, leading EEG researchers recognized that a standard electrode map (or "montage") was necessary to better compare findings across research groups. Therefore, the 10-20 international electrode map was developed to, among other advantages, provide "adequate coverage of all parts of head" (Jasper 1958). While the 10-20 montage served as a necessary standard for clinical research, this electrode layout is not optimized to capture activity from any particular cortical region. The common practice of hand-selecting electrodes or other features to target the most relevant signals demonstrates this fact. Therefore, there is an opportunity to use the forward solution to quantify how well each electrode captures activity from any cortical ROI. The ability to quantitatively assess the relationship between an ROI and electrodes leads to a number of potential research hypotheses, two of which we describe here.

First, forward modeling can predict the suitability of a montage (standard or not) for any ROI and do so on an individual basis—a goal some are already exploring (Zich et al. 2015). Quantifying the expected signal-to-noise ratio at each electrode will facilitate the BCI prototyping process while also reducing trial-and-error experimentation in selecting the best set of EEG electrodes or an optimal spatial filtering technique. For example, a few groups have developed mobile electrode montages that fit behind the ear (Debener et al. 2015; Do Valle et al. 2014). Forward modeling could be used to predict how appropriate these experimental electrode montages are for a given paradigm (e.g., SMR or P300 systems). Evaluating the overall sensitivity of an electrode montage to a given cortical ROI in a particular subject may also shed some light on why certain users are unable to control certain BCIs—a problem sometimes referred to as BCI "illiteracy." Second, the forward modeling process could be used to construct optimal electrode montage; in other words, it could be used to calculate an optimal electrode arrangement for a specific ROI rather than just quantify how receptive existing montages are. As before, this approach could take into account an individual subject's cortical geometry. The electrode arrangement might be custom tailored using an objective function that, for example, favors arrangements where electrodes are maximally influenced by a given ROI while requiring that these electrodes are separated by some minimum spatial distance. The optimal montage could then be constructed for each ROI–subject pair using techniques like 3D printing to personalize the EEG arrangement—an idea being explored by a few companies.

Given the diversity of BCI research, the methods we covered in this chapter may be more or less amenable for different researchers. Fully adopting a source imaging pipeline may be untenable for some groups, but note that the barrier for entry is lowering in the face of open source toolboxes and a focus on developing helpful tutorials. For many, a smaller but meaningful step may be to simply revisit the neuroscience literature describing BCI signal features—including the signals used in conventional BCIs. It is worth reiterating, however, that the neuroscience literature has grown considerably since the standard noninvasive BCIs were first published. This backlog of untapped insights should be investigated for new potential BCI paradigms. This chapter should also make it clear that the quantitative relationship between brain activity and EEG electrodes changes with every subject and session. Although it is tempting for experimenters to incorporate subjective choices into a processing pipeline to squeeze out every point of accuracy, these sources of variability have the potential to corrupt any resulting findings. Instead, a general goal should always be to automate BCIs as much as possible to facilitate reproducibility and scalability of any discoveries; we have shown how neuroscience offers one path to accomplishing this, and with some moderate transitions in BCI methodology, the field may again enjoy advancements at a pace not seen since its original expansion.

## ACKNOWLEDGMENTS

The authors would like to thank Nicholas Foti and the anonymous reviewers for helpful discussion and suggestions. This research was funded by the National Science Foundation Division of Graduate Education, Graduate Research Fellowship Program (DGE-1256082 to MW), the Department of Defense Air Force Office of Scientific Research Young Investigator Program (FA9550-12-1-0466 to AKCL), and the Department of Defense Office of Naval Research Young Investigator Program (N00014-15-1-2124 to AKCL).

## REFERENCES

Ahn, M., Hong, J. H. & Jun, S. C., 2012. Feasibility of approaches combining sensor and source features in brain–computer interface. *Journal of Neuroscience Methods*, 204(1), pp. 168–78.
Baillet, S., 2010. The dowser in the fields: Searching for MEG sources. In: P. C. Hansen, M. Kringelbach & R. Salmelin, eds. *MEG: An Introduction to Methods*. New York: Oxford University Press, Inc., pp. 83–123.

Baillet, S., Mosher, J. C. & Leahy, R. M., 2001. Electromagnetic brain mapping. *IEEE Signal Processing Magazine*, 18(6), pp. 14–30.

Belliveau, J. W. et al., 1991. Functional mapping of the human visual cortex by magnetic resonance imaging. *Science*, 254(5032), pp. 716–9.

Besserve, M., Martinerie, J. & Garnero, L., 2011. Improving quantification of functional networks with EEG inverse problem: Evidence from a decoding point of view. *NeuroImage*, 55(4), pp. 1536–47.

Brookes, M. J. et al., 2014. Measuring temporal, spectral and spatial changes in electrophysiological brain network connectivity. *NeuroImage*, 91, pp. 282–99.

Castaño-Candamil, S. et al., 2015. Solving the EEG inverse problem based on space-time-frequency structured sparsity constraints. *NeuroImage*, 118, pp. 598–612.

Chapman, R. M. & Bragdon, H. R., 1964. Evoked responses to numerical and non-numerical visual stimuli while problem solving. *Nature*, 203, pp. 1555–7.

Cincotti, F. et al., 2008. High-resolution EEG techniques for brain–computer interface applications. *Journal of Neuroscience Methods*, 167(1), pp. 31–42.

Dale, A. M. & Sereno, M. I., 1993. Improved localization of cortical activity by combining EEG and MEG with MRI cortical surface reconstruction: A linear approach. *Journal of Cognitive Neuroscience*, 5(2), pp. 162–76.

Darvas, F., Ermer, J. J., Mosher, J. C. & Leahy, R. M., 2006. Generic head models for atlas-based EEG source analysis. *Human Brain Mapping*, 27, pp. 129–43.

de Pasquale, F. ct al., 2010. Temporal dynamics of spontaneous MEG activity in brain networks. *PNAS*, 107(13), pp. 6040–45.

Debener, S., Emkes, R., De Vos, M. & Bleichner, M., 2015. Unobtrusive ambulatory EEG using a smartphone and flexible printed electrodes around the ear. *Scientific Reports*, 5, pp. 1–11.

Devlaminck, D. et al., 2011. Multisubject learning for common spatial patterns in motor-imagery BCI. *Computational Intelligence and Neuroscience*, 2011, pp. 1–9.

Do Valle, B., Cash, S. S. & Sodini, C. G., 2014. *Wireless behind-the-ear EEG recording device with wireless interface to a mobile device (iPhone/iPod touch)*. Chicago, IL, 2014 36th Annual International Conference on the IEEE EMBS.

Ermer, J. J., Mosher, J. C., Baillet, S. & Leahy, R. M., 2001. Rapidly recomputable EEG forward models for realistic head shapes. *Physics in Medicine and Biology*, 46, pp. 1265–81.

Farwell, L. A. & Donchin, E., 1988. Talking off the top of your head: Toward a mental prosthesis utilizing event-related brain potentials. *Electroencephalogray and Clinical Neurophysiology*, 70(6), pp. 510–23.

Fazli, S., Danóczya, M., Schelldorfer, J. & Müller, K.-R., 2011. ℓ1-penalized linear mixed-effects models for high dimensional data with application to BCI. *NeuroImage*, 56(4), pp. 2100–8.

Fazli, S. et al., 2009. Subject-independent mental state classification in single trials. *Neural Networks*, 22(9), pp. 1305–12.

Fischl, B., 2012. FreeSurfer. *NeuroImage*, 62(2), pp. 774–81.

Fischl, B., Sereno, M. & Dale, A. M., 1999a. Cortical surface-based analysis II: Inflation, flattening, and a surface-based coordinate system. *Neuroimage*, 9, pp. 195–207.

Fischl, B., Sereno, M. I., Tootell, R. B. & Dale, A. M., 1999b. High-resolution intersubject averaging and a coordinate system for the cortical surface. *Human Brain Mapping*, 8(4), pp. 272–84.

Friston, K. J., 1997. Transients, metastability, and neuronal dynamics. *NeuroImage*, 5, pp. 164–71.

Fuchs, M. et al., 2002. A standardized boundary element method volume conductor model. *Clinical Neurophysiology*, 113, pp. 702–12.

Golub, M. D., Chase, S. M., Batista, A. P. & Yu, B. M., 2016. Brain–computer interfaces for dissecting cognitive processes underlying sensorimotor control. *Current Opinion in Neurobiology*, 37, pp. 53–8.

Gramfort, A. et al., 2013. Time–frequency mixed-norm estimates: Sparse M/EEG imaging with non-stationary source activations. *NeuroImage*, 70, pp. 410–22.

Gramfort, A. et al., 2014. MNE software for processing MEG and EEG data. *NeuroImage*, 86, pp. 446–60.

Grosse-Wentrup, M., Liefhold, C., Gramann, K. & Buss, M., 2009. Beamforming in noninvasive brain-computer interfaces. *IEEE Transactions on Biomedical Engineering*, 56(4), pp. 1209–19.

Grosse-Wentrup, M. & Schölkopf, B., 2014. A brain–computer interface based on self-regulation of gamma-oscillations in the superior parietal cortex. *Journal of Neural Engineering*, 11(5), pp. 1–13.

Guger, C. et al., 2003. How many people are able to operate an EEG-based brain–computer interface (BCI)?. *IEEE Transactions on Neural Systems and Rehabilitation Engineering*, 11(2), pp. 145–147

Hämäläinen, M. et al., 1993. Magnetoencephalography—Theory, instrumentation, and applications to noninvasive studies of the working human brain. *Reviews of Modern Physics*, 65(2), pp. 413–97.

Hämäläinen, M. & Ilmoniemi, R. J., 1984. *Interpreting Measured Magnetic Fields of the Brain: Estimates of Current Distribution*, Helsinki, Finland: Helsinki University of Technology.

Hämäläinen, M., Lin, F.-H. & Mosher, J., 2010. Anatomically and functionally constrained minimum-norm estimates. In: *MEG: An Introduction to Methods*. New York: Oxford University Press, Inc., pp. 186–215.

Jasper, H. H., 1958. Report on the Committee on Methods of Clinical Examination in Electroencephalography: 1957. *Electroencephalography and Clinical Neurophysiology*, 10(2), pp. 370–5.

Jensen, O. & Hesse, C., 2010. Estimating distributed representations of evoked responses and oscillatory brain activity. In: P. C. Hansen, M. L. Kringelbach & R. Salmelin, eds. *MEG: An Introduction to Methods*. New York: Oxford University Press, pp. 156–85.

Kamousi, B., Liu, Z. & He, B., 2005. Classification of motor imagery tasks for brain–computer interface applications by means of two equivalent dipoles analysis. *IEEE Transactions on Neural Systems and Rehabilitation Engineering*, 13(2), pp. 166–71.

Kamousi, B., Nasiri, A. & He, B., 2007. Classification of motor imagery by means of cortical current density estimation and Von Neumann entropy. *Journal of Neural Engineering*, 4(2), pp. 17–25.

Kindermans, P.-J. et al., 2014. True zero-training brain–computer interfacing—An online study. *PLoS One*, 9(7), pp. 1–13.

Krauledat, M., Schroder, M., Blankertz, B. & Müller, K.-R., 2007. Reducing calibration time for brain–computer interfaces: A clustering approach. *Advances in Neural Information Processing Systems*, pp. 753–60.

Krauledat, M., Tangermann, M., Blankertz, B. & Müller, K.-R., 2008. Towards zero training for brain–computer interfacing. *PLoS One*, 3(8), pp. 1–12.

Lin, F.-H. et al., 2004. Spectral spatiotemporal imaging of cortical oscillations and interactions in the human brain. *NeuroImage*, 23(2), pp. 582–95.

Lopes da Silva, F. H., 2010. Electrophysiological basis of MEG signals. In: P. C. Hansen, M. Kringelbach & R. Salmelin, eds. *MEG: An Introduction to Methods*. New York: Oxford University Press, Inc., pp. 1–23.

Lopes da Silva, F. H. & Van Rotterdam, A., 2011. Biophysical aspects of EEG and magnetoencephalogra generation. In: D. L. Schomer & F. H. Lopes da Silva, eds. *Electroencephalography: Basic Principles, Clinical Applications, and Related Fields*. Philadelphia: Lippincott Williams & Wilkins, pp. 91–110.

Lotte, F., 2015. Signal processing approaches to minimize or suppress calibration time in oscillatory activity-based brain–computer interfaces. *Proceedings of the IEEE*, 103(6), pp. 871–90.

Lotte, F. & Guan, C., 2010. Learning from other subjects helps reducing brain–computer interface calibration time. *2010 IEEE International Conference on Acoustics Speech, and Signal Processing*, Volume 1, pp. 614–7.

Lotte, F., Lécuyer, A. & Arnaldi, B., 2009. FuRIA: An inverse solution based feature extraction algorithm using fuzzy set theory for brain–computer interfaces. *IEEE Transactions on Signal Processing*, 57(8), pp. 3253–63.

Matsuura, K. & Okabe, Y., 1995. Selective minimum-norm solution of the biomagnetic inverse problem. *IEEE Transactions on Biomedical Engineering*, 42(6), pp. 608–15.

Mattout, J., 2012. Brain–computer interfaces: A neuroscience paradigm of social interaction? A matter of perspective. *Frontiers in Human Neuroscience*, 6, pp. 1–5.

Mosher, J. C., Baillet, S. & Leahy, R. M., 2003. Equivalence of linear approaches in bioelectromagnetic inverse solutions. *2003 IEEE Workshop on Statistical Signal Processing*, pp. 294–7.

O'Connell, R. G. et al., 2009. Uncovering the neural signature of lapsing attention: Electrophysiological signals predict errors up to 20 s before they occur. *Journal of Neuroscience*, 29(26), pp. 8604–11.

Pan, S. J. & Yang, Q., 2010. A survey on transfer learning. *IEEE Transactions on Knowledge and Data Engineering*, 22(10), pp. 1345–59.

Penfield, W. & Rasmussen, T., 1950. *The Cerebral Cortex of Man*. New York, New York: The Macmillan Company.

Pfurtscheller, G. & Aranibar, A., 1979. Evaluation of event-related desynchronization (ERD) preceding and following voluntary self-paced movement. *Electroencephalography and Clinical Neurophysiology*, 46(2), pp. 138–46.

Qin, L., Ding, L. & He, B., 2004. Motor imagery classification by means of source analysis for brain–computer interface applications. *Journal of Neural Engineering*, 1(3), pp. 135–41.

Ramoser, H., Müller-Gerking, J. & Pfurtscheller, G., 2000. Optimal spatial filtering of single trial EEG during imagined hand movement. *IEEE Transactions on Rehabilitation Engineering*, 8(4), pp. 441–446.

Samek, W., Meinecke, F. C. & Müller, K.-R., 2013. Transferring subspaces between subjects in brain–computer interfacing. *IEEE Transactions on Biomedical Engineering*, 60(8), pp. 1–10.

Schalk, G. et al., 2008. Brain–computer interfaces (BCIs): Detection instead of classification. *Journal of Neuroscience Methods*, 167(1), pp. 51–62.

Sutton, S., Braren, M. & Zubin, J., 1965. Evoked-potential correlates of stimulus uncertainty. *Science*, 150(3700), pp. 1187–8.

Tikhonov, A. & Arsenin, V., 1977. *Solutions of Ill-Posed Problems*. Washington DC: Winston & Sons.

Uutela, K., Hämäläinen, M. & Somersalo, E., 1999. Visualization of magnetoencephalographic data using minimum current estimates. *NeuroImage*, 10(2), pp. 173–80.

van't Ent, D., de Munch, J. & Kaas, A. L., 2001. A fast method to derive realistic BEM models for E/MEG source reconstruction. *IEEE Transactions on Biomedical Engineering*, 48(12), pp. 1434–43.

van Veen, B. D., van Drongelen, W., Yuchtman, M. & Suzuki, A., 1997. Localization of brain electrical activity via lineraly constrained minimum variance spatial filtering. *IEEE Transactions on Biomedical Engineering*, 44(9), pp. 867–80.

Vansteensel, M. J. et al., 2010. Brain–computer interfacing based on cognitive control. *Annals of Neurology*, 67(6), pp. 809–16.

Vatta, F. et al., 2010. Realistic and spherical head modeling for EEG forward problem solution: A comparative cortex-based analysis. *Computational Intelligence and Neuroscience*, 2010, pp. 1–11.

Vidal, J. J., 1973. Toward direct brain–computer communication. *Annual Review Biophysics and Bioengineering*, 2, pp. 157–80.

Vidal, J. J., 1977. Real-time detection of brain events in EEG. *Proceedings of the IEEE*, 65(5), pp. 633–41.

Wander, J. & Rao, R. P., 2014. Brain–computer interfaces: A powerful tool for scientific inquiry. *Current Opinion in Neurobiology*, 25, pp. 70–5.

Wolpaw, J. R., McFarland, D. J., Neat, G. W. & Forneris, C. A., 1991. An EEG-based brain–computer interface for cursor control. *Electroencephalography and Clinical Neurophysiology*, 78(3), pp. 252–9.

Wolpaw, J. R. & Wolpaw, E. W., 2012. Brain–computer interfaces: Something new under the sun. In: J. R. Wolpaw & E. W. Wolpaw, eds. *Brain–Computer Interfaces: Principles and Practice*. New York: Oxford University Press, pp. 3–12.

Woolrich, M. W. et al., 2013. Dynamic state allocation for MEG source reconstruction. *NeuroImage*, 77, pp. 77–92.

Wronkiewicz, M., Larson, E. & Lee, A., 2015. Leveraging anatomical information to improve transfer learning in brain–computer interfaces. *Journal of Neural Engineering*, 12(4), pp. 1–12.

Wronkiewicz, M., Larson, E. & Lee, A., 2016. Incorporating modern neuroscience findings to improve brain–computer interfaces: Tracking auditory attention. *Journal of Neural Engineering*, 13(5), pp. 1–13.

Yuan, H., Doud, A., Gururajan, A. & He, B., 2008. Cortical imaging of event-related (de)synchronization during online control of brain–computer interface using minimum-norm estimates in frequency domain. *IEEE Transactions on Neural Systems and Rehabilitation Engineering*, 16(5), pp. 425–31.

Zich, C., De Vos, M., Kranczioch, C. & Debener, S., 2015. Wireless EEG with individualized channel layout enables efficient motor imagery training. *Clinical Neurophysiology*, 126(4), pp. 698–710.

# 3 Passive Brain–Computer Interfaces
## *A Perspective on Increased Interactivity*

*Laurens R. Krol, Lena M. Andreessen,
and Thorsten O. Zander*

## CONTENTS

3.1   Passive Brain–Computer Interfaces ....................................................................... 70
3.2   Mental State Assessment ........................................................................................ 72
   3.2.1   Introduction ................................................................................................ 72
   3.2.2   Examples from the Literature ..................................................................... 72
   3.2.3   Reflection .................................................................................................... 74
3.3   Open-Loop Adaptation ........................................................................................... 75
   3.3.1   Introduction ................................................................................................ 75
   3.3.2   Examples from the Literature ..................................................................... 75
   3.3.3   Reflection .................................................................................................... 76
3.4   Closed-Loop Adaptation ........................................................................................ 77
   3.4.1   Introduction ................................................................................................ 77
   3.4.2   Examples from the Literature ..................................................................... 77
   3.4.3   Reflection .................................................................................................... 79
3.5   Automated Adaptation ............................................................................................ 79
   3.5.1   Introduction ................................................................................................ 79
   3.5.2   Examples from the Literature ..................................................................... 80
   3.5.3   Reflection .................................................................................................... 80
3.6   Summary and Conclusion ....................................................................................... 81
Acknowledgments ............................................................................................................ 83
References ......................................................................................................................... 83

### Abstract

Passive brain–computer interfaces (passive BCI; pBCI) have been introduced and formally defined almost a decade ago and have gained considerable attention since then. In this chapter, we clarify some points of confusion and provide a perspective on the past, present, and future of the field of passive BCI. This perspective concerns a key aspect with regard to which various pBCI-based systems differ from each other: interactivity. The more interactive a system is, the more responsive it is, the more autonomous, and the better capable of adaptation. Along these lines, we identify and describe four relevant categories of systems with varying levels of interactivity: mental state assessment, open-loop adaptation, closed-loop adaptation, and automated adaptation. We give examples of past and current research for each of these categories. The latter three are collectively introduced as neuroadaptive systems. This perspective and formal categorization helps to highlight human–computer interaction aspects that are relevant for the design of pBCI-based systems and points to possibilities for future research and development into passive BCI, implicit interaction, and neuroadaptive technology.

## 3.1 PASSIVE BRAIN–COMPUTER INTERFACES

In 1977, Jacques J. Vidal demonstrated the real-time detection of "brain events" and offered an example of how these might be used to control a system. Instead of using offline, a posteriori methods to investigate neuroelectric brain activity, Vidal suggested "treating the experiment as a signal detection problem" (Vidal 1977): with continuous access to an electroencephalogram (EEG), a computer classified incoming EEG data as belonging to one of four categories, based on previously learned (and continuously updated) decision strategies. As such, the system was able to recognize specific brain activity in real time.

Although Vidal speculated upon a wide range of potential future applications of this approach, it was in a clinical context that *brain–computer interface* (BCI) methodology gained widespread attention. It was quickly realized that such direct BCIs could potentially provide a means for paralyzed or otherwise motor-impaired people to communicate with the outside world without having to use their muscles (Wolpaw et al. 2002). This resolve to help those people who stood to benefit most from this technology led to a strong focus on BCI for direct communication and control, and resulted, inter alia, in different mental speller devices (e.g., Birbaumer et al. 1999; Brouwer & Van Erp 2010; Farwell & Donchin 1988; Furdea et al. 2009; Treder et al. 2011) and brain-activated prostheses (e.g., Müller-Putz & Pfurtscheller 2008; Soekadar et al. 2016; Wessberg et al. 2000; Wolpaw & McFarland 2008). For a long time, in fact, BCI research appeared to be inseparably connected to these applications.

Improvements made over the decades have made the field more interdisciplinary and BCI methodology more reliable. Of particular significance was the introduction of machine learning techniques at the start of the current millennium (e.g., Blankertz et al. 2002a; Lotte et al. 2007; Ramoser et al. 2000). Previously, users of BCI systems were trained to generate specific machine-detectable features in their EEG, such as a specific frequency modulation at a specific electrode site (Birbaumer et al. 1999). These days, training has shifted to the machine, using supervised machine learning based on initial recordings (Blankertz et al. 2002a). As pattern recognition by the machine replaced operant conditioning of the user, the idea was rekindled that this methodology could also be applied to detect and investigate spontaneous, automatic brain activity, and that these detections could then be used as *implicit input* to a system (Rötting et al. 2009; Zander et al. 2014). (We use "spontaneous" in its biological sense, meaning automatic, instinctive, involuntary, and inattentive; see below for a further discussion.)

Early examples of this can be found in suggestions to use error-related potentials to correct classification errors of traditional BCI systems (Blankertz et al. 2002b; Ferrez & Millán 2005, 2008). This was also suggested for response errors (Parra et al. 2003) and machine errors (Zander et al. 2008a) during human–computer interaction (HCI) in general. But it was only in 2008, when BCI enjoyed increased popularity overall, that the approach gained widespread attention. The use of BCI methodology for implicit input to benefit ongoing HCI was explicitly proposed as a worthwhile research endeavor by two research groups at the same conference (CHI 2008, Florence, Italy), independently of each other (Cutrell & Tan 2008; Zander et al. 2008a). Zander et al. (2008b) subsequently presented a framework formally separating this approach from traditional BCI research and proposed a name: *passive BCI*. The concept found acceptance also among clinical BCI researchers in 2012 (Wolpaw & Wolpaw 2012).

A passive BCI (Zander et al 2008b; Zander & Kothe 2011) system derives its output from automatic, spontaneous brain activity, interpreted in the given context (Zander & Jatzev 2012). This interpreted activity is then used as implicit input to support an ongoing task (Rötting et al. 2009). Use of the word "passive" here results from a user-centered perspective on HCI. It refers to the role of the end user of a system with respect to the BCI: the underlying signals being automatic, spontaneous brain activity, it is an inherent and defining aspect that the user exerts no effort to actively, explicitly, or voluntarily elicit or modulate this activity. Instead, the user focuses on the task at hand while a passive BCI system, in the background, monitors their brain activity for informative correlates of relevant cognitive or affective states.

Zander and Kothe (2011) contrast passive BCI with *active* BCI systems, where the brain activity in question is consciously and purposefully modulated in order to control an application (e.g., motor imagery BCIs; Pfurtscheller & Neuper 2001), and with *reactive* BCI systems, which rely on brain activity that is evoked by external stimulation but indirectly modulated through voluntary attention (e.g., P300 amplitudes modulated by attention shifts; Farwell & Donchin 1988).

Care should be taken when presuming that mental states can be readily categorized as "spontaneous" versus "voluntary," as required by these definitions of BCI systems. Similarly, the activity ultimately used by any BCI system may not precisely fit one such category. A user who is aware of a passive BCI system might be influenced by the expectations they have of that system and voluntarily commit attentional resources to make sure that the "spontaneous" activity takes place. A user might also attempt to consciously modulate this activity if results are not as expected. The other way around, an active BCI might rely on, or inadvertently make use of, brain activity that is not fully voluntarily controlled by the user. Meditation, as an example, seems to present an ambiguous mixture of both: it is the voluntary attempt to induce a state that is usually only achieved when contextual factors align.

The active/reactive/passive distinction used here is a user-oriented one and focuses on conscious intentions. In meditation, the intended purpose of the activity is relaxation itself, not the communication of a state of relaxation for further processing. As a thought experiment, we could ask whether the same user behavior and brain activity would be observed if the user was not aware of their influence over a system. If the answer is "yes," then we may say that this behavior and brain activity represent "natural" human activity. The implicit input gathered from it is then dissociated from its function as input. This is taken as a core property of the technology discussed in this chapter: the underlying brain activity arises from natural human activity that is not purposefully modulated to cater to the BCI system. Note, however, that by this measure, the categorization of a BCI system as (re)active or passive ultimately depends on the individual user and not on the system itself.

Indeed, the example of meditation can in fact also be used for an active BCI—when a state of relaxation is induced with the conscious intention of influencing a BCI system—or for a reactive BCI, when, in addition, external stimuli are used to cue or achieve that state.

In the last decade, the passive BCI approach (i.e., using natural human brain activity as implicit input) has led to research into a range of different directions. Because of the general applicability of this approach to a wide variety of applications, a truly comprehensive overview is beyond the scope, and not the intention, of this chapter. Instead, we would like to discuss a trend that can be observed in recent work and thought related to passive BCI: a trend toward increased interactivity between the human user and the machine.

"Interactivity" denotes "the ability of a computer to respond to a user's input" (*Oxford English Dictionary*, Oxford University Press 2016). In the following sections, we will describe four categories of systems that all take a neurophysiological signal as their input, but respond to it with varying degrees of complexity. Each presented category represents an increase in interactivity compared to the previous one. Selected examples from past and current research are given to illustrate the different categories. A (partially) hypothetical example accompanies us throughout the chapter, suggesting how a surgeon in the operating theater might be helped by a system from each category. In sequence, the given examples thus illustrate the abovementioned trend toward increased interactivity. The chapter ends with a brief speculation of the future and a summarizing conclusion.

## 3.2 MENTAL STATE ASSESSMENT

### 3.2.1 INTRODUCTION

BCI systems in general, by one definition, consist of three components: input, output, and a translation algorithm that produces the latter based on the former (Wolpaw et al. 2000). In this definition, input focuses on the measurement of particular aspects of brain activity, which reflect or correlate to a specific mental state. The detection of such a mental state (inferred from the measured activity) is then translated into a specific computer action (output), for example, the movement of a prosthetic arm or the selection of a letter on a screen.

Passive BCIs are distinct with respect to the exact cause of the mental state that is measured, requiring it to arise automatically as the result of a natural perception, activity, or thought, without the conscious intention of influencing the BCI system (see the discussion in Section 3.1). Emotions, for example, are not usually induced voluntarily but experienced as the result of something we perceive, do, or think. Other examples include stress, workload, vigilance, arousal, and surprise.

The measurement of such mental states can be helpful and informative by itself, however, without any computer actions being initiated. Translation, in this case, merely quantifies the measurements but causes no further system changes that are reported back to the human who is being measured. A subset of traditional BCI methodology can thus be used to obtain information concerning a variety of mental states, that is, for *mental state assessment* (Müller et al. 2008; van Erp et al. 2012; Zander & Kothe 2011). The resulting state information can then be analyzed and studied further. The user is assumed to be behaving naturally, as discussed in Section 3.1.

To perform such an analysis, that is, to calibrate such a "state detector" or *classifier*, individual calibration data are usually gathered in experimental environments where an operator's mental state can be carefully controlled and induced. Signal processing, feature extraction, and classifier calibration are then performed as per the general BCI approach, in order to later be able to assess, from a new recording in a different environment, to what extent the operator's state reflected the experimentally induced one(s). If, for example, a state of engagement can reliably be induced experimentally and neurophysiological correlates of that state can robustly be detected in those recordings, then an index can be generated that quantifies, for other recordings, to what extent these engagement-related features were present. This quantification can be done for complete recordings at once, but also moment by moment, identifying, for example, at what times during the recording the features were most or least pronounced.

In brief, mental state assessment takes a recording of neurophysiological activity and interprets it by producing a quantitative measure of a given mental state.

To give a hypothetical example of how this could be used, imagine a surgeon is presented with three different designs for a new teleoperated surgical robot. The goal is to evaluate which of these designs will be most efficient under working conditions. The surgeon performs the same operation using all three designs, while her brain activity is registered. Features of this brain activity are later compared to different recordings of her brain activity, collected during carefully controlled sessions of high and low workload. Based on the gathered data, it can be determined which of the three designs evoked the least workload-correlated brain activity. Furthermore, it may even be seen what phases of the operation saw local increases or decreases in such activity.

### 3.2.2 EXAMPLES FROM THE LITERATURE

Mental state monitoring can be particularly useful where more traditional methods have clear disadvantages. In *neuroergonomics*, "the study of brain and behavior at work" (Parasuraman 2003), the use of BCI-based methods in order to assess an operator's workload levels may replace traditional ergonomics methods where the operator would need to be interrupted for data collection, for example, to fill out a workload-measuring questionnaire. Workload has been widely recognized as a fundamental issue in ergonomics (Wickens et al. 2014), but a clash of definitions and constructs and intersubjective differences prevent a uniform and objective measurement (Young et al. 2015). BCI methodology may here be able to deliver a data-driven approach that circumvents (or complements) conceptual definitions and focuses directly on the neurophysiological correlates of those conditions that are to be measured. In case of workload, a consistent finding reflects a frontal–parietal theta–alpha asymmetry in EEG activity, representing the interaction of the dorsolateral prefrontal cortex and the intraparietal sulcus, which are also described as anterior and posterior attentional systems in controlled attention tasks (Gerjets et al. 2014).

For example, Gevins and Smith (2003) used the Multi-Attribute Task Battery (Comstock & Arnegard 1992) to simulate controlled working conditions of three different load levels and found reliable differences in frontal theta and parietal alpha band power in the continuous EEG recordings. On this basis, they constructed a cognitive workload index that could then be used to analyze later recordings. It performed in line with their hypothesis on other traditional experimental workload tasks as well as during more natural HCI tasks.

Using such precalibrated indices, mental state assessment can be used to, for example, A/B test and compare alternative user interface designs or task conditions with respect to the cognitive states they induce. Frey et al. (2014) review how a number of other constructs (attention/vigilance/fatigue, error recognition, emotions, engagement/flow/immersion) can be used to evaluate user experience during HCI tasks.

Care should be taken that the recorded reference data are ecologically valid and exhibit the neurophysiological features that specifically correlate with the mental state of interest and not with other aspects of the recording's context. For example, Mühl et al. (2014) recorded both high and low workload reference data in different affective contexts and showed that cross-context training improved the classifier's robustness. See also Section 3.4.2 for another approach to make the reference data robust to unrelated influences through a careful selection of reference tasks. Gerjets et al. (2014) and Brouwer et al. (2015) present an extended discussion of pitfalls and lessons learned in mental state assessment research.

Rather than recording reference data indicating extreme ends of the spectrum (e.g., underload vs. overload conditions), reference data can also be used as a baseline indicating optimal conditions (e.g., balanced workload). Zander and Jatzev (2012) used a measure of *deviation from the baseline* as undirected measure of suboptimal performance. Such a detected divergence can then be analyzed more closely to find out the underlying factors. In their paradigm, a goal-oriented, gamified HCI task, the Kullback–Leibler divergence of recorded features, increased compared to a baseline measurement in phases where participants felt they had lost control over the interaction. This *loss of control* could perhaps constitute a mixture of workload (compensatory actions) and emotional states (frustration), contributing to the measured neurophysiological differences.

Aside from continuous, frequency-based measurements, features can also be extracted in the time domain of EEG recordings, looking at event-related potentials (ERPs).

Evoked responses to presented stimuli are said to reflect neuronal processing of those stimuli, and the ERPs' morphology may be modulated by affective and cognitive processes (Luck 2014). For example, an alternative workload measurement method is to pose an oddball paradigm as a secondary task (e.g., to count the number of relatively rare high-pitch tones among a monotonous sequence of low-pitch tones), but instruct participants to focus attention primarily on another, primary task. The more cognitive load is demanded by the primary task, the less attention can be invested in the secondary task. This decreased attention is then reflected in an amplitude decrease of the P300 component in the ERP following target stimuli in the oddball task (Kok 2001).

Frey et al. (2016) used both a continuous EEG-based measure of workload, calibrated using an experimentally controlled variant of the *n*-back task (Kirchner 1958), and a secondary oddball task to measure attention. They found that both measures differ significantly across difficulty levels in a 3D wayfinding game, albeit with different sensitivities.

ERP components may also reflect differences in higher-level cognitive processing. This assumption is the basis of ERP-based *guilty knowledge tests*, where the goal of the experiment is to find out whether or not the participant possesses any information that they wish to conceal. As such, guilty knowledge tests are a type of lie detector. Participants are shown a series of stimuli, some related to the concealed information (e.g., the used weapon in a crime), others neutral (other weapons, random objects). Should the participant exhibit deviating responses to the related stimuli compared to the neutral ones, then this could be taken as a clue that the participant does possess some information concerning the case in question. Based on differences in their ERPs, Farwell and Donchin (1991) devised a system that could accurately determine for 87.5% of participants whether or not they had information concerning mock espionage scenarios that the participants were exposed to as part of the experiment. Ongoing developments in BCI and machine learning algorithms continue to be applied to improve performance in this field (e.g., Abootalebi et al. 2009).

Similar to workload, measures of a product or service's quality, attractiveness, or potential value to the user are traditionally gauged using questionnaires or interviews, and there is difficulty with respect to conceptual definitions and objective values. In order to elucidate consumer decisions, marketing researchers have turned to neuroscientific and BCI-based methodology to investigate human consumption from a neurophysiological perspective—*neuromarketing* (Lee et al. 2007). For example, Knutson et al. (2007) investigated neural correlates of two often opposing forces in purchase decisions: a product's attractiveness and its price. In a functional magnetic resonance imaging study, they found discriminative activity in separate cortical areas for these two product attributes. Based on features extracted from the nucleus accumbens and the mesial prefrontal cortex, they were subsequently able to develop an index predicting purchase behavior as exhibited by participants during the experiment.

### 3.2.3 REFLECTION

The examples of mental state assessment given here all use an initial recording of brain activity as their basis and then apply signal processing and classification or other predictive techniques in order to obtain a continuous quantification reflecting mental states or changes in mental state. By using brain activity, these approaches exhibit a number of relevant differences compared to other methods that attempt to do the same thing (e.g., questionnaires, interviews, introspection, thinking aloud). Brain activity provides a continuous, potentially unobtrusive source of data, and its recording does not interfere with the state to be measured. It enables a functional, data-driven approach to individual, subject-specific state assessment. This can provide a possible alternative to sometimes competing and contradictory theory-driven approaches. It does, however, require special care to interpret the resulting data and validate the measures taken: in data-driven approaches, correlations that are not neurophysiologically plausible may be found—for example, co-varying neural responses to confounding variables may show up in cortical areas unrelated to the state of interest, or models may be overfitted on the available data (e.g., Babyak 2004; Haufe et al. 2014). Another reason to use neurophysiological measurements may be when the information of interest cannot be obtained otherwise, for example, when a continuous recording and quantification is required, or when the human's own indications may be biased.

Mental state monitoring is an essential element in (passive) BCI systems but does not constitute such a system in and of itself. As per the abovementioned definition of BCI systems, the third component—output—is missing: the measurement does not trigger any actions, nor does it influence any system, beyond the measurement itself. Rather, the measurement itself is the goal of the use of the technology, as an additional instrument, to be used for later post hoc analysis.

Section 3.3 will present examples of passive BCI systems that translate the measurements into system actions in real time. These actions simultaneously provide feedback to the participants, adding a first element of interactivity to the system. We will also see that this feedback has inherent advantages for the validation of the measured user state.

## 3.3 OPEN-LOOP ADAPTATION

### 3.3.1 INTRODUCTION

HCI describes the interaction between one or more human users and a technical system (Preece et al. 2015). In a typical interaction cycle, an operator (user) gives a command to a machine, which processes the command and gives corresponding feedback to the operator. "Feedback" here denotes information about an action returned to the initial causing source of the action—that is, a response from the computer back to the user. This can be either the effect of the action itself or a separate informative signal.

Even modern-day interaction techniques, for example, touch screens and virtual reality controls, in essence still rely on the same principles as traditional techniques: in order to provide input to the computer, users explicitly activate one element after another, in accordance with the computer's logic (keyboard presses, mouse clicks, virtual buttons, menus, sliders, etc.). "Explicit" here reflects that the action was voluntarily executed with the conscious and sole intention of providing input to the computer.

Passive BCI can provide a fundamentally different, *implicit* input channel. "Implicit" here is the antonym to explicit and indicates that the input in question was generated without the source's voluntary intention of doing (merely) that (Rötting et al. 2009; Schmidt 2000; Zander et al. 2016). Passive BCI can be embedded into the HCI cycle by taking mental state assessments as implicit input, processing this input accordingly, and providing corresponding feedback to the user. This feedback creates interactivity with respect to the BCI: the computer now has the ability to respond to the user's implicit input.

In the simplest case, one interaction cycle (input–processing–feedback) can be viewed in isolation, following a simple one-time stimulus–response logic. Whenever a specific input is given to the machine, it performs one and the same action. The action serves only to comply with the input as it was given. This is referred to as open-loop adaptation.

Systems from this first category of adaptive applications apply mental state assessment to obtain a measure of a mental state online and respond to certain states with specific preprogrammed actions in an open-loop fashion.

For our surgeon, the online detection of high phases of workload could, for example, automatically trigger the system to switch on an indicator light. This communicates to the other members of the surgical team that the surgeon is not to be disturbed with lower-priority interruptions (Zander et al. 2017b).

### 3.3.2 EXAMPLES FROM THE LITERATURE

One mental state that has received particular attention in the context of general HCI is the *perception of errors*. Partially due to the artificial and limited nature of traditional interaction techniques (Suchman 1987; Tufte 1990), mistakes are made during ongoing HCI, resulting in frustration, loss of productivity, or, in safety-critical environments, potentially worse (Reason 1990). Upon perceiving the feedback indicating the error, or even already upon executing the erroneous action itself, the human user recognizes that a mistake has been made. Such conscious error perception elicits a much-researched neuroelectric response known as the error-related negativity (ERN; Gehring et al. 2012). If a system could detect such a negativity in its human user, and link it to a specific action or feedback signal, it could automatically undo the apparently perceived to be erroneous action or even learn to prevent it in the future.

For example, Parra et al. (2003) report a 21.4% average reduction (albeit ranging from −6 to +49%) in errors made by the combined human–machine system on a speeded reaction task, which is the traditional experimental task to elicit response errors. Here, a passive BCI system calibrated to detect an ERN after each human response informed a decision to override the human input.

Note that, as the −6% figure for one participant indicates, this can lead to an increase in errors when the passive BCI itself makes mistakes.

Testing to what extent these findings would apply to more realistic HCI control scenarios, Iturrate et al. (2012) found similar detectable responses to errors in a series of three experiments that represent essentially a similar task but with different degrees of realism: abstract cursor control, simulated robot control, and actual robot control. Error-related responses have also been found in different HCI contexts and modalities, for example, based on auditory (Zander et al. 2011a) and tactile (Lehne et al. 2009) feedback.

Being reliable in various, realistic contexts, such responses can be used to undo or otherwise correct for errors during HCI, as, for example, Zander et al. (2010) demonstrated using passive BCI error correction support in a gaming context.

ERN detection has also been used by Kreilinger et al. (2012) to inform the continuous motion of a prosthetic arm. Blinking light-emitting diodes (LEDs) would inform the user whether the arm would continue or stop moving within the upcoming second. When a LED indicating continued movement elicited an error response in the user, this could be interpreted as a passive input command to stop moving, and vice versa.

The use of another type of cognitive state was proposed by Protzak et al. (2013) and further investigated by Shishkin et al. (2016) to support gaze-based HCI. In gaze-based HCI, an eye tracker is used to follow the user's gaze, which can thus be used to control, for example, a pointer on a screen. To select or activate an item, often a *dwell time* is used: if the cursor remains for a certain amount of time on one and the same item (i.e., if the user looks at it for that long), it is activated. This can lead to a high number of false activations, as not all gazes are intended for interaction. Both Protzak et al. (2013) and Shishkin et al. (2016) compared brain activity following gaze fixations on an item under two conditions: one where interaction was intended (gaze-based control was enabled), and one where it was not (gaze-based control was disabled). They found significant amplitude differences in the ERP following control versus no-control fixations. Shishkin et al. applied a classifier trained on these differences online, in a gaze-controlled selection task. Although their classification system achieved insufficient sensitivity values to fully replace the "click" of a mouse, this may one day be possible. A computer that can reliably detect its user's intentions in such a way could greatly reduce the amount of explicit commands required from the user.

BCI has also been used in gaming environments to effect changes in the ongoing interaction. For example, van de Laar et al. (2013) incorporated BCI into an online role-playing game. Depending on parietal alpha band power, assumed to reflect the player's state of relaxation versus tension, the character they controlled would shape-shift into either an elf (relaxation) or a bear (tension). These character forms had different functional abilities, thus affecting the user's strategy in the game. Note that, in the cited case, this was a form of *active* BCI, because the experimenters explicitly instructed the participants to control their state of mind in order to consciously shift between shapes. However, since the chosen features (parietal alpha) do naturally correlate to relaxation, this could also be an exemplary implementation of open-loop adaptation based on passive BCI. This highlights the issue discussed in Section 3.1: whether or not a system is active or passive does not depend on the implementation itself but ultimately on the user's behavior. For similar examples, see Ilstedt Hjelm and Browall (2000), Ilstedt Hjelm (2003), and Zander and Krol (2017).

### 3.3.3 REFLECTION

Open-loop adaptive systems use a measurement of the user's state as implicit input in parallel to an ongoing (inter)action. These can be transient states such as error perception or interaction intent, which should then be carefully tied to the context that evoked them, or more constant states such as moods or other psychophysical conditions, which will then also have a more constant effect on the interaction. As such, we see that the latter is used to implicitly control an application's mode, whereas the former is used to provide more timely implicit executive commands. The use of passive

BCI methodology in these interactive systems either supports the user by replacing commands that otherwise needed to be provided explicitly or provides an extra dimension of experience to the interaction that would not have been possible using traditional input modalities.

An analysis of the effects of the BCI on the interaction can also serve as a validation of the system. For example, a quantification of *errors compensated* or *correct selections* provides a clear measure of the efficacy of the system. As mentioned in Section 3.2.3, though, care should still be taken that the implicit input underlying any performance improvement is neurophysiologically plausible.

The examples mentioned here use passive BCI for implicit human-to-computer communication. The implicit input is processed immediately, corresponding actions are performed, and the feedback given to the users completes the interaction cycle. This, however, is also the full extent of the interactivity at this point: the effects do not reach beyond the current interaction cycle, as there is no closed control loop influencing the next cycle. Both the executive and mode switching actions represent open-loop control, where single, independent state detections result in single, fixed actions from the computer. More interactive applications exhibit closed-loop control, where the given feedback also influences the user, as we shall see next.

## 3.4 CLOSED-LOOP ADAPTATION

### 3.4.1 INTRODUCTION

In closed-loop systems, output is fed back to the system as new input. In other words, the generated output influences the next cycle. In case of an elementary human–machine system based on passive BCI, the ultimate source of input is the human user's mental state. One method to implement a closed loop is thus to have the produced feedback cause a change in the user state. By influencing the mental state that is measured, the system influences its own next input.

One motivation for such an implementation may be to promote and sustain a desirable psychological state; for example, an optimally supporting balance of factors, or a state of *flow* (Csikszentmihalyi 2008). The adaptive loop may, for example, be programmed to promote a state of positive engagement in order to improve performance. This type of system could modify the demands of the task to maximize the user's motivation and enjoyment. When there is a clearly defined and unambiguously operationalized psychological state that is desirable, then the system can use its adaptive logic and feedback to manipulate the state of the user until the desired target state is reached.

This increases the interactivity of the system in the sense that it is now able to respond purposefully, as well as able to monitor the effect of each response. The given response attempts to qualitatively influence the condition of the ongoing interaction.

Thus, closed-loop adaptive systems apply mental state assessment to obtain a measure of a mental state online and respond to certain states—or changes in states—with actions that influence that same mental state.

We can again turn to our earlier example of workload in the operating theater to illustrate this category of applications. When a system detects that the surgeon is currently under high load, it can attempt to directly compensate for this by assuming certain tasks on behalf of the surgeon. By relieving the surgeon from some of her tasks, the system purposefully attempts to lower her load. We will see a similar example from the literature in more detail, described next.

### 3.4.2 EXAMPLES FROM THE LITERATURE

As mentioned in Section 3.2.2, a measure of workload is important in ergonomics research in order to inform design decisions. An adaptive system, however, could contain a range of options that would otherwise be decided upon by the designers and switch between them during online operation depending on current measures of workload. One such option range is the level of automation:

a machine can be operated entirely by explicit commands from the operator, or support the human operator to various degrees, up to assuming full autonomy and leaving the user in a mere supervisory role (see Parasuraman et al. 2000 for an overview and framework describing these options). The purpose of automation is to reduce operator mental workload and alleviate fatigue during sustained performance; however, use of automation is associated with negative consequences such as the out-of-the-loop problems and decay of skilled performance (Endsley & Kiris 1995). Striking the right balance is important to the well-being and performance of the operator, but the appropriate level of automation varies with fluctuating operator capacities and varying task demands. Therefore, *adaptive automation* (Byrne & Parasuraman 1996) attempts to match the level of allocation to the current capacity of the operator, measured in real time.

Kohlmorgen et al. (2007), for example, performed EEG measurements during highway driving. Aside from controlling the vehicle, two additional tasks were given to the participants that mimic human–car interaction (an auditory response task) as well as contextual distractors during driving (a mental calculation task and a listening comprehension task). All these together defined high-workload phases, which were compared to low-workload phases, where no contextual distractors were present. A classifier calibrated to distinguish these phases was later applied in an online driving condition such that high workload detection resulted in the automatic temporary suspension of the auditory response task. The mean performance on this response task significantly improved because of this intervention.

Similar adaptive logic can be applied to intelligent tutoring systems designed to deliver educational material in a way that sustains the engagement of the student. For example, the pacing of the learning process can be adjusted dynamically in order to sustain motivation without inducing fatigue, frustration, or information overload. In particular, working memory load is said to need careful management for an optimal learning experience (Cowan 2014).

Gerjets et al. (2014) review theory and practice with respect to online working memory assessment and present two studies in the context of adaptive learning environments. Special care was taken to select experimentally controllable calibration tasks. A combination of two tasks was used, as these tasks both targeted the same cognitive resources that were to be measured during realistic learning exercises, while at the same time these tasks differed with respect to their demand on executive resources. As such, Gerjets et al. attempted to develop a classifier that could detect working memory load independent of other task properties. Using this classifier, a classification accuracy of 73% was achieved on single trials of word algebra tasks. Their aim is to apply this classifier in an online adaptive environment, catering to current cognitive abilities of the student.

Such an online application has been presented by Yuksel et al. (2016): they used functional near-infrared spectroscopy (fNIRS) first to differentiate between participants' brain activity playing easy and hard piano pieces and then to detect their cognitive workload online during the learning of a new piece. The adaptive tutor first presented only one line of musical notes and added the next line only when workload levels indicated that the previous step had been learned to a sufficient degree. Yuksel et al. report significant increases in performance and learning speed using the fNIRS-based adaptive system as compared to self-paced learning.

Ewing et al. (2016) applied the concept of closed-loop adaptation to a game, Tetris, adjusting the game's speed in order to maintain a level of optimal engagement. They implemented different adaptive behaviors (i.e., more or less responsive), but found little difference between them. They discuss the issue of finding an appropriate benchmark: taking a manual condition as control, as they did, may provide an inherent difference in user experience that is not related to the exact behavior of the closed-loop adaptive system. A better control may be to compare this adaptive system to alternative methods of adaptation, for example, preprogrammed, random, or "yoked" (responding to the user state of another individual). Similar to the earlier distinction between mode switches and executive commands, the examples given above aim to achieve a constant, optimal state in the user, but adaptive systems can also effectuate short-lived closed feedback loops in order to achieve a one-time cognitive state.

Kirchner et al. (2013) suggest closed-loop implicit control of an alarm system, making use of BCI methodology to assess whether or not the alarm has been perceived and/or the user intends to act on it. Based on this information, the system could then decide to re-sound the alarm with increased saliency until it has been perceived. A state of nonperception would thus trigger new feedback until a state of perception would be observed. Kirchner et al. report accurate classification rates of perceived versus missed alarms during a demanding robotic teleoperation scenario. In another study, they used these as measures of current load, reversing this logic: nonperception of new instructions indicated that the user was occupied with previous instructions. The new instructions were then delayed to avoid distractions and promote adequate levels of engagement and performance (Kirchner et al. 2016).

### 3.4.3 REFLECTION

Direct access to a quantification of a certain mental state enables systems to monitor and, with appropriate feedback, influence this state also in a closed loop. This approach can be used to promote and sustain desirable mental states or indeed to mitigate an undesired state. The goal of this closed-loop control can be to achieve a certain equilibrium with respect to the state of interest or to push for a given threshold. In the former case, the system's potential influence may need to be bidirectional, allowing for both changes that encourage and changes that alleviate the target state.

When considering what is a closed-loop system and what is not, special attention must be given to the exact state that is targeted, which may be related to but different from the state that is measured. For example, error perception, as a transient state in the form of an error-related potential that lasts for less than a second, cannot necessarily be used as such to define a closed-loop system. This would be different, however, if this transient mental state can be interpreted in the given context as, for example, being indicative of a more persistent state of general dissatisfaction.

A closed feedback loop represents increased interactivity because the feedback in this case does not merely function as an informative response to the user, but in fact *purposefully acts upon* the user. The feedback intends to influence the user, as the user's commands intend to influence the system. Where in our earlier examples we saw implicit human-to-computer communication, now we could speak of an *implicit dialogue* between both agents, cooperating more closely in order to achieve common goals.

This cooperation as exemplified here is still limited by the amount of information available to the system and the simplistic logic of the single loop—for example, the one-dimensional measure of workload can only have a one-dimensional adaptation of automation levels. A next step up would need to tackle the question how systems can achieve a more complex adaptive, cooperative behavior based on the limited information passive BCI methodology can obtain at any single time. One such method will be discussed next.

## 3.5 AUTOMATED ADAPTATION

### 3.5.1 INTRODUCTION

Analysis of ongoing brain activity can give insight into momentary mental states, but by itself, not into their likely causes or the appropriate responses. In the abovementioned adaptive systems, the context is controlled and specific enough to reasonably assume that, for example, workload is caused by task demands, and increased automation will lead to a reduction in measured load. The interactive functions, however, are limited to these specific conditions.

Human–human interaction, the benchmark for natural communication and cooperation, relies heavily on a shared understanding of the world, the situation, and the communication partner—a shared model of appropriate behavior and how things are (Fischer 2001). In this, however, HCI is heavily asymmetrical: the human user can potentially be appraised of all details concerning the state of the computer, but hardly any such information is available vice versa (Suchman 1987). For a computer to *understand* its user, it needs information and input that goes beyond the bare necessities for its operation. The applications discussed in this chapter so far provide such information, but use it for preprogrammed one-dimensional response logic—they do not "understand" the user, that is, they build no model of higher, more abstract aspects of the user's cognitive or affective behavior. A better-informed system has increased ability to respond appropriately to the user; even to act on the given, known information before any new input is received. This thus constitutes an additional increase in interactivity: now also the system, and not merely the human user, can autonomously decide to act.

In this final category of automated adaptive applications, the systems apply mental state assessment alongside other methods of information gathering and build a model to represent aspects of the user's cognitive or affective responses. It is this automatically generated model, finally, that serves as a basis for the system's own autonomous behavior and adaptations—not (merely) the system's current input.

Our surgeon's load may have been consistently detected to increase beyond sustainable levels after 1 h when using a specific teleoperated robot. Having learned this, a well-informed system could call for an additional assistant ahead of time.

### 3.5.2 Examples from the Literature

Zander et al. (2014) and Zander et al. (2016) used single-trial detections of error-related brain activity not to immediately correct perceived mistakes, but to learn, over time, what strategy the user followed to subjectively make the distinction between errors and non-errors. To that end, the system exhibited different behaviors and learned which behaviors evoked positive and which evoked negative responses. These responses were generated in the medial prefrontal cortex, associated with a fundamental source of human intelligence: predictive coding (Hawkins & Blakeslee 2007). It thus built a model of the user's higher-level preferences with respect to the presented behaviors. Already during this learning process, the system adapted to exhibit behavior most likely to be perceived positively.

Specifically, this approach was applied to two-dimensional cursor control. A cursor on a computer screen initially moved randomly. Movements in some directions led to positive responses, while movements in other directions evoked negative responses. Over time, the system learned the pattern behind these responses and, as such, learned where the user wanted the cursor to go. The system could thus steer the cursor toward the intended target.

Extending their earlier-mentioned experiments, Iturrate et al. (2015) demonstrated a similar principle using a robotic arm. Participants observed its movements while their error responses were tracked in order to inform the arm of appropriate and inappropriate movements.

### 3.5.3 Reflection

In the two examples given in this section, rather than either having direct consequences or not, mental state measurements were stored along with a description of the contexts (here: computer actions) during which they were observed. As such, a model that correlated user states with different contexts was created.

These examples were again limited to their respective environments, but the principle can be envisioned to apply in a broader sense. With a reliable measure of, for example, satisfaction versus dissatisfaction (as, e.g., in Zander et al. 2016), as well as an accurate recording of relevant context variables (Zander & Jatzev 2012), a hypothetical ubiquitous passive BCI system could generate such a model for a large number of aspects in a user's daily and working life. By collating contextual factors with measures of the user's mental state, the computer learns to understand this user in much the same way as we humans learn from our own experiences. Subsequently, given a known context, the ubiquitous computer could execute that action that has been observed to be most likely to satisfy the user in that context.

Although the ultimate goal of this hypothetical system would be the same as of the earlier-mentioned adaptive automation, that is, to promote and sustain a desirable state, the methods by which this can be achieved are not set: the parameters of adaptation are learned automatically by the system itself, on the basis of a continuously updated model of its user.

For a large part, it is the understanding (i.e., the models) that we have of our social and physical context that allows us humans to behave appropriately in various contexts. We have started to build these models as soon as we were born and continue to update them as long as we are capable. For this, we use all information available to us, not just the information that others have explicitly deemed relevant to us. By giving computers access to more information and giving them the freedom to build their own models of their users and the context, a form of artificial intelligence may be created that may finally be seen as an autonomous, interactive agent, just as we see ourselves.

In a far-reaching, hypothetical case of a learning, closed-loop, automatically adapting system, we could imagine a system providing what we want before we can act upon those desires ourselves. With this autonomously operating system originally having learned from our own subjective responses to various actions and contexts, it may at some point become unclear who was the ultimate initiator of the action, by whose authority the action was executed, or who, in fact, "acted." As the lines separating the two interactive agents, human and machine, become blurred, merely the interaction itself remains.

Given also ethical deliberations with respect to, for example, data ownership, informed consent, the potentially harmful influence of machine over man (the same technique could be used to promote an undesired state, resulting in the computer actively working *against* the user), and outcome responsibility, it is prudent to aim to strike a balance between the two agents' influence on each other. Users should always have access to full information concerning the system's models, processes, goals, and actions. Users should also have ultimate control over, and ownership of, data that are derived from their physiology (Fairclough 2014). From a cooperative perspective, the best balance may be one where both agents get to optimally use their strengths while their weaknesses are mitigated by the strengths of the other, while keeping these domains formally separate.

## 3.6 SUMMARY AND CONCLUSION

In this chapter we have discussed potential applications that build up on the ability to perform real-time analyses of neurophysiological data, first demonstrated as brain–computer interfacing by Jacques J. Vidal. In 1973, envisioning future progress, Vidal wrote that "mental decisions and reactions can be probed, in a dimension that both transcends and complements overt behavior" (Vidal 1973). This statement appears to accurately capture the motivation of passive BCI research today, in its various forms of applications. In this chapter, these were divided into four distinct categories, based on their level of interactivity.

One category of applications, mental state assessment, uses the quantification of state-specific brain activity as a measurement, for example, to replace or support other measurements (e.g., questionnaires, behavioral data). This approach can provide data unobtrusively, can be individually calibrated, and may be able to access information that would otherwise remain hidden. An example from this category is the generation of a workload index based on brain activity, in order to assess the amount of resources that different instruments demand from the surgeon operating them.

A second category of applications, open-loop adaptation, uses the obtained measurements to inform an open-loop adaptation of the software. Using online state assessment, these systems can respond in real time to the detection of certain states. Continuing the above example, a warning light could switch on in an operating theater when it is detected that the surgeon is currently experiencing high load.

In a further category of applications, closed-loop adaptation, the software adaptation is designed with the explicit purpose to also effect a user adaptation, creating a closed control loop. This provides the system with the ability to not merely detect but also act upon the detected mental states. To keep the surgeon's workload at a sustainable level, for example, certain systems and operations in the theater may be adaptively automated.

Finally, a category of applications was described where the control logic of the system exceeds predetermined single-loop control: automated adaptation. The system is given the autonomy to learn and adapt based on a larger amount of information, coupled with a measure of the user's mental state. This also grants the system the ability to act autonomously for, or on behalf of, the user. For the surgeon, an additional assistant may automatically be called as the system predicts workload levels that will exceed otherwise manageable levels.

The first category is neither BCI nor interactive but serves as a basis for the three following categories. Their interactivity shows in their different abilities to respond to the given input. Since effective passive BCI systems are unobtrusive and inconspicuous, these systems' responses may be similarly hidden. It is for this reason that we refer to *adaptation*, using this as a more generic term that includes traditional feedback (e.g., the movement of a prosthetic limb) but also other ways to process the given input (e.g., updating a user model) or act on the basis of previously learned information. When adaptation is ultimately based on neurophysiological measures, we refer to these systems collectively as *neuroadaptive* systems (Zander et al. 2016).

The different adaptive behaviors are not mutually exclusive. An automated adaptation system might, for example, predict what a user intends to do and execute that action in advance, but then, in an open-loop fashion, undo the action when it is detected that the prediction was in error.

The here-presented categorization emphasizes the observable path of passive BCI applications toward increased interactivity.

The investigation of truly interactive systems, in particular based on natural human brain activity, can only be properly researched and developed in natural, real-world interactive settings. The well-controlled experimental conditions will at some point no longer be sufficient to make significant progress. Luckily, easily applicable, comfortable electrodes with sufficient signal quality and stability are being developed and continue to be improved (e.g., Goverdovsky et al. 2016; Mullen et al. 2015; Zander et al. 2011b, 2017a). Increased interest from high-profile commercial ventures is currently providing an effective development infrastructure and budget, at least for specific business interests—but the field as a whole may benefit, since the underlying issues are the same. Finally, when classifiers can be constructed that are independent of the human users and applicable across contexts, their universal usability will provide easy access to mental state assessment, boosting its usage (e.g., Krol et al. 2016; Wei et al. 2015; Zander 2012). When these development reach maturity, real-world implementations of the adaptive systems discussed here may seriously and dramatically alter the many human–system interactions that dominate our everyday lives (McDowell et al. 2013).

This chapter described a trend toward increased interactivity in past and current passive BCI research and development. The history of HCI as a whole, too, can be seen in light of increased interactivity. In early computer systems, input commands were written beforehand and given to the system as complete programs. This either resulted in the successful processing of the program or, quite bluntly, it did not. It was only later that humans were given real-time control over the system, through, for example, immediate processing and interrupt options (Suchman 1987). This provided the first interactive human–computer experience, albeit with ultimate agency solely with the human user. A next step toward interactivity thus appeared to be to give agency also to the computer—allowing it to adapt itself and execute commands that the user did not explicitly ask for. Passive BCI systems, discussed here in their various forms, can provide a source of information to make this computer agency in line with the user's intentions. It can provide this next step in human–computer interactivity, and, as the categorization used here intends to show, may provide the ones after that as well, in the form of advanced neuroadaptive technology.

## ACKNOWLEDGMENTS

Part of this work was supported by the Deutsche Forschungsgemeinschaft (ZA 821/3-1). The authors thank Mahta Mousavi for her comments.

## REFERENCES

Abootalebi, V., Moradi, M. H., & Khalilzadeh, M. A. 2009. A new approach for EEG feature extraction in P300-based lie detection. *Computer Methods and Programs in Biomedicine, 94*(1), 48–57.

Babyak, M. A. 2004. What you see may not be what you get: A brief, nontechnical introduction to overfitting in regression-type models. *Psychosomatic Medicine, 66*(3), 411–421.

Birbaumer, N., Ghanayim, N., Hinterberger, T., Iversen, I., Kotchoubey, B., Kübler, A., ... Flor, H. 1999. A spelling device for the paralysed. *Nature, 398*(6725), 297–298.

Blankertz, B., Curio, G., & Müller, K.-R. 2002a. Classifying single trial EEG: Towards brain computer interfacing. In T. G. Dietterich, S. Becker, & Z. Ghahramani (Eds.), *Advances in Neural Information Processing Systems 14* (pp. 157–164). Cambridge, MA: MIT Press.

Blankertz, B., Schäfer, C., Dornhege, G., & Curio, G. 2002b. Single trial detection of EEG error potentials: A tool for increasing BCI transmission rates. In J. R. Dorronsoro (Ed.), *Artificial Neural Networks – ICANN 2002* (Vol. 2415, pp. 1137–1143). Berlin, Germany: Springer.

Brouwer, A.-M., & van Erp, J. 2010. A tactile P300 brain–computer interface. *Frontiers in Neuroscience, 4*, 19.

Brouwer, A.-M., Zander, T. O., van Erp, J. B. F., Korteling, J. E., & Bronkhorst, A. W. 2015. Using neurophysiological signals that reflect cognitive or affective state: Six recommendations to avoid common pitfalls. *Frontiers in Neuroscience, 9*, 136.

Byrne, E. A., & Parasuraman, R. 1996. Psychophysiology and adaptive automation. *Biological Psychology, 42*(3), 249–268.

Comstock, J. R. J., & Arnegard, R. J. 1992. *The Multi-Attribute Task Battery for Human Operator Workload and Strategic Behavior Research* (Tech. Rep.). Hampton, VA, United States: NASA Langley Research Center.

Cowan, N. 2014. Working memory underpins cognitive development, learning, and education. *Educational Psychology Review, 26*(2), 197–223.

Csikszentmihalyi, M. 2008. *Flow: The Psychology of Optimal Experience* (Modern Classics ed.). New York, USA: HarperCollins.

Cutrell, E., & Tan, D. 2008. BCI for passive input in HCI. In *Proceedings of the Brain–Computer Interfaces for HCI and Games Workshop at the SIGCHI Conference on Human Factors in Computing Systems (CHI).*

Endsley, M. R., & Kiris, E. O. 1995. The out-of-the-loop performance problem and level of control in automation. *Human Factors, 37*(2), 381–394.

Ewing, K. C., Fairclough, S. H., & Gilleade, K. 2016. Evaluation of an adaptive game that uses EEG measures validated during the design process as inputs to a biocybernetic loop. *Frontiers in Human Neuroscience, 10*, 223.

Fairclough, S. H. 2014. Physiological data must remain confidential. *Nature, 505*, 263.

Farwell, L. A., & Donchin, E. 1988. Talking off the top of your head: Toward a mental prosthesis utilizing event-related brain potentials. *Electroencephalography and Clinical Neurophysiology, 70*(6), 510–523.

Farwell, L. A., & Donchin, E. 1991. The truth will out: Interrogative polygraphy ("lie detection") with event-related brain potentials. *Psychophysiology, 28*(5), 531–547.

Ferrez, P. W., & Millán, J. d. R. 2005. You are wrong!—Automatic detection of interaction errors from brain waves. In *Proceedings of the 19th International Joint Conference on Artificial Intelligence* (pp. 1413–1418). San Francisco: Morgan Kaufmann.

Ferrez, P. W., & Millán, J. d. R. 2008. Error-related EEG potentials generated during simulated brain–computer interaction. *IEEE Transactions on Biomedical Engineering, 55*(3), 923–929.

Fischer, G. 2001. User modeling in human–computer interaction. *User Modeling and User-Adapted Interaction, 11*(1–2), 65–86.

Frey, J., Daniel, M., Castet, J., Hachet, M., & Lotte, F. 2016. Framework for electroencephalography-based evaluation of user experience. In *Proceedings of the 2016 CHI Conference on Human Factors in Computing Systems* (pp. 2283–2294). New York, USA: ACM.

Frey, J., Mühl, C., Lotte, F., & Hachet, M. 2014. Review of the use of electroencephalography as an evaluation method for human–computer interaction. In *Proceedings of the International Conference on Physiological Computing Systems* (pp. 214–223).

Furdea, A., Halder, S., Krusienski, D., Bross, D., Nijboer, F., Birbaumer, N., & Kübler, A. 2009. An auditory oddball (P300) spelling system for brain–computer interfaces. *Psychophysiology*, 46(3), 617–625.

Gehring, W. J., Liu, Y., Orr, J. M., & Carp, J. 2012. The error-related negativity (ERN/Ne). In S. J. Luck & E. S. Kappenman (Eds.), *Oxford Handbook of Event-Related Potential Components* (pp. 231–291). New York: Oxford University Press.

Gerjets, P., Walter, C., Rosenstiel, W., Bogdan, M., & Zander, T. O. 2014. Cognitive state monitoring and the design of adaptive instruction in digital environments: Lessons learned from cognitive workload assessment using a passive brain–computer interface approach. *Frontiers in Neuroscience*, 8, 385.

Gevins, A., & Smith, M. E. 2003. Neurophysiological measures of cognitive workload during human–computer interaction. *Theoretical Issues in Ergonomics Science*, 4(1–2), 113–131.

Goverdovsky, V., Looney, D., Kidmose, P., & Mandic, D. P. 2016. In-ear EEG from viscoelastic generic earpieces: Robust and unobtrusive 24/7 monitoring. *IEEE Sensors Journal*, 16(1), 271–277.

Haufe, S., Meinecke, F., Görgen, K., Dähne, S., Haynes, J.-D., Blankertz, B., & Bießmann, F. 2014. On the interpretation of weight vectors of linear models in multivariate neuroimaging. *NeuroImage*, 87(0), 96–110.

Hawkins, J., & Blakeslee, S. 2007. *On Intelligence*. London: Macmillan.

Ilstedt Hjelm, S. 2003. Research + design: The making of Brainball. *Interactions*, 10(1), 26–34.

Ilstedt Hjelm, S., & Browall, C. 2000. Brainball—Using brain activity for cool competition. In *Proceedings of the 1st Nordic Conference of Human–Computer Interaction (NordiCHI)*.

Iturrate, I., Chavarriaga, R., Montesano, L., Minguez, J., & Millán, J. d. R. 2012. Latency correction of error potentials between different experiments reduces calibration time for single-trial classification. In *2012 Annual International Conference of the IEEE Engineering in Medicine and Biology Society (EMBC)* (pp. 3288–3291).

Iturrate, I., Chavarriaga, R., Montesano, L., Minguez, J., & Millán, J. d. R. 2015. Teaching brain–machine interfaces as an alternative paradigm to neuroprosthetics control. *Scientific Reports*, 5, 13893.

Kirchner, E. A., Kim, S. K., Straube, S., Seeland, A., Whrle, H., Krell, M. M., ... Fahle, M. 2013. On the applicability of brain reading for predictive human–machine interfaces in robotics. *PLOS ONE*, 8(12), 1–19.

Kirchner, E. A., Kim, S. K., Tabie, M., Wöhrle, H., Maurus, M., & Kirchner, F. 2016. An intelligent man-machine interface—Multi-robot control adapted for task engagement based on single-trial detectability of P300. *Frontiers in Human Neuroscience*, 10, 291.

Kirchner, W. L. 1958. Age differences in short-term retention of rapidly changing information. *Journal of Experimental Psychology*, 55(4), 352–358.

Knutson, B., Rick, S., Wimmer, G. E., Prelec, D., & Loewenstein, G. 2007. Neural predictors of purchases. *Neuron*, 53(1), 147–156.

Kohlmorgen, J., Dornhege, G., Braun, M., Blankertz, B., Curio, G., Hagemann, K., ... Kincses, W. 2007. Improving human performance in a real operating environment through real-time mental workload detection. In G. Dornhege (Ed.), *Toward Brain–Computer Interfacing* (pp. 409–422). Cambridge, MA: MIT Press.

Kok, A. 2001. On the utility of p3 amplitude as a measure of processing capacity. *Psychophysiology*, 38(3), 557–577.

Kreilinger, A., Neuper, C., & Müller-Putz, G. R. 2012. Error potential detection during continuous movement of an artificial arm controlled by brain–computer interface. *Medical & Biological Engineering & Computing*, 50(3), 223–230.

Krol, L. R., Freytag, S.-C., Fleck, M., Gramann, K., & Zander, T. O. 2016. A task-independent workload classifier for neuroadaptive technology: Preliminary data. In *2016 IEEE International Conference on Systems, Man, and Cybernetics (SMC)* (pp. 003171–003174).

Lee, N., Broderick, A. J., & Chamberlain, L. 2007. What is 'neuromarketing'? A discussion and agenda for future research. *International Journal of Psychophysiology*, 63(2), 199–204.

Lehne, M., Ihme, K., Brouwer, A. M., van Erp, J. B. F., & Zander, T. O. 2009. Error-related EEG patterns during tactile human–machine interaction. In *2009 3rd International Conference on Affective Computing and Intelligent Interaction and Workshops* (pp. 1–9).

Lotte, F., Congedo, M., Lécuyer, A., Lamarche, F., & Arnaldi, B. 2007. A review of classification algorithms for EEG-based brain–computer interfaces. *Journal of Neural Engineering*, 4(2), 24.

Luck, S. J. 2014. *An Introduction to the Event-Related Potential Technique* (2nd ed.). Cambridge, MA: MIT Press.

McDowell, K., Lin, C.-T., Oie, K. S., Jung, T.-P., Gordon, S., Whitaker, K. W., ... Hairston, W. D. 2013. Real-world neuroimaging technologies. *IEEE Access, 1,* 131–149.

Mühl, C., Jeunet, C., & Lotte, F. 2014. EEG-based workload estimation across affective contexts. In A.-M. Brouwer, T. O. Zander, & J. B. F. van Erp (Eds.), *Using Neurophysiological Signals That Reflect Cognitive or Affective State* (pp. 227–241). Frontiers Media SA.

Mullen, T. R., Kothe, C. A. E., Chi, Y. M., Ojeda, A., Kerth, T., Makeig, S., ... Cauwenberghs, G. 2015. Real-time neuroimaging and cognitive monitoring using wearable dry EEG. *IEEE Transactions on Biomedical Engineering, 62*(11), 2553–2567.

Müller, K.-R., Tangermann, M., Dornhege, G., Krauledat, M., Curio, G., & Blankertz, B. 2008. Machine learning for real-time single-trial EEG-analysis: From brain–computer interfacing to mental state monitoring. *Journal of Neuroscience Methods, 167*(1), 82–90.

Müller-Putz, G. R., & Pfurtscheller, G. 2008. Control of an electrical prosthesis with an SSVEP-based BCI. *IEEE Transactions on Biomedical Engineering, 55*(1), 361–364.

Parasuraman, R. 2003. Neuroergonomics: Research and practice. *Theoretical Issues in Ergonomics Science, 4*(1–2), 5–20.

Parasuraman, R., Sheridan, T. B., & Wickens, C. D. 2000. A model for types and levels of human interaction with automation. *IEEE Transactions on Systems, Man, and Cybernetics—Part A: Systems and Humans, 30*(3), 286–297.

Parra, L. C., Spence, C. D., Gerson, A. D., & Sajda, P. 2003. Response error correction—A demonstration of improved human–machine performance using real-time EEG monitoring. *IEEE Transactions on Neural Systems and Rehabilitation Engineering, 11*(2), 173–177.

Pfurtscheller, G., & Neuper, C. 2001. Motor imagery and direct brain–computer communication. *Proceedings of the IEEE, 89*(7), 1123–1134.

Preece, J., Sharp, H., & Rogers, Y. 2015. *Interaction Design: Beyond Human–Computer Interaction* (4th ed.). Chichester, UK: Wiley.

Protzak, J., Ihme, K., & Zander, T. O. 2013. A passive brain–computer interface for supporting gaze-based human–machine interaction. In C. Stephanidis & M. Antona (Eds.), *Universal Access in Human–Computer Interaction. Design Methods, Tools, and Interaction Techniques for eInclusion* (Vol. 8009, pp. 662–671). Berlin Heidelberg, Germany: Springer.

Ramoser, H., Müller-Gerking, J., & Pfurtscheller, G. 2000. Optimal spatial filtering of single trial EEG during imagined hand movement. *IEEE Transactions on Rehabilitation Engineering, 8*(4), 441–446.

Reason, J. 1990. *Human Error.* Cambridge, UK: Cambridge University Press.

Rötting, M., Zander, T. O., Trösterer, S., & Dzaack, J. 2009. Implicit interaction in multimodal human–machine systems. In C. M. Schlick (Ed.), *Industrial Engineering and Ergonomics* (pp. 523–536). Berlin Heidelberg, Germany: Springer.

Schmidt, A. 2000. Implicit human computer interaction through context. *Personal and Ubiquitous Computing, 4*(2–3), 191–199.

Shishkin, S. L., Nuzhdin, Y. O., Svirin, E. P., Trofimov, A. G., Fedorova, A. A., Kozyrskiy, B. L., & Velichkovsky, B. M. 2016. EEG negativity in fixations used for gaze-based control: Toward converting intentions into actions with an eye-brain–computer interface. *Frontiers in Neuroscience, 10,* 528.

Soekadar, S. R., Witkowski, M., Gómez, C., Opisso, E., Medina, J., Cortese, M., ... Vitiello, N. 2016. Hybrid EEG/EOG-based brain/neural hand exoskeleton restores fully independent daily living activities after quadriplegia. *Science Robotics, 1*(1).

Suchman, L. A. 1987. *Plans and Situated Actions: The Problem of Human–Machine Communication.* Cambridge, UK: Cambridge University Press.

Treder, M. S., Schmidt, N. M., & Blankertz, B. 2011. Gaze-independent brain–computer interfaces based on covert attention and feature attention. *Journal of Neural Engineering, 8*(6), 066003.

Tufte, E. R. 1990. *Envisioning Information.* Cheshire, CT: Graphics Press.

van de Laar, B., Gürkök, H., Bos, D. P.-O., Poel, M., & Nijholt, A. 2013. Experiencing BCI control in a popular computer game. *IEEE Transactions on Computational Intelligence and AI in Games, 5*(2), 176–184.

van Erp, J. B., Lotte, F., & Tangermann, M. 2012. Brain–computer interfaces: Beyond medical applications. *Computer, 45*(4), 26–34.

Vidal, J. J. 1973. Toward direct brain–computer communication. *Annual Review of Biophysics and Bioengineering, 2*(1), 157–180.

Vidal, J. J. 1977. Real-time detection of brain events in EEG. *Proceedings of the IEEE, 65*(5), 633–641.

Wei, C. S., Lin, Y. P., Wang, Y. T., Jung, T. P., Bigdely Shamlo, N., & Lin, C. T. 2015. Selective transfer learning for EEG-based drowsiness detection. In *2015 IEEE International Conference on Systems, Man, and Cybernetics* (pp. 3229–3232).

Wessberg, J., Stambaugh, C. R., Kralik, J. D., Beck, P. D., Laubach, M., Chapin, J. K., ... Nicolelis, M. A. L. 2000. Real-time prediction of hand trajectory by ensembles of cortical neurons in primates. *Nature, 408*, 361–365.

Wickens, C. D., Hollands, J. G., Banbury, S., & Parasuraman, R. 2014. *Engineering Psychology and Human Performance* (4th ed.). New York: Routledge.

Wolpaw, J. R., Birbaumer, N., Heetderks, W. J., McFarland, D. J., Peckham, P. H., Schalk, G., ... Vaughan, T. M. 2000. Brain–computer interface technology: A review of the First International Meeting. *IEEE Transactions on Rehabilitation Engineering, 8*(2), 164–173.

Wolpaw, J. R., Birbaumer, N., McFarland, D. J., Pfurtscheller, G., & Vaughan, T. M. 2002. Brain–computer interfaces for communication and control. *Clinical Neurophysiology, 113*(6), 767–791.

Wolpaw, J. R., & McFarland, D. J. 2008. Brain–computer interface operation of robotic and prosthetic devices. *Computer, 41*, 52–56.

Wolpaw, J. R., & Wolpaw, E. W. 2012. Brain–computer interfaces: Something new under the sun. In *Brain–Computer Interfaces: Principles and Practice* (pp. 3–12). Oxford, UK: Oxford University Press.

Young, M. S., Brookhuis, K. A., Wickens, C. D., & Hancock, P. A. 2015. State of science: Mental workload in ergonomics. *Ergonomics, 58*(1), 1–17.

Yuksel, B. F., Oleson, K. B., Harrison, L., Peck, E. M., Afergan, D., Chang, R., & Jacob, R. J. K. 2016. Learn piano with BAch: An adaptive learning interface that adjusts task difficulty based on brain state. In *Proceedings of the 2016 CHI Conference on Human Factors in Computing Systems* (pp. 5372–5384). New York, USA: ACM.

Zander, T. O. 2012. *Utilizing Brain–Computer Interfaces for Human–Machine Systems* (Doctoral dissertation, Technische Universität Berlin, Berlin, Germany).

Zander, T. O., Andreessen, L. M., Berg, A., Bleuel, M., Pawlitzki, J., Zawallich, L., Krol, L. R., & Gramann, K. 2017a. Evaluation of a dry EEG system for application of passive brain–computer interfaces in autonomous driving. *Frontiers in Human Neuroscience, 11*, 78.

Zander, T. O., Brönstrup, J., Lorenz, R., & Krol, L. R. 2014. Towards BCI-based implicit control in human–computer interaction. In S. H. Fairclough & K. Gilleade (Eds.), *Advances in Physiological Computing* (pp. 67–90). Berlin, Germany: Springer.

Zander, T. O., & Jatzev, S. 2012. Context-aware brain–computer interfaces: Exploring the information space of user, technical system and environment. *Journal of Neural Engineering, 9*(1), 016003.

Zander, T. O., Klippel, M. D., & Scherer, R. 2011a. Towards multimodal error responses: A passive BCI for the detection of auditory errors. In *Proceedings of the 13th International Conference on Multimodal Interfaces* (pp. 53–56). New York, USA: ACM.

Zander, T. O., & Kothe, C. A. 2011. Towards passive brain–computer interfaces: Applying brain–computer interface technology to human–machine systems in general. *Journal of Neural Engineering, 8*(2), 025005.

Zander, T. O., Kothe, C. A., Jatzev, S., Dashuber, R., Welke, S., De Filippis, M., & Rötting, M. 2008a. Team PhyPA: Developing applications for brain–computer interaction. In *Proceedings of the Brain–Computer Interfaces for HCI and Games Workshop at the SIGCHI Conference on Human Factors in Computing Systems (CHI)*.

Zander, T. O., Kothe, C. A., Jatzev, S., & Gärtner, M. 2010. Enhancing human–computer interaction with input from active and passive brain–computer interfaces. In D. S. Tan & A. Nijholt (Eds.), *Brain–Computer Interfaces* (pp. 181–199). London: Springer.

Zander, T. O., Kothe, C. A., Welke, S., & Rötting, M. 2008b. Enhancing human–machine systems with secondary input from passive brain–computer interfaces. In *Proceedings of the 4th International Brain–Computer Interface Workshop & Training Course* (pp. 144–149). Graz, Austria: Verlag der Technischen Universität Graz.

Zander, T. O., & Krol, L. R. 2017. Team PhyPA: Brain–computer interfacing for everyday human–computer interaction. *Periodica Polytechnica Electrical Engineering and Computer Science, 61*(2), 209–216.

Zander, T. O., Krol, L. R., Birbaumer, N. P., & Gramann, K. 2016. Neuroadaptive technology enables implicit cursor control based on medial prefrontal cortex activity. *Proceedings of the National Academy of Sciences, 113*(52), 14898–14903.

Zander, T. O., Lehne, M., Ihme, K., Jatzev, S., Correia, J., Kothe, C. A., Nijboer, F. (2011b). A dry EEG-system for scientific research and brain–computer interfaces. *Frontiers in Neuroscience, 5*, 53.

Zander, T. O., Shetty, K., Lorenz, R., Leff, D. R., Krol, L. R., Darzi, A. W., ... Yang, G.-Z. 2017b. Automated task load detection with electroencephalography: Towards passive brain–computer interfacing in robotic surgery. *Journal of Medical Robotics Research, 2*(1), 1750003.

# Brain–Computer Interface Applications

## Section B. Therapeutic Applications

# 4 Brain–Computer Interfaces for Motor Rehabilitation, Assessment of Consciousness, and Communication

*Christoph Guger, Rossella Spataro, Jitka Annen,*
*Rupert Ortner, Danut Irimia, Brendan Allison, Vincenzo La Bella,*
*Woosang Cho, Günter Edlinger, and Steven Laureys*

## CONTENTS

4.1   Introduction ........................................................................................................... 89
4.2   Patients with DOC ................................................................................................ 90
4.3   Stroke Patients ...................................................................................................... 95
4.4   Conclusion ............................................................................................................ 97
References ....................................................................................................................... 98

**Abstract**

Brain–computer interface (BCI) technology has recently been extended to help patients with disorders of consciousness (DOC) and stroke. These two promising new directions focus on new patient groups and new applications for these groups. First, patients diagnosed with a DOC might benefit from new BCI-based systems that can help assess (or reassess) their consciousness, allow communication and even outcome prediction, and guide rehabilitation. Second, patients with motor disabilities resulting from stroke might use BCIs to facilitate rehabilitation to recover lost motor functions more quickly and completely than conventional therapy alone. Both of these directions have advanced well beyond the initial proof-of-concept stage, with dozens of publications from numerous different groups that validate methods and devices with patient groups in real-world settings. However, broader studies with patients are still needed. We briefly review these two new directions, describe the mindBEAGLE and recoveriX systems that are based on them, and present examples of results from real-world applications with patients.

## 4.1   INTRODUCTION

Early review articles focused on brain–computer interface (BCI) research correctly noted that the BCI research community was primarily focused on providing communication and control for patients who were unable to communicate through conventional means owing to severe motor disability. These target users included patients with late-stage amyotrophic lateral sclerosis and others with locked-in syndrome (LIS), meaning that they have little or no reliable voluntary muscle control (Wolpaw et al. 2002; Kübler et al. 2001). However, in the last few years, review and commentary articles have shown a different trend: helping new patient groups with BCI technology (Allison et al. 2013; Wolpaw & Wolpaw 2012; Brunner et al. 2015). Two of the most promising extensions aim to help persons with disorders of consciousness (DOC) and stroke.

## 4.2 PATIENTS WITH DOC

Patients with DOC include persons in a coma, vegetative state (also called unresponsive wakeful state or UWS), or minimally conscious state (MCS) (Giacino et al. 2012). Like patients with LIS, these patients do not have sufficient voluntary muscle control for communication, even with typical assistive technologies designed for people with limited movementt control. However, unlike LIS patients, patients diagnosed with DOC are also considered incapable of the cognitive activity necessary for communication. That is, the disorder of consciousness prevents them from understanding and remembering new information, developing new messages or commands, and executing the mental activity necessary to communicate. Thus, reassessment of their cognitive abilities, and especially the development of a communication system for these unique patients, is a major challenge.

However, the clinical observation at bedside results in diagnostic errors in up to 42% of patients, since awareness may coexist with insufficient motor control (Giacino et al. 2012). By collecting objective measures of awareness, a BCI system that does not require the patients to see may improve dramatically the diagnostic accuracy of the DOCs and, depending on the residual cognitive functioning, also enable these patients to communicate. The same approach can be used to assess awareness and allow communication for complete LIS (CLIS) patients, who are unable to communicate by any means, including visual-based BCIs (Marchetti & Priftis 2014; Guger et al. 2017). To meet the special requirements of DOCs and CLIS patients, nonconventional BCI modalities are needed, based on their residual capacity to understand instructions, perceive auditory and vibrotactile stimuli, and perform mental tasks, despite their visual impairment.

Some groups have shown that a minority of persons diagnosed with DOC are able to communicate using BCI technology (Brunner et al. 2015; Risetti et al. 2013; Schnakers et al. 2009; Lugo et al. 2014; Lulé et al. 2013). This indicates that, even if patients seem unconscious during behavioral assessment, these patients could show signs of consciousness during reassessments with a BCI.

Different approaches to consciousness assessment have been used. One of the challenges is that many patients suffer from visual deficits, and therefore conventional BCI approaches have to be adapted to be independent from visual stimuli. This means that patients must be able to understand task instructions, stimuli, and feedback even though they cannot see. To date, the auditory and tactile modalities have been employed.

Below, we introduce the mindBEAGLE system. This is a complete hardware and software platform for real-time biosignal analysis designed especially for DOC patients to assess the level of consciousness and provide communication (see Figure 4.1). It includes a laptop with preinstalled software, 16-channel EEG cap, amplifier, earbuds, and vibrotactile stimulators. All task instructions are presented auditorily in the user's native language, either through the earbuds or the experimenter's voice.

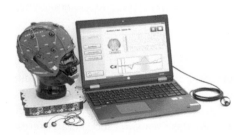 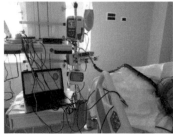

**FIGURE 4.1** Left: the mindBEAGLE system including a biosignal amplifier, computer, EEG cap, in-ear phones, and vibrotactile stimulator. Right: in usage with a patient.

This system can use four approaches for assessment:

The "Auditory Evoked Potential" or **AEP** approach is designed to elicit event-related potentials (ERPs) through auditory stimuli. mindBEAGLE uses two types of tones that are presented for 100 ms: rare target stimuli (1000 Hz) and more probable standard stimuli (500 Hz). Target tones, which are only one out of eight stimuli, are randomly interspersed among the standard tones. The user is instructed to silently count each target stimulus while ignoring other stimuli. Successful task performance will elicit an ERP with a P300 to target stimuli only.

Figure 4.2 shows an example of a UWS patient (P1) and an MCS patient (P2). The MCS patient shows a clear P300 response and an improving classification accuracy.

Figure 4.3 shows the AEPs and classification accuracy of a CLIS patient and the classification accuracy of a healthy control in sham condition. Of special interest is that the CLIS patient shows a strong ERP and perfect classification accuracy after five target tones. The accuracy looks like a healthy control person, while the EPs show a smaller amplitude and later peak compared to healthy controls. Additionally, the figure also shows the accuracy achieved with a healthy control in sham condition (in which tactors were not fixed to the arms).

The "Vibrotactile-2" or **VTP2** approach uses tactile stimuli instead of auditory stimuli, although instructions are still provided through earbuds. Vibrotactile stimulators are placed on each wrist, and the user is instructed to silently count each time the right wrist stimulator vibrates. Then, the two stimulators intermittently vibrate for 50 ms. Like the auditory paradigm, 1/8 of the stimuli are deviant stimuli (right wrist vibrations), and the stimuli are presented in random order. Thus, the VTP2 approach is also a classic oddball paradigm designed to elicit distinct ERP components that reflect the user's decision to silently count deviant stimuli.

Figure 4.4 shows the VTP2 responses and classification accuracies of P1 and of P2. There is a clear difference between the ERPs of the UWS and MCS patient. The MCS patient reached a median accuracy of 100%, while the UWS patient showed 0% accuracy.

The "Vibrotactile-3" or **VTP3** approach enables the patient to communicate in a binary fashion and differs from the VTP2 approach as follows. First, the system uses three vibrotactile

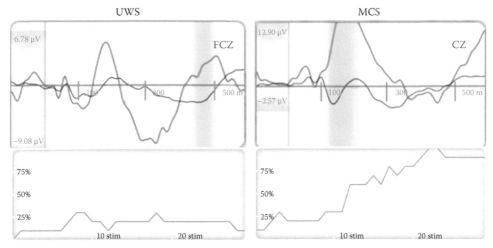

**FIGURE 4.2** Top: AEP with blue line indicating the nontargets and the green line indicating the targets. The green shaded area indicates a significant difference between targets and nontargets. The red line shows the stimulus onset. Bottom: Classification accuracy in percentage over the number of target tones. The bottom line indicates trials that were discarded from the analysis with red dots. UWS patient (P1): The AEP does not show a significant P300 response. The average accuracy of the plot is 20%, and 24 out of 480 trials contained artifacts and were rejected by the algorithm. MCS patient (P2): AEP with a clear difference between targets and nontargets. The peak amplitude of the targets reaches 12.9 μV on electrode Cz. The accuracy improves with the number of targets and reaches 100%. The average accuracy is 60% in a task with a chance accuracy of 12.5%.

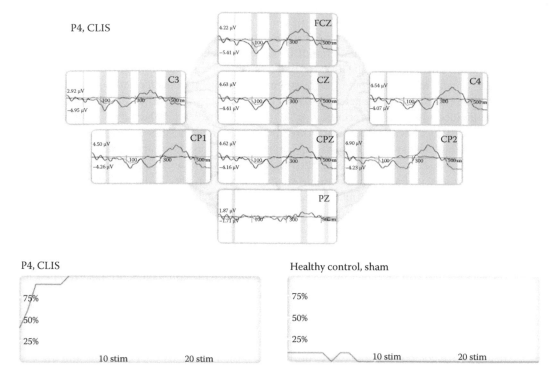

**FIGURE 4.3** Top: ERPs elicited during the AEP paradigm over eight sites. Bottom left: The accuracy for P4. Bottom right: The accuracy for a healthy control during a sham run.

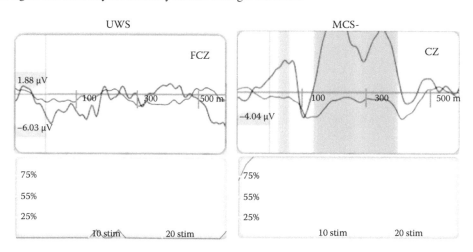

**FIGURE 4.4** Left panels: VTP2 response from an UWS patient (P1) with no significant difference between targets and nontargets. The average accuracy is 0%. Out of 480 trials, 14 contained artifacts and were excluded from analysis. Right panels: A high-amplitude P300 response with 100% classification accuracy is observed in an MCS patient. Three trials contained artifacts and were excluded from analysis.

stimulators, with the third "deviant" stimulus placed on the right ankle or chest. Second, the proportion of stimuli is different: in each sequence of eight stimuli, one is delivered to the right wrist, one is delivered to the left wrist, and six are delivered to the right ankle, in pseudorandom order. Third, the subject is instructed to silently count the stimuli to the left or right wrist, corresponding to the left or right cue. The deviant stimulus is never the target.

Last, the subject hears a cue before each sequence of pulses with the word "left" or "right." This VTP3 approach is a more complex variant of the oddball paradigm that can assess advanced cognitive function. Indeed, if the patient is performing well and above chance level during the training phase of the classifier, this paradigm can be used to test communication. The patient now does not get a cue instructing which hand is the target and instead needs to concentrate on the left hand to say yes and on the right hand to answer no.

Figure 4.5 shows the VTP3 results for a patient that seemed UWS on the behavioral level for two sessions. In the first session, no ERP was found and the average classification

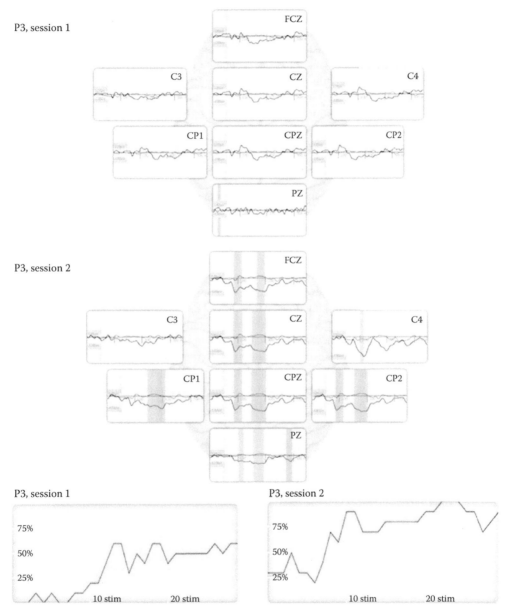

**FIGURE 4.5**    VT3 responses and classification accuracy of patient P3 for two different sessions. An improvement of the ERP and accuracy is observed from the first to the second session. Interestingly, the patient was not able to communicate during the first session, yet during the second session, the patient was able to communicate successfully. Here is an example during which the patient answered no, as shown by the higher P300 amplitude elicited by left hand stimuli.

accuracy was only 40%. The calculated classifier could not be used successfully to establish communication. In the second session, the patient was able to improve performance and a significant ERP was found, resulting in a classification accuracy of 80%. Then, the classifier was used to perform a communication run by asking yes/no questions. This patient could successfully answer 9 out of 10 questions. Figure 4.5 shows an example of a question where the known answer is NO (for which a higher-amplitude P300 is found over the left hand contralateral hemisphere) and another example for YES.

A communication run using the classifier from session 2 was employed as well (see Figure 4.6). During this session, the patient was able to answer 9 out of 10 questions correctly.

The "Motor Imagery" or **MI** approach, unlike the three preceding approaches, does not rely on the P300 and other ERPs. Instead, like most other MI BCIs, it relies on changes in EEG power in specific frequency bands that occur when a person imagines movements. These changes, called event-related (de-)synchronization or ERD/S, are typically present in the 8- to 13-Hz band over sensorimotor areas. Its specific characteristics may change in patients with brain injury. The user is instructed to imagine either left or right hand movement in response to cues that instruct "left" or "right" and a starting tone. Another cue, the word "relax," instructs the user to stop performing motor imagery. This cue occurs after eight seconds, providing eight seconds of motor imagery data.

These four assessment modes are designed to target assessment of command following and communication and to provide different approaches in case one approach is not effective. This leverages the concept of a "hybrid BCI" that can use different types of BCIs to provide the communication protocol that works best for each user (Pfurtscheller et al. 2010). If a user is successful with one or more assessment modes, then the four modes can also be used for communication. Indeed, since some DOC patients may fade in and out of command following, it seems best to switch to the communication mode as soon as the assessment reveals potential for communication. The AEP and VTP2 modes support a "quick test" of basic brain functions, while the VTP3 and MI modes support more in-depth communication options. However, mindBEAGLE can still only provide yes/no communication. We are therefore currently developing new hybrid BCI options to improve nonvisual communication.

The hybrid BCI approach may be especially important to improve the diagnostic accuracy in DOC patients, in which "BCI inefficiency" may be higher than typical patients. In a typical BCI, "BCI inefficiency" does not convey much useful information about the cognitive abilities of the user and the BCI's inability to discern relevant brain signals reflects a challenge for the system designer. However,

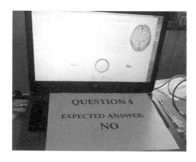 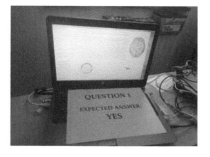

**FIGURE 4.6**    The setup to test whether the patient is able to communicate. The experimenter asks the patient question 4 (left panel) or question 1 (right panel) and then presses the communication button in mindBEAGLE. The patient begins to count the vibrotactile stimuli on the left hand (question 1) or right hand (question 4), eliciting a P300 response. Then, the classifier of the BCI system is able to identify to which stimuli the patient is attending and makes a final decision if the answer should be "yes" (right hand) or "no" (left hand). The picture on the right shows a correct answer.

if a DOC patient shows to be unable to follow commands in repetitive BCI sessions, the system might be working as expected, confirming that the patient is unaware and cannot communicate through any mechanism. Importantly, this is not the only conclusion that should result from these situations.

Two very recent developments merit attention here. First, a new publication (http://www.cnn.com/2017/06/15/politics/otto-warmbier-north-korea/index.html) showed that persons with CLIS can use BCI technology to communicate. This provides further hope for extending BCI technology to new patient groups, particularly those with the greatest need. Second, during June 2017, the popular media (such as http://www.cnn.com/2017/06/15/politics/otto-warmbier-north-korea/index.html) announced that an American student returned from North Korea with a DOC and that further details of the type of DOC were not clear. Sadly, the student died a few days after returning to the United States. If he had survived longer, might BCI technology have helped to further assess his condition, and perhaps enable him to provide information about how he was injured?

## 4.3 STROKE PATIENTS

While stroke can have many effects, we focus here on the impairment of motor function. These impairments can affect hand and arm function, speech, gait, and other motor abilities. Although stroke is very prevalent, and improved stroke treatment methods are potentially impactful and profitable, therapy outcomes remain poor. Most people who participate in therapy improve only modestly, at best.

In typical therapy, patients are asked to perform or imagine specific movements. They may receive assistance from an orthosis or functional electrical stimulator (FES) to help them complete the movements. These systems are active whenever the patient is told to perform the desired mental activity or imagery.

However, if patients are not performing the motor imagery when expected—throughout each and every trial—then the feedback they receive may often be uncorrelated with the required brain activity. Patients receive rewarding feedback when they should receive no feedback, or cues to perform the task differently. The expected pairing between brain activity and peripheral activity does not reliably occur, which violates foundational assumptions in feedback and the underlying principle of Hebbian learning (Neuper & Allison 2014). BCI technology could provide a new way to close the feedback loop by monitoring motor imagery (even if patients cannot actually move) and triggering feedback only when users are imagining movement.

This new principle, called paired stimulation (PS), has been used in recent publications (Xu et al. 2014; Pichiorri et al. 2015; Belda-Lois et al. 2011; Ortner et al. 2012). The recoveriX system (Figure 4.7) is designed to couple real-time indices of motor imagery with different types of feedback, including FES activation and the movement of a virtual avatar. By providing feedback only while

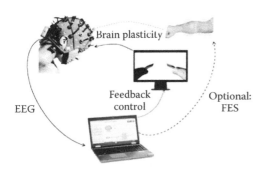
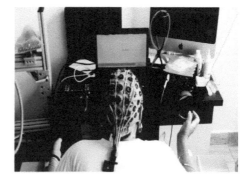

**FIGURE 4.7** The left image depicts the closed-loop feedback in recoveriX, including a 16-channel wireless system. The right image shows a patient using a recoveriX prototype to restore hand function. The system includes EEG electrodes, a biosignal amplifier, a computer, and an FES.

the user performs the expected mental activities, recoveriX creates a much more effective closed-loop paradigm that increases compliance and user engagement.

Figure 4.8 shows a 65-year-old stroke patient who began recoveriX training 3 months post-stroke. The stroke affected the functions of his left arm. A nine-hole PEG test was used to measure the time to put nine pegs into holes of a board in front of the patient. The recoveriX training was performed a total of 24 times for 30 min each (80 left hand movement imaginations, 80 right hand movement imaginations). The patient needed between 25 and 26 s to perform the task with his right hand. With the left hand, he could not do the test within the first nine sessions. Then, he improved the time of the left hand from 1 min 30 s continuously to 52 s.

Figure 4.9 shows the BCI classification error rate across 24 sessions. The patient started with a minimum error rate of 12.5% and was able to reduce the error rate to only 1.3% in session 13. Curiously, while the error rate remained low after session 13, it was always above 1.3%.

Figure 4.10 shows the changes of the common spatial pattern (CSP) filter applied to the 64 EEG electrodes. In session 2, the patterns are very fuzzy, but in session 23, clear spots around C3 (right hand representation area) and C4 (left hand representation area) can be seen.

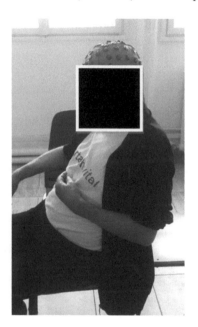 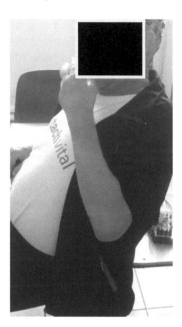

**FIGURE 4.8**  Left: Patient P5's residual arm movement before the recoveriX training (he could not lift the arm higher). Right: the same patient's arm movement after nine recoveriX sessions.

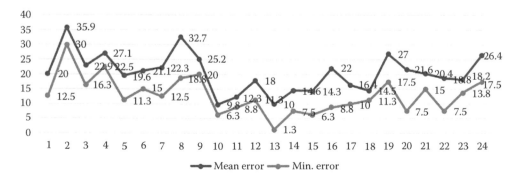

**FIGURE 4.9**  Classification error rate during the 24 recoveriX training sessions of P5.

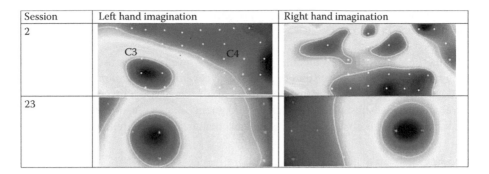

| Session | Left hand imagination | Right hand imagination |
|---|---|---|
| 2 | C3      C4 | |
| 23 | | |

**FIGURE 4.10**   Brain plasticity from session 2 to session 23. The figure shows two CSPs used to weight each electrode according to its importance for the discrimination task. Top: two most important CSP filters in session 2. Bottom: CSP filters in session 23.

recoveriX is designed to work with different movements, and we present one example based on right wrist dorsiflexion. A patient who can no longer perform this movement would typically be asked to imagine it while an FES or other mechanism tried to complete the effort by stimulating or manually manipulating relevant areas of the arm, wrist, and hand. recoveriX can add crucial information to this system: real-time measures of imagined wrist dorsiflexion based on ERD/S maps. Unlike conventional therapy, the patient would always know when dorsiflexion imagery is correctly performed. Aside from creating a more effective feedback loop during recoveriX usage, this approach is also useful for verifying compliance to therapists and doctors, who otherwise have no objective way to confirm that their patients are both trying to perform the imagined task and succeeding in their effort. Initial results have been promising, even with post-acute patients, and further research and development is ongoing.

## 4.4   CONCLUSION

The two new directions presented here could lead to new hope for patients affected by DOC and stroke. Table 4.1 summarizes the benefits that BCIs could provide, extending the classical goal of BCI research (communication for patients with LIS) with these new directions.

### TABLE 4.1
### How Different Patient Groups Might Benefit from BCI-Based Technology

| Diagnosis | Reliable Communication without a BCI? | Reliable Communication with a BCI? | Might Need BCI (re-) Assessment of Consciousness? | Might Benefit from BCI Rehabilitation? |
|---|---|---|---|---|
| Healthy | Yes | Yes | No | No |
| Most disabilities | Yes | Yes | No | Depends on disability |
| LIS | Usually | Yes | No | Being studied |
| CLIS | Very few options | See (Guger et al. 2017) | In some cases | Being studied |
| MCS | No | Depends on cognitive functioning | Yes—could lead to communication | Being studied |
| UWS | No | Depends on cognitive functioning | Yes—could lead to communication | Being studied |
| Coma | No | No | Yes—could help confirm diagnosis | No |
| Stroke that affects voluntary movement | Usually; depends on disability | Yes | No | Yes |

*Note:*   Some patients are misdiagnosed, and BCI technology can provide further information.

Table 4.1 presents nascent efforts that could inspire broader systems and applications, such as other kinds of rehabilitation (e.g., cognitive, sensory, or emotional) and extensions to other target groups (such as patients with disabilities resulting from other causes). Assessment and rehabilitation also create the new challenge of outcome prediction. Can we predict a user's likelihood of communicating with a specific approach and/or achieving a certain rehabilitation goal? How long might these challenges take, and what parameters are optimal? There are a myriad of opportunities for future development, and substantial research, development, innovation, and validation with patients will be required to see which directions are the most beneficial to different groups.

## REFERENCES

Allison, B. Z., Dunne, S., Leeb, R., Millan, J., & Nijholt, A. (2013). Recent and upcoming BCI progress: Overview, analysis, and recommendations. In: *Towards Practical BCIs: Bridging the Gap from Research to Real-World Applications*, editors: Allison, B. Z., Dunne, S., Leeb, R., Millan, J., and Nijholt, A. Springer-Verlag Berlin, 1–13.

Belda-Lois, J. M., Mena-del Horno, S., Bermejo-Bosch, I., Moreno, J. C., Pons, J. L., Farina, D., Iosa, M., Tamburella, F., Ramos Murguialday, A., Caria, A., Solis-Escalante, T., Brunner, C., & Rea, M. Rehabilitation of gait after stroke: A review towards a top-down approach. *J. Neuroeng. Rehabil.* 8 (2011) 66.

Brunner, C., Birbaumer, N., Blankertz, B., Guger, C., Kübler, A., Mattia, D., Millán, J. D. R., Miralles, F., Nijholt, A., Opisso, E., Ramsey, N., Salomon, P., & Müller-Putz, G. R. BNCI Horizon 2020: Towards a roadmap for the BCI community. *Brain–Computer Interfaces* 2(1) (2015), 1–10.

Giacino, J. T., Fins, J. J., Laureys, S., & Schiff, N. D. Disorders of consciousness after acquired brain injury: The state of the science. *Nature Review* 10 (2012) 99–114.

Guger, C., Spataro, R., Allison, B. Z., Heilinger, A., Ortner, R., Cho, W., & La Bella, V. Complete locked-in and locked-in patients: Command following assessment and communication with vibrotactile P300 and motor imagery brain–computer interface tools. *Front. Neurosci.* 11 (2017) 251.

http://www.cnn.com/2017/06/15/politics/otto-warmbier-north-korea/index.html

Kübler, A., Kotchoubey, B., Kaiser, J., Wolpaw, J., & Birbaumer, N. Brain–computer communication: Unlocking the locked-in. *Psychological Bulletin*, 127 (2001) 358–375.

Lugo, Z. R., Rodriguez, J., Lechner, A., Ortner, R., Gantner, I. S., Kübler, A., Laureys, S., Noirhomme, Q., & Guger, C. A vibrotactile P300-based BCI for consciousness detection and communication. *Clin. EEG and Neurosci.* (2014).

Lulé, D., Noirhomme, Q., Kleih, S. C., Chatelle, C., Halder, S., Demertzi, A., Bruno, M.-A., Gosseries, O., Vanhaudenhuyse, A., Schnakers, C., Thonnard, M., Soddu, A., Kübler, A., & Laureys, S. Probing command following in patients with disorders of consciousness using a brain–computer interface. *Clin. Neurophysiol.* 124 (2013) 101–106.

Marchetti, M., Priftis, K. Effectiveness of the P3-speller in brain–computer interfaces for amyotrophic lateral sclerosis patients: A systematic review and meta-analysis. *Front. Neuroeng.* 7 (2014) 12.

Neuper, C., & Allison, B. Z. (2014). The B of BCIs: Neurofeedback principles and how they can yield clearer brain signals. In: *Different Psychological Perspectives on Cognitive Processes: Current Research Trends in Alps–Adria Region*, editors: Actis, R. and Galmonte, A., Cambridge University Press, 133–153.

Ortner, R., Irimia, D. C., Scharinger, J., & Guger, C. A motor imagery based brain–computer interface for stroke rehabilitation. *Stud. Health Technol. Inform.* 181 (2012) 319–323.

Pfurtscheller, G., Allison, B. Z., Brunner, C., Bauernfeind, G., Solis-Escalante, T., Scherer, R., Zander, T. O., Mueller-Putz, G., Neuper, C., & Birbaumer, N. The hybrid BCI. *Front Neurosci.* 4 (2010) 30.

Pichiorri, F., Morone, G., Petti, M., Toppi, J., Pisotta, I., Molinari, M., Paolucci, S., Inghilleri, M., Astolfi, L., Cincotti, F., Mattia, D. Brain–computer interface boosts motor imagery practice during stroke recovery. *Ann Neurol.* 77(5) (2015) 851–865.

Risetti, M., Formisano, R., Toppi, J., Quitadamo, L. R., Bianchi, L., Astolfi, L., Cincotti, F., & Mattia, D. On ERPs detection in disorders of consciousness rehabilitation. *Front. Hum. Neurosci.* 7 (2013) 775.

Schnakers, C., Vanhaudenhuyse, A., Giacino, J., Ventura, M., Boly, M., Majerus, S., Moonen, G., Laureys, S. Diagnostic accuracy of the vegetative and minimally conscious state: Clinical consensus versus standardized neurobehavioral assessment. *BMC Neurology* 9 (2009) 35, doi: 10.1186/1471-2377-9-35.

Wolpaw, J. R., Birbaumer, N., McFarland, D. J., Pfurtscheller, G., & Vaughan, T. M. Brain–computer interfaces for communication and control. *Clin. Neurophysiol.* 113 (2002) 767–791.

Wolpaw, J. R. & Wolpaw, E. W. (2012). *Brain–Computer Interfaces: Principles & Practice.* Oxford University Press: Oxford.

Xu, R., Jiang, N., Mrachacz-Kersting, N., Lin, C., Asin, G., Moreno, J., Pons, J., Dremstrup, K., & Farina, D. A closed-loop brain–computer interface triggering an active ankle-foot orthosis for inducing cortical neural plasticity. *IEEE Trans. Biomed. Eng.* 9294 (2014) 1–1.

# 5 Therapeutic Applications of BCI Technologies

*Dennis J. McFarland*

## CONTENTS

5.1 Introduction ..................................................................................................... 101
5.2 Current BCI Rehabilitation Paradigms ........................................................... 102
5.3 Brief Overview of Research Findings .............................................................. 103
5.4 Discussion ....................................................................................................... 107
5.5 Summary .......................................................................................................... 108
References ................................................................................................................. 109

### Abstract

There has been considerable recent interest in applying brain–computer interface (BCI) technology for the rehabilitation of nervous system disorders. This survey considers possible ways that BCI technology can be applied to motor rehabilitation after stroke as well as other disorders of brain functioning. To date, there have been a number of studies demonstrating proof of principle, but definitive evidence of efficacy is lacking. This area may advance as research identifies new signals to train, more effective means of training, as well as improved paradigms for applying this technology.

## 5.1 INTRODUCTION

A brain–computer interface (BCI) is a system that measures central nervous system (CNS) activity and converts it into an artificial output that replaces, restores, enhances, supplements, or improves natural CNS output (Wolpaw & Wolpaw 2012). A number of studies have been successful in training individuals to control electroencephalogram (EEG) signals to replace lost communication or control abilities (e.g., Kostov & Polak 2000; McFarland et al. 2010; Pfurtscheller et al. 1993; Wolpaw et al. 1991). More recently, there has been increased interest in developing BCI methods for improving motor, cognitive, or emotional function (e.g., Daly & Sitaram 2012; Dobkin 2007). This chapter considers some of the possible ways that BCI technology might be applied to promote neurorehabilitation.

As noted by Dobkin (2007), both traditional rehabilitation and BCI control rely on learning to modify spared neural ensembles. Dobkin (2007) suggested that practical BCI systems could be used as a tool to reinforce the use of spared neural representations or to ensure that subjects were optimally prepared to execute a particular movement. Silvoni et al. (2011) identified three potential approaches to the use of BCI technologies for rehabilitation: the substitutive strategy, classical conditioning, and operant conditioning. The substitutive strategy refers to all technologies that bypass interrupted neural pathways. Classical conditioning promotes neuroplasticity through establishing a contingency between stimuli. Operant conditioning promotes neuroplasticity by establishing a contingency between a response and reward/feedback. Daly and Wolpaw (2008) distinguished between applications of BCI technology that bypass an impaired neuromuscular system and those that help guide activity-dependent brain plasticity to improve function. Use of BCIs to improve function more closely fits the logic of traditional rehabilitation whereas substitutive strategies correspond to providing an orthosis. Huster et al. (2014) stated that neurofeedback likely represents the earliest application of BCIs and suggest that the extent of EEG data processing is the difference between BCIs for communication and control and those for neurofeedback.

While BCI technologies have generated a considerable degree of interest as potential agents of rehabilitation, critical issues for their successful application include what signals will be used and how these signals should be used. Use of neural signals for rehabilitation involves the context in which they are used (i.e., the training paradigm), whether feedback is provided, the goal of training, and the way brain states are conceptualized. For example, traditional neurofeedback paradigms occur within a context where the task of the patient is only to regulate their brain activity based on feedback provided (Walker 2010). In contrast, if the intent of training is to ensure that patients are optimally prepared to execute a particular movement (Dobkin 2007), then BCI training should be associated with that specific movement.

In the following, we will consider some of the paradigms that have been suggested as ways to apply BCI technologies to rehabilitation. The emphasis will be on their similarities and differences. Then, we will briefly consider some of the research findings to date.

## 5.2 CURRENT BCI REHABILITATION PARADIGMS

Neurofeedback (also referred to as neurotherapy or biofeedback) has been used for many years to treat a large assortment of conditions including attention-deficit/hyperactivity disorder (ADHD; Lubar & Shouse 1976), depression (Hammond 2005), substance use disorders (Trudeau 2005), insomnia (Hammer et al. 2011), autism (Friedrich et al. 2015), and stroke (Bearden et al. 2003; Reichert et al. 2016). Neurofeedback involves providing feedback in the form of some visual or auditory stimulus based on some predetermined EEG feature (Micouland-Franchi et al. 2015). As noted above, the patient's task is only to regulate the specific brain signal and no additional behavior is required. Thus, there is no specific context in which neurofeedback occurs, other than a therapist's office. As a result, neurofeedback protocols implicitly assume that the effects of training persist as a permanent change in brain state that is sustained beyond the therapeutic context.

BCI technologies have been used for rehabilitation, for example, to enhance motor imagery. The rationale for this approach is that motor imagery may provide an effective means of therapy for stroke-related dysfunction (Sharma et al. 2006). Since brain lesions may impair imagery (McInnes et al. 2016), methods to facilitate imagery might enhance recovery. BCI-facilitated motor imagery involves providing feedback based on sensorimotor rhythms (SMRs) while users are given the task of imagining movement of affected limbs (Pichiorri et al. 2015; Prasad et al. 2010). Enhanced motor imagery training assumes that motor imagery activates some of the same neural systems as are used in actual movement. SMR training, in turn, is used as a method to enhance motor imagery. Thus, the EEG is seen as an index of a cognitive task, the rehearsal of which facilitates recovery from motor deficits after stroke.

Another paradigm for use of BCI technology to rehabilitate the motor deficits resulting from stroke involves closing the sensorimotor loop (Gomez-Rodriguez et al. 2011; Ramos-Murguialday et al. 2013). With this paradigm, SMR desynchronization is rewarded by the operation of an orthosis that produces actual movement of the affected limb. Closing the sensorimotor loop assumes that activation of motor areas will be associated with the proprioceptive feedback produced by limb movement. Several alternative explanations have been provided for the effects of closing the sensorimotor loop, including Hebbian learning (Gomez-Rodriguez et al. 2011) and priming of subsequent physiotherapy (Curado et al. 2015).

BCI technology has also been used to train users to produce brain states that ensure optimal preparation to execute a particular movement (Boulay et al. 2011; McFarland et al. 2015b). In this paradigm, users learn to modulate SMRs in advance of the motor task to be practiced. This approach assumes that advanced preparation facilitates subsequent motor performance. Therapeutic benefit

**TABLE 5.1**

**Characteristics of Several Approaches to the Use of BCI Technologies for Rehabilitation**

| Approach | Context | Feedback | Therapeutic Goal | Concept of Brain States | Range of Applications |
|---|---|---|---|---|---|
| Neurofeedback | None | Yes | Normalization of EEG | Static | Many |
| Imagery enhancement | Motor imagery | Yes | Reinforce mental imagery | Reactive | Motor tasks |
| Close sensorimotor loop | Control of orthosis | Yes | Associate intention with haptic feedback | Reactive | Motor tasks |
| Train preparation | Criterion task | Yes | Insure optimal preparation | Reactive | Many |
| State-dependent trial presentation | Criterion task | No | Insure optimal preparation | Reactive | Many |

can then result from the correct performance of the facilitated motor behavior and also from the user potentially learning task-appropriate preparatory responses.

Task-appropriate brain states have also been produced without training by making trial initiation contingent on the desired brain state (Burke et al. 2015; Griffin et al. 2004; Salari & Rose 2016). In contrast to the methods previously discussed, the state-dependent trial presentation paradigm does not provide feedback for the BCI user to learn control of the targeted brain state. It only assumes that the task-appropriate brain state facilitates performance.

Table 5.1 shows some characteristics of each of these approaches. The second column of Table 5.1 lists the context in which BCI technologies are applied. Neurofeedback has no particular context, imagery enhancement occurs in the context of practicing imagery, closing the sensorimotor loop occurs in the context of patients attempting control of an orthosis, and both trained preparation and state-dependent trial presentation occur immediately before the task to be practiced. The third column of Table 5.1 lists whether or not feedback is provided. All of the methods except state-dependent trial presentation provide feedback in order to enhance brain plasticity. While feedback will enhance learning, a method that does not provide feedback may allow for shorter training sessions. The fourth column of Table 5.1 indicates that the goal of these methods differ. Neurofeedback is generally conceptualized as a means to normalize the EEG (Walker 2010). The goal of imagery enhancement is to reinforce weak imagery (Prasad et al. 2010). Closing the sensorimotor loop strives to associate intention with haptic feedback (Gomez-Rodriguez et al. 2011). Both trained preparation and state-dependent trial presentation seek to ensure optimal preparation for the task to be practiced. Neurofeedback differs from the other approaches by implicitly assuming a static view of the EEG and the brain states it reflects. Finally, imagery enhancement and closing the sensorimotor loop are probably only applicable to the rehabilitation of motor impairments while the other methods may have broader application.

The list of methods and their characteristics shown in Table 5.1 is not exhaustive. Additional paradigms may be developed and additional ways in which paradigms differ may be identified. However, Table 5.1 provides a framework for consideration of design issues that will ultimately affect the efficiency of methods for rehabilitation.

## 5.3 BRIEF OVERVIEW OF RESEARCH FINDINGS

Neurofeedback has been a topic of extensive published research and is the only paradigm listed in Table 5.1 that is currently in widespread clinical use. In contrast, most of the research with other

BCI paradigms has been focused on rehabilitation of motor function. Perhaps the most common application of neurofeedback is for the treatment of ADHD, and this will be the focus of most of our discussion of neurofeedback.

In a review of the literature on neurofeedback for the treatment of ADHD, Monastra et al. (2005) stated that controlled group studies of ADHD have demonstrated beneficial effects on a number of outcome measures. The study by Fuchs et al. (2003) that they cite is typical. This study compared the effects of neurofeedback (SMR [12–15 Hz at C4] or beta training [15–18 Hz at C3]) and stimulant medication in children with ADHD, with treatment assignment based on the parent's preference. SMR training consisted of providing visual and auditory feedback when activity was 60% above pretraining baseline for 500 ms. Improvements were found for both groups on performance of several psychometric tests of attention and ratings of symptoms. No information was provided about the nature of changes in the EEG that might have occurred with training.

One issue with the Fuchs et al. (2003) study is that the changes observed over time could possibly be due to nonspecific effects (i.e., symptoms may get better simply with the passage of time or may be due to placebo effects). Since information was not provided about changes that occurred in the EEG in the Fuchs et al. (2003) study, it is not possible to infer what the patients in the neurofeedback group might have learned. This is a concern with the interpretation of many neurofeedback studies since the nature of the EEG changes that occur with training is typically not documented (Zuberer et al. 2015). If the effectiveness of neurofeedback is based on the premise that treatment produces a relatively permanent change in the EEG, then studies should minimally provide evidence that a change has in fact occurred. The lack of clear evidence for learned changes in the EEG may be due in part to the difficulty of doing controlled comparisons when training is in one direction only (i.e., to only increase or decrease the EEG feature in question). In contrast, the use of multiple states, as is the case with most BCI communication applications, provides a controlled within-subject comparison (McFarland et al. 2005). What is being learned with neurofeedback is important for evaluating its impact, as originally discussed by Black and Cott (1977). For example, in a double-blind study, Logemann et al. (2010) found only nonspecific effects of neurofeedback in patients with ADHD as essentially equivalent effects were observed in a sham feedback control group. These results suggest that nonspecific effects may occur with neurofeedback paradigms independent of any changes in the EEG.

Some neurofeedback studies have documented changes in the EEG that occur with training. For example, Reichert et al. (2016) trained a stroke patient and healthy controls to increase SMR (12–15 Hz at Cz) over 10 sessions on different days, each consisting of a baseline and six training runs. Feedback was also provided on the presence of artifacts, which participants were instructed to minimize. Reichert et al. (2016) showed that both the patient and controls increased the SMR signal within daily runs as compared to baseline. In addition, there were pre–post increases on several measures of cognitive performance. However, Reichert et al. (2016) did not provide information about changes in SMR across days, nor did they provide spectral and topographic information that could characterize what participants were controlling during training sessions.

EEG features targeted for a given behavioral disorder by advocates of neurofeedback vary considerably. Recommended signals for treatment of ADHD include SMR, theta/beta ratios, and slow cortical potentials (Monastra et al. 2005; Strehl et al. 2006). Specific EEG features are also recommended for multiple disorders.

The neurofeedback literature contains recommendations for signals to train that often involve elaborate schemes that have minimal empirical support. For example, Walker (2010) associates specific brain areas, behavioral functions, and corresponding clinical symptoms to each of the 19 electrode locations of the 10–20 system. These associations are not supported by citations to the scientific literature. Consider the case of electrode FP1. Walker (2010) associates activity at this electrode with left frontopolar cortex and attention. However, it is important to recognize that activity at surface electrodes does not simply reflect the activity of the neural tissue in the immediate vicinity. Rather, it is the superposition of many sources resulting from volume conduction

(Hansen et al. 2016; Srinivasan et al. 2006). In addition, attention is a complex area of study reflecting multiple processes (Posner 1975) that are associated with several distinct neural networks (Scolari et al. 2015). Realistic identification of brain signals needs to consider both the nature of the EEG and that of brain organization. Also of particular relevance is a consideration of what sorts of artifacts might be present at a particular site. For example, both eyeblinks (Picton et al. 2000) and EMG (Goncharova et al. 2003) are prominent at anterior locations such as FP1. These artifacts are of particular concern given that neurofeedback studies typically do not provide a description of what the participants are actually using for control (i.e., spectral and topographic results).

Cortese et al. (2016) concluded that evidence from a meta-analysis of randomized controlled trials does not support the effectiveness of neurofeedback for the treatment of ADHD. However, summarizing the results of a randomized controlled trial, Steiner et al. (2014) concluded that neurofeedback is a promising treatment for ADHD. In a recent review, Thibault et al. (2016) noted that the clinical effectiveness of neurofeedback remains controversial. They suggest that factors other than the feedback may be responsible for observed effects. Likewise, in their review of the literature on healthy adults, Rogala et al. (2016) conclude that there is a lack of correlation between changes induced in the trained EEG signal and targeted behaviors. They attribute this to methodology that does not allow isolation of appropriate brain regions associated with the targeted behaviors. Zuberer et al. (2015) advocate more rigorous scientific standards in this research, which makes use of devices of uncertain quality.

Several recent studies have evaluated the possibility of using BCI technology to ensure, reinforce, or enhance motor imagery. Sharma et al. (2006) have reviewed studies suggesting that motor imagery may facilitate recovery from stroke. However, they note that it is difficult to ensure compliance with motor imagery instructions. Prasad et al. (2010) suggested that EEG might prove useful to verify whether patients are actually engaging in effective motor imagery. They evaluated the use of a two-target SMR BCI task and found that all five of their stroke patients were able to achieve moderate success. Some positive results were also obtained on outcome measures of motor function. However, it was difficult to isolate the cause of these effects as all five patients received both BCI-based motor imagery training and physical practice. Furthermore, this report did not include spectral or topographic information that would allow the reader to evaluate the nature of the signals being used for BCI control.

Pichiorri et al. (2015) used BCI-based feedback consisting of SMR-dependent movement of virtual hands in patients with stroke-related motor deficits. A group of 12 patients receiving BCI-based motor imagery training was compared to a group of 11 patients receiving only motor imagery training without feedback. Both groups additionally received standard care including motor, occupational, and cognitive therapy. Pichiorri et al. (2015) found significantly greater recovery on several outcome measures in the group receiving BCI-based feedback. They also provided information about the EEG bands involved and topographic location of the signals that the BCI group used for control. These results provide stronger support for the possibility that BCI-based imagery enhancement might be therapeutically beneficial in patients with stroke-related motor deficits.

A rationale for feedback that actually moves the affected limb is the suggestion that closing the sensorimotor loop produces Hebbian plasticity owing to the pairing of intention and proprioceptive feedback (Gomez-Rodriguez et al. 2011). Although Gomez-Rodriguez et al. (2011) proposed that closing the sensorimotor loop using within-trial activation of an orthosis might prove beneficial for stroke recovery, their study only involved showing that haptic feedback facilitated classification of the EEG. Buch et al. (2008) reported that magnetoencephalography (MEG)-based BCI training paired with post-trial activation of an orthosis had no significant effect on hand function, although patients successfully learned to control the device. Using a pre–post design, Shindo et al. (2011) reported some improvement in function after EEG-based BCI operation of an orthosis. Young et al. (2015) reported an improvement in a self-reported measure of strength after training with a BCI system that produced functional electrical stimulation of the hand and tongue. No information was provided about the specific EEG features used for training. Ang et al. (2014) found no significant difference between outcome measures for stroke patients receiving BCI-controlled robotic therapy and those receiving standard robotic therapy. Ramos-Murguialday et al. (2013) reported a significant improvement in functioning of stroke patients after training with an SMR-controlled orthosis as compared to a sham control group. Both groups also received behaviorally oriented physiotherapy. Information that would characterize the EEG features used by patients for orthosis control was not provided. Ramos-Murguialday et al. (2013) suggested that BCI training may have primed the effects of physiotherapy. Using a head-mounted neurochip in monkeys, Lucas and Fetz (2013) showed that making invasive stimulation of the primary motor cortex contingent on activation of a muscle resulted in reorganization of cortical outputs. The Lucas and Fetz (2013) study illustrates the bidirectional nature of the sensorimotor loop and provides an alternative method for creating associations between motor cortex and muscles.

The evidence for beneficial effects of closing the sensorimotor loop on motor deficits after stroke is weak at present and results are inconsistent. As with neurofeedback, the designs employed often do not allow isolation of the factors that might be responsible for any observed therapeutic effects. Furthermore, there is often a lack of concern for characterizing how training affects the EEG (or MEG).

As noted earlier, Dobkin (2007) suggested that one way that BCI systems might facilitate rehabilitation is to ensure that subjects were optimally prepared to execute a particular response. The possibility of training motor preparation was demonstrated in healthy controls by Boulay et al. (2011) using a go–no-go reaction time task and McFarland et al. (2015b) using a joystick movement task. Both of these studies used a three-phase design in which subjects initially performed the criterion task to identify pre-movement EEG features predicted movement. Next, these features were trained in a bidirectional BCI task. In the third phase of the Boulay et al. (2011) study, an auditory imperative stimulus was presented cuing a button press while subjects were also controlling a cursor to hit a target on a video screen. Voluntary desynchronization in SMRs produced faster reaction times than SMR synchronization. In the third phase of the McFarland et al. (2015b) study, subjects increased or decreased SMRs according to color cues in order to initiate the joystick task. SMR desynchronization facilitated performance in subjects with lower initial performance levels. Both of these studies provided spectral and topographic information to characterize the EEG features that were used by subjects for control. The results of both the Boulay et al. (2011) and McFarland et al. (2015b) studies showed that pre-movement voluntary modulation of SMRs affects behavior. They provide a rational for the development of rehabilitation protocols that target SMRs to ensure that subjects are optimally prepared to execute a particular response.

As noted earlier, neurofeedback studies have advocated the use of SMRs for the treatment of ADHD (Monastra et al. 2005), autism (Friedrich et al. 2015), sleep disorders (Hammer et al. 2011), memory (Reichert et al. 2016), and epilepsy (Sterman 2010). In each of these applications, SMRs are treated as a unitary index of some particular brain function. However, SMRs are recording site specific. For example, SMR effects are specific to the limb involved in both movement and imagination (Pfurtscheller & Lopes da Silva 2011). Furthermore, subjects can be trained to independently modulate three different SMRs differing in location (McFarland et al. 2010). In contrast to conceptualizations of EEG rhythms reflecting global functions such as mirroring the activity of others (Pineda 2008) or behavioral inhibition (Monastra et al. 2005), activity recorded at specific locations may reflect the activity of canonical cortical circuits whose functions vary with location (Bhatt et al. 2016). From this perspective, SMRs are analogous to rhythms at similar frequencies that reflect the activity of specific brain networks such as those involved in vision and hearing (Mazaheri et al. 2014; Scheeringa et al. 2016). Thus, spatial filtering operations are important to provide more precise localization of activity as well as to improve signal-to-noise ratios (McFarland 2015). Perhaps more important is an appreciation of the anatomical specificity of brain rhythms to specific neural networks.

At the same time that SMR modulations are topographically specific to a given limb, they are also extended across multiple brain areas. For example, recording with depth electrodes implanted for deep brain stimulation reveals beta rhythm desynchronization with movement in the subthalamic nucleus (Klostermann et al. 2007). These subthalamic beta rhythms are coherent with beta rhythms recorded at the scalp (Kato et al. 2015). Likewise, beta rhythms can be recorded from specific muscles that are coherent with localized scalp beta rhythms (van de Steeg et al. 2014). Thus, SMR beta rhythms represent a resonance extended over multiple components of an effector-specific network. This provides a strong rationale for pairing specific SMR control tasks with specific movements that are targeted for therapy.

Optimal task preparation can also be produced by delaying trial onset until spontaneous fluctuations in the EEG indicate that a desired brain state is present. Griffin et al. (2004) showed that state-dependent trial presentations could affect learning of classical eyelid conditioning in rabbits. Trial presentation was contingent on the presence of hippocampal theta rhythm, as measured with implanted electrodes. A theta-contingent group learned the task much quicker than a non–theta-contingent group. State-dependent trial presentations were also used by Salari and Rose (2016) to evaluate the effects of scalp-recorded activity on memory in human subjects. EEG was recorded at frontal and temporal locations and spectral power was separately summed in theta or beta bands. Presentation of visual images in a recognition memory experiment was dependent on either high or low summed power in these bands. Subsequent recognition memory was better for high beta presentations than low beta presentations while theta-dependent presentations did not differ significantly.

## 5.4 DISCUSSION

Which of the paradigms outlined in Table 5.1 will prove most useful for rehabilitation of brain disorders is currently an empirical question. Their potential utility depends on the nature of brain states, such as whether or not these represent static traits or transient configurations of labile networks. The paradigms outlined in Table 5.1 also differ in how they conceptualize the nature of the rehabilitation process and the nervous system that is to be rehabilitated. For example, imagery enhancement implicitly assumes that the EEG provides an index of a cognitive process and that it is the strengthening of this cognitive process that is the goal of therapy. In contrast, the use of a neurochip (Lucas & Fetz 2013) has the goal of establishing simple associations between brain and muscle activity. The paradigms outlined in Table 5.1 also differ in their potential breadth of application. Although there has been great interest in the use of BCI technologies to assist recovery from the motor impairments resulting from stroke, the use of state-dependent trial presentations within classical conditioning and recognition memory paradigms shows that some of these methods may have broader application. Likewise, neurofeedback can be applied broadly as there is no dependence on context. Paradigms based on optimizing patient preparation can also be applied in any situation in which a preparatory period is feasible. However, imagery enhancement and closing the sensorimotor loop probably have less broad applicability. In addition, these methods may vary in ease of implementation. For example, state-dependent training does not require extensive training of the BCI user in brain state feature control.

Application of BCI technologies could potentially extend beyond stroke-related motor deficits to include many other disorders (Daly & Sitaram 2012). However, application to any particular disorder is dependent on identification of reliable neural signals that can be used in a suitable training paradigm. This can be challenging as not all brain states are as well characterized as those associated with movement. For example, some success has been obtained with functional magnetic resonance imaging (fMRI) detection of emotional reactivity (e.g., Martino et al. 2016). However, detection of emotional reactivity with the EEG appears to be less robust (McFarland et al. 2015a). As noted by Kragel and LaBar (2016), the brain basis of emotions is currently poorly understood. While modification of emotional reactivity might have broad clinical application, much more research will be required before this can be realized.

Selection of an appropriate brain signal is an issue facing all of the methods discussed so far, and these paradigms differ in how this has been done to date. The neurofeedback approach assumes an elaborate system that associates specific EEG features to specific functions and provides feedback accordingly (Walker 2010). Empirical support for such schemes is often not provided by those who advocate them. Selection of features for motor recovery by the other methods is generally based on the well-established association of SMRs with motor function (Pfurtscheller & McFarland 2012) but is much more limited in scope.

Even given the well-established association of SMRs with movement, there are still additional issues in selecting features for BCI systems. For example, in reviewing the use of transcranial magnetic stimulation (TMS) as a modality for motor rehabilitation, Plow et al. (2016) discuss the issue of whether ipsilesional or contralesional areas should be targeted. They suggest that the hemisphere targeted might depend on the extent of a patient's lesions. The targeted hemisphere is also relevant for BCI-based methods that might be used to enhance the activity of specific brain sites that best participate in recovery. In this sense, there are certain parallels between the logic of using TMS and that of using BCI technologies. Both technologies could work by activating task-appropriate brain networks. Use of TMS has the advantage of being quicker and probably less expensive. Use of BCI technologies may be more precise in the aspects of network function targeted since TMS is likely to activate relatively broad expanses of cortex that may be involved in multiple functions. BCI methods may be able to target more precise activation of networks associated with frequency-specific signals.

Also reviewing TMS applications for rehabilitation, Chouinard and Paus (2010) noted that there are multiple components of the motor system that could serve as targets for activation, in addition to Brodmann's area 4. This view is consistent with the results of Dum and Strick (1991) who examined the corticospinal projections to cervical segments of the spinal cord in macaques. Dum and Strick (1991) describe contributions from premotor and cingulate motor areas to the corticospinal tract. Although axons from these sites are generally smaller, they contribute a substantial portion of the pyramidal track. Dum and Strick (2005) suggested that the distinction between premotor and primary motor areas is not as clear as often supposed.

It is often assumed that SMRs arise from the primary motor cortex, but the exact neural circuitry generating SMRs are not precisely known. The hand area of the primary motor lies mainly on the anterior bank of the central fissure (Laakso et al. 2014). As such, the pyramidal cells would be aligned parallel to the scalp and would not be expected to provide a clear projection to central scalp areas. Thus, SMRs may represent the activity of areas other than the primary motor cortex. Although the motor system is perhaps better characterized than many other neural systems, much remains to be learned about how its various components generate the signals recorded from the scalp as well as their potential relevance for rehabilitation.

Although this chapter has dealt mainly with EEG, other neural signals can be used for rehabilitation. For example, Sitaram et al. (2012) used fMRI to provide real-time feedback on ventral premotor cortex activity to stroke patients and Rea et al. (2014) used fNIRS (functional near-infrared spectroscopy) to discriminate preparation of hip movement, also in stroke patients. Liew et al. (2015) provided feedback based on the correlation of fMRI activity between motor cortex and ipsilesional thalamus. This demonstrates the possibility of providing feedback on measures of connectivity. While measures of cerebral blood flow have less temporal resolution than EEG, they provide better spatial resolution. The paradigms discussed earlier (e.g., closing the sensorimotor loop or state-dependent trial presentations) could be applied to measures of cerebral blood flow just as readily as to electrophysiological indices of brain state.

## 5.5 SUMMARY

BCI methods developed for communication and control applications could also be a technology useful for rehabilitation. There are a number of different ways in which BCI technologies might be used for this purpose, depending in part on conceptualizations of nervous system functioning and therapeutic goals. Much of the work to date has been concerned with motor function after stroke, although there are many other possible applications. A number of studies have demonstrated proof of principle, but definitive evidence of efficacy is lacking. This may be partly because proof of efficacy is much more difficult to demonstrate than proof of principle. The use of BCI technology for therapeutic purposes may progress as research identifies new signals to train, more effective means of training, as well as improved paradigms for applying this technology.

# REFERENCES

Ang, K.K., Guan, C., Phua, K.S., Wang, C., Zhou, L., Tang, K.Y., Joseph, G.J.E., Kuah, C.W.K. and Chua, K.S.G. 2014, Brain–computer interface-based robotic end effector system for wrist and hand rehabilitation: Results of a three-armed randomized controlled trial for chronic stroke. *Frontiers in Neuroengineering*, 7:30.

Bearden, T.S., Cassisi, J.E. and Pineda, M. 2003, Neurofeedback training for a patient with thalamic and cortical infarctions. *Applied Psychophysiology and Biofeedback*, 28:241–252.

Bhatt, M.B., Bowen, S., Rossiter, H.E., Dupont-Hadwen, J., Moran, R.J., Friston, K.J. and Ward, N.S. 2016, Computational modelling of movement-related beta-oscillatory dynamics in human motor cortex. *Neuroimage*, 133:224–232.

Black, A.H. and Cott, A. 1977, A perspective on biofeedback. In *Biofeedback and Behavior: A NATO Symposium*, eds. J. Beatty and H. Legewie. New York, Plenum, pp. 7–19.

Boulay, C.B., Sarnacki, W.A., Wolpaw, J.R. and McFarland, D.J. 2011, Trained modulation of sensorimotor rhythm can affect reaction time. *Clinical Neurophysiology*, 122:1820–1826.

Buch, E., Weber, C., Cohen, L.G., Braun, C., Dimyan, M.A., Ard, T., Mellinger, J., Caria, A., Soekadar, S., Fourkias, A. and Birbaumer, N. 2008, Think to move: A neuromagnetic brain–computer interface (BCI) system for chronic stroke. *Stroke*, 39:910–917.

Burke, J.F., Merkow, M.B., Jacobs, J., Kahana, M.J. and Zaghloul, K.A. 2015, Brain computer interface to enhance episodic memory in human participants. *Frontiers in Human Neuroscience*, 8:1055.

Chouinard, P.A. and Paus, T. 2010, What have we learned from "perturbing" the human cortical motor system with transcranial magnetic stimulation? *Frontiers in Human Neuroscience*, 10:3389.

Cortese, S., Ferrin, M., Brandeis, D., Holtmann, M., Aggensteiner, P., Daley, D., Santosh, P., Simonoff, E., Stevenson, J., Stringaris, A. and Sonuga-Barke, E.J. 2016, Neurofeedback for attention-deficit/hyperactivity disorder: Meta-analysis of clinical neuropsychological outcomes from randomized controlled trials. *Journal of the American Academy of Child and Adolescent Psychiatry*, 55:444–455.

Curado, M.R., Cossio, E.G., Broetz, D., Agostini, M., Cho, W., Brasil, F.L., Yilmaz, O., Liberati, G., Lepski, G., Birbaumer, N. and Ramos-Murguialday, A. 2015, Residual upper arm motor function primes innervation of paretic forearm muscles in chronic stroke after brain-machine interface (BMI) training. *PLOS One*, 10:e0140161.

Daly, J.J. and Sitaram, R. 2012, BCI therapeutic applications for improving brain function. In *Brain–Computer Interfaces: Principles and Practice*, eds. J.R. Wolpaw and E.W. Wolpaw. New York: Oxford University Press, pp. 351–362.

Daly, J.J. and Wolpaw, J.R. 2008, Brain–computer interfaces in neurological rehabilitation. *Lancet Neurology*, 7:1032–1043.

Dobkin, B.H. 2007, Brain–computer interface technology as a tool to augment plasticity and outcomes for neurological rehabilitation. *Journal of Physiology* (London), 579:637–642.

Dum, R.P. and Strick, P.L. 1991, The origin of corticospinal projections from the premotor areas in the frontal lobe. *Journal of Neuroscience*, 11:667–689.

Dum, R.P. and Strick, P.L. 2005, Frontal lobe inputs to the digit representations of the motor areas on the lateral surface of the hemisphere. *Journal of Neuroscience*, 25:1375–1386.

Friedrich, E.V., Sivanathan, A., Lim, T., Suttie, N., Louchart, S., Pillen, S. and Pineda, J.A. 2015, An effective neurofeedback intervention to improve social interactions in children with autism spectrum disorder. *Journal of Autism and Developmental Disorders*, 45:4084–4100.

Fuchs, T., Birbaumer, N., Lutzenberger, W., Gruzelier, J.H. and Kaiser, J. 2003, Neurofeedback treatment for attention deficit/hyperactivity disorder in children: A comparison with methylphenidate. *Applied Psychophysiology and Biofeedback*, 28:1–12.

Gomez-Rodriguez, M., Peters, J., Hill, J., Scholkopf, B., Gharabaghi, A. and Grosse-Wentrup, M. 2011, Closing the sensorimotor loop: Haptic feedback facilitates decoding of motor imagery. *Journal of Neural Engineering*, 8:036005.

Goncharova, I.I., McFarland, D.J., Vaughan, T.M. and Wolpaw, J.R. 2003, EMG contamination of EEG: Spectral and topographical characteristics. *Clinical Neurophysiology*, 114:1580–1593.

Griffin, A.L., Asaka, Y., Darling, R.D. and Berry, S.D. 2004, Theta-contingent trial presentation accelerates learning rate and enhances hippocampal plasticity during trace eyeblink conditioning. *Behavioral Neuroscience*, 118:403–411.

Hammer, B.U., Colbert, A.P., Brown, K.A. and Ilioi, E.C. 2011, Neurofeedback for insomnia: A pilot study of Z-score SMR and individualized protocols. *Applied Psychophysiology and Biofeedback*, 36:251–264.

Hammond, D.C. 2005, Neurofeedback treatment of depression and anxiety. *Journal of Adult Development*, 12:131–137.

Hansen, S.T., Hauberg, S. and Hansen, L.K. 2016, Data-driven forward model inference for EEG brain imaging. *Neuroimage*, 139:249–258.

Huster, R.J., Mokom, Z.N., Enriquez-Geppert, S. and Herrmann, C.S. 2014, Brain–computer interfaces for EEG neurofeedback. *International Journal of Psychophysiology*, 91:36–45.

Kato, K., Yokochi, F., Taniguchi, M., Okiyama, R., Kawasaki, T., Kimura, K. and Ushiba, J. 2015, Bilateral coherence between motor cortices and subthalamic nuclei in patients with Parkinson's disease. *Clinical Neurophysiology*, 126:1941–1950.

Klostermann, F., Nikulin, V.V., Kuhn, A.A., Marzinzik, F., Wahl, M., Pogosyan, A., Kupsch, A., Schneider, G.H., Brown, P. and Curio, G. 2007, Task-related differential dynamics of EEG alpha- and beta-band synchronization in cortico-basal motor structures. *European Journal of Neuroscience*, 25:1604–1615.

Kostov, A. and Polak, M. 2000, Parallel man-machine training in development of EEG-based cursor control. *IEEE Transactions on Rehabilitation Engineering*, 8:203–205.

Kragel, P.A. and LaBar, K.S. 2016, Decoding the nature of emotion in the brain. *Trends in Cognitive Sciences*, 20:444–455.

Laakso, I., Hirata, A. and Ugawa, Y. 2014, Effects of coil orientation on the electric field induced by TMS over the hand area. *Physics in Medicine and Biology*, 59:203–218.

Liew, S.-L., Rana, M., Cornelsen, S., Fortunato de Barros Filho, M., Birbaumer, N., Sitaram, R., Cohen, L.G. and Soekadar, S.R. 2015, Improving motor corticothalamic communication after stroke using real-time fMRI connectivity-based neurofeedback. *Neurorehabilitation and Neural Repair*, 30:671–675.

Logemann, H.N.A., Lansbergen, M.M., Van Os, T.W.D.P., Bocker, K.B.E. and Kenemans, J.L. 2010, The effectiveness of EEG-feedback on attention, impulsivity and EEG: A sham feedback controlled study. *Neuroscience Letters*, 479:49–53.

Lubar, J.F. and Shouse, M.N. 1976, EEG and behavioral change in a hyperkinetic child concurrent with training of the sensorimotor rhythm (SMR): A preliminary report. *Biofeedback and Self-Regulation*, 1:293–306.

Lucas, T.H. and Fetz, E.E. 2013, Myo-cortical crossed feedback reorganizes primate motor cortex output. *Journal of Neuroscience*, 33:5274–5261.

Martino, M., Magioncaldo, P., Huang, Z., Conio, B., Piaggio, N., Duncan, N.W., Rocchi, G., Escelsior, A., Marozzi, V., Wolff, A., Inglese, A., Amore, M. and Northoff, G. 2016, Contrasting variability patterns in the default mode and sensorimotor networks balance in bipolar depression and mania. *Proceedings of the National Academy of Sciences*, 113:4824–4829.

Mazaheri, A., van Schouwenburg, M.R., Dimitrievic, A., Denys, D., Cools, R. and Jensen, O. 2014, Region-specific modulations in oscillatory alpha activity serve to facilitate processing in the visual and auditory modalities. *Neuroimage*, 87:356–362.

McFarland, D.J. 2015, The advantages of the surface Laplacian in brain–computer interface research. *International Journal of Psychophysiology*, 97:271–276.

McFarland, D.J., Parvaz, M., Sarnacki, W., Goldstein, R. and Wolpaw, J.R. 2015a, Prediction of subjective ratings of emotional pictures by features of the EEG. *Society for Neuroscience Abstracts*, Program number 410.21, http://www.abstractsonline.com/plan/ViewAbstract.aspx?cKey=83b3bda8-9bba-49e9-b85b-094a9a0d2bb7&mID=3744&mKey=d0ff4555-8574-4fbb-b9d4-04eec8ba0c84&sKey=effeacca-a492-4c6f-a9cc-cb853497a904.

McFarland, D.J., Sarnacki, W.A., Vaughan, T.M. and Wolpaw, J.R. 2005, Brain–computer interface (BCI) operation: Signal and noise during early training sessions. *Clinical Neurophysiology*, 116:56–62.

McFarland, D.J., Sarnacki, W.A. and Wolpaw, J.R. 2010, Electroencephalographic (EEG) control of three-dimensional movement. *Journal of Neural Engineering*, 7:036007.

McFarland, D.J., Sarnacki, W.A. and Wolpaw, J.R. 2015b, Effects of training pre-movement sensorimotor rhythms on behavioral performance. *Journal of Neural Engineering*, 12:066021.

McInnes, K., Friesen, C. and Boe, S. 2016, Specific brain lesions impair explicit motor imagery ability: Systematic review of the evidence. *Archives of Physical Medicine and Rehabilitation*, 97:478–489.

Micouland-Franchi, J.-A., McGonigal, A., Lopez, R., Daudet, C., Kotwas, I. and Bartolomei, F. 2015, Electroencephalographic neurofeedback: Level of evidence in mental and brain disorders and suggestions for good clinical practice. *Neurophysiologie Clinique*, 45:423–433.

Monastra, V.J., Lynn, S., Linden, M., Lubar, J.F., Gruzelier, J. and LaVaque, T.J. 2005, Electroencephalographic biofeedback in the treatment of attention-deficit/hyperactivity disorder. *Applied Psychophysiology and Biofeedback*, 30:95–114.

Pfurtscheller, G., Flotzinger, D. and Kalcher, J. 1993, Brain–computer interface—A new communication device for handicapped persons. *Journal of Microcomputer Applications*, 16:293–299.

Pfurtscheller, G. and Lopes da Silva, F.H. 2011, EEG event-related desynchronization (ERD) and event-related synchronization ERS). In *Niedermeyer's Electroencephalography 6th Edition*, eds. D. Schoner and F. Lopes da Silva. Wolters Kluver, pp. 935–948.

Pfurtscheller, G. and McFarland, D.J. 2012, BCIs that use sensorimotor rhythm. In *Brain–Computer Interfaces: Principles and Practice*, eds. J.R. Wolpaw and E.W. Wolpaw. New York: Oxford University Press, pp. 227–240.

Pichiorri, F., Morone, G., Petti, M., Toppi, J., Pisotta, I., Molinari, M., Paolucci, S., Inghilleri, M., Astolfi, L., Cincotti, F. and Mattia, D. 2015, Brain–computer interface boosts motor imagery practice during stroke recovery. *Annals of Neurology*, 77:851–865.

Picton, T.W., van Roon, P., Armilio, M.L., Berg, P., Ille, N. and Scherg, M. 2000, The correct of artifacts: A topographic perspective. *Clinical Neurophysiology*, 111:53–65.

Pineda, J.A. 2008, Sensorimotor cortex as a critical component of an "extended" mirror neuron system: Does it solve the development, correspondence, and control problems in mirroring? *Behavioral and Brain Functions*, 4:1–16.

Plow, E.B., Sankarasubramanian, V., Cunningham, D.A., Potter-Baker, K., Varnerin, N., Cohen, L.G., Sterr, A., Conforto, A.B. and Machado, A.G. 2016, Models to tailor brain stimulation therapies in stroke. *Neural Plasticity*, 4071620.

Posner, M.I. 1975, Psychobiology of attention. In *Handbook of Psychobiology*, eds. M.S. Gazzaniga and C. Blakemore. New York: Academic Press, pp. 441–480.

Prasad, G., Herman, P., Coyle, D., McDonough, S. and Crosbie, J. 2010, Applying a brain–computer interface to support motor imagery practice in people with stroke for upper limb recovery: A feasibility study. *Journal of NeuroEngineering and Rehabilitation*, 7:60.

Ramos-Murguialday, A., Broetz, D., Rea, M., Laer, L., Yilmaz, O., Brasil, F.L., Liberati, G., Curado, M.R., Garcia-Cossio, E., Vyziotis, A., Cho, W., Agostini, M., Soares, E., Soekadar, S., Caria, A., Cohen, L.G. and Birbaumer, N. 2013, Brain–machine interface in chronic stroke rehabilitation: A controlled study. *Annals of Neurology*, 74:100–108.

Rea, M., Rana, M., Lugato, N., Terekhin, P., Gizzi, L., Brotz, D., Fallgatter, A., Birbaumer, N., Sitaram, R. and Caria, A. 2014, Lower limb movement preparation in chronic stroke: A pilot study toward an fNIRS-BCI for rehabilitation. *Neurorehabilitation and Neural Repair*, 28:564–575.

Reichert, J.L., Kober, S.E., Schweiger, D., Grieshofer, P., Neuper, C. and Wood, G. 2016, Shutting down sensorimotor interference after stroke: A proof-of-principle SMR neurofeedback study. *Frontiers in Human Neuroscience*, 10:348.

Rogala, J., Jurewicz, K., Paluch, K., Kublik, E., Cetnarski, R. and Wrobel, A. 2016, The do's and don'ts of neurofeedback training: A review of the controlled studies using healthy adults. *Frontiers in Human Neuroscience*, 10:301.

Salari, N. and Rose, M. 2016, Dissociation of the functional relevance of different pre-stimulus oscillatory activity for memory formation. *Neuroimage*, 125:1013–1021.

Scheeringa, R., Koopmans, P.J., van Mourik, T., Jensen, O. and Norris, D.G. 2016, The relationship between oscillatory EEG activity and the laminar-specific BOLD signal. *Proceedings of the National Academy of Sciences*, 113:6761–6766.

Scolari, M., Seidl-Rathkopf, K.N. and Kastner, S. 2015, Functions of the human frontoparietal attention network: Evidence from neuroimaging. *Current Opinion in Behavioral Sciences*, 1:32–39.

Sharma, N., Pomeroy, V.M. and Baron, J.-C. 2006, Motor imagery: A backdoor to the motor system after stroke? *Stroke*, 37:1941–1952.

Shindo, K., Kawashima, K., Ushiba, J., Ota, N., Ito, M., Ota, T., Kimura, A. and Liu, M. 2011, Effects of neurofeedback training with an electroencephalographic-based brain–computer interface for hand paralysis in patients with chronic stroke: A preliminary case series study. *Journal of Rehabilitation Medicine*, 43:951–957.

Silvoni, S., Ramos-Murguialday, A., Cavinato, M., Volpato, C., Cisotto, G., Turolla, A., Piccione, F. and Birbaumer, N. 2011, Brain computer interface in stroke: A review of progress. *Clinical EEG and Neuroscience*, 42:245–252.

Sitaram, R., Veit, R., Stevens, B., Caria, A., Gerloff, C., Birbaumer, N. and Hummel, F. 2012, Acquired control of ventral premotor cortex activity by feedback training: An exploratory real-time fMRI and TMS study. *Neurorehabilitation and Neural Repair*, 26:256–265.

Srinivasan, R., Winter, W.R. and Nunez, P.L. 2006, Source analysis of EEG oscillations using high-resolution EEG and MEG. *Progress in Brain Research*, 159:29–42.

Steiner, N.J., Frenette, E.C., Rene, K.M., Brennan, R.T. and Perrin, E.C. 2014, In-school neurofeedback training for ADHD: Sustained improvements from a randomized control trial. *Pediatrics*, 133:483–492.

Sterman, M.B. 2010, Biofeedback in the treatment of epilepsy. *Cleveland Clinic Journal of Medicine*, 77 (Suppl 3):S60–S67.

Strehl, U., Leins, U., Goth, G., Klinger, C., Hinterberger, T. and Birbaumer, N. 2006, Self-regulation of slow cortical potentials: A new treatment for children with attention-deficit/hyperactivity disorder. *Pediatrics*, 118:1530–1540.

Thibault, R.T., Lifshitz, M. and Raz, A. 2016, The self-regulating brain and neurofeedback: Experimental science and clinical promise. *Cortex*, 74:247–261.

Trudeau, D.L. 2005, EEG biofeedback for addictive disorders—The state of the art. *Journal of Adult Development*, 12:139–146.

van de Steeg, C., Daffertshofer, A., Stegeman, D.F. and Boonstra, T.W. 2014, High-density surface electromyography improves the identification of oscillatory synaptic inputs to motoneurons. *Journal of Applied Physiology*, 116:1263–1271.

Walker, J.E. 2010, Recent advances in quantitative EEG as an aid to diagnosis and as a guide to neurofeedback training for cortical hypofunctions, hyperfunctions, disconnections, and hyperconnections: Improving efficacy in complicated neurological and psychological disorders. *Applied Psychophysiology and Biofeedback*, 35:25–27.

Wolpaw, J.R., McFarland, D.J., Neat, G.W. and Forneris, C.A. 1991, An EEG-based brain–computer interface for cursor control. *Electroencephalography and Clinical Neurophysiology*, 78:252–259.

Wolpaw, J.R. and Wolpaw, E.W. 2012, Brain–computer interfaces: Something new under the sun. In *Brain–Computer Interfaces: Principles and Practice*, eds. J.R. Wolpaw and E.W. Wolpaw. New York: Oxford University Press, pp. 3–14.

Young, B.M., Nigogosyan, Z., Walton, L.M., Remsik, A., Song, J., Nair, V.A., Tyler, M.E., Edwards, D.F., Caldera, K., Sattin, J.A., Williams, J.C. and Prabhakaran, V. 2015, Dose–response relationships using brain–computer interface technology impact stroke rehabilitation. *Frontiers in Human Neuroscience*, 9:361.

Zuberer, A., Brandeis, D. and Drechsler, R. 2015, Are treatment effects of neurofeedback training with ADHD related to the successful regulation of brain activity? A review on the learning of regulation of brain activity and a contribution to the discussion of specificity. *Frontiers in Human Neuroscience*, 2015.00135.

# 6 Advances in Neuroprosthetics
## *Past, Present, and Future*

Stuart Mason Dambrot

## CONTENTS

6.1 Introduction .................................................................................................................. 114
6.2 Evolutionary Neurobiology, Toolmaking, and Brain–Computer Interfaces ....................... 114
6.3 Current Neuroprosthetics............................................................................................... 115
    6.3.1 Neurological and Neurologically Related Disorders ............................................. 116
    6.3.2 Motor Control and Movement .............................................................................. 116
    6.3.3 Sensory Neuroprosthetics .................................................................................... 117
        6.3.3.1 Auditory ................................................................................................. 117
        6.3.3.2 Ocular .................................................................................................... 118
        6.3.3.3 Somatosensory ....................................................................................... 119
    6.3.4 Memory, Cognition, and Volition ......................................................................... 120
6.4 Microscale Brain–Computer Interfaces .......................................................................... 122
6.5 Future Neuroprosthetics ................................................................................................ 124
    6.5.1 Intelligent, Biomimetic, and Neurobiohybrid Neuroprosthetics ............................. 125
    6.5.2 Nanobiotechnology .............................................................................................. 125
    6.5.3 Synthetic Biology................................................................................................. 125
    6.5.4 Bionanoprotonics ................................................................................................ 125
6.6 Invasive versus Noninvasive Neuroprosthetics................................................................ 126
6.7 Security and Standards .................................................................................................. 126
    6.7.1 Information Security............................................................................................. 126
    6.7.2 Standards ............................................................................................................ 126
6.8 Conclusion ................................................................................................................... 126
References........................................................................................................................... 127

**Abstract**

That the *Homo sapiens* brain has structural and functional complexity, cognitive sophistication, and inventive toolmaking capabilities far beyond other known species is incontrovertible. What is debatable is who—or what—is, idiomatically, in the driver's seat. While we typically assign that role to ourselves, a closer inspection of that perspective uncovers some questionable assumptions about how we define ubiquitous concepts such as *self* and *mind*—terminological conventions that intuitively appear concrete, but have no innate physical existence; rather, these and related linguistic devices are referential descriptions of our experience as self-aware beings. Here, I propose that the self-organizing brain itself (which evolved as a result of a surprisingly limited series of genetic errors and mutations in our distant ancestors) is at the helm; that it is also the source of the intentionally generated trends in human toolmaking over the millennia; and, ultimately, that neuroprosthetics are the result of the brain applying its toolmaking acumen to treat and augment itself. I therefore present a compact history of prosthetics and early treatments that foresaw neuroprosthetics; a current review of current neuroprosthetics; and future neuroprosthetics, including neurobiohybrids and bionanoprotonics.

## 6.1  INTRODUCTION

We often have a short memory when considering the history of technology. This is not difficult to understand, given that the current state of technology has little in common with its earlier brethren. This reality is notably salient in neuroscience and prosthetics—especially so in their remarkable melding, neuroprosthetics: devices linked to the peripheral or central nervous system and enhance the cognitive, motor, or sensory abilities of an organism (*Medical Dictionary* 2009). Moreover, it is equally enlightening to glimpse the future of neuroprosthetics through the lens of its accelerating research, development, and convergence with non-neurological areas of inquiry, as is the case with several fields of science and technology currently seen as independent (National Research Council 2014; Roco 2003; Roco and Bainbridge 2003, 2013).

Within the above context, this chapter attempts to capture the toolmaking journey humans are on—from early tools, prosthetics, and surprising treatments, through today's increasingly sophisticated neuroprosthetic technologies, and looking ahead to a neurotechnological future that today may seem to confirm the late Arthur C. Clarke's observation that "any sufficiently advanced technology is indistinguishable from magic" (Clarke 1973).

## 6.2  EVOLUTIONARY NEUROBIOLOGY, TOOLMAKING, AND BRAIN–COMPUTER INTERFACES

In another point of view reminiscent to that of technology, we experience toolmaking as a series of acts—perception, ideation, planning, and physical implementation—that we accomplish by using our brain.

Perhaps a new perspective is in order.

Imagine reversing the causal direction of toolmaking—that is, defining the brain as a self-organizing, self-modifying organ with learning, memory, and categorization capabilities that recruits our sensory and motor systems in order to identify patterns in, model, and modify the external world. Given that (1) in this concept the brain might be said to categorize our body as external to itself, and (2) human technology continually increases in sophistication, complexity, and miniaturization, we should not be surprised that the brain has now engaged in applying these parameters to itself (Dambrot 2017)—the arguably inevitable result has been neuroprosthetics, enabling (for example) closed-loop, or adaptive, neurofeedback brain–computer interface (BCI) systems—those in which neural activity is used to modify an experiment in real time—that allow individuals in both clinical and private environments to directly alter their own neural activity for treatment of certain neurological conditions or the augmentation of cognition, creativity, or motor skills (Sitaram et al. 2017; Zrenner et al. 2016).

It could be equally humbling to learn that we apparently owe our uniquely complex brain to two genetic events that occurred 2–3 million years ago: (1) a partial replication of the *ARHGAP11A* gene that occurred after our ancestors diverged from *Pan troglodytes* (chimpanzees) but before diverging from *Homo neanderthalensis* (Neanderthals)—as shown in Figure 6.1—that resulted in the *ARHGAP11B* gene, which is linked to the brain's neocortical expansion and increased folding (Florio et al. 2015, 2016) that increased human brain volume by more than a factor of 3 (Vallender et al. 2008); and (2) a set of genes (*SRGAP2*, *FOXP2*, and others) that may have determined changes in both neural connectivity and the shape of our skull (and thereby our brains), giving rise to our unique cognitive and linguistic capabilities (Benítez-Burraco and Boeckx 2015). The result bestowed *Homo sapiens* with an increasingly sophisticated ability to imagine, articulate, and construct dramatically more complex, robust, and precise tools.

While we are not the only species that utilize or modify objects for specific purposes (Seed et al. 2010), evidence of our unique drive and distinctive ability to repair and enhance ourselves by devising prosthetics dates back millennia (Finch 2011): Examples include an Egyptian wood-and-leather hallux, or big toe (950–71 BC); the first prosthetic leg (~300 BC)—below-the-knee, fashioned from bronze and iron around a wood core—found in the Roman city Capua (Bliquez 1996); and the

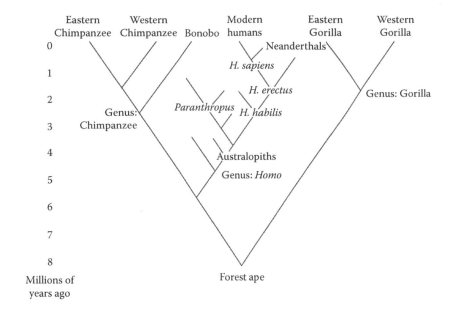

**FIGURE 6.1**   Human phylogeny. (Stephen Stearns & Rolf Hoekstra, *Evolution: An Introduction, 2nd edition*, 2005, Figure 19.1, p. 481, by permission of Oxford University Press.)

Roman General Marcus Sergius' iron right hand made during the Second Punic War (218–201 BC) (Rackham et al. 1958). Further breakthroughs did not emerge until the early 1500s with Dr. Ambroise Paré's hinged prosthetic hand and locking knee joint prosthetic leg (Thurston 2007), followed over 300 years later by a prosthetic leg with hinged joints at the knee and ankle designed and later sold by James Hanger (Lively 2013).

Perhaps surprisingly, the earliest known neural treatment modality was practiced in Antiquity as well: During the years 332 BC–395 AD, the ancient Greeks and Romans used the "invisible and seemingly magical powers of electricity" by applying shocks from electric fish to treat pain (Loeb 2011). Centuries later, the first recorded event of an electrical device—in this case, the use of a Leyden jar in 1755 by Charles Leroy as a basic ocular prosthesis—resulted in a blind patient briefly seeing a bright visual artifact when the Leyden jar was discharged (LeRoy 1755). The Leyden jar, in turn, gave way to electrostatic electricity produced by frictional machines, the first of which was constructed by Otto von Guericke in 1650) by the mid-1800s.

In the 1790s, Alessandro Volta (who developed the electric battery in 1800) connected metal probes to a 50-V source and inserted them into his ears. Upon switching the probes on, he reported an auditory sensation, described variously as "boiling soup" or "a boom within the head (American Speech-Language-Hearing Association 2004; Henkel 2013), and alternatively "The disagreeable sensation, which I apprehended being dangerous, of shock in the brain, prevented me from repeating the experiment" (Mudry and Mills 2013; Volta 1800). In 1867, Duchenne De Boulogne studied the use of electrical stimulation to restore movement to paralyzed limbs (Duchenne 1867; Parent 2014).

Ocular prosthetics are another matter: From their earliest known uses in 2900–2800 BC Iran and fifth century BC Rome and Egypt until the recent advent of functional ocular neuroprosthetics, their purpose has been aesthetic (and in Antiquity, often religious or symbolic) rather than the restoration of vision (Pine et al. 2016; Bowden et al., ongoing research).

## 6.3   CURRENT NEUROPROSTHETICS

In the early 1960s, the availability of transistors (Haviland 2002) resulted in a small number of neuroprosthetic implants by allowing portable electrical stimulation devices designed to activate muscles—the first being a stimulator with surface electrodes that counteracted foot drop (difficulty in lifting the front part of the foot and toes due to a muscular weakness or paralysis) by activating the peroneal nerve (Liberson et al. 1961). In addition, radio-frequency–controlled stimulators of the detrusor muscle of the bladder were implanted in small numbers of patients in the 1960s (Bradley et al. 1963; Stenberg et al. 1967). While bladder dysfunction is still treated with electric stimulation, modalities have become much more diverse (Jezernik et al. 2002). Small numbers of peroneal nerve stimulators to counteract hemiplegic foot drop were also implanted in the 1970s and 1980s (Jeglic et al. 1970; Strojnik et al. 1987; Waters et al. 1975).

The past two decades have seen increasing prosthetic innovation and diversity in design, biomimetic functionality (that which is based on or imitates biological structure and/or function), and advanced technology (see Chapter 1 [by Nam et al., "Brain–Computer Interface: An Emerging Interaction Technology"] and Chapter 37 [by Mikhail A. Lebedev and Alexei Ossadtchi, "Bidirectional Neural Interfaces"]). This trend continues to accelerate (DesignNews Design Hardware & Software Staff 2015), such that at this point in our scientific and technological evolution, researchers are investigating the final physiological frontier: the brain itself.

At the nexus of this challenging endeavor is the rapidly growing field of neuroengineering (also referred to as neural engineering)—a subset of biomedical engineering, which blends biology, medicine, and engineering. Neuroengineering, in turn, integrates neuroscience and biomedical engineering to produce neuroprosthetics—a driving force in BCI research and development that has been defined as a technological device integrated into the neural circuitry of a human being can be sensory, motor, or cognitive in nature (Lebedev 2014).

A profound and remarkable prosthetic technology, neuroprosthetics not only address neurological and neurologically related disorders (including Alzheimer's disease, Parkinson's disease, epilepsy, traumatic brain injury, profound depression, neurocardiac conditions, and urological illnesses) but also directly restore and augment sensory, motor, and—in what may well be our ultimate neuroprosthetic challenge and achievement—memory, cognition, and volition (see Section 6.3.4 and Chapter 4 [by Christoph Guger et al., "Brain–Computer Interfaces for Motor Rehabilitation, Assessment of Consciousness, and Communication"], Chapter 28 [by Mehdi Ordikhani-Seyedlar and Mikhail A. Lebedev, "Augmenting Attention with Brain–Computer Interfaces"], and Chapter 5 [by Dennis J. McFarland, "Therapeutic Applications of BCI Technologies"]).

### 6.3.1 Neurological and Neurologically Related Disorders

Deep brain stimulation (DBS)—the application of implantable electrical stimulation devices to treat neurological disorders (Coffey 2009)—is acknowledged to safely and effectively treat a range of symptomologies, including Parkinson's disease, dystonia, essential tremor, and (to varying degrees) other movement disorders (Gross and Lozano 2000), Alzheimer's disease (Scharre et al. 2016), epilepsy (Velasco et al. 2001), treatment-resistant obsessive–compulsive disorder (Mantione et al. 2010), intractable major depression (Mayberg et al. 2005), and other mood disorders (Downar and Daskalakis 2013). Moreover, DBS has been studied as a modality for treating chronic pain (Coffey 2001), Tourette syndrome (Kaido et al. 2011; Wårdell et al. 2015), hypertension (Das 2010), ischemic stroke (Buttaro 2012), anorexia nervosa (Lipsman et al. 2013), and addiction disorders (Müller et al. 2013).

### 6.3.2 Motor Control and Movement

Before the advent of DBS, movement disorders were treated with oral medication, physical therapy, and botulinum toxin injections. However, despite being more invasive, DBS therapy showed significantly improved physical symptoms. The subsequent introduction of feedback control theory (Todorov and Jordan 2002) provided closed-loop systems that improved Parkinson's disease symptomology management by incorporating the variable aspects of neurological movement disorders—and in a further advance, a noninvasive closed-loop framework based on force neuro-feedback suggests the possibility of personalized neurological rehabilitation (Broccard et al. 2014). Moreover, BCIs can be enhanced with artificial somatosensory feedback directed primarily to the brain's cerebellum—which regulates movement and muscular coordination—through either intra-cortical microstimulation (repetitive microelectrode application of an electrical current to stimulate a small population of neurons) or optogenetics, the use of light to modulate *in vivo* molecular events via genetically encoded proteins that respond to light by changing conformation, thereby altering cell behavior (Pastrana 2011). Scientists already envision multidisciplinary BCI research that will lead to the creation of whole-body neural prosthetic devices capable of providing paralyzed patients with fully restored mobility (Lebedev et al. 2011).

In research and development starting in the 1960s, successful but limited motor prosthetics that electrically activate skeletal muscle in order to restore paralyzed limbs with basic movement have generated demand for more sophisticated devices. In pursuing the development of neuroprosthetics to restore greater mobility and functionality to patients with spinal trauma, several avenues that seek to make use of reflexes, pattern generators, and other functional *in vivo* spinal neural pathways are being followed (Barbeau et al. 1999).

By assisting or restoring legged mobility and providing ancillary health benefits, powered exo-skeletons have increased (and promise to continue increasing) quality of life for those with spinal cord injury and its consequent lower-body paralysis or weakened legs. However, a recent litera-ture review discovered that despite significant benefits, patients using powered exoskeletons evi-denced injuries to the tenth thoracic vertebra (T10)—located in a spinal cord section vulnerable to injury—in 45.4% of the studies researched, nearly two-thirds of which were associated with gait and ambulation. In addition to improved patient selection and training criteria and safety, benefits, and usability metrics, the reviewers recommended multimodal gait intention detection systems and real-time monitoring and diagnostic capabilities (Contreras-Vidal et al. 2016).

A factor limiting neuroprosthetic utility is the absence of lifelong central nervous system neural stimulation. Toward that end, wireless multi-electrode arrays will eliminate wire interconnects, thereby extending implant longevity as well as preventing chronic tissue reactions. One candidate could be a submillimeter-size intraspinal single-channel passive microstimulator that might be pow-ered by optical, acoustic, or electromagnetic waves (Sahin and Pikov 2011)—a concept related to neural dust and similar systems (see Section 6.4).

In a proof-of-principle wireless neuroprosthetics technology study, rhesus monkeys with a spinal lesion were implanted with a wireless brain–spine interface in the leg locus of their motor cortex along with a lumbar spinal cord stimulator. Weight-bearing locomotion of the paralyzed leg was restored in 6 days post-lesion without training, suggesting the viability of applying this type of neu-roprosthetic to individuals with spinal cord injuries (Capogrosso et al. 2016).

### 6.3.3 Sensory Neuroprosthetics

Currently, most neuroprosthetics research and development efforts are focused on the auditory, ocu-lar, and haptic (touch) senses, with increasing interest in proprioception (awareness of bodily posi-tion) (Chhatbar 2009), sensorimotor (Hayashibe et al. 2015), real-time closed-loop systems (Herron et al. 2015), and cognitive restoration and augmentation (Serruya and Kahana 2008).

#### 6.3.3.1 Auditory

In 1957, Charles Eyriès implanted the first neuroprosthetic to stimulate the auditory nerve directly via a single electrode—designed by André Djourno—into a patient's temporalis (a muscle involved in mastication), with the results allowing sound perception but not speech comprehension (Eisen 2003). Four years later, William House and John Doyle surgically implanted a single-electrode gold neuroprosthetic in the cochleae of several patients, enabling limited word recognition (Henkel 2013). In 1964, F. Blair Simmons' six-electrode device (McGee 1965) demonstrated that multiple stimulation sites permitted pitch discrimination (but not speech comprehension). The first single-electrode cochlear implant was placed on the market in 1969 when House implanted a five-electrode system in three patients (Henkel 2013).

The field of cochlear (the cochlea is the inner ear organ providing hearing) implants is now well established, allowing auditory research to investigate DBS (Buell et al. 2015); speech processing (Jeyalakshmi et al. 2010); neural plasticity (the brain's abilities to self-(re)organize after trauma or environmental changes) (Grosse-Wentru et al. 2011); and various neuroprosthetic categories, including midbrain, brainstem, and thalamic implants (Atencio et al. 2014; Shannon 2014).

### 6.3.3.2 Ocular

Macular degeneration—associated with age and largely affecting those over 55—is caused by a combination of genetic and environmental factors that damage central retinal photoreceptors. Macular degeneration is the leading cause of severe loss of vision (but rarely blindness, although those with advanced macular degeneration are considered legally blind). Affecting more than 10 million individuals in the United States, macular degeneration is at this time incurable (American Macular Degeneration Foundation).

While neuroprosthetics using metallic electrodes, optical stimulation, conducting polymer and quantum dot films (sheets of nanoscale semiconductor particles), and optogenetics have made inroads into restoring vision to some degree, they face challenges that limit their efficacy. However, combining semiconductor nanorods and carbon nanotubes produced a novel wire-free, light-induced retina stimulation platform with a three-dimensional biomimetic optoelectrical interface. Stimulating a light-insensitive chick retina was successful, suggesting that the new platform may ultimately serve as an artificial retina (Bareket et al. 2014).

While rare, retinitis pigmentosa—a genetically inherited condition that causes progressive loss of vision that leads to blindness as a result of the loss of retinal photoreceptors—is incurable and (other than measures that slow the disease's progression, such as wearing ultraviolet-blocking sunglasses) untreatable. That said, restoring vision to blind or profoundly vision-impaired patients is an ongoing challenge being pursued by a range of investigations and clinical trials with retinal prostheses, gene therapy, fetal retinal cells, and other protocols. In one such effort, six legally blind retinitis pigmentosa patients received a wireless intraocular retinal implant that stimulated their retinal ganglion cells for 4 weeks. All patients reported having visual sensations—even with low levels of stimulation—and there were no surgical complications (Koch et al. 2008).

An alternate study selected a suprachoroidal implant location (illustrated in Figure 6.2), hypothesizing that doing so would allow patients with end-stage retinitis pigmentosa to both maintain preoperative residual vision and acquire prosthetic vision in a context of significant surgical and safety benefits. An associated first-in-human Phase 1 trial investigated the use of suprachoroidal retinal implants in three end-stage retinitis pigmentosa subjects, finding that the surgical approach was successful, with a 12-month period of postoperative efficacy showing potential for vision restoration (Ayton et al. 2014).

Another innovative approach used a Second Sight Argus II System—the first retinal implant for adults with advanced retinitis pigmentosa approved by the US Food and Drug Administration (FDA Press Release 2013)—that includes an electrode array prosthesis, glasses fitted with a miniature video camera, and a wearable computer. Real-time letter recognition software recognized text, converted it into the corresponding Braille letters, determined the stimulation current of each electrode in the identified text, and activated simulating visual percepts of individual Braille letters and words that subjects could then read (Lauritzen et al. 2012).

A 2006 clinical trial investigated Argus II safety and efficacy in restoring visual function to 30 blind end-stage retinitis pigmentosa patients (Ho et al. 2015). Five years after receiving the implant, 24 subjects remained functionally implanted with significantly better performance on all visual function tests and tasks (da Cruz et al. 2016).

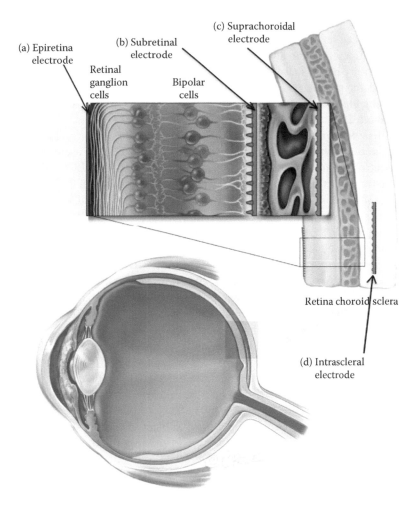

**FIGURE 6.2**  Suprachoroidal implant location. Potential anatomical locations for retinal prosthesis implantation: To date, clinical trials have been performed with devices in the (a) epiretinal position (Humayun et al. 2012), (b) subretinal space (Zrenner et al. 2011), and (c) intrascleral space (Fujikado et al. 2011). (From Ayton L.N. et al. 2014. First-in-human trial of a novel suprachoroidal retinal prosthesis. *PLoS ONE* 9(12):e115239. Creative Commons license CC BY 4.0, https://creativecommons.org/licenses/by/4.0/legalcode.)

In a pioneering blend of nanotechnology and optogenetics, researchers targeting age-related macular degeneration achieved wire-free, light-induced retina stimulation by employing a platform based on semiconductor nanorod-carbon nanotubes (which have also been studied for energy-harvesting and light-emitting applications). Their successful stimulation of a light-insensitive chick retina suggests the potential use of this novel platform in future artificial retinal applications (Bareket et al. 2014).

### 6.3.3.3  Somatosensory

The multimodal somatosensory system, which plays a perpetual and ubiquitous role in providing a range of essential bodily and environmental information—touch, pressure, pain, tickle, itch, vibration, temperature, proprioception, and bodily movement (kinesthesis), all of which interact (Rincon-Gonzalez et al. 2011)—differs from sight, hearing, taste, and smell in not being mediated by a specifically located sense organ. Since disease, trauma, and amputation can reduce or eliminate somatosensory sensation, research is pursuing the capacity to restore somatosensory awareness with neuroprosthetics.

Although two significant neuroprosthetic innovations emerged between 2000 and 2015—anthropomorphic (i.e., having human characteristics) robotic limbs implementing many primary features and functions of their human counterpart, and an improved algorithmic capability to decode brain activity-based movement intention—the haptic and proprioception somatosensory feedback needed for precise object manipulation remained. However, the situation is changing, with an increasing ability to induce relevant tactile sensations by stimulating somatosensory cortex neurons (Bensmaia 2015).

While BCI has been proposed for motor neurorehabilitation, motor replacement, and assistive technologies, the question of proprioceptive feedback affecting brain oscillation regulation—and thereby BCI control—remains open. To that end, investigators coupled BCI and online robotic hand exoskeleton for finger flexion and extension, testing the performance of 24 healthy participants on five different hand closing and opening tasks (motor imagery with and without movement and/or feedback, and passive/active hand movement). The tests showed that the proprioceptive and visual feedback (feeling and seeing the hand move, respectively) significantly improved BCI performance by closing the loop between brain, movement, and proprioception (Ramos-Murguialday et al. 2012).

In another study, pressure was directly converted into digital frequency signals using a skin-inspired mechanoreceptor with a low-power flexible organic transistor circuit. Results with mouse somatosensory neurons suggest the device's potential in designing large-area organic electronic skins with neural-integrated touch feedback for replacement limbs (Tee et al. 2015). Although replicating the mechanical and functional properties of skin remains an evasive goal, flexible electronics—the ability to create complex circuits on soft substrates, including stretchable and flexible, wearable, and epidermal sensors—is gaining momentum, due in part to developments in microcontact printing, inkjet deposition, and organic electronics (Anikeeva and Koppes 2015).

After implanting microelectrode arrays into the somatosensory cortex of an individual paralyzed by spinal cord trauma (Flesher et al. 2016), the electrodes generated microstimulation that was shown to generate tactile sensations reported by subject as taking place on his hand. Moreover, the patient experienced varying levels of pressure in relation to stimulus amplitude, suggesting the possibility that the neurotechnology reported could allow those with paralysis, amputations, or stroke could interact with objects through a system comprising a robotic hand and intracortical microstimulation neuroprosthesis (see Chapter 14 [by Melissa M. Smith et al., "Utilizing Subdermal Electrodes as a Noninvasive Alternative for Motor-Based BCIs"] and Chapter 15 [by Philip R. Kennedy et al., "Validation of Neurotrophic Electrode Long-Term Recordings in Human Cortex"]).

As depicted in Figure 6.3, timing patterns of neural action potentials, or spikes—in which the electrical membrane potential of a cell rapidly rises and falls, and propagates along neuronal connective fibers—have recently been found to have a significant impact on motor control in songbird respiration. The study, which integrated physiology, behavior, and computation, demonstrated that precise spike timing (rather than just the number of spikes, as had been thought) is also fundamental in motor behavior—suggesting that spike timing patterns may have significant relevance to neuroprosthetic and BCI design (Srivastava et al. 2017).

### 6.3.4 Memory, Cognition, and Volition

The hippocampus converts short-term memory to long-term memory in a process involving recoding sensory input and neural coding patterns. Therefore, the ability to form long-term, or episodic, memories can be diminished or eradicated if the hippocampus is damaged as a result of physical trauma, or is otherwise compromised by, for example, the brain receiving inadequate oxygen, certain forms of epilepsy, or neural tissue inflammation. However, in a significant demonstration of what neuroprosthetics can achieve, a neuroprosthesis based on hippocampal structure and function has been previously shown to effectively restore the ability to form long-term memory in laboratory

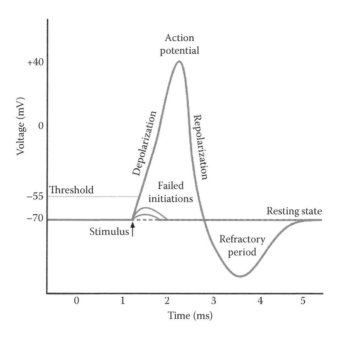

**FIGURE 6.3** Neuronal action potential. Approximate plot of a typical action potential shows its various phases as the action potential passes a point on a cell membrane. The membrane potential starts out at −70 mV at time zero. A stimulus is applied at time = 1 ms, which raises the membrane potential above −55 mV (the threshold potential). After the stimulus is applied, the membrane potential rapidly rises to a peak potential of +40 mV at time = 2 ms. Just as quickly, the potential then drops and overshoots to −90 mV at time = 3 ms, and finally the resting potential of −70 mV is reestablished at time = 5 ms. (From Wikimedia Commons. Original by en:User:Chris 73, updated by en:User:Diberri, converted to SVG by tiZom. Permission granted under the GNU Free Documentation License. Licensed under the Creative Commons Attribution-Share Alike 3.0 Unported [CC BY-SA 3.0], https://creativecommons.org/licenses/by-sa/3.0/legalcode.)

rats (Berger et al. 2011)—and subsequently demonstrated both the first successful neuroprosthesis to enhance and/or repair memory encoding in primates (Hampson et al. 2013) and, ultimately, a successful USC/DARPA trial with human patients suffering from trauma-induced hippocampal dysfunction (Reardon 2015) that led to the start-up company Kernel (kernel.co) being founded to commercialize the hippocampal prosthesis.

In a study of disrupted cognitive function (i.e., coordinating attention, decision making, and movement selection), a neuroprosthesis was used to record and analyze activity in nonhuman primate prefrontal cortex minicolumns—vertically oriented columnar groupings of interconnected networks of neurons (Casanova 2010; Opris and Casanova 2014; Schwalger et al. 2017). The recorded minicolumnar activation patterns were then replicated, demonstrating a potential protocol for restoring or repairing diminished cognitive function in humans (Hampson et al. 2012). The authors concluded that their study demonstrated "the first successful application of neuroprosthesis in the primate brain designed specifically to restore or repair the disrupted cognitive function." Two remarkable findings in rat study were as follows: (1) the unexpected ability to identify the sensory input from the associated the neural spike timing pattern encoded in the hippocampal neuroprosthesis, and (2) by transferring the VLSI device from a subject that had learned the task to one that had not, the latter subject demonstrating a functional (albeit degraded) nonexperiential memory of the task (Berger 2013).

This signal invariance across subjects (Liu et al. 2005) may also prove valuable to the elusive goal of identifying and understanding what is sometimes referred to the brain's internal language.

Specifically, in investigating the hippocampal encoding of episodic information, it had previously been found that categorically and hierarchically organized functional coding units, or *neural cliques*, countered individual cell response variability through collective cospiking, thereby generating robust real-time encoding. A previous paper (Lin et al. 2006) concludes that converting neural clique activation patterns to binary codes would allow universal categorizations of internal brain representations across individuals and species.

Using fMRI and a *de novo* natural language processing method, a recent investigation into the neural representation of narrative comprehension translated the same story into English, Mandarin, and Farsi, and presented the translations to native speakers of each language. The results showed that the neural representations imaged from a subject reading a given story identified that story in all translated languages. The researchers conclude that their findings demonstrate cross-linguistic invariance and the ability to use fMRI to predict the neural representations of unread narratives (Dehghani et al. 2017).

## 6.4  MICROSCALE BRAIN–COMPUTER INTERFACES

As shown in Table 6.1, despite recent advances in neuroprosthetics technology, a number of significant challenges—several of which are based on the response of neural tissue to implantation—await resolution (also see Chapter 29 [by Ilsun Rhiu et al., "Toward a Usability Evaluation for Brain–Computer Interfaces"] and Chapter 33 [by Md Rakibul Mowla et al., "Evaluation and Performance Assessment of Brain–Computer Interface System"]).

There are four primary challenges when considering the development of a wireless neural recording neuroprosthetic: three of the issues listed in Table 6.1—implant longevity, micromotion,

### TABLE 6.1
### Neuroprosthetics Challenges

| Factor | Challenges |
|---|---|
| Assessment improvements | Model systems |
| | Therapeutic strategies |
| | Quantitative metrics |
| Biological response initiator | CNS injury |
| | Neuroprosthetic devices that rely on implant type, location, and other factors |
| Developmental and cancer biology insights | Novel mechanisms to influence neuroprosthetic implant CNS response |
| Device design | Device/CNS cellular and molecular interface |
| | Minimized device micromotion |
| | CNS tissue mechanics in biomimetic materials |
| | Neuroprosthetics/tissue engineering/neurobiology intersection |
| Implant longevity | Long term |
| Multifactorial approaches | Drug delivery |
| | Patterning technologies |
| Tissue-mimetic model systems | Testbeds with greater physiological relevance and complexity |
| | Synergistic with animal studies |
| | Rapid identification of promising device technologies |

*Source:* Based on Leach, J.B., A.K.H. Achyuta, and S.K. Murthy. 2010. Bridging the divide between neuroprosthetic design, tissue engineering and neurobiology. *Frontiers in Neuroengineering* 2:18. Creative Commons license CC BY 4.0 (https://creativecommons.org/licenses/by/4.0/legalcode).

and CNS tissue mechanics—as well as high power requirements. Neural dust (Seo et al. 2013, 2016) is a DARPA-funded (DARPA 2016) novel implant design utilizing thousands of 10- to 100-μm independent free-floating sensor nodes that detect extracellular electrophysiological data without requiring batteries for power or communications. In addition to low-power CMOS (complementary metal-oxide semiconductor) circuits, neural dust employs ultrasonic power transmission (Arra et al. 2007) and radio-frequency–based ambient backscatter communications (Liu et al. 2013). The neural dust acquires, records, and transmits data electromyogram and electroneurogram—muscular and neuronal electrical activity, respectively—to a subdural (see Figure 6.4) transceiver implant that also provides power and communications. In conjunction with a transceiver, an external transducer is affixed to the skull surface to provide both subdural and long-range external communications (see Figure 6.5).

The in-development Free-Floating Wireless Neural Interface Wireless Implantable Neural Recording (FF-WINeR) neural recording probe also uses untethered millimeter-sized implants, citing neural tissue damage due to tethered neuroprosthesis motion—an issue associated with the current generation of invasive neuroprosthetics. Unlike neural dust, however, FF-WINeR will be powered by an electromagnetic near field (Girard et al. 2000) using magnetic resonance (Kiani and Ghovanloo 2012), the reason cited being that ultrasound induces attenuation in bone, which significantly constrains this type of BCI in terms of design, size, efficiency, and complexity (Yeon et al. 2016).

Another research effort investigating millimeter-size BCI neuroprosthetics is a first proof-of-concept 4 mm × 7.8 mm implant using ultrasonic power transfer and a hybrid (ultrasonic downlink and radio-frequency uplink) bidirectional data communication link (Charthad et al. 2015).

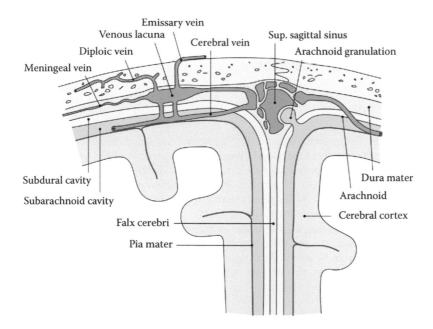

**FIGURE 6.4** Subdural cavity. Diagrammatic representation of a section across the top of the skull, showing the membranes of the brain, etc. ("Subdural cavity" visible at left.) May 30, 2010. (From Wikimedia Commons. Made by Mysid Inkscape, based on plate 769 from Gray's Anatomy [1918, public domain].)

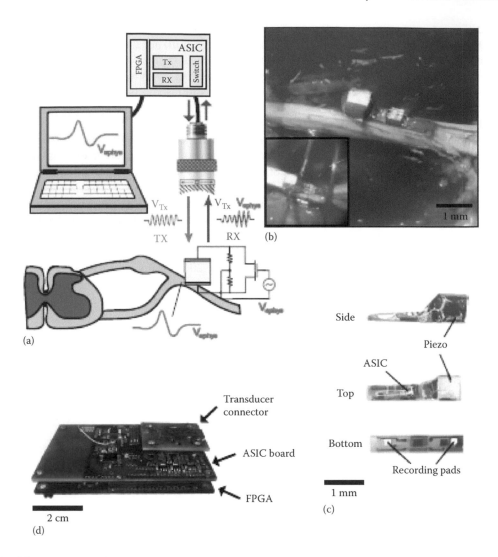

**FIGURE 6.5** Neural dust system overview. (a) An external transducer powers and communicates with a neural dust mote placed remotely in the body. Driven by a custom transceiver board, the transducer alternates between transmitting a series of pulses that power the device and listening for reflected pulses that are modulated by electrophysiological signals. (b) A neural dust mote anchored to the sciatic nerve in an anesthetized rat. Inset shows neural dust mote with optional testing leads. (c) Components of a neural dust mote. The devices were assembled on a flexible PCB and consist of a piezoelectric crystal, a single custom transistor, and a pair of recording electrodes. (d) The transceiver board consisted of an Opal Kelly FPGA board, an application-specific integrated circuit (ASIC) board (Seo et al. 2015; Tang et al. 2015), and the transducer connector board. (Reprinted from *Neuron* 91(3), Dongjin Seo et al., Wireless recording in the peripheral nervous system with ultrasonic neural dust, 529–39, 2016, with permission from Elsevier.)

## 6.5 FUTURE NEUROPROSTHETICS

A significant trend in science and technology is the progression of independent disciplines becoming multidisciplinary (draws on knowledge from different disciplines but stays within their boundaries), interdisciplinary (analyzes, synthesizes, and harmonizes links between disciplines into a coordinated and coherent whole), and ultimately transdisciplinary (integrates the natural, social, and health sciences in a humanities context, and transcends their traditional boundaries) (Choi and Pak 2006). This in-process transition is notably pronounced in the convergence of life sciences, physical sciences, and engineering (National Research Council 2014), and so encompasses neuroprosthetics.

### 6.5.1 INTELLIGENT, BIOMIMETIC, AND NEUROBIOHYBRID NEUROPROSTHETICS

Exocortical cognition (ECC) is a transdisciplinary framework designed to augment human cognition, enhance memory, and increase sensorimotor abilities. Moreover, ECC would reduce or eliminate the often-debated likelihood of an emergent cognitive gap between human and a future human-analogous Artificial General Intelligence (AGI) (Dambrot 2017).

A related concept, neurobiohybrids are a proposed future technology in which the biological brain interfaces with brain-inspired biomimetic devices, the purpose being to ensure efficient communications between living and *in vivo* artificial systems. The authors note that one consequence of their scenario is the availability of intelligent neuroprostheses that augment brain function and provide *de novo* therapeutic solutions (Vassanelli and Mahmud 2016).

### 6.5.2 NANOBIOTECHNOLOGY

A recently established discipline, nanobiotechnology—a convergence of nanotechnology and biotechnology in which tools from nanotechnology are developed and applied to study biological phenomena (e.g., nanoparticle sensors, probes, or biomolecule delivery vehicles in cellular systems)—is emerging as a source of next-generation neuroprosthetic modalities. Two of a wide range of proposed nanobiotechnology translational applications—nanoneurology, such as the use of nanoelectrodes in neurophysiology, and nano-ophthalmology—fall within the field of neuroprosthetics (Jain 2012).

There are a number of nanobiotechnology research investigations being published in peer-reviewed journals. For example, one such study (Blank et al. 2017) reports the use of engineered nanoparticles to deliver, deposit, and induce cellular uptake at a specific site (Yameen et al. 2014) to modulate pulmonary immune responses.

### 6.5.3 SYNTHETIC BIOLOGY

By designing, synthesizing, and assembling a computer-designed genome, and transplanting it into a recipient cell, researchers at the J. Craig Venter Institute created the first viable, self-replicating artificial organism in the form of a bacterium. Moreover, the bacterium's viability suggests that future research may allow synthesized genomes with preprogrammed functions to be digitally stored and expressed when required (Ahmad and Collins 2010; Gibson et al. 2010).

In addition, current studies in emergence, biologically inspired cognitive architecture, and related areas suggest that synthetic biology may elucidate cognitive processes, while AI/AGI may identify avenues of synthetic biology research that might redefine the borders of what is now considered, for example, natural and artificial (Bianchini 2016).

### 6.5.4 BIONANOPROTONICS

Memristors and memristive nanodevices—biocompatible solid-state devices that could potentially serve as both neuroprosthetic and artificial neuron—act as electrical resistance switches that, based on applied voltage and current history, can retain an internal resistance state (Yang et al. 2013). In so doing, they represent a new class of biocompatible synaptic-like solid-state devices that can control and monitor the flow of protonic current, thereby representing a step toward bionanoprotonics (Zhong et al. 2011).

## 6.6   INVASIVE VERSUS NONINVASIVE NEUROPROSTHETICS

While neuroprostheses can be classified as either invasive or noninvasive (see Chapter 2 [by Mark Wronkiewicz et al., "Facilitating the Integration of Modern Neuroscience into Noninvasive BCIs"]) depending on whether or not they penetrate the skin, their results are not identical despite measuring the same neural signals (Steyrl et al. 2016). Moreover, what is considered invasive is not consistently defined, an example being a European Space Agency report's broad definition stating that long-lived chemicals, radioactive particles, and electromagnetic energy (including infrared light) deposited on subepidermal tissue (i.e., just below the skin) could be categorized as invasive (Tonet et al. 2017).

A number of factors can conspire to form a negative bias toward invasive neuroprosthesis—even if the procedure in question is to be safe and more effective than its noninvasive counterpart (Blabe et al. 2015). Moreover, even with a favorable outcome expected, the neurosurgery was rejected as an alternative (Collinger et al. 2013). However, this is understandable given that technological and other issues are still being investigated and that intracranial neuroprosthetic implantation has only recently entered the mainstream as an approved modality for certain medical conditions. That said, once these challenges are met, invasive neuroprosthetics are likely to be preferred—especially in cases of motor function restoration (Waldert 2016).

## 6.7   SECURITY AND STANDARDS

### 6.7.1   Information Security

Information security, or InfoSec, has been defined as "The protection of information and information systems from unauthorized access, use, disclosure, disruption, modification, or destruction in order to provide confidentiality, integrity, and availability" (NIST SP 800-53 Rev. 4, 2013). For some observers, this takes on added meaning when being applied to intracortically implanted neuroprosthetics, in that the neuroprosthetic might at some point compromise the implanted person's neural environment and allow what might be termed biohacking, where physiological cognitive information may be not only accessed but modified (Gladden 2015; also see Chapter 34 [by Eran Klein and Alan Rubel, "Privacy and Ethics in Brain–Computer Interface Research"]).

### 6.7.2   Standards

While standards are relevant in all fields, they are critical in surgery and long-term implantation. In the latter case, a number of factors—biocompatibility, cognitive and sensorimotor modification, and prosthetic movement/stability, to name a few—are especially significant in biomedical engineering, neuroengineering, and neuroprosthetics. In addition, socioeconomic factors such as equal access to and affordability of neuroprosthetics are a humanitarian consideration.

## 6.8   CONCLUSION

Our self-named species, *H. sapiens* (from the Latin for *wise man*), has transformed our world and ourselves by virtue of a few genetic mutations that generated rapid changes in our brain's size, shape, and complexity. These events resulted in several abilities that set us apart from our closest nonhuman relatives, including uniquely sophisticated spoken and written languages and the curiosity and drive to investigate and understand what we perceive, which led to science and the scientific method, mathematics, and—the topic of this paper—an ability to imagine and create increasingly complex and powerful tools that have ultimately allowed us to investigate, understand, repair, and enhance the brain that made the neuroprosthetics and BCIs to do so possible. Over the next few years and certainly decades, the tools we devise and implement will allow us to increase that understanding.

There is, however, a caveat: In other ways, we have not evolved to the same degree. Our evolutionary neurobiology of our earlier-developed brain structures makes us an often-aggressive species with a hierarchical social structure and a powerful in-group/outgroup dynamic (Bos et al. 2004; Fu et al. 2012; Hewstone et al. 2002). When coupled with our toolmaking capabilities, these qualities have given us the ability to create technologies powerful enough to bring an end to not just ourselves, but with a few exceptions all other Terran lifeforms.

The hope is that BCI, neuroprosthetic, and coming generations of neuroengineering technologies will help us understand ourselves at a deeper level and thereby realize that we have the capability to envision and create a positive, constructive future.

## REFERENCES

44 U.S.C., Sec. 3542. 2013. Cited in NIST SP 800-53 Rev. 4:B-10.

Ahmad, S.K. and J.J. Collins. 2010. Synthetic biology: Applications come of age. *Nature Reviews Genetics* 11:367–379.

American Speech-Language-Hearing Association. 2004. *Cochlear Implants.* Working Group on Cochlear Implants Technical Report. Available from asha.org/policy.

Anikeeva, P. and R.A. Koppes. 2015. Restoring the sense of touch. *Science* 350(6258):274–275.

Arra, S., J. Leskinen, J. Heikkila, and J. Vanhala. 2007. *Ultrasonic Power and Data Link for Wireless Implantable Applications.* 2nd International Symposium on Wireless Pervasive Computing.

Atencio, C.A., J.Y. Shih, C.E. Schreiner, and S.W. Cheung. 2014. Primary auditory cortical responses to electrical stimulation of the thalamus. *Journal of Neurophysiology* 111(5):1077–1087.

Ayton, L.N. et al. 2014. First-in-human trial of a novel suprachoroidal retinal prosthesis. *PLoS ONE* 9(12):e115239.

Barbeau, H., D. McCrea, M. O'Donovan, S. Rossignol, W. Grill, and M. Lemay. 1999. Tapping into spinal circuits to restore motor function. *Brain Research Reviews* 30(1):27–51.

Bareket, L. et al. 2014. Semiconductor nanorod–carbon nanotube biomimetic films for wire-free photostimulation of blind retinas. *Nano Letters* 14(11):6685–6692.

Benítez-Burraco, A. and C. Boeckx. 2015. Possible functional links among brain- and skull-related genes selected in modern humans. *Frontiers in Psychology* 6:794.

Bensmaia, S.J. 2015. Biological and bionic hands: Natural neural coding and artificial perception. *Philosophical Transactions of the Royal Society B* 370(1677).

Berger, T.W. et al. 2011. A cortical neural prosthesis for restoring and enhancing memory. *J. Neural Engineering* 8:046017.

Berger, T.W. 2013. *Engineering Memories: A Cognitive Neural Prosthesis for Restoring and Enhancing Memory Function.* Presentation at GF2045 Conference, New York City.

Bianchini, F. 2016. Artificial intelligence and synthetic biology: A tri-temporal contribution. *Biosystems* 148:32–39.

Blabe, C.H., V. Gilja, C.A. Chestek, K.V. Shenoy, K.D. Anderson, and J.M. Henderson. 2015. Assessment of brain–machine interfaces from the perspective of people with paralysis. *Journal of Neural Engineering* 12:043002.

Blank, F. et al. 2017. Interaction of biomedical nanoparticles with the pulmonary immune system. *Journal of Nanobiotechnology* 15:6.

Bliquez, L.J. 1996. Prosthetics in classical antiquity: Greek, Etruscan, and Roman prosthetics. In *Aufstieg und Niedergang der römischen Welt. Teil II*: ed. Haase, Wolfgang; Temproini, Hildegard. 37.3:2640–2676. Principat, Berlin/New York: De Gruyter.

Bos, N., N.S. Shami, J.S. Olson, A. Cheshin, and N. Nan. 2004. In-group/out-group effects in distributed teams: An experimental simulation. Proceedings of the 2004 ACM conference on Computer supported cooperative work. Chicago: ACM Press 429–436.

Bowden, T., R. Brammar, J.D. Salt, E. Franks, A. Grayer, and C. Haylock. Ongoing research. *The MusEYEum Artificial Eyes Gallery.* The College of Optometrists, London, UK.

Bradley, W.E., S.N. Chou, and L.A. French. 1963. Further experience with radio transmitter receiver unit for the neurogenic bladder. *Neurosurgery* 20:953–960.

Broccard, F.D., T. Mullen, Y.M. Chi et al. 2014. Closed loop brain machine–body interfaces for noninvasive rehabilitation of movement disorders. *Annals of Biomedical Engineering* 42(8):1573–93.

Buell, T.J., A. Ksendzovsky, B.B. Shah, B.W. Kesser, and W.J. Elias. 2015. Deep brain stimulation in the setting of cochlear implants: Case report and literature review. *Stereotactic and Functional Neurosurgery* 93:245–249.

Buttaro, T.M. 2012. Neurologic disorders. In *Nursing Care of the Hospitalized Older Patient* eds. T.M. Buttaro and K.A. Barba. West Sussex, UK: John Wiley & Sons, Ltd.

Capogrosso, M., T. Milekovic, D. Borton, G. Courtine et al. 2016. A brain–spine interface alleviating gait deficits after spinal cord injury in primates. *Nature* 539:284–288.

Casanova, M.F. 2010. Cortical organization; anatomical findings based on systems theory. *Translational Neuroscience* 1(1):62–71.

Charthad, U., M.J. Weber, T.C. Chang, and A. Arbabian. 2015. A mm-sized implantable medical device (IMD) with ultrasonic power transfer and a hybrid bi-directional data link. *IEEE Journal of Solid-State Circuits* 50(8):1741–1753.

Chhatbar, P. 2009. The future of implantable neuroprosthetic devices: Ethical considerations. *Journal of Long-Term Effects of Medical Implants* 19(2):123–137.

Choi, B.C. and A.W. Pak. 2006. Multidisciplinarity, interdisciplinarity and transdisciplinarity in health research, services, education and policy: 1. Definitions, objectives, and evidence of effectiveness. *Clinical & Investigative Medicine* 29(6):351–364.

Clarke, A.C. 1973. Clarke's Third Law. In Hazards of Prophecy: The Failure of Imagination. *Profiles of the Future: An Inquiry into the Limits of the Possible*. Harper & Row 1962. Macmillan revised 1973.

Coffey, R.J. 2001. Deep brain stimulation for chronic pain: Results of two multicenter trials and a structured review. *Pain Medicine* 2:183–192.

Coffey, R.J. 2009. Deep brain stimulation devices: A brief technical history and review. *Artificial Organs* 33:208–220.

Collinger, J.L., M.L. Boninger, T.M. Bruns, K. Curley, W. Wang, and D.J. Weber. 2013. Functional priorities, assistive technology, and brain–computer interfaces after spinal cord injury. *Journal of Rehabilitation Research & Development* 50:145–160.

Contreras-Vidal, J.L. et al. 2016. Powered exoskeletons for bipedal locomotion after spinal cord injury. *Journal of Neural Engineering* 13(3).

da Cruz, L., J.D. Dorn, A.C. Ho et al. 2016. Five-year safety and performance results from the Argus II Retinal Prosthesis System Clinical Trial. *Ophthalmology* 123(10):2248–2254.

Dambrot, S.M. 2017. *Exocortical Cognition: Heads in the Cloud*. IEEE International Conference on Systems, Man, and Cybernetics (SMC), Budapest. 004007-14.

DARPA. 2016. Implantable "Neural Dust" Enables Precise Wireless Recording of Nerve Activity. News and Events. Defense Advanced Research Projects Agency. http://www.darpa.mil/news-events/2016-08-03.

Das, U.N. 2010. Is hypertension a disorder of the brain? In *Metabolic Syndrome Pathophysiology: The Role of Essential Fatty Acids*. Oxford, UK: Wiley-Blackwell.

Dehghani, M. et al. 2017. Decoding the Neural Representation of Story Meanings across Languages. *PsyArXiv Preprint*.

DesignNews Design Hardware & Software Staff. 2015. *Accelerating Medical Device Innovation Using Additive Manufacturing*. Design News.

Downar, Z. and J.Z. Daskalakis. New targets for rTMS in depression: A review of convergent evidence, 2013. In *Brain Stimulation*, 6(3):231–240.

Duchenne, G.-B. 1867. *Physiology of Motion Demonstrated by Means of Electrical Stimulation and Clinical Observation and Applied to the Study of Paralysis and Deformities* (translated from French). eds. E.B. Kaplan and W.B. Saunders. 1959 edn. Philadelphia.

Eisen, M.D. 2003. Djourno, Eyries, and the first implanted electrical neural stimulator to restore hearing. *Otology & Neurotology* 24(3):500–506.

FDA Press Release. February 15, 2013. *FDA Approves First Retinal Implant for Adults with Rare Genetic Eye Disease*.

Finch, J. 2011. The ancient origins of prosthetic medicine. *Lancet* 377(9765):548–549.

Flesher, S.N. et al. 2016. Intracortical microstimulation of human somatosensory cortex. *Sci. Transl. Med.* 8:361ra14.

Florio, M. et al. 2015. Human-specific gene ARHGAP11B promotes basal progenitor amplification and neocortex expansion. *Science* 347(6229):1465–1470.

Florio, M. et al. 2016. A single splice site mutation in human-specific ARHGAP11B causes basal progenitor amplification. *Science Advances* 2(12):e1601941.

Fu, F., C.E. Tarnita, N.A. Christakis, L. Wang, D.G. Rand, and M.A. Nowak. 2012. Evolution of in-group favoritism. *Scientific Reports* 2(460).

Fujikado, T. et al. 2011. Testing of semichronically implanted retinal prosthesis by suprachoroidal–transretinal stimulation in patients with retinitis pigmentosa. *Invest. Ophthalmol. Vis. Sci.* 52:4726–4733.

Gibson, D.G. et al. 2010. Creation of a bacterial cell controlled by a chemically synthesized genome. *Science* 329(5987):52–56.

Girard, C. et al. 2000. The physics of the near-field. *Reports on Progress in Physics* 63(6):893.

Gladden, M.E. 2015. *The Handbook of Information Security for Advanced Neuroprosthetics.* Indianapolis: Synthypnion Academic.

Gross, R.E. and A.M. Lozano. 2000. Advances in neurostimulation for movement disorders. *Neurological Research* 22(3):247–258.

Grosse-Wentru, M., D. Mattia, and K. Oweiss. 2011. Using brain–computer interfaces to induce neural plasticity and restore function. *Journal of Neural Engineering* 8(2).

Hampson, R.E. et al. 2012. Facilitation and restoration of cognitive function in primate prefrontal cortex by a neuroprosthesis that utilizes minicolumn-specific neural firing. *Journal of Neural Engineering* 9(5):056012.

Hampson, R.E. et al. 2013. Facilitation of memory encoding in primate hippocampus by a neuroprosthesis that promotes task-specific neural firing. *Journal of Neural Engineering* 10(6):066013.

Haviland, D.B. 2002. *The Transistor in a Century of Electronics.* Nobel Media AB 2014.

Hayashibe, M., D. Guiraud, J.L. Pons, and D. Farina. 2015. Editorial: Biosignal processing and computational methods to enhance sensory motor neuroprosthetics. *Frontiers in Neuroscience* 9:434.

Henkel, G. 2013. History of the cochlear implant. *ENTtoday.* Published by Triological Society (The American Laryngological, Rhinological and Otological Society, Inc.).

Herron, J., T. Denison, and H.J. Chizeck, 2015. Closed-loop DBS with movement intention. In *7th International IEEE/EMBS Conference on Neural Engineering (NER).* Montpellier. 844–847.

Hewstone, M., M. Rubin, and H. Willis. 2002. Intergroup bias. *Annual Review of Psychology* 53:575–604.

Ho, A.C. et al. 2015. Long-term results from an epiretinal prosthesis to restore sight to the blind. *Ophthalmology* 122(8):1547–1554.

Humayun, M.S. et al. 2012. Interim results from the international trial of Second Sight's visual prosthesis. *Ophthalmology* 119:779–788.

Jain, K.K. 2012. *The Handbook of Nanomedicine.* New York: Humana Press. Copyright © 2012 Springer Science+Business Media.

Jeglic, A., E. Vanken, and M. Benedik. 1970. Implantable muscle/nerve stimulator as part of an electronic brace. In *3rd International Symposium on External Control of Human Extremities.* 593–603. Nauka, Belgrade: Yugoslav Commit Jain for Electronics and Automation.

Jeyalakshmi, C., V. Krishnamurthi, and A. Revathi. 2010. Speech recognition of deaf and hard of hearing people using hybrid neural network. In *2nd International Conference on Mechanical and Electronics Engineering, Kyoto.* V1-83-V1-87.

Jezernik, S., M. Craggs, W.M. Grill, G. Creasey, and N.J.M. Rijkhoff. 2002. Electrical stimulation for the treatment of bladder dysfunction: Current status and future possibilities. *Neurological Research* 24(5).

Kaido, T., T. Otsuki, Y. Kaneko, A. Takahashi, M. Omori, and T. Okamoto. 2011. Deep brain stimulation for Tourette syndrome: A prospective pilot study in Japan. *Neuromodulation* 14:123–129.

Kiani, M. and M. Ghovanloo. 2012. The circuit theory behind coupled-mode magnetic resonance-based wireless power transmission. *IEEE Transactions on Circuits and Systems I: Regular Papers* 59(9):2065–2074.

Koch, C., M. Wilfried, M. Goertz, and P. Walter. 2008. First results of a study on a completely implanted retinal prosthesis in blind humans. In *2008 IEEE Sensors.* 1237–1240.

Lauritzen, T.Z. et al. 2012. Reading visual braille with a retinal prosthesis. *Frontiers in Neuroscience* 6:168.

Leach, J.B., A.K.H Achyuta, and S.K. Murthy. 2010. Bridging the divide between neuroprosthetic design, tissue engineering and neurobiology. *Frontiers in Neuroengineering* 2:18. Creative Commons license CC BY 4.0 (https://creativecommons.org/licenses/by/4.0/legalcode).

Lebedev, M.A. et al. 2011. Future developments in brain–machine interface research. *Clinics* 66 (Supplement 1):25–32.

Lebedev, M.A. 2014. Brain–machine interfaces: An overview. *Translational Neuroscience* 5(1):99–110.

LeRoy, C. 1755. Où l'on rend compte de quelques tentatives que l'on a faites pour guérir plusieurs maladies par l'électricité. In *Histoire de l'Academie Royale des Sciences (Paris), Mémoires de Mathematique & de Physique.* 60:87–95.

Liberson, W.T., H.J. Holmquest, D. Scott, and M. Dow. 1961. Functional electrotherapy: Stimulation of the peroneal nerve synchronized with the swing phase of the gait of hemiplegic patients. *Archives of Physical and Medical Rehabilitation* 42:101–105.

Lin, L. et al. 2005. Identification of network-level coding units for real-time representation of episodic experiences in the hippocampus. *Proc Natl Acad Sci* 102(17):6125–6130.

Lin, L. et al. 2006. Organizing principles of real-time memory encoding: Neural clique assemblies and universal neural codes. *Trends in Neurosciences* 29(1):48–57.

Lipsman, N., D.B. Woodside., P. Giacobbe, and A.M. Lozano. 2013. Neurosurgical treatment of anorexia nervosa: Review of the literature from leucotomy to deep brain stimulation. *Eur. Eat. Disorders Rev.* 21:428–435.

Liu, V., A. Parks, V. Talla, S. Gollakota, D. Wetherall, and J.R. Smith. 2013. Ambient backscatter: Wireless communication out of thin air. *ACM SIGCOMM Computer Communication Review* 43(4):39–50.

Lively, M.W. 2013. *J. E. Hanger Lost His Leg But Not His Ingenuity*. Civil War Profiles.

Loeb, G.E. 2011. Neuroprosthetic interfaces—The reality behind bionics and cyborgs. In *Human Nature and Self-Design*, eds. Schleidgen, Jungert, Bauer, and Sandow. Paderborn, Germany: Mentis Verlag GmbH.

Mantione, D.D.M. et al. 2010. Deep brain stimulation of the nucleus accumbens for treatment-refractory obsessive–compulsive disorder. *Archives of General Psychiatry* 67(10):1061–1068.

Mayberg, H.S. et al. 2005. Deep brain stimulation for treatment-resistant depression. *Neuron* (45)5:651–660.

McGee, J.R. 1965. F. Blair Simmons Press Release. Stanford Medical Center News Bureau DA 1-5310.

*Medical Dictionary*, © 2009 Farlex and Partners.

Mudry, A. and M. Mills. 2013. The early history of the cochlear implant. *JAMA Otolaryngol Head Neck Surg.* 139(5):446–453.

Müller, U.J. et al. 2013. Deep brain stimulation of the nucleus accumbens for the treatment of addiction. *Ann. N.Y. Acad. Sci.* 1282:119–128.

National Research Council 2014. *Convergence: Facilitating Transdisciplinary Integration of Life Sciences, Physical Sciences, Engineering, and Beyond*. Committee on Key Challenge Areas for Convergence and Health. Board on Life Sciences. Division on Earth and Life Studies. National Research Council. Washington DC (US): National Academies Press.

Opris, J. and M.F. Casanova. 2014. Prefrontal cortical minicolumn: From executive control to disrupted cognitive processing. *Brain* 137(7):1863–1875.

Parent, A. 2014. Duchenne De Boulogne: A pioneer in neurology and medical photography. *Canadian Journal of Neurological Sciences* 32(3):369–377.

Pastrana, E. 2011. Optogenetics: Controlling cell function with light. *Nature Methods* 8:24–25.

Pine, K., B.S. Franzco, and R. Jacobs. 2016. *A Brief History of Prosthetic Eyes*. New Zealand National Eye Centre. University of Auckland.

Pliny. Natural History. 1958. Translated by H. Rackham (vols. 1–5, 9), W.H.S. Jones (vols. 6–8), and D.E. Eichholz (vol. 10) 1949–1954. London: Harvard University Press, Massachusetts and William Heinemann.

Ramos-Murguialday, A. et al. 2012. Proprioceptive feedback and brain computer interface (BCI) based neuroprostheses. *PLoS ONE* 7(10):e47048.

Reardon, S. 2015. Memory-boosting devices tested in humans. *Nature* 527:15–16.

Rincon-Gonzalez, L., J.P. Warren, D.M. Meller, and S.H. Tillery. 2011. Haptic interaction of touch and proprioception: Implications for neuroprosthetics. *IEEE Transactions on Neural Systems and Rehabilitation Engineering* 19(5):490–500.

Roco, M.C. 2003. Converging science and technology at the nanoscale: Opportunities for education and training. *Nature Biotechnology* 21:1247–1249.

Roco, M.C. and W.S. Bainbridge. 2003. Overview converging technologies for improving human performance. In *Converging Technologies for Improving Human Performance: Nanotechnology, Biotechnology, Information Technology and Cognitive Science*. 1–27. Dordrecht: Springer Netherlands.

Roco, M.C. and W.S. Bainbridge. 2013. The new world of discovery, invention, and innovation: Convergence of knowledge, technology, and society. *Journal of Nanoparticle Research*:1946. Excerpted from *Converging Knowledge, Technology and Society: Beyond Convergence of Nano-BioInfo-Cognitive Technologies*. eds. M.C. Roco, W.S. Bainbridge, B. Tonn, and G. Whitesides. National Science Foundation/World Technology Evaluation Center report. 2013. Boston: Springer.

Sahin, M. and V. Pikov. 2011. Wireless microstimulators for neural prosthetics. *Critical Reviews in Biomedical Engineering* 39(1):63–77.

Scharre, D. et al. 2016. Deep brain stimulation of frontal lobe networks to treat Alzheimer's disease. *Neurology* 86(16) Supplement P2.222.

Schwalger, T., M. Deger, and W. Gerstner. 2017. Towards a theory of cortical columns: From spiking neurons to interacting neural populations of finite size. *PLoS Computational Biology* 13(4):e1005507.

Seed, A. et al. 2010. Animal tool-use. *Current Biology* 20(23):R1032–R1039.

Seo, D. et al. 2013. Neural dust: An ultrasonic, low power solution for chronic brain–machine interfaces. *arXiv*:1307.2196 [q-bio.NC].

Seo, D. et al. 2015. Ultrasonic beamforming system for interrogating multiple implantable sensors. In *2015 37th Annual International Conference of the IEEE Engineering in Medicine and Biology Society (EMBC), Milan*. 2673–2676.

Seo, D. et al. 2016. Wireless recording in the peripheral nervous system with ultrasonic neural dust. *Neuron* 91(3):529–539.

Serruya, M.D. and M.J. Kahana. 2008. Techniques and devices to restore cognition. *Behavioural Brain Research* 92(2):149–165.

Shannon, R.V. 2014. Advances in auditory prostheses. *Current Opinion in Neurology* 25(1):61–66.

Sitaram, R. et al. 2017. Closed-loop brain training: The science of neurofeedback. *Nature Reviews Neuroscience* 18:86–100.

Srivastava, K.H. et al. 2017. Motor control by precisely timed spike patterns. *PNAS* 114(5):1171–1176.

Stenberg, C.C., W.H. Burnett, and R.C. Bunts. 1967. Electrical stimulation of human neurogenic bladders: Experience with four patients. *Journal of Urology* 97:79–84.

Steyrl, D., R. Kobler, and G. Müller-Putz. 2016. On similarities and differences of invasive and non-invasive electrical brain signals in brain–computer interfacing. *Journal of Biomedical Science and Engineering* 9:393–398.

Strojnik, P. R. Acimovic, E. Vavken, V. Simic, and U. Stanic. 1987. Treatment of drop foot using an implantable peroneal underknee stimulator. *Scandinavian Journal of Rehabilitation Medicine* 19:37–43.

Tang, H.Y. et al. 2015. Miniaturizing ultrasonic system for portable health care and fitness. *IEEE Transactions on Biomedical Circuits and Systems* 9(6):767–776.

Tee, B.C.-K. et al. 2015. A skin-inspired organic digital mechanoreceptor. *Science* 350(6258):313–316.

Thurston, A.J. 2007. Paré and prosthetics: The early history of artificial limbs. *ANZ Journal of Surgery* 77(12):1114–1119.

Todorov, E. and M.I. Jordan. 2002. Optimal feedback control as a theory of motor coordination. *Nature Neuroscience* 5:1226–1235.

Tonet, O. et al. Accessed January 20, 2017. *Critical Review and Future Perspectives of Non-Invasive Brain–Machine Interfaces* (Final Report). European Space Agency. Adriana Study 05/6203.

Vallender, E.J., M.-B. Nitzan, and B.T. Lahn. 2008. Genetic basis of human brain evolution. *Trends in Neurosciences* 31(12):637–644.

Vassanelli, S. and M. Mahmud. 2016. Trends and challenges in neuroengineering: Toward "intelligent" neuroprostheses through brain-"brain inspired systems" communication. *Frontiers in Neuroscience* 10:438.

Velasco, M., F. Velasco, and A.L. Velasco. 2001. Centromedian-thalamic and hippocampal electrical stimulation for the control of intractable epileptic seizures. *Journal of Clinical Neurophysiology* 18:49.

Volta, A. 1800. *On the Electricity Excited by the Mere Contact of Conducting Substances of Different Kinds*. In a letter from Mr. Alexander Volta, F.R.S. Professor of Natural Philosophy in the University of Pavia, to the Right Hon. Sir Joseph Banks, Bart. K.B P.R.S.

Waldert S. 2016. Invasive vs. non-invasive neuronal signals for brain–machine interfaces: Will one prevail? *Frontiers in Neuroscience* 10:295.

Wårdell, K. et al. 2015. Deep brain stimulation of the pallidum internum for Gilles de la Tourette syndrome: A patient-specific model-based simulation study of the electric field. *Neuromodulation: Technology at the Neural Interface* 18:90–96.

Waters, R.L., D. Mcneal, and J. Perry. 1975. Experimental correction of footdrop by electrical stimulation of the peroneal nerve. *Journal of Bone and Joint Surgery* 5(57A):1047–1054.

What is Macular Degeneration? American Macular Degeneration Foundation. https://www.macular.org/what-macular-degeneration.

Yameen, B., W.I. Choi, C. Vilos, A. Swami, J. Shi, and O.C. Farokhzad. 2014. Insight into nanoparticle cellular uptake and intracellular targeting. *Journal of Controlled Release* 190(28):485–499.

Yang, J.J., D.B. Strukov, and D.R. Stewart. 2013. Memristive devices for computing. *Nature Nanotechnology* 8:13–24.

Yeon, P., S.A. Mirbozorgi, B. Ash, H. Eckhardt, and M. Ghovanloo. 2016. Fabrication and microassembly of a mm-sized floating probe for a distributed wireless neural interface. *Micromachines* 7(9):154.

Zhong, C., Y. Deng, A.F. Roudsari, A. Kapetanovic, M.P. Anantram, and M. Rolandi. 2011. A polysaccharide bioprotonic field-effect transistor. *Nature Communications* 2(476).

Zrenner, C., P. Belardinelli, F. Müller-Dahlhaus, and U. Ziemann. 2016. Closed-loop neuroscience and non-invasive brain stimulation: A tale of two loops. *Frontiers in Cellular Neuroscience* 10.92.

Zrenner, E. et al. 2011. Subretinal electronic chips allow blind patients to read letters and combine them to words. *Proc Biol Sci* 278:1489–1497.

# 7 Design and Customization of SSVEP-Based BCI Applications Aimed for Elderly People

*Piotr Stawicki, Felix Gembler, and Ivan Volosyak*

## CONTENTS

7.1 Introduction ........................................................................................................... 133
7.2 SSVEP Paradigm ................................................................................................... 134
7.3 Customization of SSVEP Parameters .................................................................... 135
    7.3.1 Stimulation Frequencies ............................................................................ 136
    7.3.2 Number of Classes ..................................................................................... 136
    7.3.3 Time Windows ............................................................................................ 137
7.4 Design of the GUI ................................................................................................. 138
7.5 Summary ............................................................................................................... 141
References ...................................................................................................................... 141

**Abstract**

In this chapter, we discuss the parameter setup for steady-state visually evoked potential (SSVEP)–based brain–computer interface (BCI) systems aimed for elderly people. In this respect, the reader is guided through the key features of SSVEP-based BCI applications. In detail, we discuss the appropriate choice of stimulation frequencies, classification time windows, and the number of selectable commands. Additionally, we list design choices for the graphical user interfaces geared to the needs of users of advanced age. The chapter summarizes results of our previous research, where age-related differences in BCI performance were investigated.

## 7.1 INTRODUCTION

Brain–computer interface (BCI) is a field of technologies that allows communication between the human brain and the computer. Brain signal data are scanned for patterns that can be interpreted as control command for external applications (Wolpaw et al. 2002).

The main BCI functions according to Wolpaw et al. include replacement, restoration, enhancement, supplement, and improvement of the central nervous system output.

For example, a BCI can be implemented as a spelling interface and has therefore the potential to become a standard tool for reestablishing communication for severely disabled people who are unable to express themselves with their traditional motor output pathway of the nervous system (Wolpaw & Wolpaw 2012).

Beside healthcare applications (see, e.g., Bamdad et al. 2015), which is the main focus of BCIs, application scenarios include computer games (Marshall et al. 2013), learning (Karkar & Mohamed 2016), and control of, for example, mobile robots (Stawicki et al. 2016).

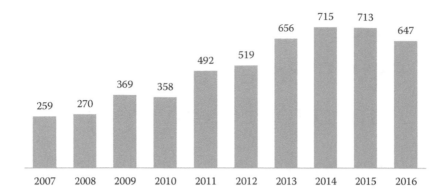

**FIGURE 7.1** Number of results for the search term "Brain–Computer Interface/Brain–Machine Interface" in the last decade (according to the PubMed database).

The most common BCI approaches in modern research are the P300 event-related potential (ERP) paradigm (Spüler et al. 2012), a BCI approach using the 300-ms component of an evoked potential, event-related desynchronization/synchronization paradigm (Hsu 2013), and the steady-state visually evoked potential (SSVEP) paradigm (Zhang et al. 2015). As can be seen in Figure 7.1, research interest in BCI is constantly growing over the last years.

However, publications about SSVEP-based BCIs are in minority when compared to, for example, P300 BCIs; the PubMed database shows for the last decade 4755 results for the search term "Brain–Computer Interface Brain–Machine Interface," but only 221 results regarding the additional phrase "SSVEP," compared to 345 when adding the phrase "P300."

In order to inspire research groups across the globe to explore the SSVEP paradigm, the instructions provided in this chapter provide helpful customization options for the SSVEP approach. The advantages of SSVEP-based BCIs include high information transfer rate (ITR) and little or no training time (Rupp 2014). Recent research demonstrated sufficient control of SSVEP-based BCIs for elderly users above 60 years (Volosyak et al. 2017).

## 7.2 SSVEP PARADIGM

The SSVEP paradigm exposes the user to a flickering visual stimulus at a constant frequency. Typical stimuli sources are light-emitting diodes (LEDs) or boxes rendered on a computer monitor, because this allows an implementation without any additional hardware. If the user gazes at the flickering stimuli, brainwaves are elicited with the corresponding frequency and its harmonics (Müller-Putz & Pfurtscheller 2008). These brainwaves can be recorded noninvasively from the scalp using an electroencephalogram (EEG). The BCI classifies the attended frequency and interprets it as control command using signal processing methods that handle data preprocessing, feature extraction, and feature classification.

There are several established signal processing methods for SSVEP-based BCIs: Feature extraction methods such as the Fourier-based transform methods discrete Fourier transformation and fast Fourier transformation; spatial filter methods such as principal component analysis, minimum energy combination, canonical correlation analysis, and maximum contrast combination; and wavelet transforms such as wavelet packet decomposition and continuous wavelet transform. Liu et al. (2013) provided a detailed review of these and other classification methods.

For the implementation of BCI systems, many research groups use software platforms such as OpenViBE (Renard et al. 2010) or BCI2000 (Schalk et al. 2004). These platforms allow easy creation and optimization of BCIs.

As the BCI relies on the user's ability to control her or his eye gaze, eye-tracking systems could provide a faster control mechanism. Eye tracking devices might as well not work properly for every user. For example, the performance can be affected by light conditions and visual aids. For some users, SSVEP-based BCIs might provide a more reliable option (Stawicki et al. 2017).

## 7.3   CUSTOMIZATION OF SSVEP PARAMETERS

It is well known that BCI performance differs among users (see, e.g., Volosyak et al. 2011b). Sometimes, the BCI even fails to classify commands reliably. This so-called BCI inefficiency (also called BCI illiteracy or BCI deficiency) also applies to the SSVEP paradigm.

Because of several system improvements, SSVEP BCI inefficiency could be reduced over time. Table 7.1 summarizes results from three larger SSVEP BCI field studies with similar hardware and experimental setup. It can be seen that BCI inefficiency occurred less often in the more recent studies and may be caused solely by the suboptimal signal processing algorithms. In a study by Gembler et al. (2015b), even all 61 participants were able to gain control over the tested system.

Apart from the utilized classification methods and data processing algorithms, there are several other factors that influence BCI performance.

In order to develop BCIs that can reliably interpret brain patterns from as many users as possible, demographic factors need to be addressed with regard to the design of the graphical user interface (GUI) and also the user-dependent parameters.

Until now, many researchers have developed communication and healthcare applications for the SSVEP paradigm that allow users to communicate with their environment by typing sentences. Though these applications are intended to work for users of all ages, some studies reported a slightly poorer BCI performance of elderly users. In an earlier study (Gembler et al. 2015a), we compared BCI performance from users of two different age groups. All participants were asked to spell a German phrase; what we found was that the classification took longer and was less accurate for the elderly participants. These preliminary results show that age is an important demographic factor that needs to be considered during the development of BCIs.

Therefore, in the succeeding paragraphs, we want to review customization options of SSVEP-based BCIs, having in mind elderly users. In this respect, we discuss key components for the SSVEP approach such as choice of frequencies, number of stimuli and classification time windows, as well as design guidelines for the GUI.

**TABLE 7.1**

**Comparison of SSVEP BCI Performance of Our Previous BCI Field Studies**

|  | Volosyak et al. 2009 | Volosyak et al. 2011 | Gembler et al. 2015b |
|---|---|---|---|
| Number of subjects | 37 | 86 | 61 |
| Mean accuracy (%) | 92.9 | 92.3 | 97.1 |
| Literacy rate (%) | 86.5 | 97.7 | 100 |
| Number of stimuli | 5 | 4 | 4 |
| Time window (s) | 2 | 2 | 0.8–8 |

*Note:* Subjects that were not able to gain control over the BCI (studies from 2009 and 2011) were excluded from calculation of mean values. The literacy rate describes the percentage of participants that achieved reliable control over the system.

### 7.3.1 STIMULATION FREQUENCIES

Stimulation frequencies are usually realized with LEDs or flickering boxes on an LCD monitor. Typically, in the latter case, the stimuli and the GUI are rendered on the same screen.

The choice of these stimulation frequencies is an important factor in BCI interface design. Two flickering targets with a frequency difference below 0.1 Hz can be reliably distinguished in the SSVEP response (Gao et al. 2003; Hwang et al. 2012; Stawicki et al. 2015). The stimulation with lower stimulation frequencies (6–12 Hz) evokes SSVEPs with larger amplitudes compared to high frequencies beyond 30 Hz (Gao et al. 2003; Zhu et al. 2010). Higher stimulation frequencies on the other hand produce less visual fatigue and show no stimulus-related seizures (Won et al. 2015).

In order to even out the imbalances in the evoked SSVEP amplitudes, each stimulus can be associated with certain individual classification thresholds. If a command is repeatedly falsely classified, without any user intention regarding this command, the threshold corresponding to the associated frequency can be increased. This might be necessary for the frequencies that elicit comparably strong SSVEP responses; for example, for a flickering at 6 Hz, the classification threshold should be set higher than for a 20-Hz target.

One should also keep in mind that the stimulation frequency elicits responses with the fundamental frequency as well as its harmonics. In order to avoid influences between frequencies, the set of stimulation frequencies should follow additional restriction rules (Volosyak et al. 2010b):

$$f_i \neq [f_j + f_k]/2, \qquad f_i \neq 2f_j - f_k, \qquad f_i \neq 2f_k - f_j, \tag{7.1}$$

for any stimulation frequency triple $f_i, f_j, f_k$. It is also important to consider that the low-frequency band usually overlaps with the alpha band (7–13 Hz). Alpha wave brain activity, typically occurring when a person closes his or her eyes, might cause false classifications (Zhu et al. 2010).

### 7.3.2 NUMBER OF CLASSES

Depending on the number of simultaneously used stimulation frequencies, applications of various complexities can be realized, but identification of the target attended by the user is usually less accurate if multiple visual stimuli are used, as they may increase the probability of false classifications.

There are several methods to generate the stimuli for SSVEP-based BCIs on LCDs.

An SSVEP stimulus can be realized as a graphics object (e.g., a box on a computer screen) with the binary states drawn/not drawn, which change at a specific rate that is dependent on the monitor's refresh rate. The number of such on/off cycles per second is then referred to as the stimulation frequency.

The frequency approximation method as proposed by Wang et al. (2010) is suitable to implement a high amount of targets on a computer monitor.

In this frame-based stimulus approximation method, a varying number of frames is used in each cycle. The stimulus signal at frequency $f$ can be generated by

$$\text{stim}(f, i) = \text{square}[2\pi f(i/r)], \tag{7.2}$$

where $r$ is the monitor refresh rate and square$[2\pi f(i/r)]$ generates the square wave with frequency $f$ and frame index $i$.

Recently, we investigated the possibilities and limitations regarding the number of targets that can be realized using this method (Gembler et al. 2016). Though some participants achieved remarkable results, the classification accuracy generally dropped with a higher number of targets, for some users to such a degree that reliable control was not possible (see Table 7.2). With increasing target number, the distance between targets and the target size needed to be lowered. The closer proximity

**TABLE 7.2**

**BCI Accuracies Achieved with Multitarget BCI Systems**

| Subject # | 15 Targets Acc (%) | ITR (bpm) | 28 Targets Acc (%) | ITR (bpm) | 60 Targets Acc (%) | ITR (bpm) | 84 Targets Acc (%) | ITR (bpm) |
|---|---|---|---|---|---|---|---|---|
| 1 | 83.33 | 31.00 | 100 | 39.37 | – | – | – | – |
| 2 | 100 | 130.15 | 100 | 120.30 | 100 | 73.65 | 91.30 | 67.03 |
| 3 | 93.75 | 29.65 | 80.00 | 22.35 | – | – | – | – |
| 4 | 93.75 | 40.25 | 84.85 | 52.02 | 93.75 | 24.51 | – | – |
| 5 | 100 | 83.63 | 90.32 | 59.30 | – | – | – | – |
| 6 | 44.12 | 7.09 | – | – | – | – | – | – |
| 7 | 83.33 | 61.79 | 82.35 | 70.92 | – | – | – | – |

*Source:* Gembler, F., Stawicki, P., & Volosyak, I. (2016). *Exploring the Possibilities and Limitations of Multitarget SSVEP-Based BCI Applications.* Orlando.

*Note:* Seven healthy participants controlled stimulation matrices with different amount of targets. The dash indicates that no control over the system was achieved.

of the target boxes influenced the classification accuracy as adjacent boxes were often falsely classified for multitarget BCIs. Some participants also expressed discomfort when using these systems.

The aspect of user friendliness has also to be considered, especially when designing a GUI for elderly people. Though generally slower, BCIs with a small number of stimuli have their advantages. Such BCIs offer more freedom in frequency selection and are less fatiguing for the visual channel of the user. If fewer targets are used, the stimulation frequencies can be selected as divisors of the vertical refresh rate of the monitor, ensuring a constant number of frames in each cycle (Volosyak et al. 2009a). Table 7.3 provides such frequencies for the most common monitor refresh rates.

Several studies reported that SSVEP also correlates with the duty cycle, which describes the percentage of the on-phase of the stimulation cycle (Shyu et al. 2013; Wu 2009). In both cited studies, the standard approach (a duty cycle of 0.5) did not yield the strongest SSVEP responses. Hence, the determination of the optimal duty cycle could be relevant, particularly for high frequencies because of their generally lower amplitudes of SSVEP responses.

### 7.3.3 TIME WINDOWS

The length of the time period between consecutive command classifications is another factor that has a high impact on the BCI performance. The classification accuracy benefits from a larger amount of collected EEG data to interpret the user intention.

Volosyak et al. (2010a) analyzed the impact of the time window used for EEG data classification in a performance comparison on eight different time segment lengths over 10 participants. Their results, displayed in Table 7.4, confirmed a close relation between the time window length and accuracy. It was also observed that some users need to gaze at the stimulation target for a comparably long period of time, before a selection was classified.

In another study (Gembler et al. 2015a), we investigated age-associated differences in SSVEP-based BCI control and found that command classifications were performed faster and more accurate for users of the younger group (see Figure 7.2). Each of the two tested age groups consisted of five participants, ranging from 19 to 27 years and 66 to 70 years. Though for some elderly users the system was slow, it interpreted the user intention reliably. Appropriate time window lengths can enable poor performers to gain accuracy and control over the BCI.

For optimal performance, the time window can be customized individually for each user. This can also be done during an automated training session as demonstrated in Gembler et al. (2015b).

**TABLE 7.3**

**Frequencies with Constant Number of Frames per Cycle for the Most Common Vertical Refresh Rates**

| Freq (Hz) | 120 | 100 | 75 | 60 |
|---|---|---|---|---|
| 6.00 | 20 | – | – | 10 |
| 6.25 | – | 16 | 12 | – |
| 6.32 | 19 | – | – | – |
| 6.67 | 18 | 15 | – | 9 |
| 6.82 | – | – | 11 | – |
| 7.06 | 17 | – | – | – |
| 7.14 | – | 14 | – | – |
| 7.50 | 16 | – | 10 | 8 |
| 7.69 | – | 13 | – | – |
| 8.00 | 15 | – | – | – |
| 8.33 | – | 12 | 9 | – |
| 8.57 | 14 | – | – | 7 |
| 9.09 | – | 11 | – | – |
| 9.23 | 13 | – | – | – |
| 9.38 | – | – | 8 | – |
| 10.00 | 12 | 10 | – | 6 |
| 10.71 | – | – | 7 | – |
| 10.91 | 11 | – | – | – |
| 11.11 | – | 9 | – | – |
| 12.00 | 10 | – | – | 5 |
| 12.50 | – | 8 | 6 | – |
| 13.33 | 9 | – | – | – |
| 14.29 | – | 7 | – | – |
| 15.00 | 8 | – | 5 | 4 |
| 16.67 | – | 6 | – | – |
| 17.14 | 7 | – | – | – |
| 18.75 | – | – | 4 | – |
| 20.00 | 6 | 5 | – | 3 |
| 24.00 | 5 | – | – | – |
| 25.00 | – | 4 | 3 | – |
| 30.00 | 4 | – | – | 2 |
| 33.33 | – | 3 | – | – |

Additionaly, adaptive methods based on the online performance can be implemented to update the time windows (da Cruz et al. 2015; Volosyak et al. 2011a). Figure 7.3 shows an illustration of an adaptive time window extension method.

## 7.4 DESIGN OF THE GUI

There are several ways to design a GUI tailored to the needs of elderly users. A low number of targets reduces the cognitive and visual load, which might result in enhanced BCI performance. In several studies, four target systems have proven to yield high classification accuracies and 100% literacy rates (see also Table 7.1). For example, in the mentioned field study with 61 participants, conducted in our laboratory, the system reliably interpreted brain signals for all participants (Gembler et al. 2015b). In the following, we provide details of a four-target BCI system, the three-step spelling application (Gembler et al. 2015a).

**TABLE 7.4**

**Mean Classification Accuracies of a BCI Online Experiment over 10 Participants for Different Time Segment Lengths**

| Time Segment (s) | Mean Accuracy (%) |
|---|---|
| 4.00 | 93.49 |
| 3.00 | 92.77 |
| 2.00 | 90.33 |
| 1.50 | 84.61 |
| 1.00 | 80.01 |
| 0.75 | 73.45 |
| 0.50 | 58.66 |
| 0.25 | 27.29 |

*Source:* Volosyak, I., Malechka, T., Valbuena, D., & Graeser, A. (2010). A novel calibration method for SSVEP based brain–computer interfaces. In *Proceedings of the 18th European Signal Processing Conference (EUSIPCO 2010)* (pp. 939–943).

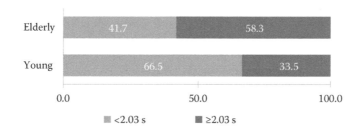

**FIGURE 7.2** Distribution of time segment window lengths for correct classifications of an online spelling experiment averaged over five young and five elderly participants. (With kind permission from Springer Science+Business Media: *Advances in Computational Intelligence*, A comparison of SSVEP-based BCI-performance between different age groups, 2015, pp. 71–77. Gembler, F., Stawicki, P., & Volosyak.) The majority of correct letter selections from elderly participants took longer than 2.03 s.

Four commands were represented on the computer screen by flickering boxes of default sizes 175 × 175 pixels (see Figure 7.4).

Three boxes were arranged horizontally in the upper part of the screen containing the letters "A–I," "J–R," and "S–_," respectively. The additional fourth box, containing the command "Löschen" (German for delete), was located on the right side of the screen.

A box for the output text was located at the center of the screen. The content of the three boxes containing the alphabet changed to more specific sets according to the first selection. At least three steps were necessary to choose a single character. The steps necessary to select the letter "E" are illustrated in Figure 7.5. Between the first and the second step and between the second and the third step, the far right box (initially "Löschen") contained the command "zurück" (German for back), which took the user to the previous step.

To increase the overall user friendliness of the GUI, additional feedback mechanisms were implemented. The size of the boxes varied in relation to the SSVEP amplitude during the experiment (Volosyak et al. 2009b). Each box was outlined by a frame, which determined the maximum size of a box before the command classification. This additional real-time visual feedback about the SSVEP signals exposes to the user what command is about to be executed.

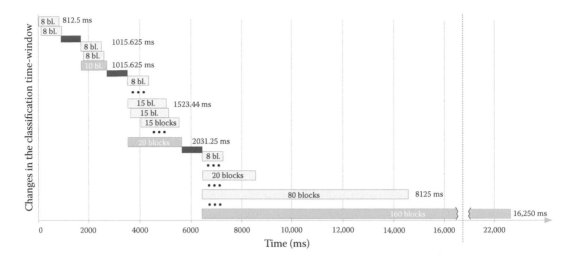

**FIGURE 7.3** Changes in the classification time window after performed classifications. (Modified from Stawicki, P., Gembler, F., & Volosyak, I. (2016). Driving a semiautonomous mobile robotic car controlled by an SSVEP-based BCI. *Computational Intelligence and Neuroscience, 2016,* 5.) Command classifications were performed with time windows of different predefined lengths. In case no command classification was executed (gray), the window slid until it could be extended to the next predefined value. For example, if no classification could be made using 8 blocks of EEG data (the smallest predefined time window length), the window slid until a classification was made or until it could be extended to the next predefined time window length, 10 blocks of EEG data. After each performed classification (green), additional time for gaze shifting was included (red). During this gaze shifting period, the classifier output was rejected.

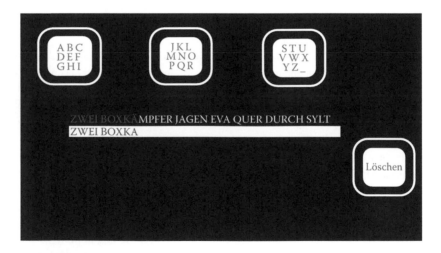

**FIGURE 7.4** Graphical user interface of the three-step spelling application. The task was to spell the German pangram "ZWEI BOXKÄMPFER JAGEN EVA QUER DURCH SYLT."

Further, in order to reduce the information load of the visual channel, every command classification was followed by an audio feedback with the name of the selected command or the letter spelled.

In addition, after each performed classification, the visual stimulation paused for approximately a second to give the user time to shift his or her gaze to the next letter.

Though the inclusion of this gaze shifting period reduces the system speed, it serves several purposes. It reduces false classifications caused by movement artifacts during the gaze shifting period.

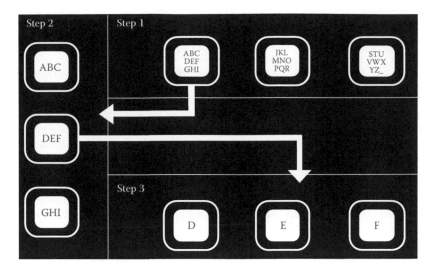

**FIGURE 7.5**    The three steps for the selection of the letter "E." Initially, the user needed to gaze at the box containing the letter group "ABC DEF GHI" (Step 1). After selection of the box containing "DEF" (Step 2), the user was able to select the desired letter "E" (Step 3).

Further, it assures that the collected EEG data are independent of the previously attended visual stimulus. This is especially helpful to prevent the subsequent classification of identical commands.

## 7.5   SUMMARY

In order to customize SSVEP-based BCIs for elderly users, several issues need to be considered. If a user interface is optimized in respect to speed only, it might lack classification accuracy and hence user friendliness. False classifications can be annoying in daily use; several participants prefer a slower BCI over a faster but less precise system (Gembler et al. 2014). Especially for elderly people, a BCI customized for high classification accuracy might be the more suitable choice. This usually means a lower number of stimuli and larger classification time windows should be used.

The topic of frequency selection still needs to be investigated further. Age-associated differences regarding optimal frequency selection need to be tested. Frequencies just below the alpha wave tend to evoke the strongest SSVEP response and yielded good performance in several studies. Some users, however, might find higher frequencies more user friendly for daily use. However, higher frequencies are generally harder to detect. Determination of frequency-specific duty cycles might enhance the SSVEP signal strength.

When designing the GUI for elderly users, the general emphasis should be put on interface simplicity, clarity of design, and intuitive control rather than speed; the visual and cognitive load should be minimized as short-term memory and episodic memory decrease when we age.

## REFERENCES

Bamdad, M., Zarshenas, H., & Auais, M. A. (2015). Application of BCI systems in neurorehabilitation: A scoping review. *Disability and Rehabilitation: Assistive Technology, 10*(5), 355–364.

da Cruz, J. N., Wan, F., Wong, C. M., & Cao, T. (2015). Adaptive time-window length based on online performance measurement in SSVEP-based BCIs. *Neurocomputing, 149*, 93–99.

Gao, X., Xu, X., Cheng, M., & Gao, S. (2003, Jun.). A BCI-based environmental controller for the motion-disabled. *IEEE Transactions on Neural Systems and Rehabilitation Engineering, 11*(2), 137–140.

Gembler, F., Stawicki, P., & Volosyak, I. (2014). Towards a user-friendly BCI for elderly people. *Proceedings of the 6th International Brain–Computer Interface Conference Graz.*

Gembler, F., Stawicki, P., & Volosyak, I. (2015a). A comparison of SSVEP-based BCI-performance between different age groups. In *Advances in Computational Intelligence* (pp. 71–77). Springer.

Gembler, F., Stawicki, P., & Volosyak, I. (2015b). Autonomous parameter adjustment for SSVEP-based BCIs with a novel BCI wizard. *Frontiers in Neuroscience, 9.*

Gembler, F., Stawicki, P., & Volosyak, I. (2016). *Exploring the Possibilities and Limitations of Multitarget SSVEP-Based BCI Applications.* Orlando.

Hsu, W.-Y. (2013). Single-trial motor imagery classification using asymmetry ratio, phase relation, wavelet-based fractal, and their selected combination. *International Journal of Neural Systems, 23*(02), 1350007.

Hwang, H.-J., Lim, J.-H., Jung, Y.-J., Choi, H., Lee, S. W., & Im, C.-H. (2012). Development of an SSVEP-based BCI spelling system adopting a QWERTY-style LED keyboard. *Journal of Neuroscience Methods, 208*(1), 59–65.

Karkar, A., & Mohamed, A. (2016). A BCI m-Learning System. *Qatar Foundation Annual Research Conference Proceedings, 2016,* p. ICTPP3331.

Liu, Q., Chen, K., Ai, Q., & Xie, S. Q. (2013). Review: Recent development of signal processing algorithms for SSVEP-based brain computer interfaces. *Journal of Medical and Biological Engineering, 34*(4), 299–309.

Marshall, D., Coyle, D., Wilson, S., & Callaghan, M. (2013). Games, gameplay, and BCI: The state of the art. *IEEE Transactions on Computational Intelligence and AI in Games, 5*(2), 82–99.

Müller-Putz, G. R., & Pfurtscheller, G. (2008, Jan.). Control of an electrical prosthesis with an SSVEP-based BCI. *IEEE Transactions on Biomedical Engineering, 55*(1), 361–364.

Renard, Y., Lotte, F., Gibert, G., Congedo, M., Maby, E., Delannoy, V. et al. (2010). Openvibe: An open-source software platform to design, test, and use brain–computer interfaces in real and virtual environments. *Presence, 19*(1), 35–53.

Rupp, R. (2014). Challenges in clinical applications of brain computer interfaces in individuals with spinal cord injury. *Front Neuroengineering.* doi: 10.3389/fneng.2014.00038

Schalk, G., McFarland, D. J., Hinterberger, T., Birbaumer, N., & Wolpaw, J. R. (2004). BCI2000: A general-purpose brain-computer interface (BCI) system. *IEEE Transactions on Biomedical Engineering, 51*(6), 1034–1043.

Shyu, K.-K., Chiu, Y.-J., Lee, P.-L., Liang, J.-M., & Peng, S.-H. (2013). Adaptive SSVEP-based BCI system with frequency and pulse duty-cycle stimuli tuning design. *IEEE Transactions on Neural Systems and Rehabilitation Engineering, 21*(5), 697–703.

Spüler, M., Bensch, M., Kleih, S., Rosenstiel, W., Bogdan, M., & Kübler, A. (2012). Online use of error-related potentials in healthy users and people with severe motor impairment increases performance of a P300-BCI. *Clinical Neurophysiology, 123*(7), 1328–1337.

Stawicki, P., Gembler, F., Rezeika. A., & Volosyak, I. (2017). A novel hybrid mental spelling application based on eye tracking and SSVEP-based BCI. *Brain Science, 7,* 35.

Stawicki, P., Gembler, F., & Volosyak, I. (2015). Evaluation of suitable frequency differences in SSVEP-based BCIs. In *Symbiotic Interaction* (pp. 159–165). Springer.

Stawicki, P., Gembler, F., & Volosyak, I. (2016). Driving a semiautonomous mobile robotic car controlled by an SSVEP-based BCI. *Computational Intelligence and Neuroscience, 2016,* 5.

Volosyak, I., Cecotti, H., & Gräser, A. (2009a). Impact of frequency selection on LCD screens for SSVEP based brain-computer interfaces. *International Work-Conference on Artificial Neural Networks* (pp. 706–713).

Volosyak, I., Cecotti, H., & Gräser, A. (2010a). Steady-state visual evoked potential response—Impact of the time segment length. *Proc. on the 7th International Conference on Biomedical Engineering BioMed2010, Innsbruck, Austria, February 17–19* (pp. 288–292).

Volosyak, I., Cecotti, H., Valbuena, D., & Gräser, A. (2009b). Evaluation of the Bremen SSVEP based BCI in real world conditions. *Proc. IEEE ICORR'09* (pp. 322–331).

Volosyak, I., Malechka, T., Valbuena, D., & Graeser, A. (2010b). A novel calibration method for SSVEP based brain–computer interfaces. In *Proceedings of the 18th European Signal Processing Conference (EUSIPCO 2010)* (pp. 939–943).

Volosyak, I., Valbuena, D., Luth, T., & Gräser, A. (2011a). *Towards an SSVEP Based BCI with High ITR.* Technical report, University of Bremen, Bremen.

Volosyak, I., Valbuena, D., Lüth, T., Malechka, T., & Gräser, A. (2011b). BCI demographics II: How many (and what kinds of) people can use an SSVEP BCI? *IEEE Transactions on Neural Systems and Rehabilitation Engineering, 19*(3), 232–239.

Volosyak, I., Gembler, F., & Stawicki, P. (2017). Age-related differences in SSVEP-based BCI performance. *Neurocomputing.* doi: 10.1016/j.neucom.2016.08.121

Wang, Y., Wang, Y.-T., & Jung, T.-P. (2010). Visual stimulus design for high-rate SSVEP BCI. *Electronics Letters, 46*(15), 1057–1058.

Wolpaw, J., Birbaumer, N., McFarland, D., Pfurtscheller, G., & Vaughan, T. (2002). Brain–computer interfaces for communication and control. *Clinical Neurophysiology, 113*, 767–791.

Wolpaw, J., & Wolpaw, E. W. (Eds.). (2012). *Brain–Computer Interfaces: Principles and Practice.* Oxford University Press.

Won, D. O., Hwang, H.-J., Dähne, S., Müller, K.-R., & Lee, S.-W. (2015). Effect of higher frequency on the classification of steady-state visual evoked potentials. *Journal of Neural Engineering, 13*(1), 016014.

Wu, Z. (2009). The difference of SSVEP resulted by different pulse duty-cycle. *International Conference on Communications, Circuits and Systems,* 2009 (pp. 605–607).

Zhang, Y., Zhou, G., Jin, J., Wang, X., & Cichocki, A. (2015). SSVEP recognition using common feature analysis in brain–computer interface. *Journal of Neuroscience Methods, 244*, 8–15.

Zhu, D., Bieger, J., Molina, G. G., & Aarts, R. M. (2010). A survey of stimulation methods used in SSVEP-based BCIs. *Computational Intelligence and Neuroscience, 1*, 702357.

# Brain–Computer Interface Applications

## Section C. Affective and Artistic Brain–Computer Interfaces

# 8 Affective Brain–Computer Interfacing and Methods for Affective State Detection

*Ian Daly*

## CONTENTS

8.1 Introduction ....................................................................................................... 147
8.2 Affective States.................................................................................................. 148
8.3 Affective State Reporting.................................................................................. 149
    8.3.1 Discrete Methods.................................................................................... 149
    8.3.2 Continuous Methods............................................................................... 150
8.4 Affective State Detection................................................................................... 151
8.5 Affective BCIs................................................................................................... 155
    8.5.1 Categories of aBCI ................................................................................. 155
    8.5.2 Use of Affect in aBCI ............................................................................ 155
8.6 Case Study: An Affective BCMI....................................................................... 156
8.7 Guide for Developing aBCIs.............................................................................. 158
8.8 Summary ............................................................................................................ 159
References..................................................................................................................... 159

**Abstract**

Affective brain–computer interfaces (aBCIs) provide a method for individuals to interact with a computer via their emotions and without needing to move.

This chapter will provide an introduction to the concept of aBCIs and their uses in applications such as music therapy and affective computing. We will first review the concept of aBCIs before going on to provide a literature review of the current state-of-the-art research in affective state detection methods and their uses in aBCI. Finally, we will describe a case study; an affective brain–computer music interface (aBCMI) and its potential for use in music therapy.

Emerging and established trends in aBCI, such as the use of prefrontal asymmetry measures of affective states, are identified. Additionally, a set of recommendations are provided for researchers seeking to work in the field of aBCI.

## 8.1 INTRODUCTION

Brain–computer interfaces (BCIs) seek to provide a channel for communication and control of a computer system that does not rely on any movement and instead uses signals recorded directly from the user's brain to achieve interaction with a computer (Wolpaw 2007). Affective BCIs (aBCIs) seek to detect a user's affective state and use that information to interact with the BCI (Zander and Jatzev 2009; Nijboer et al. 2009; Mühl et al. 2014). aBCIs may seek to detect a user's affective state either directly from their brain or via the use of a hybrid approach that combines both brain activity and measures of other physiological processes. aBCIs have a wide range of potential applications, including aiding with affective computing, entertainment, and therapy.

This chapter will first introduce affective states and how they may be categorized. It will then go on to discuss methods for individuals to report their affective states before introducing methods for affective state detection based on recordings of neurological and physiological activity. A literature review of the current-state of the art in aBCIs will then be presented before a case study, which describes a recent development in aBCIs with potential applications for music therapy. Finally, a set of guidelines will be provided to aid with the development of aBCIs.

## 8.2   AFFECTIVE STATES

An affective state is defined as a psychological construct that seeks to categorize the experience of feeling an emotion (Barrett et al. 2007). Affect is often measured along either two or three different axes, of which the most commonly used are "valance," which refers to how pleasant or unpleasant an experience is, "arousal," which refers to how exciting or unexciting an experience is, and "tension," which refers to how much or little tension is felt during an experience (Wiles and Cornwell 1991).

Taken together, these different axes may be used to model an affective space that seeks to encompass the range of human emotion. Several different models of the affective space exist, using different combinations of axes to attempt to allow all possible affective states to be collated within the model and consequently measured and analytically evaluated.

One of the more popular and frequently used such models is the valance–arousal circumplex model (Russell 1980). This model uses two axes, valance and arousal, to map the affective space onto a two-dimensional plane. A range of different discrete affective states are then mapped to this affective space by identifying their locations on the valance and arousal axes. For example, "joy" may be mapped to the upper right hand corner of the space because it corresponds to a high valance (very pleasant) state and a high arousal (very excited) state. The valence–arousal circumplex model is illustrated in Figure 8.1.

A range of other models of the affective space have also been proposed. These include the Schimack and Grob three-dimensional model, which describes the affective space via the three

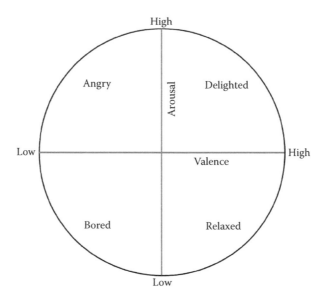

**FIGURE 8.1**   An example of the valence–arousal circumplex that may be used to model affective states along the two axes of valence and arousal.

dimensions of valence, energy–arousal, and tension–arousal (Schimmack and Grob 2000), and the Geneva Emotional Music Scale (GEMS), which seeks to describe the affective space via a set of discrete state labels that were selected for their relevance to the set of emotions commonly considered to be conveyable via music (Zentner et al. 2008).

GEMS differs from many other models of affect by utilizing labeled categories to describe an affective state in place of a continuous space. For example, the GEMS-45 system contains 45 discrete labels, grouped under nine categories, that describe affective states such as "wonder" or "joyful activation." Different combinations of labels or individual labels may be used to describe a single affective state.

Although affect may be described by discrete states or labels, the actual processes involved in the experience of affect are widely understood to be multimodal and involve multiple different neurological and physiological processes. Specifically, when you feel an emotion, this is the result of a complex interaction of multiple neurological and physiological processes acting at different time scales and influencing one another to together result in the embodied feeling of an affect (Pantic and Rothkrantz 2003).

For example, your heart rate changes with differing levels of arousal (Brosschot and Thayer 2003; Appelhans and Luecken 2006; Agrafioti et al. 2012), while skin conductivity (measured by galvanic skin response) has been reported to change with changing levels of arousal, valence, and tension (Landis and Hunt 1935; Villarejo et al. 2012; Daly et al. 2015). Additionally, respiration rate has been reported to change in response to changing levels of both valence and arousal (Etzel et al. 2006; Jones and Troen 2007). Thus, an individual's affective state may be understood to be a combination of their brain and body responding to changes in their situation (either triggered by external stimuli or internal processes such as memory recall of emotive events) (Barrett et al. 2007; Ekman 1993).

With regard to external stimuli, affect can either be felt or perceived (Gabrielsson 2001). Perceived affect is an individual's understanding of the affective state a stimuli is attempting to convey, while felt affect refers to the actual affective state experienced by the individual when exposed to the stimuli. An illustrative example of this is the enjoyment of "sad" music. A listener may perceive that a piece of music is attempting to convey sadness and yet derive considerable pleasure from listening to it (Gabrielsson 2001).

## 8.3 AFFECTIVE STATE REPORTING

When studying affect (e.g., the affective response of an individual or group to stimuli), it is often necessary to provide some mechanism for the individual to report their current felt or perceived affective state. Consequently, a variety of tools have been developed to allow the recording of users' reports of their affective states.

These tools are useful to consider in the development of aBCIs as, when developing tools and component parts of an aBCI, it is often necessary to have a ground truth measure of an individual's current affective state. For example, when developing a classifier to detect a user's current felt affective state in an aBCI user, it may often be necessary to train the classifier on some ground truth measure.

Affective state reporting tools may be described as either discrete or continuous tools. Discrete tools are used for recording single discrete snapshots of a user's affective state at one particular moment in time or over one discrete time window. By way of contrast, continuous affect reporting tools allow users to provide a moment-by-moment report of their affective state as it changes over time.

### 8.3.1 DISCRETE METHODS

There are a variety of discrete affective state reporting tools available. Two of the most widely used in psychological studies of affect are the self-assessment manikin (SAM) and the GEMS.

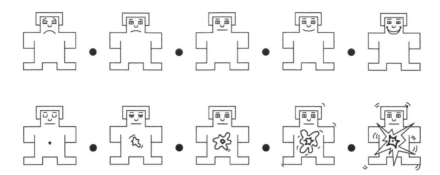

**FIGURE 8.2** SAM method of affective state reporting.

The SAM provides a set of figures depicting different positions within the valence arousal space (Bradley and Lang 1994). These are illustrated in Figure 8.2. Participants are asked to select different positions on the space that match the affective state they wish to report.

The SAM is able to provide a discrete snapshot of affect at a single moment in time. Furthermore, it does so via the use of pictographic representations of affect, which may be less susceptible to interpersonal differences in understanding of linguistics descriptors of affect in different languages (Morris 1995). Thus, there is no need to translate the SAM scale into different languages. However, the use of SAM does require participants to understand the concepts of the valence and arousal scales that are employed before they can use it effectively.

By way of contrast, the GEMS is composed of a set of text labels describing different regions of the affective space (Zentner et al. 2008; Vuoskoski and Eerola 2011). Individuals are asked to select specific labels that correspond to the regions matching how they wish to report their affective state. For example, they may be asked to select labels corresponding to feelings of nostalgia after hearing a piece of music. This allows for more immediate understanding by participants in an experiment but requires the GEMS to be translated into a language the participant is able to understand.

### 8.3.2 CONTINUOUS METHODS

Several tools are available for continuous reporting of affective states; some examples include FEELTRACE and GTRACE.

The FEELTRACE tool allows participants to report an affective state on a continuous basis (Cowie et al. 2000). The tool comprises a two-dimensional on-screen interface with valence mapped to the horizontal axis and arousal mapped to the vertical axis. Participants can report their current affective state by moving a mouse, joystick, or other input system to position a cursor at a position on the space that best matches the affective state they wish to report.

An example of the FEELTRACE reporting tool is illustrated in Figure 8.3. The tool allows individuals to report their affective state via a relatively simple representation of the valence–arousal space, but can cause confusion in some less computer-literate individuals.

To resolve this, a new version of FEELTRACE has recently been developed known as GTRACE (Cowie et al. 2012). GTRACE provides two one-dimensional reporting systems to allow individuals to report an affective state on either the valence or arousal scales independently By separating the valence and arousal axes, it has also been reported that GTRACE can act to remove some potential sources of confusion that are related to the simultaneous reporting of different axes in the affective space (Cowie et al. 2012).

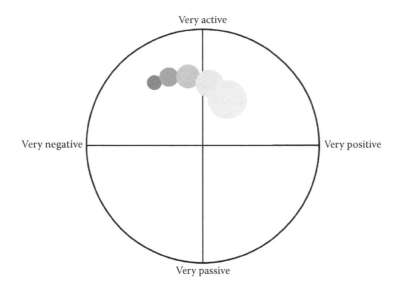

**FIGURE 8.3** The FEELTRACE interface for continuous reporting of affective states. The user controls the position of the cursor via a mouse or joystick and positions it at a location in the valence–arousal circumplex that best matches how they are feeling at that moment in time.

## 8.4 AFFECTIVE STATE DETECTION

A key component of aBCI systems is the ability to identify a user's current affective state (Mühl et al. 2014). By detecting a user's affective state, it is possible for BCIs to respond to a user's changing emotions. However, this provides a potentially very personal insight into how an individual is feeling and it is important to consider related privacy and ethical issues (see Chapter 34). To detect affective states, a variety of different approaches have been developed. These can be based on either just neurophysiological activity or a combination of neurophysiological activity and other physiological activity (a hybrid BCI approach Pfurtscheller et al. 2010; Müller-Putz et al. 2011).

BCIs (and by extension aBCIs) can be developed using a variety of different neurological signal types such as functional near-infrared spectroscopy (fNIRS), magnetic encephlography (MEG), or functional magnetic resonance imaging (fMRI) (Min et al. 2010). However, one of the most frequently used methods for measuring neurological activity used in BCI is the electroencephalogram (EEG) (Graimann et al. 2010). Consequently, the majority of affective state detection methods developed for aBCIs have been developed for EEG, with relatively fewer affective state detection methods for aBCI developed for use with other modalities, such as fMRI (Liberati et al. 2013).

When considering only the EEG as the signal from which to detect affective states, the affective state detection methods that have been developed for aBCI systems and other affective computing applications use a range of different types of features. These features may be grouped into the following categories:

1. Band-power–based features
2. Asymmetry features
3. Network features
4. Event-related potentials

The first three feature types are not phase locked to the stimulus and can be used on a continuous basis, while event-related potentials (ERPs) are phase locked to a particular stimuli presentation time. Thus, the first three feature types can be used with either synchronous or asynchronous BCI, while ERPs can only be used with synchronous (cue-based) BCIs (Müller-Putz et al. 2006). These different types of features and their use in affective state detection are detailed in Table 8.1, along with references to studies that employ these features for identifying an individual's affective state.

Band-power–based features measure changes in ongoing oscillatory activity within the EEG. They are not phase locked to a stimulus and, consequently, may be used to measure ongoing changes in affective states in response to continuously changing stimuli. They are most frequently measured via a fast Fourier transform (FFT) or a wavelet decomposition of the EEG signals. The specific frequency and spatial regions over which these band-powers may be measured differ from study to study. However, there are common regions over which they are most frequently measured.

Table 8.2 lists the spatial and frequency regions that band-power features are measured over and lists the number of participants over which these features have been demonstrated to relate to changes in affective states. It may be observed that the EEG band-powers over the prefrontal cortex in a wide range of frequency bands and the band-powers in the parietal cortex in the alpha band are most often reported to relate to affective state changes.

Asymmetry features make use of a difference in the relative intensity of activity, typically between the left and right hemispheres when experiencing different affective states. Specifically, when experiencing changing levels of valence or arousal, the mean amplitude of EEG recorded over the right hemisphere differs significantly from the left hemisphere (Fox 1991). This effect is most pronounced in the prefrontal cortex (Daly et al. 2014).

## TABLE 8.1
### Different Types of Features That May Be Used in Identifying Affective States in aBCIs

| Feature Type | Description | Measured by | References |
|---|---|---|---|
| Band power features | Relative or absolute changes in the magnitude of ongoing non–phase-locked oscillatory activity within one or more frequency bands over specific cortical regions | FFT, wavelets etc. | (Daly et al. 2015; Reuderink et al. 2009; Makeig et al. 2011; AlZoubi et al. 2009; Koelstra and Patras 2013; Petrantonakis and Hadjileontiadis 2010; Mauri et al. 2010; Khosrowabadi et al. 2009; Stikic et al. 2014; Müller et al. 1999; Mühl et al. 2011; Walpulski 2008; Aftanas et al. 2001; Krause et al. 2000; Dennis and Solomon 2010; Soleymani et al. 2014; Reuderink et al. 2012; Rogenmoser et al. 2016) |
| Asymmetry features | Relative differences in neural activity between different regions of the cortex, most typically between the left and right hemispheres | FFT, wavelets, absolute or relative magnitude differences, etc. | (AlZoubi et al. 2009; Koelstra and Patras 2013; Mauri et al. 2010; Walpulski 2008; Reuderink et al. 2012; Cavazza et al. 2014; Schmidt and Trainor 2001; Canli et al. 1998; Kirke and Miranda 2011; Aftanas et al. 2006; Cacioppo 2004; Daly et al. 2014) |
| Network features | Connectivity or associativity between different regions of the cortex | PLV, coherence, etc. | (Daly et al. 2014; Rutkowski et al. 2011; Bakardjian et al. 2011; Chanel et al. 2009) |
| Event-related potentials | Phase-locked changes in EEG amplitude | Amplitude averaging | (Olofsson et al. 2008; Frantzidis et al. 2010; Briggs and Martin 2009; Schupp et al. 2000) |

**TABLE 8.2**
**Use of EEG Band-Power Features to Identify an Individual's Affective State in Different Frequency Bands and Spatial Regions of the Cortex**

| | | Regions | | | | | | | |
|---|---|---|---|---|---|---|---|---|---|
| | | **Front.** | **Cent.** | **Occip.** | **Temp.** | **Pari.** | **Left** | **Right** | **All** |
| Frequency bands | Delta (0–4 Hz) | 93 (Daly et al. 2015; AlZoubi et al. 2009; Mauri et al. 2012; Walpulski 2008) | 20 (Reuderink et al. 2009; AlZoubi et al. 2009; Walpulski 2008) | 79 (Stikic et al. 2014; Walpulski 2008) | | 39 (AlZoubi et al. 2009; Walpulski 2008; Reuderink et al. 2012) | 1 (Reuderink et al. 2009) | 51 (Daly et al. 2015; Reuderink et al. 2012) | 63 (Stikic et al. 2014) |
| | Theta (4–8 Hz) | 241 (AlZoubi et al. 2009; Koelstra and Patras 2013; Petrantonakis and Hadjileontiadis 2010; Mauri et al. 2010; Khosrowabadi et al. 2009; Stikic et al. 2014; Walpulski 2008; Aftanas et al. 2001; Krause et al. 2000; Reuderink 2012) | 77 (AlZoubi et al. 2009; Koelstra and Patras 2013; Khosrowabadi et al. 2009; Walpulski 2008; Krause et al. 2009) | 97 (Stikic et al. 2014; Walpulski 2008; Krause et al. 2000) | | 81 (AlZoubi et al. 2009; Koelstra and Patras 2013; Khosrowabadi 2009; Walpulski 2008; Aftanas et al. 2001) | | 22 (Aftanas et al. 2001) | 22 (Rogenmoser et al. 2016) |
| | Alpha (8–13 Hz) | 329 (Makeig et al. 2011; AlZoubi et al. 2009; Koelstra and Patras 2013; Petrantonakis and Hadjileontiadis 2010; Mauri et al. 2010; Khosrowabadi et al. 2009; Stikic et al. 2014; Mühl et al. 2011; Walpulski 2008; Krause et al. 2000; Dennis and Solomon 2010; Reuderink 2012) | 141 (Makeig et al. 2011; AlZoubi et al. 2009; Koelstra and Patras 2013; Khosrowabadi et al. 2009; Stikic et al. 2014; Mühl et al. 2011; Walpulski 2008; Krause et al. 2000) | 35 (Makeig et al. 2011; Walpulski 2008; Krause et al. 2000) | 63 (Stikic et al. 2014) | 153 (Makeig et al. 2011; AlZoubi et al. 2009; Koelstra and Patras 2013; Khosrowabadi et al. 2009; Mühl et al. 2011; Walpulski 2008; Dennis and Solomon 2010) | 1 (Makeig et al. 2011) | 92 (Makeig et al. 2011; Aftanas et al. 2001; Dennis and Solomon 2010) | 22 (Rogenmoser et al. 2016) |

*(Continued)*

**TABLE 8.2 (CONTINUED)**
**Use of EEG Band-Power Features to Identify an Individual's Affective State in Different Frequency Bands and Spatial Regions of the Cortex**

| | Regions | | | | | | | |
| --- | --- | --- | --- | --- | --- | --- | --- | --- |
| | Front. | Cent. | Occip. | Temp. | Pari. | Left | Right | All |
| Beta (13–30 Hz) | 218 (Daly et al. 2015; AlZoubi et al. 2009; Koelstra and Patras 2013; Petrantonakis and Hadjileontiadis 2010; Mauri et al. 2010; Stikic et al. 2014; Walpulski 2008) | 77 (AlZoubi et al. 2009; Koelstra and Patras 2013; Walpulski 2008; Soleymani et al. 2014) | 16 (Walpulski 2008) | 63 (Stikic et al. 2014) | 112 (AlZoubi et al. 2009; Koelstra and Patras 2013; Stikic et al. 2014; Walpulski 2008) | | 31 (Daley et al. 2015) | |
| Gamma (30+ Hz) | 213 (Daly et al. 2015; AlZoubi et al. 2009; Koelstra and Patras 2013; Petrantonakis and Hadjileontiadis 2010; Mauri et al. 2010; Stikic et al. 2014; Müller et al. 1999; Walpulski 2008) | 140 (AlZoubi et al. 2009; Koelstra and Patras 2013; Mauri et al. 2010; Stikic et al. 2014, Walpulski 2008; Dennis and Solomon 2010) | 79 (Stikic et al. 2014; Walpulski 2008) | 74 (Stikic et al. 2014; Müller et al. 1999) | 49 (AlZoubi et al. 2009; Koelstra and Patras 2013; Walpulski 2008) | | 94 (Daly et al. 2015; Stikic et al. 2014) | 63 (Stikic et al. 2014) |

*Note:* For each region of the cortex and EEG frequency band, the total number of participants involved in all studies providing evidence of an involvement of that cortical region is listed, along with references to the supporting studies.

Network features are used to provide a measure of the amount of communication between different cortical regions (Varela et al. 2001; Lachaux et al. 1999; Daly et al. 2012). This gives an indication of which cortical regions are either in direct communication with one another or are influenced by a common (but potentially unobserved) neural generator (Lachaux et al. 2000). Changes in ongoing neural network activity have been observed to reflect changes in both valence and arousal and may be exploited for use in aBCIs (Daly et al. 2014).

ERPs provide a phase-locked measure of a change in amplitude of ongoing oscillatory activity in the EEG that relates to a time-locked event (Handy 2005). They may only be used with synchronous BCIs (BCIs that rely on a stimulus presentation at a specific time) (Müller-Putz et al. 2006). Thus, they are most commonly used in conjunction with emotive images to improve classification accuracies in BCIs designed to allow selection between different choices (Olofsson et al. 2008; Briggs and Martin 2009; Schupp et al. 2000).

An alternative approach to affective state detection is to use a hybrid approach that combines EEG-based features with one or more other physiological features (Pfurtscheller et al. 2010). Examples of this approach include the use of ECG and EEG for improved classification accuracies (Daly et al. 2016b) and the combination of EEG and fNIRS to understand affective responses to speech (Rutkowski et al. 2011).

## 8.5 AFFECTIVE BCIS

### 8.5.1 CATEGORIES OF aBCI

BCIs, and by extension aBCIs, may be categorized as being either passive BCIs or active BCIs.

Passive BCIs use some measure of the user's neurological activity to affect passive control over a system (Cutrell and Tan 2007; Zander et al. 2010; Zander and Kothe 2011). Thus, the BCI responds to the user's current state without the user actually actively intending or willing the control to happen. An example of this may be a pBCI that uses a measure of the user's current level of frustration to adjust the type of options presented to them (Reuderink et al. 2012). A more frustrated user may be making lots of errors and may benefit from a reduced number of control options, which can lead to increased control accuracies.

By contrast, active BCIs allow the user to actively effect control over the system via their affective state. An example of this is the use of affective imagery to select between different control options (Makeig et al. 2011). For example, participants may be asked to imagine either low or high valence affective states in order to select between two control options.

### 8.5.2 USE OF AFFECT IN aBCI

Affect may be employed in many different ways within both active and passive aBCIs. These different approaches may be grouped into the following categories:

1. Boosting classification performance
2. Understanding the user's emotions
3. Modulating the user's emotions

Classification boosting refers to the use of affect to improve the classification accuracy of an active BCI that is intended for aiding a user's ability to communicate or control their environment. For example, affect may be employed to identify incorrect selections (by identifying increases in user frustration). Alternatively, affect may be used directly to allow the user to select different options, for example, affective imagery may be used to select between different choices made available to the user (Makeig et al. 2011).

Understanding of user emotions can allow both active and passive aBCIs to respond better to a user's needs (Mühl et al. 2014). For example, an understanding of a user's current affective state can be used to modulate the contents of an aBCI controlled game (Reuderink et al. 2009).

Finally, a measurement of affect in an aBCI can be used to allow a passive aBCI to modulate the user's emotions. This allows the aBCI system to potentially be used for therapeutic purposes, where the aBCI is used to attempt to produce either short- or long-term improvements in an individual's emotions or moods (Daly et al. 2016a). An example of this approach is presented in the case study in Section 8.6.

There are several different potential applications of these various categories and types of aBCI. Specifically, aBCIs have been proposed for use in the following areas:

1. Therapy
2. Affective computing
3. Entertainment
4. Communication and control

Therapeutic uses of BCI are diverse and range from rehabilitation of motor control after stroke through to treatment of attention-deficit/hyperactivity disorder. Chapter 5 provides an overview of the range of different therapeutic uses of BCI systems.

aBCIs have potential applications as aids and assistive tools in therapy. Specifically, by identifying and responding to an individual's current affective state, an aBCI has the potential to be able to deliver stimuli to that user that are therapeutically beneficial. An example of this potential use in the case of a passive aBCI is discussed in Section 8.6.

Affective computing is the development of computer systems that can respond to a user's affective state (D'Mello et al. 2011). This allows a computer system to dynamically change its operating principles in order to meet the affective needs of a user. For example, an affective computing system may be used in e-learning applications in order to detect changes in a user's affective state related to boredom (when the material is already known) or frustration (when the material is poorly understood) (Tao and Tan 2005). The system could then respond to these changes in affect by adapting the material presented to the student.

aBCIs have also been proposed for use in entertainment devices. For example, by identifying a user's current affective state, a passive aBCI is able to more effectively adapt an entertainment media (such as film, music, or stories) to better entertain the user. An example of this is described by Brouwer et al., who have developed an aBCI that responds to changes in user affect while they read passages from a novel (Brouwer et al. 2015). The novel was written to contain multiple branching sections and different routes through the story that were selected depending on the user's changing affective state as the story progresses.

Finally, active aBCIs may also be used for communication and control. In this application type, the user may attempt to actively modulate their affective state or engage in affective state imagery in order to select between different control options. Alternatively, affective states may be detected and used to inform the selection of control options via other means, such as ERP-based BCI.

## 8.6   CASE STUDY: AN AFFECTIVE BCMI

We describe one example of an aBCI system developed for use as a passive BCI that uses a measure of a user's current affective state in order to attempt to modulate their future affective state. Specifically, we describe an affective brain–computer music interface (aBCMI) developed by Daly et al. (2016b). This aBCMI system is designed to detect a user's current affective state and, given that affective state and a target affective state, use a music generator in order to modulate the user's affective state.

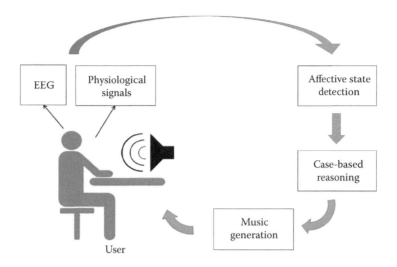

**FIGURE 8.4**   An aBCMI.

The aBCMI provides a potential tool for use in music therapy by utilizing the feedback loop provided by the BCI system to allow modulation of a user's affective state. BCMIs are an emerging form of BCI system designed to allow their users to interact with or create music. Chapter 10 provides an overview of the history and current state of the art in the development of BCMI systems. The aBCMI system we describe here (illustrated in Figure 8.4) includes four stages.

First, EEG and other physiological signals are recorded from the user and preprocessed to remove artifacts. Second, these preprocessed signals are used to identify the user's current affective state. The third step is then a case-based reasoning system, which is used to identify the specific modulations of the music played to the user in order to move them from their current affective state to a new target affective state. Finally, the fourth stage of the system is a music generator, which is used to generate music in order to attempt to move the user closer to the target affective state.

This aBCMI system was evaluated on a population of 20 healthy participants in order to determine whether it was able to successfully modulate their current affective states. Participants were asked to attend five separate sessions, the first four of which were used to train the aBCMI system and the fifth of which was used to evaluate the system's ability to achieve four key targets:

1. Make the user happier (increase the valence they report)
2. Make the user calmer (decrease arousal)
3. Reduce the user's stress (increase valence and decrease arousal)
4. Excite the user (increase arousal)

The success of the system was evaluated by measuring participants' self-reports of their current felt emotions, which were reported on a continuous basis using the FEELTRACE reporting tool (Cowie et al. 2000). Participant reports during trials in which the aBCMI attempted to achieve each of the four goals were compared against the trajectory of the change in affective state that is intended during each of the key system goals. For example, in trials for which the goal of the aBCMI was to induce an increase in the user's valence (make the user happier), the valence reported by the users was evaluated to determine whether it significantly increased over the course of the trial.

This is illustrated in Figure 8.5, which shows the mean FEELTRACE reports from all aBCI users during the "make happier" condition. Note that the report of valence increases over the course of the trial, a change that was observed to be statistically significant ($p < 0.01$).

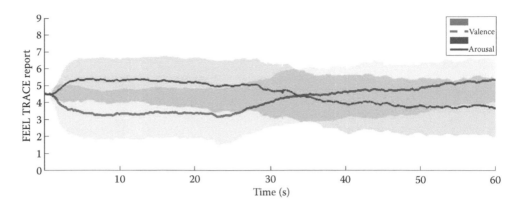

**FIGURE 8.5** Mean FEELTRACE reports from all users of the aBCMI under the "make happier" condition.

The aBCMI was able to significantly increase the valence reported by its users during online evaluation. It was also able to significantly decrease user's arousal and reduce the reported stress of its users (simultaneously decreasing arousal and increasing valence). However, it was unable to increase the arousal reported by its users, which may be due to the type of music generated by the aBCMI. Specifically, classic monophonic piano music was generated by the system, and this genre of music may be less likely to induce excitement and, therefore, increases in arousal levels in listeners.

## 8.7   GUIDE FOR DEVELOPING aBCIs

Based on our observations from the literature, a set of guidelines are provided to highlight key considerations when developing an aBCI.

First, **identify the purpose of the aBCI**. There are a wide range of different possible application areas for aBCI, such as aiding with communication or movement, therapy, or aiding with artistic expression, as well as new and previously unexplored areas. The first step in developing the aBCI should be to clearly identify the application area and the purpose of the aBCI.

Second, **the category the aBCI falls into should be identified**. aBCIs can be categorized as either active or passive (or a hybrid approach that combines both) and determining this category significantly affects how it is designed.

Third, **identify how affect will be used within the aBCI**. Measures of affect can be used in a wide range of different ways in aBCI, from aiding with communication/control accuracy, to providing a form of therapeutic feedback to the user. Additionally, affect may be the only control signal in your aBCI or it may be used in combination with other signals (such as ERPs).

Fourth, **define how affect will be categorized and measured within the aBCI**. Affect can be described within a range of different frameworks and measured via a variety of different metrics and it is important to identify which framework is to be used before constructing an aBCI.

Fifth, **identify the affective state detection method** to use in the aBCI and verify that it works correctly. This may involve offline studies, simulations, or pilot experiments, depending on the type of affective state detection method employed.

Sixth, **it is important to consider intertrial and interuser variability** in affective state responses. Affect is a fluid process that changes nonlinearly over time and with respect to multiple factors. It also varies hugely between people. Thus, an affective stimulus may have very different effects on different users.

Seventh, **it is also important to consider nonstationarity of affect**. Affective state changes are not stationary over time and such nonstationarity needs to be considered when designing an aBCI.

For example, in the case study described in Section 8.6, the aBCMI uses generated music to avoid the well-known effects of repeat exposure to the same stimuli on affective responses.

Eighth, **it is important to remove artifacts from the neurological data used to control the aBCI**. Artifacts are a problem for all BCI systems and need to be removed to ensure intention/affective state detection is accurate. However, they can be more of a problem for aBCIs where the most frequently used affective state detection methods are based on the prefrontal asymmetry, a measure recorded from the EEG electrodes positioned closest to the eyes, and therefore the most susceptible to interruption by blink artifacts.

Finally, **it is important to plan an appropriate testing strategy**. Validating the efficacy of an aBCI can be more challenging than other types of BCI because of the inherent challenges in identifying a user's "ground truth," a measure of their actual affective state. Thus, experiments need careful designing in order to allow the aBCI to be rigorously evaluated.

## 8.8 SUMMARY

aBCIs incorporate a measure of the user's affective state in order to provide a method for either improving BCI performance or widening the range of applications to which BCI can be applied. Specifically, aBCIs have been developed as tools for entertainment, aids to communication, and therapeutic devices.

By including an understanding of affect, an aBCI has the potential to respond more dynamically to a user's needs. This allows BCI applications to be expanded in scope and variety and, ultimately, has the potential to lead to improvements in the quality of life for a large number of people.

## REFERENCES

Aftanas, L. I., Reva, N. V., Savotina, L. N., and Makhnev, V. P. Neurophysiological correlates of induced discrete emotions in humans: An individually oriented analysis. *Neuroscience and Behavioral Physiology*, vol. 36, no. 2, pp. 119–130, Mar 2006. [Online]. Available: http://www.ncbi.nlm.nih.gov/pubmed/16380825

Aftanas, L., Varlamov, A., Pavlov, S., Makhnev, V., and Reva, N. Event-related synchronization and desynchronization during affective processing: Emergence of valence-related time-dependent hemispheric asymmetries in theta and upper alpha band. *The International Journal of Neuroscience*, vol. 110, no. 3–4, pp. 197–219, 2001. [Online]. Available: http://www.ncbi.nlm.nih.gov/pubmed/11912870

Agrafioti, F., Hatzinakos, D., and Anderson, A. K. ECG pattern analysis for emotion detection. *IEEE Transactions on Affective Computing*, vol. 3, no. 1, pp. 102–115, Jan 2012. [Online]. Available: http://ieeexplore.ieee.org/document/5999653/

AlZoubi, O., Calvo, R. A., and Stevens, R. H. Classification of EEG for affect recognition: An adaptive approach, in *AI 2009: Advances in Artificial Intelligence*. Springer Berlin Heidelberg, 2009, pp. 52–61. [Online]. Available: http://link.springer.com/10.1007/978-3-642-10439-8_6

Appelhans, B. M., and Luecken, L. J., Heart rate variability as an index of regulated emotional responding. *Review of General Psychology*, vol. 10, no. 3, pp. 229–240, 2006. [Online]. Available: http://doi.apa.org/getdoi.cfm?doi=10.1037/1089-2680.10.3.229

Bakardjian, H., Tanaka, T., and Cichocki, A. Emotional faces boost up steady-state visual responses for brain–computer interface. *NeuroReport*, vol. 22, no. 3, pp. 121–125, Feb 2011. [Online]. Available: http://content.wkhealth.com/linkback/openurl?sid=WKPTLP:landingpage&an=00001756-201102160-00005

Barrett, L. F., Mesquita, B., Ochsner, K. N., and Gross, J. J. The experience of emotion. *Annual Review of Psychology*, vol. 58, pp. 373–403, 2007. [Online]. Available: http://www.ncbi.nlm.nih.gov/pubmed/17002554 http://www.pubmedcentral.nih.gov/articlerender.fcgi?artid=PMC1934613

Bradley,M. M., and Lang, P. J. Measuring emotion: The Self-Assessment Manikin and the Semantic Differential. *Journal of Behavior Therapy and Experimental Psychiatry*, vol. 25, no. 1, pp. 49–59, Mar 1994. [Online]. Available: http://www.ncbi.nlm.nih.gov/pubmed/7962581

Briggs, K. F., and Martin, F. H. Affective picture processing and motivational relevance: Arousal and valence effects on ERPs in an oddball task. *International Journal of Psychophysiology*, vol. 72, no. 3, pp. 299–306, 2009.

Brosschot, J. F., and Thayer, J. F. Heart rate response is longer after negative emotions than after positive emotions. *International Journal of Psychophysiology*, vol. 50, no. 3, pp. 181–187, 2003.

Brouwer, A.-M., Hogervorst, M., Reuderink, B., van der Werf, Y., and van Erp, J. Physiological signals distinguish between reading emotional and non-emotional sections in a novel. *Brain–Computer Interfaces*, vol. 2, no. 2–3, pp. 76–89, Apr 2015. [Online]. Available: http://www.tandfonline.com/doi/full/10.1080/2326263X.2015.1100037

Cacioppo, J. T. Feelings and emotions: Roles for electrophysiological markers. *Biological Psychology*, vol. 67, no. 1–2, pp. 235–243, Oct 2004. [Online]. Available: http://www.ncbi.nlm.nih.gov/pubmed/15130533

Canli, T., Desmond, J. E., Zhao, Z., Glover, G., and Gabrieli, J. D. Hemispheric asymmetry for emotional stimuli detected with fMRI. *Neuroreport*, vol. 9, no. 14, pp. 3233–3239, Oct 1998. [Online]. Available: http://www.ncbi.nlm.nih.gov/pubmed/9831457

Cavazza, M. M., Aranyi, G. G., Charles, F. F., Porteous, J. J., Gilroy, S. W. S., Jackont, G. G., Klovatch, I. I., Raz, G. G., Keynan, N. J. N. J., Cohen, A. A., and Hendler, T. T. Frontal alpha asymmetry neurofeedback for brain–computer interfaces, 2014.

Chanel, G., Kierkels, J. J., Soleymani, M., and Pun, T. Short-term emotion assessment in a recall paradigm. *International Journal of Human–Computer Studies*, vol. 67, no. 8, pp. 607–627, 2009.

Cowie, R., Douglas-Cowie, E., Savvidou, S., McMahon, E., Sawey, M., and Schröder, M. 'FEELTRACE': An instrument for recording perceived emotion in real time, in *Proceedings of the ISCA Workshop on Speech and Emotion*, 2000, pp. 19–24. [Online]. Available: http://citeseerx.ist.psu.edu/viewdoc/summary?doi=10.1.1.58.7528

Cowie, R., McKeown, G., Douglas-Cowie, E., Caridakis, G., Karpouzis, K., Wallace, M., Kessous, L., Amir, N., Cowie, R., Cornelius, R., Cowie, R., Douglas-Cowie, E., Tsapatsoulis, N., Votsis, G., Kollias, S., Fellenz, W., Taylor, J. G., Douglas-Cowie, E., Campbell, N., Cowie, R., Roach, P., Barrett, L. F., Russell, J. A., Fontaine, J. R., Scherer, K. R., Roesch, E. B., Ellsworth, P., Forgas, J., Bower, G. H., Ioannou, S., Raouzaiou, A., Tzouvaras, V., Mailis, T., Karpouzis, K., Kollias, K., Krumhansl, C., Levenson, R. W., Gottman, J. M., Luck, G., Toiviainen, P., Erkkila, J., Lartillot, O., Riikkila, K., Makela, A., Mayer, J., Caruso, D., Salovey, P., Mehrabian, A., Messinger, D. S., Cassel, T., Acosta, S., Ambadar, Z., Cohn, J. F., Nagel, F., Kopiez, R., Grewe, O., Altenmüller, E., Reisenzein, R., Russell, J., Russell, J. A., Sander, D., Grandjean, D., Scherer, K., Schlosberg, H., Schubert, E., Shriberg, E., Stolcke, A., Hakkani-Tur, D., Tur, G., Sneddon, I., McKeown, G., McRorie, M., Vukicevic, T., Stevens, C., Schubert, E., Morris, R., Frear, M., Stevens, S., and Sutton, J. Tracing emotion. *International Journal of Synthetic Emotions*, vol. 3, no. 1, pp. 1–17, Jan 2012. [Online]. Available: http://services.igi-global.com/resolvedoi/resolve.aspx?doi=10.4018/jse.2012010101

Cutrell, E., and Tan, D. BCI for passive input in HCI, in *Proc. ACM CHI 2008 Conference on Human Factors in Computing Systems Workshop on Brain–Computer Interfaces for HCI and Games*, 2007.

D'Mello, S., Graesser, A., Schuller, B., and Martin, J.-C., Eds., *Affective Computing and Intelligent Interaction*, ser. Lecture Notes in Computer Science. Berlin, Heidelberg: Springer Berlin Heidelberg, 2011, vol. 6975. [Online]. Available: http://link.springer.com/10.1007/978-3-642-24571-8

Daly, I., Malik, A., Hwang, F., Roesch, E., Weaver, J., Kirke, A., Williams, D., Miranda, E., and Nasuto, S. J. Neural correlates of emotional responses to music: An EEG study. *Neuroscience Letters*, vol. 573, pp. 52–57, May 2014.

Daly, I., Nasuto, S. J., and Warwick, K. Brain computer interface control via functional connectivity dynamics. *Pattern Recognition*, vol. 45, no. 6, pp. 2123–2136, Jun 2012. [Online]. Available: http://dx.doi.org/10.1016/j.patcog.2011.04.034

Daly, I., Williams, D., Hallowell, J., Hwang, F., Kirke, A., Malik, A., Weaver, J., Miranda, E., and Nasuto, S. J. Music-induced emotions can be predicted from a combination of brain activity and acoustic features. *Brain and Cognition*, vol. 101, pp. 1–11, Dec 2015. [Online]. Available: http://www.sciencedirect.com/science/article/pii/S0278262615300142

Daly, I., Williams, D., Kirke, A., Weaver, J., Malik, A., Hwang, F., Miranda, E., and Nasuto, S. Affective brain–computer music interfacing. *Journal of Neural Engineering*, vol. 13, no. 4, 046022, 2016a.

Daly, I., Williams, D., Kirke, A., Weaver, J., Malik, A., Hwang, F., Wairagkar, M., Miranda, E., and Nasuto, S. An affective brain–computer music interface, in *Proceedings of the 6th International Brain–Computer Interface Meeting, organized by the BCI Society*, 2016b.

Dennis, T. A., and Solomon, B. Frontal EEG and emotion regulation: Electrocortical activity in response to emotional film clips is associated with reduced mood induction and attention interference effects. *Biological Psychology*, vol. 85, no. 3, pp. 456–464, Dec 2010.

Ekman, P. Facial expression and emotion. *American Psychologist*, vol. 48, no. 4, pp. 384–392, 1993.

Etzel, J. A., Johnsen, E. L., Dickerson, J., Tranel, D., and Adolphs, R. Cardiovascular and respiratory responses during musical mood induction. *International Journal of Psychophysiology: Official Journal of the International Organization of Psychophysiology*, vol. 61, no. 1, pp. 57–69, Jul 2006. [Online]. Available: http://www.ncbi.nlm.nih.gov/pubmed/16460823

Fox, N. A. If it's not left, it's right. Electroencephalograph asymmetry and the development of emotion. *The American Psychologist*, vol. 46, no. 8, pp. 863–872, Aug 1991. [Online]. Available: http://www.ncbi.nlm.nih.gov/pubmed/1928939

Frantzidis, C. A., Bratsas, C., Papadelis, C. L., Konstantinidis, E., Pappas, C., and Bamidis, P. D. Toward emotion aware computing: An integrated approach using multichannel neurophysiological recordings and affective visual stimuli. *IEEE Transactions on Information Technology in Biomedicine: A Publication of the IEEE Engineering in Medicine and Biology Society*, vol. 14, no. 3, pp. 589–597, May 2010. [Online]. Available: http://www.ncbi.nlm.nih.gov/pubmed/20172835

Gabrielsson, A. Emotion perceived and emotion felt: Same or different? *Musicae Scientiae*, vol. Spec Issue, pp. 123–147, 2001.

Graimann, B., Pfurtscheller, G., Allison, B., and Neuper, C. *Brain–Computer Interfaces*, ser. The Frontiers Collection, B. Graimann, G. Pfurtscheller, and B. Allison, Eds. Berlin, Heidelberg: Springer, 2010. [Online]. Available: http://www.springerlink.com/content/k5x8743w21p8rx50/

Handy, T. C. *Event-Related Potentials: A Methods Handbook*. MIT Press, 2005. [Online]. Available: http://books.google.com/books?hl=en&lr=&id=OQyZEfgEzRUC&pgis=1

Jones, C. M., and Troen, T. Biometric valence and arousal recognition, in *Proceedings of the 2007 Conference of the Computer–Human Interaction Special Interest Group (CHISIG) of Australia on Computer–Human Interaction: Design: Activities, Artifacts and Environments—OZCHI '07*. New York, New York, USA: ACM Press, 2007, p. 191. [Online]. Available: http://portal.acm.org/citation.cfm?doid=1324892.1324929

Khosrowabadi, R., Wahab, A., Ang, K. K., and Baniasad, M. H. Affective computation on EEG correlates of emotion from musical and vocal stimuli, in *2009 International Joint Conference on Neural Networks*. IEEE, Jun 2009, pp. 1590–1594. [Online]. Available: http://ieeexplore.ieee.org/lpdocs/epic03/wrapper.htm?arnumber=5178748

Kirke, A., and Miranda, E. Combining EEG frontal asymmetry studies with affective algorithmic composition and expressive performance models, pp. 1–4, 2011.

Koelstra, S., and Patras, I. Fusion of facial expressions and EEG for implicit affective tagging. *Image and Vision Computing*, vol. 31, no. 2, pp. 164–174, 2013.

Krause, C. M., Viemerö, V., Rosenqvist, A., Sillanmäki, L., and Aström, T. Relative electroencephalographic desynchronization and synchronization in humans to emotional film content: An analysis of the 4–6, 6–8, 8–10 and 10–12 Hz frequency bands. *Neuroscience Letters*, vol. 286, no. 1, pp. 9–12, May 2000. [Online]. Available: http://www.ncbi.nlm.nih.gov/pubmed/10822140

Lachaux, J. P., Rodriguez, E., Martinerie, J., and Varela, F. J. Measuring phase synchrony in brain signals. *Human Brain Mapping*, vol. 8, no. 4, pp. 194–208, Jan 1999.

Lachaux, J. P., Rodriguez, E., Quyen, M. L. V., Lutz, A., Martinerie, J., and Varela, F. J. Studying singletrials of phase synchronous activity in the brain. *International Journal of Bifurcation and Chaos*, vol. 10, no. 10, pp. 2429–2439, 2000.

Landis, C., and Hunt, W. A. The conscious correlates of the galvanic skin response. *Journal of Experimental Psychology*, vol. 18, no. 5, pp. 505–529, 1935. [Online]. Available: http://content.apa.org/journals/xge/18/5/505

Liberati, G., Veit, R., Kim, S., Birbaumer, N., von Arnim, C., Jenner, A., Lule, D., Ludolph, A. C., Raffone, A., Belardinelli, M. O., da Rocha, J. D., and Sitaram, R., Development of a binary fMRI-BCI for Alzheimer patients: A semantic conditioning paradigm using affective unconditioned stimuli, in *2013 Humaine Association Conference on Affective Computing and Intelligent Interaction*. IEEE, Sep 2013, pp. 838–842. [Online]. Available: http://ieeexplore.ieee.org/document/6681549/

Makeig, S., Leslie, G., Mullen, T., Sarma, D., Bigdely-Shamlo, N., and Kothe, C. First demonstration of a musical emotion BCI. *Affecti. Comput. and Int. Interact. Lect. Notes in Comp. Sci.*, vol. 6975, pp. 487–496, 2011.

Mauri, M., Magagnin, V., Cipresso, P., Mainardi, L., Brown, E. N., Cerutti, S., Villamira, M., and Barbieri, R. Psychophysiological signals associated with affective states, in *2010 Annual International Conference of the IEEE Engineering in Medicine and Biology*. IEEE, Aug 2010, pp. 3563–3566. [Online]. Available: http://ieeexplore.ieee.org/document/5627465/

Min, B.-K., Marzelli, M. J., and Yoo, S.-S. Neuroimaging-based approaches in the brain–computer interface. *Trends in Biotechnology*, vol. 28, no. 11, pp. 552–560, Nov 2010. [Online]. Available: http://dx.doi.org/10.1016/j.tibtech.2010.08.002

Morris, J. Observations: SAM: The Self-Assessment Manikin; an efficient cross-cultural measurement of emotional response. *Journal of Advertising Research*, vol. 35, no. 8, 1995.

Mühl, C., Allison, B., Nijholt, A., and Chanel, G. A survey of affective brain computer interfaces: Principles, state-of-the-art, and challenges. *Brain–Computer Interfaces*, vol. 1, no. 2, pp. 66–84, Apr 2014. [Online]. Available: http://www.tandfonline.com/doi/abs/10.1080/2326263X.2014.912881

Mühl, C., Brouwer, A.-M., van Wouwe, N., van den Broek, E., Nijboer, F., and Heylen, D. Modality-specific affective responses and their implications for affective BCI, in *Fifth International Brain–Computer Interface Conference*. Verlag der Technischen Universität, 2011, pp. 22–24.

Müller, M. M., Keil, A., Gruber, T., and Elbert, T. Processing of affective pictures modulates righthemispheric gamma band EEG activity. *Clinical Neurophysiology: Official Journal of the International Federation of Clinical Neurophysiology*, vol. 110, no. 11, pp. 1913–1920, Nov 1999. [Online]. Available: http://www.ncbi.nlm.nih.gov/pubmed/10576487

Müller-Putz, G. R., Breitwieser, C., Cincotti, F., Leeb, R., Schreuder, M., Leotta, F. et al., Tools for brain–computer interaction: A general concept for a hybrid BCI. *Front Neuroinform*, vol. 5, p. 30, Jan 2011.

Müller-Putz, G. R., Scherer, R., Pfurtscheller, G., and Rupp, R. Brain–computer interfaces for control of neuroprostheses: From synchronous to asynchronous mode of operation. *Biomed Tech (Berl)*, vol. 51, no. 2, pp. 57–63, Jul 2006. [Online]. Available: http://www.degruyter.com/view/j/bmte.2006.51.issue-2/bmt.2006.011/bmt.2006.011.xml http://www.ncbi.nlm.nih.gov/pubmed/16915766

Nijboer, F., Morin, F. O., Carmien, S. P., Koene, R. A., Leon, E., and Hoffmann, U. Affective brain–computer interfaces: Psychophysiological markers of emotion in healthy persons and in persons with amyotrophic lateral sclerosis, in *2009 3rd International Conference on Affective Computing and Intelligent Interaction and Workshops*. Sep 2009, pp. 1–11. [Online]. Available: http://ieeexplore.ieee.org/document/5349479/

Olofsson, J. K., Nordin, S., Sequeira, H., and Polich, J. Affective picture processing: An integrative review of ERP findings. *Biological Psychology*, vol. 77, no. 3, pp. 247–265, Mar 2008. [Online]. Available: http://www.ncbi.nlm.nih.gov/pubmed/18164800; http://www.pubmedcentral.nih.gov/articlerender.fcgi?artid=PMC2443061 http://linkinghub.elsevier.com/retrieve/pii/S0301051107001913

Pantic, M., and Rothkrantz, L. Toward an affect-sensitive multimodal human–computer interaction. *Proceedings of the IEEE*, vol. 91, no. 9, pp. 1370–1390, Sep 2003. [Online]. Available: http://ieeexplore.ieee.org/document/1230215/

Petrantonakis, P., and Hadjileontiadis, L. Emotion recognition from EEG using higher order crossings. *IEEE Transactions on Information Technology in Biomedicine*, vol. 14, no. 2, pp. 186–197, Mar 2010. [Online]. Available: http://ieeexplore.ieee.org/document/5291724/

Pfurtscheller, G., Allison, B. Z., Brunner, C., Bauernfeind, G., Solis-Escalante, T., Scherer, R., Zander, T. O., Müller-Putz, G., Neuper, C., and Birbaumer, N. The hybrid BCI. *Frontiers in Neuroprosthetics*, vol. 4, no. 30, 2010.3

Reuderink, B., Mühl, C., and Poel, M., Valence, arousal and dominance in the EEG during game play. *International Journal of Autonomous and Adaptive Communications Systems*, vol. 6, no. 1, Dec 2012. [Online]. Available: http://www.inderscienceonline.com/doi/abs/10.1504/IJAACS.2013.050691

Reuderink, B., Nijholt, A., and Poel, M. *Affective Pacman: A Frustrating Game for Brain–Computer Interface Experiments*. Springer Berlin Heidelberg, 2009, pp. 221–227. [Online]. Available: http://link.springer.com/10.1007/978-3-642-02315-6_23

Rogenmoser, L., Zollinger, N., Elmer, S., and Jäncke, L. Independent component processes underlying emotions during natural music listening. *Social Cognitive and Affective Neuroscience*, vol. 7, no. 37, pp. 1–12, Apr 2016. [Online]. Available: http://www.ncbi.nlm.nih.gov/pubmed/27217116

Russell, J. A. A circumplex model of affect. *Journal of Personality and Social Psychology*, vol. 39, no. 6, pp. 1161–1178, 1980.

Rutkowski, T. M., Zhao, Q., Cichocki, A., Tanaka, T., and Mandic, D. P. Towards affective BCI/BMI paradigms—Analysis of fEEG and fNIRS brain responses to emotional speech and facial videos, in *Advances in Cognitive Neurodynamics (II)*. Dordrecht: Springer Netherlands, 2011, pp. 671–675. [Online]. Available: http://www.springerlink.com/index/10.1007/978-90-481-9695-1_100

Schimmack, U., and Grob, A. Dimensional models of core affect: A quantitative comparison by means of structural equation modeling. *European Journal of Personality*, vol. 14, no. 4, p. 21, 2000.

Schmidt, L. A., and Trainor, L. J. Frontal brain electrical activity (EEG) distinguishes valence and intensity of musical emotions. *Cognition & Emotion*, vol. 15, no. 4, pp. 487–500, Jul 2001. [Online]. Available: http://dx.doi.org/10.1080/02699930126048

Schupp, H. T., Cuthbert, B. N., Bradley, M. M., Cacioppo, J. T., Ito, T., and Lang, P. J. Affective picture processing: The late positive potential is modulated by motivational relevance. *Psychophysiology*, vol. 37, no. 2, pp. 257–261, Mar 2000. [Online]. Available: http://www.ncbi.nlm.nih.gov/pubmed/10731776

Soleymani, M., Asghari-Esfeden, S., Pantic, M., and Fu, Y. Continuous emotion detection using EEG signals and facial expressions, in *2014 IEEE International Conference on Multimedia and Expo (ICME)*. IEEE, Jul 2014, pp. 1–6. [Online]. Available: http://ieeexplore.ieee.org/lpdocs/epic03/wrapper.htm ?arnumber=6890301

Stikic, M., Johnson, R. R., Tan, V., and Berka, C. EEG-based classification of positive and negative affective states. *Brain Computer Interfaces*, vol. 1, no. 2, pp. 99–112, May 2014. [Online]. Available: http://www .tandfonline.com/doi/abs/10.1080/2326263X.2014.912883

Tao, J., and Tan, T. *Affective Computing: A Review*. Springer Berlin Heidelberg, 2005, pp. 981–995. [Online]. Available: http://link.springer.com/10.1007/11573548_125

Varela, F., Lachaux, J. P., Rodriguez, E., and Martinerie, J. The brainweb: Phase synchronization and large-scale integration. *Nature Reviews. Neuroscience*, vol. 2, no. 4, pp. 229–239, Apr 2001. [Online]. Available: http://dx.doi.org/10.1038/35067550

Villarejo, M. V., Zapirain, B. G., and Zorrilla, A. M. A stress sensor based on Galvanic Skin Response (GSR) controlled by ZigBee. *Sensors (Basel, Switzerland)*, vol. 12, no. 5, pp. 6075–101, Jan 2012. [Online]. Available: http://www.pubmedcentral.nih.gov/articlerender.fcgi?artid=3386730&tool=pmcentrez&render type=abstract

Vuoskoski, J. K., and Eerola, T. Measuring music-induced emotion: A comparison of emotion models, personality biases, and intensity of experiences. *Musicae Scientiae*, vol. 15, no. 2, pp. 159–173, Jul 2011. [Online]. Available: http://msx.sagepub.com/content/15/2/159.short

Walpulski, M. EEG representation of emotion evoking pictures, 2008.

Wiles, J. A., and Cornwell, T. B. A review of methods utilized in measuring affect, feelings, and emotion in advertising. *Current Issues and Research in Advertising*, vol. 13, no. 1–2, pp. 241–275, Mar 1991. [Online]. Available: http://www.tandfonline.com/doi/abs/10.1080/01633392.1991.10504968

Wolpaw, J. R. Brain–computer interfaces as new brain output pathways. *The Journal of Physiology*, vol. 579, no. Pt 3, pp. 613–619, Mar 2007.

Zander, T. O., and Kothe, C. Towards passive brain–computer interfaces: Applying brain–computer interface technology to human–machine systems in general. *Journal of Neural Engineering*, vol. 8, no. 2, p. 025005, Apr 2011. [Online]. Available: http://www.ncbi.nlm.nih.gov/pubmed/21436512

Zander,T. O., and Jatzev, S. Detecting affective covert user states with passive brain–computer interfaces, in *2009 3rd International Conference on Affective Computing and Intelligent Interaction and Workshops*. IEEE, Sep 2009, pp. 1–9. [Online]. Available: http://ieeexplore.ieee.org/document/5349456/

Zander, T. O., Kothe, C., Jatzev, S., and Gaertner, M. Enhancing human–computer interaction with input from active and passive brain–computer interfaces, in *Proc. 4th Int. BCI Workshop and Training Course*. Springer London, 2010, pp. 181–199. [Online]. Available: http://link.springer.com/10.1007/978-1-84996-272-8_11

Zentner, M., Grandjean, D., and Scherer, K. R. Emotions evoked by the sound of music: Characterization, classification, and measurement. *Emotion*, vol. 8, no. 4, pp. 494–521, 2008. [Online]. Available: http:// doi.apa.org/getdoi.cfm?doi=10.1037/1528-3542.8.4.494

# 9 Toward Practical BCI Solutions for Entertainment and Art Performance

*Paruthi Pradhapan, Ulf Großekathöfer,*
*Giuseppina Schiavone, Bernard Grundlehner,*
*and Vojkan Mihajlović*

## CONTENTS

9.1 Introduction: Practical BCI Solutions for Masses .................................................. 166
9.2 Technology Required for Practical BCI Solutions .................................................. 167
    9.2.1 Convenient EEG Electrodes ......................................................................... 167
    9.2.2 Active Sensors .............................................................................................. 168
    9.2.3 Electronic Design ......................................................................................... 168
    9.2.4 EEG Headset ................................................................................................. 169
    9.2.5 Data Processing ............................................................................................ 170
    9.2.6 Actuation/Information Communication ........................................................ 170
9.3 Competitive Toy Car Racing Using Motor Imagery BCI ...................................... 171
    9.3.1 Study Population ........................................................................................... 171
    9.3.2 Experimental Protocol .................................................................................. 172
        9.3.2.1 Cue-Based Measurements .............................................................. 173
        9.3.2.2 Self-Paced Measurements .............................................................. 173
    9.3.3 Data Analysis ............................................................................................... 174
        9.3.3.1 Preprocessing ................................................................................. 174
        9.3.3.2 Feature Extraction and Classification ............................................ 174
        9.3.3.3 Evaluation ...................................................................................... 174
    9.3.4 Results .......................................................................................................... 174
    9.3.5 Application Example ..................................................................................... 175
9.4 Enriching Performance of a Juggler by Brain and Body Sonification .................... 176
    9.4.1 Study Population ........................................................................................... 177
    9.4.2 Experimental Protocol .................................................................................. 177
    9.4.3 Data Analysis ............................................................................................... 179
        9.4.3.1 Preprocessing ................................................................................. 179
        9.4.3.2 Data Analysis ................................................................................. 179
    9.4.4 Results .......................................................................................................... 179
    9.4.5 Application Example ..................................................................................... 180
9.5 Monitoring Vigilance in Children during Entertainment and Learning .................. 181
    9.5.1 Study Population ........................................................................................... 182
    9.5.2 Experimental Protocol .................................................................................. 182
    9.5.3 Data Analysis ............................................................................................... 184
        9.5.3.1 Preprocessing ................................................................................. 184
        9.5.3.2 Data Analysis ................................................................................. 184

9.5.4   Results.................................................................................................................... 185
9.5.5   Application Example ............................................................................................. 186
9.6   Discussion............................................................................................................................ 186
Acknowledgments............................................................................................................................ 188
References......................................................................................................................................... 189

**Abstract**

To facilitate wider adoption of brain–computer interface (BCI), we need ergonomic and user-friendly BCI solutions that provide high-quality brain signal acquisition and robust and reliable information extraction. Such BCI solutions require addressing all aspects of the design and development for the targeted application, including sensor and electronics design, headset integration and ergonomics, data acquisition, signal cleaning and analysis, extraction of meaningful information, intuitive user interfaces, and effective information communication methods. These aspects are addressed through the analysis of three use cases, all having in common practical electroencephalogram (EEG)-based BCI able to achieve reliable real-time interaction in ecological, real-life scenarios. The use cases include using a four-channel dry electrode EEG solution to control a toy car based on motor imagery BCI, transforming jugglers' brain activity into a sonic experience for the audience, and monitoring the cognitive state of a child during gaming/training. Special attention is given to improving the experience of a user (e.g., using flexible electrodes, ergonomic headsets, seamless feedback methods) and to approaches that allow for best possible signal quality (e.g., using active electrodes, careful system integration, optimal signal conditioning methods). Critical overview of existing solutions is given, speculating how they can be improved such that we could see BCI solutions as essential components of future products not only in gaming and arts performance but also in medical fields.

## 9.1   INTRODUCTION: PRACTICAL BCI SOLUTIONS FOR MASSES

Most brain–computer interface (BCI) solutions used in research laboratories or clinical environments are designed to measure brain activity in a reliable and robust way, with the rationale of exploring real-world applications or assessing status of a patient. Suitability of these systems for the end user and applicability to the use case in question are seldom drivers for the design and development of BCI systems. Thus, these systems are far from practical if we consider users' perspective and end application's point of view. One may ask whether BCI systems need to be tailored toward different use cases, keeping in mind the demands of the user and the applications it is intended to be used for now. We can only speculate about the future developments of BCIs, but we can identify two application areas where practicality of BCI solutions is a critical component: entertainment and artistic performances. For exploring these application areas, we focus on surface electroencephalogram (EEG) measurements, since it is the dominant modality for studying brain dynamics and performance in real-life interaction of humans with their environment. The use of EEG for art and entertainment has a long history starting in the 1960s (Rosenboom 1976), but has only recently gained wider popularity (Wadeson et al. 2015). Most of the work in this domain has been focusing on visualizing and sonifying brain activity of an individual or a group without considering the convenience and the need of a performer. In our effort to develop intelligent, practical, wearable, and wireless EEG solution suitable for art and entertainment applications, we follow the guidelines for application and end user–driven development (Mihajlović et al. 2015). Having users perceive these devices as unobtrusive tools to enhance their performance and facilitate experience is our goal.

Conventional EEG systems used in research and clinical environments have a dense net of electrodes (20 or more) connected to a nonportable unit. In addition, traditional conductive gel-based electrodes are used because of the high signal-to-noise ratio and low susceptibility to noise and artifacts.

However, dense gel electrode systems pose several drawbacks, such as long and cumbersome preparation procedure, need for expert assistance, inconvenience to users, and varying impedance during long-term measurements requiring frequent calibration (Falco et al. 2005). These EEG systems lack mobility and robustness, restricting the use of EEG monitoring and BCI to controlled laboratory environments. As a result, most BCI applications are inconvenient or unfeasible for entertainment or enhancing user experience. Recent advancements in terms of miniaturization have made it possible to move toward wearable and mobile EEG systems suitable also for "out of the lab" environments. Given that EEG headsets have to be convenient to mount and comfortable to wear on a regular basis, recent EEG headset designs use a lower number (up to 16) of dry contacts, that is, dry EEG electrodes, between the electrode and the skin, with only a few systems exceeding this range (e.g., Cognionics, Inc., San Diego). To facilitate robust signal acquisition using dry electrodes, several enhancements of EEG systems, ranging from active sensors and shielding to robust algorithms, are used to tackle interferences from the environment in real-world applications. Despite having immediate benefits of using active-dry electrodes in BCI applications (Fonseca et al. 2007; Saab et al. 2011; Zander et al. 2011), BCI systems with dry electrodes are seldom used for entertainments and art performances, barring a few notable exceptions (Hamano et al. 2013; Mullen et al. 2015; Zioga et al. 2014).

Here, we present an investigation that determines whether current, cumbersome, and inconvenient conductive gel electrode systems with high-density EEG channels can be replaced by an intelligent, wearable, dry electrode EEG solution for BCI applications without compromising on performance. The BCI solutions presented here follow design and development guidelines for the targeted application, including sensor and electronics design, headset integration and ergonomics, data acquisition, signal cleaning and analysis, extraction of meaningful information, intuitive user interfaces, and effective information communication methods (Mihajlović et al. 2015). In this chapter, we discuss how these aspects have been addressed by analyzing three use cases, all having in common the desire to provide practical EEG-based BCI, able to achieve reliable real-time interaction in ecological, real-life scenarios. Before discussing these use cases, details on the technological aspects for wearable and wireless EEG applications are presented in Section 9.2.

The first use case, presented in Section 9.3, investigates a combination of a motor imagery/movement prediction BCI with a relaxation/concentration paradigm to operate remote-controlled cars in a gaming application. A minimalistic BCI approach that uses two low-power wireless EEG headsets developed by IMEC, with four active-dry EEG channels each (Patki et al. 2012), is realized. Two players are engaged in a BCI-controlled racing game, choosing the directions of their cars with motor imagery, while controlling the car's speed by relaxing/concentrating. In the second use case, we show how the same wearable and wireless EEG system can be used to enrich the artistic performance of a juggler (Section 9.4). Data from the EEG headset and motion sensors are used to transform the juggler's brain and body activity into a sonic experience, such that the audience has a richer impression of different aspects of the juggler's performance. The third use case, described in Section 9.5, illustrates how these intricate design and development aspects are beneficial when developing a BCI solution that monitors the cognitive state of a child during gaming or training. A new ergonomic eight-channel EEG headset containing conductive polymer electrodes is designed specifically for this exploration. Although the study was originally designed to assess the feasibility of estimating vigilance level of autistic children, it enabled us to implement a use case of online co-registration of vigilance levels of several persons through cloud-based interface.

## 9.2  TECHNOLOGY REQUIRED FOR PRACTICAL BCI SOLUTIONS

### 9.2.1  Convenient EEG Electrodes

EEG recordings are typically performed with the use of silver/silver chloride (Ag/AgCl) electrodes that are in contact with the scalp through conductive electrolytic gel. The electrolyte bridges the ionic current flow from the scalp and the electron flow in the electrode, in addition to increasing adhesion of the electrode to the scalp (Webster 2009). To further improve signal quality, the scalp is frequently cleaned and, especially in clinical applications, skin on the scalp is abraded. This results in a stable electrical contact with impedances typically lower than 10 k$\Omega$ (if measured below 100 Hz) over several hours (Tallgren et al. 2005). However, the abrasion process, as well as the use of conductive gel, makes the whole EEG setup inconvenient for practical applications. The application of electrolyte and the electrodes requires expert assistance and the setup process is lengthy. Moreover, the cleaning process, including removing the electrolyte substance from the scalp of the participant and preparing the electrodes for reuse, is cumbersome. This is the primary reason why recent EEG headset solutions rely on the so-called dry (or dry-contact) electrodes that include pin-like structures to penetrate the hairy regions (Chi et al. 2010).

While EEG systems with dry electrodes have a short setup time, they are often faced with decreased signal quality compared to ambulatory EEG systems. The low signal quality is mainly caused by the fragile electrical contact interface and changes in the contact properties. The contact impedance of dry electrodes is in the order of few tens to few hundreds of kilohms (if measured below 100 Hz), given the absence of electrolyte (Mihajlović et al. 2015). In real-life situations when a person is freely moving, the artifacts stemming even from slight movements are substantially enlarged. To cope with such challenges, special care is taken in the system design, including active sensors and active shielding, monitoring contact properties, and developing algorithms to cope with noise and artifacts (see below). Furthermore, given that most of these first-generation dry electrodes are made of rigid material (metal), they are usually perceived uncomfortable by users, especially when worn for long periods. To improve user comfort and electrode-skin contact, spring mechanism or flexible support is often used, as in the case of the IMEC EEG headsets discussed in this chapter. The silver/silver chloride (Ag/AgCl) electrodes have 12 posts, each 2 mm deep and produce a 10 mm$^2$ surface contact area with the scalp during measurements. Although beneficial, having electrodes with rigid metal pins still brings higher risk of injury. Using flexible electrodes made of conductive polymer material (Chen et al. 2014; Chi et al. 2013) is the latest trend in the dry electrode EEG recordings. These electrodes can be considered most suitable for entertainment and art performance applications as their flexible properties add comfort to the users. At IMEC, we use such electrodes coated with Ag/AgCl layer on the tips to improve conductivity. Each polymer electrode consists of 15 pins of either 5 or 8 mm length. The short and long pin electrodes are interchangeable based on the morphology of subjects' scalp.

### 9.2.2 Active Sensors

Active sensors are typically used to prevent the noise (including power line noise) entering the signal chain (Chimeno and Pallas-Areny 2000). This is achieved by placing the first amplification stage very close to the electrode itself, a concept followed in all IMEC EEG solutions. In addition, IMEC's active sensors are capable of continuously measuring electrode-tissue impedance (ETI) signals along with EEG (Patki et al. 2012). ETI information is extremely useful for continuous assessment of signal quality and for reducing the impact of motion artifacts on EEG (Bertrand et al. 2013; Mihajlović et al. 2014). To what degree they can be utilized in these applications is beyond the scope of this chapter.

### 9.2.3 Electronic Design

EEG systems are designed using a combination of discrete components and integrated circuits that are performing analog and digital signal acquisition and processing. Apart from providing proper signal paths, systems built with these components also minimize the impact of any kind of noise that can hamper the signal. This is typically done through adequate patient grounding, common-mode rejection solutions (for power line noise), and proper shielding of analog lines and board ground planes. Proper shielding is crucial in preventing radio transmission interferences, which is nowadays mainly done using Bluetooth (Ferree et al. 2011). Such signal protection methods are also part of the headsets developed at IMEC, used in the studies discussed. Furthermore, special care is taken to miniaturize electronic designs and ensure they consume the lowest power possible to facilitate long operating hours with the ergonomic headset design (Patki et al. 2012).

### 9.2.4 EEG HEADSET

Two types of IMEC EEG headsets are used in the studies presented in this chapter. A rigid headset (Patki et al. 2012), shown in Figure 9.1, comprises six reusable Ag/AgCl electrodes with rigid pins, which are discussed in Section 9.2.1. The electrodes are mounted on a spring-loaded support to ensure good contact with the skin while providing increased comfort to the user. Active electrode chips that buffer the electrical signal are placed directly on top of the spring-loaded contact to prevent noise from entering the EEG system as much as possible. The four active channels are positioned at $C_3$, $C_4$, $C_z$, and $P_z$ of the International 10–20 system. The headset measures the potential difference between measurement electrodes at these locations and the reference electrode positioned at the right mastoid. The subject bias/ground electrode is located on the left mastoid. The electrodes that cover central positions record EEG activity at the primary motor cortex, the region of the brain responsible for control and execution of movement. The parietal electrode covers the region responsible for motor coordination and planning of movement execution. Both areas are crucial for capturing movement intention/motor imagery activity in the brain as well as activity related to planning and execution of coordinated hand movements during juggling. This headset can measure continuous EEG and ETI signals at up to 1024 Hz (Patki et al. 2012). In the two studies presented here, a sampling rate of 256 Hz was used. Mounting of this EEG headset typically requires less than a minute, allowing for easy setup. The headset transfers the acquired data over Bluetooth to a workstation running an in-house developed EEG acquisition and visualization software.

A flexible EEG headset supports up to eight measurement channels, designed to be used for EEG measurements on children (Pradhapan et al. 2017). The headset (shown in Figure 9.2) is a highly integrated EEG acquisition device, with measurement electrodes positioned at $F_z$, $F_3$, $F_7$, $F_4$, $F_8$, $P_3$, $P_4$, and $A_1$ of the International 10–20 electrode positioning system. Patient ground is placed at $P_z$ and the reference electrode is at $A_2$ (right mastoid). Electrode positions in this headset are suitable for cognition and emotion monitoring and hence are used in the study on vigilance in children. The electronics integrated is the same as in the rigid headset. The flexible headset configuration allows re-referencing each of the channels to a specific reference (if required). The headset can be mounted easily, taking approximately 2 min to position, without the need of expert intervention, and is fitted with conductive polymer electrodes

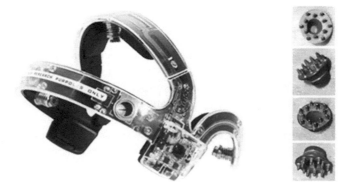

**FIGURE 9.1** A rigid EEG headset designed by IMEC for monitoring activity related to motor planning and execution. Figures on the right show the rigid Ag/AgCl electrodes with pins.

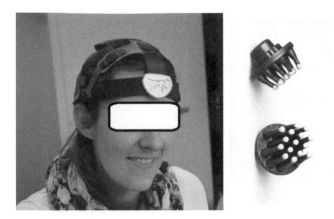

**FIGURE 9.2** A flexible EEG headset designed by IMEC for cognition monitoring studies. Figure on the right shows the flexible polymer electrodes with silver/silver chloride coating used for data acquisition.

introduced above. Overall, for both headset solutions, the use of a wireless and dry electrode EEG system minimized setup time and made it possible for measurements to be performed in an uncontrolled setting.

### 9.2.5 DATA PROCESSING

The IMEC EEG software enables real-time visualization of EEG traces from all channels, along with spectral information. As mentioned, the contact impedance of each channel is continuously monitored and displayed along with EEG traces. This enables proper inspection of the signal at the beginning of the recording/interaction session and optional readjustment of the headset whenever a noisy EEG channel is observed. Furthermore, impedance information is used to identify electrodes/ segments with lower signal quality during EEG monitoring.

Apart from the impedance, statistical properties of the EEG signal in each of the channels are used to assess the signal quality. In the software, visual feedback is given in real time whenever the signal quality level drops below the acceptable level for that specific application. The signal quality levels are defined based on prespecified thresholds derived from clean segments of EEG recordings. Typical EEG features that are required for the three example application cases discussed include spectral power across different frequency bands and output of the (personalized) common special pattern filters and linear discriminant analysis (LDA). Data processing for offline signal analysis is done differently in each of the cases we studied and is discussed in detail in the following sections.

### 9.2.6 ACTUATION/INFORMATION COMMUNICATION

For the three use cases discussed, three different actuation techniques are implemented. For motor imagery BCI, the actuation is done by using a toy car that was steered by the user. The communication between the EEG software and the car was established via Bluetooth. The outcome of the car control efforts of the user was directly visible and the speed, navigation, and audio and visual effects of the car are set such as to maximize the entertainment quotient for both users and spectators. Sonification of brain and body activity was chosen as the actuation method for juggling performance enhancement. The information about the brain state of a juggler is sent from the EEG software to the sonification unit that translated it into different sound effects. Finally, in case of vigilance monitoring, the information about vigilance status of several persons is sent to the cloud, where the data are collected, visualized, and compared in near real time. This enables monitoring of a user group while they are engaged in an interaction.

## 9.3 COMPETITIVE TOY CAR RACING USING MOTOR IMAGERY BCI

BCIs have traditionally been developed for communication or rehabilitation of patients who cannot interact naturally because of brain or muscle disorders. Only recently, healthy users have been subjects to BCI methods, using it as a supplement to existing interfaces or additional mode of communication with the environment (Allison and Neuper 2010), and patients with disability have started using BCIs for expressing their artistic skills through, for example, painting (Münßinger et al. 2010). However, the system and setup complexity of EEG-based BCIs discussed earlier have limited its use to specific clinical and controlled environments. EEG has shown promising results in characterizing brain activity related to motor planning and execution (Ahmedian et al. 2013; Nakayashiki et al. 2014). The earliest evidence of neural correlates to voluntary movement intention through EEG monitoring was presented by Kornhuber and Deecke (1965). They identified a slow cortical potential in the negative direction starting about 1.5 s before voluntary movement. These potentials also came to be known as bereitschaftspotential or readiness potentials. The readiness potential is marked by two components: a slow negative potential starting 1.5 s before voluntary movement (predominantly over central medial scalp) and a late component with steeper slope over the contralateral primary motor area occurring 0.4 s before movement (Shibasaki and Hallett 2006). In addition to readiness potentials, event-related power fluctuations in different frequency bands, better known as event-related desynchronization (ERD) and event-related synchronization (ERS), are observed in EEG (Kilavik et al. 2013; Neuper et al. 2009). ERD is an EEG correlate of movement preparation, imagination, and execution, marked by a significant reduction in the mu and beta power (8–30 Hz) over the contralateral primary motor cortex (Pfurtscheller et al. 1999). More information on motor imagery brain activity correlates and methods used to capture those can be found in Chapter 23.

EEG-based BCI studies often include dense electrode arrays to accurately identify movement intention immediately before the actual movement. In a review by Ahmedian et al. (2013), it was found that almost the entirety of research studying movement onset or direction prediction used high-density electrode placements, the number of measurement channels ranging between 27 and 128. Although maximum binary (e.g., left arm vs. right arm) classification accuracy of over 90% was achieved on a single subject (Morash et al. 2008; Santana et al. 2014), accuracies over the general population were much lower—in the order of 65% to 80% (Christoforou et al. 2010; Lew et al. 2012; Morash et al. 2008; Santana et al. 2014). One of the reasons for lower performance over a number of users could be cumbersome setup and inconvenience of traditional systems. To prove the feasibility of detecting motor intention and motor imagery using a minimalistic approach and assess whether more convenient EEG monitoring would help, we used a low-power wireless EEG headset developed at IMEC that has four active-dry EEG channels (Patki et al. 2011). Furthermore, to make users less inhibited by the setup and EEG monitoring itself, the experiments were performed in an uncontrolled setting, that is, regular office environment, prone to interferences of electrical, physiological, and psychological origin. With such a setup, we also explored the robustness of motor imagery BCI. The results demonstrated that the use of a wearable dry electrode EEG system combined with suitable signal processing techniques matched the performance of traditional BCI approaches, albeit without the need for complex systems or setup. Given that the proposed setup does not require expert intervention for mounting or electrode placement, it can deliver to wider application space in a real-life setting than the traditional gel-based EEG setup. We demonstrated this by having two people mounting the headsets by themselves and participating in an entertainment-like scenario during a public event (Großekathöfer et al. 2016), where they raced against each other using a toy car that was steered by imagined movements and paced by their state of relaxedness.

### 9.3.1 STUDY POPULATION

Ten healthy volunteers (mean ± SD age: 30.1 ± 5.4 years) with no history of neurological disorders were recruited for the study. To avoid variability in primary cortex activation patterns, only participants with an Edinburgh Handedness Inventory (Oldfield 1971) score greater than 0.7 (right hand dominance) were included. None of them had undergone any prior BCI or neurofeedback training. All participants gave written informed consent for the study.

### 9.3.2 EXPERIMENTAL PROTOCOL

The experimental protocol was reviewed and approved by IMEC's ethical review committee. Both cue-based and self-paced paradigms have been evaluated in this study. We used visual cues to adhere to a simplistic and straightforward setup and use. All measurements were performed in a normal office environment, during regular work hours, between 8 a.m. and 5 p.m. The measurement location was situated adjacent to a corridor with a sliding glass wall in between (layout shown in Figure 9.3). There was frequent and uncontrolled movement of people near the location of the experiment. In addition, other colleagues seated in the same room where the experiments took place continued their regular workday without being cautioned or advised to refrain from any kind of activities. Time of the day when experiments were performed was not controlled.

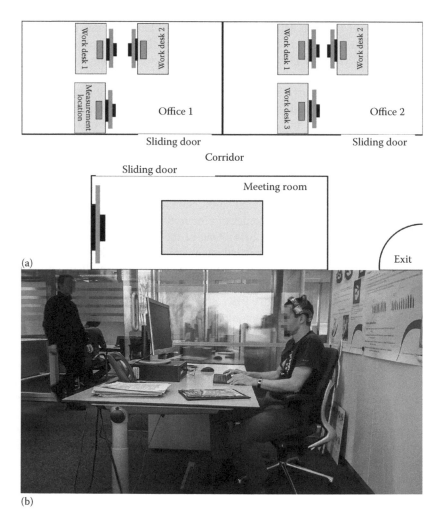

**FIGURE 9.3** Experimental setup and environment. (a) Room plan of the experiment location and (b) photograph during a measurement session.

Participants were comfortably seated at approximately 1 m away from the monitor. They were asked to relax and avoid voluntary movements, except those required by the measurement protocol. IMEC's wireless EEG headset was then placed on the participant's scalp and adjusted until proper contact was achieved. The electrodes are mounted on magnetic holders and they could rotate in all directions (up to approximately 30°), making adjustments easy to perform by the users themselves. To guarantee excellent signal quality, all signals were visually inspected by the experimenter before recording was initiated. The average duration of measurement preparation, from mounting the headset to achieving good quality signals, took approximately 2 min. To gauge the user response, each participant was asked to hold down the left Control (by left arm index finger), number-pad key 0 (by right arm index finger), and the Spacebar (by right foot) on the additional keyboard placed at the feet of the participant. The software was designed to record key release timing information, depending on whether the left arm, right arm, or right foot movement was executed by the user. Measurements were divided into four sessions, each consisting of one cue-based and one self-paced recording. One session lasted approximately 35 min and sessions were distributed over several days.

### 9.3.2.1 Cue-Based Measurements

A single cue-based measurement session consisted of 100 cues generated in a random order and equally distributed between four different movements, namely, left arm, right arm, right foot, and tongue movements. Each cue-based trial was divided into four phases, that is, cue, motor imagery, relaxation, and activity phases, respectively. The cue phase lasts 3 s, beginning when the cue is generated. At the end of the cue phase, participants are prompted to imagine the movement they needed to perform, marking the start of the motor imagery phase. They were specifically instructed not to perform any physical movements during this phase. This phase lasted 3 s followed by a short pause. The activity phase was marked by a command asking the participant to perform the movement instructed during the cue phase of the trial. During this phase, the user released either the Control, number-pad key 0, or the Spacebar, depending on the type of cue that was generated. The event breakup of the cue-based trial and interim duration are depicted in Figure 9.4.

### 9.3.2.2 Self-Paced Measurements

During the self-paced measurements, participants performed random movements in a self-paced manner, subsequently releasing the Control, number-pad key 0, or the Spacebar based on the movement executed. Tongue movements were excluded from self-paced measurements. Participants were instructed to complete the movement and return to the original position (key-press state) within 3 s from the start of the movement. After each movement, they were asked to relax for a short duration (at least 2 s) before the next self-paced movement was initiated.

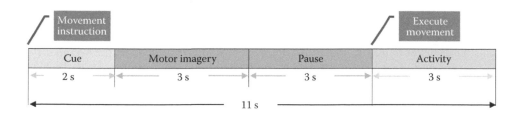

**FIGURE 9.4** Timing information for cue-based measurements.

### 9.3.3 Data Analysis

#### 9.3.3.1 Preprocessing

The raw EEG signals were bandpass filtered (third-order Butterworth) between 0.2 and 100 Hz frequency band. In addition, a notch filter between 49 and 51 Hz (fifth-order Butterworth) was used to remove the power line component. Data are segmented such that epochs of 2 s preceding the cue-based and self-paced movement onset and 3-s motor imagery segments are extracted. After segmentation, epochs in which the generated cue did not match the type of movement executed were excluded from the analysis. Each of the four measurement sessions in cue-based recording consisted of 100 trials, equally distributed among the four different movement types. After trial exclusion, mean (±SD) of successfully completed trials among all subjects during cue-based measurements was 396.7 ± 1.3. During self-paced measurements, the mean number of trials during each session across subjects was 32.6 ± 6.1 for right-hand, 30:6 ± 6.8 for left-hand, and 31.2 ± 5.4 for foot movements.

#### 9.3.3.2 Feature Extraction and Classification

Common spatial pattern (CSP) filtering is a method often used in identifying similar patterns in the signal across different electrode locations (Dornhege et al. 2003; Gerking et al. 1999). CSP uses a linear transformation to project a multichannel signal to a lower-dimensional spatial subspace by means of a projection matrix. The algorithm used in this study finds directions (i.e., filters) that maximize the variance for one class while simultaneously minimizing variance for the other class, and thereby maximizing variance ratio of both classes. In this way, the CSP extracts components from the EEG signal that differ maximally between distinct conditions. A detailed description of the CSP method can be found in Chapter 23. The performance of various classifiers on the current data set was evaluated and presented elsewhere (Großekathöfer et al. 2015). Based on these results, LDA was chosen for the current study. LDA is obtained by deriving the classifier that minimizes the risk of misclassification under the assumption that the class distributions obey known Gaussian distributions with equal covariances.

#### 9.3.3.3 Evaluation

Since CSP is a method for two-class classification by design, in the evaluation, we divided the classes corresponding to different movement types into class combinations of two classes. This resulted in six combinations for cue-based and three combinations for self-paced measurements. As the brain works differently for motor execution and imagination of different body parts, this also gives insight into the class combination that produced the best classification performance in each individual. The maximum classification accuracy achieved by each participant for cue-based (both movement prediction and motor imagery) and self-paced paradigms was determined.

### 9.3.4 Results

The average two-class classification accuracy reached 77.5% ± 3.5% and 76.1% ± 4% for movement prediction in cue-based and self-paced paradigms, and 80.4% ± 7.1% for motor imagery, over all possible class combinations from all subjects, respectively. Although cue-based intention detection yielded slightly better results in 7 out of 10 subjects for movement prediction, the overall differences in classification performance was marginal. Overall, motor imagery paradigm yielded substantially better performance, indicating that motor imagery paradigm is better suited for BCI applications. In addition, the intrasubject classification accuracies between different paradigms were consistent, with an intersubject maximum of 86.00% and 82.23% (Participant 9) and a minimum of 73.46% and 72.41% (Participant 2) for cue-based and self-paced measurements, respectively. Table 9.1 summarizes classification results for all subjects who participated in the study.

**TABLE 9.1**

**Maximum Two-Class Classification Accuracy over All Trials for Each Participant for Cue-Based, Self-Paced, and Motor Imagery BCI**

| Participant | Cue-Based | Self-Paced | Motor Imagery |
|---|---|---|---|
| 01 | 75.7 | 73.4 | 77.4 |
| 02 | 73.4 | 72.4 | 79.1 |
| 03 | 75.9 | 75.4 | 72.3 |
| 04 | 77.6 | 68.8 | 77.6 |
| 05 | 76.0 | 76.7 | 75.9 |
| 06 | 80.0 | 78.1 | 88.2 |
| 07 | 75.0 | 76.9 | 73.4 |
| 08 | 77.8 | 75.6 | 78.9 |
| 09 | 86.0 | 82.2 | 96.8 |
| 10 | 78.0 | 81.4 | 84.3 |
| **Mean ± SD** | 77.5 ± 3.5 | 76.1 ± 4.0 | 80.4 ± 7.1 |

The maximum and average accuracies reached in the analysis are in line with the values reported in the literature (see above). Given that in this study we used an ergonomic headset that users could mount themselves and only four channels of EEG, these results demonstrate that it is viable to use convenient dry electrode EEG monitoring in motor imagery BCI. We expect that having more EEG channels at relevant position using, for example, a headset similar to the one described in Section 9.5 could lead to further improvement in the performance as well as increase of user comfort and acceptability of such a solution. To demonstrate the feasibility, we have translated the offline data analysis algorithms into a real-time toy car racing application.

### 9.3.5 APPLICATION EXAMPLE

An application example is realized such that BCI commands are interpreted from imagined movements of the user and actuate Zen Wheels micro cars (Zen Wheels 2016) via Bluetooth. The cars were steered with the goal of completing a lap on a racing track model, as shown in Figure 9.5. The application is implemented using IMEC's EEG software, by extracting the car steering direction through monitoring motor imagery and car speed (stopping) by using spectral power levels across all electrodes. Motor imagery from imagined limb movements (personalized combination of classes) by means of pretrained classifiers for the two best performing subjects (mean classification accuracy over 85%) is used. The classification is performed in two steps: CSP filtering and LDA score computation. The LDA output is used to steer the car to the left or right if the score values exceeded a predefined threshold. The actuation is implemented by steering the front wheels at 45° for 2 s such that the cars are navigated in the direction of the detected motor imagery class, with direction indicators adding to the entertainment experience. Relaxation level in terms of the mean spectral power in the theta, alpha, and beta frequency bands over the central and parietal cortex (Zao et al. 2014) is used to control the speed. The relaxation ranges are calibrated beforehand for each participant, such that the car would stop and all the lights would be switched on in case of brain relaxation; in case of typical brain activity, the car would move at a constant speed of approximately 1 cm/s with lights switched off. Although both subjects had similar performance according to the classification results, one of them achieved substantially better control during the race (achieving on average four correct steering commands out of five) in front of a number of spectators. This indicates that more challenges exist when translating off-line BCI-based interaction to real-time

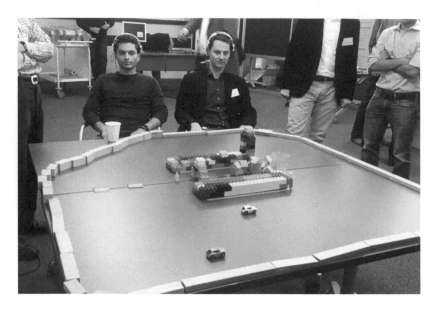

**FIGURE 9.5** A picture taken during the BCI racing game. The two opponents wearing the wireless headset are in the upper left corner, and the two remote-controlled cars are driving on a racetrack on the table.

application than what is represented in the classification results. Despite this difference in actual performance on the track, the spectators were thrilled by the racing event.

## 9.4 ENRICHING PERFORMANCE OF A JUGGLER BY BRAIN AND BODY SONIFICATION

Professional juggling involves complex technical and aesthetic visuomotor skills that are acquired through rigorous practice and exercise over the course of months and years. Surpassing the initial "wow" effect of a complex juggling trick and producing long-lasting engaging performances are the main goals of any juggling act. Conveying to the audience the skill and the effort required for a performance is often difficult. To capture these hidden aspects of juggling, jugglers have introduced auxiliary means of performing the art in recent years. These means are typically presented as artistic concepts based on synergic interaction between body movements and objects in the 3D space (Bovermann et al. 2007; Reynolds et al. 2001; Willier and Marque 2002). While these interpretations of a juggler's performance can illustrate the complexity of aspects of juggling, the skill required for these routines remains unseen. To tap into this hidden legacy of a juggler, one must capture brain dynamics during the act of juggling. Attentive screening of literature on this topic failed to find studies where EEG activity was recorded during execution of juggling performances. The most trivial reason preventing studies is the delicate nature of EEG systems in contrast to requirements of the artists to be able to freely move while juggling. Cumbersome EEG systems that require the use of conductive gel and wires that connect electrodes to the EEG acquisition system, which are highly sensitive to motion-induced noise, are among the main obstacles. Furthermore, experiments confined to a limited working space are unsuitable for encompassing juggling posture and movements.

Here, we summarize how a wearable EEG system can be used for investigating the neuronal mechanisms that underlie visuomotor processing during juggling, explored in detail in Schiavone et al. (2015). We demonstrate how BCI can provide alternative opportunities for training and for enhancement of juggling performances. Two experimental conditions were designed. The first one was intended to characterize brain activity and connectivity during three-ball cascade juggling compared to conditions such as rest, imagery juggling, and juggling movements without balls in both intermediate and expert juggler. The second experimental condition was intended to investigate whether the difficulty of a juggling trick was reflected in the EEG of the expert juggler while performing a juggling cascade with three, five, and seven balls. We observed characteristic brain activity and synchronization while juggling in both an expert and an intermediate juggler. We also found that processing of visuomotor skills and memory retention can be distinguished during motor imagery and simulated juggling conditions. This was the first experiment reported in literature to monitor a juggler's brain in action. We have shown that using EEG while juggling could both improve our understanding of neuronal mechanisms governing visuomotor control and, importantly, represent a potential to enrich artistic performance and increase audience engagement. To demonstrate the possibility of actuating brain activity of a juggler in a way that reflects the complexity of the executed act, which we believe can help in increasing the engagement and tuning the audience during a show, we converted the juggler's brain dynamics into sound. The actuation is motivated by the number of successful brain sonification examples demonstrated by Eduardo R. Miranda and his team (Miranda 2010), Wu et al. (2013), and Mullen et al. (2015), explored in more detail in Chapter 10. We demonstrated how EEG signal as well as the movement of both arm-wrists, captured by wearable sensors, can be used for enhancing art performance. Signals coming from the juggler's brain and body are sonified in real time, thus allowing the audience to experience the interaction of a juggler's body movements and their underlying neuronal mechanisms in novel ways (Schiavone et al. 2016).

### 9.4.1 STUDY POPULATION

Two subjects participated in our study, an intermediate juggler (left-handed male, 40 years old) and an expert juggler (right-handed male, 22 years old). The intermediate amateur juggler was recruited among colleagues, while the expert was a professional juggler with more than 10 years of juggling experience. We consider the difference between the intermediate and expert juggler in line with previous definitions: experts are defined as those who could juggle five or more balls; intermediate jugglers are defined as those who could comfortably maintain a three-ball juggle for more than a minute (Schiavone et al. 2015).

### 9.4.2 EXPERIMENTAL PROTOCOL

Two experimental protocols were imposed on both intermediate and expert jugglers. The first one consisted of the following five conditions:

- Rest: rest and think of something not related to juggling
- Imagery: imagine juggling
- Juggle: perform a three-ball cascade pattern
- ImageryHands: move arms without balls in a juggle-like fashion and imagine juggling
- NoBalls: move arms in a juggle-like fashion and think of something not related to juggling

An illustration of juggling performance of an expert juggler is depicted in Figure 9.6. Each condition lasted 20 s and was repeated 15 times (trials) for the intermediate juggler and 10 times (trials) for the expert juggler. The number of trials was less in the expert juggler because of time constraints. In each trial, the sequence of conditions was randomized. For all conditions, the subjects had their eyes open. They were asked to keep their head as still as possible and to limit overall upper body movement to reduce the impact of motion on the EEG signal. While juggling, whenever

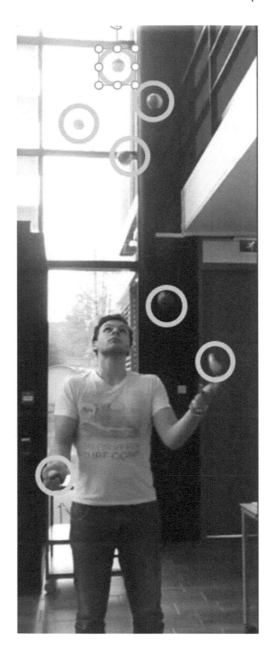

**FIGURE 9.6** An illustration of a juggling performance.

a ball fell down before the established execution time was reached, the trial was discarded and the condition was repeated. There were pauses of a few minutes between trials whenever requested by the subjects.

The second protocol involved only the expert juggler and consisted of three conditions with incremental difficulty:

- 3 Balls: perform a three-ball cascade pattern
- 5 Balls: perform a five-ball cascade pattern
- 7 Balls: perform a seven-ball cascade pattern

Each condition was repeated three times (trials) in a randomized order at each trial. Because of the difficulty of sustaining the seven-ball game for longer periods, a duration threshold of 15 s was defined for each trial. If a ball fell down within this threshold, the trial was discarded and repeated; if the juggler was able to sustain the game for a longer period, the recording was continued until the first ball dropped. The cascade pattern (Beek and Santvoord 1992) was chosen because of the consistency of the ball pattern across task difficulties induced by increasing the number of props (horizontal figure-eight above the hands, produced by throwing one prop in an arc-like fashion before catching another on its way down).

### 9.4.3 DATA ANALYSIS

#### 9.4.3.1 Preprocessing

To ensure the integrity of the data, we initially visually inspected all signals and manually removed segments containing spike-like artifacts that are representative of nonphysiological signal disturbances. Segments containing ETI higher than 40 kΩ were also considered as artifact segments and discarded. We then band-pass filtered the EEG signal with a third-order Butterworth filter in a 3–70 Hz frequency band and applied a 50-Hz notch filter. Considering that juggling movement can reach up to 2–3 Hz for intermediate and advanced jugglers (Mapelli et al. 2012), we chose a high-pass cutoff frequency of 3 Hz to remove EOG and other movement artifacts. Our empirical evaluation showed that in all cases in this study (except for juggling with seven balls), motion artifacts mostly affected EEG content below 4 Hz. Given that the impact of automatic motion artifact reduction on the EEG content is unknown (Mihajlović et al. 2015), we decided not to use any motion artifact reduction methods, but instead excluded the delta band (1–4 Hz) from our analysis. It is worth mentioning that, according to observations from a previous study in which the impact of head movements on EEG spectral content was investigated (Mihajlović et al. 2014), we expected that motion artifacts could cause increases in the EEG power spectrum for a frequency range lower than 20 Hz. Artifact removal processing resulted in a total of about 31 min of recording for each EEG channel [(15 for intermediate +10 for expert) trials * 15 s (clean signal) * 5 conditions] for the first experiment and a total of about 1.5 min for each EEG channel [3 trials * 10 s (clean signal) * 3 conditions] for the second experiment. For the latter, signals in $P_z$ were excluded from further analysis because of the high ETI signal, caused by skin-electrode contact loss.

#### 9.4.3.2 Data Analysis

We used the Welch method to compute EEG power spectra in the predefined frequency bands: theta (4–8 Hz), alpha (8–13 Hz), beta (13–30 Hz), and gamma (30–40 Hz). Spectral coherence between pairs of EEG channels was considered to measure synchrony of oscillations between electrodes in each frequency band, as defined for the spectral analysis. The *mscohere* MATLAB® function, which computes the magnitude squared coherence estimate of the two EEG signals using Welch's averaged modified periodogram method and measures linear synchronization between two series, was used. A value of 1 indicates a perfect linear relationship, meaning perfect agreement in phase difference, while a value of 0 denotes that the series are uncorrelated, meaning completely random phase differences. We used analysis of variance for testing differences in power spectra and coherence between conditions.

### 9.4.4 RESULTS

While comparing Juggle versus other conditions, we found that, for the expert juggler, the power under juggling conditions was significantly higher than that under other conditions across all frequency bands. For the intermediate juggler, this was only the case in high gamma and theta bands. In the Rest versus Imagery conditions comparison, we found overall significantly higher power in

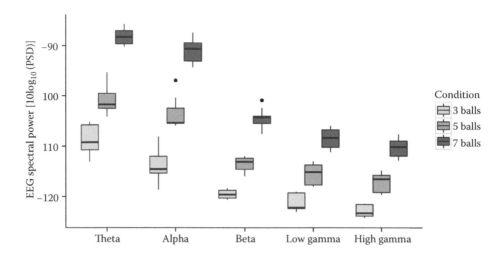

**FIGURE 9.7** Boxplot of log power spectral density averaged across electrodes and trials for each frequency band and condition in the second experimental protocol.

the alpha band for the Rest condition compared to the Imagery condition for the expert juggler. For the intermediate juggler, no significant differences between these two conditions were found.

Also, we found significant difference in the alpha power in the NoBalls condition compared to the ImageryHands condition for the intermediate juggler and no significant differences for the expert juggler. For the expert juggler, the theta coherence during Juggle is significantly different from the theta coherence in the ImageryHands condition and the alpha coherence in Juggle significantly differs from other conditions. For the intermediate juggler, gamma-band coherence during Juggle is overall significantly higher than that under other conditions. In the Rest versus Imagery conditions comparison, no significant differences in coherence across frequencies were found for both expert and intermediate juggler.

Grand averages of power spectra across trial repetitions (Figure 9.7) show that increasing difficulty due to increased number of balls for the cascade pattern is reflected in an increase of power across all frequency bands and channels. Grand averages of coherence across trial repetitions show similar behavior, with strong increase for the seven-ball cascade compared to the three- and five-ball cascade. This was particularly the case for theta band coherence across all electrode pairs.

Overall, these results demonstrate the feasibility of monitoring brain activity of a juggler in action and potential of capturing the impact of visuomotor coordination challenges on a juggler's brain. We have shown that for elementary characterization of brain activity, an ergonomic and wireless EEG headset with four dry electrode channels will suffice. The latest results indicate that we can use overall power and coherence captured by such easy-to-use headset to indicate difficulty of a trick performed by a juggler. Given that lower-frequency bands (theta and alpha) can still contain traces of motion-induced activity in our application example, we used gamma frequency band as an indicator of complex juggling performance.

### 9.4.5 APPLICATION EXAMPLE

For the application example, we developed a brain and body computer interaction approach (B²CI) that enriches jugglers' performance using wearable sensors and real-time sonification of brain activity and arm movements, and hence can be considered as a representative of hybrid BCI discussed in Chapter 27. Besides the rigid IMEC's EEG headset and EEG software application, two ergonomic IMEC wrist-based activity monitors were used (CHILL Band 2016). They are low-power,

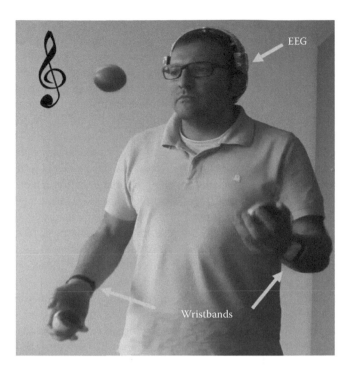

**FIGURE 9.8** Amateur juggler in sonified juggling action, wearing IMEC's EEG headset and two IMEC EEG wristbands.

miniaturized devices that monitor 3D acceleration among other modalities. Two such sensors were mounted on the arms, and the acceleration magnitude is extracted using a custom-developed MATLAB script, which read the Bluetooth information transmitted from these devices and sent the acceleration magnitude over TCP/IP to a SuperColider (SuperCollider 2016) software using an Open Sound Control (OSC) protocol (OSC 2016). The EEG software sent information on gamma band spectral power (and coherence) using the same protocol to the SuperColider software.

Dedicated scripts are used in the SuperColider engine to translate these features such that they affect the tempo and volume of a music piece and adjust the duration of a tone. Such an application was demonstrated, among others, to an audience without special tuning of the audio performance and it was well received (Schiavone et al. 2016). One of the performances is illustrated in Figure 9.8. We can envision that proper music adjustment for such $B^2CI$ would yield more effective performance of a juggler in which audience can tune to his or her artistic and skillful tricks. The actuation could be further enriched by introducing other sensing modalities, the most representative being visual.

## 9.5 MONITORING VIGILANCE IN CHILDREN DURING ENTERTAINMENT AND LEARNING

One of the important aspects in a child's performance is related to their ability to be attentive to certain stimuli over a long period of time. This is relevant not only for healthy children but also for children with cognitive deficits, which are a result of cognitive impairments such as attention-deficit/hyperactivity disorder or autism spectrum disorder (Bink et al. 2015; Johnson et al. 2007; Lansbergen et al. 2011; Mathewson et al. 2012), as also emphasized in Chapter 28. Sustained attention/vigilance is defined as the ability to sustain conscious processing of random, repetitive stimuli without succumbing to habituation or distraction by other trivial stimuli. The ability to measure sustained attention/vigilance in response to events or tasks is essential in determining cognitive state and memory processes associated with the brain. Baseline shifts in EEG spectral response, in combination with phasic activity, can result in poor performance in sustaining attention. Researchers have explored a range of EEG features derived from data collected during experimental paradigms that involve cued responses to trials while anticipating a target stimulus. Orienting responses (phasic neurophysiological processes), which is described as the immediate, short-term response elucidated in the brain as a result of target stimulus, are often investigated to understand the cognitive processes related to attention. However, it has been reported that EEG changes cycle at lengths in the order of 15 s to minutes (i.e., tonic response) (Makeig and Inlow 1993), which leads to the hypothesis that poor tonic activity, in combination to phasic processes, might result in poor task performance. Observed tonic changes include increased low frequency activity during decreasing attention and attenuation of alpha frequencies during maximal attention (Oken et al. 2006), as well as relative increase in theta band power 10 s before stimulus onset (Makeig and Jung 1996; Makeig et al. 2000). The often-encountered limitations in assessing these changes is the intersubject variability of spectral responses, especially in children, since the alpha peak frequency matures progressively with age (Niedermeyer and da Silva 2005). Moreover, these evaluations are performed in a clinical setting, which does not truly reflect the cognitive state in an uncontrolled environment where other external stimuli could dissolve the attention process.

The fact that the traditional EEG devices use wired systems limits the possibilities of conducting experiments that elucidate natural brain processes. Furthermore, monitoring brain activity of children poses serious challenges, mainly in their acceptance of wearing a headset with electrodes and in adhering to the protocol such that reliable data can be acquired. To overcome these measurement challenges, we designed a flexible eight-channel headset with conductive polymer electrodes, as described in Section 9.2.4. We explored metrics that indicate tonic differences in spectral response between error and no-error trials while performing a Sustained Attention to Response Task (SART) in a nonclinical setting. To estimate the contribution of tonic response changes, we studied the 10-s segments preceding cues of correct and incorrect responses during target stimuli of an attention paradigm. In addition to fixed frequency bands, personalized bands based on individual alpha peak frequencies (IAF) were computed to account for intersubject variability. The results indicate that relative theta and alpha power, along with their ratios, is a reliable metric indicating periods of attention or its lapses. To demonstrate a real-time application scenario, we developed a cloud-based solution that monitors vigilance level of a number of subjects, in terms of relative theta and alpha power, and compares subjects' mental state in real time. More information on the study can be found in Pradhapan et al. (2017).

### 9.5.1 Study Population

Nine children (age range, 6–18 years; mean ± SD = 12.4 ± 3.5 years; three male) without any history of neurological disorders participated in the study. Since the subjects were below 18 years of age, measurements were performed only after written informed consent was obtained from their parent/guardian. Two subjects (female) could not complete the data acquisition because of improper fitting of the headset and were, therefore, excluded from analyses. Two subjects (one male and one female; 10 years) completed two measurements during different sessions, as described below.

### 9.5.2 Experimental Protocol

SART, a GO/NO-GO paradigm, was chosen as the voluntary attention task to determine metrics for sustained attention. SART protocol is a computer-based user response task designed to measure a person's ability to withhold responses to infrequent and unpredictable target stimuli while responding as quickly and accurately as possible. Traditionally, the SART protocol involves flashing numbers between 1 and 9 on a screen for a short and fixed duration for which the user responds, depending on the type of cue (target or non-target stimulus). To motivate the young subjects of the current study, traditional SART was modified to include pictures of cartoon characters instead of numbers. The cue duration, that is, duration for which the cue appears on the screen, was set at 0.30 s for subjects between 6 and 12 years of age and at 0.15 s for older subjects. The inter-cue interval was between 1 and 1.5 s, inclusive of cue duration. Subjects were asked to respond to the cues by mouse button click for GO trials (nontarget stimuli; probability of occurrence, 87.5%) using the index finger of the dominant arm and refrain from producing any response when the NO-GO trials (target stimulus; probability of occurrence, 12.5%) appeared. The picture that represented the NO-GO trial was shown to the subjects before the start of the measurement. The subjects were specifically instructed to give equal importance to accuracy and speed while performing the tasks. The protocol was implemented in the data acquisition software used to record EEG data from the headset. Timing information of cues and user responses (mouse button clicks) were recorded as events on the software. This information was later used for segmenting trials and determining correct and incorrect responses.

Figure 9.9 summarizes a sample sequence of events during SART. Each measurement session involved 300 cues appearing in random sequence. Baseline recording, each comprising 90 s of eyes-closed and eyes-open recording, was performed before and after each SART measurement to determine the IAF of each subject for personalization of frequency bands. In between two SART tasks, the subjects participated in either an interactive on-screen dolphin game or a dog training session that lasted about 10 min. The sequence of activities during the measurement sessions is described in Figure 9.10. Participants were instructed not to remove the headset until the entire measurement phase was completed. Two subjects (one male and one female) participated in both sessions and therefore have recorded two sets of SART measurements. The measurements, including the intersession activities, were performed under normal room conditions. Children also filled in the questionnaire where they

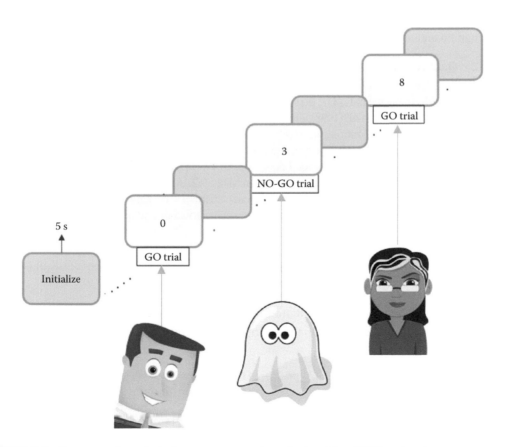

**FIGURE 9.9**  Sequence of events during a measurement session involving SART protocol.

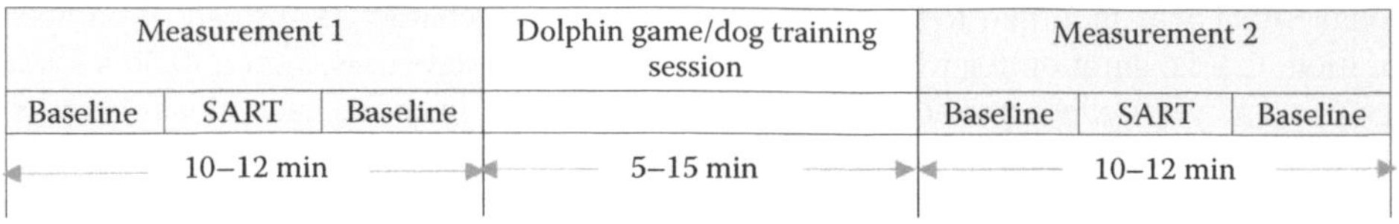

| Measurement 1 | | | Dolphin game/dog training session | Measurement 2 | | |
|---|---|---|---|---|---|---|
| Baseline | SART | Baseline | | Baseline | SART | Baseline |
| ◄———— 10–12 min ————► | | | ◄———— 5–15 min ————► | ◄———— 10–12 min ————► | | |

**FIGURE 9.10** Sequence of events during a measurement session involving SART protocol.

assessed the experimental aspects on a scale of 1–5, along the following factors: convenience of the setup, comfort of electrodes, headset mounting procedure, ease of following the protocol, and experiment duration. A score of 1 denotes the most negative side and a score of 5 denotes the most positive side of the scale. The protocol was approved and executed by the SAM Foundation (the Netherlands).

### 9.5.3 DATA ANALYSIS

#### 9.5.3.1 Preprocessing

The preprocessing step involved band-pass filtering (third-order Butterworth) in the 1–45 Hz frequency band and the use of 49–51 Hz notch filter (fifth-order Butterworth). Epochs of NO-GO trials starting 10 s before the cue and until the cue onset were segmented based on cue timing information. An automatic artifact rejection method based on standard deviation and min–max of the signals within an epoch was used. By applying statistics-based artifact rejection in the data analyses, epochs corrupted by noise and motion artifacts were automatically discarded from analysis. After segmentation and artifact data exclusion, the epochs were classified as no-error or error trials.

#### 9.5.3.2 Data Analysis

Power spectral densities were calculated using the Welch method based on either fixed frequency bands or personalized frequency bands. The personalized frequency bands were computed based on methods described by Doppelymayr et al. (1998), distributed around the IAF in order to account for the intersubject variability. For personalization, the IAF was identified by analyzing 10-s epochs data from eyes-closed baseline measurements. The spectral features were represented as both absolute and relative (ratio of power in specific frequency band to total power in the 1–30 Hz range) powers. The frequency bands for both feature extraction methods are described in Table 9.2. After spectral analyses, ratios between theta/alpha and theta/beta bands were computed for each channel. The statistical analysis was performed using Mann–Whitney $U$ tests, and the differences between erroneous and correct trials were explored.

**TABLE 9.2**
**Frequency Band Boundaries for Standard and Personalized Frequency Ranges**

| Bands | Frequencies (Hz) | |
|---|---|---|
| | Fixed | Personalized |
| Theta | 4–7.99 | $(0.4–0.6) \times IAF$ |
| Alpha | 8–12.99 | $(0.6–1.2) \times IAF$ |
| Beta | 13–19.99 | $1.2 \times IAF–19.99$ |

### 9.5.4 RESULTS

In fixed frequency band analysis, significant differences in relative theta power and alpha power in the frontal midline for fixed frequency bands was observed when comparing erroneous to correct NO-GO trials. This contributed to the theta/alpha and theta/beta ratio being significant indicators of a vigilance status at the $F_z$ channel. The personalized frequency bands revealed a significant difference in relative alpha power across the frontal positions of $F_z$, $F_3$, and $F_4$ with respect to vigilance level. Similarly, the theta/alpha ratios were significant indicators of differences across the same frontal electrodes. The theta/beta ratio exhibited significant change only at electrode $F_3$. An example of power distribution differences across scalp locations when personalized frequency bands are used is shown in Figure 9.11.

The average feedback score given by users for headset and electrode comfort was 3.3 and 3.1 (out of 5), respectively, indicating that the children perceived the headset to be comfortable and convenient to wear during the course of the measurements. None of the participants complained about discomfort or wanted to discontinue the experiment. Study participants evaluated headset mounting as particularly good (3.67). Following the protocol was not an issue for participants, having an average score of 3.1. Finally, they were accepting well the duration of the experiment, which was typically around 1 h, having the same evaluation score. After observing the positive reaction of participants and obtaining acceptable usability scores, we could infer that the flexible EEG system with eight comfortable dry electrodes is a suitable solution for capturing the vigilance level of children. Given that we also identified statistically significant differences in the spectral power across several electrode locations, we designed and developed a multi-user solution for monitoring vigilance level.

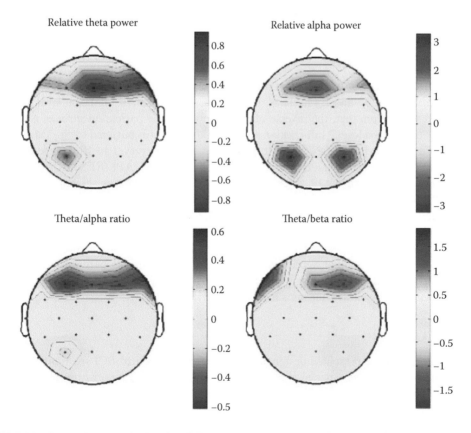

**FIGURE 9.11** Spectral power distribution differences across the scalp when comparing correct and erroneous trials.

```
METHOD: POST
Content-Type: application/json
Body:

{
"sessionId":        "session1",
"dataType":         "concentration",
"values":
[
        {
        "timestamp":        "2015-07-23 21:20:34",
        "value":            "0.4"
        },
        {
        "timestamp":        "2015-07-23 21:20:44",
        "value":            "0.56"
        },

        ...

        {
        "timestamp":        "2015-07-23 21:22:14",
        "value":            "0.761"
        }
]
}
```

**FIGURE 9.12** Request message used to send vigilance level information. The message is formatted using JSON array and is sent using REST API.

### 9.5.5 Application Example

Existing IMEC's EEG Software was modified such that it extracts 10-s theta/alpha ratios from frontal electrodes ($F_3$, $F_4$, and $F_z$) in the form of a tonic estimation of vigilance level and sends it to the cloud. Aside from that, the inverse of alpha power in the parietal electrodes is used as an indication of "relaxation level." Information about vigilance level is buffered by the IMEC software and sent, as a JSON array (JSON 2016), to the Cloud Service every 1 to 10 s (depending on the settings). The communication interface is implemented as a REST API (REST 2016). The request message is depicted in Figure 9.12, where *sessionId* identifies the training session, *dataType* specifies if the "values" array contains information about vigilance or relaxation, and *values* contains the vigilance/relaxation level data itself. On the cloud, the vigilance and relaxation level of several persons is captured at the same time and visualized on the monitoring interface, as illustrated in Figure 9.13. As an additional option, comparison of vigilance/relaxation statistics for these persons could also be displayed. Such an application demonstrates the feasibility of real-time monitoring of attention level of children when they are interacting in a playful environment or observing art and entertainment performances or during a learning experience.

## 9.6 DISCUSSION

In this chapter, we have presented design and application of practical BCI solutions for entertainment and art performances. Special attention was given to improving user experience in terms of convenience and comfort on one side and suitable information extraction and feedback on the other. Through three use cases, we have demonstrated how practical BCI solutions can be developed using flexible electrode (support) designs, active sensors, careful system integration, ergonomic headsets, signal quality estimators, artifact handling methods, and proper actuation methods.

Reliability and robustness of a practical BCI solution can be seen from the motor imagery and movement intention detection case. The proposed solution can identify two classes of movement

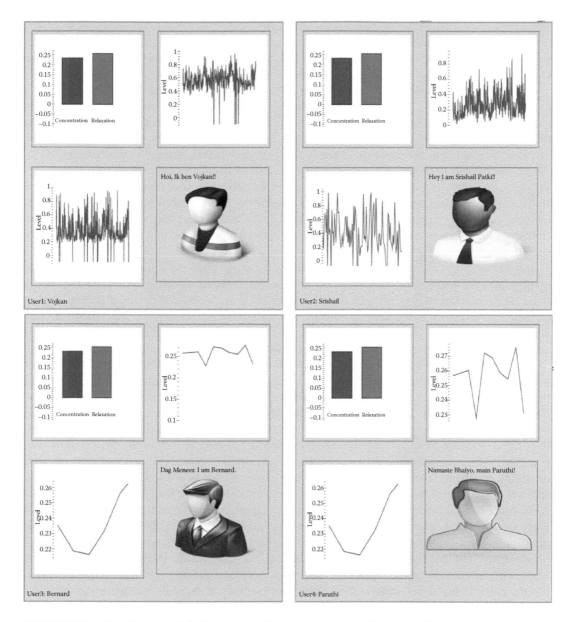

**FIGURE 9.13** Visualization of vigilance level of four persons in real time in the cloud.

intention with sufficient accuracy. Although measurement sessions from each participant were spread across different days, cross-validation revealed a stable performance. This indicates that the signal quality and movement prediction features were consistent and reproducible across sessions. This is true despite the fact the small variability in electrode positioning was inevitable since no special care was taken to ensure same positioning of the headset during different days. Given that all measurements in our study were performed in an office environment and during regular office hours, achieving mean accuracies higher than 75% across 10 subjects using only four dry electrode channels shows great promise that such a BCI setup can be used in normal day-to-day life applications. We have demonstrated this by successfully applying a BCI setup that uses motor imagery paradigm in an entertainment scenario, involving two participants steering a toy car in a simulated race. We expect that the robustness and accuracy could be further improved by using more electrodes at the relevant position such as the (pre-)motor cortex. Still, we see that the main challenge for practical use of the presented motor imagery BCI is that it requires a long training procedure (about 1 h in our case). Hence, reducing learning time overall or allowing for intra- and interpersonal transfer learning would substantially increase the chance of wider adoption of such applications.

Suitability of a proposed EEG solution for enhancing art performances was showcased on a use case of juggling. In our approach, the user is allowed to freely move and perform juggling activities, while his or her EEG is recorded with a wireless dry electrode EEG headset. From the experimental evaluation, we discovered that the increase in difficulty in performing cascade juggling from three to five and seven balls is reflected in the EEG of the experienced juggler. We found that the power of neuronal oscillations across all frequency bands generally increases with the task difficulty. Also, synchronous activity across four channels was found to increase across all frequencies when passing from the three-ball to the five-ball condition. While synchronization and increase in power was more obvious in lower-frequency bands (theta and alpha), we used gamma frequency band as the most reliable estimator of brain changes, given that the former can be corrupted by motion artifacts.

Interpretations of the reported results are still speculative, given the limited number of jugglers involved and the simplistic methods used. More sustained considerations can be achieved by involving a larger number of jugglers with different skill levels and/or by comparing different juggling techniques. Nevertheless, the analysis outcome was utilized in a successfully demonstrated use case where the brain and body activity of a juggler was transformed into sonic experience capable of articulating better mental state of a juggler when performing a juggling act to the audience.

Real-time monitoring in interactive scenarios is proven to be challenging in adults and inherently more difficult in children. Here, we have presented a new wearable and wireless EEG system that can be used to monitor brain activity while performing cognitive tasks in a regular home or classroom environment. We successfully applied this headset for monitoring sustained attention in children aged 8–18 years. To assess the attention level changes in healthy children, differences in spectral features computed for 10-s epochs preceding correct and incorrect SART trials were compared. The interindividual differences in spectral response were accounted for by normalizing the frequency bands based on the IAF. The results have demonstrated that consistent differences in spectral power distribution can be observed between periods of sustained attention and its lapses. Although EEG mounting setup was substantially simplified, the mounting procedure required a person experienced in EEG measurements to perform this process. This indicates that the headset design improvements and better assistance in headset mounting are required such that the naive experimenter could mount the headset and execute the experiment. Furthermore, a substantial amount of data was corrupted because of the presence of noise and artifacts in the data. This signifies the need to implement signal quality estimation methods in the real-time application software to reject all the corrupt segments from vigilance estimation. Finally, multi-user real-time vigilance level estimation through the cloud service presented in this chapter showcases great potential such a solution can have in various applications related to monitoring attention in humans.

Despite suffering from several shortcomings, we believe that the three EEG solutions presented here give a good indication that application of BCI in entertainment and art performances is viable. If we continue to improve the three mentioned design aspects (or alike) of EEG solutions, namely, ergonomic wearable headset, usage of necessary data analysis methods for providing reliable data, and proper actuation method required for the application, we will see a rapid increase of BCI solutions applied in these domains.

## ACKNOWLEDGMENTS

This study involving children (discussed in Section 9.5) was supported by the EIT Digital Program (Activity no. A15257) of the Playful Supervised Smart Spaces (P3S) project.

# REFERENCES

Ahmedian, P., Cagnoni, S., and Ascari, L. 2013. How capable is non-invasive EEG data of predicting the next movement? A mini review. *Front. Hum. Neurosci.* 7 (124).

Allison, B. Z., and Neuper, C. 2010. Could anyone use a BCI? In *Brain–Computer Interfaces*. 35–54. London: Springer-Verlag.

Beek, P. J., and Santvoord, A. V. 1992. Learning the cascade juggle: A dynamical systems analysis. *J. Motor Behav.* 4 (1): 85–94.

Bertrand, A., Mihajlović, V., Grundlehner, B., Van Hoof, C., and Moonen, M. 2013. Motion artifact reduction in EEG recordings using multi-channel contact impedance measurements. *IEEE Biomedical Circuits and Systems Conference (BioCAS)* 258–261.

Bink, M., van Boxtel, G., Popma, A., Bongers, I., Denissen, A., and van Nieuwenhuizen, C. 2015. EEG theta and beta power spectra in adolescents with ADHD versus adolescents with ASD + ADHD. *Eur. Child Adolesc. Psychiatry* 24: 873–886.

Bovermann, T., Groten, J., De Campo, A., et al. Juggling sounds. 2007. *Proceedings of the 2nd International Workshop on Interactive Sonification.*

Chen, Y. H., Op de Beeck, M., Vanderheyden, L., Carrette, E., Mihajlović, V., Vanstreels, K., Grundlehner, B., Gadeyne, S., Boon, P., and Van Hoof, C. 2014. Soft, comfortable polymer dry electrodes for high quality ECG and EEG recording. *Sensors* 14: 23758–23780.

Chi, Y. M., Jung, T.-P., and Cauwenberghs, G. 2010. Dry-contact and noncontact biopotential electrodes: Methodological review. *IEEE Rev. Biomed. Eng.* 3 (1): 106–119.

Chi, Y. M., Wang, Y., Wang, Y.-T., Jung, T.-P., Kerth, T., and Cao, Y. 2013. A practical mobile dry EEG system for human computer interfaces. *Foundations of Augmented Cognition.* 8027: 649–655.

CHILL Band. 2016. IMEC, http://www.imec-nl.nl/content/user/File/Brochures/ip2016/CHILL%20BAND .pdf.

Chimeno, M. F., and Pallas-Areny, R. 2000. A comprehensive model for power line interference in biopotential measurements. *IEEE Trans. Instrum. Meas.* 49 (3): 535–540.

Christoforou, C., Haralick, R., Sajda, P., and Parra, L.C. 2010. Second-order bilinear discriminant analysis. *J. Mach. Learn Res.* 11: 665–685.

Doppelymayr, M., Klimesch, W., Pachinger, T., and Ripper, B. 1998. Individual differences in brain dynamics: Important implications for the calculation of event-related band power. *Biol. Cybern.* 79: 49–57.

Dornhege, G., Blankertz, B., Curio, G., and Müller, K.-R. 2003. Increase information transfer rates in BCI by CSP extension to multi-class. *Adv. Neural Inf. Process. Syst.* 16: 733–740.

Falco, C., Sebastiano, F., Cacciola, L., Orabona, F., Ponticelli, R., Stirpe, P., and Di Gennaro, G. 2005. Scalp electrode placement by EC2 adhesive paste in long-term video-EEG monitoring. *Clin. Neurophysiol.* 116 (8): 1771–1773.

Ferree, T. C., Luu, P. L., Russel, G. S., and Tucker, D. M. 2011. Scalp electrode impedance, infection risk, and EEG data quality. *Clin. Neurophysiol.* 112 (3): 536–544.

Fonseca, C., Silva Cunha, J. P., Martins, R. E., Ferreira, V. M., Marques de Sa, J. P., Barbosa, M. A., and Martin da Silva, A. 2007. A novel dry electrode for EEG recording. *IEEE Trans. Biomed. Eng.* 54 (1): 162–165.

Gerking, J. M., Pfurstscheller, G., and Flyvbjerg, H. 1999. Designing optimal spatial filters for single-trial EEG classification in a movement task. *Clin. Neurophsyiol.* 110 (5): 787–798.

Großekathöfer, U., Pradhapan, P., Grundlehner, B., and Mihajlović, V. 2016. Motor imagery based BCI racing: Challenge a friend with 4 channel dry electrode EEG. *International Brain–Computer Interface (BCI) Meeting.*

Großekathöfer, U., Pradhapan, P., and Mihajlović, V. 2015. Predicting intentions in an uncontrolled environment using 4-channel dry electrode EEG. *5th NIPS Workshop on Machine Learning and Interpretation in Neuroimaging.*

Johnson, K. A., Robertson, I. H., Kelly, S. P., Silk, T. J., Barry, E., Daibhis, A., Watchorn, A., Keavey, M., Fitzgerald, M., Gallagher, L., Gill, M., and Bellgrove, M. A. 2007. Dissociation in performance of children with ADHD and high-functioning autism on a task of sustained attention. *Neuropsycholgia* 45: 2234–2245.

JSON. 2016. JavaScript Object Notation. *http://www.json.org/.*

Hamano, T., Rutkowski, T. M., Terasawa, H., Okanoya, K., and Furukawa, K. 2013. Generating an integrated musical expression with a brain–computer interface. *Proceedings of the 13th International Conference on New Interfaces for Musical Expression (NIME).* 49–54.

Kilavik, B. E., Zaepffel, M., Brovelli, A., MacKay, W. A., and Riehle, A. 2013. The ups and downs of oscillations in sensorimotor cortex. *Exp. Neurol.* 245: 15–26.

Kornhuber, H., and Deecke, L. 1965. Changes in the brain potential in voluntary movements and passive movements in man: Readiness potentials and reafferent potentials. *Pflugers Arch Gesamte Physiol Menchen.* Tiere, 10 (284): 1–17.

Lansbergen, M., Arns, M., van Dongen-Boomsma, M., Spronk, D., and Buitelaar, J. K. 2011. The increase in theta/beta ratio on resting-state EEG in boys with attention-deficit/hyperactivity disorder is mediated by slow alpha peak frequency. *Prog. Neuropsychopharmacol. Biol. Psychiatry* 35: 47–52.

Lew, E., Chavarriaga, R., Silvoni, S., and del Millán, J. R. 2012. Detection of self-paced reaching movement intention from EEG signals. *Front. Neuroeng.* 5 (13).

Makeig, S., and Inlow, M. 1993. Lapses is alertness: Coherence of fluctuations in performance and EEG spectrum. *Electroencephalogr. Clin. Neurophysiol.* 86: 23–35.

Makeig, S., and Jung, T. P. 1996. Tonic, phasic, and transient EEG correlates of auditory awareness in drowsiness. *Cogn. Brain. Res.* 4: 15–25.

Makeig, S., Jung, T. P., and Sejnowski, T. J. 2000. Awareness during drowsiness: Dynamics and electrophysiological correlates. *Can. J. Exp. Psychol.* 54: 266–273.

Mathewson, K. J., Jetha, M. K., Drmic, I. E., Bryson, S. E., Goldberg, J. O., and Schmidt, L. A. 2012. Regional EEG alpha power, coherence, and behavioral symptomatology in austism spectrum disorder. *Clin. Neurophysiol.* 123: 1798–1809.

Mapelli, A., Galante, D., Paganoni, S., Fusini, L., Forlani, G., and Sforza, C. 2012. Three-dimensional hand movements during the execution of ball juggling: Effect of expertise in street performers. *J. Electromyogr. Kinesiol.* 2 (6): 859–865.

Mihajlović, V., Grundlehner, B., Vullers, R., and Penders, J. 2015. Wearable, wireless EEG solutions in daily life applications: What are we missing? *J. Biomed. Health Inform.* 19 (1): 6–21.

Mihajlović, V., Patki, S., and Grundlehner, B. 2014. The impact of head movements on EEG and contact impedance: An adaptive filtering solution for motion artifact reduction. *36th Annual International Conference of the IEEE Engineering in Medicine and Biology Society (EMBC).* 5064–5067.

Miranda, E. R. 2010. Plymouth brain–computer music interfacing project: From EEG audio mixers to composition informed by cognitive neuroscience. *International Journal of Arts and Technology* 3 (2/3): 154–176.

Morash, V., Bai, O., Furlani, S., Lin, P., and Hallett, M. 2008. Classifying EEG signals preceding right hand, left hand, tongue, and right foot movements and motor imageries. *Clin. Neurophysiol.* 119 (11): 2570–2578.

Mullen, T., Khalil, A., Ward, T., Iversen, J., Leslie, G., Warp, R., Whitman, M., Minces, V., McCoy, A., Ojeda, A., Bigdely-Shamlo, N., Chi, M., and Rosenboom, D. 2015. MindMusic: Playful and social installations at the interface between music and the brain. In *Gaming Media and Social Effects.* Springer. 197–229.

Münßinger, J. I., Halder S., Kleih, S. C., Furdea, A., Raco, V., Hösle, A., and Kübler, A. 2010. Brain painting: First evaluation of a new brain–computer interface application with ALS-patients and healthy volunteers. *Front. Neurosci.* 4: 182.

Nakayashiki, K., Saeki, M., Takata, Y., Hayashi, Y., and Kondo, T. 2014. Modulation of event-related desynchronization during kinematic and kinetic hand movements. *J. Neuroeng. Rehabil.* 11 (90).

Neuper, C., Scherer, R., Wriessnegger, S., and Pfurtscheller, G. 2009. Motor imagery and action observation: Modulation of sensorimotor brain rhythms during mental control of a brain–computer interface. *Clin. Neurophysiol.* 120 (2): 239–247.

Niedermeyer, E., and Lopes da Silva, F. H. 2005. *Electroencephalography: Basic Principles, Clinical Applications, and Related Fields.* Lippincott Williams & Wilkins.

Oken, B., Salinsky, M., and Elsas, S. 2006. Vigilance, alertness, or sustained attention: Physiological basis and measurement. *Clin. Neurophysiol.* 117: 1885–1901.

Oldfield, R. C. 1971. The assessment and analysis of handedness: The Edinburgh inventory. *Neuropsychologia* 9 (1): 97–113.

OSC. 2016. Open Sound Control. http://opensoundcontrol.org/.

Patki, S., Grundlehner, B., Nakada, T., and J. Penders. 2011. Low power wireless EEG headset for BCI applications. *14th International Conference on Human–Computer Interaction.* 6762: 481–490.

Patki, S., Grundlehner, B., Verwegen, A., Mitra, S., Xu, J., Matsumoto, A., Yazacioglu, R. F., and Penders, J. 2012. Wireless EEG system with real time impedance monitoring and active electrodes. *Biomedical Circuits and Systems Conference (BioCAS).* 108–111.

Pfurtscheller, G., and Lopes da Silva, F. H. 1999. Event-related EEG/MEG synchronization and desynchronization: Basic principles. *Clin. Neurophysiol.* 110 (11): 1842–1857.

Pradhapan, P., Clerx, M., Griffioen, R., and Mihajlović, V. 2017. Personalized characterization of sustained attention/vigilance in healthy children. *eHealth 360°*. 271–281.

REST. 2016. REpresentation State Transfer. https://en.wikipedia.org/wiki/Representational_state_transfer.

Reynolds, M., Schoner, B., Richards, J., Dobson, K., and Gershenfeld, N. 2001. An immersive, multi-user, musical stage environment. *28th Annual Conference on Computer Graphics and Interactive Techniques.* 553–560.

Rosenboom, D., 1976. *Biofeedback and the Arts: Results of Early Experiments.* Vancouver: A.R.C. Publications.

Saab, J., Battles, B., and Grosse-Wentrup, M. 2011. Simultaneous EEG recordings with dry and wet electrodes in motor-imagery. *5th International Brain–Computer Interface Conference.* 312–315.

Santana, E., Brockmeier, A. J., and Principe, J. C. 2014. Joint optimization of algorithmic suites for EEG analysis. *Annual International Conference of IEEE Eng. Med. Biol. Soc. (EMBC).* 2997–3000.

Schiavone, G., Großekathöfer, U., à Campo, S., and Mihajlović, V. 2015. Towards real-time visualization of a juggler's brain. *Brain–Computer Interfaces* 2 (2–3): 90–102.

Schiavone, G., Großekathöfer, U., à Campo, S., and Mihajlović, V. 2016. The sonified juggling brain. *International Brain–Computer Interface (BCI) Meeting.*

Shibasaki, H., and Hallett, M. 2006. What is Bereitschaftspotential? *Clin. Neurophysiol.* 117 (11): 2341–2356.

SuperCollider. 2016. http://supercollider.github.io/.

Tallgren, P., Vanhatalo, S., Kaila, K., and Voipio, J. 2005. Evaluation of commercially available electrodes and gels for recording of slow EEG potentials. *Clin. Neurophysiol.* 116 (4): 799–806.

Wadeson, A., Nijholt, A., and Nam, C. S. 2015. Artistic brain–computer interfaces: State-of-the-art of control mechanisms. *Brain–Computer Interfaces* 2 (2–3): 70–75.

Webster, J. G. Ed. 2009. *Medical Instrumentation: Application and Design.* 4th ed. Wiley.

Willier, A., and Marque, C. 2002. Juggling gestures analysis for music control. *Gesture and Sign Language in Human Computer Interaction.* 296–306.

Wu, D., Li, C., and Dezhong, Y. 2013. Scale-free brain quartet: Artistic filtering of multi-channel brainwave music. *PLoS ONE* 1–7.

Zander, T. O., Lehne, M., Ihme, K., Jatzev, S., Correia, J., Kothe, C., Picht, B., and Nijboer, F. 2011. A dry EEG-system for scientific research and brain–computer interfaces. *Front. Neurosci.* 5 (53).

Zao, J. K., Gan, T. T., You, C. K., Chung, C. E., Wang, Y. T., Rodríguez Méndez, S. J., Mullen, T., Yu, C., Kothe, C., Hsiao, C. T., Chu, S. L., Shieh, C. K., and Jung, T. P. 2014. Pervasive brain monitoring and data sharing based on multi-tier distributed computing and linked data technology. *Front. Hum. Neurosci.* 8 (370).

Zen Wheels. 2016. Zen Wheels Micro Cars. http://zenwheels.com/.

Zioga, P., Chapman, P., Ma, M., and Pollick, F. 2014. Wireless future: Performance art, interaction and the brain–computer interfaces. *INTER-FACE: International Conference on Live Interfaces.*

# 10 BCI for Music Making
## Then, Now, and Next

*Duncan A.H. Williams*
*and Eduardo R. Miranda*

## CONTENTS

10.1 Introduction ........................................................................................................ 193
10.2 BCI and Music, An Overview .......................................................................... 194
10.3 Historical Approaches ...................................................................................... 196
10.4 Current: Hybrid Systems and Affective State Control .................................... 199
10.5 Next Steps.......................................................................................................... 201
References................................................................................................................... 202

**Abstract**

Brain–computer music interfacing (BCMI) is a growing field with a history of experimental applications derived from the cutting edge of BCI research as adapted to music making and performance. BCMI offers some unique possibilities over traditional music making, including applications for emotional music selection and emotionally driven music creation for individuals as communicative aids (either in cases where users might have physical or mental disabilities that otherwise preclude them from taking part in music making or in music therapy cases where emotional communication between a therapist and a patient by means of traditional music making might otherwise be impossible). This chapter presents an overview of BCMI and its uses in such contexts, including existing techniques as they are adapted to musical control, from P300 and SSVEP (steady-state visually evoked potential) in EEG (electroencephalogram) to asymmetry, hybrid systems, and joint fMRI (functional magnetic resonance imaging) studies correlating affective induction (by means of music) with neurophysiological cues. Some suggestions for further work are also volunteered, including the development of collaborative platforms for music performance by means of BCMI.

## 10.1 INTRODUCTION

The expression brain–computer music interfacing, or BCMI, was coined by Plymouth University's Interdisciplinary Centre for Computer Music Research team to denote BCI systems for Musical applications, and it has since been generally adopted by the research community (Miranda and Castet 2014). Research into BCMI involves three major challenges: the extraction of meaningful control information from signals emanating from the brain, the design of generative music techniques that respond to such information, and the definition of ways in which such technology can be deployed effectively, for example, to improve the lives of people with special needs, to address therapeutic applications, or for artistic purposes. BCMI is a growing field, with a history of experimental applications derived from the cutting edge of BCI research as adapted to music making and performance. BCMI offers some unique possibilities over traditional music making, including applications for emotional music selection and emotionally driven music creation for individuals as communicative aids. Examples of this include cases where users might have physical or mental disabilities that otherwise preclude them from taking part in music making or in music therapy cases where emotional communication between a therapist and a patient by means of traditional music making might otherwise be impossible. We assume that the reader will already have a strong understanding of the particular BCI methods documented in this chapter and their uses in other types of control signal generation. Therefore, we present an overview of BCMI and its uses in explicitly musical contexts, including existing techniques as they are adapted to musical control, from P300 and steady-state visually evoked potential (SSVEP) in electroencephalogram (EEG) to asymmetry, hybrid systems, and joint functional magnetic resonance imaging (fMRI) studies correlating affective induction by means of music with neurophysiological cues. Some suggestions for further work are also volunteered, including development of collaborative platforms for music performance by means of BCMI. The field, though small at first glance, is steadily growing, and this chapter focuses on a discrete group of research in the context of the field—inclusive but by no means exhaustive—a great variety of existing work is taking place at the time of writing. Music remains an exciting and challenging application, particularly at this time, for the BCI community.

## 10.2 BCI AND MUSIC, AN OVERVIEW

Music can be considered the language of emotion (Lin and Cheng 2012) and shares two fundamental properties with BCI, more generally, communication and interaction. Music facilitates communication from the composer to the audience of listener/s, and interaction between an individual performer and other musicians, as well as interaction between the performer/s and the audience of listener/s. Listeners do not need any special musical education to understand communication made by musical means (Bailes and Dean 2009; Bigand and Poulin-Charronnat 2006). The dream of many musicians, particularly musicians who also engage in composition activity, is to be able to bypass the physical intermediary in the process; that of notation or transcribing ideas for subsequent performance. Highly talented musicians are able to do this to some extent through improvisation; they create and perform at the same impulse. However, this requires a significant degree of musical training and becomes infinitely more complex when other musicians are also involved. BCI offers the possibility of directly translating thought to performance in music making. We consider this *mapping* and will refer to it throughout this chapter according to the definition that mapping encompasses the process of bridging particular BCI data with auditory cues. These cues might be musical notes, complete pieces of prerendered music, smaller sound stimuli such as noises or test tones, or specific auditory filtering processes (frequency or time domain-based effects, such as frequency equalization, phasing, reverberation, dynamic time warping, etc.). An overview of different types of music mapping from complex biomedical data and subsequent evaluation strategies is given in Williams (2016). In layman's terms, one might consider a BCMI goal to be, for the user, "Think of a tune," and as you do so, the BCMI mapping would transcribe your thoughts into musical notation, or perhaps synthesize them directly as audio. Therefore, the evaluation strategy can be relatively simple in such a case. A further level of complexity might be achieved if the system could automatically generate accompaniment or other instrumentation on the fly, requiring more complex evaluation. Beyond traditional music making (i.e., composition and performance), the possibility of adapting BCMI to patients with physical disabilities who might otherwise be unable to participate in music making is clear (Miranda et al. 2011). However, BCMI systems remain a long way from this goal at the time of writing.

The use of BCI for music has steadily been gaining traction over the past three decades. Yet, before this, early pioneers made use of the EEG to generate control data for musical performance. Alvin Lucier's 1965 piece *Music for Solo Performer* (Lucier 1976) distributes amplified alpha waves around a real-world performance space, in which various types of percussion are triggered or stimulated by the amplified waves as the performer mediates their mental state by meditating and increasing the corresponding alpha wave output. The otherworldly effect was well suited to the experimental avant-garde composition movement of the time, such as the work of John Cage and contemporaries, whom Lucier had seen some years prior and would have likely been influenced by. David Rosenboom continued the early exploration with the release of *Brainwave Music* (1974), adapting the sensor/mapping strategy to incorporate biofeedback in the compositional process (Rosenboom 1990; Teitelbaum 1976). Much of this period of BCMI evolution can be characterized by the realization of the control of alpha in a participant and the subsequent adaptation of this control to music creation. The concept of adaptive biofeedback was explored by Eaton (1971), who combined visual and auditory stimuli in a manner that facilitated much of the later design of BCMI. Historically, BCMI systems would not seek to extrapolate direct meaning from brainwaves but rather force a semantic mapping between the stimulus and the generated musical output. The principal distinction is that the influence of music on brainwaves and other physiological readings might also be harnessed as some form of control signal to facilitate musical interaction. Should the system for musical interaction be designed with this in mind, the subsequent feedback loop could create useful applications in and of itself, for example, in the context of music therapy. Music therapy is a psychological therapy technique that aims to facilitate communication and improve the emotional state of a patient via musical interaction with the therapist (Aigen 2005). A typical session might involve a patient performing on an instrument in solo or in a duet with the therapist. A BCMI system might be useful for such work by facilitating patients who are not musically confident or competent enough to engage in traditional music-making activities as part of the therapeutic process, for example, performing or improvising new music that might otherwise be restricted by age or previous experience (Clair and Memmott 2008; Fagen 1982; Hanser 1985).

Significant progress toward functional BCMI was made in the 1990s in systems such as *Biomuse* (Knapp and Lusted 1990), which mapped the acquisition of low-level neuroelectric and myoelectric signals to the generation of musical structure in MIDI format in real time, after applying statistical feature extraction to the captured signals. This system also used other physiological readings, including eye tracking, muscle tension, and real-time audio input, and as such could be considered a "hybrid BCMI."* At the time of publication, the creators of Biomuse directly acknowledged the possibility of adapting this technology to paralyzed or otherwise movement-impaired individuals, in order to give them access to music making—which in and of itself has been known to be a therapeutic process (Aldridge 2005; Hanser 1985)—and thus the importance of BCMI systems that only require brainwave control becomes clear in cases where the intended end user might be physically paralyzed such as "locked-in" patients (victims of amyotrophic lateral sclerosis or motor neurone disease).

Figure 10.1 shows an overview of a generic BCMI. This signal flow diagram can be applied to most BCMIs. Typically, a real-time input is analyzed and subjected to some signal processing. The exact processing varies; it could be as simple as filtering or a more complicated statistical reduction such as principal component analysis. Machine learning techniques are now becoming common for adaptive processing of control signals for music generation and performance (AlZoubi et al. 2008, 2009; Kirke et al. 2012, 2013). In such cases, the processed signal is used as a control signal to inform mapping to musical structure, or a specific range of musical features that might combine to make a musical structure of some description (note that this is not necessarily "music" at this stage of the process). An overview of specific mapping techniques for digital instrument design is given by Goudeseune (2002). Various combinations of mapping strategies exist, including one-to-one, one-to-many, and many-to-many combinations (Hunt and Kirk 2000). Typically, the mapping is predetermined at the stage of system design, but an adaptive mapping is indicated in this figure by the dashed lines (systems that use neurofeedback to adapt in this manner are discussed later in this chapter). It is in the mapping stage that most BCMIs derive their variety. Both the format of the output and the particular individual musical features and ratios between filtered control signal

---

* See Section 10.4 for the distinction between this and a BCMI that combines both active and passive control solely from brainwave input.

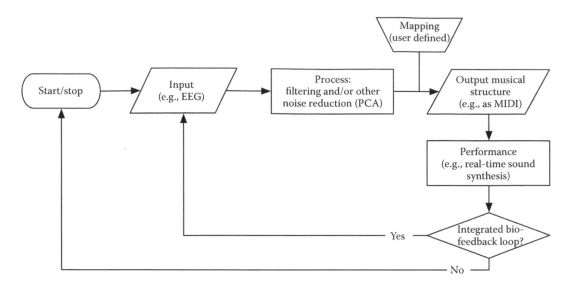

**FIGURE 10.1**  Overview of a generic BCMI. Most systems are differentiated by the mapping, which is typically fixed at the point of system design but in the future might be adaptable to neurofeedback.

and given musical feature are valid, and many different types of mappings have been experimented with (Brouwer and van Erp 2010; Chew and Caspary 2011; Daly et al. 2014c). The linear mapping of alpha waves to particular acoustic instruments in *Music for Solo Performer* is significantly different to the mapping in later systems such as Miranda's BCMI, which maps the control signal to the control of amplitude of specific musical sequence playback (Miranda 2010). Further variety can be given at the performance stage; oftentimes, BCMI systems have been married with sound synthesis to facilitate real-time performance (Hinterberger and Baier 2005). These systems have been used to generate musical scores for human performers or to trigger playback of pre-recorded musical material from a database or library (Eaton et al. 2014). The use of the resulting musical stimulus to mediate or entrain the listeners' brain activity (i.e., neurofeedback) is also a fertile area for research activity (Daly et al. 2014a, 2016; Hinterberger and Baier 2005) and forms the last generic functionality shown in Figure 10.1.

Neurofeedback is becoming increasingly common in the design of BCMI for specific purposes such as the therapeutic applications described above. Recent advances in electroencephalography have made these platforms more affordable and accessible to BCMI designers. Next, we might expect to see fully realized BCMI systems that provide full control over the generation and playback of electronic music, the creation of the score for acoustic instrumental music, or multibrain systems facilitating the kinds of interactions that musicians who are used to performing in groups can already experience. This chapter will explore historical approaches first, before illustrating some of these applications to music creation and offering some suggestions as to what might happen next in the field.

## 10.3  HISTORICAL APPROACHES

Three types of BCMI approaches have been formally documented: user oriented, computer oriented, and mutually oriented approaches (Miranda et al. 2003). User-oriented approaches attempt to derive meaning directly from the input, giving the user complete control within the boundaries of the mapping. This often relies on a one-to-one mapping, as more complex mappings can be less readily interpretable by a casual user assuming the user is not also the determiner of the mapping in question. As well as the early experiments documented in the introduction to this chapter by Lucier and Rosenboom, Richard Teitelbaum demonstrated the use of a user-oriented one-to-one mapping in a BCMI in his 1967 piece *Spacecraft* (Teitelbaum 1976), which used amplified EEG as a control signal for an analog sound synthesizer in an improvised performance. Classification of meaning from EEG can be technically challenging, though as many chapters of this book explore this classification process has advanced significantly in recent years. Computer-oriented systems require the user to adapt their own interactions toward the functions of the computer to achieve musical control. Most BCMI systems fall into this category. Particular frequencies might be mapped to fixed musical parameters, so that the forms are required to mediate their own brainwave frequencies to achieve the desired musical output from the system (e.g., meditating or otherwise actively controlling the state of mind to change the brainwave amplitudes and frequencies as collected by the EEG). This approach is exemplified by *Music for Solo Performer* as discussed in the introduction of this chapter, or more latterly by ensemble performance in examples by the *Biomuse Trio* (Knapp et al. 2009; Lyon et al. 2014) (see, e.g., their 2011 piece *Music for Sleeping and Waking Minds*). The third category, mutually oriented, combines both the user-oriented and computer-oriented functions, allowing a more complex degree of user control over the resulting music. Mutually oriented systems combine the functions of both user and computer orientation whereby the two elements adapt to each other, so that more sophisticated musical mappings can be inferred from the EEG data. The mutually oriented system learns an individual's responses over a time series and then creates primary and secondary mappings. This increases the likelihood of useable and accurate EEG as the input and output effectively calibrates for an individual. This was the approach used in Eaton's *The Warren*. Here, the system requires the user to learn how to generate specific commands and features mappings that adapt depending on the behavior of the user (Miranda and Castet 2014).

Various commercially available systems allow EEG detection to command musical functions, albeit often with rudimentary mapping. Two types of EEG data are common in BCMI systems, event-related potentials (ERP) and spontaneous input. The P300 ERP (or "oddball paradigm") has been used to allow active control over note selection for real-time synthesis (Grierson 2008; Grierson and Kiefer 2011) using methods that are not dissimilar to the ERP typing or spelling systems that have become more common in the BCI world but adapted to musical notes rather than text input. Stimulus-responsive input measures, for example, the SSVEP (Middendorf et al. 2000), have been adapted to real-time score selection and other controls of musical features such as volume (Miranda 2010). One system developed by Miranda and colleagues made use of such measurement from the visual cortex in response to flashing stimuli and subsequently mapped these to particular selections of pre-composed musical score. Users were able to make the selection by focusing their gaze on a particular icon flashing at a given rate. The system looked for amplitude changes across the four frequencies presented as visual stimuli and then correlated these amplitude changes to musical feature selection. A second level of control was also shown to be useful and possible in the system as the amplitude response in the corresponding wave could gradually increase in proportion to the duration of the viewers' gaze, thereby giving mapping control for musical features that were not linear (e.g., volume control of a particular passage or instrument). This combination represented a breakthrough in that real-time explicit control of a BCMI was shown to be practical, albeit with a limited selection of musical mappings. A photograph of the system in performance is shown in Figure 10.2. For a full treatment of this process, and others like it, the reader is referred to Eaton and Miranda (2014). Whether this specific example should be classified as a "pure" BCI or not could be the subject of some debate as the interface required an EEG interpretation of eye position, rather than explicit brainwave-only measurement.

There is a marked difference between systems for direct musical control by means of BCI, as documented above, and systems for *sonification* or *musification* of brainwave data (typically EEG)

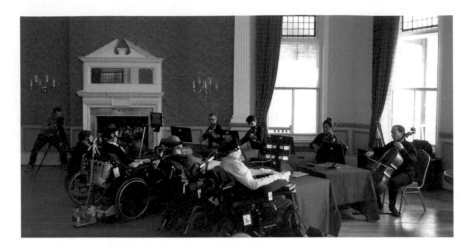

**FIGURE 10.2** SSVEP-based performance of a string quartet, under the active control of four patients with varying degrees of locked-in syndrome. Here, the patients perform "Activating Memory" (Eduardo Reck Miranda), a composition for eight performers: a string quartet and a BCMI quartet. In this performance, four severely motor-impaired patients at the Royal Hospital for Neurodisability (RHN), London, UK, use BCMI technology to generate musical scores in real time for the string quartet to play.

(Baier et al. 2007a,b; Hinterberger and Baier 2005). Sonification is a process whereby data are directly transmitted by auditory means:

> Sonification conveys information by using non-speech sounds. To listen to data as sound and noise can be a surprising new experience with diverse applications ranging from novel interfaces for visually impaired people to data analysis problems in many scientific fields. (Toharia et al. 2014)

Sonification in biomedical applications is a growing and progressive field, with many existing mappings from EEG (Väljamäe et al. 2013). The distinction between *sonification* and *musification*, both related forms of auditory display, is that in a *musification*, the data are not just auralized linearly, but instead, various constraints are created and applied in order to create a musical performance of the sonic data. This is an indistinct line and not easily delineated, but essentially the complexity and intent of the mapping involved determine whether the BCMI system is sonifying or musifying in its output. One example of EEG musification applied the rate of alpha to the cadence of the rhythm structure in a music segment, while mapping the variance of EEG to chords in a bar and the amplitude of waves to the note position of a melody (Wu et al. 2010). Rhythm is an interesting musical property with specific brain cortex associations (Baier et al. 2007a) and, as such, has also been utilized in EEG analysis of musical rhythm, for example, in the evoked gamma band (20–60 Hz) by rhythmic tone sequences (Snyder and Large 2005). However, evaluation strategies for such mappings, and musification in general, are not universally agreed upon and remain a significant area for further work. Nevertheless, musification allows the listener to engage with complex data in an intuitive way by exploiting their everyday listening experiences in the real world. This philosophy is common to many auditory display projects making use of multimodal techniques in the biomedical arena.

> The idea behind sonification is that synthetic non-verbal sounds can represent numerical data and provide support for information processing activities of many different kinds. (Mihalas et al. 2012)

The limitation is somewhat dependent on the complexity of the mappings and the number of meaningful, controllable features that might be extracted from the EEG. This might include overall EEG amplitude, the amplitude of specific frequencies, or the amplitude of frequencies at specific

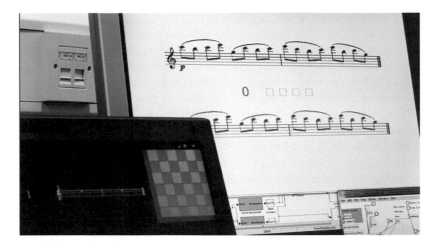

**FIGURE 10.3**   Score being generated in real time according to SSVEP selection. Taken from the documentary film of "Activating Memory" by the Paramusical Ensemble at the RHN on July 17, 2015, directed by Tim Grabham.

electrode placements on the scalp including dependent measures such as the level of asymmetry between electrodes on opposite sides of the cortex (Kirke and Miranda 2011).

The simplistic level of control available with direct mapping has led to the adoption of more complicated mapping strategies—that is, many-to-many—where algorithmic composition techniques are correlated with specific control signals. Melodies might be controlled by comparing alpha and beta amplitudes across given electrodes, or rhythmic properties adapted from a probabilistic algorithmic composition system (Miranda and Soucaret 2008). This mapping has also been reversed, wherein the rhythmic properties of the resulting material are directly controlled by the BCMI (Daly et al. 2014c). In such systems, there is a separation between cognitive control and the deliberate mapping of algorithmic composition techniques or other generative music techniques in semantic response to this control. Music is perhaps particularly well suited to the presentation of brainwave states in this manner, given the parallels in temporal nature between the two mediums. See Figure 10.3 for an example of SSVEP in use for score selection in real time.

## 10.4   CURRENT: HYBRID SYSTEMS AND AFFECTIVE STATE CONTROL

The historic systems presented in the section above can be broadly separated into two types: those that offer active control, wherein the user makes deliberate cognitive choices that are then mapped to musical features, and passive control, wherein BCI is used to determine subconscious mental states that are then used to inform the musical feature mapping. Hybrid systems combining both approaches simultaneously are also possible, though it is important to make a clear distinction between these types of hybrid systems and hybrid systems that combine different types of input sensors, for example, combining acoustic features with EEG, or combining other biophysiological readings such as heart rate or galvanic skin response with EEG (Daly et al. 2014b, 2015b). One of the earliest examples of such a performance can be seen in Richard Tietelbaum's *In Tune* (1967), which combined two EEG inputs with heartbeat and breathing sensors, to create one-to-one computer-oriented mappings for a musical performance (giving the users control of on and off switches and amplitude envelopes as they were passed to an analog sound synthesizer). Systems that combine both active and passive control might use passive affective state detection in combination with a degree of active control, for example, as afforded by the linear amplitude response of SSVEP as described above.

Collaborative music generation has a rich history (Le Groux and Verschure 2009; Manzolli and Verschure 2005). The ability of BCI to determine affective states and the ability of music to communicate emotions suggest that affect-driven BCMI (aBCMI) could be a logical multidisciplinary application toward collaborative music making. One such example provides the ability for two users to collaborate—collaboration is one of the central tenets of ensemble music performance—by mapping BCI measures of affect to the control of amplitude of two separate musical features (Leslie and Mullen 2012). This aspect of collaboration is perhaps one of the most exciting outcomes of BCMI. Subsequent measures of detecting different levels of emotional states have been adapted to musical control by Ramirez and Vamvakousis (2012), who evaluated a database of emotionally charged sound stimuli by means of EEG analysis across a two-dimensional affect space. Russel's two-dimensional space (Russell 1980) is commonly, but not exclusively, used in emotional assessment of musical stimuli. These mappings have also been exploited by computer-aided composition systems, with the suggestion that such systems could be driven by neurophysiological readings from BCI in aBCMI implementations (Williams et al. 2014).

Measurement of affective state changes in response to music takes its lead, as in most other cases of BCMI development, from the startling advances in BCI, in this case in defining affective (emotional) states from EEG (Chanel et al. 2006, 2007). The distinction is that emotional responses to music can be state dependent or independent in the same way that BCMI systems might be user or computer oriented—in other words, an emotional response *to music* (Lin et al. 2010). The ability of music to communicate emotions makes affective state measurement in order to inform musical feature selection a particularly strong candidate for BCMI applications. Recent research has highlighted a number of benefits when emotionally charged music is used to improve the listeners' cognitive performance (Franco et al. 2014). A significant amount of further work remains in quantifying listener responses to affectively charged music and in measuring the impact on a given affective state that music might have, as individual preferences and other environmental factors such as cultural expectations and musical training make emotional responses to musical stimuli highly variable (Scherer 2004). Nevertheless, the possibility of developing affectively responsive BCMI means that these individual variations might be mediated by BCI technology in ways that had previously been thought impossible by musicologists and music psychologists.

An example of affective state mapping to musical feature selection can be seen in the world of musical information retrieval (Eaton et al. 2014; Lin and Cheng 2012). Here, affective state measures are adopted from the mainstream BCI world and used to select music from a database that has already been tagged with emotional descriptors ("calm," "energetic," "happy," "sad," etc.). There is an interesting point to be made while determining listeners' emotional responses to certain types of music, because "sad" music has been shown to be enjoyable in some cases (Vuoskoski and Eerola 2012; Vuoskoski et al. 2012) and indeed to have similar neural correlates when measured by EEG (Daly et al. 2014b). It is also important in such work to acknowledge the difference between "perceived" and "induced" emotions. *Perceived* emotions refer to the emotional meaning the listener *understands* the music is supposed to convey, while *induced* responses refer to the emotion, or emotions, actually *felt* by the listener while listening (Juslin and Laukka 2004). In this manner, a piece of music may be perceived as intending to communicate "sadness" by the listener, while at the same time giving them a pleasurable feeling (i.e., they enjoy listening to the sad music). This seeming paradox has been well explored in musicological research (Hunter et al. 2010; Huron 2011; Manuel 2005). The ability of music to match or influence a listener's emotions has been exploited by, among other disciplines, music therapy, facilitating communication and improving the emotional state of a patient via musical interaction with the therapist. By enabling the generation of music that matches the emotional state of a patient, an aBCMI might potentially be of use as an expressive tool for patients to express their emotional state to the therapist regardless of physical ability or communicative handicap, for example, patients with autism, Asperger's syndrome, or even locked-in patients with little or no physical mobility.

The theoretical advantage of this approach over conventional music therapy approaches is that the BCMI is able to directly monitor the users' emotional state via physiological indices of emotion, which have the potential to be more robust and objective measures of emotion than user reports or even the expertise of the music therapist. Finally, the design and implementation of a successful aBCMI for music therapy might also facilitate modulation of a user's emotion by means of an affective feedback loop. This application would be unique to an aBCMI—which might, for example, generate music that gradually improves the mood of the patient in an autonomic process without the need for a therapist (Daly et al. 2014b, 2016).

## 10.5  NEXT STEPS

This chapter has presented a brief overview of the growing field of applications harnessing the power of BCI for music. From a somewhat fantastical science-fiction plot just a few decades ago to real-time control of musical feature generation for synthesis or playback by real musicians, the dream of going from imagining music to hearing it performed instantly, along with all of the benefits that such a realization might bring for patients with particular physical disabilities or those in music therapy practice, is drawing ever closer.

Tentative steps toward biofeedback from the 1960s and 1970s where alpha band control from EEG was exploited for one-to-one computer-centered BCMIs have exploded after the advances in other BCI technology, to accommodate affective state measurement, multiple user interfaces, a degree of live performance, and hybrid systems that combine both active and passive control, as well as hybrid systems that accommodate other physiological readings. A move toward aBCMI, affectively driven brain computer music interfacing, suggests that a freedom to explore the creative possibilities afforded by music, including emotional contagion, communication, and perhaps, most importantly, *interaction* with others, is on the near horizon in a developmental and commercial sense. It is fair to say that BCMI does not contribute enormously to the development of new BCI technologies in the main, being an engineering problem of implementation rather than advancement. On the other hand, significant advances in understanding particular responses that are only inherent in listening—for example, the emotional difference in 2D between "angry" and "afraid" sounding music, both of which would be classified traditionally as high arousal and low valence, yet both of which would encapsulate markedly different types of music regardless of an individual's listening preferences—suggest that BCMI still has something to offer to both neuroscience and the BCI community in general. The distinction between perceived and induced emotion is one that is still challenging. While visual examples can help differentiate this, music offers perhaps one of the strongest ways to explore this affective phenomenon. The temporal nature of music also lends itself well to illustrating the changing pattern and transient nature of emotions and many neurophysiological responses in general.

A tangential, but very related area to this chapter is the burgeoning field of work using non-nervous physiological signals, such as heart rate, galvanic skin response, and so on. It would be remiss not to speculate on the possibility of combining such work with BCMI in a sensor-fusion setting, especially given recent advances in biosignal interfacing for music making (Daly et al. 2015a; Nirjon et al. 2012; Pérez and Knapp 2008). However, it would be almost impossible here to explore the full range of possibilities afforded by BCI for music making as conducted to date, without looking to other biosignal interfacing. Nevertheless, looking to the future, one area that this chapter has not yet been able to explore in the context of neurophysiological interfacing is the future application of joint studies combining fMRI with EEG. This is particularly relevant to music given the spatial resolution issues that are currently inherent with EEG work. fMRI studies have been shown, in the context of affect measurement and, thus, subsequent aBCMI design, to be particularly useful in measuring and estimating induced affective states; yet, in a standalone context, they are not often employed by BCMI research. This is partly a practical concern of course not only because of the cost and size of facilities required but also partly because of the temporal resolution being inherently problematic when specific listening tasks are concerned. Musical features can often change radically in the duration of a second or two, which can be the smallest possible frame size afforded by some fMRI studies. Nevertheless, despite these concerns, fMRI does provide for a much greater spatial resolution for real-time musical control and adaptation. A combined approach comparing EEG and fMRI results to the adaptive control of music generation for affective induction has been proposed and is the subject of recent trials (Daly et al. 2016; Miranda 2010). We may then, in the future, see these trials and other work like them be adapted to more generalizable portable models that might be controlled by EEG, using adaptive mappings derived by machine learning rather than prescribed by the designers of such systems, for musical collaboration regardless of physical ability or previous musical training. Anyone who has played an instrument in isolation will know that here, in the process of *collaboration*, might BCMI's real future lie.

## REFERENCES

Aigen, Kenneth. 2005. *Music-Centered Music Therapy*. Barcelona Pub.

Aldridge, David. 2005. *Music Therapy and Neurological Rehabilitation: Performing Health*. Jessica Kingsley Publishers.

AlZoubi, Omar, Rafael A. Calvo, and Ronald H. Stevens. 2009. Classification of EEG for affect recognition: An adaptive approach. In *Australasian Joint Conference on Artificial Intelligence*, 52–61. Springer.

AlZoubi, Omar, Irena Koprinska, and Rafael A. Calvo. 2008. Classification of brain–computer interface data. In *Proceedings of the 7th Australasian Data Mining Conference—Volume 87*, 123–131. Australian Computer Society, Inc.

Baier, Gerold, Thomas Hermann, and Ulrich Stephani. 2007a. Event-based sonification of EEG rhythms in real time. *Clinical Neurophysiology* 118: 1377–1386.

Baier, Gerold, Thomas Hermann, and Ulrich Stephani. 2007b. Multi-channel sonification of human EEG. In *Proceedings of the 13th International Conference on Auditory Display*.

Bailes, Freya, and Roger T. Dean. 2009. Listeners discern affective variation in computer-generated musical sounds. *Perception* 38: 1386–1404. doi:10.1068/p6063.

Bigand, Emmanuel, and Bénédicte Poulin-Charronnat. 2006. Are we "experienced listeners"? A review of the musical capacities that do not depend on formal musical training. *Cognition* 100: 100–130.

Brouwer, Anne-Marie, and Jan van Erp. 2010. A tactile P300 brain–computer interface. *Frontiers in Neuroscience*. doi:10.3389/fnins.2010.00019.

Chanel, Guilliame, Ansari-Asl, Karim, and Pun, Thierry. 2007. Valence-arousal evaluation using physiological signals in an emotion recall paradigm. In *Systems, Man and Cybernetics, 2007. ISIC. IEEE International Conference on*, 2662–2667. doi:10.1109/ICSMC.2007.4413638.

Chanel, Guilliame, Kronegg, Julien, Grandjean, Didier, and Pun, Thierry. 2006. Emotion assessment: Arousal evaluation using EEG's and peripheral physiological signals. *Multimedia Content Representation, Classification and Security*: 530–537.

Chew, Yee Chieh (Denise), and Eric Caspary. 2011. MusEEGk: A brain computer musical interface. In *Proceedings of the 2011 Annual Conference Extended Abstracts on Human Factors in Computing Systems*, 1417–1422. New York: ACM Press. doi:10.1145/1979742.1979784.

Clair, Alicia Ann, and Jenny Memmott. 2008. *Therapeutic Uses of Music with Older Adults*. ERIC.

Daly, Ian, James Hallowell, Faustina Hwang, Alexis Kirke, Asad Malik, Etienne Roesch, James Weaver, Duncan Williams, Eduardo Miranda, and Slawomir J. Nasuto. 2014a. Changes in music tempo entrain movement related brain activity. In *2014 36th Annual International Conference of the IEEE Engineering in Medicine and Biology Society*, 4595–4598. IEEE.

Daly, Ian, Asad Malik, Faustina Hwang, Etienne Roesch, James Weaver, Alexis Kirke, Duncan Williams, Eduardo Miranda, and Slawomir J. Nasuto. 2014b. Neural correlates of emotional responses to music: An EEG study. *Neuroscience Letters* 573: 52–57.

Daly, Ian, Asad Malik, James Weaver, Faustina Hwang, Slawomir J. Nasuto, Duncan Williams, Alexis Kirke, and Eduardo Miranda. 2015a. Towards human–computer music interaction: Evaluation of an affectively-driven music generator via galvanic skin response measures. In, 87–92. IEEE. doi:10.1109/CEEC.2015.7332705.

Daly, Ian, Duncan Williams, James Hallowell, Faustina Hwang, Alexis Kirke, Asad Malik, James Weaver, Eduardo Miranda, and Slawomir J. Nasuto. 2015b. Music-induced emotions can be predicted from a combination of brain activity and acoustic features. *Brain and Cognition* 101: 1–11. doi:http://dx.doi.org/10.1016/j.bandc.2015.08.003.

Daly, Ian, Duncan Williams, Faustina Hwang, Alexis Kirke, Asad Malik, Etienne Roesch, James Weaver, Eduardo Miranda, and Slawomir J Nasuto. 2014c. Brain–computer music interfacing for continuous control of musical tempo.

Daly, Ian, Duncan Williams, Alexis Kirke, James Weaver, Asad Malik, Faustina Hwang, Eduardo Miranda, and Slawomir J. Nasuto. 2016. Affective brain–computer music interfacing. *Journal of Neural Engineering* 13: 46022–46035.

Eaton, Joel, and Eduardo Reck Miranda. 2014. On mapping EEG information into music. In *Guide to Brain–Computer Music Interfacing*, 221–254. Springer.

Eaton, Joel, Duncan Williams, and Eduardo Miranda. 2014. Affective jukebox: A confirmatory study of EEG emotional correlates in response to musical stimuli. In *ICMC/SMC 2014 Conference*.

Eaton, Manford L. 1971. *Bio-Music: Biological Feedback Experimental Music Systems*. Orcus.

Fagen, Trudy Shulman. 1982. Music therapy in the treatment of anxiety and fear in terminal pediatric patients. *Music Therapy* 2: 13–23.

Franco, Fabia, Joel S. Swaine, Shweta Israni, Katarzyna A. Zaborowska, Fatmata Kaloko, Indu Kesavarajan, and Joseph A. Majek. 2014. Affect-matching music improves cognitive performance in adults and young children for both positive and negative emotions. *Psychology of Music* 42: 869–887.

Goudeseune, Camille. 2002. Interpolated mappings for musical instruments. *Organised Sound* 7: 85–96.

Grierson, Mick. 2008. Composing with brainwaves: Minimal trial P300b recognition as an indication of subjective preference for the control of a musical instrument. In *Proceedings of International Cryogenic Materials Conference (ICMC'08)*.

Grierson, Mick, and Chris Kiefer. 2011. Better brain interfacing for the masses. In *1681*. ACM Press. doi:10.1145/1979742.1979828.

Hanser, Suzanne B. 1985. Music therapy and stress reduction research. *Journal of Music Therapy* 22: 193–206.

Hinterberger, Thilo, and Gerold Baier. 2005. Poser: Parametric orchestral sonification of EEG in real-time for the self-regulation of brain states. *IEEE Trans. Multimedia* 12: 70.

Hunt, Andy, and Ross Kirk. 2000. Mapping strategies for musical performance. *Trends in Gestural Control of Music* 21: 231–258.

Hunter, Patrick G., E. Glenn Schellenberg, and Ulrich Schimmack. 2010. Feelings and perceptions of happiness and sadness induced by music: Similarities, differences, and mixed emotions. *Psychology of Aesthetics, Creativity, and the Arts* 4: 47.

Huron, David. 2011. Why is sad music pleasurable? A possible role for prolactin. *Musicae Scientiae* 15: 146–158.

Juslin, Patrik N., and Petri Laukka. 2004. Expression, perception, and induction of musical emotions: A review and a questionnaire study of everyday listening. *Journal of New Music Research* 33: 217–238.

Kirke, Alexis, and Eduardo Miranda. 2011. Combining EEG Frontal Asymmetry Studies with Affective Algorithmic Composition and Expressive Performance Models. In *International Computer Music Conference (ICMC 2011), Huddersfield, UK*.

Kirke, Alexis, Eduardo Miranda, and Slawomir J. Nasuto. 2013. Artificial affective listening towards a machine learning tool for sound-based emotion therapy and control. In *Proceedings of the Sound and Music Computing Conference*, 259–265. Stockholm, Sweden: SMC Network.

Kirke, Alexis, Eduardo Reck Miranda, and Slawomir Nasuto. 2012. Learning to make feelings: Expressive performance as a part of a machine learning tool for sound-based emotion therapy and control. In *Cross-Disciplinary Perspectives on Expressive Performance Workshop*. London.

Knapp, R. Benjamin, Javier Jaimovich, and Niall Coghlan. 2009. Measurement of motion and emotion during musical performance. In *Proceedings of the 3rd International Conference on Affective Computing and Intelligent Interaction and Workshops*, Amsterdam, Netherlands.

Knapp, R. Benjamin, and Hugh S. Lusted. 1990. A bioelectric controller for computer music applications. *Computer Music Journal* 14: 42–47.

Le Groux, Sylvain, and Paul Verschure. 2009. Neuromuse: Training your brain through musical interaction. In *Proceedings of the International Conference on Auditory Display, Copenhagen, Denmark*.

Leslie, Grace, and Tim Mullen. 2012. MoodMixer: EEG-based collaborative sonification. In *Proceedings of the International Conference on New Interfaces for Musical Expression*, 296–299, http://www.nime.org/proceedings/2011/nime2011_296.pdf. Accessed November 19.

Lin, Chih-Yi, and Stone Cheng. 2012. Multi-theme analysis of music emotion similarity for jukebox application. In *Audio, Language and Image Processing (ICALIP), 2012 International Conference on*, 241–246. IEEE.

Lin, Yuan-Pin, Chi-Hong Wang, Tzyy-Ping Jung, Tien-Lin Wu, Shyh-Kang Jeng, Jeng-Ren Duann, and Jyh-Horng Chen. 2010. EEG-based emotion recognition in music listening. *IEEE Transactions on Biomedical Engineering* 57: 1798–1806. doi:10.1109/TBME.2010.2048568.

Lucier, Alvin. 1976. Statement on: Music for solo performer. *Biofeedback and the Arts, Results of Early Experiments. Vancouver: Aesthetic Research Center of Canada Publications*: 60–61.

Lyon, Eric, R. Benjamin Knapp, and Gascia Ouzounian. 2014. Compositional and performance mapping in computer chamber music: A case study. *Computer Music Journal*.

Manuel, Peter. 2005. Does sad music make one sad? An ethnographic perspective. *Contemporary Aesthetics* 3.

Manzolli, Jonatas, and Paul Verschure. 2005. Roboser: A real-world composition system. *Computer Music Journal* 29: 55–74.

Middendorf, Matthew, Grant McMillan, Gloria Calhoun, Keith S. Jones, and others. 2000. Brain–computer interfaces based on the steady-state visual-evoked response. *IEEE Transactions on Rehabilitation Engineering* 8: 211–214.

Mihalas, Georges I., Sorin Paralescu, Nicoleta Mirica, Danina Muntean, Mircea Hancu, Anca Tudor, and Minodora Andor. 2012. Sonic representation of information: Application for heart rate analysis. In *Proceedings MIE*.

Miranda, Eduardo R, and Vincent Soucaret. 2008. Mix-it-yourself with a brain–computer music interface. *Proceedings of 7th ICDVRAT with ArtAbilitation*.

Miranda, Eduardo R. 2010. Plymouth brain–computer music interfacing project: From EEG audio mixers to composition informed by cognitive neuroscience. *International Journal of Arts and Technology* 3: 154–176.

Miranda, Eduardo R., Wendy L. Magee, John J. Wilson, Joel Eaton, and Ramaswamy Palaniappan. 2011. Brain–computer music interfacing (BCMI) from basic research to the real world of special needs. *Music and Medicine* 3: 134–140.

Miranda, Eduardo Reck, and Julien Castet, ed. 2014. *Guide to Brain–Computer Music Interfacing*. London: Springer.

Miranda, Eduardo Reck, Ken Sharman, Kerry Kilborn, and Alexander Duncan. 2003. On Harnessing the Electroencephalogram for the Musical Braincap. *Computer Music Journal* 27: 80–102. doi:10.1162/014892603322022682.

Nirjon, Shahriar, Robert F. Dickerson, Qiang Li, Philip Asare, John A. Stankovic, Dezhi Hong, Ben Zhang, Xiaofan Jiang, Guobin Shen, and Feng Zhao. 2012. Musicalheart: A hearty way of listening to music. In *Proceedings of the 10th ACM Conference on Embedded Network Sensor Systems*, 43–56. ACM.

Pérez, Miguel Angel Ortiz, and R. Benjamin Knapp. 2008. BioTools: A biosignal toolbox for composers and performers. In *Computer Music Modeling and Retrieval. Sense of Sounds*, 441–452. Springer.

Ramirez, Rafael, and Zacharias Vamvakousis. 2012. Detecting emotion from EEG signals using the emotive epoc device. In *Brain Informatics*, ed. Fabio Massimo Zanzotto, Shusaku Tsumoto, Niels Taatgen, and Yiyu Yao, 7670: 175–184. Lecture Notes in Computer Science. Springer Berlin Heidelberg.

Rosenboom, David. 1990. The performing brain. *Computer Music Journal* 14: 48–66.

Russell, James. 1980. A circumplex model of affect. *Journal of Personality and Social Psychology* 39: 1161.

Scherer, Klaus R. 2004. Which emotions can be induced by music? What are the underlying mechanisms? And how can we measure them? *Journal of New Music Research* 33: 239–251.

Snyder, Joel S., and Edward W. Large. 2005. Gamma-band activity reflects the metric structure of rhythmic tone sequences. *Cognitive Brain Research* 24: 117–126. doi:10.1016/j.cogbrainres.2004.12.014.

Teitelbaum, Richard. 1976. In tune: Some early experiments in biofeedback music (1966–1974). In *Biofeedback and the Arts, Results of Early Experiments*. Vancouver: Aesthetic Research Center of Canada Publications.

Toharia, Pablo, Juan Morales, Octavio Juan, Isabel Fernaud, Angel Rodríguez, and Javier DeFelipe. 2014. Musical representation of dendritic spine distribution: A new exploratory tool. *Neuroinformatics*: 1–13. doi:10.1007/s12021-013-9195-0.

Väljamäe, Anastasiia, Steffert, Tony, Holland, Simon, Marimon, Xavier, Benitez, Rafael Mealla, Sebastian, Oliveira, Aluizio, and Sergio Jordà. 2013. A review of real-time EEG sonification research. In *International Conference on Auditory Display 2013 (ICAD 2013)*, July 6–10, 2013, Lodz, Poland, pp. 85–93.

Vuoskoski, Jonna K., and Tuomas Eerola. 2012. Can sad music really make you sad? Indirect measures of affective states induced by music and autobiographical memories. *Psychology of Aesthetics, Creativity, and the Arts* 6: 204.

Vuoskoski, Jonna K., William F. Thompson, Doris McIlwain, and Tuomas Eerola. 2012. Who enjoys listening to sad music and why? *Music Perception* 29: 311–317.

Williams, Duncan, Kirke, Alexis, Miranda, Eduardo, Roesch, Etienne Daly, Ian, and Slawomir Nasuto. 2014. Investigating affect in algorithmic composition systems. *Psychology of Music.* doi:10.1177/0305735614543282.

Williams, Duncan. 2016. Utility versus creativity in biomedical musification. *Journal of Creative Music Systems* 1.

Wu, Dan, Chaoyi Li, Yu Yin, Changzheng Zhou, and Dezhong Yao. 2010. Music composition from the brain signal: Representing the mental state by music. *Computational Intelligence and Neuroscience* 2010: 14.

# Brain–Computer Interface Applications

*Section D. BCI Control of Entertainment and Multimedia*

# 11 BCI and Games: Playful, Experience-Oriented Learning by Vivid Feedback?

*Silvia E. Kober, Manuel Ninaus, Elisabeth V.C. Friedrich, and Reinhold Scherer*

## CONTENTS

11.1 Overview ................................................................................................................. 210
11.2 Need for New Feedback Designs? ......................................................................... 210
11.3 Summary of BCI/NF Studies Using Games as Feedback ...................................... 211
11.4 Potential Value of Using Game-Like FB ............................................................... 212
    11.4.1 Motivation and Interest ............................................................................... 212
    11.4.2 Flow, Immersion, and Presence ................................................................. 224
    11.4.3 Attract Users' Attention and Reduce Mind Wandering ............................. 224
    11.4.4 Intuitive Feedback and Interactions ........................................................... 225
    11.4.5 Activating the Mirror Neuron System ....................................................... 226
    11.4.6 Transfer to Real-World Behavior ............................................................... 226
    11.4.7 Increasing BCI/NF Performance and Consequently Its Outcome ............. 227
11.5 Drawbacks—Lack of Evaluation of Effects .......................................................... 227
11.6 Conclusion ............................................................................................................. 228
Acknowledgments ............................................................................................................ 229
References ......................................................................................................................... 229

### Abstract

Play, that is, self-motivated activities for enjoyment, is a significant aspect for human development and essential to learning and skill acquisition. Games, the structured form of play, are increasingly being used in brain–computer interface (BCI) and neurofeedback (NF) applications. In BCI and NF applications, patterns of the users' brain activation are assessed in real time and fed back to the users. When users become successful in modulating their own brain activation, improvements in behavior, cognition, or motor function follow or they are able to control external devices such as a computer, wheelchair, or neuroprosthesis. In electroencephalogram-based applications, however, a large number of users cannot attain control over their own brain signals. Current approaches to attaining control require lengthy repetitive trainings. The use of games and game-like feedback aims at keeping user motivation and engagement high over time. This chapter provides an overview of existing game-like feedback modalities and critically discusses their potential value and also possible drawbacks in BCI and NF applications.

## 11.1  OVERVIEW

A recent trend in brain–computer interface (BCI) and neurofeedback (NF) applications is to use games and game-like feedback scenarios with the aim of increasing training motivation, interest, and engagement and to provide a more intuitive and meaningful feedback compared to traditional two-dimensional and relatively monotonous feedback modalities. In the present chapter, we first give an overview of existing game-like feedback modalities (e.g., ping-pong, puzzle games, racing games, and role-play games) including serious games as well as virtual reality (VR) technology and discuss their potential value in BCI and NF applications. In the second part of the chapter, we discuss possible drawbacks of game-like feedback modalities. Although the number of BCI and NF studies using game-like feedback is steadily increasing, the effects on BCI/NF performance are mostly unknown. The assumed positive effects of game-like feedback on users' motivation, engagement, and interest are scarcely investigated as well as its outcome measures such as motor/cognitive performance improvements in comparison to traditional feedback modalities. Hence, there is a lack of empirical evidence of the supposed value of games in BCI and NF applications. In conclusion, we propose possible indications and contraindications of game-like feedback scenarios for BCI and NF applications.

## 11.2  NEED FOR NEW FEEDBACK DESIGNS?

In BCI and NF applications, patterns of the users' brain activation are assessed in real time and fed back to the users via sensory stimulation. Commonly, auditory, visual, or tactile feedback and combinations thereof are presented. When users become successful in modulating their own brain activation, generally improvements in behavior, cognition, or motor function follow or they are able to control external devices such as a computer, wheelchair, or neuroprosthesis (Gruzelier 2014; Millán et al. 2010; Neuper et al. 2006; Scherer et al. 2009). However, reliable online assessment of brain activation patterns is challenging. As a consequence, a large portion of BCI and NF users fail to gain voluntary control over their brain activity. In electroencephalogram (EEG)-based (bioelectrical potentials recorded from the scalp) applications, about 30% of potential BCI or NF users cannot attain control over their own brain signals (Allison and Neuper 2010; Blankertz et al. 2010a; Kober et al. 2015). Usually, functional magnetic resonance imaging (fMRI)–based BCI or NF applications report a lower percentage of users who fail to gain voluntary control over their brain signals (e.g., Haller et al. 2010; Johnston et al. 2011; Zhang et al. 2015). The relatively high number of nonresponders in EEG-based BCI and NF applications is a crucial issue since it prevents a large number of people from benefitting from highly innovative and alternative communication and therapy options (Kober et al. 2016). EEG recording technology is widely available, portable, and, compared to fMRI, affordable (Thibault et al. 2015). In the BCI community, the inability to use BCI applications is called "BCI-illiteracy phenomenon" (Blankertz et al. 2010a). There are different attempts to explain this phenomenon. For instance, in some BCI/NF users, cortical neuronal networks involved in voluntary control might generate electrical activity that is not detectable on the scalp (e.g., electrodes placed on iospotential surface). Other users might produce excessive artifacts (interference signals that lead to erroneous translation of brain activity patterns), which disturb the feedback signal and hamper the learning effect (Allison and Neuper 2010). The definite reason why so many people cannot benefit from BCI and NF technology remains elusive.

A few studies report on a relationship between neurophysiological parameters such as resting-state EEG or brain volumetry and successful BCI and NF performance (Blankertz et al. 2010a; Halder et al. 2013; Kübler et al. 2004; Ninaus et al. 2013a, 2015a; Reichert et al. 2015). Furthermore, there is evidence that more subjective psychological factors such as control beliefs, mood, mastery confidence, motivation, or the used mental strategy (Friedrich et al. 2013, 2015a; Hammer et al. 2012; Kleih et al. 2010; Kober et al. 2013; Nijboer et al. 2008; Scherer et al. 2015a; Witte et al. 2013) also correlate with BCI/NF success rates. In this context, the feedback design, which might influence psychological variables, could play a crucial role (Neuper et al. 2009). The design of the training protocol also seems to be important (Jeunet et al. 2016; Lotte et al. 2013). Learning to control BCI or NF applications is relatively time consuming. The number of BCI and NF training sessions necessary to obtain significant effects on different outcome measures varies between 1 and more than 100 sessions (Arns et al. 2009; McFarland et al. 2010; Müller-Putz et al. 2005; Pfurtscheller et al. 2003; Tan et al. 2009). Such a high number of repeated BCI and NF training sessions can make users bored and tired, and even result in high costs (Cho et al. 2004). Furthermore, successful BCI and NF performance requires top-down cognitive control (Emmert et al. 2016; Lacroix and Gowen 1981; Lacroix et al. 1986; Ninaus et al. 2013a, 2015a; Wood et al. 2014), so that the user can stay focused and concentrated on the BCI or NF task over a long training period. Monotonous or boring feedback modalities might increase the occurrence of mind-wandering episodes and task-irrelevant thoughts, leading to reduced task performance (Mrazek et al. 2011; Ros et al. 2013; Smallwood and Schooler 2006). Such monotonous feedback methods might not attract users to focus on them (Yan et al. 2008), leading to decreased motivation, interest, concentration, and finally to a lower performance and success rate (Keller 2010; Kleih et al. 2010). Importantly, games (Koepp et al. 1998) or game-based serious applications (Cole et al. 2012) act on the mesolimbic and mesocortical dopaminergic reward system of the brain (for a review, see, e.g., Howard-Jones et al. 2011) and thereby might promote user performance, learning rates, and cognitive performance (e.g., Mekler et al. 2015; Ninaus et al. 2015b; for a review, see Lumsden et al. 2016). Hence, introducing more attractive, interesting, engaging, and entertaining game-like feedback modalities might lead to increased motivation and compliance to training and finally to an improved BCI/NF performance outcome.

## 11.3 SUMMARY OF BCI/NF STUDIES USING GAMES AS FEEDBACK

The traditional visualization of the feedback in BCI and NF paradigms ranges from controlling a simple bar graph to more sophisticated visual renditions. Usually, an object (e.g., bar graph, circle, car, or rocket ship) moves along the screen or increases/decreases in size depending on the brain activity level. Some studies also use auditory feedback in which a tone is changing in its volume or pitch according to the brain activity shown. These traditional feedback implementations are very simple and easy to understand but at the same time extremely prosy. This is especially problematic for BCI and NF studies as they rely on the repetition of numerous trials and sessions.

Thus, an increasing number of studies use game-like feedback. Early attempts to use simple visualizations in a game-like setup were inspired by basket, ping-pong, or Tetris games (e.g., Blankertz et al. 2010b; Krausz et al. 2003; Müller and Blankertz 2006; Scherer et al. 2015b). Figure 11.1 shows examples of how game-related feedback evolved over time. With upcoming VR technology such as head-mounted displays or three-dimensional (3D) projection systems including stereoscopic glasses, the number of BCI and NF studies that use 3D VR-based game-like feedback scenarios is also expanding. VR games include car driving games, virtual flight simulators, or navigation and interaction tasks in virtual environments such as virtual apartments (e.g., Leeb et al. 2005; Royer et al. 2010; Scherer et al. 2008). Role-play games such as World of Warcraft are also used as feedback scenario (e.g., Scherer et al. 2013a; Van De Laar et al. 2013). Role-play mechanisms are not only a powerful tool toward boosting motivation to learn controlling a BCI or NF, but have also been shown to successfully intervene on behavior (Friedrich et al. 2014). This indicates that game-like interactions and role-playing improve the learning experience. Table 11.1 summarizes BCI and NF studies that use game-like feedback modalities.

Generally, key components of games are goals, rules, challenge, and interaction.* "Serious games" are defined as games that are designed for a primary purpose other than pure entertainment (Carter et al. 2014). The critical reader might maintain that traditional feedback modalities as described above might also fulfill these criteria. Traditional 2D feedback screens used in BCI

---

* https://en.wikipedia.org/wiki/Game

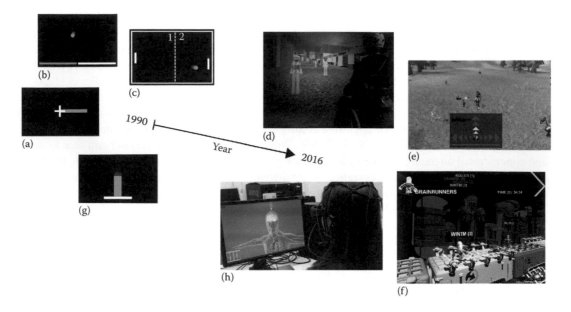

**FIGURE 11.1**   Evolution of BCI and NF feedback. Initially, feedback was presented in the form of a basic geometric shape, such as a bar graph. Brain activation was typically mapped to change direction (a) and/or length of the bar graph (g). First game-like feedbacks included the Basket [(b) hit the correct basket with the ball] and Pong (c) game. In modern days, feedback includes immersive 3-D Virtual Reality (d and h) and commercial computer games such as the MMRPG *World of Warcraft* (e). Commonly special applications are developed and adapted for BCI, such as the (f) BCI Race game *BrainRunners* for the first international Cybathlon competition.

or NF applications, such as vertically moving bars (Figure 11.1g), might also fulfill these criteria. There are goals (e.g., increasing the bar and getting as much reward points as possible), rules (e.g., the bar in the middle of the screen should increase while the bars on the left and right side of the screen should be as low as possible so as to earn reward points), challenge (e.g., adaptive individual thresholds that should be exceeded), and interaction (direct real-time feedback of one's own brain activity), and they have an educational purpose, which is learning to voluntarily modulate one's own brain activity. So can we consider these traditional feedback modalities as "games"?

We maintain that compared to traditional feedback modalities, the additional value of using game-like feedback scenarios, in which often an advanced technique (e.g., VR equipment) is used to present the game in a more immersive way, is that games might increase motivation, interest, and compliance, and are more intuitive, self-explanatory, and engaging. Moreover, transfer of the acquired skill to real-world situations might be enhanced because of more realistic and context-specific feedback. Meaningful feedback that is specific to the signal being trained might also foster intended behavioral changes in NF (Friedrich et al. 2014, 2015b).

In Section 11.4, we describe studies that directly investigate the effects of game-like feedback modalities on these factors.

## 11.4   POTENTIAL VALUE OF USING GAME-LIKE FB

### 11.4.1   MOTIVATION AND INTEREST

Kleih et al. (2010) provided evidence that motivation can influence the NF/BCI performance. They experimentally manipulated the level of motivation of the BCI users by monetary reward. Highly motivated BCI users showed a superior BCI performance compared to users with a lower motivation (Kleih et al. 2010). Hence, increasing motivation by introducing more interesting game-like feedback might also positively affect BCI/NF performance.

## TABLE 11.1
## Journals

| Reference | Method | NF/BCI | Physiological Parameters Used in FB Signal | Mental Task | Game-Like Feedback | Study Design and Participants | Feedback Presentation | Outcome Measures | Main Finding | UX[1] |
|---|---|---|---|---|---|---|---|---|---|---|
| Ron-Angevin and Díaz-Estrella (2009) | EEG | BCI | EEG power in different frequency bands | Mental relaxation vs. motor imagery (right hand) | Virtual car driving game (visual) | $N = 16$ (age= mean 24.4 years) 2 groups (control group = CG; virtual reality = VR, each $N = 8$), between-subject design | VR: Head-mounted display (HMD) CG: computer screen | BCI performance | Feedback control VR > conventional feedback Subjective reports of the VR group indicated a motivational effect | ✓ |
| Zhao et al. (2009) | EEG | BCI | EEG power in different frequency bands | Motor imagery (left hand, right hand, and foot) vs. resting period | Virtual car driving game (visual) | $N = 4$ (age= 24–30 years) | Conventional computer monitor | BCI performance | 2 of 4 participants were able to drive the car along predefined pathways | |
| Cho et al. (2004) | EEG | NF | Controlling EEG beta wave ratio | Concentration | Virtual classroom gradual completion of a puzzle (visual) | $N = 28$ (age = 14–18 years) with social problems 3 groups: control group (CG; $n = 9$); VR-NF group (3D, $n = 10$); non-VR NF group (2D; $n = 9$); between-subject design | VR: HMD Non-VR: conventional computer monitor | NF performance Attention and impulsiveness (pre/post with a continuous performance task [CPT]) | Performance improvement in CPT CG < non-VR-NF < VR-NF NF performance: VR group > non-VR group | ✓ |

*(Continued)*

**TABLE 11.1 (CONTINUED)**
Journals

| Reference | Method | NF/ BCI | Physiological Parameters Used FB Signal | Mental Task | Game-Like Feedback | Study Design and Participants | Feedback Presentation | Outcome Measures | Main Finding | UX[1] |
|---|---|---|---|---|---|---|---|---|---|---|
| Wang et al. (2011) | EEG | NF | EEG power in different frequency bands theta/beta ratio | Relaxation vs. concentration | 2D and 3D NF games (visual) | N = 5 (age = 22–30 years) | Conventional computer monitor | Comparison of different fractal dimension algorithms to quantify concentration levels (relaxation vs. concentration) | Results in effectiveness of the proposed fractal dimension approach to differentiate relaxation and concentration Fractal dimension algorithms were embedded in the neurofeedback games | |
| Doud et al. (2011) | EEG | BCI | Controlling EEG SMR (12–15 Hz) frequency | Motor imagery (rest vs. arm vs. hand vs. tongue) | Navigating a 3D virtual helicopter through a virtual space (visual) | N = 3 (age = 20–23 years) Within-subject design | Conventional computer monitor | BCI performance | Effective, three-dimensional control with motor imagery based BCI system | |
| Gruzelier et al. (2010) | EEG | NF | Controlling different EEG frequency bands (increasing SMR while inhibiting theta and high beta) | No specific task—learning with the provided feedback | Interaction with virtual theater auditorium (visual) | N = 15 (age = 20–23 years) 3 groups: 2D NF (n = 6) vs. 3D NF (n = 5) vs. no-NF CG (n = 4); drama students; between-subject design | VR: CAVE-like system, with surrounding image projection seen through glasses CG: Conventional computer monitor | NF performance Acting performance Flow and presence | NF performance 2D = 3D Acting performance 3D > 2D transfer to real world, ecologically relevant learning context Flow 3D > 2D > CG | ✓ |

*(Continued)*

**TABLE 11.1 (CONTINUED)**
Journals

| Reference | Method | NF/BCI | Physiological Parameters Used FB Signal | Mental Task | Game-Like Feedback | Study Design and Participants | Feedback Presentation | Outcome Measures | Main Finding | UX[1] |
|---|---|---|---|---|---|---|---|---|---|---|
| Kober et al. (2016) | EEG | NF | Controlling EEG SMR (12–15 Hz) frequency | No specific task—learning with the provided feedback | Virtual 3D semitransparent stereoscopic render of a human body | N = 9 (age = 37–76 years) 2 groups: 3D NF group (n = 2); 2D NF-group (n = 7) stroke patients; between-subject design | VR: stereoscopic 24" display + stereoscopic glasses 2D: conventional computer screen settings | NF performance Interest, challenge, perceived feeling of control, motivation, mood, incompetence fear, mastery confidence | NF performance 2D = 3D Interest, perceived feeling of control, and motivation 3D > 2D Higher incompetence fear and lower values in mastery confidence in 3D than in 2D | ✓ |
| Yan et al. (2008) | EEG | NF | EEG power in different frequency bands | Concentration | Virtual reality games (e.g., flying spaceships) 30 VR games available including sports, puzzle, building block, and teaching games | N = 12 (age 8–12 years) ADHD | Conventional computer monitor | NF performance Visual and auditory-continuous performance test (IVA-CPT) to assess attention | NF training was successful Attention measures improved Subjective reports: VR more interesting and attractive than traditional graphical presentations (2D games) used in previous system | ✓ |
| Benedetti e. al. (2014) | EEG | BCI | EEG power in different frequency bands | Use of distinct mental states | 3D video game, move objects, erotic kind of reward | N = 1 (age = 36 years) TBI patient, frontal lobe syndrome | Conventional computer monitor | Attentional performance (Posner, CPT, d2) | Attentional improvement BCI > rest | |

(Continued)

**TABLE 11.1 (CONTINUED)**
Journals

| Reference | Method | NF/BCI | Physiological Parameters Used FB Signal | Mental Task | Game-Like Feedback | Study Design and Participants | Feedback Presentation | Outcome Measures | Main Finding | UX[1] |
|---|---|---|---|---|---|---|---|---|---|---|
| Friedman et al. (2007) | EEG | BCI | EEG power in different frequency bands | Motor imagery (hand/foot movement) | 3D virtual bar, 3D virtual street | $N = 3$ (age: no information provided) VR CAVE (vs. VR HMD and traditional BCI experiences recorded from previous measurement) Within-subject design | CAVE-like VR system, and shutter glasses | Presence experience and interview BCI performance | Presence: no differences between VR and traditional BCI BCI performance was relatively high, CAVE > HMD | ✓ |
| Bayliss and Ballard (2000) | EEG | BCI | Evoked potentials (P300) | Focus on a specific visual stimulus (red light), while ignoring other visual stimuli (green and yellow lights) | Virtual car driving game (visual) | $N = 5$ (age = no information provided) | HMD | BCI performance | Single trial accuracy of 85% | |
| Bayliss (2003) | EEG | BCI | Evoked potentials (P300) | Focus on several objects or commands in a virtual apartment | Control objects in virtual apartment | $N = 9$; age = no information provided Several non-immersive conditions vs. VR | HMD | BCI performance | BCI performance VR > 2D Most participants preferred VR | ✓ |
| Middendorf et al. (2000) | EEG | BCI | SSVEP | Focus on virtual buttons | Flight simulator, control plane via button selection (roll left or right) | $N = 8$ (age = no information provided) Continuous vs. discrete FB; between-subject design | Projected onto a large screen | BCI performance | Accuracy of 85%–90% | |

*(Continued)*

**TABLE 11.1 (CONTINUED)**

Journals

| Reference | Method | NF/ BCI | Physiological Parameters Used FB Signal | Mental Task | Game-Like Feedback | Study Design and Participants | Feedback Presentation | Outcome Measures | Main Finding | UX¹ |
|---|---|---|---|---|---|---|---|---|---|---|
| Lalor et al. (2005) | EEG | BCI | SSVEP | Focus on one of two checkerboards (right vs. left) | 3D game; players had to intervene when a character walking on a thin rope lost balance | $N = 6$ (age = 23–27 years) | Conventional computer monitor | BCI performance | Accuracy of 89% | |
| Mercier-Ganacy et al. (2014) | EEG | BCI | EEG power in different frequency bands (theta and alpha) | Concentration vs. relaxation | Augmented reality (AR) Mind-Mirror; subjects' brain activity is displayed | $N = 12$ (age = 21–30 years) 2 conditions: temporal gauge (2D) vs. AR brain Mind-Mirror, within-subject design | AR, semitransparent mirror positioned in front of a computer screen. A virtual brain is displayed on screen and automatically follows the head movements using an optical face-tracking system | BCI performance Subjective user experience | BCI performance 2D = AR Participants found the Mind-Mirror less simple, less clear but more innovative and more original than the gauge representation | ✓ |
| Hwang et al. (2009) | EEG | BCI | EEG power mu (8–12 Hz) | Motor imagery (left or right hand) | 3D brain: real-time cortical activation maps | $N = 10$ (age = mean 25.1 years) $n = 5$ BCI training (BCI), $n = 5$ no training (CG), between-subjects design | Conventional computer monitor | EEG signal during MI before and after training BCI performance | BCI group showed changes in EEG signal during MI, CG did not show changes Classification accuracy in BCI group after training better than before | |

*(Continued)*

**TABLE 11.1 (CONTINUED)**
Journals

| Reference | Method | NF/BCI | Physiological Parameters Used FB Signal | Mental Task | Game-Like Feedback | Study Design and Participants | Feedback Presentation | Outcome Measures | Main Finding | UX[1] |
|---|---|---|---|---|---|---|---|---|---|---|
| Leeb et al. (2007) | EEG | BCI | EEG power in different frequency bands | Motor imagery (left or right hand) | Navigate freely through 3D virtual apartment | N = 10 (age = mean 24.7 years) Within-subject design | Desktop VR and immersive VR used (single-wall system, shutter glasses) vs. standard BCI paradigm | BCI performance Motivation | BCI enables subjects to freely navigate in VR (with neutral cues) Cognitive load higher in navigation paradigm than in standard BCI paradigm Motivated subjects perform much better than unmotivated ones Motivation: VR > standard BCI | ✓ |
| Leeb et al. (2006) | EEG | BCI | EEG power in different frequency bands (SMR) | Motor imagery (foot and hand) | Navigate through virtual 3D street/city environment | N = 3 (age = 23–30 years) Conventional monitor (2D moving bars) vs. 3D city HMD vs. 3D city CAVE, within-subject design | 2D: Conventional computer monitor 3D: HMD and CAVE | BCI performance | BCI performance best in CAVE condition Subjective experience: CAVE more comfortable than HMD, VR preferred over standard 2D BCI paradigm | ✓ |

*(Continued)*

## TABLE 11.1 (CONTINUED)
Journals

| Reference | Method | NF/BCI | Physiological Parameters Used FB Signal | Mental Task | Game-Like Feedback | Study Design and Participants | Feedback Presentation | Outcome Measures | Main Finding | UX[1] |
|---|---|---|---|---|---|---|---|---|---|---|
| van Aart et al (2008) | EEG | NF | EEG power in different frequency bands | Concentration vs. rest | 3D VR environment; different visualizations of brain activity (e.g., a fire intensity is related to level of concentration) | N = 20 (age = 20–24 years) | Conventional computer monitor | EEG data quality (impedances) | EEG data quality is good | |
| Friedrich et al. (2015b) | EEG | NF | Mu rhythm | Being social active vs. relaxing | Game character imitates social expression of friend when accurate brain response is shown | N = 13 (age = 12 years) Autism spectrum disorder (ASD); two training groups (unidirectional vs. bidirectional) | Conventional computer monitor | Pre/post test with behavioral measures EEG tasks Emotional responsiveness with facial EMG NF performance and mu levels | Overall, positive effects on all measures; in both groups reduced symptoms in children with ASD | |
| Krausz et al. (2003) | EEG | BCI | EEG power in different frequency bands | Motor imagery (left or right hand) | Basket paradigm; a falling ball had to be led into a randomly marked target halfway down the screen | N = 4 (age = 19–27 years) Young paraplegic patients | Conventional computer monitor | BCI performance; information transfer rate | Three out of four participants showed reliable results to control the BCI | |
| Müller-Putz et al. (2010) | EEG | BCI | EEG power in different frequency bands mu and beta | Motor imagery (left or right hand, foot) | Platform game; controlling a jumping ball and control of an artificial arm | N = 8 (age = mean 28 years) Within-subject design | Conventional computer monitor and artificial arm | BCI performance | Mental imagery pattern was successfully used to control an artificial arm | |

(Continued)

**TABLE 11.1 (CONTINUED)**
Journals

| Reference | Method | NF/BCI | Physiological Parameters Used FB Signal | Mental Task | Game-Like Feedback | Study Design and Participants | Feedback Presentation | Outcome Measures | Main Finding | UX[1] |
|---|---|---|---|---|---|---|---|---|---|---|
| Scherer et al. (2013a) | EEG | BCI | EEG power in different frequency bands | Motor imagery (left hand, right hand and feet motor imagery versus rest) | Interacting with a 3D massive multiplayer online role playing game (MMORPG) | N = 1 (age = no information provided) | Conventional computer monitor | BCI performance | Successful interaction with MMORPG via BCI | |
| Scherer et al. (2015c) | EEG | BCI | EEG power in different frequency bands | Motor imagery | Row–column communication board | N = 11 (age = no information provided); patients with cerebral palsy | Conventional computer monitor | BCI performance | Seven out of 11 users performed better than chance and were consequently able to communicate by using the developed system | |
| Scherer et al. (2015d) | EEG | BCI | EEG power in different frequency bands | Right hand motor imagery; word generation | Jigsaw puzzle; arranging pieces to form a puzzle | N = 4 (age = 42 years) patients with cerebral palsy | Tablet computer | BCI performance User acceptance | Four CP users suggest high user acceptance Three out of the four users achieved better than chance accuracy in arranging pieces to form the puzzle | ✓ |
| Scherer et al. (2016) | EEG | BCI | EEG power in different frequency bands | Motor imagery | Tic-Tac-Toe | N = 1 (age = 34 years) Individual with cerebral palsy | Tablet computer | BCI performance; game moves meaningful or not | User liked the game and would play it more often when available. Game most likely difficult for some of the users friends | ✓ |

*(Continued)*

## TABLE 11.1 (CONTINUED)
### Journals

| Reference | Method | NF/BCI | Physiological Parameters Used FB Signal | Mental Task | Game-Like Feedback | Study Design and Participants | Feedback Presentation | Outcome Measures | Main Finding | UX[1] |
|---|---|---|---|---|---|---|---|---|---|---|
| Schwarz et al. (2016) | EEG | BCI | EEG power in different frequency bands | Motor imagery; mental subtraction; rest | Brainrunners: 3D jump-and-run game | N = 1 (age = 36 years) locked-in syndrome—stroke patient | Conventional computer monitor | BCI performance | Successful interaction with the BCI race game at the Cybathlon competition | |
| Scherer et al. (2013b) | EEG | BCI | EEG power in different frequency bands | Motor imagery | Virtual ball game using Kinect motion tracking sensor (Microsoft, Inc., Redmond, WA, USA) | N = 8 (age = 23 years) | Kinect motion tracking sensor (Microsoft, Inc., Redmond, WA, USA) | ERD/ERS time–frequency analysis | Interaction with a game to map motor activity while moving | |
| Tangermann et al. (2008) | EEG | BCI | EEG power in different frequency bands | Motor imagery (left hand and right hand) | Controlling real-world pinball machine | N = 6 (age = no information provided) | Real-world pinball machine | BCI performance | Three out of six participants enjoyed experience and played very successfully | |
| Ayaz et al. (2011) | NIRS | BCI | Relative concentration changes in oxy-Hb | Intention-related cognitive activity | Controlling of objects in 3D virtual environment (visual); navigating through virtual maze with keyboard, open doors with BCI control | N = 10 (age = no information provided) | Conventional computer monitor | BCI performance | Overall, subjects had success with the BCI and volitionally increased their cerebral oxygenation level | |

*(Continued)*

**TABLE 11.1 (CONTINUED)**
Journals

| Reference | Method | NF/BCI | Physiological Parameters Used FB Signal | Mental Task | Game-Like Feedback | Study Design and Participants | Feedback Presentation | Outcome Measures | Main Finding | UX[1] |
|---|---|---|---|---|---|---|---|---|---|---|
| Coyle et al. (2007) | NIRS | BCI | Relative concentration changes in oxy-Hb | Motor imagery (MI; right hand) vs. rest | *Mindswitch* game (visual); binary switching action | $N = 3$ (age = mean 35 years) | Conventional computer monitor | BCI performance | Basic "on/off" switching were successfully used with NIRS based MI vs. rest | |
| Matsuyama et al. (2009) | NIRS | BCI | Relative concentration changes in oxy-Hb | Mental arithmetic task vs. resting period | Moving a real humanoid robot (visual; brain–machine interface, BMI) | $N = 7$ (age = no information provided) | Humanoid robot | BMI performance | NIRS-based BMI can serve as stable controller of a robot | |
| Ninaus et al. (2013b) | NIRS | BCI | Relative concentration changes in oxy-Hb | Motor imagery (left or right hand) | Navigate a penguin either to the left or to the right side of a feedback screen to catch a fish and avoid crashing into a barrier | 10 feedback sessions (no further information provided) | Conventional computer monitor | NF performance | Participants successfully learned to control the penguin | |
| Power et al. (2012) | NIRS | BCI | Relative concentration changes in oxy-Hb | Mental arithmetic task vs. mental singing task vs. "no-control" state | Answer multiple choice questions (visual) | $N = 7$ (age = mean 26 years) | Conventional computer monitor | BCI performance | Three-class discrimination was unsuccessful for three participants | |

*(Continued)*

**TABLE 11.1 (CONTINUED)**
Journals

| Reference | Method | NF/BCI | Physiological Parameters Used FB Signal | Mental Task | Game-Like Feedback | Study Design and Participants | Feedback Presentation | Outcome Measures | Main Finding | UX[1] |
|---|---|---|---|---|---|---|---|---|---|---|
| deCharms et al. (2005) | fMRI | BCI | BOLD signal | Different strategies to increase and decrease activation in targeted brain area (Attention, Stimulus quality, Stimulus severity, Control) | Brightness of virtual fire image and movement of scrolling line graph (visual) | N = 36 (age = 24 years) Healthy participants and chronic pain patients (N = 12; age = 36.7 years); between-subject design | MRI-compatible screen | BCI performance Pain perception (noxious thermal stimulus) | Subjects learned to regulate activation in the rostral anterior cingulate cortex (rACC) Pain perception was reduced after rtfMRI of rACC | |
| Sorger et al. (2009) | fMRI | BCI | BOLD signal | Motor imagery, mental calculation, inner speech | Answer multiple choice questions (visual) | N = 8 (mean age = 28 years) | MRI-compatible screen | BCI performance | Participants were able to select answers to multiple choice questions with their brain activity with an high accuracy | |
| Yoo et al. (2004) | fMRI | BCI | BOLD signal | Mental calculation, mental speech generation, left and right hand motor imagery | Navigation through a simple 2D maze (visual) | N = 3 (age = 21–24 years) | MRI-compatible screen | BCI performance | The proposed rtfMRI-BCI method allowed volunteer subjects to navigate through a simple 2D maze | |

*Note:* This table includes BCI/NF papers detailing the brain signal recording technique, the physiological parameters, the mental tasks, the type of feedback, the feedback device, the study design and participants, the outcome measure, the main findings, and the user experience assessment. Papers are sorted by brain signals.

[1] User Experience: In studies with a check mark, the researcher assessed the user experience in game-like and VR-based NF/BCI scenarios.

Kober et al. (2016) investigated the effects of traditional feedback (2D vertically moving bars) and 3D VR-based game-like feedback (virtual 3D semitransparent stereoscopic render of a human body) on the NF training performance and user experience in stroke patients (Figure 11.1h). They could not find any beneficial effects of the game-like feedback scenario on NF performance. The NF performance was comparable between conditions. However, interest, perceived feeling of control, and motivation were higher in patients using the VR game-like feedback compared to the traditional feedback condition. Hence, these results indicate that NF can be improved with the implementation of VR scenarios, especially with regard to users' interest and motivation (Kober et al. 2016).

Yan et al. (2008) also investigated effects of game-like feedback scenarios on users' levels of interest. Although the authors did not directly assess the level of interest and motivation of the participants during game-like NF training, they mentioned that most of their participants admitted that the game-like feedback was more interesting and attractive than traditional feedback presentations used in previous studies (Yan et al. 2008).

Leeb et al. (2006) also reported that motivated BCI users performed much better than unmotivated ones in a VR-based feedback paradigm. Furthermore, motivation was higher in a VR-based game-like feedback paradigm than in a traditional BCI paradigm.

### 11.4.2 FLOW, IMMERSION, AND PRESENCE

Flow is defined as a mental state in which a person performing an activity is fully immersed in a feeling of energized focus, full involvement, and enjoyment in the process of the activity. This mental state is associated with complete absorption in what one is doing (Csikszentmihályi 1990). Immersion and the presence experience ("sense of being there") in game-like environments (Witmer and Singer 1998) might play an important role for NF/BCI applications, because immersion and the sense of presence in virtual environments are generally considered as the propensity of users to respond to virtually generated sensory data as if they were real (Slater et al. 2009). In this context, Gruzelier et al. (2010) used a virtual theater auditorium for a sensorimotor rhythm NF in drama students. They compared the effects of a highly immersive 3D feedback scenario (CAVE-like system) with a less immersive 2D feedback (computer screen). The 3D feedback scenario led to the highest flow experience and NF learning was also improved in the 3D scenario compared to the 2D feedback condition.

Friedman et al. (2007) also investigated the effect of a highly immersive VR CAVE-like system on BCI performance. Importantly, the highest level of BCI accuracy was achieved in the CAVE-like VR environment, compared to less immersive conditions. Moreover, in a post-questionnaire interview, participants reported that after a while they gradually felt more absorbed by the VR and, as a result, felt more present in the virtual environment.

### 11.4.3 ATTRACT USERS' ATTENTION AND REDUCE MIND WANDERING

More interesting and immersive feedback modalities might also attract users' attention and might reduce the number of task-irrelevant thoughts or mind-wandering episodes, which often occur in monotonous and boring tasks and reduce task performance (Mrazek et al. 2011; Ros et al. 2013; Smallwood and Schooler 2006). Generally, there is evidence that an increased ability to focus on the BCI/NF task leads to an improved BCI/NF performance (Tan et al. 2014). In this context, Tan et al. (2014) demonstrated that mindfulness meditation training led to higher BCI accuracy rates than other interventions such as a music intervention or no interventions. Mindfulness is defined as a cognitive state of being attentive to and aware of what is happening in the present moment, inside as well as outside one's own body, without judging it (Lu et al. 2014). It is associated with self-regulation and attentional control (Lu et al. 2014; Tan et al. 2014). Improved self-regulation and attentional focus improves cognitive performance in general and consequently BCI/NF performance (Tan et al. 2014).

Cho et al. (2004) show that a 3D VR game-like feedback scenario not only improves NF training performance compared to traditional feedback; participants who receive the 3D VR game-like feedback also show more improvement in attentional functions due to NF training compared to participants who receive traditional feedback (Cho et al. 2004).

## 11.4.4 INTUITIVE FEEDBACK AND INTERACTIONS

Intuitive feedback and intuitive interaction are essential from a user experience perspective. BCIs are complex systems. User-specific BCI parameter calibration seems vital to achieve optimal control. User compliance with the calibration protocol and an elementary understanding of basic function principles are crucial for calibration. Explaining basic details can be challenging, depending on the user group. Games are ideal means for telling stories. Game play and feedback design can be used to educate users on the use of the system, just like computer game tutorials teach the player how to play the game. Scherer et al. (2015b) introduced a row–column scanning communication board for end users with cerebral palsy. Cerebral palsy is a nonprogressive condition caused by damage to the brain during early developmental stages. Individuals with cerebral palsy may have a broad range of problems related to motor control,

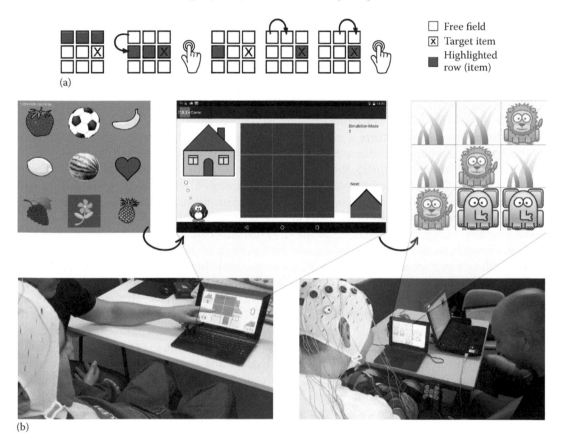

**FIGURE 11.2** One-switch row–column scanning communication board. (a) Example of single-switch row–column scanning selection. Items are arranged in a grid. Each item is associated to a command (e.g., "Turn the light in the room on" or tell the computer to say the sentence "I have pain"). To select the target item ("X"), first the row and then the column have to be selected by activating a switch. (b) To familiarize end users with the communication board, a puzzle game and a Tic-Tac-Toe game were implemented. The pictures show end users with cerebral palsy who use the games. (Based on Scherer, R. et al., 2015c. *Ann Phys Rehabil Med* 58, 14–22. doi:10.1016/j.rehab.2014.11.005; Scherer, R. et al., 2015d. Game-based BCI training: Interactive design for individuals with cerebral palsy. In: *2015 IEEE International Conference on Systems, Man, and Cybernetics*. IEEE, pp. 3175–3180. doi:10.1109/SMC.2015.551; Scherer, R. et al., 2016. Let's play Tic-Tac-Toe: A brain–computer interface case study in cerebral palsy. In: *IEEE International Conference on Systems, Man, and Cybernetics (SMC)*, pp. 3736–3741. doi:10.1109/SMC.2016.784415.)

speech, comprehension, or mental retardation. Because of lack of movement and posture control, many affected individuals cannot use standard human–computer interaction devices. Figure 11.2a illustrates the row–column scanning selection process. To speed up familiarization with the communication board, a jigsaw puzzle and a Tic-Tac-Toe game were introduced. The aim of the former game is to piece together a puzzle to unmask the selected puzzle image. By assembling images, users learned the control mechanism and became familiar with the BCI dynamics. Personalized audio cues served as the narrator and guided the user step by step through the process. Four users with cerebral palsy participated in a pilot study. User acceptance was high (Pammer et al. 2015). Three out of the four users gained minimum BCI control and managed to complete puzzles (Scherer et al. 2015d). The Tic-Tac-Toe game introduced competitive elements, allowing the BCI user to play against another human player (Scherer et al. 2016). Competition is a motivator and guarantees engagement (Bonnet et al. 2013). The user successfully played the game and was visibly enjoying engaging in competition. For the first time in a long while, the user was able to play a computer game with his friend (Scherer et al. 2016). Figure 11.2b shows the prototype communication board, the puzzle, and the Tic-Tac-Toe graphical user interfaces. By playing, users became acquainted with BCI control. Moreover, what they learned was directly relevant for controlling the communication board. The transition to real-world applications is straightforward.

### 11.4.5 Activating the Mirror Neuron System

Using virtual models of real-world scenarios might directly affect brain structures (Cameirão et al. 2007). In this context, several VR systems have been developed and evaluated for the rehabilitation of motor deficits after stroke, with particular emphasis on the rehabilitation of the upper extremities. Virtual limbs are used since there is evidence that movement observation also affects motor areas in the brain by recruiting the mirror neuron system, probably boosting the rehabilitation success (Mulder 2007; Pichiorri et al. 2015; Rizzolatti and Craighero 2004; Sollfrank et al. 2015).

NF to activate the mirror neuron system is also a viable strategy to reduce symptoms in children with autism spectrum disorder (ASD). The Social Mirroring Game incorporates role-playing game mechanics that allow the temporal dynamics of the player to be recorded to track behavior changes, accommodate game mechanic changes, and help direct the player (Friedrich et al. 2014). It encourages children with ASD to engage in social interactions and requires them to modulate their mu power in the EEG (i.e., 8–12 Hz oscillation over somatosensory cortex, which is assumed to be an indicator of mirror neuron activity). Mu power needs to be modulated in gaming parts as well as in social situations between the child's avatar and his friend (i.e., a non-player character) in order to get rewarded. The rewarding feedback involves the child's avatar imitating the facial emotions of the non-player character. Using meaningful feedback (i.e., showing the control of imitation behavior in a game character instead of a race car on the screen) for specific signals being trained (i.e., training the mu rhythm to engage the mirror neuron system) might be more effective in linking brain activation and anticipated behavior (i.e., improved imitation behavior) (Friedrich et al. 2014, 2015b). This game-based NF was shown to activate the mirror neuron system (i.e., increase mu suppression), to improve emotion recognition and spontaneous imitation, and to significantly reduce the symptoms of children with ASD in everyday life (Friedrich et al. 2015b).

Using virtual models of the humans' brain might be also used as feedback scenario to provide the BCI/NF user with explanatory feedback, informing the user about what is going on in his or her brain, as well as with engaging and entertaining feedback (Kober et al. 2016; Mercier-Ganady et al. 2014).

### 11.4.6 Transfer to Real-World Behavior

Some studies use virtual copies of real-world scenarios as feedback modality to foster the transfer of the learned skill to real-world situations (e.g., Gruzelier et al. 2010). Leeb et al. (2007) reported on a spinal cord–injured tetraplegic individual who used a BCI to control the movements of his wheelchair in VR. The tetraplegic was asked to move the wheelchair in a populated area, stop in front of virtual avatars, and talk to them. The virtual street was diversified, engaging, and contained distractions like real streets have. VR technology allowed this individual to experience—as close as possible—to move a real wheelchair in a real street, however, in a safe environment.

Moreover, games aiming to enhance social behavior demonstrated that role-play mechanics transferred to a virtual agent can be used to increase learned social skills from the game to the real world for children with ASD (Friedrich et al. 2014).

Cho et al. (2004) used a virtual classroom as a feedback scenario for children having problems in school and thereby provided a more realistic and context-specific feedback. After eight sessions of NF training over 2 weeks, the children showed an improved attentional performance compared to a control group that received no training.

Highly immersive game-like feedback scenarios might also foster the transfer of knowledge/skills acquired in the virtual environment to corresponding real-world behavior due to an increased flow and/or presence experience (Slater et al. 1996). Gruzelier et al. (2010) demonstrated that using a virtual theater auditorium as feedback scenario during NF training improved real-world acting perfromance. Furthermore, real-world acting performance was superior in a highly immersive 3D condition compared to a less immersive 2D condition after NF training. The higher efficacy of the 3D feedback scenario was attributed to a higher psychological engagement to the ecologically relevant learning context of the acting space, which might have fostered the transfer to real-world acting performance.

### 11.4.7 INCREASING BCI/NF PERFORMANCE AND CONSEQUENTLY ITS OUTCOME

Some studies also investigate the effects of game-like feedback on behavioral measures such as cognitive performance (Benedetti et al 2014; Cho et al. 2004), acting performance (Gruzelier et al. 2010), pain perception (deCharms et al. 2004), and so on. Game-like feedback often leads to stronger improvements in these behavioral measures compared to traditional feedback modalities.

Studies that found an increased BCI/NF performance in game-like feedback scenarios compared to traditional feedback paradigms (e.g., Bayliss 2003; Cho et al. 2004; Leeb et al. 2006; Ron-Angevin and Díaz-Estrella 2009) highlight the potential of immersive and motivating learning environments for NF/BCI learning. However, so far, only a few studies explicitly assessed the likely beneficial effects of game-based NF/BCI training as compared to a non–game-based equivalent (see Table 11.1).

## 11.5 DRAWBACKS—LACK OF EVALUATION OF EFFECTS

Game-like or 3D/VR feedback is mainly used to increase motivation, interest, and engagement, which are assumed to have a positive impact on compliance and performance. Nevertheless, only a few studies have actually investigated the user experience, that is, whether the game-like feedback really is motivating, interesting, and engaging and leads to a better outcome. The user experience is mainly assessed by subjective reports of the users if assessed at all. The use of questionnaires, rating scales, or structured interviews is rare and thus comprehensive objective evaluation of the game-like feedback effects is missing.

Kober et al. (2016) reported a positive effect of a game-like VR feedback scenario on interest, perceived feeling of control, and motivation in stroke patients (37–76 years old) compared to a traditional NF design. Besides these positive effects of game-like feedback, stroke patients who performed the game-like NF training showed higher values in incompetence fear and lower values in mastery confidence compared to patients who performed the traditional NF training. These results indicate that stroke patients might be more skeptical concerning the VR technique and less self-confident in using it (Kober et al. 2016).

Mercier-Ganady et al. (2014) used an augmented reality paradigm, in which the own brain activity was processed in real time and displayed on the mirrored head of the user. They also compared NF training effects between this augmented reality scenario and a traditional feedback modality

(2D moving bars). Although the NF users particularly appreciated the innovation and originality of this novel augmented reality approach as assessed with subjective questionnaires, participants rated the augmented reality condition as less simple and less clear (Mercier-Ganady et al. 2014).

Thus, using game-like or 3D/VR feedback not only has positive effects but also can lead to difficulties such as cognitive overload or incompetence fear. In this context, there might be some kind of technology gap, which is generally strongly pronounced in the elderly, increasing resistance to or fear of computer-based applications, especially of "unusual" computer techniques such as the VR technique. Older individuals are generally not familiar with computer technology (Morganti 2004). Studies on people older than 40 years provide evidence that as age increases, attitudes toward computer technique tend to become more negative and increasing age is associated with increased computer anxiety. Older people have more negative emotional reactions to making errors using computers (Wagner et al. 2010) and are generally not familiar with VR interfaces (Morganti 2004), which might explain increases in incompetence fear in elderly users (Kober et al. 2016). However, most existing studies were performed with young and middle-aged adults (see Table 11.1). Thus, it remains unclear whether elderly users are willing to adapt to such new immersive and game-based training methods over the long term or whether they are more comfortable with conventional training approaches. The same is also true for some end users with cognitive impairments. The inability to explain game dynamics and mechanisms or the use of "unusual" equipment may cause unexpected difficulties.

Besides psychological and cognitive strain, using an advanced technology such as VR to present the game-like feedback can cause physical side effects including ocular problems, disorientation, and nausea, which is called simulator sickness or cybersickness. Approximately 25% of participants interacting in VR report such cybersickness symptoms, which can potentially confound data and undo the potential value of game-like feedback using VR technology in BCI/NF applications (Brooks et al. 2010).

## 11.6 CONCLUSION

Summing up, there is some evidence of the potential positive effects of using games and game-like feedback on BCI/NF performance, outcome measures, as well as user experience. Overall, there is agreement between BCI/NF users that motivation, interest, and engagement are increased. A significant broad-scale performance improvement, however, is not documented in the literature. By examining the data in Table 11.1, several weaknesses of current studies can be identified. Weaknesses include the small number of study participants, the fact that mainly young and healthy people participate in studies, missing control groups, missing comparison between conventional and novel game-like feedback designs, and missing user experience evaluation. There is lack of empirical evidence that confirms that the use of games has a significant impact on outcome. Different age groups have different preferences, skills, and capabilities. These have to be considered when designing games. Young persons may like complex role-playing games in VR better than the elderly, who may be overwhelmed by technology. Likewise, young people may get bored when playing Tic-Tac-Toe. Children, the elderly, or individuals with cerebral palsy may like to play the game on a conventional computer screen. Thus, the possibility to have an individual configuration and the opportunity to define an individual level of difficulty are key requirements to keep motivation high and the player in the flow (Keller 2010).

It is interesting to note that the large majority of BCI/NF studies used visually appealing games as a substitute for the graphically less exciting "bar" feedback. Users already need BCI/NF control to be able to play the game. However, if BCI performance is close to random levels, not allowing the user to have minimum level of control, then users will not be able to play the game. Motivation ends in frustration. One major aim in BCI is to reduce the number of users that are not able to use a BCI, that is, to find solutions for the "BC illiteracy phenomenon." The approach to substitute feedback technology alone seems to be of limited usefulness toward this aim. The example of the Puzzle game app developed for users with cerebral palsy shows that games have much more potential than just serving as a colorful visualization tool. Games can tell stories, educate users about specific topics, and much more. Moving forward these ideas and exploring novel ways on how to combine BCI/NF technology, teaching and learning methods, and interactive games and entertainment seem very promising. Although evidence is very limited at this moment, a bright future lies ahead.

## ACKNOWLEDGMENTS

This work was supported by the Leibniz-Competition Fund (SAW; SAW-2016-IWM-3, Dr. Manuel Ninaus), the FP7 Framework EU Research Project ABC (No. 287774, Dr. Reinhold Scherer), the FP7 Framework EU Research Project CONTRAST (No. 287320, Dr. Silvia E. Kober), and the LMUexcellent (Dr. Elisabeth Friedrich). This chapter reflects only the authors' views, and funding agencies are not liable for any use that may be made of the information contained herein.

## REFERENCES

Allison, B., Neuper, C., 2010. Could anyone use a BCI? In: Tan, D., Nijholt, A. (Eds.), *Brain–Computer Interfaces*. Human–Computer Interaction Series, Springer-Verlag, London, pp. 35–54.

Arns, M., Ridder, S. de, Strehl, U., Breteler, M., Coenen, T., 2009. Efficacy of neurofeedback treatment in ADHD: The effects on inattention, impulsivity and hyperactivity: A meta-analysis. *Clin EEG Neurosci* 40(3), 180–189.

Ayaz, H., Shewokis, P., Bunce, S., Onaral, B., 2011. An optical brain computer interface for environmental control. In: *Conference Proceedings—IEEE Engineering in Medicine and Biology Society*, pp. 6327–6330.

Bayliss, J., Ballard, D., 2000. A virtual reality testbed for brain computer interface research. *IEEE Trans Rehabil Eng* 8, 188–190.

Bayliss, J.D., 2003. Use of the evoked potential P3 component for control in a virtual apartment. *IEEE Trans Rehabil Eng* 11(2), 113–116.

Benedetti, F., Catenacci Volpi, N., Parisi, L., Sartori, G., 2014. Attention training with an easy-to-use brain–computer interface. In: Shumaker, R., Lackey, S. (Eds.), *Virtual, Augmented and Mixed Reality. Applications of Virtual and Augmented Reality: 6th International Conference, VAMR 2014*, Held as Part of HCI International 2014, Heraklion, Crete, Greece, June 22–27, 2014, Proceedings, Part II. Springer International Publishing, Cham, pp. 236–247. doi:10.1007/978-3-319-07464-1_22

Blankertz, B., Sannelli, C., Halder, S., Hammer, E.M., Kübler, A., Müller, K.-R., Curio, G., Dickhaus, T., 2010a. Neurophysiological predictor of SMR-based BCI performance. *NeuroImage* 51(4), 1303–1309. doi:10.1016/j.neuroimage.2010.03.022

Blankertz, B., Tangermann, M., Vidaurre, C., Fazli, S., Sannelli, C., Haufe, S., Maeder, C., Ramsey, L., Sturm, I., Curio, G., Müller, K.R., 2010b. The Berlin brain–computer interface: Non-medical uses of BCI technology. *Front Neurosci* doi:10.3389/fnins.2010.00198

Bonnet, L., Lotte, F., Lecuyer, A., 2013. Two brains, one game: Design and evaluation of a multiuser BCI video game based on motor imagery. *IEEE Transactions on Computational Intelligence and AI in Games* 5(2), 185–198.

Brooks, J.O., Goodenough, R.R., Crisler, M.C., Klein, N.D., Alley, R.L., Koon, B.L., Logan, W.C., JR, Ogle, J.H., Tyrrell, R.A., Wills, R.F., 2010. Simulator sickness during driving simulation studies. *Accident; analysis and prevention*, 42(3), 788–796. doi:10.1016/j.aap.2009.04.013

Cameirão, M., Bermúdez i Badia, S., Zimmerli, L., Oller, E.D., Verschure, P., 2007. A virtual reality system for motor and cognitive neurorehabilitation. *Challenges for Assistive Technology* 20, 393–397.

Carter, M., Downs, J., Nansen, B., Harrop, M., Gibbs, M., 2014. Paradigms of games research in HCI: A review of 10 years of research at CHI. In: *Proceedings of the First ACM SIGCHI Annual Symposium on Computer–Human Interaction in Play —CHI PLAY '14*. ACM Press, New York, New York, USA, pp. 27–36. doi:10.1145/2658537.2658708

Cho, B.-H., Kim, S., Shin, D.I., Lee, J.H., Lee, S.M., Kim, I.Y., Kim, S.I., 2004. Neurofeedback training with virtual reality for inattention and impulsiveness. *Cyberpsychology & Behavior* 7(5), 519–526. doi:10.1089/cpb.2004.7.519

Cole, S.W., Yoo, D.J., Knutson, B., 2012. Interactivity and reward-related neural activation during a serious videogame. *PLoS ONE* 7, e33909. doi:10.1371/journal.pone.0033909

Coyle, S.M., Ward, T.E., Markham, C.M., 2007. Brain–computer interface using a simplified functional near-infrared spectroscopy system. *J Neural Eng* 4, 219–226. doi:10.1088/1741-2560/4/3/007

Csikszentmihályi, M., 1990. *Flow: The Psychology of Optimal Experience.* Harper & Row. ISBN 978-0-06-016253-5.

deCharms, R.C., Christoff, K., Glover, G.H., Pauly, J.M., Whitfield, S., Gabrieli, J.D.E., 2004. Learned regulation of spatially localized brain activation using real-time fMRI. *NeuroImage* 21(1), 436–443.

deCharms, R.C., Maeda, F., Glover, G.H., Ludlow, D., Pauly, J.M., Soneji, D., Gabrieli, J.D.E., Mackey, S.C., 2005. Control over brain activation and pain learned by using real-time functional MRI. *Proc. Natl. Acad. Sci. U. S. A.* 102, 18626–18631. doi:10.1073/pnas.0505210102

Doud, A.J., Lucas, J.P., Pisansky, M.T., He, B., 2011. Continuous three-dimensional control of a virtual helicopter using a motor imagery based brain–computer interface. *PLoS ONE* 6, e26322. doi:10.1371/journal.pone.0026322

Emmert, K., Kopel, R., Sulzer, J., Brühl, A.B., Berman, B.D., Linden, D.E., Horovitz, S.G., Breimhorst, M., Caria, A., Frank, S., Johnston, S., Long, Z., Paret, C., Robineau, F., Veit, R., Bartsch, A., Beckmann, C.F., van de Ville, D., Haller, S., 2016. Meta-analysis of real-time fMRI neurofeedback studies using individual participant data: How is brain regulation mediated? *NeuroImage* 124, 806–812. doi:10.1016/j.neuroimage.2015.09.042.

Friedman, D., Leeb, R., Guger, C., Steed, A., Pfurtscheller, G., Slater, M., 2007. Navigating virtual reality by thought: What is it like? *Presence: Teleoperators Virtual Environ* 16, 100–110. doi:10.1162/pres.16.1.100

Friedrich, E.V.C., Neuper, C., Scherer, R., 2013. Whatever works: A systematic user-centered training protocol to optimize brain–computer interfacing individually. *PLoS ONE* 8(9), e76214. doi:10.1371/journal.pone.0076214

Friedrich, E.V.C., Sivanathan, A., Lim, T., Suttie, N., Louchart, S., Pillen, S., Pineda, J.A., 2015b. An effective neurofeedback intervention to improve social interactions in children with autism spectrum disorder. *J Autism Dev Disord* 45, 4084–4100. doi:10.1007/s10803-015-2523-5

Friedrich, E.V.C., Suttie, N., Sivanathan, A., Lim, T., Louchart, S., Pineda, J.A., 2014. Brain–computer interface game applications for combined neurofeedback and biofeedback treatment for children on the autism spectrum. *Front Neuroeng* 7, 21. doi: 10.3389/fneng.2014.00021

Friedrich, E.V.C., Wood, G., Scherer, R., Neuper, C., Eds., 2015a. *Mind Over Brain, Brain Over Mind: Cognitive Causes and Consequences of Controlling Brain Activity.* Lausanne: Frontiers Media. doi: 10.3389/978-2-88919-663-0

Gruzelier, J., Inoue, A., Smart, R., Steed, A., Steffert, T., 2010. Acting performance and flow state enhanced with sensory-motor rhythm neurofeedback comparing ecologically valid immersive VR and training screen scenarios. *Neuroscience Letters* 480(2), 112–116. doi:10.1016/j.neulet.2010.06.019.

Gruzelier, J.H., 2014. EEG-neurofeedback for optimising performance. I: A review of cognitive and affective outcome in healthy participants. *Neuroscience & Biobehavioral Reviews* 44, 124–141. doi:10.1016/j.neubiorev.2013.09.015

Halder, S., Varkuti, B., Bogdan, M., Kübler, A., Rosenstiel, W., Sitaram, R., Birbaumer, N., 2013. Prediction of brain–computer interface aptitude from individual brain structure. *Front Hum Neurosci* 7, 1–9. doi:10.3389/fnhum.2013.00105.

Haller, S., Birbaumer, N., Veit, R., 2010. Real-time fMRI feedback training may improve chronic tinnitus. *Eur. Radiol* 20, 696–703. doi:10.1007/s00330-009-1595-z

Hammer, E.M., Halder, S., Blankertz, B., Sannelli, C., Dickhaus, T., Kleih, S., Müller, K.-R., Kübler, A., 2012. Psychological predictors of SMR-BCI performance. *Biological Psychology* 89(1), 80–86. doi:10.1016/j.biopsycho.2011.09.006

Howard-Jones, P., Demetriou, S., Bogacz, R., Yoo, J.H., Leonards, U., 2011. Toward a science of learning games. *Mind, Brain, Educ* 5, 33–41. doi:10.1111/j.1751-228X.2011.01108.x

Hwang, H.-J., Kwon, K., Im, C.-H., 2009. Neurofeedback-based motor imagery training for brain–computer interface (BCI). *J Neurosci Methods* 179, 150–156. doi:10.1016/j.jneumeth.2009.01.015

Jeunet, C., Jahanpour, E., Lotte, F., 2016. Why standard brain–computer interface (BCI) training protocols should be changed: An experimental study. *J Neural Eng* 13, 36024. doi:10.1088/1741-2560/13/3/036024

Johnston, S., Linden, D.E.J., Healy, D., Goebel, R., Habes, I., Boehm, S.G., 2011. Upregulation of emotion areas through neurofeedback with a focus on positive mood. *Cogn Affect Behav Neurosci* 11, 44–51. doi:10.3758/s13415-010-0010-1

Keller, J.M., 2010. *Motivational Design for Learning and Performance—The ARCS Model Approach.* Springer: New York.

Kleih, S., Nijboer, F., Halder, S., Kübler, A., 2010. Motivation modulates the P300 amplitude during brain–computer interface use. *Clinical Neurophysiology* 121(7), 1023–1031. doi:10.1016/j.clinph.2010.01.034.

Kober, S., Reichert, J., Schweiger, D., Neuper, C., Wood, G., 2016. Effects of a 3D virtual reality neurofeedback scenario on user experience and performance in stroke patients. *GALA Conference 2016 Proceedings.*

Kober, S.E., Schweiger, D., Witte, M., Reichert, J.L., Grieshofer, P., Neuper, C., Wood, G., 2015. Specific effects of EEG based neurofeedback training on memory functions in post-stroke victims. *Journal of Neuroengineering and Rehabilitation* 12, 107. doi:10.1186/s12984-015-0105-6

Kober, S.E., Witte, M., Ninaus, M., Neuper, C., Wood, G., 2013. Learning to modulate one's own brain activity: The effect of spontaneous mental strategies. *Front Hum Neurosci* 7. doi:10.3389/fnhum.2013.00695

Koepp, M.J., Gunn, R.N., Lawrence, A.D., Cunningham, V.J., Dagher, A., Jones, T., Brooks, D.J., Bench, C.J., Grasby, P.M., 1998. Evidence for striatal dopamine release during a video game. *Nature* 393, 266–268. doi:10.1038/30498

Krausz, G., Scherer, R., Korisek, G., Pfurtscheller, G., 2003. Critical decision-speed and information transfer in the "Graz brain–computer interface". *Appl Psychophysiol Biofeedback* 28, 233–240. doi:10.1023/A:1024637331493

Kübler, A., Neumann, N., Wilhelm, B., Hinterberger, T., Birbaumer, N., 2004. Predictability of brain–computer communication. *Journal of Psychophysiology* 18, 121–129.

Lacroix, J., Shapiro, D., Schartz, G., 1986. Mechanisms of biofeedback control. In: *Consciousness and Self-Regulation: Vol. 4,* Plenum, New York.

Lacroix, J.M., Gowen, A.H., 1981. The acquisition of autonomic control through biofeedback: Some tests of discrimination theory. *Psychophysiology* 18(5), 559–572.

Lalor, E.C., Kelly, S.P., Finucane, C., Burke, R., Smith, R., Reilly, R.B., McDarby, G., 2005. Steady-state VEP-based brain–computer interface control in an immersive 3D gaming environment. *EURASIP J Adv Signal Process* 2005, 3156–3164. doi:10.1155/ASP.2005.3156

Leeb, R., Keinrath, C., Friedman, D., Guger, C., Scherer, R., Neuper, C., Garau, M., Antley, A., Steed, A., Slater, M., Pfurtscheller, G., 2006. Walking by thinking: The brainwaves are crucial, not the muscles! *Presence: Teleoperators Virtual Environ* 15, 500–514. doi:10.1162/pres.15.5.500

Leeb, R., Lee, F., Keinrath, C., Scherer, R., Bischof, H., Pfurtscheller, G., 2007. Brain–computer communication: Motivation, aim, and impact of exploring a virtual apartment. *IEEE Trans Neural Syst Rehabil Eng* 15, 473–482. doi:10.1109/TNSRE.2007.906956

Leeb, R., Scherer, R., Keinrath, C., Guger, C., Pfurtscheller, G., 2005. Exploring virtual environments with an EEG-based BCI through motor imagery. *Biomed Tech (Berl)* 50, 86–91. doi:10.1515/BMT.2005.012

Lotte, F., Larrue, F., Mühl, C., 2013. Flaws in current human training protocols for spontaneous brain–computer interfaces: Lessons learned from instructional design. *Front Hum Neurosci* 7, 568. doi:10.3389/fnhum.2013.00568

Lu, H., Song, Y., Xu, M., Wang, X., Li, X., Liu, J., 2014. The brain structure correlates of individual differences in trait mindfulness: A voxel-based morphometry study, *Neuroscience* 272, 21–28.

Lumsden, J., Edwards, E.A., Lawrence, N.S., Coyle, D., Munafò, M.R., 2016. Gamification of cognitive assessment and cognitive training: A systematic review of applications and efficacy. *JMIR Serious Games* 4, e11. doi:10.2196/games.5888

Matsuyama, H., Asama, H., Otake, M., 2009. Design of differential near-infrared spectroscopy based brain machine interface. *RO-MAN 2009—18th IEEE Int. Symp. Robot Hum. Interact. Commun.*, pp. 775–780. doi:10.1109/ROMAN.2009.5326215

McFarland, D.J., Sarnacki, W.A., Wolpaw, J.R., 2010. Electroencephalographic (EEG) control of three-dimensional movement. *J Neural Eng* 7, 36007.

Mekler, E.D., Brühlmann, F., Tuch, A.N., Opwis, K., 2015. Towards understanding the effects of individual gamification elements on intrinsic motivation and performance. *Comput Human Behav* 1–10. doi:10.1016/j.chb.2015.08.048

Mercier-Ganady, J., Lotte, F., Loup-Escande, E., Marchal, M., Lecuyer, A., 2014. The Mind-Mirror: See your brain in action in your head using EEG and augmented reality. In: *2014 IEEE Virtual Reality (VR),* Minneapolis, MN, USA, pp. 33–38.

Middendorf, M., McMillan, G., Calhoun, G., Jones, K.S., 2000. Brain–computer interfaces based on the steady-state visual-evoked response. *IEEE Trans Rehabil Eng* 8, 211–214.

Millán, J.D.R., Rupp, R., Müller-Putz, G.R., Murray-Smith, R., Giugliemma, C., Tangermann, M., Vidaurre, C., Cincotti, F., Kübler, A., Leeb, R., Neuper, C., Müller, K.R., Mattia, D., 2010. Combining brain–computer interfaces and assistive technologies: State-of-the-art and challenges. *Front Neurosci* 4. doi:10.3389/fnins.2010.00161

Morganti, F., 2004. Virtual interaction in cognitive neuropsychology. *Studies in Health Technology and Informatics* 99, 55–70.

Mrazek, M.D., Chin, J.M., Schmader, T., Hartson, K.A., Smallwood, J., Schooler, J.W., 2011. Threatened to distraction: Mind-wandering as a consequence of stereotype threat. *Journal of Experimental Social Psychology* 47(6), 1243–1248. doi:10.1016/j.jesp.2011.05.011

Mulder, T., 2007. Motor imagery and action observation: Cognitive tools for rehabilitation. *Journal of Neural Transmission* 114(10), 1265–1278. doi:10.1007/s00702-007-0763-z

Müller-Putz, G.R., Scherer, R., Pfurtscheller, G., Neuper, C., 2010. Temporal coding of brain patterns for direct limb control in humans. *Front Neurosci* 4, 1–11. doi:10.3389/fnins.2010.00034

Müller, K.-R., Blankertz, B., 2006. Toward noninvasive brain–computer interfaces. *IEEE Signal Process Mag* 23, 128–126. doi:10.1109/MSP.2006.1708426

Müller-Putz, G.R., Scherer, R., Pfurtscheller, G., Rupp, R., 2005. EEG-based neuroprosthesis control: A step towards clinical practice. *Neurosci Lett* 382, 169–174. doi:10.1016/j.neulet.2005.03.021

Neuper, C., Müller-Putz, G.R., Scherer, R., Pfurtscheller, G., 2006. Motor imagery and EEG-based control of spelling devices and neuroprostheses. *Prog Brain Res* 159, 393–409. doi:10.1016/S0079-6123(06)59025-9

Neuper, C., Scherer, R., Wriessnegger, S., Pfurtscheller, G., 2009. Motor imagery and action observation: Modulation of sensorimotor brain rhythms during mental control of a brain–computer interface. *Clin Neurophysiol* 120, 239–247. doi:10.1016/j.clinph.2008.11.015

Nijboer, F., Furdea, A., Gunst, I., Mellinger, J., McFarland, D.J., Birbaumer, N., Kübler, A., 2008. An auditory brain–computer interface (BCI). *Journal of Neuroscience Methods* 167(1), 43–50. doi:10.1016/j.jneumeth.2007.02.009

Ninaus, M., Kober, S., Witte, M., Koschutnig, K., Neuper, C., Wood, G., 2015a. Brain volumetry and self-regulation of brain activity relevant for neurofeedback. *Biological Psychology* 110, 126–133. doi:10.1016/j.biopsycho.2015.07.009

Ninaus, M., Kober, S., Witte, M., Koschutnig, K., Stangl, M., Neuper, C., Wood, G., 2013a. Neural substrates of cognitive control under the belief of getting neurofeedback training. *Frontiers in Human Neuroscience* 7(914), 1–10.

Ninaus, M., Pereira, G., Stefitz, R., Prada, R., Paiva, A., Wood, G., 2015b. Game elements improve performance in a working memory training task. *Int J Serious Games* 2, 3–16. doi:10.17083/ijsg.v2i1.60

Ninaus, M., Witte, M., Kober, S.E., Friedrich, E.V.C., Kurzmann, J., Hartsuiker, E., Neuper, C., Wood, G., 2013b. Neurofeedback and serious games. In: Connolly, T.M., Boyle, E., Hainey, T., Baxter, G., Moreno-ger, P. (Eds.), *Psychology, Pedagogy, and Assessment in Serious Games*. IGI Global, Hershey, PA, pp. 82–110. doi:10.4018/978-1-4666-4773-2.ch005

Pammer, V., Simon, J., Wilding, K., Keller, S., Scherer, R., 2015. Designing for engaging BCI training. In: *Proceedings of the 2015 Annual Symposium on Computer–Human Interaction in Play—CHI PLAY '15*. ACM Press, New York, New York, USA, pp. 667–672. doi:10.1145/2793107.2810290

Pfurtscheller, G., Müller, G.R., Pfurtscheller, J., Gerner, H.J., Rupp, R., 2003. Thought—Control of functional electrical stimulation to restore hand grasp in a patient with tetraplegia. *Neurosci Lett* 351, 33–36. doi:10.1016/S0304-3940(03)00947-9

Pichiorri, F., Morone, G., Petti, M., Toppi, J., Pisotta, I., Molinari, M., … Mattia, D., 2015. Brain–computer interface boosts motor imagery practice during stroke recovery. *Annals of Neurology* 77(5). http://doi.org/10.1002/ana.24390

Power, S.D., Kushki, A., Chau, T., 2012. Automatic single-trial discrimination of mental arithmetic, mental singing and the no-control state from prefrontal activity: Toward a three-state NIRS-BCI. *BMC Res Notes* 5, 141. doi:10.1186/1756-0500-5-141

Reichert, J.L., Kober, S.E., Neuper, C., Wood, G., 2015. Resting-state sensorimotor rhythm (SMR) power predicts the ability to up-regulate SMR in an EEG-instrumental conditioning paradigm. *Clin Neurophysiol* 126(11), 2068–2077. doi:10.1016/j.clinph.2014.09.032.

Rizzolatti, G., Craighero, L., 2004. The mirror–neuron system. *Annual Review of Neuroscience* 27, 169–192. doi:10.1146/annurev.neuro.27.070203.144230

Ron-Angevin, R., Díaz-Estrella, A., 2009. Brain–computer interface: Changes in performance using virtual reality techniques. *Neurosci Lett* 449, 123–127. doi:10.1016/j.neulet.2008.10.099

Ros, T., Théberge, J., Frewen, P.A., Kluetsch, R., Densmore, M., Calhoun, V.D., Lanius, R.A., 2013. Mind over chatter: Plastic up-regulation of the fMRI salience network directly after EEG neurofeedback. *NeuroImage* 65, 324–335. doi:10.1016/j.neuroimage.2012.09.046.

Royer, A.S. , Doud, A.J., Rose, M.L., He, B., 2010. EEG control of a virtual helicopter in 3-dimensional space using intelligent control strategies. *IEEE Transactions on Neural Systems and Rehabilitation Engineering* 18(6), 581– 589, doi:10.1109/TNSRE.2010.2077654.

Scherer, R., Billinger, M., Wagner, J., Schwarz, A., Hettich, D.T., Bolinger, E., Lloria Garcia, M., Navarro, J., Müller-Putz, G., 2015c. Thought-based row-column scanning communication board for individuals with cerebral palsy. *Ann Phys Rehabil Med* 58, 14–22. doi:10.1016/j.rehab.2014.11.005

Scherer, R., Faller, J., Balderas, D., Friedrich, E.V.C., Pröll, M., Allison, B., Müller-Putz, G., 2013a. Brain–computer interfacing: More than the sum of its parts. *Soft Comput* 17, 317–331. doi:10.1007/s00500-012-0895-4

Scherer, R., Faller, J., Friedrich, E.V.C., Opisso, E., Costa, U., Kübler, A., Müller-Putz, G.R., 2015a. Individually adapted imagery improves brain–computer interface performance in end-users with disability. *PLoS ONE* 10(5), e0123727. http://doi.org/10.1371/journal.pone.0123727

Scherer, R., Lee, F., Schlögl, A., Leeb, R., Bischof, H., Pfurtscheller, G., 2008. Toward self-paced brain–computer communication: Navigation through virtual worlds. *IEEE Trans Biomed Eng* 55, 675–682. doi:10.1109/TBME.2007.903709

Scherer, R., Moitzi, G., Daly, I., Müller-Putz, G.R., 2013b. On the use of games for noninvasive EEG-based functional brain mapping. *IEEE Trans Comput Intell AI Games* 5, 155–163. doi:10.1109/TCIAIG.2013.2250287

Scherer, R., Müller-Putz, G.R., Friedrich, E.V.C., Pammer-Schindler, V., Wilding, K., Keller, S., Pirker, J., 2015b. Games for BCI skill learning. In: *Handbook of Digital Games and Entertainment Technologies*. Springer Science+Business Media Singapore. doi:10.1007/978-981-4560-52-8_6-1

Scherer, R., Müller-Putz, G.R., Pfurtscheller, G., 2009. Flexibility and practicality graz brain–computer interface approach. *Int Rev Neurobiol* 86, 119–131. doi:10.1016/S0074-7742(09)86009-1

Scherer, R., Schwarz, A., Müller-Putz, G.R., Pammer-Schindler, V., Garcia, M.L., 2015d. Game-based BCI training: Interactive design for individuals with cerebral palsy. In: *2015 IEEE International Conference on Systems, Man, and Cybernetics*. IEEE, pp. 3175–3180. doi:10.1109/SMC.2015.551

Scherer, R., Schwarz, A., Müller-Putz, G.R., Pammer-Schindler, V., García, M.L., 2016. Let's play Tic-Tac-Toe: A brain–computer interface case study in cerebral palsy. In: *IEEE International Conference on Systems, Man, and Cybernetics (SMC)*, pp. 3736–3741. doi:10.1109/SMC.2016.784415

Schwarz, A., Steyrl, D., Müller-Putz, G.R., 2016. Brain-computer interface adaptation for an end user to compete in the Cybathlon. *In: IEEE International Conference on Systems, Man, and Cybernetics (SMC)*, pp. 1803–1808. doi: 10.1109/SMC.2016.7844499

Slater, M., Linakis, V., Usoh, M., Kooper, R., 1996. Immersion, presence and performance in virtual environments: An experiment with tri-dimensional chess. In: Green, M. (Ed.), *ACM Virtual Reality Software and Technology (VRST)*, pp. 163–172.

Slater, M., Lotto, B., Arnold, M.M., Sanchez-Vives, M.V., 2009. How we experience immersive virtual environments: The concept of presence and its measurement. *Anuario de Psicología* 40(2), 193–210.

Smallwood, J., Schooler, J.W., 2006. The restless mind. *Psychological Bulletin* 132(6), 946–958. doi:10.1037/0033-2909.132.6.946

Sollfrank, T., Hart, D., Goodsell, R., Foster, J., Tan, T., 2015. 3D visualization of movements can amplify motor cortex activation during subsequent motor imagery. *Frontiers in Human Neuroscience* 9, 463. doi:10.3389/fnhum.2015.00463

Sorger, B., Dahmen, B., Reithler, J., Gosseries, O., Maudoux, A., Laureys, S., Goebel, R., 2009. Another kind of "BOLD Response": Answering multiple-choice questions via online decoded single-trial brain signals. *Prog Brain Res* 177, 275–292. doi:10.1016/S0079-6123(09)17719-1

Tan, G., Thornby, J., Hammond, D.C., Strehl, U., Canady, B., Arnemann, K., Kaiser, D.A., 2009. Meta-analysis of EEG biofeedback in treating epilepsy. *Clin EEG Neurosci* 40(3), 173–179.

Tan, L.F., Dienes, Z., Jansari, A., Goh, S.Y., 2014. Effect of mindfulness meditation on brain–computer interface performance. *Consciousness and Cognition* 2, 12–21.

Tangermann, M., Krauledat, M., Grzeska, K., Sagebaum, M., Blankertz, B., Vidaurre, C., Müller, K.-R., 2008. Playing pinball with non-invasive BCI. *Adv Neural Inf Process Syst (NIPS 2008)* 21, 1–8.

Thibault, R.T., Lifshitz, M., Birbaumer, N., Raz, A., 2015. Neurofeedback, self-regulation, and brain imaging: Clinical science and fad in the service of mental disorders. *Psychotherapy and Psychosomatics* 84(4), 193–207. doi:10.1159/000371714

van Aart, J., Klaver, E.R.G., Bartneck, C., Feijs, L.M.G., Peters, P.J.F., 2008. EEG headset for neurofeedback therapy: Enabling easy use in the home environment. *Proc. Biosignals 2008 Int. Conf. Bio-inspired Signals Syst* Funchal, pp. 23–30. doi:citeulike-article-id:8184469

Van De Laar, B., Gürkök, H., Plass-Oude Bos, D., Poel, M., Nijholt, A., 2013. Experiencing BCI control in a popular computer game. *IEEE Trans Comput Intell AI Games* 5, 176–184. doi:10.1109/TCIAIG.2013.2253778

Wagner, N., Hassanein, K., Head, M., 2010. Computer use by older adults: A multi-disciplinary review. *Computers in Human Behavior* 26(5), 870–882. doi:10.1016/j.chb.2010.03.029

Wang, Q., Sourina, O., Nguyen, M.K., 2011. Fractal dimension based neurofeedback in serious games. *Vis Comput* 27, 299–309. doi:10.1007/s00371-011-0551-5

Witmer, B.G., Singer, M.J., 1998. Measuring presence in virtual environments: A presence questionnaire. *Presence: Teleoperators and Virtual Environments* 7(3), 225–240.

Witte, M., Kober, S.E., Ninaus, M., Neuper, C., Wood, G., 2013. Control beliefs can predict the ability to up-regulate sensorimotor rhythm during neurofeedback training. *Front Hum Neurosci* 7(478), 1–8. doi:10.3389/fnhum.2013.00478

Wood, G., Kober, S.E., Witte, M., Neuper, C., 2014. On the need to better specify the concept of "control" in brain–computer-interfaces/neurofeedback research. *Frontiers in Systems Neuroscience* 8(171). doi:10.3389/fnsys.2014.00171

Yan, N., Wang, J., Liu, M., Zong, L., Jiao, Y., Yue, J., Lv, Y., Yang, Q., Lan, H., Liu, Z., 2008. Designing a brain–computer interface device for neurofeedback using virtual environments. *Journal of Medical and Biological Engineering* 28(3), 167–172.

Yoo, S.-S., Fairneny, T., Chen, N.-K., Choo, S.-E., Panych, L.P., Park, H., Lee, S.-Y., Jolesz, F.A., 2004. Brain–computer interface using fMRI: Spatial navigation by thoughts. *Neuroreport* 15, 1591–1595. doi:10.1097/01.wnr.0000133296.39160.fe

Zhang, G., Yao, L., Shen, J., Yang, Y., Zhao, X., 2015. Reorganization of functional brain networks mediates the improvement of cognitive performance following real-time neurofeedback training of working memory. *Hum Brain Mapp*. doi:10.1002/hbm.22731

Zhao, Q., Zhang, L., Cichocki, A., 2009. EEG-based asynchronous BCI control of a car in 3D virtual reality environments. *Chinese Sci Bull* 54, 78–87. doi:10.1007/s11434-008-0547-3

# 12 Brain–Computer Interfaces for Mediating Interaction in Virtual and Augmented Reality

*Josef Faller, Neil Weiss, Nicholas Waytowich, and Paul Sajda*

## CONTENTS

12.1 Virtual and Augmented Reality..................................................................................236
    12.1.1 What Makes VR/AR Interesting for Research? .....................................................236
    12.1.2 Measures of VR/AR Fidelity: Immersion and Presence ........................................236
    12.1.3 How VR/AR Setups Work.....................................................................................237
12.2 General Research Applications for VR/AR....................................................................238
12.3 VR and BCIs...............................................................................................................238
    12.3.1 Control and Exploration.......................................................................................238
    12.3.2 Therapeutic Intervention......................................................................................242
12.4 AR and BCIs...............................................................................................................243
12.5 Example Architecture for BCI/VR Setup .....................................................................244
12.6 Validation of Example Architecture..............................................................................245
    12.6.1 Technical Validation—Latency and Jitter of Processing .......................................245
    12.6.2 Experimental Validation.......................................................................................246
12.7 Limitations of VR and AR in the Context of BCI..........................................................246
12.8 Future Developments...................................................................................................246
    12.8.1 Novel Interfaces between User and VR/AR...........................................................246
    12.8.2 Novel Paradigms—Opportunistic Sensing...........................................................246
12.9 Conclusion .................................................................................................................247
Acknowledgments.................................................................................................................247
References.............................................................................................................................247

**Abstract**

Virtual and augmented reality (VR/AR) are immersive and potentially multimodal sensory experiences that augment or completely replace real-world sensory input with artificial content. Outside commercial applications in entertainment, VR and AR can be used to create controlled, yet ecologically valid experimental paradigms for research in cognitive science or related fields. Here, we review how brain–computer interfaces (BCIs) are being integrated with VR/AR to rehabilitate and assist the injured and disabled, improve interaction between human and computer, and provide us more insight into how our brains process and evaluate complex environments and events. We also describe a concrete example architecture for conducting BCI/VR experiments and conclude our review with a discussion on limitations and potential future developments on BCI-based interaction with VR and AR.

## 12.1  VIRTUAL AND AUGMENTED REALITY

Virtual and augmented reality (VR/AR) are immersive and multimodal sensory experiences that augment, or completely replace, our regular, real-world sensory input with artificial content. Key to the VR/AR experience is the interaction between the human and the computer-generated/ augmented environment. VR/AR are not simply display modalities but experiential modalities that will potentially change the way we interact with virtual content and even our "real" world. The potential for VR/AR is so great that the last several years have seen dramatic increases in investment in the potential commercial applications of VR/AR, with major tech companies such as Google, Microsoft, Facebook, and Tesla having their own products and platforms.

In this chapter, we look at how VR/AR might be used together with recordings of brain activity, to better understand how we interact with the world. We describe how brain–computer interfaces (BCIs) are being integrated with VR/AR to rehabilitate and assist the injured and disabled, improve interaction between human and computer, and provide us more insight into how our brains process and evaluate complex environments and events.

### 12.1.1  What Makes VR/AR Interesting for Research?

In any experiment, as scientists, we try to isolate variables so as to detect differences in these variables across conditions. This requires tight control of the environment, often at the cost of oversimplifying the experiment. On the other hand, in cognitive neuroscience, we are interested in how our brains parse and interact with complex scenes and situations. This, of course, is best done if presented in a way that is similar to the real world (i.e., has ecological validity) so that we can generalize from the experiment to relevant real-life situations. These two goals—tight control of the environment and authenticity to reality—are often at tension with one another.

In considering such a trade-off, VR allows for a high level of control while maintaining an immersive, naturalistic environment. This level of control facilitates acquisition and synchronization of experimental data, which is especially important for relating events in the environment to neurophysiological signals. The naturalistic environment is important for building a scientific understanding of how human perception, cognition, and emotion operate in a complex environment.

AR can be viewed as a step in between the real world and virtual worlds, where real-world sensory input is overlaid with artificial stimuli, allowing the experimenter to leverage both ecological validity and tight control. Finally, another considerable advantage of VR and AR is that they allow one to realize experimental setups that might otherwise be infeasible, unethical, and/or too difficult or expensive.

Neurophysiological measures of interest in VR/AR are usually varied and differ in their temporal and spatial resolution. Compatible types of measures of brain activity include, but are not limited to, the electroencephalogram (EEG; Schomer and Da Silva 2012), the electrocorticogram (ECoG; Moran 2010), functional magnetic resonance imaging (fMRI; Sitaram et al. 2008), or functional near-infrared spectroscopy (fNIRS; Sitaram et al. 2007).

### 12.1.2  Measures of VR/AR Fidelity: Immersion and Presence

"Immersion" in the context of VR/AR can be defined as the "extent and fidelity of sensory stimulation" and the responsiveness of the system to user action (Bohil et al. 2011). A more sophisticated sensory illusion will have a higher level of immersion. A more immersive system in turn will give the user a stronger sense of presence, the "feeling of being there" (Biocca 1997). Presence can be defined more formally as "the perceptual illusion of nonmediation" (Bohil et al. 2011; Lombard and Ditton 1997). Presence is commonly quantified through self-reporting, for example, through the Slater–Usoh–Steed questionnaire (Slater et al. 1994).

## 12.1.3  How VR/AR Setups Work

At a minimum, most VR/AR setups manipulate the input to the user's sense of vision. The least immersive technique is "desktop-based VR," where three-dimensional (3D) objects are rendered to a 2D computer monitor (e.g., Scherer et al. 2012). This technique has the advantage of being the least expensive and simplest to implement. Some 2D monitors support the use of shutter-glasses or other techniques to create a 3D illusion by presenting an adjusted image for both the left and right eyes (Marathe et al. 2008). 3D projection walls typically create a 3D illusion in a similar way, but offer a larger field of view (Slobounov et al. 2015). Head-mounted displays (HMDs) generally have a higher level of immersion. They are fixed to the user's head and present separately rendered images for each eye. HMDs track the movement of the user's head so that the images adapt to the orientation of the head (e.g., Faller et al. 2016; see also Figure 12.1a). At a similar, high level of immersion, CAVE audiovisual experience automatic virtual environments (CAVE; Cruz-Neira et al. 1992; see also Figure 12.1b) position the user in a box, where images are projected onto each wall. Like with HMDs, the images are dynamically rendered and take into account head orientation.

Visual, auditory (Begault and Trejo 2000), and somatosensory (Lee et al. 2004) stimulation are often combined to create a more immersive experience, while other stimulation modalities like olfaction (Barfield and Danas 1996) or gustation (Narumi et al. 2011) have received less attention so far, especially in the context of BCI.

Similar to the fidelity of sensory stimulation, interactivity is another key component for creating highly immersive VR/AR systems. Non-naturalistic interfaces, such as a keyboard or a computer mouse, despite being easier to work with, are typically less immersive. Other interfaces, such as joysticks, wands, gloves that track finger movement (Bowman et al. 2002), and head, eye, extremity, or body trackers (Zhou et al. 2008), are more naturalistic forms of interaction that provide a higher sense of presence.

BCIs, which decode brain activity for real-time communication and control (Wolpaw and Wolpaw 2012), are potentially the most naturalistic form of interaction with the VR/AR environment, as they aim to establish a direct link between the brain and system. From the perspective of the user, the nature of this interaction can be characterized in the following ways:

- **Conscious and spontaneous interaction: Active BCI** (Zander and Kothe 2011)
  Active BCIs rely on signals that are generated when the user actively modulates their brain activity as the basis of control, for example, using movement imagery, cognitive tasks, or other control strategies to modulate the sensorimotor rhythms (SMRs).

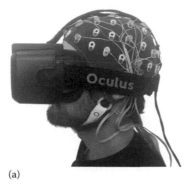
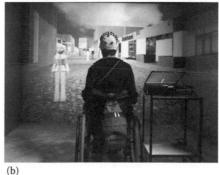

(a)                              (b)

FIGURE 12.1  (a) A healthy user wearing an EEG electrode cap and a head-mounted device (HMD). (b) A disabled individual moving through an immersive CAVE environment only by imagining movement of the feet. (From Leeb, R., Friedman, D., Müller-Putz, G.-R., Scherer, R., Slater, M., and Pfurtscheller, G. 2007c. Self-paced (asynchronous) BCI control of a wheelchair in virtual environments: A case study with a tetraplegic. *Computational Intelligence and Neuroscience.* 2007.)

- **Directing attention to external stimuli: Reactive BCI** (Zander and Kothe 2011)

  Reactive BCIs utilize brain signals that are elicited in response to external stimuli. In the oddball paradigm, for example, a set of stimuli (e.g., visual, auditory, or tactile) is presented and the user pays attention to one stimulus that occurs less frequently. In the EEG, this task causes a measurable positive deflection (P300) in evoked potentials (EP). This deflection can be measured and used for interaction through what is referred to as a P300-based BCI.

  As another example, stimulation in the range of 5 to 30 Hz causes a measureable modulation in brain activity, the steady-state evoked potential (SSEP). If the stimulation is visual, the signal is referred to as a steady-state visual evoked potential (SSVEP).

- **Subconscious, seamless interaction: Opportunistic BCI** (Saproo et al. 2016a) **or Passive BCI** (Zander and Kothe 2011)

  Passive (or opportunistic) BCIs passively monitor brain activity for indirect control. Based on changes in brain signals, such BCIs could, for example, track fatigue or other mental states, or detect when the user's expectation is violated.

Another increasingly studied concept is that of hybrid BCIs (Pfurtscheller et al. 2010). A hybrid BCI uses at least one CNS signal and at least one additional CNS or non-CNS signal, either sequentially or in parallel. The aim of combining a BCI signal with other signals is to improve information throughput and/or robustness of the interaction.

## 12.2  GENERAL RESEARCH APPLICATIONS FOR VR/AR

Outside the context of BCI, VR has been used in basic research on spatial cognition and navigation, social sciences, or multisensory integration like for investigating the phenomenon of the body-transfer illusion (Slater et al. 2010). VR has also been widely used in research on therapeutic applications like pain remediation, neurorehabilitation, and the treatment of psychiatric disorders, for instance, treating anxiety through exposure therapy (Bohil et al. 2011). Finally, VR has been used where a virtual simulation of an environment, procedure, or scenario is more effective than standard instructional training, like, for example, simulations of procedures and surgeries for training medical personnel (e.g., Seymour et al. 2002).

AR has also been used for improving training effectiveness. For example, healthy individuals were made to show symptoms of specific ailments through the use of AR so that medical professionals could train in diagnosis and treatment (Ikeda et al. 2008). In military aviation, HMDs have long been used to project critical information such as air speed, altitude, and so on, into the field of view of pilots in fighter jets (Wood and Howells 2016).

## 12.3  VR AND BCIs

VR has been used extensively in the field of BCIs. VR provides a novel feedback modality for BCIs that allows for increased immersion and presence for direct-control BCIs as well as therapeutic intervention. This section gives an overview of notable contributions using VR with BCIs. Several VR-BCI–based applications will be discussed such as VR-BCIs for direct control and exploration, for augmented human–machine interaction, and for therapeutic intervention.

### 12.3.1  CONTROL AND EXPLORATION

BCI researchers have investigated numerous ways of incorporating VR into BCIs for direct control and exploration of a user's environment. Such work has primarily been applied to active, reactive, and hybrid BCIs, with passive BCIs receiving much less attention so far.

There are numerous examples of VR being applied to active BCIs, where users consciously modulate an endogenous signal that can be used to control a computer or peripheral device. The most commonly used modality for active BCI is the voluntary modulation of the SMR. By increasing immersion and presence, VR has been used largely to give richer feedback, to thereby enhance subject's control of SMR signals. In one such example from 2003, Pineda and others sought to improve SMR BCI efficacy through VR-enhanced training of the participants (Pineda et al. 2003). The authors were able to show an increase in maximum mu rhythm amplitude after 10 h of training sessions, in which subjects would control turning left and right through imagined movement of the hands in a 3D shooter presented in a desktop-based VR system. Over the next few years, Leeb and colleagues gradually increased the level of immersion to HMD-mediated VR and demonstrated that healthy subjects were able to turn left or right in immersive VR using a more challenging synchronized SMR BCI interface in which a user had to control the BCI at the pace of the system (Leeb et al. 2004a, 2005). Using the same HMD-based VR setup, Leeb also showed that healthy subjects were able to successfully move down a virtual street via imagined "foot" movement (Leeb et al. 2004b). Later, Leeb and colleagues examined the differences between different types of VR feedback for control of an SMR BCI. Using three healthy volunteers, Leeb et al. compared SMR performance using standard bar feedback with a desktop monitor, virtual world feedback with an HMD, and virtual world feedback using a CAVE. The authors found that both users' BCI performance and preference were highest in CAVE-based VR, lowest in desktop VR, and in between with HMD-based VR (Leeb et al. 2006).

Friedman and colleagues investigated perceptual differences between the three VR feedback modalities (desktop, HMD, and CAVE) for SMR BCI in experiments also reported in Leeb et al. (2004a,b, 2006). Friedman and others found that when using VR over desktop-based feedback, subjects' BCI performance improved, and their sense of presence and body representation were increased (Friedman et al. 2007). The three subjects in this study reported more natural interactions with the BCI when using VR than with desktop-based feedback. Additionally, these subjects also reported increased motivation when VR was used for feedback, which is of particular importance since motivation has been shown to influence BCI performance (Baykara et al. 2016; Kleih et al. 2011). Similar to the previous studies performed by Leeb and colleagues, Friedman and colleagues found that CAVE-based VR led to greater BCI performance as well as a higher sense of presence when compared to the HMD-based VR. This may be attributed to the reported irritancy in HMD-based VR as well as the narrower field of view.

In 2007, Leeb and colleagues further advanced VR-based BCI for navigation by implementing a self-paced SMR BCI with VR feedback where subjects were free to navigate a virtual environment at their own pace. Using 10 healthy participants, Leeb et al. showed that self-paced SMR control could be achieved using a 3D wall VR system (Leeb et al. 2007a), and later, with 5 healthy participants, they showed that a similar level of control could be achieved using a CAVE VR (Leeb et al. 2007b). In the same year, Leeb and colleagues demonstrated self-paced SMR control in a case study using a tetraplegic volunteer who was able to control a wheelchair in a virtual environment (Leeb et al. 2007c; see also Figure 12.1b).

In 2008, Scherer et al. and Zhao et al. independently showed successful control of a highly complex self-paced SMR BCI–based navigation in a virtual environment using desktop VR (Scherer et al. 2008; Zhao et al. 2008). Using different signal processing approaches, both groups demonstrated four-class SMR control that supported a noncontrol state, turning left, turning right, and moving forward.

Before this point, the majority of self-paced SMR-based BCIs typically required extensive training for both the user and the machine (i.e., training of the user to modulate their SMR and training of the machine to recognize that modulation). In 2008, Lotte and colleagues developed a desktop VR game for an SMR-based BCI that required zero calibration from the computer and showed that without any training, half of the 21 subjects were able to control the BCI with real foot movements and a quarter were able to control it using imagined foot movements (Lotte et al. 2008).

Despite the advances in SMR BCI approaches, a major challenge that still exists today is that SMR-based BCIs do not work well for all users. In 2009, Ron-Angevin and colleagues aimed to address this problem with a systematic comparison between feedback modalities for SMR BCIs (Ron-Angevin and Díaz-Estrella 2009). The study consisted of two groups of eight healthy participants who trained to use an SMR-based BCI using either a 2D bar on a computer screen or an HMD VR for feedback. Over multiple sessions, Ron-Angevin et al. showed that classification error rates could be significantly reduced, indicating that interfaces based on VR can improve BCI control specifically for untrained subjects. Later that year, another approach to improve BCI usability by the same group utilized a low-bandwidth user interface for virtual navigation using a 3D wall VR. Their approach, which mapped an SMR control signal from only two mental states (imagined right hand movement and rest) onto four navigation commands (forward, back, left, and right), showed that six out of the seven subjects who participated in the exploration of a virtual environment could improve their performance after each experimental run (Ron-Angevin et al. 2009). Velasco-Alvarez and colleagues, in 2010, further demonstrated the efficacy of this approach using a 3D wall–based VR environment for wheelchair control in three healthy participants (Velasco-Alvarez et al. 2010).

Most of the SMR BCI–based VR interactions described so far have used low-level commands for virtual navigation, where SMR control signals are translated into incremental movement commands such as "rotate left" or "take one step forward." Each decoded command can take on the order of a few seconds and trajectories must be accumulated through successive low-level commands. Furthermore, the user might be required to correct occasional misclassifications by sending further BCI commands. All this leads to rather slow navigation speeds. To address this issue, Lotte et al. (2010) showed that an alternative interaction modality based on high-level commands, such as moving to a waypoint, allowed participants to increase their speed and significantly reduce the time required to navigate through a virtual environment from a first-person perspective.

Expanding on the idea of using more intelligent control strategies for SMR BCI–based navigation, Royer et al. (2010) demonstrated that four healthy subjects were able to fly a virtual helicopter through rings in a desktop-based VR system by thoughtfully mapping BCI output signals to flight control inputs (Royer et al. 2010). In this case, the helicopter moved forward at a constant velocity while the subjects controlled the altitude (up/down translation) and yaw (left/right rotation). In a more complex version of this setup, Doud et al. (2011) proved that simultaneous control of forward/backward movement, altitude, and yaw was possible using an SMR BCI with a desktop VR (Doud et al. 2011). Furthermore, in 2013, LaFleur and colleagues from the same group demonstrated SMR BCI–based control of a real-world drone through rings suspended from the ceiling of a gymnasium. These studies illustrate how VR can be used as a test-bed for novel applications in a safe and controlled environment before they are tested in reality (LaFleur et al. 2013).

A novel aspect of the opportunities that are afforded with BCI-based VR interaction is highlighted independently by Hazrati and Hofmann (2013) and Scherer et al. (2012). They each demonstrated that SMR-based BCIs can be used to interact with massively multiplayer online (MMO) gaming platforms such as Second Life and World of Warcraft (Hazrati and Hofmann 2013; Scherer et al. 2012). This work illustrates possible applications of SMR-based BCIs as entertainment for healthy users as well as the possibility of increasing social inclusion for individuals with severe functional disability, as was the aim in related projects (Faller et al. 2013).

Similar to the work in incorporating VR into active BCIs, reactive BCIs, which rely on brain signals elicited from exogenous stimuli, have also been used heavily with VR technology. Unlike active BCIs, which do not require any external stimuli, reactive BCIs have a unique constraint in that the external stimuli must be incorporated into the VR system. The two most widely studied reactive BCIs are the P300 and steady-state visual evoked potential (SSVEP)–based BCIs, both of which have used VR for stimulus generation as well as for BCI feedback.

In pioneering work, Bayliss et al. showed in 1999 and 2000 that P300-based responses can be elicited in a visual oddball task mediated via traffic lights in a natural HMD-based VR driving task (Bayliss and Ballard 1999, 2000). Additionally, Bayliss et al. showed offline that these HMD-elicited

P300 responses can be accurately detected and classified. In 2003, the same group developed a more elaborate P300 BCI-based VR to interact with a virtual apartment via either HMD or a desktop monitor. Unlike the results shown by Leeb et al. with SMR BCIs, Bayliss et al. found no differences in performance between using the HMD and the desktop monitor for P300-based BCI, suggesting that the increased level of presence provided by the VR has less of an effect for P300-based BCIs (Bayliss 2003; Bayliss et al. 2004). Building on this as well as work from Piccione et al. (2008), Donnerer and Steed (2010) studied the effect of different stimulation modalities for the P300 BCI using a CAVE VR system. In a study involving seven healthy individuals, the authors found that P300 stimuli that were either embedded as objects in the virtual scene or were overlaid on top of the virtual scene had no significant difference in selection accuracy, illustrating the flexibility with which P300 stimuli can be utilized in virtual and possibly real-world environments (Donnerer and Steed 2010).

In a recent study from 2015 involving 15 healthy users and 1 locked-in user, Käthner and colleagues used an HMD VR to explore different stimulation techniques for a P300 BCI. They displayed a standard speller matrix instead of a virtual environment in the HMD (Käthner et al. 2015). In one condition, the entire $5 \times 5$ matrix of letters was visible and users visually attended to the target letter to spell. In the second condition, the same $5 \times 5$ matrix was zoomed in such that only a single letter could be viewed in the HMD at a time depending on the user's head orientation. The authors found no significant difference in P300 detection performance between the two conditions.

Most BCI VR research for direct control has focused on spatial navigation and exploration applications where an avatar moves through a virtual environment. In 2009, Edlinger et al. developed a BCI VR task in which the user controls a virtual "smart home" using a desktop-based P300 BCI setup (Edlinger et al. 2009). In a small study of three healthy users, the authors achieved accurate control of various aspects of the virtual home, such as turning on/off lights and appliances.

As explained earlier, SSVEP-based BCIs use stimuli that flash at distinct frequencies for tagging different classes or actions. Like the P300-based BCI, SSVEP-based BCIs have also been used in VR where flashing stimuli must be incorporated in the virtual environment in some fashion. After Middendorf and colleagues first used virtual SSVEP buttons to control a physical flight simulator in 2000 (Middendorf et al. 2000), Lalor and colleagues were the first to overlay SSVEP stimuli onto an actual VR environment (desktop based) and demonstrate successful SSVEP BCI control for six healthy individuals. The participants' task was to focus attention on one of two SSVEP stimuli (representing "move left" or "move right") in a synchronized BCI setup with the goal of balancing a 3D avatar on a tightrope (Lalor et al. 2005). In a more complex setup using a desktop-based VR, Faller et al. (2010a) demonstrated that seven healthy individuals were able to control an avatar's movement with a self-paced SSVEP BCI in multiple conditions from just controlling the avatar's arms to guiding the avatar through a slalom and a virtual apartment (Faller et al. 2010a). The authors subsequently extended their earlier work showing that three healthy volunteers were able to guide an avatar through an HMD-based VR slalom task by using a self-paced SSVEP BCI system that relied on stimuli in the VR environment (Faller et al. 2010b,c, 2017).

Similar to the P300 work presented earlier, research on optimal methods for integrating flashing stimuli within a VR system has also been explored using SSVEP. One attempt by Legény et al. in 2011 experimented with using naturally integrated stimuli as a way to improve SSVEP stimulus presentation within VR (Legény et al. 2011). In their study, they used the flickering of butterfly wings moving in a virtual environment as the basis for SSVEP–BCI interaction for virtual navigation and compared it to a standard 2D overlay of stimuli and found that even though the subjects felt a greater sense of presence when using natural stimuli, the overall SSVEP performance was lower compared to standard stimuli. This is in contrast to the findings with P300 of Donnerer and Steed in 2010, suggesting that the SSVEP responses are potentially more vulnerable to visual discrepancies potentially caused by a VR system. Despite the degradation in performance, this study demonstrates that SSVEP stimuli can be integrated in an ecological way to create a more natural interaction. Other attempts to improve the integration of flashing stimuli within VR, such as the work done by

Waytowich and Krusienski, spatially decouple targets from flashing stimuli in a desktop-based VR. This showed that it is possible to obtain BCI control without the need to directly fixate on rapidly flashing visual stimuli. The authors hypothesize that this may reduce visual fatigue and allow users to better attend to the task on hand (Waytowich 2015; Waytowich and Krusienski 2015).

As mentioned above, hybrid BCIs combine BCI with other BCI or non-BCI interaction modalities to achieve a higher fidelity of interaction or control (Pfurtscheller et al. 2010). In one of the earliest attempts of using VR and BCI from 1997, Nelson et al. conducted a study using 12 subjects and demonstrated successful control of a virtual airplane displayed within a VR dome using a mix of EEG and EMG signals (Nelson et al. 1997). In another hybrid BCI approach that used both EEG and motor movement, Leeb and colleagues showed that half of 14 healthy subjects were able to simultaneously use joystick input and an SMR-based BCI to control a virtual penguin in CAVE-based VR (Leeb et al. 2013).

Using a hybrid BCI composed solely of EEG-based signals, Su et al. (2011) demonstrated the effectiveness of a sequential hybrid BCI that leverages both SMR and P300 signals to both navigate through a desktop-based VR apartment and interact with devices within the virtual environment (Su et al. 2011).

Unlike the well-researched classes of BCI VR above, there has been relatively little research using passive BCIs with VR. To date, the majority of work has used desktop-based VR in video game applications. Two notable examples use a passive BCI to gather implicit information from the user to change the state of a video game. Mühl and colleagues developed a game called *Bacteria Hunt* in which the level of alpha power of the player affected the controllability of the player's avatar (Mühl et al. 2010). Similarly, in *Alpha WoW*, based on the popular MMO *World of Warcraft*, Bos and colleagues passively monitored the EEG of the player to transform the player's avatar into an animal based on alpha activity (Bos et al. 2010). Additional work using passive BCIs with VR games have explored changing the state of the game environment (Girouard et al. 2013) as well as monitoring content that has been perceived by the player (Reissland and Zander 2009).

Some more recent approaches have moved beyond direct control and instead used BCI-enabled VR to improve human–machine interaction. For example, Faller et al. (2016) showed that neurologically healthy participants were able to improve their performance in an HMD-mediated VR flight task relative to control conditions when they performed audio-mediated BCI-based down-regulation of their arousal while flying. Additional details of this study and the BCI VR setup and configuration are presented in Section 12.6.2.

## 12.3.2 Therapeutic Intervention

In recent years, researchers have begun exploring BCI as a rehabilitation tool to treat stroke and traumatic brain injury. It is thought that BCI can help in rehabilitation because it increases immersion and motivation relative to other classic rehabilitation methods like imagined movements. Furthermore, the combination of VR and BCI allows subjects to actually observe their imagined movements, creating "motor resonance," which may increase plasticity (Van Dokkum et al. 2015).

Holper, in 2010, laid the groundwork for building an fNIRS-based BCI for neurorehabilitation. fNIRS is a brain imaging modality that monitors the blood oxygenation near the surface of the brain, reflecting activity in those regions. Holper et al. used a (desktop-based) VR avatar and had subjects perform four grasping-related tasks: (1) observe it, (2) imagine performing the action, (3) both observe and imagine the action simultaneously, and (4) imitate the action. With this experimental setup, the authors demonstrated that activations in the primary and secondary motor areas occur during both overt motor execution and observation or imagery of the same motor action, thus illustrating the potential for fNIRS-based BCI for neurorehabilitation.

Rehabilitation after damage to motor regions of the brain generally involves exercises previously mediated by the damaged brain tissue. This recruits healthy regions of secondary motor areas to take over the function of the damaged regions. In severe cases, though, a patient may not be able to perform these exercises at all (Holper et al. 2010). In 2013, Bermudez i Badia et al. developed a BCI system whereby a patient paralyzed in an upper limb can play a game in which a virtual avatar intercepts spheres with its arms (Bermudez i Badia et al. 2013). The patient controls the arms with imagined movements and sees those movements carried out on the screen in a first-person perspective. This recruits the mirror neurons and activates the motor system more extensively than if the task was performed without a BCI. The experiment was carried out in nine healthy subjects as a proof of concept. Subjects achieved a successful functional performance rate of 85%. In a separate experiment in the same study, Bermudez i Badia found that by having subjects simultaneously mimic the actions of an onscreen avatar and imagine the movement (i.e., motor activity and motor imagery), they were able to recruit more task-related networks than by doing either activity alone.

In 2015, Pichiorri et al. performed a randomized clinical trial, testing the functional benefits of stroke rehabilitation with a BCI (Pichiorri et al. 2015). They divided 28 hospitalized, subacute stroke patients into a BCI group and a control motor imagery group. For the BCI group, patients were seated at a table where their hands were covered in a white sheet. A BCI was set up so that when they imagined movement of their affected hand, a hand projected onto the sheet would perform the imagined movement. The motor imagery group underwent a comparable therapy routine except they were instructed to imagine the movements without any BCI feedback. After a month of therapy, the BCI group performed better on the Fugl–Meyer Assessment (an assessment of motor function, balance, sensation, and joint function), the Medical Research Council scale for muscle strength, and the National Institutes of Health Stroke Scale. They also found that the BCI group had a significantly more robust desynchronization in the alpha and beta bands of the centroparietal regions of the ipsilesional hemisphere. The authors attribute the difference to the visual feedback given to the BCI group, allowing patients to continuously improve their task performance.

In the past few years, researchers have carried out proof-of-concept experiments that incorporate BCI and VR into more sophisticated rehabilitation regimens. In 2016, Luu and colleagues showed that BCI can provide an alternative to rehabilitative exoskeletons in the field of gait rehabilitation (Luu et al. 2016). They created a VR avatar whose gait was controlled by a BCI and showed that subjects could control the gait even under perturbations. In another study in 2015, Brauchle and colleagues sought to enhance exoskeleton-based therapy (Brauchle et al. 2015). They were concerned that exoskeletons provide too much support during exercise. To address this issue, the authors developed a BCI–exoskeleton system that only provided support when the subject was making an effort to move and his brain was responsive to peripheral input. The BCI was simultaneously used to generate visual feedback via an avatar (desktop VR). Finally, in 2016, Grimm and colleagues built a proof-of-concept rehabilitation system that combined neurofeedback, neuromuscular electric stimulation (to restore muscle strength), and an exoskeleton (to improve range of motion and intensity of training) (Grimm et al. 2016). In his system, the joint angles of the exoskeleton were used to generate a 3D avatar that was displayed to the subject (desktop-based VR). They found that by combining these three methods of therapy, they were able to augment upper limb function and brain activity during rehabilitation.

In more basic research, Perez-Marcos et al. (2009) showed that healthy subjects were able to feel "ownership" of a virtual hand if it responded to motor imagery, which, as they argue, might aid in rehabilitation applications.

## 12.4  AR AND BCIs

AR, where sensory input is only partially replaced or augmented, has recently been applied to BCIs to develop novel feedback interfaces that uniquely blend the user's reality with VR. In 2010, Faller and colleagues showed that three healthy subjects were able to guide an avatar along a course in HMD-mediated AR using an SSVEP control signal. The avatar appeared in the AR surrounded by three flickering SSVEP icons. Using this setup, the subjects were able to successfully guide the avatar through a course of obstacles constructed in the AR (Faller et al. 2010b,c, 2017).

Also in 2010, Kansaku and colleagues were concerned that successful BCI paradigms may not translate to VR and AR settings. Neuroscientists found that when humans look through new visual perspectives (i.e., through a monitor), their body scheme changes. The usual experience of being located inside one's own body is disturbed, and there is an illusion of swapping bodies with another (Botvinick and Cohen 1998; Petkova and Ehrsson 2008). Kansaku and colleagues studied whether this would affect the P300 signal by having 10 subjects control a robot in a separate environment. A video feed from the perspective of a camera mounted on the robot was displayed to subjects on a monitor, and a modified P300 speller was overlaid. They found that the subjects were able to control the robot despite the changed perspective (Kansaku et al. 2010).

In 2015, Petit and colleagues built a BCI-based robotic control system that compensates for the low frequency and accuracy of BCI signals. They took the video feed from cameras mounted on a robot and overlaid flickering icons to be recognized in the SSVEP signal. They used object recognition, mapping techniques, and shared control to augment the BCI control signal (Petit et al. 2015).

Finally, Kim et al. (2016) used BCI and AR to explore human–animal interaction, creating a BCI-controlled "cyborg-turtle." They mounted an apparatus onto four turtles that included a camera as well as a rotating cylinder that could obstruct the turtle's view and thereby guide it in the opposite direction. Five users wore HMDs in which they could see the video stream from the turtle and juxtaposed flickering SSVEP stimuli. Subjects successfully guided the turtle using the SSVEP-based control signal.

## 12.5 EXAMPLE ARCHITECTURE FOR BCI/VR SETUP

Apart from custom software, there are several openly available platforms that can be used to implement BCI VR/AR experiments (cf. Brunner et al. 2012), for example, OpenVibe (Renard et al. 2010), an integrated environment that features visual programming, or BCI2000 (Schalk et al. 2004), a particularly thoroughly tested BCI platform. We review a setup that allows researchers to flexibly interconnect functionality from different software packages and toolboxes, allowing for a highly customizable, extensible, cross-platform setup that is particularly well suited for rapid prototyping of VR/AR experiments. At the core of this approach lies a software package called Labstreaming Layer (LSL; Kothe 2013), that relies on software-based, distributed signal acquisition and synchronization at sub-millisecond precision. It consists of a cross-platform library that can be used by any application written in C, C++, Python, Java, C#, and MATLAB®. LSL facilitates the streaming of data to and from any application or device on a network. With LSL, applications can easily record, store, process, or visualize any number of bio-signals from one or more subjects with accurate time stamping and synchronization including experimental events. LSL comes preloaded with dozens of applications, and new applications can be easily created as communicating data via the LSL library is a matter of only few lines of code in any of the supported languages. In this BCI/VR approach, LSL is used to network together the various experimental modules and components as shown in Figure 12.2.

Using LSL, signals from different sources (i.e., EEG, eye-tracker, mouse, keyboard, joystick, video, etc.) can have completely different meta-information and sampling rates (including an option for nonequidistant sampling). The LSL application LabRecorder can save any set of such streams into files of the recently introduced extensible file format (XDF; Kothe and Brunner 2015). Such multirate signals in XDF can then be seamlessly displayed in the cross-platform visualization application SigViewer (Schlögl and Brunner 2008).

For VR visualization, this experimental setup relies on the openly available software framework NEDE (Jangraw et al. 2014), which runs in Unity 3D, a cross-platform 3D environment (Unity Technologies, San Francisco, CA, USA).

As for processing of the signals, the present setup uses BCILAB, a thoroughly documented MATLAB toolbox, that supports relevant procedures for all major steps in BCI processing, from

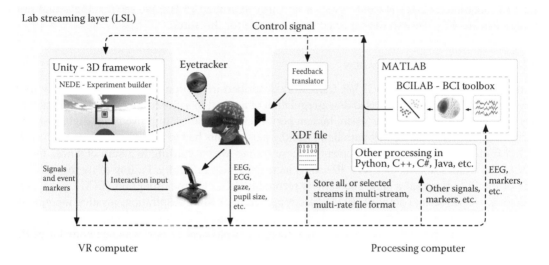

**FIGURE 12.2** Architecture overview diagram for the presented exemplary BCI VR/AR framework. The VR experiment (NEDE/Unity-3D) is displayed via HMD (Oculus) while signals are simultaneously recorded and processed via BCILAB for real-time feedback. The oculus rift head-mounted device in this setup is retrofitted with an eye-tracker by SMI (SensoMotoric Instruments GmbH, Teltow, Germany). This setup allows for both open- and closed-loop experiments.

preprocessing, over feature extraction, to classification for all major BCI approaches (Kothe and Makeig 2013). Figure 12.2 shows a general system architecture overview diagram for the presented setup.

## 12.6 VALIDATION OF EXAMPLE ARCHITECTURE

### 12.6.1 Technical Validation—Latency and Jitter of Processing

LSL was developed and tested at Swartz Center for Computational Neuroscience at University of California San Diego, and, according to the authors, the precision of its timing can be assumed to be at the sub-millisecond level in a local network (Kothe 2013). LSL records a time stamp for every acquired sample. This allows one to debug systems and perform post hoc validation in terms of sampling jitter and delay on recorded data. In Figure 12.3, we show histograms of sample frequencies

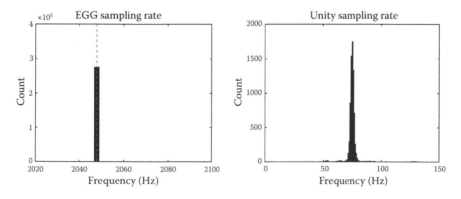

**FIGURE 12.3** Histograms for sample times for EEG (peak at 2048 Hz) and for signals from within Unity (peak at 75 Hz). The screen refresh rate in Unity is not fixed, which explains the absence of the vertical line indicating the nominal sampling rate.

for EEG acquired at 2048 Hz and signals from Unity at around 75 Hz. We see that the actual sampling rates are very close to the expected sampling rate for this setup.

### 12.6.2 Experimental Validation

Faller et al. (2016) used the BCI VR framework described in Section 12.5 for a preliminary study into the hypothesis that BCI-based down-regulation of arousal in a closed-loop setup could increase decision flexibility to a degree where human performance could be improved in a flight task with increasing difficulty. In the VR paradigm, healthy participants had to fly a plane through a corridor of red frames. The vertical arrangement of these frames was according to a sum of sines, and the size of the frames decreased every 30 s, thus increasing task difficulty. Failing to fly through only one of the frames ended a run. The authors recorded EEG, electrocardiogram (ECG), gaze, pupil diameter, electrodermal activity (EDA), electromyogram (EMG), respiration, joystick input, plane movement, head orientation, and paradigm-specific markers.

The nature of the flight task requires that there exist physical or performance boundaries that are task-critical, simulating what is referred to as a boundary avoidance task (BAT) (Saproo et al. 2016b). The BAT is often used as a surrogate task to investigate human–machine interaction that is the basis for pilot-induced oscillations (PIOs). The more realistic the BAT task, the greater the likelihood of generating a neurophysiological state that captures the real-world scenario, namely, a pilot losing control of their aircraft via destructive man–machine coupling.

This study found that the BAT employed in this VR environment strongly elicited PIO-like behavior and that a closed-loop BCI that tracked neurophysiological signatures of arousal and cognitive flexibility could be used to develop an intervention that improved flight performance relative to control and sham conditions.

## 12.7 LIMITATIONS OF VR AND AR IN THE CONTEXT OF BCI

Creating VR or AR scenarios typically requires 3D modeling and/or programming skills, as well as unique knowledge and understanding of the environment to be simulated. This problem is mitigated, when using specialized frameworks like NEDE, where tools and existing code already handle most routine tasks. This allows the scientist to focus on experimental design. A remaining problem is that some VR/AR users experience nausea in VR, which is believed to be related to a sensitivity of these users to incongruencies between the inputs to visual and vestibular system. Thus, some populations may not be a good match for VR/AR experiments.

## 12.8 FUTURE DEVELOPMENTS

### 12.8.1 Novel Interfaces between User and VR/AR

Future technological improvements to VR and AR could involve virtual retinal displays that project images directly onto the retina, thus producing a sharp, high-contrast picture (Pryor et al. 1998). Another approach, which is currently under development, is bionic contact lenses that receive both power and information wirelessly to display images to the user via a contact lens (Parviz 2009). Other potential approaches aim to completely bypass the input sensory pathways of the peripheral nervous system, those normally responsible, for example, for feeling the texture of objects, by stimulating the brain directly (O'Doherty et al. 2011).

### 12.8.2 Novel Paradigms—Opportunistic Sensing

As we have said, integration of BCI with VR offers a convenient and promising platform to investigate basic questions in cognitive neuroscience using more naturalistic and complex, yet controlled environments. For example, future paradigms, some of which would employ closed-loop neurofeedback, could investigate cognitive phenomena ranging from emotional regulation to dynamic decision-making. The collection of neurophysiological data across multiple subjects interacting with each other in virtual worlds may provide new insight into social cognition. In fact, opportunistic sensing of cognitive state using BCI platforms within complex virtual environments is one avenue for potentially integrating noninvasive human neuroscience with big data analytics. The level of immersion and entertainment value of VR potentially enables collection of massive EEG and physiological data both longitudinally and across large and diverse subject populations. New neural correlates may be revealed by using machine learning and big data tools to discover relationships between the neurophysiological data and the complex events and interactions in these environments.

Integrated BCI and AR systems hold promise for new ways we will interact with the real world. Instead of recommender systems and user models being developed by monitoring what we click on when using our computer or smartphone, opportunistic sensing of cognitive data, via BCI-enabled AR, could be used to label elements in the world that we find interesting. By combining opportunistically sensed signals with metadata in the environment, one can provide immediate information to the individual, including a model that provides insightful recommendations. (Did you just see someone walking down the street that caught your attention?) By opportunistically sensing the orienting response and snapping a photo with your built-in AR camera, that image can be sent to the cloud, compared against a database, and up pops her name on your AR display. It jogs your memory and you remember you went to school with her! This type of "just in time" metadata derived from linking opportunistic sensing and cloud-based analytics has applications that are not just a social network novelty but could enable new classes of cognitive orthotics. As the population ages, new type of platforms will be needed to help us maintain our cognitive capabilities, for example, "putting a name to a face." Opportunistically sensing neurophysiological correlates of orienting and familiarity, and using these to inform computer vision and machine learning analytics so that they can provide individuals with metadata and context, is just one such way that BCI AR systems will change how we interact with our world.

## 12.9  CONCLUSION

The current state of research indicates that BCIs can facilitate natural, seamless, and intuitive interaction with VR and AR, and preliminary attempts to use VR and AR for clinical purposes like stroke rehabilitation also appear promising. Future technological improvements like bionic lenses and concepts like opportunistic sensing will likely make BCI VR/AR systems even more immersive and pervasive.

## ACKNOWLEDGMENTS

The authors thank Jennifer Cummings for her help with editing and formatting the text. This work was funded by the Defense Advanced Research Projects Agency (DARPA) and Army Research Office (ARO) under grant number W911NF-11-1-0219, the Army Research Laboratory under Cooperative agreement number W911NF-10-2-0022, the U.K. Economic and Social Research Council under grant number ES/L012995/1, and the National Science Foundation under grant no. IIS-1527747.

## REFERENCES

Barfield, W., and Danas, F. 1996. Comments on the use of olfactory displays for virtual environments. *Presence: Teleoperators and Virtual Environments.* 5(1): 109–121.

Baykara, E., Ruf, C. A., Fioravanti, C., Käthner, I., Simon, N., Kleih, S. C., Kübler, A., and Halder, S. 2016. Effects of training and motivation on auditory P300 brain–computer interface performance. *Clinical Neurophysiology.* 127(1): 379–387.

Bayliss, J. D., and Ballard, D. H. 1999. Single trial P300 recognition in a virtual environment. *Computational Intelligence: Methods & Applications Proceedings, Soft Computing in Biomedicine.*

Bayliss, J. D., and Ballard, D. H. 2000. A virtual reality testbed for brain–computer interface research. *IEEE Transactions on Rehabilitation Engineering.* 8(2): 188–190.

Bayliss, J. D. 2003. Use of the evoked potential P3 component for control in a virtual apartment. *IEEE Transactions on Neural Systems and Rehabilitation Engineering.* 11(2): 113–116. doi:10.1109/TNSRE .2003.814438.

Bayliss, J. D, Inverso, S. A., and Tentler, A. 2004. Changing the P300 brain computer interface. *CyberPsychology & Behavior.* 7(6): 694–704. doi:10.1089/cpb.2004.7.694.

Begault, D. R., and Trejo, L. J. 2000. 3-D sound for virtual reality and multimedia. *NASA, Technical Report.*

Bermudez i Badia, S., Morgade, A. G., Samaha, H., and Verschure, P. F. M. J. 2013. Using a hybrid brain computer interface and virtual reality system to monitor and promote cortical reorganization through motor activity and motor imagery training. *IEEE Transactions on Neural Systems and Rehabilitation Engineering.* 21(2): 174–181.

Biocca, F. 1997. The cyborg's dilemma: Progressive embodiment in virtual environments. *Journal of Computer-Mediated Communication,* 3. doi:10.1111/j.1083–6101.1997.tb00070.x.

Bohil, C. J., Alicea, B., and Biocca, F. A. 2011. Virtual reality in neuroscience research and therapy. *Nature Reviews Neuroscience,* 1–11. doi:10.1038/nrn3122.

Bos, D. P. O., Reuderink, B., van de Laar, B., Gürkök, H., Mühl, C., Poel, M., Nijholt, A., and Heylen, D. 2010. Brain–computer interfacing in games. In *Brain–Computer Interfaces,* pp. 149–178. Springer London.

Botvinick, M., and Cohen, J. 1998. Rubber hands "feel" touch that eyes see. *Nature.* 391(6669): 756.

Bowman, D. A., Wingrave, C. A., Campbell, J. M., Ly, V. Q., and Rhoton, C. J. 2002. Novel uses of Pinch Gloves™ for virtual environment interaction techniques. *Virtual Reality.* 6(3): 122–129.

Brauchle, D., Vukelić, M., Bauer, R., and Gharabaghi, A. 2015. Brain state-dependent robotic reaching movement with a multi-joint arm exoskeleton: Combining brain–machine interfacing and robotic rehabilitation. *Frontiers in Human Neuroscience.* 9: 564.

Brunner, C., Andreoni, G., Bianchi, L., Blankertz, B., Breitwieser, B., Kanoh, S., Kothe, C. A., Lécuyer, A., Makeig, S., Mellinger, J., Perego, P., Renard, Y., Schalk, G., Susila, P., Venthur, B., and Müller-Putz, G. R. 2012. BCI software platforms. In Allison, B. Z. A., Dunne, S., Leeb, R. and Millán, J. d. R. (Eds.) *Towards Practical Brain–Computer Interfaces,* pp. 303–331. Springer Berlin Heidelberg.

Cruz-Neira, C, Sandin, D. J., DeFanti, T. A., Kenyon, R. V., and Hart, J. C. 1992. The CAVE: Audio visual experience automatic virtual environment. *Communications of the ACM.* 35(6): 64–72. doi:10.1145/129888.129892.

Donnerer, M., and Steed, A. 2010. Using a P300 brain–computer interface in an immersive virtual environment. *Presence: Teleoperators and Virtual Environments.* 19(1): 12–24.

Doud, A. J., Lucas, J. P., Pisansky, M. T., and He, B. 2011. Continuous three-dimensional control of a virtual helicopter using a motor imagery based brain–computer interface. *PLoS One.* 6(10): e26322.

Edlinger, G., Holzner, C., Groenegress, C., Guger, C., and Slater, M. 2009. Goal-oriented control with brain–computer interface. In *International Conference on Foundations of Augmented Cognition,* pp. 732–740. Springer Berlin Heidelberg.

Faller, J., Allison, B. Z., Brunner, C. et al. 2017. A feasibility study on SSVEP-based interaction with motivating and immersive virtual and augmented reality. *arXiv preprint arXiv:1701.03981.*

Faller, J., Allison, B. Z., Brunner, C., Scherer, R., Schmalstieg, D., Pfurtscheller, G., and Neuper, C. 2010c. A feasibility study on SSVEP-based interaction with motivating and immersive virtual and augmented reality. *Technical Report, Institute for Knowledge Discovery, Graz University of Technology.*

Faller, J., Leeb, R., Pfurtscheller, G., and Scherer, R. 2010b. Avatar navigation in virtual and augmented reality environments using an SSVEP BCI. In *International Conference on Applied Bionics and Biomechanics (ICABB),* pp. 1–4.

Faller, J., Müller-Putz, G., Schmalstieg, D., and Pfurtscheller, G. 2010a. An application framework for controlling an avatar in a desktop-based virtual environment via a software SSVEP brain–computer interface. *Presence: Teleoperators and Virtual Environments.* 19(1): 25–34.

Faller, J., Saproo, S., Shih, V., and Sajda, P. 2016. Closed-loop regulation of user state during a boundary avoidance task. In *Proceedings of the International Conference on Systems, Man, and Cybernetics (SMC) 2016, Budapest, Hungary.*

Faller, J., Torrellas, S., Costa, U. et al. 2013. Autonomy and social inclusion for the severely disabled: The BrainAble Prototype. In *Proceedings of the BCI Meeting 2013, Asilomar, CA, USA.*

Friedman, D., Leeb, R., Guger, C., Steed, A., Pfurtscheller, G., and Slater, M. 2007. Navigating virtual reality by thought: What is it like? *Presence: Teleoperators and Virtual Environments.* 16(1): 100–110.

Girouard, A., Solovey, E. T., and Jacob, R. J. 2013. Designing a passive brain computer interface using real time classification of functional near-infrared spectroscopy. *International Journal of Autonomous and Adaptive Communications Systems*. 6(1), 26–44.

Grimm, F., Walter, A., Spüler, M., Naros, G., Rosenstiel, W., and Gharabaghi, A. 2016. Hybrid neuroprosthesis for the upper limb: Combining brain-controlled neuromuscular stimulation with a multi-joint arm exoskeleton. *Frontiers in Neuroscience*. 10.

Hazrati, M. K., and Hofmann, U. G. 2013. Avatar navigation in Second Life using brain signals. In *Intelligent Signal Processing (WISP), 2013 IEEE 8th International Symposium on*, pp. 1–7.

Holper, L., Muehlemann, T., Scholkmann, F., Eng, K., Kiper, D., and Wolf, M. 2010. Testing the potential of a virtual reality neurorehabilitation system during performance of observation, imagery and imitation of motor actions recorded by wireless functional near-infrared spectroscopy (fNIRS). *Journal of Neuroengineering and Rehabilitation*. 7(1): 57.

Ikeda, S., Villagran, C. T., Fukuda, T. et al. 2008. Patient-specific IVR endovascular simulator with augmented reality for medical training and robot evaluation. *Journal of Robotics and Mechatronics*. 20(3): 441.

Jangraw, D. C, Johri, A., Gribetz, M., and Sajda, P. 2014. NEDE: An open-source scripting suite for developing experiments in 3D virtual environments. *Journal of Neuroscience Methods*. 235: 245–251. doi:10.1016/j.jneumeth.2014.06.033.

Kansaku, K., Hata, N., and Takano, K. 2010. My thoughts through a robot's eyes: An augmented reality-brain–machine interface. *Neuroscience Research*. 66(2): 219–222. doi:10.1016/j.neures.2009.10.006.

Käthner, I., Kübler, A., and Halder, S., 2015. Rapid P300 brain–computer interface communication with a head-mounted display. *Frontiers in Neuroscience*. 9, 207.

Kim, C.-H., Choi, B., Kim, D.-G., Lee, S., Jo, S., and Lee, P.-S. 2016. Remote navigation of turtle by controlling instinct behavior via human brain–computer interface. *Journal of Bionic Engineering*. 13(3): 491–503.

Kleih, S. C., Riccio, A., Mattia, D., Schreuder, M., Tangermann, M., Zickler, C., Neuper, C., and Kübler, A. 2011. Motivation affects performance in a P300 brain computer interface. *International Journal of Bioelectromagnetism*. 13(1): 46–47.

Kothe, C. A. 2013. Labstreaming layer (LSL): A system for unified collection of measurement time series in research experiments. *Swartz Center for Computational Neuroscience (SCCN), University of California San Diego, CA, USA*. [Online]. Available: https://github.com/sccn/labstreaminglayer/

Kothe, C. A., and Brunner, C. 2015. Extensible data format (XDF)—A simple extensible storage format for time series and associated data. *Swartz Center for Computational Neuroscience (SCCN), University of California San Diego, CA, USA*. [Online]. Available: https://github.com/sccn/xdf/wiki/Specifications

Kothe, C. A., and Makeig, S. 2013. BCILAB: A platform for brain–computer interface development. *Journal of Neural Engineering*. 10(5): 056014. [Also Online]. Available: https://sccn.ucsd.edu/wiki/BCILAB/

LaFleur, K., Cassady, K., Doud, A., Shades, K., Rogin, E., and He, B. 2013. Quadcopter control in three-dimensional space using a noninvasive motor imagery-based brain–computer interface. *Journal of Neural Engineering*. 10(4): 046003.

Lalor, E. C., Kelly, S. P., Finucane, C. et al. 2005. Steady-state VEP-based brain–computer interface control in an immersive 3D gaming environment. *EURASIP Journal on Applied Signal Processing*. 2005: 3156–3164.

Lee, H.-Y., Cherng, R.-J., and Lin, C.-H. 2004. Development of a virtual reality environment for somatosensory and perceptual stimulation in the balance assessment of children. *Computers in Biology and Medicine*. 34(8): 719–733.

Leeb, R., Friedman, D., Müller-Putz, G.-R., Scherer, R., Slater, M., and Pfurtscheller, G. 2007c. Self-paced (asynchronous) BCI control of a wheelchair in virtual environments: A case study with a tetraplegic. *Computational Intelligence and Neuroscience*. 2007.

Leeb, R., Keinrath, C., Friedman, D., Guger, C., Scherer, R., Neuper, C., Garau, M. et al. 2006. Walking by thinking: The brainwaves are crucial, not the muscles! *Presence: Teleoperators and Virtual Environments*. 15(5): 500–514.

Leeb, R., Lancelle, M., Kaiser, V., Fellner, D. W., and Pfurtscheller, G. 2013. Thinking penguin: Multimodal brain computer interface control of a VR game. *IEEE Transactions on Computational Intelligence and AI in Games*. 5(2): 117–128.

Leeb, R., Lee, F., Keinrath, C., Scherer, R., Bischof, H., and Pfurtscheller, G. 2007a. Brain–computer communication: Motivation, aim, and impact of exploring a virtual apartment. *IEEE Transactions on Neural Systems and Rehabilitation Engineering*. 15(4): 473–482.

Leeb, R., and Pfurtscheller, G. 2004b. Walking through a virtual city by thought. In *Engineering in Medicine and Biology Society, 2004. IEMBS'04. 26th Annual International Conference of the IEEE*. 2: 4503–4506.

Leeb, R., Scherer, R., Keinrath, C., Guger, C., and Pfurtscheller, G. 2005. Exploring virtual environments with an EEG-based BCI through motor imagery/Erkundung von virtuellen Welten durch Bewegungsvorstellungen mit Hilfe eines EEG-basierten BCI. *Biomedizinische Technik/Biomedical Engineering*. 50(4): 86–91.

Leeb, R., Scherer, R., Lee, F., Bischof, H., and Pfurtscheller, G. 2004a. Navigation in virtual environments through motor imagery. In *9th Computer Vision Winter Workshop, CVWW*, vol. 4, pp. 99–108.

Leeb, R., Settgast, V., Fellner, D., and Pfurtscheller, G. 2007b. Self-paced exploration of the Austrian National Library through thought. *International Journal of Bioelectromagnetism*. 9(4): 237–244.

Legény, J., Abad, R. V., and Lécuyer, A. 2011. Navigating in virtual worlds using a self-paced SSVEP-based brain–computer interface with integrated stimulation and real-time feedback. *Presence: Teleoperators and Virtual Environments*. 20(6): 529–544.

Lombard, M., and Ditton, T. 1997. At the heart of it all: The concept of presence. *Journal of Computer-Mediated Communication*. 3(2).

Lotte, F., Renard, Y., and Lécuyer, A. 2008. Self-paced brain–computer interaction with virtual worlds: A quantitative and qualitative study "out of the lab". In *4th International Brain Computer Interface Workshop and Training Course* 2008, Graz, Austria.

Lotte, F., Van Langhenhove, A., Lamarche, F., Ernest, T., Renard, Y, Arnaldi, B., and Lécuyer, A. 2010. Exploring large virtual environments by thoughts using a brain–computer interface based on motor imagery and high-level commands. *Presence*. 19(1): 54–70.

Luu, T. P., He, Y., Brown, S., Nakagame, S., and Contreras-Vidal, J.-L. 2016. Gait adaptation to visual kinematic perturbations using a real-time closed-loop brain–computer interface to a virtual reality avatar. *Journal of Neural Engineering*. 13(3): 036006.

Marathe, A. R., Carey, H. L., and Taylor, D. M. 2008. Virtual reality hardware and graphic display options for brain–machine interfaces. *Journal of Neuroscience Methods*. 167(1): 2–14. doi:10.1016/j.jneumeth.2007.09.025.

Middendorf, M., McMillan, G., Calhoun, G., and Jones, K. A. 2000. Brain–computer interfaces based on the steady-state visual-evoked response. *IEEE Transactions on Rehabilitation Engineering*. 8(2): 211–214.

Moran, D. 2010. Evolution of brain–computer interface: Action potentials, local field potentials and electrocorticograms. *Current Opinion in Neurobiology*. 20(6): 741–745.

Mühl, C., Gürkök, H., Bos, P.-O. D., Thurlings, M. E., Scherffig, L., Duvinage, M., Elbakyan, A. A., Kang, S., Poel, M., and Heylen, D. 2010. Bacteria hunt. *Journal of Multimodal Interfaces*. 4(1): 11–25.

Narumi, T., Nishizaka, S., Kajinami, T., Tanikawa, T., and Hirose, M. 2011. Augmented reality flavors: Gustatory display based on edible marker and cross-modal interaction. In *Proceedings of the SIGCHI Conference on Human Factors in Computing Systems, ACM*. pp. 93–102.

Nelson, W. T., Hettinger, L. J., Cunningham, J. A. et al. 1997. Navigating through virtual flight environments using brain-body-actuated control. In *Virtual Reality Annual International Symposium, 1997, IEEE*, pp. 30–37.

O'Doherty, J. E., Lebedev, M. A., Ifft, P. J., Zhuang, K. Z., Shokur, S., Bleuler, H., and Nicolelis, M. A. L. 2011. Active tactile exploration using a brain–machine–brain interface. *Nature*. 479(7372): 228–231.

Parviz, B. A. 2009. For your eye only. *IEEE Spectrum*. 46(9).

Perez-Marcos, D., Slater, M., and Sanchez-Vives, M. V. 2009. Inducing a virtual hand ownership illusion through a brain–computer interface. *NeuroReport*. 20(6): 589–594. doi:10.1097/WNR.0b013e32832a0a2a.

Petit, D., Gergondet, P., Cherubini, A., and Kheddar, A. 2015. An integrated framework for humanoid embodiment with a BCI. In *IEEE International Conference on Robotics and Automation (ICRA) 2015*. pp. 2882–2887.

Petkova, V. I., and Ehrsson, H. H. 2008. If I were you: Perceptual illusion of body swapping. *PLoS One*. 3(12): e3832.

Pfurtscheller, G., Allison, B. Z., Bauernfeind, G. et al. 2010. The hybrid BCI. *Frontiers in Neuroscience*. 4: 3.

Piccione, F., Priftis, K., Tonin, P. et al. 2008. Task and stimulation paradigm effects in a P300 brain computer interface exploitable in a virtual environment: A pilot study. *PsychNology Journal*. 6(1): 99–108.

Pichiorri, F., Morone, G., Petti, M. et al. 2015. Brain–computer interface boosts motor imagery practice during stroke recovery. *Annals of Neurology*. 77(5): 851–865.

Pineda, J. A., Silverman, D. S., Vankov, A., and Hestenes, J. 2003. Learning to control brain rhythms: Making a brain–computer interface possible. *IEEE Transactions on Neural Systems and Rehabilitation Engineering*. 11(2): 181–184. doi:10.1109/TNSRE.2003.814445.

Pryor, H. L., Furness, T. A. III, and Viirre, E. III. 1998. The virtual retinal display: A new display technology using scanned laser light. In *Proceedings of the Human Factors and Ergonomics Society Annual Meeting*, Sage, CA, USA. 42(22): 1570–1574.

Reissland, J., and Zander, T. O. 2009. Automated detection of bluffing in a game—Revealing a complex covert user state with a passive BCI. In *Proceedings of the Human Factors and Ergonomics Society Europe Chapter Annual Meeting*, Linkoeping, Sweden.

Renard, Y., Lotte, F., Gibert, G. et al. 2010. Openvibe: An open-source software platform to design, test, and use brain–computer interfaces in real and virtual environments. *Presence: Teleoperators and Virtual Environments*. 19(1): 35–53.

Ron-Angevin, R., and Díaz-Estrella, A. 2009. Brain–computer interface: Changes in performance using virtual reality techniques. *Neuroscience Letters*. 449(2): 123–127.

Ron-Angevin, R., Díaz-Estrella, A., and Velasco-Alvarez, F. 2009. A two-class brain computer interface to freely navigate through virtual worlds/Ein zwei-klassen-brain–computer-interface zur freien navigation durch virtuelle welten. *Biomedizinische Technik/Biomedical Engineering*. 54(3): 126–133.

Royer, A. S., Doud, A. J., Rose, M. L., and He, B. 2010. EEG control of a virtual helicopter in 3-dimensional space using intelligent control strategies. *IEEE Transactions on Neural Systems and Rehabilitation Engineering*. 18(6): 581–589.

Saproo, S., Faller, J., Shih, V., Sajda, P., Waytowich, N. R., Bohannon, A., Lawhern, V. J., Lance, B. J., and Jangraw, D. 2016a. Cortically coupled computing: A new paradigm for synergistic human–machine interaction. *IEEE Computer*. 49(9): 60–68.

Saproo, S., Shih, V., Jangraw, D. C., and Sajda, P. 2016b. Neural mechanisms underlying catastrophic failure in human–machine interaction during aerial navigation. *Journal of Neural Engineering*. 13(6): 066005.

Schalk, G., McFarland, D. J., Hinterberger, T., Birbaumer, N., and Wolpaw, J. 2004. BCI2000: A general-purpose brain–computer interface (BCI) system. *IEEE Transactions on Biomedical Engineering*. 51(6): 1034–1043.

Scherer, R., Faller, J., Balderas, D. et al. 2012. Brain–computer interfacing: More than the sum of its parts. *Soft Computing*. 17(2): 317–331. doi:10.1007/s00500-012-0895-4.

Scherer, R., Lee, F., Schlogl, A., Leeb, R., Bischof, H., and Pfurtscheller, G. 2008. Toward self-paced brain–computer communication: Navigation through virtual worlds. *IEEE Transactions on Biomedical Engineering*. 55(2): 675–682.

Schlögl, A., and Brunner, C. 2008. BioSig: A free and open source software library for BCI research. *Computer*. 41(10).

Schomer, D. L., and da Silva, F. L. 2012. Niedermeyer's electroencephalography: Basic principles, clinical applications, and related fields. *Lippincott Williams & Wilkins*.

Seymour, N. E., Gallagher, A. G., Roman, S. A. et al. 2002. Virtual reality training improves operating room performance: Results of a randomized, double-blinded study. *Annals of Surgery*. 236(4): 458–464.

Sitaram, R., Weiskopf, N., Caria, A., Veit, R., Erb, M., and Birbaumer, N. 2008. fMRI brain–computer interfaces. *IEEE Signal Processing Magazine*. 25(1): 95–106.

Sitaram, R., Zhang, H., Guan, C. et al. 2007. Temporal classification of multichannel near-infrared spectroscopy signals of motor imagery for developing a brain–computer interface. *NeuroImage*. 34(4): 1416–1427.

Slater, M., Spanlang, B., Sanchez-Vives, M. V., and Blanke, O. 2010. First person experience of body transfer in virtual reality. *PLoS One* 5: e10564.

Slater, M., Usoh, M., and Steed, A. 1994. Depth of presence in virtual environments. *Presence: Teleoperators and Virtual Environments*. 3(2): 130–144.

Slobounov, S. M., Ray, W., Johnson, B., Slobounov, E., and Newell, K. M. 2015. Modulation of cortical activity in 2D versus 3D virtual reality environments: An EEG study. *International Journal of Psychophysiology*. 95(3): 254–260.

Su, Y., Qi, Y., Luo, J.-X. et al. 2011. A hybrid brain–computer interface control strategy in a virtual environment. *Journal of Zhejiang University SCIENCE*. 12(5): 351.

Van Dokkum, L. E. H., Ward, T., and Laffont, I. 2015. Brain computer interfaces for neurorehabilitation—Its current status as a rehabilitation strategy post-stroke. *Annals of Physical and Rehabilitation Medicine*. 58(1): 3–8.

Velasco-Alvarez, F., Ron-Angevin, R., and Blanca-Mena, M. J. 2010. Free virtual navigation using motor imagery through an asynchronous brain–computer interface. *Presence: Teleoperators and Virtual Environments*. 19(1): 71–81.

Waytowich, N. R. 2015. Development of a practical visual-evoked potential-based brain–computer interface. Ph.D. Thesis, Old Dominion University, 2015.

Waytowich, N. R., and Krusienski, D. J. 2015. Spatial decoupling of targets and flashing stimuli for visual brain–computer interfaces. *Journal of Neural Engineering.* 12(3): 036006.

Wolpaw, J., and Wolpaw, E. W. 2012. Brain–computer interfaces: Principles and practice. Oxford University Press, USA.

Wood, R. B., and Howells, P. J. 2016. Head-up displays. CRC Press LLC, URL: http://www.davi.ws/avionics /TheAvionicsHandbook_Cap_4.pdf [cited 3 February 2017].

Zander, T. O., and Kothe, C. 2011. Towards passive brain–computer interfaces: Applying brain–computer interface technology to human–machine systems in general. *Journal of Neural Engineering.* 8(2): 025005.

Zhao, Q., Zhang, L., and Cichocki, A. 2008. EEG-based asynchronous BCI control of a car in 3D virtual reality environments. *Chinese Science Bulletin.* 54(1): 78–87.

Zhou, F., Duh, H. B.-L., and Billinghurst, M. 2008. Trends in augmented reality tracking, interaction and display: A review of ten years of ISMAR. In *Proceedings of the 7th IEEE/ACM International Symposium on Mixed and Augmented Reality,* IEEE Computer Society, pp. 193–202.

# 13 Brain–Computer Interfaces and Haptics
## *A Literature Review*

*Jan B.F. van Erp*

## CONTENTS

13.1 Introduction .................................................................................................253
    13.1.1 Introduction to Haptics ......................................................................254
        13.1.1.1 Cutaneous or Tactile Sensing..............................................254
    13.1.2 The Potential of Haptics for HCI and BCI .........................................254
13.2 Haptic Feedback in Active BCIs...................................................................256
    13.2.1 Haptic Feedback in Active BCIs in a Nutshell ..................................257
13.3 Haptic Cues in Reactive BCIs .......................................................................257
    13.3.1 ERP-Based BCIs.................................................................................258
        13.3.1.1 Tactile ERP-Based Reactive BCIs in a Nutshell................259
    13.3.2 SSSEP-Based BCIs.............................................................................259
        13.3.2.1 SSSEP-Based BCIs in a Nutshell........................................260
    13.3.3 Other BCI Paradigms Including Haptics.............................................260
13.4 Conclusions and Recommendations ...............................................................261
References...............................................................................................................261

### Abstract

This review discusses the potential use of the sense of touch (haptics) in brain–computer interfaces (BCIs) that commenced a decade ago. In motor imagery BCIs, haptics can be used to provide feedback, which feels more intuitive to users and obtains results comparable to visual feedback. In event-related potential BCIs, haptic stimuli (mainly in the form of vibration to the torso, wrists, or fingers) are used to present the user with options. Spatial, selective tactile attention increases specific components of the ERP in a similar way visual attention does. Performance of these tactile ERPs has improved rapidly over the past few years and surpasses that of gaze-independent visual BCIs. This gaze independence is of interest to specific users who may not have full control over their eye movements or whose visual channel is under the threat of overload. Haptic stimuli are also investigated with steady-state evoked potential BCIs. So far, this BCI paradigm has not been very successful using haptic stimuli. Recent reports, however, show that adding haptic steady-state stimuli to a motor imagery BCI may improve overall performance. To progress haptic BCIs, we should further optimize hardware, BCI paradigms, and classification algorithms tuned to the characteristics of haptics.

## 13.1 INTRODUCTION

This chapter discusses the potential of haptics for brain–computer interfaces (BCIs). We start with introducing haptics and the potential of touch for the different BCI paradigms. Next, we review and discuss the available literature for each of the relevant BCI paradigms separately. We end by identifying general issues that deserve our attention to improve haptic BCIs.

### 13.1.1 Introduction to Haptics

Haptics is an overarching term combining the sense of kinesthesis and of touch. Kinesthesis refers to perception of, among others, body position, joint angles, and forces. Touch (also referred to as tactile or cutaneous) comprises (mechanical, thermal, chemical, or electrical) stimulation of the skin (ISO 9241-910 2011). The human haptic sense is a very complex system with receptors in the skin, joints, and muscles and is able to process large amounts of (abstract) information. The bandwidth of the tactile sense is estimated to be in the order of 125 MB/s which is an order of magnitude smaller than vision, and an order of magnitude larger than audition. To illustrate the high bandwidth of the sense of touch, people who are trained in reading Braille are able to read at speeds of 100 words per minute or more using just their fingertips (a grown human has about 2 $m^2$ of skin surface, albeit large parts have a much lower information processing capacity than the fingertips).

Although not as widely used as visual and auditory displays, haptic displays are starting to become more common in human–computer interaction (HCI). This development is partly attributed to the threat of visual and auditory overload (e.g., in car driving) and to the fact that haptic feedback may be the most natural option (e.g., when using gesture or touch-based input). The growth of haptic displays accelerated in the mid-1990s with the introduction of the vibration function on mobile phones, and currently, the displays come in many different forms tapping into the different subsystems that comprise the haptic sense. With respect to BCIs, tactile displays presenting mechanical stimulation to the skin (including pressure and vibration) are the most relevant.

#### 13.1.1.1 Cutaneous or Tactile Sensing

For the skin to sense a stimulus, the stimulus must evoke a response in at least one receptor. There are several types of receptors in the skin and each of them has a distinctive structure and reacts differently to different characteristics of the stimulus. In general, four physiological channels are discerned, which are assumed to have a one-to-one link with mechanoreceptor types in glabrous skin ("glabrous skin" is non-hairy skin and mainly found in the palms of the hands and on the sole of the feet; most other skin areas are called "hairy skin"). The superficial skin contains rapidly adapting Meissner corpuscles and slowly adapting Merkel receptors. Deeper tissue contains rapidly adapting Pacinian corpuscles and slowly adapting Ruffini endings or corpuscles (see Figure 13.1). Slowly adapting means that the mechanoreceptor's response does not change for stimulus durations longer than 1 s, while rapidly adapting means that it does. However, the time scale of rapidly adapting is not strictly defined (e.g., in the order of hundreds of milliseconds). More information of cutaneous sensing can be found in, for example, Kandel and Jessell (1991) and Cheung et al. (2008).

Like other modalities, the cutaneous system cannot process information with an unlimited accuracy. Stimulus information is lost in the different stages of cutaneous processing that act as a spatiotemporal filter upon the stimulus that is applied to the skin. Generally, the skin receptors are sensitive to vibration in the 0.4–800 Hz frequency range with a detection threshold at 200 Hz of 2 µm. Spatial acuity differs largely across the body and is highest for the fingertips (1 mm or better) and lowest on the torso and the legs (4 cm). The cutaneous sense has a high temporal sensitivity, which is in the order of 5 ms. For more information, see Van Erp (2002, 2007).

### 13.1.2 The Potential of Haptics for HCI and BCI

A key question here is if and how the haptic sense is of relevance to BCIs. Within HCI, the sense of touch is often used as an additional or alternative sensory channel to present information when the visual and auditory channels are not available or overloaded (Prewett et al. 2012). We see this in many application domains including aviation, transport, and health care. Of course, the potential to mitigate the risk of sensory overload is also relevant for BCI applications (e.g., Gwak et al. 2013), especially when designing applications for specific user groups that may suffer from, for example, lack of gaze control like people with amyotrophic lateral sclerosis (ALS) may have in the course of

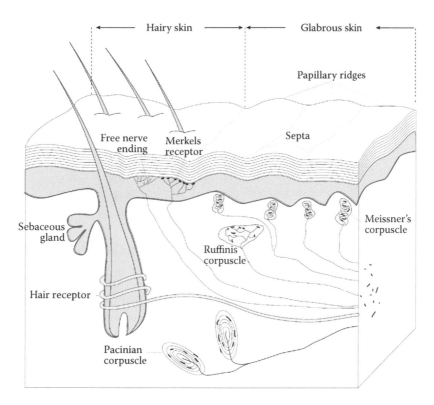

**FIGURE 13.1**  Mechanoreceptors in the human skin. (Artwork licensed by Thomas Haslwanter under Creative Commons license.)

their disease. Furthermore, haptics may be the preferred sensory channel for motor imagery BCIs because it can close the perception–action loop in motor control (e.g., Gomez-Rodriguez et al. 2011). We will explore the potential for different BCIs in the remainder of this section.

BCIs are a specific class of devices within HCI. According to a recent definition (Van Erp et al. 2012), "a BCI uses brain signals to control a device or to adjust the communication between user and device." BCIs basically come in three different types (Zander et al. 2008): active, reactive, and passive (see Figure 13.2). Active BCIs are based on brain patterns (e.g., power in specific frequency bands at a specific electrode location) that are actively generated by the user, for instance, through imagining a left-hand movement to go left and a right-hand movement to go right, or through performing specific mental calculations or language processing tasks. Reactive BCIs measure the brain responses to specific stimuli or cues. These patterns include event-related potentials (ERPs) (specific peaks in the EEG signal) and steady-state evoked potentials (SSEPs; power in the frequency

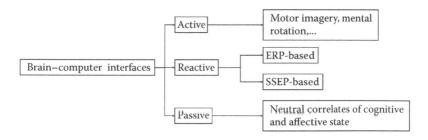

**FIGURE 13.2**  BCI classes and paradigms.

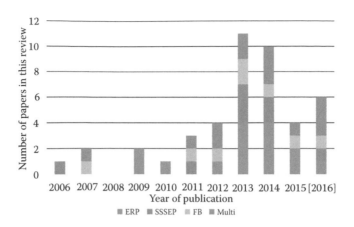

**FIGURE 13.3** The 44 papers used in this review as a function of year of publication and BCI paradigm employed. The data of 2016 represent only the first half of 2016.

corresponding to that of the stimulus). Brain patterns to cues that the user attends to differ from patterns to cues that are ignored. These differences in brain patterns are large and robust and can relatively easily be picked up by the BCI, although classification will not be perfect because of user variability and other factors. This means that the BCI user can select one stimulus among a multitude of stimuli by selectively attending to it while ignoring irrelevant stimuli. Finally, the third class called passive BCIs measure the cognitive or emotional state of the user from brain patterns without any need for specific user activity (for instance, power in specific EEG frequency bands). Examples of these states are workload, frustration, attention, and drowsiness (Coffey et al. 2010; Van Erp et al. 2015; Zander & Kothe 2011).

Passive BCIs use information about cognitive or emotional state to improve human–machine interaction and have no direct link to haptics. Active and reactive BCI approaches are relevant with respect to the involvement of haptics. For active BCIs, haptic displays can provide feedback on the output of the BCI, while in reactive BCIs, haptic stimuli can be employed as options for the user to choose from. The latter is of specific interest with respect to applications in the assistive technology domain. Specific BCI target groups like people with ALS suffer from a decreasing ability to focus their gaze as their disease progresses, ultimately making vision-based BCIs ineffective. The development of gaze-independent reactive BCIs is progressing, albeit slowly. In a 2012 review (Riccio et al. 2012), only six articles on auditory BCIs and three on touch-based BCIs were reported. In this review, we discuss 44 papers on haptic BCIs only. These papers were the result of a database search using Scopus performed on July 1, 2016. Additional papers were selected based on the references in the original data set. Papers were included only when original experimental data were presented. Figure 13.3 provides the spread of the papers over the years and as a function of employed BCI paradigm.

## 13.2 HAPTIC FEEDBACK IN ACTIVE BCIs

One of the first involvements of touch in BCI systems concerned applications in which the BCI was actively controlled by imagined movement and feedback was provided through the sense of touch. This approach seems very promising in BCI-controlled prostheses where tactile and haptic feedback can potentially mimic the natural representation of limb state variables (London et al. 2011) and may facilitate correct decoding of motor imagery or movement intention (Gomez-Rodriguez et al. 2011). Badakva et al. (2016) performed a review of invasive BCIs and conclude that invasive BCIs have to be based on a bidirectional system, that is, including tactile, proprioceptive, and other useful feedback.

Murguialday et al. (2007) tested a BCI-controlled prosthetic hand with force and angle sensors that provided haptic feedback and showed that users were able to control the grasping force with accuracies comparable to an electromyography-based control scheme. Similar encouraging results were reported for cursor control. Chatterjee et al. (2007) showed that users can control a BCI using only vibrotactile feedback and Wilson et al. (2012), Leeb et al. (2013), and Jeunet et al. (2015) demonstrated that task performance with tactile feedback was comparable to or, in a multitask situation, even outperformed visual feedback. In an extended experiment with 30 healthy and 3 spinal cord injury participants, Cincotti et al. (2007) using a simulated BCI system conclude that the vibrotactile channel can function as a valuable feedback modality, especially when the visual channel is loaded by a secondary task. In addition, they report that vibrotactile feedback felt more natural than visual feedback.

Ahn et al. (2014) and Yao et al. (2013a,b) designed a new so-called hybrid BCI paradigm by combining motor imagery with an SSSEP (steady-state somatosensory evoked potential) paradigm. In this paradigm, SSSEP stimuli were presented to the wrists while the motor imagery was based on imagined hand movements. In other words, tactile cues were not used as a post-stimulus to provide feedback on the resulting motion but as a pre-stimulus to aid the user in producing a stronger motor imagery (or, more specifically, an event-related desynchronization) signal. They report an increase in performance in a two-class motor imagery BCI from 60% to 80% for some participants when the SSSEP signal was added. A similar approach applied to upper limb rehabilitation was described by Saetang et al. (2013).

### 13.2.1 Haptic Feedback in Active BCIs in a Nutshell

Example of haptic feedback in a BCI is touch feedback in a prosthetic hand. Research by Chatterjee et al. (2007), Cincotti et al. (2007), and Wilson et al. (2012) shows that tactile feedback is as good as visual feedback, tactile feedback is better in the presence of a visual distractor, and tactile feedback feels more natural in imagined movement BCIs. Recent research shows that adding a steady-state somatosensory stimulus as a pre-stimulus can increase performance of a motor imagery BCI.

## 13.3 HAPTIC CUES IN REACTIVE BCIs

While touch can be used as feedback channel in active BCIs, touch cues can be the main modality of actual control in reactive BCIs. Two main paradigms have been used in reactive BCIs. The first is based on the so-called P300 ERP. The P300 occurs about 300 ms after the presentation of a relevant stimulus and can be easily detected using EEG sensors that measure the brain's electrical signals on the outside of the skull. P300 BCIs can be used to spell words or to navigate through a menu (Farwell & Donchin 1988). For instance, in a P300 visual speller, letters or other possible options are displayed in a matrix of which rows and columns are flashed sequentially and in random order. The row and column that contain the option attended to by the user results in a larger P300 compared to the rows and columns that contain only nontargets. The second paradigm is the SSEP. In this paradigm, options are presented in parallel but with different frequencies. In the case of visual stimuli, this is done by presenting stimuli that flash at different frequencies. All frequencies are reflected in the resulting brain pattern, but the frequency of the attended stimulus is more pronounced than the frequencies of the ignored stimuli. For instance, in a navigation BCI, four arrows indicating four directions may flash with a different frequency. The user directs his or her visual attention to the arrow of choice and the flashing frequency of this selected arrow will be more strongly reflected in the brain's pattern and can be picked up by the BCI.

As the name already implies, reactive BCIs depend on the brain's reaction to stimuli. Or in other words, a reactive BCI is independent of body motions as output but still requires sensory input. Touch-based BCIs, based on both the P300 signal and the steady state signal (SSSEP) are gaining interest. We will describe the state of the art in the next sections.

### 13.3.1 ERP-Based BCIs

ERP BCIs are by far the most popular and successful touch-based BCIs. The first description of a touch-based P300 BCI is from 2008 (Van Erp et al. 2008) in which the authors present a system based on two to six vibrating elements or tactors around the waist that are activated in a random pattern (see Figure 13.4). The user attends to one of the tactors while ignoring the others, which increases the brain response (i.e., the amplitude of the associated P300 brain potential) to this particular tactor. The BCI system identifies this particular signal and therewith the chosen option. This approach is further validated in Van Erp et al. (2009) and Brouwer and Van Erp (2010) and compared to a similar visual BCI in Thurlings et al. (2012a). The authors conclude that the system shows potential for users who can benefit from vision-independent BCIs like specific patient groups and in situations with a risk of visual overload. A spelling application with the use of tactile stimulation on the fingertips was developed by Van der Waal et al. (2012). When comparing the tactile speller with a visual speller (Hex-o-Spell), average performance was lower with the tactile speller (Severens et al. 2014) for both healthy and ALS users with mild to moderate disabilities. However, contrary to the Hex-o-Spell, the developed tactile speller is gaze-independent and therefore less prone to degradation of gaze control that occurs in later stages of ALS. Other authors specifically compared performance with a gaze-independent visual BCI (Herweg & Kübler 2016; Thurlings et al. 2014) and conclude that under these conditions, the tactile BCI performs at least as good as the (gaze-independent) visual BCI.

Kaufmann et al. (2014) described an experiment in which they tested healthy users steering a virtual wheelchair through a building. The four navigation directions were associated with different tactor locations on the body (left upper leg: move left; right upper leg: move right; belly: move forward; lower neck: move backward). Out of the 15 participants, 11 successfully navigated a route along four waypoints. Ortner et al. (2013a) introduced a system based on 2 (wrists), 3 (wrists and neck), or 8 (fingers) tactors. Evaluation with 12 healthy participants showed fairly good classification rates (between 70% for the eight tactor system and 100% for the two tactor system). The

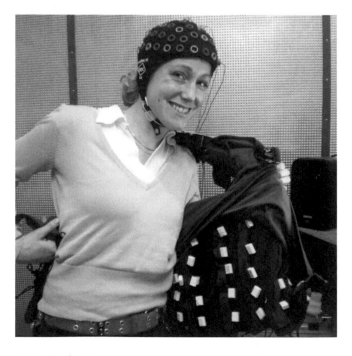

**FIGURE 13.4** Small vibrating boxes worn on the torso as used in the first experiments on tactile ERP-based BCIs (TNO, The Netherlands).

system's usefulness was also shown for people with Locked-in syndrome (Ortner et al. 2013b, 2014). Mori et al. experimented with the body loci that can be used for stimulation in a tactile P300 BCI. Besides the torso (Mori et al. 2013a) as used in the first BCI described, they reported systems based on 10 tactors on the 10 fingertips (Mori et al. 2013b) and based on 6 tactors mounted on the head resulting in combined tactile and auditory cues (Rutkowski & Mori 2015). The latter system was tested by 11 healthy participants showing a large variation in classification rates (from 0% to 100%) but with an acceptable overall score.

Generally, there is an increasing interest in multisensory BCIs combining tactile cues with visual and/or auditory cues. Yin et al. (2016) combined tactile and auditory cues and reported bitrates above 10 bits/min for the bimodal BCI, substantially above the rates reached for each modality alone. Thurlings et al. (2014) reported increased classification rates for bimodal visual/tactile cues as compared to the unimodal conditions. They also tested a tactile ERP BCI under dual-task conditions and although the size of the P300 and the BCI bitrate were reduced under dual-task conditions, the authors concluded that the BCI was still usable, that is, complied with the minimal requirements for adequate BCI control (Thurlings et al. 2013). Although the majority of the experiments were done employing vibrotactile stimuli, the haptic cues for the ERP-based BCI could also consist of pressure like that shown by Shimizu et al. (2014) or forces delivered to the hand through a joystick as shown by Kono and Rutkowski (2015). The potential of these haptic BCI has not been thoroughly explored.

Taking these results into account, we can conclude that tactile P300 BCIs are feasible, and although they are not as advanced as visual BCIs yet, they show performance within or above the range reported for gaze-independent vision-based systems, also under dual task conditions. It is important to notice that brain responses to tactile stimuli are not affected by ALS as recently shown by Silvoni et al. (2016) comparing a group of 14 participants with ALS with a control group of 10 healthy volunteers.

### 13.3.1.1 Tactile ERP-Based Reactive BCIs in a Nutshell

Example of a tactile ERP BCI is presenting vibration to two or more fingers in random order. Cincotti et al. (2007) and Van Erp et al. (2008) reported a first proof of concept and Brouwer and Van Erp (2010) a first operational version. Van der Waal et al. (2012) described the first tactile ERP speller, and Kaufman et al. (2014) and Herweg and Kübler (2016) described simulated wheelchair control. The results of the recent studies show that performance with a tactile ERP BCI is as good as with a visual ERP BCI and outperforms SSSEP BCIs as illustrated in Section 13.3.2.

## 13.3.2  SSSEP-Based BCIs

The first preliminary study into the use of SSSEP BCIs was reported in 2006 by Müller-Putz et al. (2006). They tested four users with vibration stimuli on both index fingers. Of these four users, two reached accuracies well above chance (70%–80% accuracy) and two did not, which was not overwhelming but showed the feasibility of the paradigm. In a study by Breitwieser et al. (2011), accuracies above chance were only reached by 2 out of the 14 tested users. Later studies showed that SSSEP BCIs are not as successful as their visual counterparts (if eye movements are allowed) and performance is also generally lower than with tactile P300 BCIs (see also Ahn et al. 2016 for a recent mini-review). For instance, Severens et al. (2013) designed stimuli to evoke both tactile P300s and SSSEPs and found that P300s outperformed SSSEPs and the combination of both did not result in better performance than P300s alone. Smith et al. (2014) directly compared visual and somatosensory SSEPs for six participants and found effects to be stronger and more consistently for the steady-state visually evoked potentials (SSVEPs). This leads to the conclusion that SSSEP-based BCIs may be feasible but have not reached an acceptable performance level yet.

There may be several causes for the relatively poor performance of SSSEP BCIs compared to SSVEP BCIs. First, users may have difficulties in focusing tactile spatial attention. Some paradigms even include transient tactile patterns into their continuous vibration streams to help users keep their focus, also known as twitches, which, in themselves, may reduce the classification (Pokorny et al. 2016). Reduced ability of sustained spatial selective attention will decrease the difference in brain pattern between targets and nontargets and hamper classification performance. Another cause may be related to the complex way the tactile sensory system codes vibration frequencies. In the visual system, the rhythm of stimulation is preserved between the peripheral receptors and the visual cortex, resulting in a direct link between flashing frequency and activation pattern in the visual cortex. However, in the tactile system, this link is less clear (Gardner & Palmer 1989). The different types of vibrotactile peripheral receptors (see Section 13.1) already perform complex spatiotemporal processing before signals are transported to the primary sensory cortex (Valbo et al. 1995; Van Erp 2007) while preserving spatial (i.e., body locus) information. This may mean that classification algorithms that only use features based on frequency information are suboptimal. Adding spatial information as, for instance, the common spatial pattern method does may improve classification performance as shown by Nam et al. (2013, 2014).

As described in Section 13.2, preliminary studies on using steady-state somatosensory stimuli to guide spatial attention may increase motor imagery BCIs (e.g., Ahn et al. 2014; Saetang et al. 2013; Yao et al. 2013a,b). Ahn and Jun (2012) combined the SSSEP (left and right finger) with an imagined movement BCI paradigm. In a preliminary study, it appeared that the SSSEP could reveal patterns not visible in the imagined movement signals but performance was again not very high and probably too low to be applied in an assistive technology device.

### 13.3.2.1 SSSEP-Based BCIs in a Nutshell

SSEP BCIs are based on power spectra evoked by external stimuli. An example is an SSSEP based on different vibration frequencies on two or more fingers. Müller-Putz et al. (2006) report a first proof of principle but with low performance. More recent research by Nam et al. (2013), Smith et al. (2014), and Ahn and Jun (2012) indicate that SSSEP performance increased over the years but SSSEPs have a lower signal-to-noise ratio than SSVEPs and also a lower accuracy and bitrate than tactile ERP BCIs.

### 13.3.3 OTHER BCI PARADIGMS INCLUDING HAPTICS

In the search to increase the reliability and bandwidth of BCI systems, new paradigms are designed, such as systems that combine two BCI paradigms and multisensory BCIs (Van Erp et al. 2011). Some of those also employ haptics. For example, Schreuder et al. (2012) developed an auditory P300 BCI that provided feedback on performance through touch cues in order not to load the auditory channel too heavily. Multisensory visual–tactile BCIs were investigated by Thurlings et al. (2012b) and Brouwer et al. (2010) who found somewhat better performance of multisensory over unisensory stimulation. Multisensory stimuli also allow the user to switch attention between modalities and use this attentional switch to communicate. This approach was described by Zhang et al. (2007) who found distinguishable differences in brain patterns as a function of attentional switching that could potentially be used.

Yet another approach was taken by Lehne et al. (2009) who focused on so-called error potentials in the brain (specific patterns that signify a mistake or error) to correct wrong interpretations of the system in a tactile task. Users controlled a tactile cursor using button presses. Tactile feedback that was not intended or expected (due to an error generated by either the user or the system) resulted in distinctive error-related potentials, as found before for the visual and auditory modality. As suggested previously (Zander et al. 2008), these error-related potentials could (potentially) be used to improve human–machine interaction. The results of Lehne et al. (2009) indicate that these error signals are modality independent, allowing the transfer of vision-based BCI paradigms to touch-based BCIs.

## 13.4 CONCLUSIONS AND RECOMMENDATIONS

The current review shows that the BCI community has long been focusing on vision-based systems and started to explore the potential of the tactile modality only in the last decade. The first publications on SSSEP-based BCIs, tactile feedback BCIs, and tactile P300-based BCIs appeared in 2006, 2007, and 2008, respectively. The number of touch-based BCI studies is still very limited but increases steadily and doubled compared to a review presented 2 years ago (Van Erp & Brouwer 2014). Taken together, the picture arises that touch-based BCIs are feasible, that the potential of touch-based P300 BCIs is not less than that of vision-based gaze-independent P300 BCIs, but that SSSEP BCIs are less successful than their visual counterparts, at least those that allow eye movements (SSVEP BCIs). In addition, touch-based BCIs may enhance vision-based BCIs using a multisensory paradigm. An encouraging result, especially for users or situations that require a system that does not depend on vision and steady state somatosensory stimuli, may increase performance of active BCIs.

To bring touch-based BCIs further, we recommend research in the following four areas:

- Hardware. So far, the BCI community employed relatively simple and standard hardware that is not specifically designed to be used in a BCI context (see Pokorny et al. 2013 for an exception). For BCIs, it is important that the tactile hardware does not electrically interfere with the EEG sensor system. Furthermore, predictable and sudden onsets of tactile stimuli will improve performance of tactile P300 BCIs.
- Touch-based BCI paradigms. Based on neurophysiological and psychophysical knowledge on, for instance, sensitivity to certain types of touch of different body locations, stimulus presentation rate, stimulus duration, and attentional switching, we must develop BCI paradigms that are optimal for touch (Van Erp 2007). The paradigms currently employed often start from vision-based BCIs without specific adjustments.
- Classification algorithms. The vast majority of the (EEG) classification algorithms are developed for vision-based BCIs while the neurophysiological responses to tactile stimuli may differ from those to visual stimuli in, for instance, (electrode) location and temporal pattern (e.g., compared to the visual P300, the tactile P300 starts later and has a less sharper peak). Although many classification algorithms are general in nature, specific tuning and adjustments are required for optimal performance. Specific tactile features must be identified to improve the classifiers. For instance, common spatial filter techniques may be beneficial because spatial relations are, to a large extent, preserved during tactile processing.
- Multisensory integration. As in many more general HCI systems, haptic displays are often not applied as stand-alone devices but rather as parts of a multimodal system. This will also be the case for touch-based BCIs, which makes multisensory integration a relevant topic, not only from a perceptual and cognitive perspective but also from a neurophysiological perspective. Knowledge on neurophysiological features related to multisensory processing is needed to optimize multisensory BCI systems.
- Testing in special user groups. Touch-based BCIs should be tested in the user groups that would be among the first to benefit from touch-based BCIs like people with ALS. The first case studies are available (e.g., Kaufmann et al. 2013), but more data are needed to draw conclusions and improve systems.

## REFERENCES

Ahn, S., Ahn, M., Cho, H., Chan Jun, S. (2014). Achieving a hybrid brain–computer interface with tactile selective attention and motor imagery. *Journal of Neural Engineering*, 11 (6), art. no. 066004. DOI: 10.1088/1741-2560/11/6/066004.

Ahn, S., Jun, S.C. (2012). Feasibility of hybrid BCI using ERD- and SSSEP- BCI. *International Conference on Control, Automation and Systems*, art. no. 6393191, pp. 2053–2056.

Ahn, S., Kim, K., Jun, S.C. (2016). Steady-state somatosensory evoked potential for brain–computer interface-present and future. *Frontiers in Human Neuroscience*, 9 (JAN2016), art. no. 716. DOI: 10.3389/fnhum.2015.00716.

Badakva, A.M., Miller, N.V., Zobova, L.N. (2016). Artificial feedback for invasive brain–computer interfaces. *Human Physiology*, 42 (1), 111–118. DOI: 10.1134/S0362119716010023.

Breitwieser, C., Pokorny, C., Neuper, C., Muller-Putz, G.R. (2011). Somatosensory evoked potentials elicited by stimulating two fingers from one hand Usable for BCI? *Proceedings of the Annual International Conference of the IEEE Engineering in Medicine and Biology Society, EMBS*, art. no. 6091573, pp. 6373–6376.

Brouwer, A.-M., Van Erp, J.B.F. (2010). A tactile P300 brain–computer interface. *Frontiers in Neuroscience*, 4 (19), 1–12. DOI: 10.3389.

Brouwer, A.-M., Van Erp, J.B.F., Aloise, F., Cincotti, F. (2010). Tactile, visual and bimodal P300s: Could bimodal P300s boost BCI performance? *SRX Neuroscience*, 2010, 1–9. Article ID 967027. DOI: 10.3814/2010/967027.

Chatterjee, A., Aggarwal, V., Ramos, A., Acharya, S., Thakor, N.V. (2007). A brain–computer interface with vibrotactile biofeedback for haptic information. *Journal of NeuroEngineering and Rehabilitation*, 4, art. no. 40.

Cheung, B., Van Erp, J.B.F., Cholewiak, R.W. (2008). Anatomical, neurophysiological and perceptual issues of tactile perception. In: *Tactile Displays for Orientation, Navigation and Communication in Air, Sea and Land Environments*. Neuilly-sur-Sein Cedex (France): NATO Research and Technology Organisation, pp. 1–18.

Cincotti, F., Kauhanen, L., Aloise, F., Palomäki, T., Caporusso, N., Jylänki, P., Mattia, D., Babiloni, F., Vanacker, G., Nuttin, M., Marciani, M.G., Millán, J.D.R. (2007). Vibrotactile feedback for brain–computer interface operation. *Computational Intelligence and Neuroscience*, 2007, art. no. 48937.

Coffey, E.B.J., Brouwer, A.-M., Wilschut, E.S., van Erp, J.B.F. (2010). Brain–machine interfaces in space: Using spontaneous rather than intentionally generated brain signals. *Acta Astronautica*, 67, 1–11.

Farwell, L.A., Donchin, E. (1988). Talking off the top of your head: A mental prosthesis utilizing event-related brain potentials. *Electroencephalogr Clin Neurophysiol*, 70, 510–523.

Gardner, E.P., Palmer, C.I. (1989). Simulation of motion on the skin. I. Receptive fields and temporal frequency coding by cutaneous mechanorecptors of OPTACON pulses delivered to the hand. *J Neurophysiol*, 62 (6), 1410–1436.

Gomez-Rodriguez, M., Peters, J., Hill, J., Schölkopf, B., Gharabaghi, A., Grosse-Wentrup, M. (2011). Closing the sensorimotor loop: Haptic feedback facilitates decoding of motor imagery. *Journal of Neural Engineering*, 8 (3), art. no. 036005. DOI: 10.1088/1741-2560/8/3/036005.

Gwak, K., Leeb, R., Millán, J.D.R., Kim, D.-S. (2013). A novel tactile stimulation system for BCI feedback. *International Winter Workshop on Brain–Computer Interface, BCI 2013*, art. no. 6506619, pp. 29–31. DOI: 10.1109/IWW-BCI.2013.6506619.

Herweg, A., Kübler, A. (2016). High performance with tactile P300 BCIs. *4th International Winter Conference on Brain–Computer Interface, BCI 2016*, art. no. 7457442. DOI: 10.1109/IWW-BCI.2016.7457442.

ISO 9241-910 (2011). Ergonomics of human-system interaction—Part 910: Framework for tactile and haptic interaction.

Jeunet, C., Vi, C., Spelmezan, D., N'Kaoua, B., Lotte, F., Subramanian, S. (2015). Continuous tactile feedback for motor-imagery based brain–computer interaction in a multitasking context. *Lecture Notes in Computer Science* (including subseries Lecture Notes in Artificial Intelligence and Lecture Notes in Bioinformatics), 9296, 488–505. DOI: 10.1007/978-3-319-22701-6_36.

Kandel, E.R., Jessell, T.M. (1991). Touch. In: E.R. Kandel, J.H. Schwartz, T.M. Jessell (Eds.), *Principles of Neural Science*, pp. 367–384. Amsterdam: Elsevier.

Kaufmann, T., Herweg, A., Kübler, A. (2014). Toward brain–computer interface based wheelchair control utilizing tactually-evoked event-related potentials. *Journal of NeuroEngineering and Rehabilitation*, 11 (1), art. no. 7. DOI: 10.1186/1743-0003-11-7.

Kaufmann, T., Holz, E.M., Kübler, A. (2013). Comparison of tactile, auditory and visual modality for brain–computer interface use: A case study with a patient in the locked-in state. *Frontiers in Neuroscience*, 7, article 00129.

Kono, S., Rutkowski, T.M. (2015). Tactile-force brain–computer interface paradigm: Somatosensory multimedia neurotechnology application. *Multimedia Tools and Applications*, 74 (19), pp. 8655–8667. DOI: 10.1007/s11042-014-2351-1.

Leeb, R., Gwak, K., Kim, D.-S., Millan, J.D.R. (2013). Freeing the visual channel by exploiting vibrotactile BCI feedback. *Proceedings of the Annual International Conference of the IEEE Engineering in Medicine and Biology Society, EMBS*, art. no. 6610195, pp. 3093–3096. DOI: 10.1109/EMBC.2013.6610195.

Lehne, M., Ihme, K., Brouwer, A.-M., Van Erp, J.B.F., Zander, T.O. (2009). Error-related EEG patterns during tactile human–machine interaction. *Proceedings—2009 3rd International Conference on Affective Computing and Intelligent Interaction and Workshops, ACII 2009*, art. no. 5349480.

London, B.M., Torres, R.R., Slutzky, M.W., Miller, L.E. (2011). Designing stimulation patterns for an afferent BMI: Representation of kinetics in somatosensory cortex. *Proceedings of the Annual International Conference of the IEEE Engineering in Medicine and Biology Society, EMBS*, art. no. 6091854, pp. 7521–7524.

Mori, H., Makino, S., Rutkowski, T.M. (2013a). Multi-command chest tactile brain computer interface for small vehicle robot navigation. *Lecture Notes in Computer Science* (including subseries Lecture Notes in Artificial Intelligence and Lecture Notes in Bioinformatics), 8211 LNAI, pp. 469–478. DOI: 10.1007/978-3-319-02753-1_47.

Mori, H., Matsumoto, Y., Kryssanov, V., Cooper, E., Ogawa, H., Makino, S., Struzik, Z.R., Rutkowski, T.M. (2013b). Multi-command tactile brain computer interface: A feasibility study. *Lecture Notes in Computer Science* (including subseries Lecture Notes in Artificial Intelligence and Lecture Notes in Bioinformatics), 7989 LNCS, pp. 50–59. DOI: 10.1007/978-3-642-41068-0_6.

Müller-Putz, G.R., Scherer, R., Neuper, C., Pfurtscheller, G. (2006). Steady-state somatosensory evoked potentials: Suitable brain signals for brain–computer interfaces? *IEEE Transactions on Neural Systems and Rehabilitation Engineering*, 14 (1), 30–37.

Murguialday, A.R., Aggarwal, V., Chatterjee, A., Cho, Y., Rasmussen, R., O'Rourke, B., Acharya, S., Thakor, N.V. (2007). Brain–computer interface for a prosthetic hand using local machine control and haptic feedback. *IEEE 10th International Conference on Rehabilitation Robotics, ICORR'07*, art. no. 4428487, pp. 609–613.

Nam, Y., Cichocki, A., Choi, S. (2013). Common spatial patterns for steady-state somatosensory evoked potentials. *Proceedings of the Annual International Conference of the IEEE Engineering in Medicine and Biology Society, EMBS*, art. no. 6609986, pp. 2255–2258. DOI: 10.1109/EMBC.2013.6609986.

Nam, Y., Koo, B., Choi, S. (2014). Spatial patterns of SSSEP under the selective attention to tactile stimuli in each hand. *2014 International Winter Workshop on Brain–Computer Interface, BCI 2014*, art. no. 6782563. DOI: 10.1109/iww-BCI.2014.6782563.

Ortner, R., Kapeller, C., Prückl, R., Guger, C. (2013a). A tactile P300-based BCI. *Proceedings of the Fifth International Brain–Computer Interface Meeting 2013*. DOI:10.3217/978-4-83452-381-5/098.

Ortner, R., Lugo, Z., Noirhomme, Q., Laureys, S., Guger, C. (2014). A tactile brain–computer interface for severely disabled patients. *IEEE Haptics Symposium, HAPTICS*, art. no. 6775460, pp. 235–237. DOI: 10.1109/HAPTICS.2014.6775460.

Ortner, R., Lugo, Z., Pruckl, R., Hintermuller, C., Noirhomme, Q., Guger, C. (2013b). Performance of a tactile P300 speller for healthy people and severely disabled patients. *Proceedings of the Annual International Conference of the IEEE Engineering in Medicine and Biology Society, EMBS*, art. no. 6609987, pp. 2259–2262. DOI: 10.1109/EMBC.2013.6609987.

Pokorny, C., Breitwieser, C., Müller-Putz, G.R. (2016). The role of transient target stimuli in a steady-state somatosensory evoked potential-based brain–computer interface setup. *Frontiers in Neuroscience*, 10 (APR), art. no. 152. DOI: 10.3389/fnins.2016.00152.

Pokorny, C., Breitwieser, C., Muller-Putz, G.R.A. (2013). Tactile stimulation device for EEG measurements in clinical use. *IEEE Transactions on Biomedical Circuits and Systems*.

Prewett, M.S., Elliott, L.R., Walvoord, A.G., Coovert, M.D. (2012). A meta-analysis of vibrotactile and visual information displays for improving task performance. *IEEE Transactions on Systems, Man and Cybernetics Part C: Applications and Reviews*, 42 (1), art. no. 5710431, pp. 123–132.

Riccio, A., Mattia, D., Simione, L., Olivetti, M., Cincotti, F. (2012). Eye-gaze independent EEG-based brain–computer interfaces for communication. *Journal of Neural Engineering*, 9 (4), art. no. 045001.

Rutkowski, T.M., Mori, H. (2015). Tactile and bone-conduction auditory brain computer interface for vision and hearing impaired users. *Journal of Neuroscience Methods*, 244, 45–51. DOI: 10.1016/j.jneumeth.2014.04.010.

Saetang, J., Punsawad, Y., Wongsawat, Y. (2013). Real-time hybrid SSSEP-MI based brain computer interface system for upper limb rehabilitation. *I-CREATe 2013—International Convention on Rehabilitation Engineering and Assistive Technology, in Conjunction with SENDEX 2013*.

Schreuder, M., Thurlings, M.E., Brouwer, A.-M., Van Erp, J.B.F. Tangermann, M. (2012). Exploring the use of tactile feedback in an ERP-based auditory BCI. *Proceedings of the Annual International Conference of the IEEE Engineering in Medicine and Biology Society, EMBS*, art. no. 6347533, pp. 6707–6710.

Severens, M., Farquhar, J., Duysens, J., Desain, P. (2013). A multi-signature brain–computer interface: Use of transient and steady-state responses. *Journal of Neural Engineering*, 10 (2), art. no. 026005.

Severens, M., Van der Waal, M., Farquhar, J., Desain, P. (2014). Comparing tactile and visual gaze-independent brain–computer interfaces in patients with amyotrophic lateral sclerosis and healthy users. *Clinical Neurophysiology*, 125 (11), 2297–2304. DOI: 10.1016/j.clinph.2014.03.005.

Shimizu, K., Mori, H., Makino, S., Rutkowski, T.M. (2014). Tactile pressure brain–computer interface using point matrix pattern paradigm. *2014 Joint 7th International Conference on Soft Computing and Intelligent Systems, SCIS 2014 and 15th International Symposium on Advanced Intelligent Systems, ISIS 2014*, art. no. 7044756, pp. 473–477. DOI: 10.1109/SCIS-ISIS.2014.7044756.

Silvoni, S., Konicar, L., Prats-Sedano, M.A., Garcia-Cossio, E., Genna, C., Volpato, C., Cavinato, M., Paggiaro, A., Veser, S., De Massari, D., Birbaumer, N. (2016). Tactile event-related potentials in amyotrophic lateral sclerosis (ALS): Implications for brain–computer interface. *Clinical Neurophysiology*, 127 (1), 936–945. DOI: 10.1016/j.clinph.2015.06.029.

Smith, D.J., Varghese, L.A., Stepp, C.E., Guenther, F.H. (2014). Comparison of steady-state visual and somatosensory evoked potentials for brain–computer interface control. *36th Annual International Conference of the IEEE Engineering in Medicine and Biology Society, EMBC 2014*, art. no. 6943820, pp. 1234–1237. DOI: 10.1109/EMBC.2014.6943820.

Thurlings, M.E., Brouwer, A.-M., van Erp, J.B.F., Blankertz, B. & Werkhoven, P.J. (2012a). Does bimodal stimulus presentation increase ERP components usable in BCIs? *Journal of Neural Engineering*, 9 (4), 045005. DOI:10.1088/1741-2560/9/4/045005.

Thurlings, M.E., Brouwer, A.-M., van Erp, J.B.F., Werkhoven, P. (2014). Gaze-independent ERP-BCIs: Augmenting performance through location-congruent bimodal stimuli. *Frontiers in Systems Neuroscience*, 8 (SEP), art. no. 143. DOI: 10.3389/fnsys.2014.00143.

Thurlings, M.E., Van Erp, J.B.F., Brouwer, A.-M., Blankertz, B. Werkhoven, P.J. (2012b). Control-display mapping in brain–computer interfaces. *Ergonomics*, 55 (5), 1–17. DOI:10.1080/00140139.2012.661085.

Thurlings, M.E., Van Erp, J.B.F., Brouwer, A.-M., Werkhoven, P. (2013). Controlling a tactile ERP-BCI in a dual task. *IEEE Transactions on Computational Intelligence and AI in Games*, 5 (2), art. no. 6461930, pp. 129–140. DOI: 10.1109/TCIAIG.2013.2239294.

Valbo, Å.B., Olausson, H., Wessberg, J., Kakuda, N. (1995). Receptive field characteristics of tactile units with myelinated afferents in hairy skin of human subjects. *Journal of Physiology*, 483 (3), 783–795.

Van der Waal, M., Severens, M., Geuze, J., Desain, P. (2012). Introducing the tactile speller: An ERP-based brain–computer interface for communication. *Journal of Neural Engineering*, 9 045002.

Van Erp, J.B.F. (2002). Guidelines for the use of vibro-tactile displays in human computer interaction. *Proceedings of Eurohaptics*, 2002, 18–22.

Van Erp, J.B.F. (2007). Tactile displays for navigation and orientation: Perception and behavior. Utrecht University, The Netherlands.

Van Erp, J.B.F., Brouwer, A.-M. (2014). Touch-based brain computer interfaces: State of the art. *IEEE Haptics Symposium, HAPTICS*, art. no. 6775488, pp. 397–401. DOI: 10.1109/HAPTICS.2014.6775488.

Van Erp, J.B.F., Brouwer, A.M., Aloise, F., Cincotti, F. (2008). Navigation BCI based on touch evoked potentials. *Revista Espagnola de Neuropsicologia*, 10 (1), 89.

Van Erp, J.B.F., Brouwer, A.-M., Zander, T.O. (2015). Editorial: Using neurophysiological signals that reflect cognitive or affective state. *Frontiers in Neuroscience*, 9, 00193.

Van Erp, J.B.F., Lotte, F., Tangermann, M. (2012). Brain–computer interfaces: Beyond medical applications. *IEEE Computer*, 45 (4), 26–34.

Van Erp, J.B.F., Thurlings, M.E., Brouwer, A.-M., Werkhoven, P.J. (2011). BCIs in multimodal interaction and multitask environments: Theoretical issues and initial guidelines. HCI International. In: Stephanidis, C. (Ed.), *Universal Access in Human–Computer Interaction. Users Diversity*. LNCS6766, pp. 610–619. Berlin/Heidelberg: Springer.

Van Erp, J.B.F., Werkhoven, P.J., Thurlings, M.E., Brouwer, A.-M. (2009). Navigation with a passive brain based interface. *ICMI-MLMI'09—Proceedings of the International Conference on Multimodal Interfaces and the Workshop on Machine Learning for Multimodal Interfaces*, pp. 225–226. DOI: 10.1145/1647314.1647357.

Wilson, J.A., Walton, L.M., Tyler, M., Williams, J. (2012) Lingual electrotactile stimulation as an alternative sensory feedback pathway for brain–computer interface applications. *Journal of Neural Engineering*, 9 (4), art. no. 045007.

Yao, L., Meng, J., Zhang, D., Sheng, X., Zhu, X. (2013a). Selective sensation based brain–computer interface via mechanical vibrotactile stimulation. *PLoS ONE*, 8 (6), art. no. e64784. DOI: 10.1371/journal .pone.0064784.

Yao, L., Sheng, X., Meng, J., Zhang, D., Zhu, X. (2013b). Mechanical vibrotactile stimulation effect in motor imagery based brain–computer interface. *Annual International Conference of the IEEE Engineering in Medicine and Biology Society*, 2013, pp. 2772–2775. DOI: 10.1109/EMBC.2013.6610115.

Yin, E., Zeyl, T., Saab, R., Hu, D., Zhou, Z., Chau, T. (2016). An auditory–tactile visual saccade-independent P300 brain–computer interface. *International Journal of Neural Systems*, 26 (1), art. no. 1650001. DOI: 10.1142/S0129065716500015.

Zander, T.O., Kothe, C. (2011). Towards passive brain–computer interfaces: Applying brain–computer interface technology to human–machine systems in general. *Journal of Neural Engineering*, 8, 025005.

Zander, T.O., Kothe, C., Welke, S. Rötting, M. (2008). Enhancing human–machine systems with secondary input from passive brain–computer interfaces. *Proc. of the 4th Int. BCI Workshop & Training Course, Graz, Austria*, 2008. Graz University of Technology Publishing House.

Zhang, D., Wang, Y., Maye, A., Engel, A.K., Gao, X., Hong, B., Gao, S. (2007). A brain–computer interface based on multi-modal attention. *Proceedings of the 3rd International IEEE EMBS Conference on Neural Engineering*, art. no. 4227302, pp. 414–417.

# Part II

---

*Signal Acquisition and Open Source Platform in BCI*

# 14 Utilizing Subdermal Electrodes as a Noninvasive Alternative for Motor-Based BCIs

*Melissa M. Smith, Jared D. Olson,*
*Felix Darvas, and Rajesh P.N. Rao*

## CONTENTS

14.1 Introduction .................................................................................................. 270
14.2 Materials and Methods .................................................................................. 270
    14.2.1 Subjects ................................................................................................ 270
    14.2.2 Electrodes and Electrode Placement .................................................... 270
    14.2.3 Task ...................................................................................................... 271
    14.2.4 Data Acquisition .................................................................................. 272
    14.2.5 Data Preprocessing .............................................................................. 272
        14.2.5.1 Comparing Mu, Beta, and High Gamma Band Power Changes
                 in Subdermal and Surface Electrode Recordings ..................... 272
        14.2.5.2 Comparing Magnitude Squared Coherence between Subdermal
                 and Surface Electrode Recordings ............................................ 272
14.3 Results ............................................................................................................ 273
    14.3.1 Comparison of Low- and High-Frequency Band Power Changes in Subdermal
         and Surface Electrode Recordings ....................................................... 273
    14.3.2 Comparison of Magnitude Squared Coherence between Subdermal
         and Surface Electrode Recordings ....................................................... 274
14.4 Discussion ...................................................................................................... 275
References ............................................................................................................. 276

**Abstract**

Continuous, long-term scalp electroenchephalogram (EEG) monitoring of brain activity is difficult to perform on awake, ambulatory patients because of increased artifacts from muscles and electronic interference, as well as frequent electrode replacement over time. Prior research has shown that subdermal wire electrodes placed below the scalp maintain good recording characteristics with stable impedances for long-term monitoring of EEG signals. This chapter provides evidence that an implanted subdermal recording electrode system may provide a reliable, long-term, portable method for recording motor-related signals from the brain. This chapter outlines a study that found that neural recordings that used subdermal electrodes were comparable to those of scalp surface recordings, particularly in the low-frequency bands (8–30 Hz). The coherence results indicate that there appears to be mutual information between the subdermal and surface electrode signals in the low-frequency signal, but many of signals in the higher frequencies (>40 Hz) may be unique to each surface and subdermal electrode. These results further support the idea that an implantable subdermal electrode system may provide reliable, long-term motor control signals for brain–computer interface control.

## 14.1 INTRODUCTION

Long-term electroenchephalogram (EEG) monitoring is useful for monitoring physiological changes in brain function, such as epileptic seizures, as well as changes in brain signals that can be used to control brain–computer interface (BCI) devices. However, continuous, long-term EEG monitoring is difficult to perform on awake, ambulatory patients because of increased artifacts from muscles and electronic interference. Current surface EEG systems require continuous supervision with frequent electrode readjustments to acquire quality data over extended periods of time (days to months). In addition, common artifacts generated by these recording systems during movement can lead to misleading clinical diagnosis and suboptimal control signals for BCI systems. An implanted, stable, subdermal electrode system could provide the high-fidelity signals necessary for the long-term control of a BCI device (Leuthardt et al. 2004; Ojemann et al. 2007; Wang et al. 2013).

Prior research has shown that subdermal wire electrodes maintain good recording characteristics with stable impedances for long-term monitoring of EEG signals (Martz et al. 2009). In addition, subdermal wire electrodes have been found to be less susceptible to artifacts than surface electrodes (Young et al. 2006). A study comparing the alpha attenuation over the occipital lobe during eye closure in an implanted subcutaneous system to a surface EEG system found the recordings of both systems to be similar (Duun-Henriksen et al. 2015). The investigators also concluded that the subcutaneous recording system provides a stable signal with long-term use (26 days). Subdermal electrodes have also been used by clinicians in the intensive care unit (Ives 2005; Vulliemoz et al. 2009), in healthcare settings (Schneider 2006), as well as for extended monitoring (Martz et al. 2009).

Research comparing subgaleal and electrocorticography (ECoG) recordings have shown that neural signals outside of the skull are attenuated linearly and can be recorded up to 110 Hz (Olson et al. 2015). Their study indicated that subgaleal electrodes could record high gamma (HG; 70–110 Hz) signals without frequency distortion from the skull. In addition, Olson et al. (2017) have reported activity-dependent changes in beta and HG frequency bands recorded with subdermal electrodes during the same finger-tapping task outlined in this chapter. They observed decreases in the beta frequency band power (12–30 Hz) over motor areas of the cortex that preceded and coincided with movement. In addition, they were able to spatially localize high gamma activity that preceded movement by implementing a spatial beamformer over all subjects to increase the signal-to-noise ratio (SNR) of the HG band.

The aim of this study was to investigate the motor-related brain activity of healthy subjects in the mu (8–12 Hz), beta (12–30 Hz), and high gamma (70–110 Hz) frequency bands recorded using subdermal EEG electrodes. Cortical activity was recorded over the motor regions of the cortex while healthy subjects participated in a finger-tapping task. To assess the quality of these subdermal recordings, they were compared to recordings performed simultaneously using surface EEG electrodes. This study found that neural recordings using subdermal electrodes were comparable to those of surface recordings, and thus these subdermally detected motor-related brain signals may prove to be used for the development of BCIs that can be used reliably for long-term outpatient use.

## 14.2 MATERIALS AND METHODS

### 14.2.1 SUBJECTS

Data were recorded from eight healthy subjects who provided their informed consent according to the protocol approved by the Institutional Review Board at the University of Washington.

### 14.2.2 ELECTRODES AND ELECTRODE PLACEMENT

To detect movement onset, surface electromyography (EMG) electrodes were placed over the forearm flexor with reference and ground electrodes placed on bony prominences at the wrist to minimize electrocardiogram artifacts.

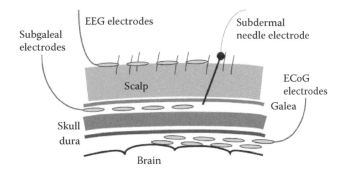

**FIGURE 14.1** Schematic of subdermal needle electrode depths relative to other common recording locations and relevant layers of anatomy. Not to scale. (Adapted from Olson, J.D., Wander, J.D., Johnson, L., Sarma, D., Weaver, K., Novotny, E.J., Ojemann, J.G., Darvas, F. 2015. Comparison of subdural and subgaleal recordings of cortical high gamma activity in humans. *Clinical Neurophysiology.* International Federation of Clinical Neurophysiology. doi:10.1016/j.clinph.2015.03.014.)

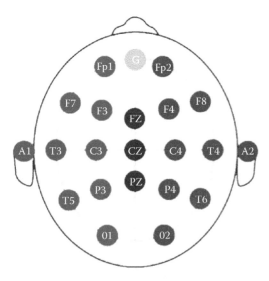

**FIGURE 14.2** Location of needle electrodes relative to the accepted 10–20 EEG system. Electrodes were placed around C3/C4, with one reference at Cz and one ground at G.

Using a clean technique, bare-metal FDA-approved subdermal needle electrodes (Rochester Electro-Medical, Lutz, Florida) were placed at the bone–scalp interface depicted in Figure 14.1, with two electrodes around C3/C4, one reference at Cz, and one ground at G using the standard scalp EEG 10–20 system (Niedermeyer and Lopes da Silva 2004) as in Figure 14.2. Surface electrodes were placed directly above subcutaneous electrodes. Subcutaneous electrodes were placed directly under the surface electrodes. Electrode pairs were placed approximately 1 inch apart from each other.

### 14.2.3 TASK

Subjects were cued to move either their left or right forefinger once per trial. Subjects were seated in a recliner and four blocks of 25 right- and 25 left-hand trials were recorded (only left-hand trials were recorded and executed from Subject 2), totaling 100 trials per hand. The subjects had their eyes open and fixated on a cross or cue. Each trial consisted of a rest period of 2 s, during which a fixation cross was shown. At the end of that rest period, the fixation cross was changed to a written instruction, which indicated either "right" for right finger movement or "left" for left finger movement. The cue was shown for 3 s and then changed back to a fixation cross, which concluded the trial. During each block, "left" and "right" cues were presented in random order, for a total of 50 cues per block.

### 14.2.4 DATA ACQUISITION

Surface and subdermal EEG data were continuously recorded during each block. Data were sampled at 1200 Hz using two GugerTec (GugerTec, Graz, Austria) EEG amplifiers recorded in DC from −250 to +250 mV. Impedance values were below 20 kΩ for all subdermal and surface electrodes. In parallel, EMG activity was recorded at the same sampling rate from the flexor indices from both hands. Data were high pass filtered at 2 Hz using an eighth-order Butterworth filter, as well as notch filtered from 58 to 62 Hz using a fourth-order Butterworth filter to remove any line noise.

### 14.2.5 DATA PREPROCESSING

Trials were inspected for artifacts (excessive EMG, eye blinks, etc.) and rejected if any channels showed artifact contamination. Both surface and subdermal EEG data were re-referenced to a common average reference to eliminate any common noise introduced by activity recorded at the reference electrode. Data were then segmented from continuously recorded EEG data into 5-s-long segments for each block, with time 0 s centered at the onset of movement (detected by EMG), resulting in a within-trial axis ranging from −2 to 3 s (rest being between −2 and 0 s).

#### 14.2.5.1 Comparing Mu, Beta, and High Gamma Band Power Changes in Subdermal and Surface Electrode Recordings

In order to compare the strength of the signals recorded with subdermal versus surface electrodes, power spectra were generated using a windowed fast Fourier transform (FFT). Specifically, a hanning window was applied to each trial, and FFT and squared absolute value were then computed. These results were then averaged over all trials. Data were divided into rest (−1.5 to −0.5 s) and movement (0 to 1 s) periods. The spectra were normalized by dividing by the mean power across all trials at each frequency and the log of the values were determined. To determine the degree of separation in the low-frequency (mu/beta; 8–30 Hz) and high-frequency (70–100 Hz) band powers between rest and movement tasks, the area between the curves in each corresponding frequency range was calculated.

#### 14.2.5.2 Comparing Magnitude Squared Coherence between Subdermal and Surface Electrode Recordings

To determine the similarity between subdermal and surface electrode recordings, the magnitude squared coherence spectrum was calculated for movement states. The coherence spectrum was computed using Welch's averaged periodogram method (a function of the power spectral densities $P_{xx}(f)$, $P_{yy}(f)$, and the cross power spectral density, $P_{xy}(f)$):

$$C_{xy}(f) = \frac{\left| P_{xy}(f) \right|^2}{P_{xx}(f) \cdot P_{yy}(f)} \tag{14.1}$$

## 14.3  RESULTS

### 14.3.1  COMPARISON OF LOW- AND HIGH-FREQUENCY BAND POWER CHANGES IN SUBDERMAL AND SURFACE ELECTRODE RECORDINGS

We found that the power spectra of subdermal electrodes provide similar signals to those of surface electrodes. Current motor-based BCIs typically rely on the change in spectral power in the low- or high-frequency ranges, and in order to assess the degree of differentiation of the change in spectral band powers during a movement task, power spectra during rest and movement periods were compared. Two frequency bands were considered: the low-frequency band (mu/beta; 8–30 Hz) and the high-frequency band (70–100 Hz). Figures 14.3 and 14.4 show that the subcutaneous electrodes provide similar differentiation between rest and movement periods, in each of the designated frequency bands, when compared to surface electrodes recorded simultaneously. Table 14.1 shows a comparison between the areas between the movement and rest power spectra.

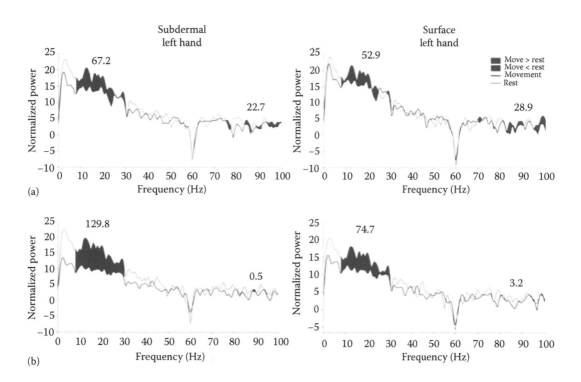

**FIGURE 14.3**  A comparison of power spectral densities for subdermal and surface recordings during rest and left-hand movement periods recorded from electrode pairs 2 (a) and 4 (b). Spectra are for recordings over C4. Blue power spectra are representative of the normalized power over frequencies 3–100 Hz during the rest period (−1.5 to −0.5 s before movement onset). Red power spectra are representative of the normalized power over the same frequency range during the movement period (0 to 1 s, with 0 s being the onset of movement). Blue fill between rest and movement power spectra represents the area between the two curves in the low-frequency band of 8–30 Hz. Red fill between rest and movement power spectra represents the area between the two curves in the high-frequency band of 70–100 Hz. Numerical values above each of the low- and high-frequency bands indicate the value of the area between the two curves in each frequency range.

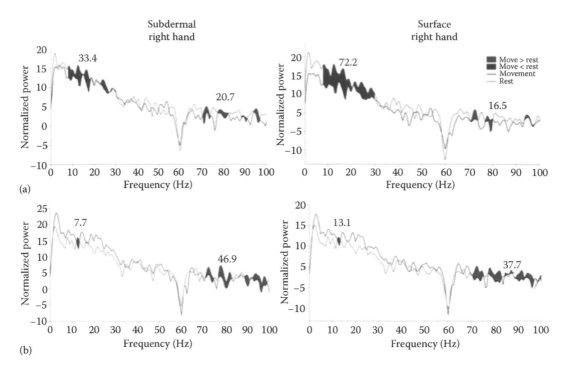

**FIGURE 14.4** A comparison of power spectral densities for subdermal and surface recordings during rest and right-hand movement periods recorded from electrode pairs 1 (a) and 3 (b). Spectra are for recordings over C4. Blue power spectra are representative of the normalized power over frequencies 3–100 Hz during the rest period (−1.5 to −0.5 s before movement onset). Red power spectra are representative of the normalized power over the same frequency range during the movement period (0 to 1 s, with 0 s being the onset of movement). Blue fill between rest and movement power spectra represents the area between the two curves in the low-frequency band of 8–30 Hz. Red fill between rest and movement power spectra represents the area between the two curves in the high-frequency band of 70–100 Hz. Numerical values above each of the low- and high-frequency bands indicate the value of the area between the two curves in each frequency range.

**TABLE 14.1**

**Area between Movement and Rest Power Spectra in Low-Frequency (8–32 Hz) and High-Frequency (70–100 Hz) Bands**

| Location/Pair # | Low Frequency (8–32 Hz) | | High Frequency (70–100 Hz) | |
|---|---|---|---|---|
| | Subdermal | Surface | Subdermal | Surface |
| C3/1 | 33.4 | 72.2 | 20.7 | 16.5 |
| C3/2 | 7.7 | 13.1 | 46.9 | 37.7 |
| C4/3 | 67.2 | 52.9 | 22.7 | 29.0 |
| C4/4 | 129.8 | 74.7 | 0.5 | 3.2 |

## 14.3.2 COMPARISON OF MAGNITUDE SQUARED COHERENCE BETWEEN SUBDERMAL AND SURFACE ELECTRODE RECORDINGS

To assess the similarities between the signals recorded from subdermal and surface electrodes, the magnitude squared coherence spectrum between each electrode pair was computed. The coherence spectra in Figure 14.5 show that the lower frequencies (<30 Hz) in each electrode pair have greater coherence than the higher frequencies (2–30 Hz). These coherence results indicate that there

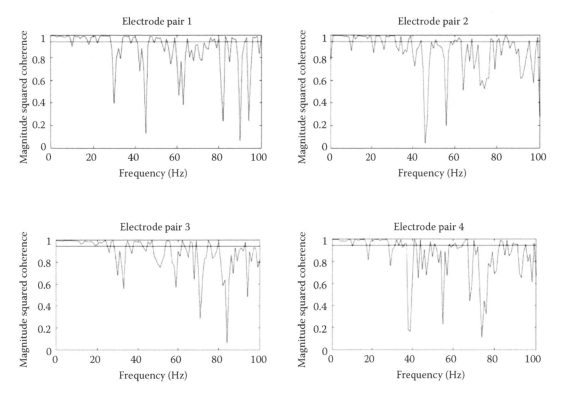

**FIGURE 14.5** Magnitude squared coherence spectrum of electrode pairs 1–4 over C3 during right-hand movements and C4 during left-hand movements. Black line indicates 95% confidence interval.

appears to be mutual information between the subdermal and surface electrode signals in the low-frequency signals, but many of signals in the higher frequencies may be unique to each surface and subdermal electrode.

## 14.4 DISCUSSION

The goal of this study was to characterize the movement-related cortical signals recorded over the motor cortex using subdermal EEG electrodes. Brain signals were recorded over the contralateral motor cortex while healthy subjects performed a finger-tapping task. Our analysis focused on frequency bands that are frequently used for motor-related BCI control signals (mu, beta, and high gamma). Overall, the signals recorded using subdermal needle electrodes were found to be comparable to those recorded simultaneously with surface EEG electrodes.

The spectral and coherence analyses showed that subdermal and surface recording electrodes provide very similar signals, especially in the low-frequency bands. Considering that the degree of separation between the power in the low-frequency bands during rest and movement in subdermal recordings is similar to that of surface recordings, these results further support the idea that an implantable subdermal electrode system may be able to provide reliable, long-term motor control signals for BCI control.

Several limitations of this study should be noted. The first limitation being that sources of noise could have been introduced owing to the instability of the electrode connections to the skin or from induced currents owing to movement of the electrodes. These sources of noise may be reduced and the SNR of the system could be improved if the subdermal electrodes are fully implanted with a rigid connection. Second, because high gamma band activity is spatially focal on the cortex compared to the beta band activity, it is possible that our single electrode placements could have missed the cortical location of high gamma band activity. Using a high-density electrode array could potentially improve the SNR in the high gamma band. Third, in order to determine the usefulness of subdermally driven BCI, real-time control of a BCI using these motor-related signals needs to be studied. Last, in order to provide reliable, long-term monitoring and BCI control, the subdermal recording device must provide a high SNR with little data loss with long-term use. An extension of this work could assess the fidelity of the signals in longitudinal studies.

This research was based on the knowledge that electrodes placed closer to the brain provide greater signal than those that are placed further away on top of the scalp. As a general rule, the amplitude of recorded brain signals decreases proportionally to the inverse square of the distance from the source. Therefore, ECoG electrodes provide a signal that is many degrees of magnitude larger than the signal recorded from surface EEG electrodes. However, ECoG electrodes are considered invasive, as they require surgery to place the electrodes on the surface of the brain. Subdermal electrodes placed below the scalp may provide an intermediate option in regard to the degree of invasiveness and signal quality when compared to surface EEG electrodes. Several studies have shown that subdermal electrodes enhance the precision and accuracy of EEG measurements compared to scalp EEG electrodes (Wendel et al. 2010; Subramaniyam et al. 2011). The data analysis outlined in this chapter was intended to determine the capacity to record brain signals with subdermal electrodes, focusing on characterizing the movement-related cortical signals that are relevant to BCI research recorded over the motor cortex. Our results show that the motor-related signals recorded with subdermal electrodes are comparable to scalp EEG electrodes. While the intent of the data analysis did not include a comparison of the SNR between subdermal and scalp EEG electrodes, our results, in conjunction with previous studies showing an improved SNR in subdermal electrodes when compared to scalp EEG electrodes (Subramaniyam et al. 2011; Wendel et al. 2010), show that subdermal electrodes may provide an intermediate option between scalp and ECoG electrodes when studying motor-related brain signals. While invasive recordings such as ECoG still provide a greater SNR than subdermal electrodes, it is possible that the SNR of the subdermal system could be improved if the subdermal electrodes were fully implanted with a rigid connection. In addition, a fully implanted subcutaneous system with wireless telemetry could provide a long-term option for a BCI device or clinical monitoring.

## REFERENCES

Duun-Henriksen, J., Kjaer, T.W., Looney, D., Atkins, M.D., Sørensen, J.A., Rose, M., Mandic, D.P., Madsen, R.E., Juhl, C.B., 2015. EEG signal quality of a subcutaneous recording system compared to standard surface electrodes. *Journal of Sensors* 2015, 1–9. doi:10.1155/2015/341208.

Ives, J.R., 2005. New chronic EEG electrode for critical/intensive care unit monitoring. *J Clin Neurophysiol* 22, 119–123.

Leuthardt, E.C., Schalk, G., Wolpaw, J.R., Ojemann, J.G., Moran, D.W., 2004. A brain–computer interface using electrocorticographic signals in humans. *J Neural Eng* 1, 63–71. 10.1088/1741-2560/1/2/001

Martz, G.U., Hucek, C., Quigg, M., 2009. Sixty day continuous use of subdermal wire electrodes for EEG monitoring during treatment of status epilepticus. *Neurocritical Care* 11 (2), 223–227. doi:10.1007/s12028-009-9215-y.

Niedermeyer, E., Lopes da Silva, F., 2004. *Electroencephalography: Basic Principles, Clinical Applications, and Related Fields.*

Ojemann, J.G., Leuthardt, E.C., Miller, K.J., 2007. Brain–machine interface: Restoring neurological function through bioengineering. *Clin Neurosurg* 54, 134–136.

Olson, J.D., Wander, J.D., Darvas, F., 2017. Demonstration of motor-related beta and high gamma brain signals in subdermal electroencephalography recordings. *Clinical Neurophysiology: Official Journal of the International Federation of Clinical Neurophysiology*, 128(3), 395–396.

Olson, J.D., Wander, J.D., Johnson, L., Sarma, D., Weaver, K., Novotny, E.J., Ojemann, J.G., Darvas, F. 2015. Comparison of subdural and subgaleal recordings of cortical high-gamma activity in humans. *Clinical Neurophysiology*. International Federation of Clinical Neurophysiology. doi:10.1016/j.clinph.2015.03.014.

Schneider, A.L., 2006. Subdermal needle electrodes: An option for emergency ("stat") EEGs. *Am J Electroneurodiagnostic Technol* 46, 363–368.

Subramaniyam, N.P., Wendel, K., Joutsen, A., Hyttinen, J., 2011. Investigating the measurement capability of densely-distributed subdermal EEG electrodes. *2011 8th International Symposium on Noninvasive Functional Source Imaging of the Brain and Heart and the 2011 8th International Conference on Bioelectromagnetism, NFSI and ICBEM 2011* 0 (3), 109–13. doi:10.1109/NFSI.2011.5936830.

Vulliemoz, S., Perrig, S., Pellise, D., Vargas, M.I., Gasche, Y., Ives, J.R., Seeck, M., 2009. Imaging compatible electrodes for continuous electroencephalogram monitoring in the intensive care unit. *J Clin Neurophysiol* 26, 236–243. 10.1097/WNP.0b013e3181af1c95

Wang, W., Collinger, J.L., Degenhart, A.D., Tyler-Kabara, E.C., Schwartz, A.B., Moran, D.W., Weber, D.J., Wodlinger, B., Vinjamuri, R.K., Ashmore, R.C., Kelly, J.W., Boninger, M.L., 2013. An electrocorticographic brain interface in an individual with tetraplegia. *PloS one* 8, e55344. 10.1371/journal.pone.0055344

Wendel, K., Väisänen, J., Seemann, G., Hyttinen, J., Malmivuo, J., 2010. The influence of age and skull conductivity on surface and subdermal bipolar EEG leads. *Computational Intelligence and Neuroscience* 2010. doi:10.1155/2010/397272.

Young, G.B., Ives, J.R., Chapman, M.G., Mirsattari, S.M., 2006. A comparison of subdermal wire electrodes with collodion-applied disk electrodes in long-term EEG recordings in ICU. *Clinical Neurophysiology: Official Journal of the International Federation of Clinical Neurophysiology* 117(6), 1376–1379. doi:10.1016/j.clinph.2006.02.006.

# 15 Validation of Neurotrophic Electrode Long-Term Recordings in Human Cortex


*Philip R. Kennedy, Dinal S. Andreasen,*
*Jess Bartels, Princewill Ehirim, Edward Joe Wright,*
*Steven Seibert, and Andre Joel Cervantes*

## CONTENTS

15.1 Introduction ...................................................................................................279
15.2 Methods .......................................................................................................280
15.3 Results..........................................................................................................280
15.4 Four Years after Implantation.....................................................................283
15.5 Nine Years after Implantation ....................................................................286
15.6 Functional Studies at Year 9 ......................................................................289
15.7 Discussion....................................................................................................292
References.............................................................................................................293
Glossary ...............................................................................................................294
Acknowledgments................................................................................................295
Institutional Review Board Approval ..................................................................295
Federal Drug Administration Approval................................................................295
Conflicts of Interest.............................................................................................295

**Abstract**

The development of a reliable neural interface is essential for lifetime cortical control of prosthetic devices such as robotic arms, paralyzed limbs, or speech. Standard tine or wire electrodes are not long lasting, surviving a few years with very few remaining useful signals. The neurotrophic electrode engages radically different methodology that allows the brain's neuropil to grow into the electrode tip. Successful anchoring of the electrode tip within the neuropil has resulted in functionally usable single-unit recordings for over a decade. Tine- and wire-type electrodes lose units over months and years unlike the neurotrophic electrode described here. These data demonstrate that stable recordings can be accomplished in humans by *allowing neuropil to grow into the electrode, rather than by inserting the electrode into the neuropil.* This is the first electrode methodology to produce such long-lasting signals that remain functional for over a decade.

## 15.1 INTRODUCTION

For the development of long-term neural prosthetics that require cortical control signals, it is essential to develop an electrode that can continuously record these cortical signals over the lifetime of the subject. Over the past several decades, different types of long-term electrodes have been developed. Tine-type electrodes (Rousche and Normann 1998), wire electrodes (Presacco et al. 2011), and many other electrode types (Ward et al. 2009) have successfully recorded signals for months or years. However, signal quality declines gradually, with only 43% of electrodes producing usable single-unit recordings at 3 years with the Utah array (Simeral et al. 2011) and with only 15% of signals remaining in humans (from 96 original signals) (Hochberg et al. 2011). These signal losses did result in serious degradation of function (Perge et al. 2013) though some function remained (Hochberg et al. 2011). Over the past decade, major efforts have been undertaken to understand the factors that lead to loss of signal. These factors include micro-movements that result in fluctuating signal amplitudes and glial scars that separate the recording tip from the recorded neurons resulting in loss or destructive degradation of the signal. Despite extensive efforts, satisfactory solutions for these problems remain elusive (Ward et al. 2009).

A different approach to chronic recordings of brain signals began in 1986. Instead of inserting an electrode into the brain's neuropil, the neuropil is grown into the hollow, cone-shaped, glass tip of a coiled wire electrode (Kennedy 1989). This tip is impregnated with trophic factors to induce growth into the tip. In the weeks and months following insertion, the neural tissue grows into and through the 2-mm glass tip forming a bridge of neuropil. This anchors the electrode within the cortex (Bartels et al. 2008). This chapter focuses on the longevity of this type of electrode in humans. It describes and references how it is constructed and provides tests of impedance, quality of signals, and function of signal over the 10 years in the, so far, longest surviving implant.

## 15.2 METHODS

Assembly of the electrode has been described in great detail previously (Bartels et al. 2008). Briefly, the 2-mm glass conical-shaped tip contains two to eight 2-mil Teflon-insulated gold wires that record the axonal firings of the ingrown neurites. As shown in Figure 15.1a, the wires are first coiled for strain relief and then bent appropriately to produce a shelf that lies along the surface of the cortex to prevent too deep a penetration (Bartels et al. 2008). The tip consists of a glass pipette drawn to produce a tip diameter of 25 to 50 μm, and an upper opening several hundred microns in diameter that provides space for placement of the recording wires. As many as seven wires have been placed within the glass cone secured with methyl methacrylate glue (Figure 15.1b) (Bartels et al. 2008). The wire tips are spaced several hundred microns apart. During human surgery, after placement of the (proprietary) growth factors, the 5-mm-long tip (measured from the angle of the wire) is inserted at a 45° angle to reach the layer 5 corticospinal tract neurons in motor cortex (Figure 15.1c). The trophic factors are drawn into the glass tip by capillary action. Then, the tip is left to dry so the factors are mainly on the inside of the glass tip. After insertion, the factors diffuse into the neuropil.

For recordings in humans, a power-inducted pair of amplifiers (typical gain ×800, band pass 5 to 5000 Hz) are implanted above the skull under the scalp, connected to the electrode, and secured to the skull with acrylic cement. The amplified neural signals are transmitted through the scalp using a frequency-modulated transmitter operating in the 42 ± 8 MHz range for external processing (Kennedy et al. 1992b). During the recording sessions, the power induction coil and the FM receiving coils are secured to the scalp, using EEG paste to provide stability (Figure 15.1g). The demodulated signals are passed through CWE amplifiers (Ardmore, PA; 20× gain, band pass filtered 3–10 kHz). After A/D conversion, the digital filters are set at 300 Hz to 6 KHz for single units and 1 Hz to 6 KHz for continuous recordings. Trauma to the electronics due to handling of the head during hygiene has led to replacement of the units. The electrodes have never needed replacement. The electronic units are protected by Elvax and Silastic for insulation and trauma protection. The recording electronics are totally passive, contain no batteries, and are not used for stimulation, so there is so danger of electrical discharge.

## 15.3 RESULTS

Following implantation under full sterile protocol, neurites are induced to grow into the tip from layers 5 and upper layers 2 and 3 where interneurons reside. Growth into the tip begins within a

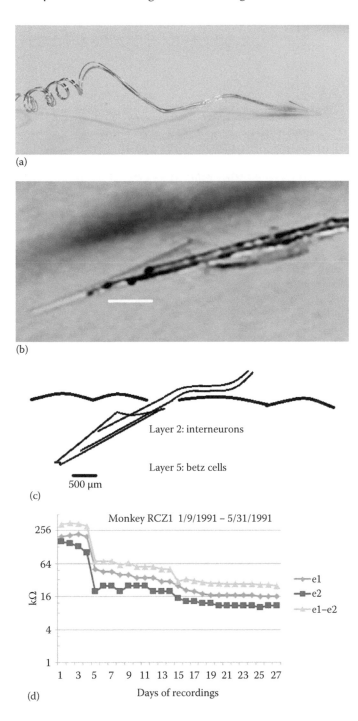

**FIGURE 15.1** Neurotrophic electrode design and characteristics. (a) Two-mil, Teflon-insulated coiled gold wires are shown on the left of the figure with the 5-mm shelf of wire that limits implantation depth, and to the right, the glass tip. (b) The glass tip contains four gold wires whose black shadowed tips are visible. The calibration bar is 500 µm. (c) The 5- to 6-mm-long tip is inserted into the cortex at a 45° angle to reach the corticospinal tract layer. Trophic factors encourage neurites to grow into and through the tip, thus anchoring it within the neuropil. (d) Impedances remain stable over months as measured in early monkey recordings. e1 and e2 refer to the wires inside the glass cone with recordings referred to a ground electrode on the rat's skull. e1–e2 refers to impedance measurements between e1 and e2. *(Continued)*

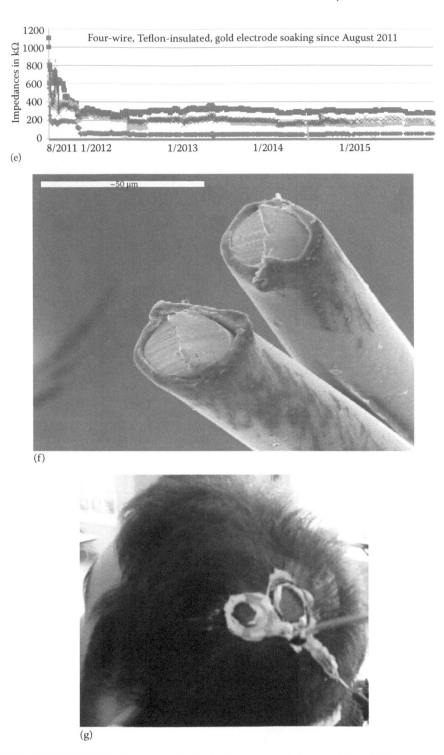

(e)

(f)

(g)

**FIGURE 15.1 (CONTINUED)**   Neurotrophic electrode design and characteristics. (e) Impedances in saline remain stable over 4 years so far. Note the initial drop in impedance for both in vivo and in vitro measurements. (f) Electron-microscopic images of the Teflon coating near the tips demonstrating the peeling back of the Teflon that may explain the drop in impedances. (g) Recordings are obtained from implanted wireless systems transmitted using FM carriers. The receiving coils are temporarily fixed to the scalp using water-soluble EEG paste. Power is provided by induction via a coil on the opposite side of the head (not seen).

week or two (Kennedy 1989) and it takes as long as 3 months before signals stabilize. Control placements of electrodes without the trophic factors in rats resulted in no recordings (Kennedy 1989).

Histological analysis of the tissue inside the recording tip has shown that there is normal neuropil except for the lack of neurons. Non-myelinated axons appear during the first few weeks and myelinated axons are abundant after 3 weeks. Blood vessels and axo-dendritic synapses are seen, but no microglial cells (that would indicate gliosis are found) and no gliosis is seen. These results have been described and illustrated in detail (Kennedy et al. 1992b). Stable impedances seen after several months coincide with signal stability as shown in Figure 15.1d for recordings in primates. After an initial drop in impedance, signals from this animal and others were stable and functional, being related to arm movements throughout the nearly 6 months of study (Kennedy et al. 1992a; Kennedy and Bakay 1997). We have seen an initial similar gradual drop in impedance with the four-wire electrode tested in saline over 4 years as shown in Figure 15.1e (still stable after 5.5 years). The initial reduced impedance is attributed to retraction of the Teflon insulation of the recording wires as shown (Figure 15.1f). Impedance measurements in humans during follow-on surgery for replacing the implanted electronics revealed impedances of 70 to 100 k$\Omega$ similar to non-human primate measurements A photo of ER's two recording coils are shown in Figure 15.1g. The white substance is water-soluble EEG paste used to attach and stabilize the coils.

## 15.4 FOUR YEARS AFTER IMPLANTATION

Recording stability over long time periods is addressed by the following data. The two channels of continuous recordings shown in Figure 15.2a are from the same subject (ER). This subject is "locked-in" following a brainstem stroke at age 16. He was implanted in December 2004. His electrode has three wires inside the cone, the center wire acting as reference for the other two, thus creating two bipolar recording channels. The figure illustrates labeled multi-units, some with matching peak amplitudes. Since these are recorded from myelinated axons, these are really action potentials and not somatic recordings, and thus there may be some differences between these axonal recordings and somatic single-unit recordings. Somatic recordings have a deeper after-hyperpolarization, whereas the axonal spikes do not and hence appear sharper. Furthermore, the neuron is refractory to firing during this time for about 1 ms, so with the axonal spikes, this refractory period is shorter (between 0.5 and 1 ms). These continuously recorded multi-units are cluster cut into single units by using Neuralynx Inc.'s (Bozeman MT) convex hull technique (see examples in Figure 15.2b). The technique uses simple parameters such as total height, peak, valley, spike width, and energy. These are used to cut the continuous signals into single units.

To assess whether the separated wave shapes reflect the activity of single units, interspike interval distributions are constructed as shown under each single unit in Figure 15.2b from post-implant day 1582. These histograms demonstrate single peaks as expected for single units. It is observed that units of different amplitudes have vastly different firing rates as shown in Figure 15.2c. The larger units have the slowest modulating (or firing) rates and are likely related to corticospinal tract neurons, whereas the rapidly modulating small-amplitude units likely originate from interneurons. These data were recorded and archived in 2009, *4.4 years after implantation*. The units shown here have been used in functional studies involving the development of the speech prosthesis (Brumberg et al. 2011; Guenther et al. 2009).

To further assess for single units, interspike interval histograms are constructed as shown in Figure 15.2d for data recorded on post-implant day 1556 (2009). If the interspike interval histogram is constructed by using data from individual neurons, it ought not to contain firing activity at very short interspike intervals, because action potentials during these times would fall into the cell's refractory period. (Note the software retrigger time after a threshold crossing is a quarter millisecond so it will not blank out this time.) If such short intervals of no firings (minus the quarter millisecond) are identified, there is a high probability that the firings came from single units. A similar analysis of data containing multiple cells did contain data at short intervals so there was no "gap" near time zero because firings of multiple cells overlapped as shown previously [Kennedy et al. 2011 (fig 5b)].

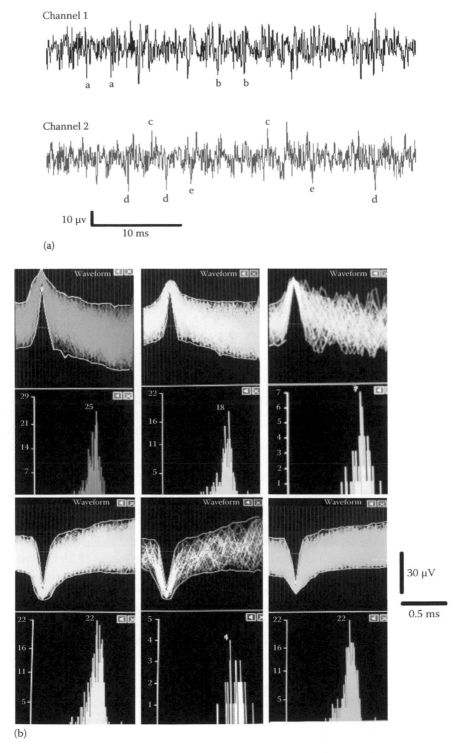

**FIGURE 15.2** Multi-unit data are received and analyzed in real time. (a) Two channels of data from the three wires within the electrode demonstrate units of similar amplitude as labeled by letters. Voltage levels (not shown) above and below the data stream separate the single un its from the multi-units. (b) Examples of units cluster cut from the multi-unit data are shown along with interspike interval distributions that demonstrate a single peak, strongly suggesting a single unit (June 22, 2009, post-implant day 1582).                    (*Continued*)

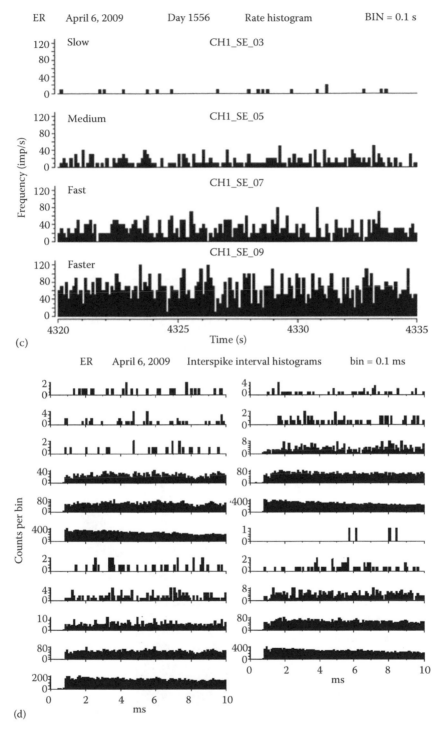

**FIGURE 15.2 (CONTINUED)**    Multi-unit data are received and analyzed in real time. (c) Unit firing rates shown over a 15-s range from less than 1 Hz to 100 Hz or more. The largest units have the slowest rates, suggesting that they originate from corticospinal tract neurons. The smallest units have the fastest rates, suggesting that they origi-nate from interneurons (April 6, 2009, post-implant day 1556). Units are labeled ch1_SE_0* meaning they originate from channel 1, single electrode, and number 0*. (d) Interspike interval histograms demonstrate no firing at less than 1 ms, strongly suggesting that these are single units. Multi-units would fill in the 1-ms gap. The non-trigger time applied to the voltage threshold is 250 μs, so only a quarter of the gap could be caused by non-triggering.

## 15.5   NINE YEARS AFTER IMPLANTATION

Data recorded in October 2013, *nine years after implantation*, are shown in Figure 15.3a. Examples in the top row demonstrate single wave shapes, and interspike interval distributions are shown in the next row, indicating a high probability of single units. Further examples are shown in the next two rows. Interspike interval histograms are shown in Figure 15.3b, strongly suggesting the presence of single units. To provide further evidence, cross-correlation analyses were performed with the aim of determining if units were related to each other during rest and during task performance. An example is shown in Figure 15.3c during rest and in Figure 15.3d during activity. During rest, all units indicated little if any correlation with the index unit (SE1-se-01: abbreviated to 1-1 in the text). However, during activity, increased correlation was evident between unit 1-1 and units 1-5,

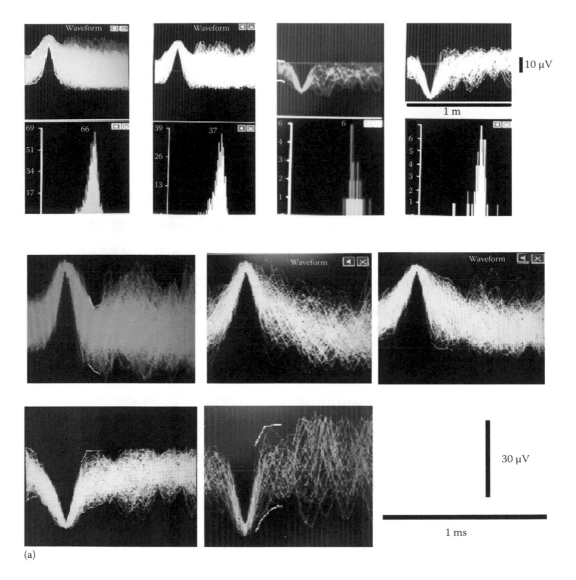

(a)

**FIGURE 15.3** Ensemble activity almost nine years post implant. (a) Single units along with interspike interval distributions are shown along with individual examples in the lower two rows.                    (*Continued*)

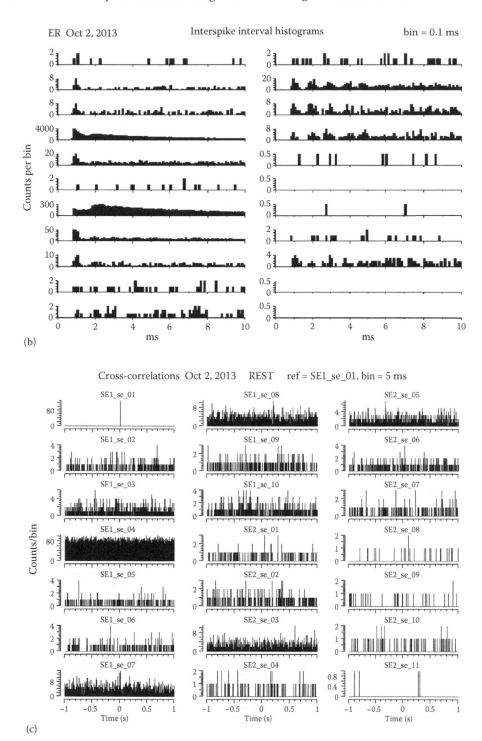

**FIGURE 15.3 (CONTINUED)**  Ensemble activity almost nine years post implant. (b) Interspike interval histograms are shown for data recorded October 2, 2013 (post-implant day 3081). (c) During quiet resting, minimal if any cross-correlation of units is demonstrated using unit 1-1 as the index unit (also from October 2, 2013).                                                                                                            *(Continued)*

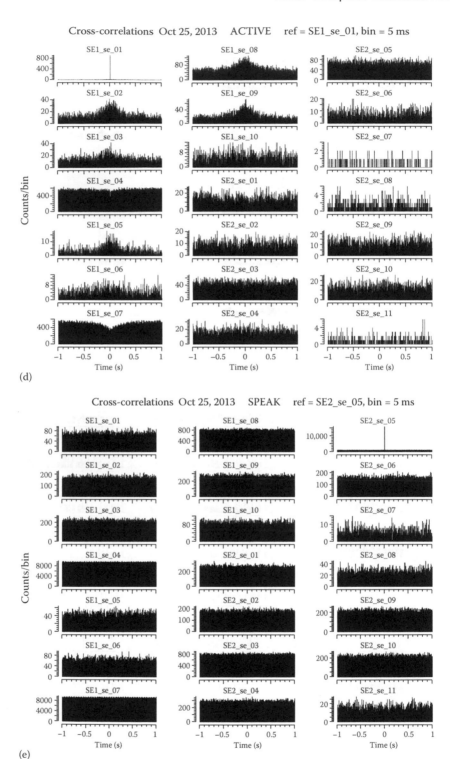

**FIGURE 15.3 (CONTINUED)** Ensemble activity almost nine years post implant. (d) However, during activity, using the same 1-1 index unit, cross-correlations appear only on channel (wire) 1, such as SE1_se_02, SE1_se_03, SE1_se_05, SE1_se_08, and SE1_se_09. (e) Some units during activity such as SE2_se_05, on the other hand, display no cross-correlations with other units.                                                    (*Continued*)

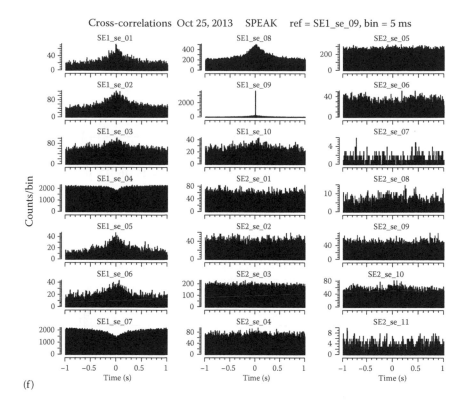

(f)

**FIGURE 15.3 (CONTINUED)**   Ensemble activity almost nine years post implant. (f) Units such as SE1_ se_09, however, display extensive cross-correlations during task performance. All data in (c) through (f) were recorded on October 2 (b and c) or October 25, 2013.

1-8, and 1-9, and weak correlations with units 1-2 and 1-3. It is noteworthy that only some units demonstrate cross-correlations, while others do not. An example of noncorrelation is shown in Figure 15.3e where unit 2-5 does not cross-correlate with other units during task performance (task described below). In contrast, Figure 15.3f illustrates the correlations between the index unit 1-9 and units 1-1, 1-2, 1-3, 1-5, 1-8, and inverse correlations with units 1-4 and 1-7. Thus, these units are active as an *ensemble* after almost 9 years of implantation.

## 15.6   FUNCTIONAL STUDIES AT YEAR 9

To further examine the question of functionality after almost 9 years of implantation, we used these units in conditioning experiments as part of a speech prosthesis development project (Brumberg et al. 2011; Guenther et al. 2009). An audible guitar chord, "D7," was tagged to unit 2-7 so that every time unit 2-7 fired, the guitar chord sounded through the computer speakers. The subject was asked to sing the guitar sound in his head by firing the unit, a task he performed many years before (Kennedy 2011). Average unit activities 10 s before and after the request to sing were compared. This comparison revealed a ratio of firing rates for each unit: when the rates before and after the "go" signals were equal, the ratio was 1, whereas an increase in the firing rate increases the ratio during singing. The ratio for recording day 3135 is illustrated in Figure 15.4a. Two epochs of conditioning during the same session (gray and dark gray bars) demonstrated little effect on the ratio for most of the units with a few exceptions such as number 18 (unit 2 7), which is the unit being conditioned. Four days later, this study is repeated as shown in Figure 15.4b. An effect on most ratios was now evident with a larger ratio increase during the second (dark gray) and third (white) epochs

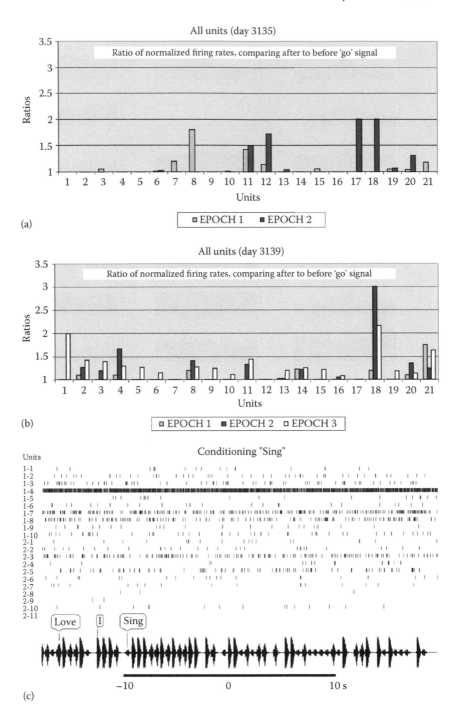

**FIGURE 15.4** Examples of conditioning of units. (a) Normalized firing rates of unit SE2_se_07 (#18 in the figure) on day 3135 after implantation (October 25, 2013). All 21 units are shown. To normalize the different firing rates, the ratio of task-related firings (averaged over 10 s) after the "go" signal are compared with 10-s averages before the signal. The ratio does not increase for most units. (b) Four days later, the same paradigm suggested that unit SE2_se_07 (the conditioned unit, #18) did dramatically increase its ratio on the second set (dark gray bar) and maintained this increase on the third set (white bar). Most other units also increased their ratios, at least by the third set. (c) All units are shown as time stamps over 30 s of data. The lower trace shows the wave files of the words "I," "Love," and "Sing."                                          (*Continued*)

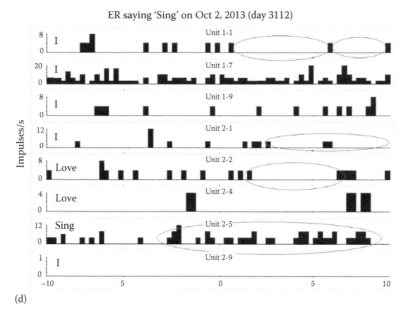

(d)

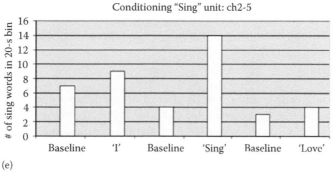

(e)

**FIGURE 15.4 (CONTINUED)** Examples of conditioning of units. (d) The words were attached to specific units as shown. Note the increase in unit 2-5 (SE2_se_05, attached to "Sing") and the decreased firing in other units allowing the word "Sing" to be emitted by the computer speaker. (e) A complete session demonstrates the frequency of the word "Sing" in 20-s time bins. During "I," the subject was requested to produce "I" not "Sing," and during "Love," the subject was requested to produce "Love." Baselines were 2 min in duration. Chi-square test value was 0.44 for "I" and 0.25 for "Love," but when asked to say "Sing," the number of "Sing" words above baseline was statistically significant (chi-square test value of 7.14). Note the expected shifting baselines.

indicating a learning effect in some of the units. Of most importance was the large effect seen with unit 2-7 (#18 in Figure 15.4), which was the unit being conditioned. *Thus, these data suggested that functional conditioning of units was possible even after 9 years of implantation.*

The above data illustrate increases in averaged firing rates after the "go" signal compared with before the signal. Sometimes, however, the rate decreased. To determine if increases and/ or decreases of unit activity were important in the development of a speech prosthetic, a different paradigm was examined. Figure 15.4c illustrates that audible wave files containing the words "I," "Love," and "Sing" are illustrated by their spectrograms and tagged to single units. Above the spectrograms for "Love," "I," and "Sing," the firing frequencies of all the units are illustrated as time stamps. Units were chosen based on previously determined strong modulation during time periods when the subject attempted to speak these three words in his head (inaudible as the subject is mute).

During the present task shown in Figure 15.4c, production of the word from the speakers was triggered by unit firings in a "winner-take-all" paradigm. The successfully emitted word was contained in a wave file so that it could be identified by its frequency spectrogram illustrated along the bottom of the 30-s data segment in the figure. The illustrated task required the subject to produce the word "Sing," and not "I" or "Love." The "go" signal is marked at the approximate time the word was requested (time "0"). The spectrogram for the requested word "Sing" is rarely seen before the "go" signal. After the "go" signal, he did not initially produce the word "Sing" more frequently than the other words, as illustrated. However, after about 5 s, the word "Sing" appeared more frequently.

To understand why and how the word "Sing" appeared when it did, the specific single units attached to the three wave files are shown over a ±10-s time period in Figure 15.4d centered on the "go" signal. Only unit 2-5 is attached to the word "Sing." It appeared to *increase* its firing rate near time zero but the word "Sing" was not produced. The explanation is likely seen in the suppression of firing of the other units attached to the other two words. Units 1-1 and 2-1 (attached to "I") and unit 2-2 (attached to "Love") *decreased* their firing rates, thus allowing unit 2-5 to be the "winner" and produce the word "Sing."

To illustrate this point further over a complete session, the conditioning of the word "Sing" is illustrated in Figure 15.4e. During requests to produce "Sing," the subject could produce "Sing" significantly above baseline (14 compared to 4 words per 20-s bin). Even more telling is that the production of "Sing" was restrained during requests to produce "I" and "Love." The chi-square test values 0.44 for "I" and 0.25 for "Love" were not significant, but when asked to say "Sing," the number of "Sing" words above baseline was statistically significant with a chi-square test value of 7.14. Note the expected shifting baseline (going from 7 to 4 to 3) previously documented (Kennedy 2011).

## 15.7  DISCUSSION

Recording functionally active neural signals after almost a decade of implantation in the human cortex strongly suggests that the neurotrophic electrode fulfills the requirement for a reliable neural interface. The examples of cross-correlation data and the conditioning data strongly suggest that units remain individual and functional after almost 9 years. In fact, the electrode and electronics were implanted in 2004 with signals recorded in 2015, producing 11 years of recording. The subject is too ill to record functional activity. Attempts to record on January 1, 2016, resulted in no evidence of the FM transmitter signal. The electrode is likely intact, but the electronics has failed.

The chronic recording over a decade implies that even longer time periods are likely. The design of the electrode tip is crucial to providing a firm attachment to the neuropil to ensure longevity. This design allows the neuropil to grow into and through the tip and thus anchors it in place. A second important feature is the strain relief provided by coiling the delicate 2-mil gold wires. After the neurites have grown into the tip, they become myelinated and electrically active, with stability occurring at about 3 months. Examples of functional single unit activity at 4 years and 9 years after implantation are described above and provide strong evidence that this neural interface is reliable. After implantation in December 2004, data have been obtained on a continuing basis. For example, data obtained in 2005, 2006, and 2007 indicate that half the English 39 phonemes can be identified as confirmed by using multiple decoding paradigms (Brumberg et al. 2011); data in 2009 indicate that vowel production can be produced using a linear discriminant analysis decoding paradigm and controlled by the subject (Guenther et al. 2009); data recorded in 2008, 2009, and 2010 describe the effect of emotional state on background firing rates (Kennedy 2011); data recorded in 2007, 2008, and 2009 indicate that pure tones are associated with synchronized firing of single units, but not multi-units (Kennedy et al. 2011); data collected over the 2008 and 2009 periods indicate that vocalization onset could be detected by analyzing the pattern of activation in the low beta frequency range (Sarmah and Kennedy 2013); and conditioning of unit firings was undertaken in 2013, an example of which is described above. Such single-unit conditioning was originally successfully demonstrated in 1973 by Fetz and Baker in monkeys (Fetz and

Baker 1973). These authors demonstrated that monkeys could control firing rates of more than one unit by increasing the firing of one and decreasing the firing of the other. This is broadly similar to the data presented in Figure 15.4d and e and is the first such demonstration in humans of reciprocal conditioning.

So where does that leave the field of brain–machine/computer interfacing? First and most obvious, the field must overcome the fear of implantation, just as the cardiovascular field overcame the fear of cardiac pacemaker implantations. In experienced hands, brain surgery is safe. It has the usual risks of bleeding, infection, seizures, and damage to the underlying brain. In the case of electrode implantation, any damage is done to the functional cortex that is not being used because of the paralysis or loss of output. With modern sterilization techniques and careful surgical technique, the questions of infection and hemorrhage are minimized. Seizures can be controlled with medication. So the question becomes which electrode to implant? For short-term usage, the tine-type electrodes are excellent choices, but for long-term implantation, the data show that their signals do not persist and their utility ends (Ward et al. 2009; Simeral et al. 2011; Hochberg et al. 2011; Perge et al. 2013). Therefore, the neurotrophic electrode or some variation thereof is the choice for long term survival of the signal. The aim is at least 50 years of recording. The disadvantages of the neurotrophic electrode are that it is bulky and damages the cortex. However, the cortex is not useful anyway because the individual is paralyzed or locked-in so the damage is not relevant especially since function can be obtained from the implanted cortex. This electrode has been studied in rats (Kennedy 1989) and has been found to record from a radius at least 600 μm of cortex, thus covering a relatively wide area. In fact, in the most recent implantation (Kennedy et al. 2016), four electrodes were implanted 6 mm apart with no ill effects long term. However, the principle of using trophic factors to ensure a long-lasting tight binding between the neuropil and the electrodes is mandatory for long-term signal stability and functionality. The present results strongly imply that the most reliable neural interface can be produced by *growing the neuropil into the electrode rather than by inserting the electrode into the neuropil.*

# REFERENCES

Bartels, J., Andreasen, D., Ehirim, P., Mao, H., Seibert, S., Wright, E. J., Kennedy, P. R. Neurotrophic electrode: Method of assembly and implantation into human motor speech cortex. *J. Neurosci. Methods* 174(2), 168–176 (2008).

Brumberg, J. S., Wright, E. J., Andreasen, D., Guenther, F. H., Kennedy, P. R. Classification of intended phoneme production from chronic intracortical microelectrode recordings in speech motor cortex. *Front. Neurosci.* 5(65) (2011).

Fetz, E. E., Baker, M. A. Operantly conditioned patterns on precentral unit activity and correlated responses in adjacent cells and contralateral muscles. *J. Neurophysiology* 36(2), 179–204 (1973).

Guenther, F. H., Brumberg, J. S., Wright, E. J., Nieto-Castanon, A., Tourville, J. A., Panko, M., Law, R., Siebert, S. A., Bartels, J. L., Andreasen, D., Ehirim, P., Mao, H., Kennedy, P. R. A wireless brain–machine interface for real-time speech synthesis. *PLoS One* 4(12), 8218 (2009).

Hochberg, L. R., Bacher, D., Barefoot, L., Berhanu, E., Black, M. J., Cash, S. S., Feldman, J. M., Gallivan, E. M., Homer, M., Jarosiewicz, B., King, B., Liu, J., Malik, W. Q., Masse, N. Y., Perge, J. A., Rosler, D. M., Schmansky, N., Simeral, J. D., Travers, B., Truccolo, W., Donoghue, J. P. *Soc. Neurosci. Abstr.* 2011.

Kennedy, P. R. A long-term electrode that records from neurites grown onto its recording surface. *J. Neuroscience Methods* 29, 181–193 (1989).

Kennedy, P. R., Andreasen, D. S., Bartels, J., Ehirim, P., Mao, H., Velliste, M., Wichmann, T., Wright, E. J. Making the lifetime connection between brain and machine for restoring and enhancing function. *Prog. Brain Res.* 194, 1–25 (2011).

Kennedy, P. R., Bakay, R. A. E. Activity of single action potentials in monkey motor cortex during longterm task learning. *Brain Res.* 760, 251–254 (1997).

Kennedy, P. R., Bakay, R. A. E., Sharpe, S. M. Behavioral correlates of action potentials recorded chronically inside the Cone Electrode. *NeuroReport* 3, 605–608 (1992a).

Kennedy, P. R. Changes in emotional state modulate neuronal firing rates of human speech motor cortex: A case study in long-term recording. *Neurocase* 17(5), 381–393 (2011).

Kennedy, P. R., Gambrell, C., Shih, N. Detection of phonemes, short words and phrases from single units and 12-20 Hz frequency beta band data during overt and covert speech recorded chronically from a speaking human. *SFN Abstracts* 439.04 (2016).

Kennedy, P. R., Mirra, S., Bakay, R. A. E. The Cone Electrode: Ultrastructural studies following longterm recording. *Neurosci. Let.* 142, 89–94 (1992b).

Perge, J. A., Homer, M. L., Malik, W. Q., Cash, S., Eskandar, E., Friehs, G., Donoghue, J. P., Hochberg, L. R. Intra-day signal instabilities affect decoding performance in an intracortical neural interface system. *J. Neural Eng.* 10(3), 036004 (2013).

Presacco, A., Forrester, L., Contreras-Vidal, J. L. Towards a non-invasive brain-machine interface system to restore gait function in humans. *IEEE Eng. Med. Biol. Soc.* 45, 88–91 (2011).

Rousche, P. J., Normann, R. A. Chronic recording capability of the Utah Intracortical Electrode Array in cat sensory cortex. *J. Neurosci. Methods* 82(1), 1–15 (1998).

Sarmah, E., Kennedy, P. R. Detecting silent vocalizations in a locked-in subject. *Neuroscience Journal* 2013, Article ID 594624 (2013).

Simeral, J. D., Kim, S. P., Black, M. J., Donoghue, J. P., Hochberg, L. R. Neural control of cursor trajectory and click by a human with tetraplegia 1000 days after implant of an intracortical microelectrode array. *J. Neural Eng.* 8(2), 025027 (2011).

Ward, M. P., Rajdev, P., Ellison, C., Irazoqui, P. P. Toward a comparison of microelectrodes for acute and chronic recordings. *Brain Res.* 1282, 183–200 (2009).

## GLOSSARY

**Cross-correlations:** The firing rate of one single unit is correlated with the firing rates of all the others. If some or all of the other units fire at the same time as the single unit fires, then they are related.

**Ensemble:** Units act together like a crowd, for example, clapping a speaker all together.

**Histogram:** A bar graph with bar heights indicating the frequency of a variable, in our case firing rate, depicted over time.

**Impedance:** The resistance of the tip of the electrode when measured using an AC versus a DC source.

**Interspike interval histogram:** The time between firings of the units is plotted as a histogram over time.

**Microns:** One micron is one-thousandth of a meter.

**Mil:** There are 39.37 mils in 1 mm; 1 mm = 0.0254 mils.

**Neurites:** A general term for any outgrowth from a neuron. When a neurite becomes myelinated, it is called an axon or dendrite depending on its location with respect to the neuronal body.

**Neuropil:** The neural tissue that makes up the brain and consists of neurons, axons, dendrites, glial cells, and interneurons. It also includes blood vessels such as capillaries.

**Polarization and after polarization:** Polarization refers to the abrupt change in membrane potential that generates the spike, and "after polarization" refers to the brief period after the main spike.

**Refractory period:** A short period (less than 1 ms usually) during which the neuron will not fire (depolarize).

**Spikes:** This term refers to action potentials that are discharges from neurons or axons that exceed a baseline membrane potential that results in a sudden sharp increase in the potential, and hence the (somewhat slang) term "spike" or action potential.

**Tines:** Tiny, sharp needles that penetrate the brain and made of a metal (platinum or iridium for example) that is insulated except at its tip. The impedance of the de-insulated tip is of the order of a few tens of ohms or a mohm (rarely more).

**Trophic factors:** Substances such as nerve growth factor, ciliary nerve growth factor, and so on, attract and nourish neurites and neurons.

## ACKNOWLEDGMENTS

Roy A.E. Bakay, Rush Presbyterian Medical Center, Chicago, IL, USA, is posthumously acknowledged as being a key person in the early and most recent study. Thanks also to the many people who participated over the years in these studies: Frank Guenther, Boston University, Boston, MA, USA; Jonathan Brumberg, 1450 Jayhawk Boulevard, Lawrence, KS, USA; and Edward Joe Wright, formerly at Neural Signals Inc. Grateful thanks to the subject and his parents for their enthusiastic participation and support.

Funded by NIDCD grant R44DC007050, NINDS grant R44NS36913, and funds from Community Neurological Clinic.

## INSTITUTIONAL REVIEW BOARD APPROVAL

All studies were approved by the institutional review board of Neural Signals Inc.; Gwinnett Medical Center, Lawrenceville, GA; and Emory University, Atlanta, GA (earlier studies). Studies were carried out in accordance with the Helsinki declarations.

## FEDERAL DRUG ADMINISTRATION APPROVAL

Study was approved by the FDA G960032.

## CONFLICTS OF INTEREST

P.R. Kennedy owns 98% and D. Andreasen owns 2% of the stock of Neural Signals Inc.

# 16 ECoG-Based BCIs

*Aysegul Gunduz and Gerwin Schalk*

## CONTENTS

16.1 Introduction..................................................................................................................297
16.2 ECoG Signal Acquisition............................................................................................298
16.3 ECoG Signal Physiology.............................................................................................299
16.4 Current ECoG-Based BCIs.........................................................................................303
    16.4.1 ECoG BCIs for Control....................................................................................303
    16.4.2 ECoG BCIs for Communication.......................................................................304
    16.4.3 ECoG BCIs for Neuromodulation...................................................................305
16.5 Current Implantable Devices......................................................................................309
16.6 Open Questions and Directions for Further Research.................................................312
16.7 Summary.....................................................................................................................314
Acknowledgment..................................................................................................................314
References..............................................................................................................................315

**Abstract**

This chapter reviews the state of the art of brain–computer interfaces (BCIs) that use electrocorticography (ECoG) signals as an input. We first present the clinical settings and signal acquisition systems, including subdural grid electrodes, that lend themselves to ECoG data collection. Second, we discuss the current understanding of ECoG signal physiology and ECoG features that cannot be captured by noninvasive electrophysiology or imaging, and how this knowledge can be translated to signal features that can control BCIs. Next, we review ECoG-based BCIs in the literature that enable control, communication, and therapeutic neuromodulation. This is followed by a review of current implantable ECoG device technologies approved or available for investigational use in humans. Finally, we present and discuss various open questions in the field of ECoG BCIs and future research directions that may lead to the translation of these technologies into clinical practice.

## 16.1 INTRODUCTION

Electrocorticography (ECoG) is an electrophysiological technique that utilizes electrodes placed intracranially on the surface of the brain. ECoG has been employed in humans clinically for over six decades for the localization of epileptic zones and for functional brain mapping. However, its value for basic human neuroscientific research and its potential to enable new translational applications had not been widely recognized until recently. ECoG signals are captured either above (epidural) or below (subdural) the dura mater, but not within the brain tissue itself (see Figure 16.1). Many studies over the last decade have demonstrated the functional specificity, signal fidelity, and long-term stability of ECoG activity in behavioral and cognitive tasks (Schalk 2010). Together with its spatial and temporal resolution and coverage of distant areas of the brain, these unique qualities suggest that ECoG elucidates brain function in ways that cannot be achieved by other electrophysiological or neuroimaging techniques. For instance, intracortical electrode recordings usually have issues with long-term stability; scalp-recorded EEG lacks functional specificity and is very prone to artifacts; and metabolic responses captured via neuroimaging may be too slow for practical applications.

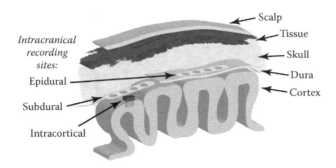

**FIGURE 16.1** Intracranial neural signal modalities and their respective signal acquisition methodologies.

This chapter focuses on ECoG-based brain–computer interface (BCI) development as an exciting and important area in clinical translation in humans. It has four major sections. The first section addresses signal acquisition methods to capture ECoG signals. The second section examines the emerging understanding of ECoG physiology and the ECoG signal features that form the basis for BCI applications. The third section examines current BCI applications that utilize ECoG signals for computer/machine control, for communication, and for neuromodulation in neurological disorders. The fourth and final section discusses the limitations of and open questions in ECoG-based BCI development and suggests how ongoing ECoG studies, such as investigations of optimal electrode configurations (size and spacing) and investigations of signal quality of epidurally recorded ECoG, are likely to facilitate the feasibility of ECoG-based BCIs outside the clinic.

## 16.2 ECoG SIGNAL ACQUISITION

Penfield's pioneering work in the 1950s with epilepsy patients represented the first comprehensive ECoG-based effort to study the neural basis of human behavior (Penfield and Rasmussen 1950). To this date, the large majority of human ECoG studies have been restricted to neurosurgical patients since the collection of ECoG signals requires surgery that consists of a craniotomy, followed by an incision to the protective dura matter for the placement of electrode arrays on the cortical surface. ECoG electrodes for human use are commonly made of platinum, platinum-iridium, stainless steel, or silver, and embedded into a thin flexible silastic sheet. The diameter of conventional clinical electrodes is typically 4 mm, with 2.3 mm of the contact exposed, and the interelectrode distance is usually 10 mm from center to center (see Figure 16.2). Electrode arrays can be arranged in square, rectangular,

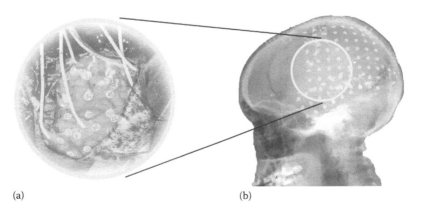

(a)                                                              (b)

**FIGURE 16.2**  (a) ECoG array in situ. (b) Postoperative CT highlighting electrode locations. (From P. Brunner, A. L. Ritaccio, J. F. Emrich, H. Bischof, and G. Schalk. Rapid communication with a "P300" matrix speller using electrocorticographic signals (ECoG). *Front in Neuroprosthet*, 5(5):1–9, 2011.)

or L-shaped configurations. In the United States, the implantation duration is limited by the U.S. Food and Drug Administration (FDA) to a maximum of 28 days, and the typical implant duration is about 1 week. All relevant implant parameters (duration of the implant and size of the craniotomy) are determined solely by the clinical needs of the patients and without any regard for research interests.

After the implantation of the electrodes, bioamplifiers with high temporal resolution (i.e., an adequate sampling rate) and with sufficient range and resolution in voltage (i.e., an adequate quantization level) are required to capture all important features of ECoG signals. In practice, a sampling rate of 1 kHz or higher, a voltage range of at least several dozens of µV, and a digital resolution of 24 bits are recommended. These are good recording practices, as the spectral bandwidth of ECoG signals extends to ~250 Hz, and voltage amplitudes attenuate inversely with increasing frequency (i.e., from several hundred microvolts at low frequencies to several hundred nanovolts at higher frequencies). Ideally, the bioamplifier should minimize the amount of analog filtering: high-pass filters can remove evoked potentials of interest, whereas low-pass filters with too low of a cutoff frequency will remove important high-frequency content of ECoG signals. The physiological basis of these signals and the most relevant features for BCI applications are discussed in Section 16.3.

## 16.3 ECoG SIGNAL PHYSIOLOGY

Macroscale field potentials are generated by current dipoles between cortical laminae (Nunez and Srinivasan 2006). The physiological underpinnings of the current source density (CSD) in cortical laminae that give rise to these potentials were established experimentally in the late 1970s and early 1980s (Mitzdorf 1985). These studies demonstrated that propagating action potentials in axons and axonal terminals do not contribute strongly to the CSD at spatial scales of ~50–300 µm or greater, which suggests that ECoG signals comprise dendritic synaptic current exchange (i.e., influx and efflux) that modulates the CSD. This has recently been substantiated by simultaneous in vivo recordings of the intracellular potential and local field potentials over which ECoG signals are averaged, showing tight temporal coupling that is independent of the spiking pattern of the neuron (Miller 2010; Miller et al. 2009a; Okun et al. 2009). Thus, ECoG signals can be explained by synchronous synaptic inputs from large ensembles underlying the electrode. If this synchronization/desynchronization occurs rhythmically, it can be observed as rhythmic amplitude modulations in the time series (Figure 16.3a) and as a peak in the frequency domain (Figure 16.3b) (Ritaccio et al. 2011). If the synchronization is related to a stimulus (e.g., a visual cue) or an event (e.g., movement onset), the time series may reflect a multiphasic, time-locked response, known as an "event-related potential" (ERP).

In addition to ERPs, whose physiological origin is complex and unresolved (Kam et al. 2016; Makeig et al. 2002; Mazaheri and Jensen 2006, 2008), ECoG signals also contain two components that are particularly relevant to BCIs: broadband gamma and low-frequency oscillations. ECoG broadband gamma activity (often measured in the 70–170 Hz range) has been suggested by many studies to be the key indicator of cortical population-level activity (Aoki et al. 1999; Canolty et al. 2007; Chang et al. 2011; Crone et al. 2001a,b, 1998a; Darvas et al. 2010; Edwards et al. 2010, 2005, 2009; Freeman et al. 2000; Jensen et al. 2007; Kubánek et al. 2009; Lachaux et al. 2007; Leuthardt et al. 2007, 2004; Maris et al. 2011; Menon et al. 1996; Miller et al. 2007, 2010b; Pei et al. 2010; Pfurtscheller et al. 2003; Ray et al. 2008; Sanchez et al. 2008; Schalk et al. 2007; Sinai et al. 2005; Tort et al. 2008; Voytek et al. 2010; Wang et al. 2010). Broadband gamma has been shown to be a direct reflection of the level of *cortical excitation*, that is, a reflection of the average firing rate of neurons directly underneath the electrode (Manning et al. 2009; Miller et al. 2009b; Ray and Maunsell 2011; Whittingstall and Logothetis 2009), and has been shown to drive the BOLD signal identified using fMRI (Lachaux et al. 2007; Engell et al. 2012; Logothetis et al. 2001; Mukamell et al. 2005; Niessing et al. 2005). Thus, the use of broadband gamma (which is not readily available in scalp-recorded EEG) provides a link between ECoG-based research and work using single-neuron recordings and fMRI. Broadband gamma activity usually presents itself as a broad spectral distribution above 60 Hz that follows a $1/f$ trend in the frequency domain (Miller et al. 2009a,c). Most relevant to BCI development, many studies have reported that topographically

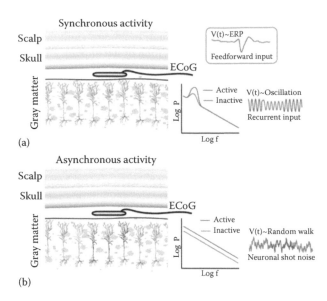

**FIGURE 16.3** ECoG potential time series $V(t)$ is modulated by various synaptic input. (a) Synchronized activity or event-related potential changes are revealed by changes in peaked aspects of the logarithmic power spectrum. (b) Asynchronous, local activity is revealed by broadband changes in the logarithmic power spectrum. P, power; f, frequency; ERP, event-related potential. (From A. Ritaccio, D. Boatman-Reich, P. Brunner, M. C. Cervenka, A. J. Cole, N. Crone, R. Duckrow, A. Korzeniewska, B. Litt, K. J. Miller, D. W. Moran, J. Parvizi, J. Viventi, J. Williams, and G. Schalk. Proceedings of the Second International Workshop on Advances in Electrocorticography. *Epilepsy behav: E&B*, 22(4):641–650, Dec 2011.)

focused broadband gamma activity correlates closely with specific aspects of behavior such as the direction of limb movements (Kubánek et al. 2009; Leuthardt et al. 2004; Schalk et al. 2007; Miller et al. 2009c; Acharya et al. 2010; Gunduz et al. 2016; Pistohl et al. 2008; Wang et al. 2012) (see Figure 16.4).

In contrast to broadband gamma, low-frequency oscillatory activity provides an index of *cortical excitability* (Fitzgibbon et al. 2004; Haegens et al. 2011; Howard et al. 2003; Kubanek et al. 2015, 2013; Miltner et al. 1999; Sederberg et al. 2003; Singer and Gray 1995; Szczepanski et al. 2014; Womelsdorf et al. 2006) and plays a central role in the dynamic modulation of cortical function in response to varying task demands (Fries 2005; Jensen and Mazaheri 2010; Schalk 2015). Thus, even though low-frequency activity is likely produced by electrical events in certain (putatively subcortical) populations of neurons, it has proven to be a useful metric of the modulation of the cortex that is different from cortical excitation indexed by broadband gamma. Oscillations at different frequencies subserve different cortical regions. For example, activity in the alpha (8–12 Hz) band is prevalent throughout the sensorimotor system (e.g., Kubanek et al. 2015, 2013) where it is usually referred to as the mu rhythm that is well described in the classical EEG literature (Chatrian 1976) (see Figure 16.5 Brunner et al. 2009). Typically, the mu rhythm and the closely associated beta (18–26 Hz) rhythm are relatively focused spectrally and appear as peaks in the power spectrum but are relatively widespread spatially (see Figure 16.5a, bottom). Although their peak amplitude modulates with actual or imagined movements (Crone et al. 1998b; Pfurtscheller and Cooper 1975) (see Figure 16.6 Schalk 2006), activity in mu or beta bands appears to reveal only modest information about localized differential cortical processing (Toro et al. 1994). Outside the sensorimotor system, alpha oscillations are also prevalent in the visual system (e.g., Van Dijk et al. 2008) and auditory system (e.g., Potes et al. 2014, 2012). In contrast, oscillations in the theta (4–8 Hz) band are pervasive in prefrontal and hippocampal networks (Anderson et al. 2009; Dürschmid et al. 2014; Fujisawa and Buzsáki 2011). Across all these types of systems and oscillations, oscillatory amplitude is typically large during rest, and reduced while the subject is engaging in corresponding function (e.g., Figure 16.6).

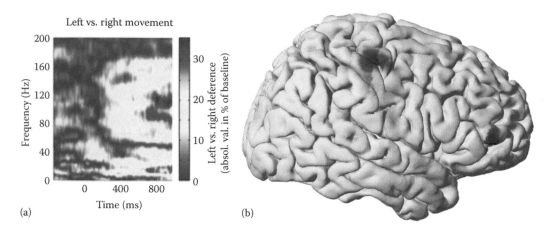

(a)                                                                           (b)

**FIGURE 16.4**  ECoG recording reveals information about the direction of a hand movement. (a) ECoG signal in different frequency bands recorded at one location in the contralateral hand area of motor cortex from one subject differentiates left and right movement directions. (From E. Leuthardt, G. Schalk, J. Wolpaw, J. Ojemann, and D. Moran. A brain–computer interface using electrocorticographic signals in humans. *J Neural Eng*, 1(2):63–71, 2004.) (b) Color-coded shading of average data from five subjects illustrates the information about hand movement direction provided by ECoG recorded over different cortical areas. Most of the information is captured over the hand representations of motor cortex. (Modified from G. Schalk, J. Kubánek, K. J. Miller, N. R. Anderson, E. C. Leuthardt, J. G. Ojemann, D. Limbrick, D. Moran, L. A. Gerhardt, and J. R. Wolpaw. Decoding two-dimensional movement trajectories using electrocorticographic signals in humans. *J Neural Eng*, 4(3):264–275, Sep 2007.)

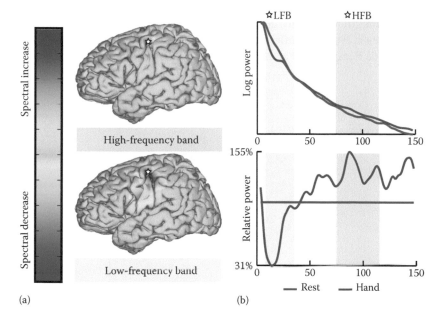

(a)                                                                           (b)

**FIGURE 16.5**  Example of ECoG during the task of repetitively opening and closing the hand and during rest. (a) Signals in the mu/beta band (5–30 Hz) decrease with the task and are spatially less specific (i.e., they are broadly distributed topographically), whereas signals in the gamma band (i.e., 70–116 Hz as measured here) increase with the task and are spatially more specific (i.e., they are sharply focused topographically). (b) The power spectrum on a logarithmic scale for the electrode marked with a star in the topographies illustrates the decrease in the mu/beta band (marked by the green bar) and increase in the gamma band (orange bar). (From P Brunner, A. L. Ritaccio, T. M. Lynch, J. F. Emrich, J. A. Wilson, J. C. Williams, E. J. Aarnoutse, N. F. Ramsey, E. C. Leuthardt, H. Bischof, and G. Schalk. A practical procedure for real-time functional mapping of eloquent cortex using electrocorticographic signals in humans. *Epilepsy Behav*, 15(3):278–286, Apr 2009.)

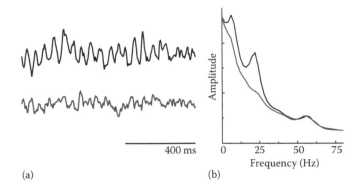

(a)                                                                     (b)

**FIGURE 16.6**  Example of ECoG signals during a task and rest. (a) Raw ECoG signals from one subject during rest (black trace) and while imagining saying the word "move" (red trace). The amplitude of the oscillation associated with rest decreases with imagery. (b) Frequency spectra for the corresponding conditions. Imagery is associated with decrease in the mu (8–12 Hz) and beta (18–26 Hz) frequency bands. (From G. Schalk. *Towards a Clinically Practical Brain–Computer Interface*. PhD thesis, Rensselaer Polytechnic Institute, Troy, Dec 2006.)

Cortical excitability and cortical excitation (as measured by oscillatory and broadband gamma activity, respectively) are intrinsically linked: cortical activity is usually highest during periods when oscillatory power is low or when oscillations are in their trough. The latter relationship between the phase of low-frequency oscillations and the amplitude envelope of the signal in the broadband gamma range is usually referred to as phase–amplitude coupling (PAC; see Figure 16.7 Schalk and Leuthardt 2011) (Canolty et al. 2006). Recent research has increasingly pointed to a link between changes in PAC and different neurological or psychiatric disorders (Allen et al. 2011; Crowell et al. 2012; de Hemptinne et al. 2013; Shute et al. 2015; Uhlhaas and Mishara 2007; Uhlhaas and Singer 2010).

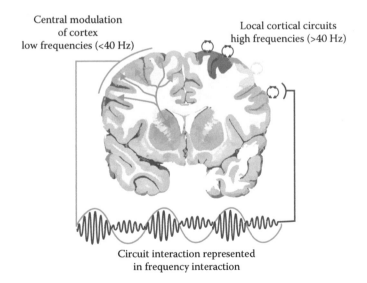

**FIGURE 16.7**  Schematic of current and emerging understanding of the physiological origin of ECoG signals. The amplitude of low-frequency oscillatory activity represents the level of cortical excitability. Broadband gamma activity represents the degree of cortical excitation. Oscillatory phase modulates cortical excitation. (From G. Schalk and E. C. Leuthardt. Brain–computer interfaces using electrocorticographic signals. *IEEE Rev Biomed Eng*, 4:140–154, 2011.)

In addition to ECoG potentials that are evoked by discrete motor movements or sensory stimuli, and to oscillatory and broadband activity, recent studies (Kubánek et al. 2009; Schalk et al. 2007; Acharya et al. 2010; Gunduz et al. 2016; Pistohl et al. 2008) describe a continuous time-domain ECoG feature called the *local motor potential (LMP)* that encodes different aspects of movements. LMPs are observed mainly in the prefrontal cortex (Schalk et al. 2007; Gunduz et al. 2016). The physiological origin of the LMP remains unknown and its potential value for ECoG-based BCIs has not been explored beyond these studies.

Because of its closer proximity to the neurons producing electrical modulations, ECoG has larger signal amplitude and broader bandwidth compared to EEG. In addition to these advantages of signal quality, ECoG electrodes may provide greater long-term functional stability (Bullara et al. 1979; Loeb et al. 1977; Margalit et al. 2003; Pilcher and Rusyniak 1993; Yuen et al. 1987) than intracortical electrodes, which induce tissue responses that may degrade or prevent neuronal recordings. A study by Chao et al. (2010) in primates showed that the signal-to-noise ratio of ECoG signals and the BCI features of motor function are stable over several months (Schalk 2010). Thus, there is strong support that ECoG-based BCIs provide high functional specificity and are less susceptible to the problems of reliability and long-term stability that often affect other electrophysiological signal-acquisition methodologies.

## 16.4 CURRENT ECoG-BASED BCIs

### 16.4.1 ECoG BCIs FOR CONTROL

BCI systems based on ECoG have advanced well beyond initial proof of concept. As of 5 years ago, ECoG BCIs had been extensively validated across numerous different labs (Leuthardt et al. 2004, 2006; Miller et al. 2007; Blakely et al. 2009; Brunner et al. 2011; Felton et al. 2007; Hinterberger et al. 2008; Rouse and Moran 2009; Schalk 2008; Vansteensel et al. 2010; Wilson et al. 2006). In the first paper reporting an ECoG BCI with humans (Leuthardt et al. 2004), four participants could move a cursor up or down by performing or imagining different movements. Overall, the four subjects attained 74%–100% accuracy (with 50% chance accuracy) in the task of moving the cursor to a target on the top or bottom of the monitor. This real-time control required only 3–24 min of training (see Figure 16.8a for learning curves). This performance is difficult to compare to BCIs based on EEG because of the limited amount of data from only four subjects, but the training required for such control does appear to be shorter than that for EEG-based BCIs based on motor imagery (see Figure 16.8a). The authors also conducted offline analyses of data from all four subjects while they moved a cursor in two dimensions using a joystick. Their results showed that ECoG features as high as 180 Hz encoded movement direction (see also Figure 16.4a).

Subsequent work included several improvements that extended this study beyond one-dimensional control. Schalk et al. (Schalk et al. 2008) presented a BCI that allowed five subjects to control two-dimensional movement in real time based on ECoG measures of imagined or actual movements. A more recent study presented offline decoding of three-dimensional movements in humans (Bundy et al. 2016). Actual two- and three-dimensional control was shown in a patient with tetraplegia resulting from a C4 spinal injury (Wang et al. 2013). This was the first publication that reported real-time ECoG-based robotic arm control in a tetraplegic patient (see Section 16.5). Despite this successful demonstration of improved control, the ECoG array had to be explanted within 28 days of implantation to comply with requirements from the FDA. In a different direction based on ipsilateral ECoG activity from four chronic stroke patients with severe paralysis, Spueler et al. successfully discriminated seven distinct hand movement intentions (Spueler et al. 2014). This research direction could go beyond high-dimensional control to allow more natural control based on hand movement imagination.

While improving the number of dimensions of movement is important, other work has instead focused on making ECoG BCIs more flexible by supporting control from other brain regions. Two studies (Yuen et al. 1987; Wilson et al. 2006) conducted research based on ECoG activity that reflected sensory (not motor) function, with an electrode spacing of about 5 (not 10) mm, resulting in

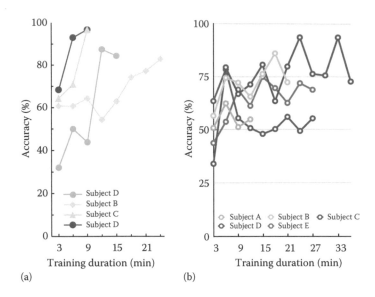

**FIGURE 16.8** (a) Learning curves for ECoG control of vertical cursor movement using motor imagery to move up and rest to move down. (Accuracy in absence of control would be 50%.) Subject B (green trace) imagined opening and closing the right hand. Subjects C (yellow trace) and D (red trace) imagined saying the word "move." Subject D (blue trace) imagined protruding the tongue. (Modified from E. Leuthardt, G. Schalk, J. Wolpaw, J. Ojemann, and D. Moran. A brain–computer interface using electrocorticographic signals in humans. *J Neural Eng*, 1(2):63–71, 2004.) (b) Learning curves for ECoG control of two-dimensional cursor movement. (Accuracy in absence of control would be 25%.) (Modified from G. Schalk, K. J. Miller, N. R. Anderson, J. A. Wilson, M. D. Smyth, J. G. Ojemann, D. W. Moran, J. R. Wolpaw, and E. C. Leuthardt. Two-dimensional movement control using electrocorticographic signals in humans. *J Neural Eng*, 5(1):75–84, Mar 2008.)

control that was roughly comparable to Ref. (Leuthardt et al. 2004). Related work showed that primates could learn to control one-dimensional cursor movement via broadband gamma hand activity by modulating activity of any ECoG electrode in motor or premotor areas (Rouse and Moran 2009), further extending the potential flexibility of ECoG BCIs. Slightly later research showed that humans can quickly learn to direct movement through ECoG activity from the left dorsolateral prefrontal cortex, associated with working arithmetic memory (Vansteensel et al. 2010). Collectively, these studies suggest that patients could attain control from a wide variety of ECoG locations while performing tasks beyond motor control.

Human ECoG BCIs were shown to provide a stable signal across 5 days of recording (Blakely et al. 2009). Slightly later work showed that motor imagery BCIs produced more pronounced changes in ECoG activity over the motor cortex than actual movements (Miller et al. 2010).

Collectively, these results from ECoG BCI research with humans and primates have provided the motivation and potential for improved systems that could use a variety of options for electrode positions and associated mental tasks. For the minority of BCIs that do require significant training (typically based on motor imagery), ECoG BCIs should entail less training and provide improved control. The improved spatial resolution (and in particular the use of broadband gamma that is not readily detectable in EEG recordings) should provide the foundation for new directions with ECoG BCIs for control, as well as other goals such as communication that is addressed in Section 16.4.2.

### 16.4.2  ECoG BCIs for Communication

During early BCI research, most work was focused on providing communication for severely disabled users through BCI paradigms involving visual attention or imagined movements (Wolpaw et al. 2002). One common approach used the P300 and other EEG activity associated with voluntary selective attention to spell or select other items from a matrix of choices, and this paradigm is still widely employed (Fazel-Rezai et al. 2012; Powers et al. 2015). In 2011, the first matrix speller using ECoG was reported (Brunner et al. 2011). One subject with ECoG electrodes implanted in the occipital lobe used P300 and visual evoked potentials to spell very effectively, attaining 17 characters/min (69 bits/min) over sustained BCI operation and 22 characters/min (113 bits/min) at peak. These rates are considerably higher than those reported for EEG-based P300 spellers at that time and are still higher than typical EEG-based P300 BCIs today. Two additional studies also achieved encouraging results with a similar approach (Krusienski and Shih 2011a, b). Another study (Krusienski and Shih 2011c) defined the spectral components involved in such ECoG-based BCIs.

Other groups have explored paradigms to select characters and/or other items using ECoG measures of motor imagery. For example, Hinterberger et al. (2008) presented a two-class ECoG BCI based on imagination of either tongue or hand movement. Using these two commands, participants could select characters through a sequence of binary selections. The subject with the best performance required about 3 min to convey one character.

A more recent study provided communication for a patient with amyotrophic lateral sclerosis (Vansteensel et al. 2016). The study utilized a fully implanted ECoG-based BCI device (Activa PC+S, Medtronic, Minneapolis, Minnesota (Afshar et al. 2012; Rouse et al. 2011; Stanslaski et al. 2012)) with subdural ECoG electrodes over cortical motor areas and a subcutaneously placed transmitter in the thorax. The patient could convey about two letters per minute by imagining hand movement. The patient also used the BCI with their eye-tracking system, both simultaneously and as an alternate communication tool (see Section 16.5). The BCI provided communication through an implanted device designed for chronic recording and remained effective 28 weeks after electrode placement. This study showed that an ECoG BCI can provide practical communication, even in a hybrid environment with an eye-tracker, for about 7 months after implantation surgery.

In addition to working with selective attention and imagined movement, several ECoG studies have introduced communication options that may not be readily viable with EEG BCIs or any current noninvasive imaging method. For example, ECoG signals may be employed to decode phonemes or words that a subject speaks or even simply imagines (Pei et al. 2010, 2011; Kellis et al. 2010; Leuthardt et al. 2011; Martin et al. 2016; Mugler et al. 2015, 2014). These approaches generally rely on ECoG electrodes placed on the temporal lobe since this region includes Wernicke's area and earlier auditory processing areas over superior temporal gyrus. ECoG activity reflecting speech processing has also been explored over Broca's area and nearby motor areas involved in speech. One study used ECoG to explore vocal track kinematics as six participants articulated nine vowels. The authors could predict lip kinematics based on ECoG activity from ventral sensorimotor cortical areas (Bouchard et al. 2016). Advancing beyond isolated phonemes or words, Brumberg et al. (Brumberg et al. 2016) explored ongoing spatiotemporal changes in cortical activity while people overtly or covertly read sentences continuously, and Martin et al. (2014) and Herff et al. (2015) decoded complete spectro-temporal representations and even whole sentences from ECoG, respectively. Another study explored ECoG activity while 10 patients listened to a rock song or spoken narrative (Sturm et al. 2014). The authors could precisely and reliably identify the moments when spoken lyrics began and ended within the rock song, and showed that broadband gamma power over temporal areas reflected processing dynamics relating to different aspects of sound such as pitch and timbre. These new approaches could lead to BCIs based on words, sentences, or other speech-related activity that people simply imagine. BCIs that can directly interpret imagined words, sentences, or related mental activities could lead to major advances for BCIs in terms of ease of use, practicality, flexibility, bandwidth, and other factors.

### 16.4.3  ECoG BCIs for Neuromodulation

Over the past several years, human and animal neurophysiologists have begun to increasingly explore ECoG to explain neurophysiological correlates of disease. Intraoperative studies during deep brain stimulation (DBS) electrode implantation surgeries (during which the patients remain awake) provide a particularly opportune window for these studies. Acute intraoperative ECoG strips can be implanted during these surgeries to study thalamocortical or basal ganglia–cortical pathways of disease. Many studies in the literature point to pathologically high beta band activity in the basal ganglia–cortical network in Parkinson's disease (PD) (Bronte-Stewart et al. 2009; Brown et al. 2001; Levy et al. 2002). Moreover, the amplitude of the beta rhythm correlates with clinical measures of symptom severity in PD (Bronte-Stewart et al. 2009; Brown et al. 2001; Levy et al. 2002). In a similar intraoperative study of essential tremor (ET), which consists mostly of slow tremors (4–8 Hz) of the upper extremities, Air et al. (2012) reported high coherence with the primary motor cortex ECoG activity and an accelerometer placed on the tremor dominated hands of patients. Studying the neural correlates of neurological disorders not only contributes to our understanding of the pathophysiologies, but may also allow us to develop better treatment strategies.

DBS, which has been an FDA-approved treatment for PD and ET since the early 1990s (Okun 2014a), aims to suppress pathophysiological activity that leads to symptoms by delivering electrical pulses to target deep-brain structures (such as the basal ganglia nuclei or thalamic subregions). The clinical personnel that program the stimulation settings (amplitude, frequency, and pulse width of the electrical current), however, do not necessarily have a scientific understanding of the underlying pathology or the physiological response to the adjustments to various stimulation parameters. Instead, they base their decisions on the observable behavioral responses and verbal response of patients. This is known as an *open-loop DBS* system. Studying the neurophysiological signatures of neurological disorders and the after-effects of brain stimulation would enable direct interpretation of the disorder and provide insight into treatment options that can be tailored to the current clinical condition of the patient. A DBS system that responsively stimulates when pathological signals are present or adaptively modifies stimulation parameters to match the degree of pathology is called a *closed-loop DBS* system. Although the clinical value of a DBS system that can initiate stimulation and/or adapt its stimulation parameters to the input received from the brain signals has long been recognized within the neuromodulation community (McIntyre 2015), the proof of concept has been lacking and the clinical efficacy of closed-loop DBS remains to be demonstrated in movement disorders.

One of the barriers to this goal has been the fact that these studies were thus far limited to the operating rooms. Recently, next generation bidirectional devices capable of performing chronic brain recordings in humans have emerged, and we present examples of these systems in Section 16.5. These devices allow for studying and tracking of the pathophysiological neural signals that can drive therapeutic stimulation. However, tracking a neuromarker on the electrode array used for stimulation is usually challenging in these implantable devices owing to amplifier saturation or significant stimulation artifacts. Thus, many groups are now seeking FDA investigational device exemption (IDE) to implant an ECoG strip from which they can extract the pathophysiological neuromarker and deliver stimulation to deep brain structures. The ECoG strip is far enough from the subcortically implanted electrodes and is not significantly affected by the stimulation artifact because of this distance and the much higher signal amplitudes in ECoG. For instance, the pathological beta rhythms in PD that are present in the basal ganglia are also present in motor cortex and thus can be used as a marker to drive closed-loop DBS (Little et al. 2013; Rosa et al. 2015).

Moreover, an additional ECoG strip allows researchers to study basal ganglia–cortical networks or thalamocortical networks of disease in humans when stimulation is temporarily turned off. Shute et al. (2015) studied the thalamocortical network of Tourette syndrome (TS) with Activa PC+S devices. TS is a highly complex neuropsychiatric disorder characterized by involuntary motor and vocal tics. Figure 16.9 shows data recorded chronically in two patients with TS with bilateral implants in the centromedian-parafascicular (Cm-Pf) complex of the thalamus, which is the most common DBS target for TS, and bilateral ECoG strips over their hand motor cortices. Figure 16.9 shows the differences in signal modulations during involuntary hand motor tics and voluntary hand movements. During both types of movement, beta desynchronization is evident in motor cortex. Only during involuntary tics is there a deviation from the baseline in the raw Cm-Pf recordings that is reflected as increase in the low-frequency activity in the spectrogram.

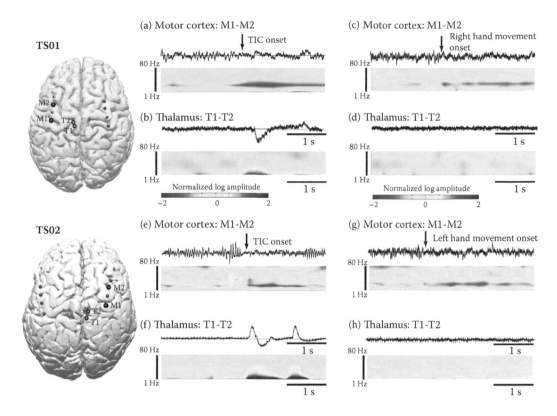

**FIGURE 16.9** Time series and spectrograms for motor cortical and thalamic recordings. Panels (a) to (d) correspond to Subject TS01, and panels (e) to (h) correspond to Subject TS02. (b and f) Increases in Cm-Pf low-frequency activity are concurrent with (a and e) motor cortex beta desynchronization at the onset of tics. (d and h) No increases in low-frequency Cm-Pf local field potentials are observed during volitional movements such as grasping (shown), but (c and g) motor cortex beta desynchronization is still observed. (From J. Shute, P. Rossi, C. de Hemptinne, K. Foote, M. Okun, and A. Gunduz. Neural correlates of tourette syndrome within the centromedian thalamus, premotor and primary motor cortices. *Movement Disord*, 30:S492–S493, 2015.)

In addition to studying disease biomarkers, bidirectional neural implants could enable studying the neural correlates of DBS therapy and could uncover how DBS modulates neural networks to bring about symptom relief. As discussed above, recent evidence supports the argument that local neuronal population activity, as detected via broadband gamma amplitude shifts, is co-modulated with the phase of lower frequencies (Voytek et al. 2010; Canolty et al. 2006; Miller et al. 2010). In an intraoperative study, de Hemptinne et al. (2013) showed pathologically high coupling between beta phase-broadband gamma in the motor cortex of PD patients compared to epilepsy and dystonia patients. The signals as captured through ECoG strip electrodes placed over the hand motor cortex intraoperatively (see Figure 16.10). The same group recently also showed that optimal DBS stimulation that brought symptom relief also decreased this coupling (see Figure 16.11) (de Hemptinne et al. 2015). In a similar study in TS, Shute et al. showed that there was no significant coupling in the motor cortices of TS patients and that optimal DBS increased this coupling (see Figure 16.12 Okun 2014b). These results are interesting, as they provide an ECoG biomarker that is exaggerated for a hypokinetic disorder (PD) and is absent for a hyperkinetic disorder (TS). Moreover, through ECoG, these studies present how DBS brings these patients to a healthier, less symptomatic state through stimulation of different nodes in the motor network. This ECoG biomarker can be used to adaptively change DBS parameters in both disorders and to develop adaptive closed-loop DBS systems in the future.

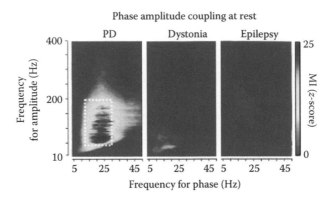

**FIGURE 16.10** Comparison of phase–amplitude coupling in the three different disease states showing pathological patterns in motor cortex in Parkinson's disease compared to dystonia and epilepsy. (From C. de Hemptinne, E. S. Ryapolova-Webb, E. L. Air, P. A. Garcia, K. J. Miller, J. G. Ojemann, J. L. Ostrem, N. B. Galifianakis, and P. A. Starr. Exaggerated phase–amplitude coupling in the primary motor cortex in Parkinson disease. *Proc Nat Acad Sci*, 110(12):4780–4785, 2013.)

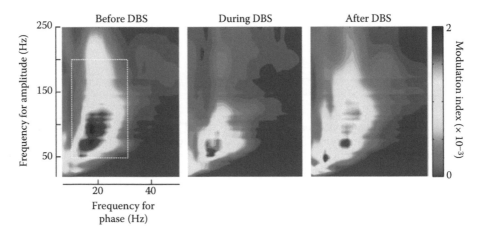

**FIGURE 16.11** Representative example of coupling observed in motor cortex of a Parkinson's disease patient before (left), during (middle), and after STN stimulation (right). (From C. de Hemptinne, N. C. Swann, J. L. Ostrem, E. S. Ryapolova-Webb, M. San Luciano, N. B. Galifianakis, and P. A. Starr. Therapeutic deep brain stimulation reduces cortical phase–amplitude coupling in Parkinson's disease. *Nat Neurosci*, 18(5), Apr 2015.)

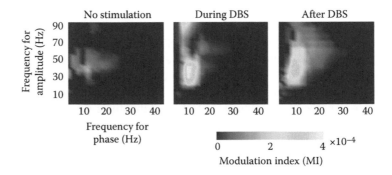

**FIGURE 16.12** Representative example of coupling observed in motor cortex of a Tourette syndrome patient before (left), during (middle), and after Cm-Pf stimulation (right). (From M. Okun. Tourette syndrome deep brain stimulation, clinicaltrials.gov identifier:nct02056873. https://clinicaltrials.gov/ct2/show/NCT02056873, 2014.)

## 16.5   CURRENT IMPLANTABLE DEVICES

Recent years have seen an increase in the development, testing, and regulatory approval of implantable recording and stimulation systems for BCI use. We introduced the Activa PC+S system (Afshar et al. 2012; Rouse et al. 2011; Stanslaski et al. 2012) in Section 16.4. The system has received FDA IDE; however, clinical investigations are currently clinician initiated with a right of reference from Medtronic. The Activa PC+S is the same form factor and has the equivalent capability as the commercially available Activa PC, which connects to two four-contact electrode arrays (commonly referred to as leads by DBS clinicians) for stimulation delivery. The device is implanted in the chest cavity, similar to a pacemaker. In addition to providing predicate therapy capabilities, the Activa PC+S adds key elements to facilitate chronic research, such as two channels of ECoG or LFP amplification and spectral analysis, algorithm processing, event-based data logging, and wireless telemetry for data uploads and algorithm/configuration updates (Rouse et al. 2011). The device is capable of recording time-domain brain signals from one bipolar electrode configuration from each lead simultaneously at sampling rates of 200, 422, or 800 Hz (Rouse et al. 2011). It can also record the desired spectral power of a frequency band in four channels at 5 Hz (Rouse et al. 2011). Data can be streamed to a computer for algorithm development (Afshar et al. 2012), or an embedded linear discriminant analysis classifier can be used to detect events (Stanslaski et al. 2012). Figure 16.13 shows the schematic presented in the Vansteensel et al. study with a locked-in patient (Vansteensel et al. 2016). Data are streamed out to control a speller. If a study involves stimulation (which is not the case in Figure 16.13), stimulation parameters are set using a separate clinical stimulation programmer. The patient receives a programmer to switch between open- and closed-loop settings and an event marker, which triggers a recording. A second-generation rechargeable device with higher channel counts and better stimulation artifact rejection, the Activa RC+S, is currently being developed (Bourget et al. 2015). These two devices are registered with the BRAIN Initiative Public-Private Partnership Program.

A system that has received approval from the FDA is the NeuroPace (Mountain View, California) Responsive Neurostimulator (RNS) for the treatment of intractable epilepsy (Morrel and RNS System in Epilepsy Study Group 2011). The RNS System provides responsive cortical stimulation via a cranially implanted programmable neurostimulator connected to one or two recording and stimulating four-contact depth or subdural cortical strip leads that are surgically placed in the brain according to the seizure focus (see Figure 16.14 Heck et al. 2014). The neurostimulator continually senses ECoG or LFP activity and is programmed by the physician to detect abnormal neural activity and then provide stimulation. The physician adjusts detection and stimulation parameters for each patient to optimize control of seizures. The device is fully implanted in the skull (see Figure 16.14). Other components include a physician programmer, a patient remote monitor and a magnet for marking events. A multicenter, double-blind, randomized controlled trial assessing the safety and effectiveness of responsive cortical stimulation study as an adjunct therapy for partial onset seizures was conducted in 191 adults with medically refractory epilepsy. The study is registered on ClinicalTrials.gov (NCT00264810), and the results of the study are publically available. The RNS system is registered with the BRAIN Initiative Public-Private Partnership Program.

The French WIMAGINE system is capable of real-time recording and wireless transmission of the ECoG signals from 64 electrodes at a sampling rate of 600 Hz to an external computer housing the control software (see Figure 16.15) (Mestais et al. 2015). The hermetic housing and the antennae have been designed and optimized to ease the surgical implantation in the skull. The software system is designed for BCI use.

The Australian NeuroVista device was an implantable seizure advisory system for patients with intractable epilepsy. Two silicon implantable lead assemblies, each with eight platinum iridium contacts distributed across two electrode arrays, collect ECoG at a sampling rate of 400 Hz (Cook et al. 2013) and the system wirelessly transmits these data to an external, handheld personal advisory

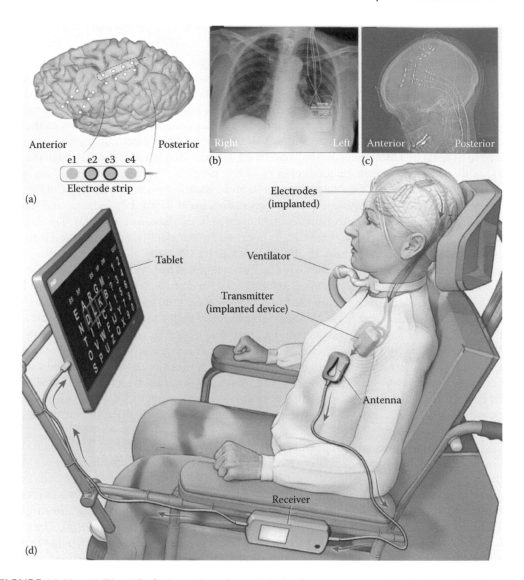

**FIGURE 16.13** (a) The ECoG electrode strips and their placement over patient brain model (coverage is over the sensorimotor and dorsolateral prefrontal cortex). (b) Postoperative chest x-ray displaying the Activa PC+S implant. (c) Postoperative CT scan with the locations of four electrode strips. (d) The brain–computer interface system, including the Activa PC+S, receiving antenna, receiver, and tablet. (From M. Vansteensel, E. Pels, M. Bleichner, M. Branco, T. Denison, Z. Freudenberg, P. Gosselaar, S. Leinders, T. Ottens, M. VandenEboom, P. van Rijen, E. Aarnoutse, and N. Ramsey. Fully implanted brain–computer interface in a locked-in patient with ALS. *N Engl Med*, 375(21):2060–2066, 2016.)

device (see Figure 16.16). The implantable telemetry unit is inductively recharged through an external charging accessory. A terminated clinical trial for safety and efficacy with 15 patients is registered with ClinicalTrials.gov (NCT01043406).

The German BrainInterchange system by CorTec (see Figure 16.17) is based on a fully implantable device for recording and stimulation in humans. It provides 32 electrode contacts, all of which can be used for signal recording (1 kHz sampling rate at 16 bit dynamic range) or brain stimulation (maximum 6 mA/2.5 ms). The system consists of (a) the electrodes; (b) a hermetically encapsulated

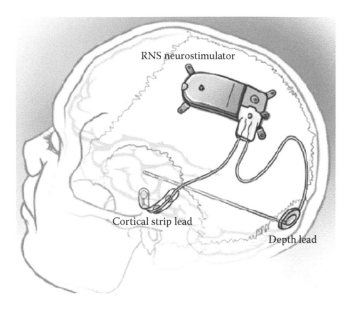

**FIGURE 16.14** Schematic of an implanted Neuropace RNS system with one ECoG strip and one depth lead. (From C. N. Heck, D. King-Stephens, A. D. Massey, D. R. Nair, B. C. Jobst, G. L. Barkley, V. Salanova, A. J. Cole, M. C. Smith, R. P. Gwinn et al. Two-year seizure reduction in adults with medically intractable partial onset epilepsy treated with responsive neurostimulation: Final results of the RNS system pivotal trial. *Epilepsia*, 55(3):432–441, 2014.)

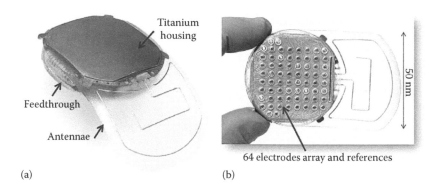

(a)                                                                                        (b)

**FIGURE 16.15** WIMAGINE ECoG recording implant: (a) top and (b) bottom view. (From C. S. Mestais, G. Charvet, F. Sauter-Starace, M. Foerster, D. Ratel, and A.-L. Benabid. WIMAGINE: Wireless 64-channel ECoG recording implant for long term clinical applications. *IEEE Trans Neural Syst Rehabil Eng: A Publication of the IEEE Engineering in Medicine and Biology Society*, 23(1):10–21, Jan 2015.)

electronic unit that amplifies, digitizes, and broadcasts brain signals and directs electrical stimuli to selected electrodes; (c) a telemetric unit that is placed outside the body on the skin; and (d) a wearable controller unit. The telemetric unit communicates with the implant and provides it wirelessly with energy. The controller unit (laptop PC) runs a software interface to custom-specific application software. The application software that controls the brain signal data stream, analyzes the data, takes decisions, and sends commands to the implant that can be customized for a specific application by the user in C++, Python II, or MATLAB.

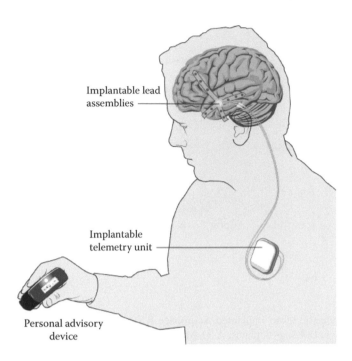

**FIGURE 16.16**   Schematic of the Neurovista seizure advisory system. Sixteen electrodes are connected to a subclavicularly placed implanted telemetry unit, which transmits data to an external handheld device. (From M. J. Cook, T. J. O'Brien, S. F. Berkovic, M. Murphy, A. Morokoff, G. Fabinyi, W. D'Souza, R. Yerra, J. Archer, L. Litewka, S. Hosking, P. Lightfoot, V. Ruedebusch, W. D. Sheffield, D. Snyder, K. Leyde, and D. Himes. Prediction of seizure likelihood with a long-term, implanted seizure advisory system in patients with drug-resistant epilepsy: A first-in-man study. *Lancet Neurol*, 12(6):563–571, June 2013.)

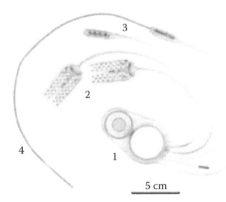

**FIGURE 16.17**   The implantable part of CorTec's Brain Interchange system: (1) hermetically packaged electronics; (2) grid electrodes; (3) connectors for deep brain stimulation (DBS) leads; (4) DBS lead. (Figure courtesy of CorTec.)

## 16.6   OPEN QUESTIONS AND DIRECTIONS FOR FURTHER RESEARCH

At present, most ECoG-based BCI research is still performed in human subjects who have been temporarily implanted with an ECoG array for the purpose of presurgical assessments. Thus, substantial practical constraints and challenges affect the design of ECoG-based BCI studies. Perhaps the most hindering issue is the limited amount of time that is available with these subjects. This may be the main reason that there are still relatively few online human ECoG-based BCI studies in the literature today (Leuthardt et al. 2004, 2006; Miller et al. 2010b; Blakely et al. 2009; Brunner et al. 2011; Felton et al. 2007; Hinterberger et al. 2008; Rouse and Moran 2009; Schalk 2008; Vansteensel et al. 2010; Wilson et al. 2006; Wang et al. 2013). At the same time, together with the many offline BCI-related studies, this work strongly encourages further investigations of ECoG BCI technology.

Another limitation of ECoG studies performed with this patient population is the electrode size and interelectrode distance of the clinical arrays that are currently being used. As discussed in previous subsections, conventional clinical grids are often configured as an 8-by-8 array with 1 cm interelectrode spacing and an exposed contact diameter of 2–3 mm. These arrays are designed with such large contact area surfaces to yield low impedance values (around several hundred ohms), which prove to be advantageous in the noisy environment of a hospital room. A grid can spatially cover a large area of a lateral hemisphere but samples sparsely because of the large interelectrode distance, typically from only a few electrodes on a given gyrus (Chang 2015). The optimal electrode size and interelectrode distance to maximize the amount of information extracted through ECoG is one of the most important open questions in the field. While smaller electrodes, sometimes referred to as micro-ECoG, can bring about improved spatial selectivity, this comes at the expense of increased impedance. Moreover, while more channels may promise increased spatial sampling, an increased number of channels provides practical and clinical challenges. Some studies have utilized micro-ECoG arrays to show higher information extraction in the superior temporal gyrus to study speech generation (Bouchard et al. 2016; Chang et al. 2010; Mesgarani et al. 2014) and to show improved BCI performance (Kellis et al. 2010, 2016; Leuthardt et al. 2009). A computational finite element modeling study that predicted the biophysical correlation between electrodes at various distances suggested a minimum spacing of 1.7–1.8 mm for subdural recordings (Slutzky et al. 2010), which is still larger than the size of cortical ocular dominance columns in the human visual cortex that are about 1 mm wide (Adam and Horton 2008). It should be noted that correlation between electrode recordings, and thus optimal electrode spacing, is dependent on frequency. As discussed earlier, lower frequencies are more broadly distributed while high frequencies are spatially more focal. Thus, it is not surprising that when Chang (2015) computed the correlation of different spectral bands as a function of electrode distance, correlation was lowest for the broadband gamma band at the lowest electrode spacing and higher for lower frequencies (see Figure 16.18).

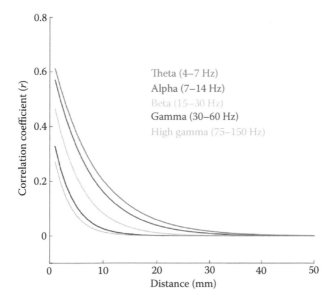

**FIGURE 16.18** Human cortical recordings obtained on a 4-mm-spaced ECoG grid. Significant differences in spatial resolution, especially at less than 1 cm, can be observed depending on the frequency band of interest. Correlations for distances less than 4 mm are extrapolated. (From E. F. Chang. Towards large-scale, human-based, mesoscopic neurotechnologies. *Neuron*, 86(1):68–78, Apr. 2015.)

Rouse et al. (Rouse et al. 2016) utilized micro-ECoG electrodes with 300 m diameter for one-dimensional and two-dimensional BCI tasks in primates. They tested the effect of interelectrode distance on BCI control between 3 and 15 mm. The primates achieved successful BCI control with two electrodes separated by 9 and 15 mm. Performance decreased and the signals became more correlated when the electrodes were only 3 mm apart. Overall, more systematic studies informed by computational models are imperative to determine the optimal electrode design for BCI utility.

It should be noted that in the study by Rouse et al. (2016), the electrode arrays were placed epidurally, that is, on top of the dura, which does not require a dural incision. Given that most complications involved in epilepsy surgery are related to infections due to incisions to the dura (Van Gompel et al. 2008), studying the signal fidelity of epidural ECoG could lead to a potentially less invasive BCI system and a justification for BCI users to undergo implantation of such systems with benefits potentially outweighing the risks. For instance, Spueler et al. (2014) temporally implanted ECoG strips epidurally in chronic stroke patients with paresis. In this study, the authors were able to decode seven imagined hand movements from the ipsilateral hemisphere. In another study, Bundy et al. (2014) utilized simultaneously acquired epidural and subdural ECoG signals while the patients were at rest. Both macro-scale (2-mm-diameter electrodes with 1-cm interelectrode distance, one patient) and micro-scale (75-μm-diameter electrodes with 1-mm interelectrode distance, four patients) ECoG electrodes were tested. While subdural micro-ECoG contacts have significantly higher spectral amplitudes and reached the noise floor around 150–200 Hz, epidural micro-ECoG contacts reached the noise floor around 80 Hz. Epidural placement of macroelectrode grids did not affect the noise floor significantly. More studies are needed to confirm these results in behaviorally modulated signals and BCI tasks.

## 16.7 SUMMARY

With its unique characteristics, ECoG is producing strong support and growing excitement for its potential as a BCI signal modality. ECoG is likely to be an integral part of foreseeable chronic neural implants because of its high signal fidelity, long-term stability, and relatively low demands on sampling rate, thus greatly reducing the power requirements of the implantable system.

Using similar signal-processing techniques, ECoG BCIs can make use of similar features used in EEG-based BCIs, mainly the mu and beta rhythm bands prominent in the scalp-recorded EEG over sensorimotor cortex. In addition, it also yields higher-frequency broadband gamma activity and, with depth electrodes, activity from subcortical structures that cannot be captured over the scalp. ECoG high-frequency activity reflects asynchronous synaptic activity, demonstrates greater functional localization than the low-frequency synchronized rhythms, and thus may be particularly beneficial to improve the performance of a BCI system. In addition, ECoG also detects the LMP, which has been shown to have a differential role in decoding motor execution and planning.

ECoG-based BCI studies to date have been limited primarily to people temporarily implanted with ECoG recording arrays before epilepsy surgery. However, with increased interest and investment in implantable technologies, ECoG arrays are being implanted chronically and in various disease conditions. In this case, it can provide an interface to stably record from and stimulate both cortical and subcortical neuronal populations. Thus, compared to scalp-recorded EEG, its use should enable an array of new neuromodulation applications. At the same time, to maximize the benefit and the utility of ECoG, the following open questions need to be addressed: can signal acquisition be improved through optimal electrode design or optimal electrode placement; can epidural ECoG yield acceptable BCI performance? Also, can BCI performance be improved by optimizing feature selection or through a combination of features (such as broadband gamma and LMP)? These questions should keep the field active and vibrant for the decade ahead.

## ACKNOWLEDGMENT

We are grateful to Dr. Brendan Z. Allison for his help editing this chapter.

# REFERENCES

Acharya, S., Fifer, M. S., Benz, H. L., Crone, N. E., and Thakor, N. V. Electrocorticographic amplitude predicts finger positions during slow grasping motions of the hand. *J Neural Eng*, 7(4):046002–046002, Aug 2010.

Adams, D. L., and Horton, J. C. Ocular dominance columns: Enigmas and challenges. *Neuroscientist*, 15(1):62–77, Nov 2008.

Afshar, P., Khambhati, A., Stanslaski, S., Carlson, D., Jensen, R., Linde, D., Dani, S., Lazarewicz, M., Cong, P., Giftakis, J., Stypulkowski, P., and Denison, T. A translational platform for prototyping closedloop neuromodulation systems. *Front Neural Circ*, 6:117, 2012.

Air, E. L., Ryapolova-Webb, E., de Hemptinne, C., Ostrem, J. L., Galifianakis, N. B., Larson, P. S., Chang, E. F., and Starr, P. A. Acute effects of thalamic deep brain stimulation and thalamotomy on sensorimotor cortex local field potentials in essential tremor. *Clin Neurophysiol*, 123(11):2232–2238, Nov 2012.

Allen, E. A., Liu, J., Kiehl, K. A., Gelernter, J., Pearlson, G. D., Perrone-Bizzozero, N. I., and Calhoun, V. D. Components of cross-frequency modulation in health and disease. *Front Syst Neurosci*, 5:59, 2011.

Aoki, F., Fetz, E. E., Shupe, L., Lettich, E., and Ojemann, G. A. Increased gamma-range activity in human sensorimotor cortex during performance of visuomotor tasks. *Clin Neurophysiol*, 110(3):524–537, Mar 1999.

Anderson, K. L., Rajagovindan, R., Ghacibeh, G. A., Meador, K. J., and Ding, M. Theta oscillations mediate interaction between prefrontal cortex and medial temporal lobe in human memory. *Cereb Cortex*, 20(7):1604–1612, 2009.

Blakely, T., Miller, K., Zanos, S., Rao, R., and Ojemann, J. Robust, long-term control of an electrocorticographic brain–computer interface with fixed parameters. *J Neurosurg Pediatr*, 27(1), 2009.

Bouchard, K. E., Conant, D. F., Anumanchipalli, G. K., Dichter, B., Chaisanguanthum, K. S., Johnson, K., and Chang, E. F. High-resolution, non-invasive imaging of upper vocal tract articulators compatible with human brain recordings. *PloS One*, 11(3):e0151327, 2016.

Bourget, D., Bink, H., Stanslaski, S., Linde, D., Arnett, C., Adamski, T., and Denison, T. An implantable, rechargeable neuromodulation research tool using a distributed interface and algorithm architecture. *7th, International IEEE EMBS Conference on Neural Engineering*, pages 1–5, Oct 2015.

Bronte-Stewart, H., Barberini, C., Koop, M. M., and Hill, B. C. The STN beta-band profile in Parkinson's disease is stationary and shows prolonged attenuation after deep brain stimulation. *Exp Neurol*, 2009.

Brown, P., Oliviero, A., Mazzone, P., Insola, A., Tonali, P., and Di Lazzaro, V. Dopamine dependency of oscillations between subthalamic nucleus and pallidum in Parkinson's disease. *Neurosci*, 21(3):1033–1038, Feb 2001.

Brumberg, J. S., Krusienski, D. J., Chakrabarti, S., Gunduz, A., Brunner, P., Ritaccio, A. L., and Schalk, G., Spatio-temporal progression of cortical activity related to continuous overt and covert speech production in a reading task. *PloS One*, 11(11):e0166872, 2016.

Brunner, P., Ritaccio, A. L., Emrich, J. F., Bischof, H., and Schalk, G. Rapid communication with a "P300" matrix speller using electrocorticographic signals (ECoG). *Front Neuroprosthet*, 5(5):1–9, 2011.

Brunner, P., Ritaccio, A. L., Lynch, T. M., Emrich, J. F., Wilson, J. A., Williams, J. C., Aarnoutse, E. J., Ramsey, N. F., Leuthardt, E. C., Bischof, H., and Schalk, G. A practical procedure for real-time functional mapping of eloquent cortex using electrocorticographic signals in humans. *Epilepsy Behav*, 15(3):278–286, Apr 2009.

Bullara, L. A., Agnew, W. F., Yuen, T. G., Jacques, S., and Pudenz, R. H. Evaluation of electrode array material for neural prostheses. *Neurosurgery*, 5(6):681–686, Dec 1979.

Bundy, D. T., Pahwa, M., Szrama, N., and Leuthardt, E. C. Decoding three-dimensional reaching movements using electrocorticographic signals in humans. *J Neural Eng*, 13(2):026021, 2016.

Bundy, D. T., Zellmer, E., Gaona, C. M., Sharma, M., Szrama, N., Hacker, C., Freudenburg, Z. V., Daitch, A., Moran, D. W., and Leuthardt, E. C. Characterization of the effects of the human dura on macro- and micro-electrocorticographic recordings. *J Neural Eng*, 11(1):016006, Jan 2014.

Canolty, R. T., Edwards, E., Dalal, S. S., Soltani, M., Nagarajan, S. S., Kirsch, H. E., Berger, M. S., Barbaro, N. M., and Knight, R. T. High gamma power is phase-locked to theta oscillations in human neocortex. *Science*, 313(5793):1626–1628, Sep 2006.

Canolty, R., Soltani, M., Dalal, S., Edwards, E., Dronkers, N., Nagarajan, S., Kirsch, H., Barbaro, N., and Knight, R. Spatiotemporal dynamics of word processing in the human brain. *Front Neurosci*, 1(1):185, 2007.

Chang, E. F., Edwards, E., Nagarajan, S. S., Fogelson, N., Dalal, S. S., Canolty, R. T., Kirsch, H. E., Barbaro, N. M., and Knight, R. T. Cortical spatio-temporal dynamics underlying phonological target detection in humans. *J Cogn Neurosci*, 23(6):1437–1446, 2011.

Chang, E. F., Rieger, J. W., Johnson, K., Berger, M. S., Barbaro, N. M., and Knight, R. T. Categorical speech representation in human superior temporal gyrus. *Nat Neurosci*, 13(11):1428–1432, Nov 2010.

Chang, E. F. Towards large-scale, human-based, mesoscopic neurotechnologies. *Neuron*, 86(1):68–78, Apr 2015

Chao, Z. C., Nagasaka, Y., and Fujii, N. Long-term asynchronous decoding of arm motion using electrocorticographic signals in monkeys. *Front Neuroeng*, 3:3–3, 2010.

Chatrian, G. *Handbook of Electroencephalography and Clinical Neurophysiology*. Elsevier, Amsterdam, 1976.

Cook, M. J., O'Brien, T. J., Berkovic, S. F., Murphy, M., Morokoff, A., Fabinyi, G., D'Souza, W., Yerra, R., Archer, J., Litewka, L., Hosking, S., Lightfoot, P., Ruedebusch, V., Sheffield, W. D., Snyder, D., Leyde, K., and Himes, D. Prediction of seizure likelihood with a long-term, implanted seizure advisory system in patients with drug-resistant epilepsy: A first-in-man study. *Lancet Neurol*, 12(6):563–571, June 2013.

Crone, N. E., Boatman, D., Gordon, B., and Hao, L. Induced electrocorticographic gamma activity during auditory perception. *J Clin Neurophysiol*, 112(4):565–582, Apr 2001a.

Crone, N. E., Hao, L., Hart, J., Boatman, D., Lesser, R. P., Irizarry, R., and Gordon, B. Electrocorticographic gamma activity during word production in spoken and sign language. *Neurology*, 57(11):2045–2053, Dec 2001b.

Crone, N. E., Miglioretti, D. L., Gordon, B., and Lesser, R. P. Functional mapping of human sensorimotor cortex with electrocorticographic spectral analysis. II. Event-related synchronization in the gamma band. *Brain*, 121 (Pt 12):2301–2315, Dec 1998a.

Crone, N. E., Miglioretti, D. L., Gordon, B., Sieracki, J. M., Wilson, M. T., Uematsu, S., and Lesser, R. P. Functional mapping of human sensorimotor cortex with electrocorticographic spectral analysis. I. Alpha and beta event-related desynchronization. *Brain*, 121 (Pt 12):2271–2299, Dec 1998b.

Crowell, A. L., Ryapolova-Webb, E. S., Ostrem, J. L., Galifianakis, N. B., Shimamoto, S., Lim, D. A., and Starr, P. A. Oscillations in sensorimotor cortex in movement disorders: An electrocorticography study. *Brain*, 135 (Pt 2):615–630, 2012.

Darvas, F., Scherer, R., Ojemann, J. G., Rao, R., Miller, K. J., and Sorensen, L. B. High gamma mapping using EEG. *NeuroImage*, 49(1):930–938, 2010.

de Hemptinne, C., Ryapolova-Webb, E. S., Air, E. L., Garcia, P. A., Miller, K. J., Ojemann, J. G., Ostrem, J. L., Galifianakis, N. B., and Starr, P. A. Exaggerated phase–amplitude coupling in the primary motor cortex in Parkinson disease. *Proc Nat Acad Sci*, 110(12):4780–4785, 2013.

de Hemptinne, C., Swann, N. C., Ostrem, J. L., Ryapolova-Webb, E. S., San Luciano, M., Galifianakis, N. B., and Starr, P. A. Therapeutic deep brain stimulation reduces cortical phase–amplitude coupling in Parkinson's disease. *Nat Neurosci*, 18(5), Apr 2015.

Dürschmid, S., Quandt, F., Krämer, U. M., Hinrichs, H., Heinze, H.-J., Schulz, R., Pannek, H., Chang, E. F., and Knight, R. T. Oscillatory dynamics track motor performance improvement in human cortex. *PloS One*, 9(2):e89576, 2014.

Edwards, E., Nagarajan, S. S., Dalal, S. S., Canolty, R. T., Kirsch, H. E., Barbaro, N. M., and Knight, R. T. Spatiotemporal imaging of cortical activation during verb generation and picture naming. *NeuroImage*, 50(1):291–301, Mar 2010.

Edwards, E., Soltani, M., Deouell, L. Y., Berger, M. S., and Knight, R. T. High gamma activity in response to deviant auditory stimuli recorded directly from human cortex. *J Neurophysiol*, 94(6):4269–4280, 2005.

Edwards, E., Soltani, M., Kim, W., Dalal, S. S., Nagarajan, S. S., Berger, M. S., and Knight, R. T. Comparison of time-frequency responses and the event-related potential to auditory speech stimuli in human cortex. *J Neurophysiol*, 102(1):377–386, 2009.

Engell, A. D., Huettel, S., and McCarthy, G. The fMRI BOLD signal tracks electrophysiological spectral perturbations, not event-related potentials. *NeuroImage*, 59(3):2600–2606, 2012.

Fazel-Rezai, R., Allison, B. Z., Guger, C., Sellers, E., Kleih, S., and Kuebler, A. P300 brain–computer interface: Current challenges and emerging trends. *Front Neuroeng*, 5(14), 2012.

Felton, E. A., Wilson, J. A., Williams, J. C., and Garell, P. C. Electrocorticographically controlled brain–computer interfaces using motor and sensory imagery in patients with temporary subdural electrode implants. Report of four cases. *J Neurosurg*, 106(3):495–500, Mar 2007.

Fitzgibbon, S. P., Pope, K. J., Mackenzie, L., Clark, C. R., and Willoughby, J. O. Cognitive tasks augment gamma EEG power. *Clin Neurophysiol*, 115(8):1802–1809, 2004.

Freeman, W. J., Rogers, L. J., Holmes, M. D., and Silbergeld, D. L. Spatial spectral analysis of human electrocorticograms including the alpha and gamma bands. *J Neurosci Methods*, 95(2):111–121, Feb 2000.

Fries, P. A mechanism for cognitive dynamics: neuronal communication through coherence. *Trends Cogn Sci*, 9(10):474–480, Oct 2005.

Fujisawa, S., and Buzsáki, G. A 4 Hz oscillation adaptively synchronizes prefrontal, VTA, and hippocampal activities. *Neuron*, 72(1):153–165, 2011.

Gunduz, A., Brunner, P., Sharma, M., Leuthardt, E. C., Ritaccio, A. L., Pesaran, B., and Schalk, G. Differential roles of high gamma and local motor potentials for movement preparation and execution. *Brain–Comput Interf*, 3(2):88–102, 2016.

Haegens, S., Nácher, V., Luna, R., Romo, R., and Jensen, O. α-Oscillations in the monkey sensorimotor network influence discrimination performance by rhythmical inhibition of neuronal spiking. *Proc Natl Acad Sci U S A*, 108(48):19377–19382, 2011.

Heck, C. N., King-Stephens, D., Massey, A. D., Nair, D. R., Jobst, B. C., Barkley, G. L., Salanova, V., Cole, A. J., Smith, M. C., Gwinn, R. P. et al. Two-year seizure reduction in adults with medically intractable partial onset epilepsy treated with responsive neurostimulation: Final results of the rns system pivotal trial. *Epilepsia*, 55(3):432–441, 2014.

Herff, C., Heger, D., De Pesters, A., Telaar, D., Brunner, P., Schalk, G., and Schultz, T. Brain-to-text: Decoding spoken phrases from phone representations in the brain. *Front Neurosci*, 9:217, 2015.

Hinterberger, T., Widman, G., Lal, T., Hill, J., Tangermann, M., Rosenstiel, W., Schölkopf, B., Elger, C., and Birbaumer, N. Voluntary brain regulation and communication with electrocorticogram signals. *Epilepsy Behav*, 13(2):300–306, 2008.

Howard, M. W., Rizzuto, D. S., Caplan, J. B., Madsen, J. R., Lisman, J., Aschenbrenner-Scheibe, R., Schulze-Bonhage, A., and Kahana M. J. Gamma oscillations correlate with working memory load in humans. *Cereb Cortex*, 13(12):1369–1374, 2003.

Jensen, O., and Mazaheri, A. Shaping functional architecture by oscillatory alpha activity: Gating by inhibition. *Front Hum Neurosci*, 4, 2010.

Jensen, O., Kaiser, J., and Lachaux, J.-P. Human gamma-frequency oscillations associated with attention and memory. *Trends Neurosci*, 30(7):317–324, 2007.

Kam, J., Szczepanski, S., Canolty, R., Flinker, A., Auguste, K., Crone, N., Kirsch, H., Kuperman, R., Lin, J., Parvizi, J. et al. Differential sources for 2 neural signatures of target detection: An electrocorticography study. *Cereb Cortex*, 1–12, 2016.

Kellis, S., Miller, K., Thomson, K., Brown, R., House, P., and Greger, B. Decoding spoken words using local field potentials recorded from the cortical surface. *J Neural Eng*, 7(5):056007, 2010.

Kellis, S., Sorensen, L., Darvas, F., Sayres, C., O'Neill, K., Brown, R. B., House, P., Ojemann, J., and Greger, B. Multi-scale analysis of neural activity in humans: Implications for micro-scale electrocorticography. *Clin Neurophysiol*, 127(1):591–601, Jan 2016.

Krusienski, D., and Shih, J. J. Control of a brain–computer interface using stereotactic depth electrodes in and adjacent to the hippocampus. *J Neural Eng*, 8(2):025006, 2011a.

Krusienski, D. J., and Shih, J. J. Control of a visual keyboard using an electrocorticographic brain–computer interface. *Neurorehabil Neural Repair*, 25(4):323–331, 2011b.

Krusienski, D. J., and Shih, J. J. Spectral components of the p300 speller response in electrocorticography. In *Neural Engineering (NER), 2011 5th International IEEE/EMBS Conference on*, pages 282–285. IEEE, 2011c.

Kubanek, J., Hill, N. J., Snyder, L. H., and Schalk, G. Cortical alpha activity predicts the confidence in an impending action. *Front Neurosci*, 9, 2015.

Kubánek, J., Miller, K. J., Ojemann, J. G., Wolpaw, J. R., and Schalk, G. Decoding flexion of individual fingers using electrocorticographic signals in humans. *J Neural Eng*, 6(6):066001–066001, Dec 2009.

Kubanek, J., Snyder, L. H., Brunton, B. W., Brody, C. D., and Schalk, G. A low-frequency oscillatory neural signal in humans encodes a developing decision variable. *NeuroImage*, 83:795–808, 2013.

Lachaux, J. P., Fonlupt, P., Kahane, P., Minotti, L., Hoffmann, D., Bertrand, O., and Baciu, M. Relationship between task-related gamma oscillations and bold signal: New insights from combined fMRI and intracranial EEG. *Hum Brain Mapp*, 28(12):1368–1375, Dec 2007.

Leuthardt, E. C., Freudenberg, Z., Bundy, D., and Roland, J. Microscale recording from human motor cortex: Implications for minimally invasive electrocorticographic brain–computer interfaces. *dx.doi.org*, 27(1):E10, July 2009.

Leuthardt, E. C., Gaona, C., Sharma, M., Szrama, N., Roland, J., Freudenberg, Z., Solis, J., Breshears, J., and Schalk, G. Using the electrocorticographic speech network to control a brain–computer interface in humans. *J Neural Eng*, 8(3):036004, 2011.

Leuthardt, E., Miller, K., Anderson, N., Schalk, G., Dowling, J., Miller, J., Moran, D., and Ojemann, J. Electrocorticographic frequency alteration mapping: A clinical technique for mapping the motor cortex. *Neurosurgery*, 60:260–70; discussion 270–1, Apr 2007.

Leuthardt, E., Miller, K., Schalk, G., Rao, R., and Ojemann, J. Electrocorticography-based brain computer interface—The Seattle experience. *IEEE Trans Neur Sys Rehab Eng*, 14:194–8, Jun 2006.

Leuthardt, E., Schalk, G., Wolpaw, J., Ojemann, J., and Moran, D. A brain–computer interface using electrocorticographic signals in humans. *J Neural Eng*, 1(2):63–71, 2004.

Levy, R., Hutchison, W. D., Lozano, A. M., and Dostrovsky, J. O. Synchronized neuronal discharge in the basal ganglia of parkinsonian patients is limited to oscillatory activity. *Neurosci*, 22(7):2855–2861, Apr 2002.

Little, S., Pogosyan, A., Neal, S., Zavala, B., Zrinzo, L., Hariz, M., Foltynie, T., Limousin, P., Ashkan, K., FitzGerald, J., Green, A. L., Aziz, T. Z., and Brown, P. Adaptive deep brain stimulation in advanced Parkinson disease. *Ann Neurol*, 74(3):449–457, Sept 2013.

Loeb, G. E, Walker, A. E., Uematsu, S., and Konigsmark, B. W. Histological reaction to various conductive and dielectric films chronically implanted in the subdural space. *J Biomed Mater Res*, 11(2):195–210, Mar 1977.

Logothetis, N. K., Pauls, J., Augath, M., Trinath, T., and Oeltermann, A. Neurophysiological investigation of the basis of the fMRI signal. *Nature*, 412(6843):150–157, 2001.

Makeig, S., Westerfield, M., Jung, T.-P., Enghoff, S., Townsend, J., Courchesne, E., and Sejnowski, T. J. Dynamic brain sources of visual evoked responses. *Science*, 295(5555):690–694, 2002.

Manning, J., Jacobs, J., Fried, I., and Kahana, M. Broadband shifts in local field potential power spectra are correlated with single-neuron spiking in humans. *J Neurosci*, 29(43):13613, 2009.

Margalit, E., Weiland, J., Clatterbuck, R., Fujii, G., Maia, M., Tameesh, M., Torres, G., D'Anna, S., Desai, S., Piyathaisere, D., Olivi, A., de Juan, E. J., and Humayun, M. Visual and electrical evoked response recorded from subdural electrodes implanted above the visual cortex in normal dogs under two methods of anesthesia. *J Neurosci Methods*, 123(2):129–137, 2003.

Maris, E., van Vugt, M., and Kahana, M. Spatially distributed patterns of oscillatory coupling between high-frequency amplitudes and low-frequency phases in human iEEG. *NeuroImage*, 54(2):836–850, 2011.

Martin, S., Brunner, P., Holdgraf, C., Heinze, H.-J., Crone, N. E., Rieger, J., Schalk, G., Knight, R. T., and Pasley, B. N. Decoding spectrotemporal features of overt and covert speech from the human cortex. *Front Neuroeng*, 7:14, 2014.

Martin, S., Brunner, P., Iturrate, I., Millán, J. d. R., Schalk, G., Knight, R. T., and Pasley, B. N. Word pair classification during imagined speech using direct brain recordings. *Sci Rep*, 6, 2016.

Mazaheri, A., and Jensen, O. Asymmetric amplitude modulations of brain oscillations generate slow evoked responses. *J Neurosci*, 28(31):7781–7787, 2008.

Mazaheri, A., and Jensen, O. Posterior $\alpha$ activity is not phase-reset by visual stimuli. *Proc Natl Acad Sci U S A*, 103(8):2948–2952, 2006.

McIntyre, C. C., Chaturvedi, A., Shamir, R. R., and Lempka, S. F. Engineering the next generation of clinical deep brain stimulation technology. *Brain Stimul*, 8(1):21–26, Jan 2015.

Menon, V., Freeman, W. J., Cutillo, B. A., Desmond, J. E., Ward, M. F., Bressler, S. L., Laxer, K. D., Barbaro, N., and Gevins, A. S. Spatio-temporal correlations in human gamma band electrocorticograms. *Electroencephalogr Clin Neurophysiol*, 98(2):89–102, Feb 1996.

Mesgarani, N., Cheung, C., Johnson, K., and Chang, E. F. Phonetic feature encoding in human superior temporal gyrus. *Science (New York, NY)*, 343(6174):1006–1010, Feb 2014.

Mestais, C. S., Charvet, G., Sauter-Starace, F., Foerster, M., Ratel, D., and Benabid, A.-L. WIMAGINE: Wireless 64-channel ECoG recording implant for long term clinical applications. *IEEE Trans Neural Syst Rehabil Eng*, 23(1):10–21, Jan 2015.

Miller K. Broadband spectral change: Evidence for a macroscale correlate of population firing rate? *J Neurosci*, 30(19):6477, 2010.

Miller, K., Hermes, D., and Honey, C. Dynamic modulation of local population activity by rhythm phase in human occipital cortex during a visual search task. *Front Hum Neurosci*, 29(4):197,2010a.

Miller, K., Leuthardt, E., Schalk, G., Rao, R., Anderson, N., Moran, D., Miller, J., and Ojemann, J. Spectral changes in cortical surface potentials during motor movement. *J Neurosci*, 27:2424–2432, Mar 2007.

Miller, K. J., Sorensen, L. B., Ojemann, J. G., and den Nijs, M. Power-law scaling in the brain surface electric potential. *PLoS Comput Biol*, 5(12):e1000609, Dec 2009a.

Miller, K., Schalk, G., Fetz, E., den Nijs, M., Ojemann, J., and Rao, R. Cortical activity during motorexecution, motor imagery, and imagery-based online feedback. *Proc Nat Acad Sci*, 107(9):4430, 2010b.

Miller, K., Sorensen, L., Ojemann, J., and Den Nijs, M. Power-law scaling in the brain surface electricpotential. *PLoS Comput Biol*, 5:e1000609, 2009b.

Miller, K., Zanos, S., Fetz, E., den Nijs, M., and Ojemann, J. Decoupling the cortical power spectrum reveals real-time representation of individual finger movements in humans. *J Neurosci*, 29(10):3132, 2009c.

Miltner, W. H., Braun, C., Arnold, M., Witte, H., and Taub, E. Coherence of gamma-band EEG activity as a basis for associative learning. *Nature*, 397(6718):434–436, 1999.

Mitzdorf U. *Current Source-Density Method and Application in Cat Cerebral Cortex: Investigation of Evoked Potentials and EEG Phenomena.* American Physiological Society, 1985.

Morrell M. J., and RNS System in Epilepsy Study Group. Responsive cortical stimulation for the treatment of medically intractable partial epilepsy. *Neurology*, 77(13):1295–1304, Sept 2011.

Mugler, E. M., Goldrick, M., Rosenow, J. M., Tate, M. C., and Slutzky, M. W. Decoding of articulatory gestures during word production using speech motor and premotor cortical activity. In *Engineering in Medicine and Biology Society (EMBC), 2015 37th Annual International Conference of the IEEE*, pages 5339–5342. IEEE, 2015.

Mugler, E. M., Patton, J. L., Flint, R. D., Wright, Z. A., Schuele, S. U., Rosenow, J., Shih, J. J., Krusienski, D. J., and Slutzky, M. W. Direct classification of all american english phonemes using signals from functional speech motor cortex. *J Neural Eng*, 11(3):035015, 2014.

Mukamel, R., Gelbard, H., Arieli, A., Hasson, U., Fried, I., and Malach, R. Coupling between neuronal firing, field potentials, and fMRI in human auditory cortex. *Science*, 309(5736):951–954, Aug 2005.

Niessing, J., Ebisch, B., Schmidt, K., Niessing, M., Singer, W., and Galuske, R. Hemodynamic signals correlate tightly with synchronized gamma oscillations. *Science*, 309(5736):948, 2005.

Nunez, L., and Srinivasan, R. *Electric Fields of the Brain: The Neurophysics of EEG*. Oxford University Press, USA, 2006.

Okun, M., Naim, A., and Lampl, I. Intracellular recordings in awake rodent unveil the relation between local field potential and neuronal firing. In *Abstracts, Society for Neuroscience Meeting*, 2009.

Okun, M. S. Deep-Brain Stimulation—Entering the Era of Human Neural-Network Modulation. *The N Engl Med*, Sept 2014a.

Okun, M. Tourette syndrome deep brain stimulation, clinicaltrials.gov identifier:nct02056873. https://clinicaltrials.gov/ct2/show/NCT02056873, 2014b.

Pei, X., Barbour, D. L., Leuthardt, E. C., and Schalk, G. Decoding vowels and consonants in spoken and imagined words using electrocorticographic signals in humans. *J Neural Eng*, 8(4):046028, 2011.

Pei, X., Leuthardt, E. C., Gaona, C. M., Brunner, P., Wolpaw, J. R., and Schalk, G. Spatiotemporal dynamics of electrocorticographic high gamma activity during overt and covert word repetition. *NeuroImage*, Oct 2010.

Penfield, W., and Rasmussen, T. editors. *The Cerebral Cortex of Man. MacMillan*, New York, 1950.

Pfurtscheller, G., and Cooper, R. Frequency dependence of the transmission of the EEG from cortex to scalp. *Electroenceph Clin Neurophysiol*, 38:93–96, 1975.

Pfurtscheller, G., Graimann, B., Huggins, J. E., Levine, S. P., and Schuh, L. A. Spatiotemporal patterns of beta desynchronization and gamma synchronization in corticographic data during self-paced movement. *Clin Neurophysiol*, 114(7):1226–1236, Jul 2003.

Pilcher, W. and Rusyniak, W. Complications of epilepsy surgery. *Neurosurg Clin N Am*, 4(2):311–325, 1993.

Pistohl, T., Ball, T., Schulze-Bonhage, A., Aertsen, A., and Mehring, C. Prediction of arm movement Trajectories from ECoG-recordings in humans. *J Neurosci Methods*, 167(1):105–114, 2008.

Potes, C., Brunner, P., Gunduz, A., Knight, R. T., and Schalk, G. Spatial and temporal relationships of electrocorticographic alpha and gamma activity during auditory processing. *NeuroImage*, 97:188–195, Apr 2014.

Potes, C., Gunduz, A., Brunner, P., and Schalk, G. Dynamics of electrocorticographic (ECoG) activity in human temporal and frontal cortical areas during music listening. *NeuroImage*, 61(4):841–848, Jul 2012.

Powers, J. C., Bieliaieva, E., Wu, S., and Nam, C. S. The human factors and ergonomics of P300-based brain–computer interfaces. *Brain Sci*, 5(3):318–56, 2015.

Ray, S., and Maunsell, J. Different origins of gamma rhythm and high-gamma activity in macaque visual cortex. *PLoS Biol*, 9(4):e1000610, 2011.

Ray, S., Niebur, E., Hsiao, S. S., Sinai, A., and Crone, N. E. High-frequency gamma activity (80–150 Hz) is increased in human cortex during selective attention. *Clin Neurophysiol*, 119(1):116–133, 2008.

Ritaccio, A., Boatman-Reich, D., Brunner, P., Cervenka, M. C., Cole, A. J., Crone, N., Duckrow, R., Korzeniewska, A., Litt, B., Miller, K. J., Moran, D. W., Parvizi, J., Viventi, J., Williams, J., and Schalk, G. Proceedings of the Second International Workshop on Advances in Electrocorticography. *Epilepsy Behav*, 22(4):641–650, Dec 2011.

Rosa, M., Arlotti, M., Ardolino, G., Cogiamanian, F., Marceglia, S., Di Fonzo, A., Cortese, F., Rampini, P. M., and Priori, A. Adaptive deep brain stimulation in a freely moving parkinsonian patient. *Movement Disord*, May 2015.

Rouse, A., and Moran, D. Neural adaptation of epidural electrocorticographic (EECoG) signals during closed-loop brain computer interface (BCI) tasks. In *Engineering in Medicine and Biology Society, 2009. EMBC 2009. Annual International Conference of the IEEE*, pages 5514–5517. IEEE, 2009.

Rouse, A. G., Stanslaski, S. R., Cong, P., Jensen, R. M., Afshar, P., Ullestad, D., Gupta, R., Molnar, G. F., Moran, D. W., and Denison, T. J. A chronic generalized bi-directional brain–machine interface. *J Neural Eng*, 8(3):036018, June 2011.

Rouse, A. G., Williams, J. J., Wheeler, J. J., and Moran, D. W. Spatial co-adaptation of cortical control columns in a micro-ECoG brain–computer interface. *J Neural Eng*, 13(5), Oct 2016.

Sanchez, J. C., Gunduz, A., Carney, P. R., and Principe, J. C. Extraction and localization of mesoscopic motor control signals for human ECoG neuroprosthetics. *J Neurosci Methods*, 167(1):63–81, Jan 2008.

Schalk, G. A general framework for dynamic cortical function: The function-through-biased-oscillations (FBO) hypothesis. *Front Hum Neurosci*, 9, 2015.

Schalk, G., and Leuthardt, E. C. Brain–computer interfaces using electrocorticographic signals. *IEEE Rev Biomed Eng*, 4:140–154, 2011.

Schalk, G. Brain–computer symbiosis. *J Neural Eng*, 5(1):1–1, Mar 2008.

Schalk, G. Can electrocorticography (ECoG) support robust and powerful brain–computer interfaces? *Front Neuroeng*, 3:9–9, 2010.

Schalk, G., Kubánek, J., Miller, K. J., Anderson, N. R., Leuthardt, E. C., Ojemann, J. G., Limbrick, D., Moran, D., Gerhardt, L. A., and Wolpaw, J. R. Decoding two-dimensional movement trajectories using electro-corticographic signals in humans. *J Neural Eng*, 4(3):264–275, Sep 2007.

Schalk, G., McFarland, D., Hinterberger, T., Birbaumer, N., and Wolpaw, J. BCI2000: A general-purpose brain–computer interface (BCI) system. IEEE Trans Biomed Eng, 51:1034–1043, 2004. 145. E. F. Chang. Towards large-scale, human-based, mesoscopic neurotechnologies. *Neuron*, 86(1):68–78, Apr 2015.

Schalk, G., Miller, K. J., Anderson, N. R., Wilson, J. A., Smyth, M. D., Ojemann, J. G., Moran, D. W., Wolpaw, J. R., and Leuthardt, E. C. Two-dimensional movement control using electrocorticographic signals in humans. *J Neural Eng*, 5(1):75–84, Mar 2008.

Schalk, G. *Towards a Clinically Practical Brain–Computer Interface.* PhD thesis, Rensselaer Polytechnic Institute, Troy, Dec 2006.

Sederberg, P. B., Kahana, M. J., Howard, M. W., Donner, E. J., and Madsen, J. R. Theta and gamma oscillations during encoding predict subsequent recall. *J Neurosci*, 23(34):10809–10814, 2003.

Shute, J., Rossi, P., de Hemptinne, C., Foote, K., Okun, M., and Gunduz, A. Neural correlates of tourette syndrome within the centromedian thalamus, premotor and primary motor cortices. *Movement Disord*, 30:S492–S493, 2015.

Sinai, A., Bowers, C. W., Crainiceanu, C. M., Boatman, D., Gordon, B., Lesser, R. P., Lenz, F. A., and Crone, N. E. Electrocorticographic high gamma activity versus electrical cortical stimulation mapping of naming. *Brain*, 128(Pt 7):1556–1570, Jul 2005.

Singer, W., and Gray, C. M. Visual feature integration and the temporal correlation hypothesis. *Annu Rev Neurosci*, 18(1):555–586, 1995.

Slutzky, M. W., Jordan, L. R., Krieg, T., Chen, M., Mogul, D. J., and Miller, L. E. Optimal spacing of surface electrode arrays for brain–machine interface applications. *J Neural Eng*, 7(2):26004, Apr 2010.

Spueler, M., Walter, A., Ramos-Murguialday, A., Naros, G., Birbaumer, N., Garabaghi, A., Rosenstiel, W., and Bogdan, M. Decoding of motor intentions from epidural ECoG recordings in severely paralyzed chronic stroke patients. *J Neural Eng*, 11(6):066008, 2014.

Stanslaski, S., Afshar, P., Cong, P., Giftakis, J., Stypulkowski, P., Carlson, D., Linde, D., Ullestad, D., Avestruz, A., and Denison, T. Design and validation of a fully implantable, chronic, closed-loop neuromodulation device with concurrent sensing and stimulation. *IEEE Trans Neural Syst Rehabil Eng*, 20(4):410–421, July 2012.

Sturm, I., Blankertz, B., Potes, C., Schalk, G., and Curio, G. ECoG high gamma activity reveals distinct cortical representations of lyrics passages, harmonic and timbre-related changes in a rock song. *Front Hum Neurosci*, 8:798, 2014.

Szczepanski, S. M., Crone, N. E., Kuperman, R. A., Auguste, K. I., Parvizi, J., and Knight, R. T. Dynamic changes in phase–amplitude coupling facilitate spatial attention control in fronto-parietal cortex. *PLoS Biol*, 12:e1001936, 2014.

Toro, C., Cox, C., Friehs, G., Ojakangas, C., Maxwell, R., Gates, J. R., Gumnit, R. J., and Ebner, T. J. 8-12 Hz rhythmic oscillations in human motor cortex during two-dimensional arm movements: Evidence for representation of kinematic parameters. *Electroencephalogr Clin Neurophysiol*, 93(5):390–403, Oct 1994.

Tort, A. B., Kramer, M. A., Thorn, C., Gibson, D. J., Kubota, Y., Graybiel, A. M., and Kopell, N. J. Dynamic cross-frequency couplings of local field potential oscillations in rat striatum and hippocampus during performance of a t-maze task. *Proc Natl Acad Sci U S A*, 105(51):20517–20522, 2008.

Uhlhaas, P. J., and Mishara, A. L. Perceptual anomalies in schizophrenia: Integrating phenomenology and cognitive neuroscience. *Schizophr Bulletin*, 33(1):142–156, 2007.

Uhlhaas, P. J., and Singer, W. Abnormal neural oscillations and synchrony in schizophrenia. *Nature Rev Neurosci*, 11(2):100–113, 2010.

Van Dijk, H., Schoffelen, J.-M., Oostenveld, R., and Jensen, O. Prestimulus oscillatory activity in the alpha band predicts visual discrimination ability. *J Neurosci*, 28(8):1816–1823, 2008.

Van Gompel, J. J., Worrell, G. A., Bell, M. L., Patrick, T. A., Cascino, G. D., Raffel, C., Marsh, W. R., and Meyer, F. B. Intracranial electroencephalography with subdural grid electrodes: Techniques, complications, and outcomes. *Neurosurgery*, 63(3):498–505; discussion 505–6, Sept 2008.

Vansteensel, M., Hermes, D., Aarnoutse, E., Bleichner, M., Schalk, G., van Rijen, P., Leijten, F., and Ramsey, N. Brain–computer interfacing based on cognitive control. *Ann Neurol*, 67(6):809–816, 2010.

Vansteensel, M., Pels, E., Bleichner, M., Branco, M., Denison, T., Freudenberg, Z., Gosselaar, P., Leinders, S., Ottens, T., VandenEboom, M., van Rijen, P., Aarnoutse, E., and Ramsey, N. Fully implanted brain–computer interface in a locked-in patient with ALS. *N Engl Med*, 375(21):2060–2066, 2016.

Voytek, B., Secundo, L., Bidet-Caulet, A., Scabini, D., Stiver, S. I., Gean, A. D., Manley, G. T., and Knight, R. T. Hemicraniectomy: A new model for human electrophysiology with high spatio-temporal resolution. *J Cogn Neurosci*, 22(11):2491–2502, 2010.

Wang, W., Collinger, J. L., Degenhart, A. D., Tyler-Kabara, E. C., Schwartz, A. B., Moran, D. W., Weber, D. J., Wodlinger, B., Vinjamuri, R. K., Ashmore, R. C. et al. An electrocorticographic brain interface in an individual with tetraplegia. *PloS One*, 8(2):e55344, 2013.

Wang, W., Collinger, J. L., Perez, M. A., Tyler-Kabara, E. C., Cohen, L. G., Birbaumer, N., Brose, S. W., Schwartz, A. B., Boninger, M. L., and Weber, D. J. Neural interface technology for rehabilitation: Exploiting and promoting neuroplasticity. *Phys Med Rehabil Clin N Am*, 21(1):157–178, Feb 2010.

Wang, Z., Gunduz, A., Brunner, P., Ritaccio, A. L., Ji, Q., and Schalk, G. Decoding onset and direction of movements using electrocorticographic (ECoG) signals in humans. *Front Neuroeng*, 5(15), 2012.

Whittingstall, K., and Logothetis, N. K. Frequency-band coupling in surface EEG reflects spiking activity in monkey visual cortex. *Neuron*, 64(2):281–289, 2009.

Wilson, J., Felton, E., Garell, P., Schalk, G., and Williams, J. ECoG factors underlying multimodal control of a brain–computer interface. *IEEE Trans Neur Sys Rehab Eng*, 14:246–250, Jun 2006.

Wolpaw, J. R., Birbaumer, N., McFarland, D. J., Pfurtscheller, G., and Vaughan, T. M. Brain–computer interfaces for communication and control. *Electroenceph Clin Neurophysiol*, 113(6):767–791, June 2002.

Womelsdorf, T., Fries, P., Mitra, P. P., and Desimone, R. Gamma-band synchronization in visual cortex predicts speed of change detection. *Nature*, 439(7077):733–736, 2006.

Yuen, T. G., Agnew, W. F., and Bullara, L. A. Tissue response to potential neuroprosthetic materials implanted subdurally. *Biomaterials*, 8(2):138–141, Mar 1987.

# 17 BCI Software

*Peter Brunner and Gerwin Schalk*

## CONTENTS

17.1 Introduction ....................................................................................................323
    17.1.1 Technical Demands .................................................................................324
    17.1.2 Scope of Investigation.............................................................................325
17.2 Implementation................................................................................................325
    17.2.1 BCI Software Platforms Using Commercial High-Level Platforms ........327
        17.2.1.1 MATLAB.................................................................................327
        17.2.1.2 SIMULINK.............................................................................327
        17.2.1.3 LabVIEW ...............................................................................329
    17.2.2 Self-Contained BCI Software Platforms .................................................330
        17.2.2.1 OpenViBE ..............................................................................331
        17.2.2.2 BCI2000..................................................................................331
17.3 Impact of BCI Software...................................................................................335
17.4 Summary and Conclusions ..............................................................................335
References.................................................................................................................336

### Abstract

In this chapter, we highlight relevant characteristics of BCI software, discuss the importance of these characteristics in different contexts of BCI research, and document the important impact of BCI software on productivity. The central purpose of BCI software is to facilitate implementation, verification, and dissemination of a wide range of BCI approaches. To do this, BCI software needs to satisfy complex technical demands across a wide array of scientific, clinical, and commercial investigations. BCI software can be implemented either from scratch, using low- or high-level programming environments and toolboxes, or on top of pre-existing BCI software platforms. We assign contemporary BCI software into these categories and investigate their impact on the field of BCI research. Our results demonstrate that only BCI2000 and OpenViBE have enjoyed sustained development and widespread dissemination and have had a strong impact on productivity of the whole field of BCI research.

## 17.1 INTRODUCTION

It is becoming increasingly clear that BCI systems will eventually realize important new technologies that replace, restore, supplement, or improve function in people affected by neurological disorders. The extent to which these possibilities are realized, that is, the extent to which BCI technologies achieve substantial practical impact, is critically dependent on the ability to effectively and efficiently implement and test different BCI approaches. The purpose of BCI software is to facilitate such implementation and testing across the whole range of research and development, that is, from basic research to clinical translation and, in some cases, even to commercialization. For BCI software to fulfill this purpose, it needs to satisfy two important requirements.

The first requirement, satisfying the technical demands of a particular BCI system, is daunting. An effective BCI must perform three major functions: (1) acquire signals from the brain and/or other physiological or behavioral sources; (2) analyze these signals to produce output commands; and (3) produce the output and associated feedback. It most often must interact with several different devices (e.g., a biosignal amplifier and an eye tracker) simultaneously, and it must do all this in real time with minimal delays and stable timing. Implementation and integration of these three functions are difficult and time consuming, and require substantial competence in different areas of science and engineering. Thus, unlike in other fields of research in which limited expertise in software engineering can suffice (e.g., implementation of a mathematical algorithm), the design of BCI systems requires individuals who are highly qualified not only in one subject area (e.g., signal processing) but also in other areas.

The second requirement for BCI software is to readily facilitate the implementation, verification, and dissemination of any and all BCI experiments planned in a particular laboratory. Implementation of any specific BCI design, and any subsequent modification, should be relatively easy and should not require extensive reprogramming. This principle is particularly important for human BCI studies since they usually test many different BCI approaches. The ease at which any BCI software can be modified depends mainly on the BCI framework's architecture, that is, the flexibility, capacity, and practicality of the BCI system's components and their interactions. This architecture must be general enough to accommodate changes to particular BCI system configurations. As an example, BCI software should not be limited to a certain number of signal channels, a specific sampling rate, or a specific signal analysis method. To facilitate the dissemination of the BCI system among a group of researchers or to other scientists in the field, it should also be possible and practical that system or experimental development, data collection, and data analysis can be performed by different personnel in different locations and with varying hardware. In addition, data stored during online operation should include all meta information (e.g., recording or stimulation parameters) that is necessary for interpretation by personnel other than those individuals who collected the data.

In summary, implementation of BCI software that functions properly, that can be easily adapted to different experimental situations, and that can facilitate operation of whole research programs rather than execution of an individual study, is complex, difficult, and costly. The premise of existing open-source or commercial BCI software is to reduce this complexity, difficulty, and cost.

### 17.1.1 TECHNICAL DEMANDS

BCI systems depend on hardware and software to acquire, synchronize, and process electrophysiological signals (electroencephalography/magnetoencephalography [EEG/MEG], electrocorticography [ECoG], or single-neuron activity) and behavioral data (e.g., finger movements, eye-gaze) in real time. The acquisition of these signals is accomplished using specialized hardware devices and requires the implementation of proprietary software interfaces to configure the device and acquire data in real time. Both configuration and type of interface can vary substantially across different devices. Some devices are directly supported by the operating system and require no configuration (keyboard, mouse, etc.), but others require the use of application programming interfaces (APIs) provided by the manufacturer and extensive configuration to define complex parameters of signal acquisition. These APIs can vary substantially in their suitability to provide the acquired data in real time. For example, while some APIs provide the acquired signal data in precise intervals, for example, through call-back notifications, others may not support such notifications or may have imprecise timing owing to limitations in the underlying data connection to the hardware (as is the case with most wireless connections). BCI software may account for these shortcomings, but doing so typically requires the use of substantial processing resources and additional buffers that entail additional acquisition delays.

As an additional complication, to properly relate physiological and behavioral signals, they need to be synchronized with each other. This can be technically difficult, because it may require adjustments for differences in sampling rates and acquisition delays across these signals.

BCI systems that provide continuous feedback have further requirements. To enable users to naturally regulate their neural activity, a BCI system must compute and output feedback within a short period of time (~100 ms or less). In addition, this feedback must be perceived as continuous, which requires BCI software to update the output signal rapidly (>20 times per second). At this rate, the BCI software has less than 50 ms to perform signal acquisition, processing, and feedback calculations.

Demanding BCI configurations (e.g., including high channel counts/sampling rates, complex signal processing algorithms) may require more than that brief time period, thus necessitating highly optimized coding.

### 17.1.2 SCOPE OF INVESTIGATION

For BCI systems, the scope of investigation is determined by its functional, scientific, and experimental complexity. Understanding these three factors is critical to selecting proper BCI software.

Functional complexity depends on the nature of the investigated BCI problem and is influenced by signal and stimulus modalities, online processing, and feedback and timing requirements. For example, a study in which a single type of brain signal is acquired while visual stimuli are presented at a predetermined timing and sequence could be considered to have relatively low functional complexity. In contrast, a study in which auditory or visual stimuli are presented, and in which their timing or other properties depend on signals acquired from multiple physiological or behavioral signal modalities, could be considered to have relatively high functional complexity.

Scientific complexity increases with the number of different experiments, personnel, and institutions. For example, a study performed by one investigator and one student at one institution could be considered to have low scientific complexity. In contrast, a program project that is performed by multiple investigators and students located at different institutions (with associated variations in experiments and equipment) could be considered to have high scientific complexity. In the first example, the BCI software needs to support a particular experiment executed by one person using one particular kind of equipment. In the latter example, the BCI software needs to support a wide range of experiments executed by many people using diverse equipment in different environments. The difference in technical requirements for BCI software implied by this difference in scientific complexity is enormous but not widely recognized.

Experimental complexity increases with varying experimental situations. For example, a study may conduct a reaction-time experiment to investigate the relationship between sensory stimulus duration and the delay of the neural and behavioral responses for different sensory stimulus modalities (e.g., auditory, visual, or tactile). Investigating this relationship requires post hoc analysis of neural signals (e.g., EEG) and behavioral signals (e.g., button press) for the different experimental conditions under consideration. Properly facilitating not only the conduct of the experiment but also the requisite corresponding offline analyses requires that the BCI software store all signals and experimental parameters in a cohesive and general fashion, and that they can be readily made available to third-party applications (such as MATLAB®) for offline analysis.

Functional, scientific, and experimental complexity typically decreases as a BCI system moves from basic scientific endeavors to a commercial clinical application, concomitant with an increase in technological, scientific, and regulatory maturity and a sharp decrease in variations in experimental or other parameters. Ideally, a BCI software system can accommodate the differing requirements of these different stages of development.

## 17.2 IMPLEMENTATION

Once investigators have identified the technical demands and scope of their investigation, they are in a good position to select the proper BCI software to implement a specific BCI system (Figure 17.1). The initial and important choice is whether to implement their BCI software from scratch using low- or high-level programming environments, or whether to proceed with a preexisting BCI software platform (see Table 17.1).

Given the limited human and financial resources in most academic laboratories, implementing BCI software from scratch is often only practical if the technical demands and the scope of investigation are limited, such as for early-stage technical demonstrations.

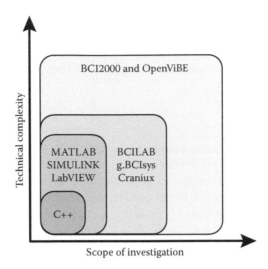

**FIGURE 17.1** Technical complexity and scope of investigation. This figure highlights the capabilities of different BCI software to implement BCI systems of varying technical complexity and scope of investigation.

In this case, BCI software may be implemented using open-source or commercial programming platforms such as Python, MATLAB, SIMULINK, or LabVIEW. These platforms provide the ability to rapidly prototype BCI systems, but, without complex additions, with only limited technical complexity.

Some commercial or academic BCI software platforms are implemented on top of these programming languages. For example, BCILAB and g.BCIsys expand MATLAB/SIMULINK with a wide range of BCI-specific functionality and with the convenience of implementing the BCI system

## TABLE 17.1
## BCI Software Overview

|  | Language | License | Website |
|---|---|---|---|
| **Self-Contained BCI Software Platforms** | | | |
| BCI2000 | C++ | GPL GNU | http://www.bci2000.org |
| OpenViBE | C++ | GPL Affero | http://openvibe.inria.fr |
| **Commercial High-Level Platforms** | | | |
| MATLAB | MATLAB | Commercial | http://www.mathworks.com |
| SIMULINK | SIMULINK | Commercial | http://www.mathworks.com/simulink |
| LabVIEW | G | Commercial | http://www.ni.com/labview |
| **Toolboxes** | | | |
| EEGLab | MATLAB | GPL GNU | http://sccn.ucsd.edu/eeglab |
| BCILAB | MATLAB | GPL GNU | http://sccn.ucsd.edu/wiki/BCILAB |
| PsychoPy | Python | GPL GNU | http://www.psychopy.org |
| BioSig | MATLAB | GPL GNU | http://biosig.sourceforge.net |
| rtsBCI | MATLAB | GPL GNU | http://biosig.sourceforge.net |
| FieldTrip | MATLAB | GPL GNU | http://www.fieldtriptoolbox.org |
| MNE | MATLAB | BSD | http://martinos.org/mne |
| Psychophysics | MATLAB | MIT | http://psychtoolbox.org |
| g.HIsys | LabVIEW | Commercial | http://www.gtec.at/Products/Software |
| g.BCIsys | SIMULINK | Commercial | http://www.gtec.at/Products/g.BCIsys |

using visual data flow programming. This convenience allows for rapid prototyping and verification of a specific BCI approach. At the same time, the underlying platform (i.e., MATLAB, SIMULINK, or LabVIEW) usually imposes important limitations in system performance or technical complexity (e.g., processing rate and latency, limited ability to simultaneously acquire signals from different devices). It also impedes commercialization because of prohibitive licensing costs.

In contrast, self-contained BCI software platforms do not depend on underlying commercial software and do not have their limitations. For example, BCI2000 and OpenViBE are based on standard C++ and provide general-purpose BCI functionality at high performance and without depending on other software. The modular and general-purpose nature of these software packages lends itself well to a wide scope of systematic BCI investigations. For example, the support for a wide range of data acquisition systems in BCI2000 and OpenViBE facilitates the use of the BCI system in other environments. These systems also facilitate translating the BCI system into a clinical (and eventually commercial) application. OpenViBE is focused on providing visual data flow programming to facilitate the rapid prototyping of BCI systems. In contrast, BCI2000 is focused on providing a highly stable and performant general-purpose BCI software infrastructure that facilitates systematic and large-scale investigations.

## 17.2.1 BCI Software Platforms Using Commercial High-Level Platforms

Commercial high-level platforms (MATLAB, SIMULINK, or LabVIEW) have been used in the development of early real-time BCI demonstrations (Lauer et al. 1999; Guger et al. 1999). The sections below give an overview of their impact on BCI research.

### 17.2.1.1 MATLAB

MATLAB (MATrix LABoratory) is a commercial programming language for numerical computing that supports Linux, Windows, and Mac OS X and that has been continuously developed by Mathworks Inc. since 1984. MATLAB is principally focused on supporting the development of mathematical algorithms but can also plot data and create user interfaces. Because of its ease of use and expansive functionality, MATLAB has become popular with scientists and engineers. MATLAB is relatively affordable for students and faculty (e.g., $100 for the basic functionality and $29 for each additional toolbox) but carries a steep price tag for commercial users (e.g., $2150 for the basic functionality and $1000 for each additional toolbox). Thus, MATLAB is mostly used within the academic setting and in a limited fashion (for rapid prototyping) in the industrial setting. The high cost of MATLAB has motivated the development of the open-source GNU Octave software, which replicates large portions of the basic MATLAB functionality.

MATLAB's popularity among scientists and engineers has led to the development of specialized toolboxes for the presentation of behavioral paradigms (e.g., Psychophysics Toolbox Brainard 1997) and the post hoc analysis and visualization of biosignals (e.g., EEGLab Delorme and Makeig 2004, BioSig Vidauure et al. 2011, FieldTrip Oostenveld et al. 2011, and MNE Gramfort et al. 2014).

EEGLab, BioSig, and FieldTrip have recently been extended into MATLAB toolboxes for the rapid prototyping and evaluation of online BCIs, called BCILAB, rtsBCI, and FieldTrip buffer, respectively. These extended toolboxes make use of MATLAB functionality to process, classify, and visualize signals in real time (see Figures 17.2 and 17.3). The capabilities of BCILAB have been illustrated in several real-time demonstrations that range from EEG signal visualization (Mullen et al. 2013) to EEG state classification (Mullen et al. 2015) and the decomposition of EEG signals into independent components (Hsu et al. 2016).

### 17.2.1.2 SIMULINK

SIMULINK is a commercial graphical user interface that expands MATLAB with a graphical block programming interface. Each block in this interface can contain either custom or preexisting code. The ability to seamlessly combine preexisting code into new applications makes SIMULINK well suited for users

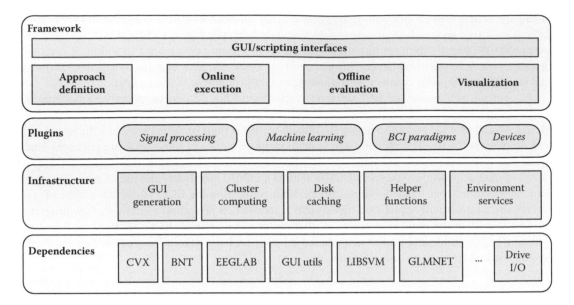

**FIGURE 17.2**  Basic architecture of BCILAB. It is based on four layers: (1) The dependency layer provides external functionality, for example, MATLAB and required toolboxes, machine learning toolboxes, and user interfaces. (2) The infrastructure layer provides functionality for GUIs, parallel computing, disk caching, and helper functions for testing and deployment. (3) The plugin layer provides BCI-specific signal processing and machine learning functionality. (4) The framework layer provides the scripting interface to interact with the first layers of the BCILAB toolbox.

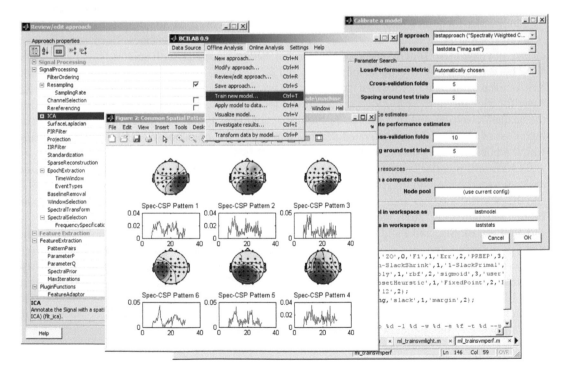

**FIGURE 17.3**  User interface of BCILAB. This screenshot shows the main menu (top center), a model visualization (bottom), a model configuration dialog (left), an evaluation setup dialog (top right), and the script editor (bottom right).

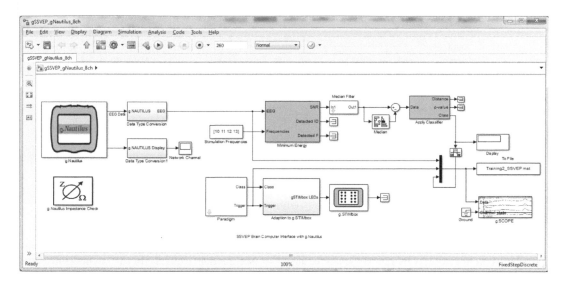

**FIGURE 17.4** User interface of g.BCIsys. This screenshot shows the implementation of a simple SSVEP-based BCI within SIMULINK. The parameters of this paradigm (e.g., stimulation frequency) can be changed by clicking at the appropriate block.

with limited programming skills. The g.BCIsys software,[*] a commercial SIMULINK-based software package, makes use of this functionality to provide a front-end interface for rapid BCI research and development to users of g.tec hardware (see Figure 17.4). The capacities of g.BCIsys have been demonstrated in several real-time demonstrations (Guger et al. 2012a,b; Ortner et al. 2013; Kapeller et al. 2013).

### 17.2.1.3 LabVIEW

LabVIEW (Laboratory Virtual Instrument Engineering Workbench) is a commercial graphical block programming interface software for data acquisition, signal processing, visualization, and controlling of instrumentation. The most recent version of LabVIEW (2016) runs on Windows 7, 8.1, and 10 and, with limited functionality, on Mac OS X (10.10, 10.11) and Linux (Red Hat, Scientific, openSUSE). National Instruments has been developing LabVIEW since 1983, mainly to serve as a real-time processing frontend for their NI-DAQ (Data Acquisition) series hardware. This type of hardware provides affordable analog and digital input/output at relatively high sampling rates (e.g., 100 kHz) and resolution (e.g., ±500 mV dynamic range, 3 μV resolution at 16 bits). In combination with appropriate pre-amplifiers, NI-DAQ hardware is suitable for a wide range of biosignal applications. While these boards lack regulatory approval for clinical use in humans, their affordable price (e.g., 1/10th of a comparable biosignal acquisition system approved for human use) made them popular with animal experiments. The ability to interface with external instrumentation through analog and digital NI-DAQ board inputs and outputs, together with an increased availability of data acquisition modules for third-party biosignal acquisition systems (e.g., g.HIsys, g.tec, Austria[†]; OpenEEG[‡]; OpenBCI[§]), has led to some adoption of LabVIEW within the BCI community. In this context, LabVIEW has been the basis for several BCI demonstrations that range from EMG-based assistive technology (Huang et al. 2006), to NIRS-based communication (Matthew et al. 2008),

---

[*] g.BCIsys—g.tec's brain–computer interface research environment.  http://www.gtec.at/Products/Complete-Solutions/g .BCIsys-Specs-Features.

[†] g.HIsys—g.tec's high-speed online processing under LabVIEW. http://www.gtec.at/Products/Software/Software -options/ (show)/1711/#p1711.

[‡] OpenEEG for LabVIEW. https://sourceforge.net/projects/ openeeglabview.

[§] OpenBCI Toolkit. http://forums.ni.com/t5/Example-Program-Drafts/LabVIEW-OpenBCI-Toolkit/ta-p/3495333.

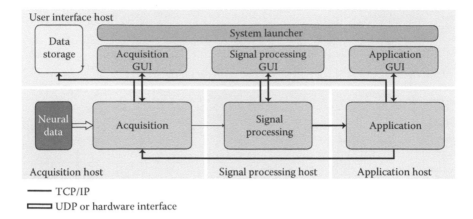

**FIGURE 17.5** LabVIEW-based system architecture of Craniux. The Craniux system implements the same distributed architecture as BCI2000 (Schalk et al. 2004) (see Section 17.2.2.2). In this architecture, three interchangeable modules (Source, Signal Processing, and User Application) are controlled by a user interface host that facilitates the configuration and communication across all modules.

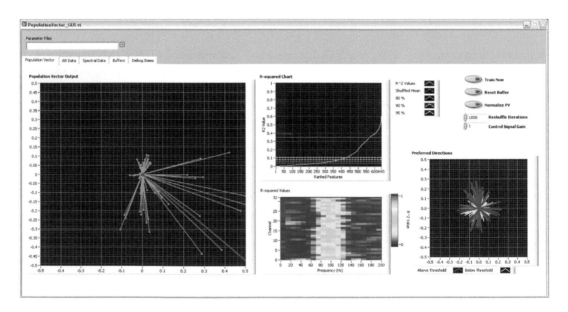

**FIGURE 17.6** LabVIEW-based user interface of Craniux. The user interface presents several data visualizations along with buttons to control the system.

to steady-state visual evoked potential (SSVEP)–based wheelchair control (Singla et al. 2014). In addition to these demonstrations, LabVIEW has been used to implement the BCI system Craniux (Degenhart et al. 2011), which is illustrated in Figures 17.5 and 17.6. Craniux has been used for BCI studies in monkeys and for humans with tetraplegia (Wang et al. 2013; Collinger et al. 2013, 2014).

## 17.2.2 Self-Contained BCI Software Platforms

Self-contained BCI software platforms are implemented in low-level programming languages (e.g., C++), compiled into native machine code, and executed without dependencies on commercial libraries. This makes these platforms ideal for supporting systematic scientific and clinical studies

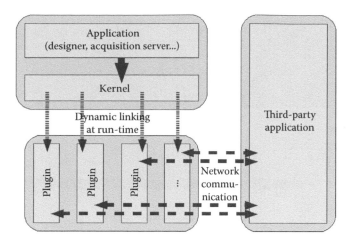

**FIGURE 17.7** Software architecture of OpenViBE. The architecture of OpenViBE is centered around boxes that are combined into scenarios. The boxes provide modular functionality that is supported by global functionality by the kernel. Each box is defined by its input, functionality, and output. Several managers (scenario, player, visualization, type, and plugin) manage the interplay between this functionality. Certain functionalities can be seamlessly expanded through a plugin system, for example, to implement a new classification algorithm that retains the same input–output characteristics.

that entail complex experiments with high technical demands (e.g., high channel count or sampling rate, low latencies) as well as a wide scope of investigation (e.g., the economical deployment across many laboratories and users). While many self-contained BCI software platforms have been proposed (e.g., BCI++ Perego et al. 2009, xBCI Susila et al. 2010, and TOBI Breitwieser et al. 2012), only BCI2000 and OpenViBE have enjoyed significant adoption beyond the authors' own laboratory. Sections 17.2.2.1 and 17.2.2.2 describe and summarize these two platforms.

### 17.2.2.1 OpenViBE

The OpenViBE software platform has been developed since 2007 (Reynard et al. 2010). The most recent version of OpenViBE (1.3.0) is licensed under the GNU Affero General Public License, a copyleft license that provides the right to freely distribute copies and modified versions of a work with the stipulation that the same rights be preserved in derivative works. OpenViBE is implemented in C++ and compiled into binaries that run on Windows 7 and 10, as well as on several Linux distributions (Ubuntu 12.04, 14.04, and 16.04; Fedora 20 and 21). The recently founded start-up Mensia Technologies is translating OpenViBE's core into CertiViBE, a hardened and medically certifiable BCI software platform for clinical applications.

OpenViBE is based on an architecture that facilitates the integration, expansion, and configuration of modular functionality (Figure 17.7), while the graphical interface makes OpenViBE easy to use for a wide range of investigators, including engineers, scientists, and clinicians (Figure 17.8). These two factors make OpenViBE well suited to supporting the implementation of different BCI approaches. The capabilities of OpenViBE have been demonstrated in several publications, including EEG-based workload estimation (Mühl et al. 2014; Frey et al. 2016), SSVEP-based BCIs (Zhao et al. 2015; Martisius and Damasevičius 2016), and motor imagery BCIs (Jeunet et al. 2015, 2016a,b).

### 17.2.2.2 BCI2000

The BCI2000 software platform has been developed since 1998 (Schalk et al. 2004; Schalk and Mellinger 2010). Its development is a major component of the recently established NIH-funded National Center for Adaptive Neurotechnologies.* The most recent version of BCI2000 (3.6) is

---

\* http://www.neurotechcenter.org

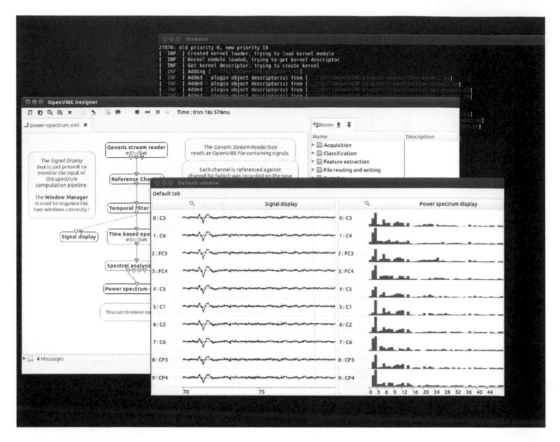

**FIGURE 17.8**   User interface of OpenViBE. This screenshot shows the implementation of a simple power-spectrum visualization in OpenViBE. The designer application facilitates the authoring of this scenario.

licensed under version 3 of the GNU General Public License, a copyleft license that is compatible with other open-source licenses (e.g., LGPLv3, Apache 2.0, XFree 1.1). GPL v3 facilitates the integration of functionality from other open-source projects. BCI2000 is implemented in C++ and compiled into binaries that run on Windows 7, 8.1, and 10. Its implementation is based on a model that can describe any BCI system (Schalk et al. 2004; Mason and Birch 2003). In accord with this model, and as shown in Figure 17.9, BCI2000 has four modules that communicate with each other: Source (data acquisition and storage), Signal Processing, User Application, and Operator Interface. The modules communicate through a documented network-capable protocol based on TCP/IP.

The implementation of BCI2000 is highly optimized, so that it can support even very demanding BCI configurations with good timing characteristics (Wilson et al. 2010).

The BCI2000 data storage format accommodates variations in the digitized signals (e.g., in number of channels, sampling rate), defines the operating protocol, and includes a record of all events (e.g., feedback to user, device control, artifact detection) that occur during operation. BCI2000 has a roster of existing implementations with primarily technical documentation. These implementations can realize different BCI designs and methods that are readily usable and employ readily available and relatively inexpensive hardware components (Figure 17.10). BCI2000 is described in detail in a book [38], as well as in multiple book chapters (Melllinger and Schalk 2007, 2010; Wilson and Schalk 2010; Wilson et al. 2012; Allison et al. 2012; Brunner et al. 2013) and peer-reviewed articles (Schalk et al. 2004; Wilson et al. 2010, 2009; Schalk 2009).

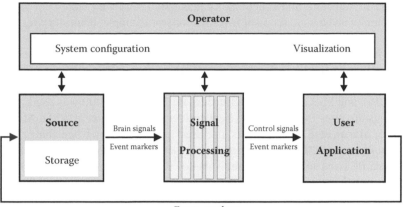

**FIGURE 17.9** Basic structure of BCI2000. It has three interchangeable modules (Source, Signal Processing, and User Application) and an Operator module that facilitates the configuration and communication across all modules.

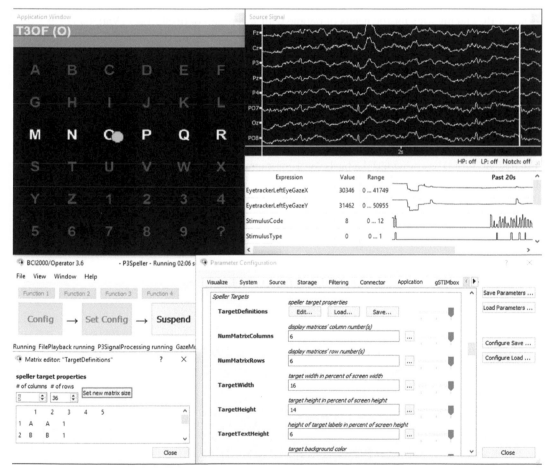

**FIGURE 17.10** User interface of BCI2000. This screenshot shows the use of BCI2000 in a P300 speller study that acquires EEG signals along with eye gaze. The user is presented with a P300 speller window (top left), while the operator monitors the user's EEG (top right) and eye gaze as presented as an overlay over a copy of the P300 speller window (green dot, top left) and as a time trace (center right). The configuration of this experiment can be changed through a parameter window (bottom).

The software architecture and functionality make BCI2000 well suited for studies with high technical complexity and a wide scope of investigation, for example, laboratory research conducted across multiple laboratories. The utility of BCI2000 is documented by the more than 1000 published studies that have used it for BCI-related experimentation. These studies include cursor control using EEG (Wolpaw and McFarland 2004; McFarland et al. 2008, 2010), ECoG (Leuthardt et al. 2004, 2006; Wilcon and Lacoboni 2006; Felton et al. 2007; Blakely et al. 2009; Miller et al. 2010; Bundy et al. 2016), and MEG signals (Mellinger et al. 2007). BCI2000 was used to work toward a speech prosthesis that uses ECoG signals (Leuthardt et al. 2011; Pei et al. 2011; Mugler et al. 2014; Herf et al. 2015; Martin et al. 2016). It was also used for control of a wheelchair (Kaufmann et al. 2014), a humanoid robot (Bell et al. 2008), and a quad-copter (Doud et al. 2011; LaFleur et al. 2013) by a noninvasive BCI and for exploring the value of P300 evoked potentials (Sellers et al. 2006, 2010; Vaughan et al. 2006; Nijboer et al. 2008; Furdea et al. 2009; Kübler et al. 2009; Townsend et al. 2010, 2016; Cecotti and Gräser 2011; Kaufmann et al. 2011, 2013; Brunner et al. 2011; Aloise et al. 2012; Käthner et al. 2013), steady-state auditory evoked potentials (SSAEPs) (Hill and Schölkopf 2012), SSVEP (Allison et al. 2008; Yin et al. 2013), and the combination of P300 with SSVEP signals (Yin et al. 2014) for BCI purposes. BCI2000 has been used to implement real-time BCIs for high-resolution EEG techniques (Mattia et al. 2008) and for BCI control of assistive technologies (Cincotti et al. 2008). BCI2000 has also provided the basis for the first large-scale clinical evaluations of BCI technology for the needs of people with severe motor disabilities (Vaughan et al. 2006; Nijboer et al. 2008; Kübler et al. 2005; Spüler et al. 2012; Kaufmann et al. 2013; Zickler et al. 2012, Holz et al. 2015; Vansteensel et al. 2016) and the first applications of BCI technology to functional restoration in patients with chronic stroke (Buch et al. 2008; Daly et al. 2009; Wisneski et al. 2008; Cincotti et al. 2012). Finally, several studies have used BCI2000 for purposes other than online BCI control, for example, the optimization of BCI signal processing routines (Fuentes Cabrera and Dremstrup 2008; Royer and He 2009; Yamawaki et al. 2006) and the mapping of cortical function using ECoG (Leuthardt et al. 2007; Miller et al. 2007a, b; Schalk et al. 2007, 2008; Kubanek et al. 2009; Brunner et al. 2009; Roland et al. 2010; Gupta et al. 2014; Korostenskaja et al. 2014). Finally, BCI2000 has provided the basis for a commercial functional mapping system called cortiQ (Prueckl et al. 2013).

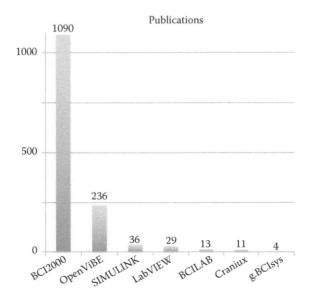

**FIGURE 17.11**    Impact of BCI software platforms as measured by scientific publications.

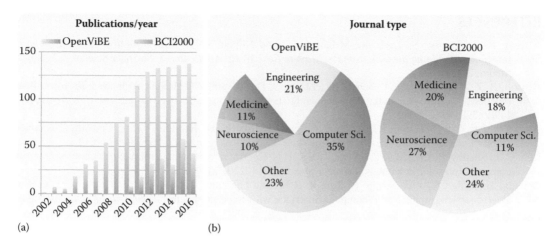

**FIGURE 17.12** Number (a) and journal type (b) of publications using OpenViBE and BCI2000. To date, OpenViBE has supported the studies in more than 230 publications. Their focus on engineering and computer science indicates that OpenViBE is mostly used within these disciplines. By comparison, BCI2000 has supported the studies in more than 1000 publications, and the composition of scientists from different fields is more diverse. For both OpenViBE and BCI2000, the apparent recent slower growth of publications per year suggests that the range of applications within these disciplines is limited.

## 17.3 IMPACT OF BCI SOFTWARE

The ultimate purpose of BCI software is to facilitate implementation and testing of different BCI approaches. Thus, the success of BCI software in achieving this purpose can be measured by the number of scientific studies that they have supported. The illustration in Figure 17.11 indicates the number of publications that have been supported by different BCI software packages. Among these software packages, OpenViBE and BCI2000 together account for 93% of all publications. Additional analyses demonstrate evidence (Figure 17.12b) that the user base of OpenViBE and BCI2000 is substantially different: users of OpenViBE are likely to be active in the computer science and engineering domains, whereas BCI2000 appears to primarily cater to scientists in the neuroscience and medicine domains.

The benefit of the use of BCI software is a reduction in the time, risk, and cost associated with BCI system development. The large number of BCI studies enabled by existing BCI software implies that many of these studies have likely only been possible because of existing BCI software and that the accumulated economic benefits of using existing BCI software are likely in the range of tens of millions of US dollars.

## 17.4 SUMMARY AND CONCLUSIONS

Systematic research and development of BCIs is critically facilitated by existing BCI software platforms that support the ability to effectively and efficiently implement and verify BCI systems. To fulfill this promise, BCI software platforms need to satisfy complex technical demands and support the implementation, verification, and dissemination of many different BCI approaches. Two fundamental types of BCI software platforms exist, those implemented using existing high-level platforms, and those implemented using low-level programming languages. Over the past two decades, many BCI software platforms have been developed, but only two of them have enjoyed sustained development and widespread dissemination and have succeeded in making a strong impact on productivity of the whole field of BCI research. The increasing complexity of BCI approaches (e.g., multimodal signal acquisition and processing) will likely further increase the value of BCI software and will place new demands on their capacities.

## REFERENCES

Allison, B. Z., Dunne, S., Leeb, R., Millán, J. R., and Nijholt, A. *Towards Practical Brain–Computer Interfaces: Bridging the Gap from Research to Real-World Applications.* Springer Science & Business Media, 2012.

Allison, B. Z., McFarland, D. J., Schalk, G., Zheng, S. D., Jackson, M. M., and Wolpaw, J. R. Towards an independent brain–computer interface using steady state visual evoked potentials. *Clin Neurophys,* 119(2):399–408, 2008.

Aloise, F., Aricò, P., Schettini, F., Riccio, A., Salinari, S., Mattia, D., Babiloni, F., and Cincotti, F. A covert attention P300-based brain–computer interface: Geospell. *Ergonomics,* 55:538–551, 2012.

Bell, C. J., Shenoy, P., Chalodhorn, R., and Rao, R. P. N. Control of a humanoid robot by a noninvasive brain-computer interface in humans. *J Neural Eng,* 5(2):214–220, 2008.

Blakely, T., Miller, K. J., Zanos, S. P., Rao, R. P. N., and Ojemann, J. G. Robust, longterm control of an electrocorticographic brain–computer interface with fixed parameters. *Neurosurg Focus,* 27(1):E13, 2009.

Brainard, D. H. The psychophysics toolbox. *Spatial Vis,* 10(4):433–436, 1997.

Breitwieser, C., Daly, I., Neuper, C., and Müller-Putz, G. R. Proposing a standardized protocol for raw biosignal transmission. *IEEE Trans BME,* 59(3):852–859, 2012.

Brunner, C., Andreoni, G., Bianchi, L., Blankertz, B., Breitwieser, C., Kanoh, S., Kothe, C. A., Lécuyer, A., Makeig, S., Mellinger, J., Perego, P., Renard, Y., Schalk, G., Susila, I. P., Venthur, B., and Müller-Putz, G. R. BCI Software Platforms. In Brendan Z. Allison, Stephen Dunne, Robert Leeb, José Del R Millán, and Anton Nijholt, editors, *Toward Practical BCIs: Bridging the Gap from Research to Real-World Applications,* pages 303–331. Springer, 2013.

Brunner, P., Ritaccio, A. L., Emrich, J. F., Bischof, H., and Schalk, G. Rapid communication with a "P300" matrix speller using electrocorticographic signals (ECoG). *Front Neurosci,* 5:5, 2011.

Brunner, P., Ritaccio, A. L., Lynch, T. M., Emrich, J. F., Wilson, J. A., Williams, J. C., Aarnoutse, E. J., Ramsey, N. F., Leuthardt, E. C., Bischof, H., and Schalk, G. A practical procedure for real-time functional mapping of eloquent cortex using electrocorticographic signals in humans. *Epilepsy Behav,* 15(3):278–286, 2009.

Buch, E., Weber, C., Cohen, L. G., Braun, C., Dimyan, M. A., Ard, T., Mellinger, J., Caria, A., Soekadar, S., Fourkas, A., and Birbaumer, N. Think to move: A neuromagnetic brain–computer interface (BCI) system for chronic stroke. *Stroke,* 39(3):910–917, 2008.

Bundy, D. T., Pahwa, M., Szrama, N., and Leuthardt, E. C. Decoding three-dimensional reaching movements using electrocorticographic signals in humans. *J Neural Eng,* 13(2):026021, 2016.

Cecotti, H., and Gräser, A. Convolutional neural networks for P300 detection with application to brain–computer interfaces. *IEEE Trans Pattern Anal Mach Intell,* 33(3):433–445, 2011.

Cincotti, F., Mattia, D., Aloise, F., Bufalari, S., Schalk, G., Oriolo, G., Cherubini, A., Marciani, M. G., and Babiloni, F. Non-invasive brain-computer interface system: Towards its application as assistive technology. *Brain Res Bull,* 75(6):796–803, 2008.

Cincotti, F., Pichiorri, F., Aricò, P., Aloise, F., Leotta, F., Fallani, d. V., F., Millán, J., Molinari, M., and Mattia, D. EEG-based brain–computer interface to support post-stroke motor rehabilitation of the upper limb. *Conf Proc IEEE Eng Med Biol Soc,* 2012:4112–4115, 2012.

Collinger, J. L., Kryger, M. A., Barbara, R., Betler, T., Bowsher, K., Brown, E. H. P., Clanton, S. T., Degenhart, A. D., Foldes, S. T., Gaunt, R. A., Gyulai, F. E., Harchick, E. A., Harrington, D., Helder, J. B., Hemmes, T., Johannes, M. S., Katyal, K. D., Ling, G. S. F., McMorland, A. J. C., Palko, K., Para, M. P., Scheuermann, J., Schwartz, A. B., Skidmore, E. R., Solzbacher, F., Srikameswaran, A. V., Swanson, D. P., Swetz, S., Tyler-Kabara, E. C., Velliste, M., Wang, W., Weber, D. J., Wodlinger, B., and Boninger, M. L. Collaborative approach in the development of high-performance brain–computer interfaces for a neuroprosthetic arm: Translation from animal models to human control. *Clin Transl Sci,* 7(1):52–59, 2014.

Collinger, J. L., Wodlinger, B., Downey, J. E., Wang, W., Tyler-Kabara, E. C., Weber, D. J., McMorland, A. J. C., Velliste, M., Boninger, M.L., and Schwartz, A. B. Highperformance neuroprosthetic control by an individual with tetraplegia. *Lancet,* 381(9866):557–564, 2013.

Daly, J. J., Cheng, R., Rogers, J., Litinas, K., Hrovat, K., and Dohring, M. Feasibility of a new application of noninvasive brain computer interface (BCI): A case study of training for recovery of volitional motor control after stroke. *J Neurol Phys Ther,* 33(4):203–211, 2009.

Degenhart, A. D., Kelly, J. W., Ashmore, R. C., Collinger, J. L., Tyler-Kabara, E. C., Weber, D. J., and Wang, W. Craniux: A LabVIEW-based modular software framework for brain–machine interface research. *Comput Intell Neurosci,* 2011:363565, 2011.

Delorme, A., and Makeig, S. EEGLAB: An open source toolbox for analysis of single-trial EEG dynamics including independent component analysis. *J Neurosci Methods*, 134(1):9–21, 2004.

Doud, A. J., Lucas, J. P., Pisansky, M. T., and He, B. Continuous three-dimensional control of a virtual helicopter using a motor imagery based brain–computer interface. *PLoS One*, 6(10):e26322, 2011.

Felton, E. A., Wilson, J. A., Williams, J. C., and Garell, P. C. Electrocorticographically controlled brain–computer interfaces using motor and sensory imagery in patients with temporary subdural electrode implants. Report of four cases. *J Neurosurg*, 106(3):495–500, 2007.

Frey, J., Appriou, A., Lotte, F., and Hachet, M. Classifying EEG signals during stereoscopic visualization to estimate visual comfort. *Comput Intell Neurosci*, 2016:2758103, 2016.

Fuentes Cabrera, A. and Dremstrup, K. Auditory and spatial navigation imagery in brain–computer interface using optimized wavelets. *J Neurosci Methods*, 174(1):135–146, 2008.

Furdea, A., Halder, S., Krusienski, D. J., Bross, D., Nijboer, F., Birbaumer, N., and Kübler, A. An auditory oddball (P300) spelling system for brain–computer interfaces. *Psychophysiology*, 46(3):617–625, 2009.

Gramfort, A., Luessi, M., Larson, E., Engemann, D. A., Strohmeier, D., Brodbeck, C., Parkkonen, L., and Hämäläinen, M. S. MNE software for processing MEG and EEG data. *NeuroImage*, 86:446–460, 2014.

Guger, C., Allison, B., Grosswindhager, B., Prückl, R., Hintermüller, C., Kapeller, C., Bruckner, M., Krausz, G., and Edlinger, G. How many people could use an SSVEP BCI? *Front Neurosci*, 6:169, 2012a.

Guger, C., Allison, B., Hintermueller, C., Prueckl, R., Grosswindhager, B., Kapeller, C., and Edlinger, G. Poor performance in SSVEP BCIs: Are worse subjects just slower? *Conf Proc IEEE Eng Med Biol Soc*, 2012:3833–3836, 2012b.

Guger, C., Schlögl, A., Walterspacher, D., and Pfurtscheller, G. Design of an EEG-based brain–computer interface (BCI) from standard components running in real-time under Windows. *Biomedizinische Technik*, 44(1–2):12–16, 1999.

Gupta, D., Hill, N. J., Brunner, P., Gunduz, A., Ritaccio, A. L., and Schalk, G. Simultaneous real-time monitoring of multiple cortical systems. *J Neural Eng*, 11(5):056001, 2014.

Herff, C., Heger, D., de Pesters, A., Telaar, D., Brunner, P., Schalk, G., and Schultz, T. Brain-to-text: Decoding spoken phrases from phone representations in the brain. *Front Neurosci*, 9:217, 2015.

Hill, N. J., and Schölkopf, B. An online brain–computer interface based on shifting attention to concurrent streams of auditory stimuli. *J Neural Eng*, 9(2):026011, 2012.

Holz, E. M., Botrel, L., Kaufmann, T., and Kübler, A. Long-term independent brain–computer interface home use improves quality of life of a patient in the locked-in state: A case study. *Arch Phys Med*, 96(3 Suppl):S16–S26, 2015.

Hsu, S.-H., Mullen, T. R., Jung, T.-P., and Cauwenberghs, G. Real-time adaptive EEG source separation using online recursive independent component analysis. *IEEE T Neur Sys Reh*, 24(3):309–319, 2016.

Huang, C.-N., Chen, C.-H., and Chung, H.-Y. Application of facial electromyography in computer mouse access for people with disabilities. *Disabil Rehabil*, 28(4):231–237, 2006.

Jeunet, C., Jahanpour, E., and Lotte, F. Why standard brain–computer interface (BCI) training protocols should be changed: An experimental study. *J Neural Eng*, 13(3):036024, 2016a.

Jeunet, C., N'Kaoua, B., and Lotte, F. Advances in user-training for mental-imagerybased BCI control: Psychological and cognitive factors and their neural correlates. *Prog Brain Res*, 228:3–35, 2016b.

Jeunet, C., N'Kaoua, B., Subramanian, S., Hachet, M., and Lotte, F. Predicting mental imagery-based BCI performance from personality, cognitive profile and neurophysiological patterns. *PLoS One*, 10(12):e0143962, 2015.

Kapeller C., Hintermuller C., Abu-Alqumsan M., Pruckl R., Peer A., and Guger C.. A BCI using VEP for continuous control of a mobile robot. *Conf Proc IEEE Eng Med Biol Soc*, 2013:5254–5257, 2013.

Käthner, I., Ruf, C. A., Pasqualotto, E., Braun, C., Birbaumer, N., and Halder, S. A portable auditory P300 brain–computer interface with directional cues. *Clin Neurophys*, 124(2):327–338, 2013.

Kaufmann, T., Herweg, A., and Kübler, A. Toward brain–computer interface based wheelchair control utilizing tactually-evoked event-related potentials. *J Neuroeng Rehabil*, 11:7, 2014.

Kaufmann, T., Holz, E. M., and Kübler, A. Comparison of tactile, auditory, and visual modality for brain–computer interface use: A case study with a patient in the locked-in state. *Front Neurosci*, 7:129, 2013.

Kaufmann, T., Schulz, T., Grünzinger, C., and Kübler, A. Flashing characters with famous faces improves ERP-based brain–computer interface performance. *J Neural Eng*, 8(5):056016, 2011.

Kaufmann, T., Schulz, S. M., Köblitz, A., Renner, G., Wessig, C., and Kübler, A. Face stimuli effectively prevent brain–computer interface inefficiency in patients with neurodegenerative disease. *Clin Neurophys*, 124(5), 2013.

Kubanek, J., Miller, K. J., Ojemann, J. G., Wolpaw, J. R., and Schalk, G. Decoding flexion of individual fingers using electrocorticographic signals in humans. *J Neural Eng*, 6(6):066001, 2009.

Kübler, A., Furdea, A., Halder, S., Hammer, E. M., Nijboer, F., and Kotchoubey, B.. A brain–computer interface controlled auditory event-related potential (P300) spelling system for locked-in patients. *Ann N Y Acad Sci*, 1157:90–100, 2009.

Kübler, A., Nijboer, F., Mellinger, J., Vaughan, T. M., Pawelzik, H., Schalk, G., McFarland, D. J., Birbaumer, N., and Wolpaw, J. R. Patients with ALS can use sensorimotor rhythms to operate a brain–computer interface. *Neurology*, 64(10):1775–1777, 2005.

Korostenskaja, M., Chen, P.-C., Salinas, C. M., Westerveld, M., Brunner, P., Schalk, G., Cook, J. C., Baumgartner, J., and Lee, K. H. Real-time functional mapping: Potential tool for improving language outcome in pediatric epilepsy surgery. *J Neurosurg*, 14(3):287–295, 2014.

LaFleur, K., Cassady, K., Doud, A., Shades, K., Rogin, E., and He, B. Quadcopter control in three-dimensional space using a noninvasive motor imagery-based brain–computer interface. *J Neural Eng*, 10(4):046003, 2013.

Lauer, R. T., Peckham, P. H., and Kilgore, K. L. EEG-based control of a hand grasp neuroprosthesis. *Neuroreport*, 10(8):1767–1771, 1999.

Leuthardt, E. C., Gaona, C., Sharma, M., Szrama, N., Roland, J., Freudenberg, Z., Solis, J., Breshears, J., and Schalk, G. Using the electrocorticographic speech network to control a brain–computer interface in humans. *J Neural Eng*, 8(3):036004, 2011.

Leuthardt, E. C., Miller, K., Anderson, N. R., Schalk, G., Dowling, J., Miller, J., Moran, D. W., and Ojemann, J. G. Electrocorticographic frequency alteration mapping: A clinical technique for mapping the motor cortex. *Neurosurgery*, 60(4 Suppl 2):260–270, 2007.

Leuthardt, E. C., Miller, K. J., Schalk, G., Rao, R. P. N., and Ojemann, J. G. Electrocorticography-based brain computer interface—The Seattle experience. *IEEE Trans Neural Syst Rehabil Eng*, 14(2):194–198, 2006.

Leuthardt, E. C., Schalk, G., Wolpaw, J. R., Ojemann, J. G., and Moran, D. W. A brain–computer interface using electrocorticographic signals in humans. *J Neural Eng*, 1(2):63–71, 2004.

Martin, S., Brunner, P., Iturrate, I., Millán, JR., Schalk, G., Knight, R. T., and Pasley, B. N. Word pair classification during imagined speech using direct brain recordings. *Sci Rep*, 6:25803, 2016.

Martisius, I., and Damasevičius, R. A prototype SSVEP based real time BCI gaming system. *Comput Intell Neurosci*, 2016:3861425, 2016.

Mason, S. G., and Birch, G. E. A general framework for brain–computer interface design. *IEEE Trans Neur Syst Rehabil Eng*, 11(1):70–85, 2003.

Matthews, F., Soraghan, C., Ward, T. E., Markham, C., and Pearlmutter, B. A. Software platform for rapid prototyping of NIRS brain computer interfacing techniques. *Conf Proc IEEE Eng Med Biol Soc*, 2008:4840–4843, 2008.

Mattia, C. F., Aloise, D., Bufalari, F. S., Astolfi, L., De Vico Fallani, F., Tocci, A., Bianchi, L., Marciani, M. G., Gao, S., Millan, J., and Babiloni, F. High-resolution EEG techniques for brain–computer interface applications. *J Neurosci Methods*, 167(1):31–42, 2008.

McFarland, D. J., Krusienski, D. J., Sarnacki, W. A., and Wolpaw, J. R. Emulation of computer mouse control with a noninvasive brain–computer interface. *J Neural Eng*, 5(2):101–110, 2008.

McFarland, D. J., Sarnacki, W. A., and Wolpaw, J. R. Electroencephalographic (EEG) control of three-dimensional movement. *J Neural Eng*, 7(3):036007–036007, 2010.

Mellinger, J., and Schalk, G. BCI2000: A general-purpose software platform for BCI. In Guido Dornhege, José del R. Millán, Thilo Hinterberger, Dennis J. McFarland, and Klaus-Robert Müller, editors, *Toward Brain–Computer Interfacing*, pages 359–367. MIT Press, Cambridge, MA, USA, 2007.

Mellinger, J., Schalk, G., Braun, C., Preissl, H., Rosenstiel, W., Birbaumer, N., and Kübler, A. An MEG-based brain–computer interface (BCI). *NeuroImage*, 36(3):581–593, 2007.

Mellinger, J., and Schalk, G. Using BCI2000 in BCI Research. In Bernhard Graimann, Gert Pfurtscheller, and Brendan Z. Allison, editors, *Brain–Computer Interfaces: Revolutionizing Human–Computer Interaction*, pages 259–279. Springer, 2010.

Miller, K. J., Leuthardt, E. C., Schalk, G., Rao, R. P. N., Anderson, N. R., Moran, D. W., Miller, J. W., and Ojemann, J. G. Spectral changes in cortical surface potentials during motor movement. *J Neurosci*, 27(9):2424–2432, 2007a.

Miller, K. J., den Nijs, M., Shenoy, P., Miller, J. W., Rao, R. P. N., and Ojemann, J. G. Real-time functional brain mapping using electrocorticography. *NeuroImage*, 37(2):504–507, 2007b.

Miller, K. J., Schalk, G., Fetz, E. E., den Nijs, M., Ojemann, J. G., and Rao, R. P. N. Cortical activity during motor execution, motor imagery, and imagery-based online feedback. *Proc Natl Acad Sci USA*, 107(9):4430–4435, 2010.

Mullen, T. R., Kothe, C. A. E., Chi, Y. M., Ojeda, A., Kerth, T., Makeig, S., Cauwenberghs, G., and Jung, T.-P. Real-time modeling and 3D visualization of source dynamics and connectivity using wearable EEG. *Conf Proc IEEE Eng Med Biol Soc*, 2013:2184–2187, 2013.

Mullen, T. R., Kothe, C. A. E., Chi, Y. M., Ojeda, A., Kerth, T., Makeig, S., Jung, T.-P., and Cauwenberghs, G. Real-time neuroimaging and cognitive monitoring using wearable dry EEG. *IEEE Trans Biomed Eng*, 62(11):2553–2567, 2015.

Mühl, C., Jeunet, C., and Lotte, F. EEG-based workload estimation across affective contexts. *Front Neurosci*, 8:114, 2014.

Mugler, E. M., Patton, J. L., Flint, R. D., Wright, Z. A., Schuele, S. U., Rosenow, J., Shih, J. J., Krusienski, D. J., and Slutzky, M. W. Direct classification of all American English phonemes using signals from functional speech motor cortex. *J Neural Eng*, 11(3):035015, 2014.

Nijboer, F., Sellers, E. W., Mellinger, J., Jordan, M. A., Matuz, T., Furdea, A., Halder, S., Mochty, U., Krusienski, D. J., Vaughan, T. M., Wolpaw, J. R., Birbaumer, N., and Kubler, A. A P300-based brain–computer interface for people with amyotrophic lateral sclerosis. *Clin Neurophysiol*, 119(8):1909–1916, 2008.

Oostenveld, R., Fries, P., Maris, E., and Schoffelen, J.-M. Field-Trip: Open source software for advanced analysis of MEG, EEG, and invasive electrophysiological data. *Comput Intell Neurosci*, 2011:156869, 2011.

Ortner, R., Ram, D., Kollreider, A., Pitsch, H., Wojtowicz, J., and Edlinger, G. *Human–Computer Confluence for Rehabilitation Purposes after Stroke*, pages 74–82. Springer Berlin Heidelberg, Berlin, Heidelberg, 2013.

Pei, X., Barbour, D. L., Leuthardt, E. C., and Schalk, G. Decoding vowels and consonants in spoken and imagined words using electrocorticographic signals in humans. *J Neural Eng*, 8(4):046028, 2011.

Perego, P., Maggi, L., Parini, S., and Andreoni, G. BCI++: A new framework for brain computer interface application. In *Proceedings of the 18th International Conference on Software Engineering and Data Engineering, Las Vegas*, pages 37–41, 2009.

Prueckl, R., Kapeller, C., Potes, C., Korostenskaja, M., Schalk, G., Lee, K. H., and Guger, C. CortiQ-Clinical software for electrocorticographic real-time functional mapping of the eloquent cortex. *Conf Proc IEEE Eng Med Biol Soc*, 2013:6365–6368, 2013.

Renard, Y., Lotte, F., Gibert, G., Congedo, M., Maby, E., Delannoy, V., Bertrand, O., and Lécuyer, A. OpenViBE: An open-source software platform to design, test, and use brain–computer interfaces in real and virtual environments. *Presence: Teleoperators and Virtual Environments*, 19(1):35–53, 2010.

Roland, J., Brunner, P., Johnston, J., Schalk, G., and Leuthardt, E. C. Passive real-time identification of speech and motor cortex during an awake craniotomy. *Epilepsy Behav*, 18(1–2):123–128, 2010.

Royer, A. S., and He, B. Goal selection versus process control in a brain–computer interface based on sensorimotor rhythms. *J Neural Eng*, 6(1):16005, 2009.

Schalk, G., and Mellinger, J. *A Practical Guide to Brain–Computer Interfacing with BCI2000*. Springer, London, UK, 1st edition, 2010.

Schalk, G., Brunner, P., Gerhardt, L. A., Bischof, H., and Wolpaw, J. R. Brain–computer interfaces (BCIs): Detection instead of classification. *J Neurosci Meth*, 167(1):51–62, 2008a.

Schalk, G. Effective brain–computer interfacing using BCI2000. In *Conf Proc IEEE Eng Med Biol Soc*, pages 5498–5501. IEEE, 2009.

Schalk, G., Kubanek, J., Miller, K. J., Anderson, N. R., Leuthardt, E. C., Ojemann, J. G., Limbrick, D., Moran, D., Gerhardt, L. A., and Wolpaw, J. R. Decoding two-dimensional movement trajectories using electrocorticographic signals in humans. *J Neural Eng*, 4(3):264, 2007.

Schalk, G., Leuthardt, E. C., Brunner, P., Ojemann, J. G., Gerhardt, L. A., and Wolpaw, J. R. Real-time detection of event-related brain activity. *NeuroImage*, 43(2):245–249, 2008b.

Schalk, G., McFarland, D. J., Hinterberger, T., Birbaumer, N., and Wolpaw, J. R. BCI2000: A general-purpose brain–computer interface (BCI) system. *IEEE Trans Biomed Eng*, 51(6):1034–1043, 2004.

Sellers, E. W., Krusienski, D. J., McFarland, D. J., Vaughan, T. M., and Wolpaw, J. R. A P300 event-related potential brain-computer interface (BCI): The effects of matrix size and inter stimulus interval on performance. *Biol Psychol*, 73(3):242–252, 2006.

Sellers, E. W., Vaughan, T. M., and Wolpaw, J. R. A brain–computer interface for longterm independent home use. *Amyotroph Lateral Scler*, 11(5):449–455, 2010.

Singla, R., Khosla, A., and Jha, R. Influence of stimuli colour in SSVEP-based BCI wheelchair control using support vector machines. *J Med Eng Technol*, 38(3):125–134, 2014.

Spüler, M., Bensch, M., Kleih, S., Rosenstiel, W., Bogdan, M., and Kübler, A. Online use of error-related potentials in healthy users and people with severe motor impairment increases performance of a P300-BCI. *Clin Neurophys*, 123(7):1328–1337, 2012.

Susila, I. P., Kanoh, S., Miyamoto, K., and Yoshinobu, T. xBCI: A generic platform for development of an online BCI system. *IEEJ Trans Electr Electron Eng*, 5:467–473, 2010.

Townsend, G., and Platsko, V. Pushing the P300-based brain–computer interface beyond 100 bpm: Extending performance guided constraints into the temporal domain. *J Neural Eng*, 13(2):026024, 2016.

Townsend, G., LaPallo, B. K., Boulay, C. B., Krusienski, D. J., Frye, G. E., Hauser, C. K., Schwartz, N. E., Vaughan, T. M., Wolpaw, J. R., and Sellers, E. W. A novel P300-based brain–computer interface stimulus presentation paradigm: Moving beyond rows and columns. *Clin Neurophysiol*, 121(7):1109–1120, 2010.

Vansteensel, M. J., Pels, E. G. M., Bleichner, M. G., Branco, M. P., Denison, T., Freudenburg, Z. V., Gosselaar, P., Leinders, S., Ottens, T. H., Van Den Boom, M. A., Van Rijen, P. C., Aarnoutse, E. J., and Ramsey, N. F. Fully implanted brain–computer interface in a locked-in patient with ALS. *N Engl J Med*, 375(21):2060–2066, 2016.

Vaughan, T. M., McFarland, D. J., Schalk, G., Sarnacki, W. A., Krusienski, D. J., Sellers, E. W., and Wolpaw, J. R. The Wadsworth BCI Research and Development Program: At home with BCI. *IEEE Trans Neural Syst Rehabil Eng*, 14(2):229–233, 2006.

Vidaurre, C., Sander, T. H., and Schlögl, A. Biosig: The free and open source software library for biomedical signal processing. *Comput Intell Neurosci*, 2011:935364, 2011.

Wang, W., Collinger, J. L., Degenhart, A. D., Tyler-Kabara, E. C., Schwartz, A. B., Moran, D. W., Weber, D. J., Wodlinger, B., Vinjamuri, R. K., Ashmore, R. C., Kelly, J. W., and Boninger, M. L. An electrocorticographic brain interface in an individual with tetraplegia. *PLoS One*, 8(2):e55344, 2013.

Wilson, A., and Schalk,G. Using BCI2000 for HCI-centered BCI research. In *Brain–Computer Interfaces*, pages 261–274. Springer, 2010.

Wilson, A., Guger, C., and Schalk, G. BCI hardware and software. In *Brain–Computer Interfaces: Principles and Practice*, pages 165–188. Oxford, 2012.

Wilson, A. J., Mellinger, J., Schalk, G., and Williams, J. A procedure for measuring latencies in brain–computer interfaces. *IEEE Trans Biomed Eng*, 57(7):1785–1797, 2010.

Wilson, A. J., Schalk, G., Walton, L. M., and Williams, J. C. Using an EEG-based brain–computer interface for virtual cursor movement with BCI2000. *JoVE (J Vis Exp)*, (29):e1319–e1319, 2009.

Wilson, S. M., and Iacoboni, M. Neural responses to non-native phonemes varying in producibility: Evidence for the sensorimotor nature of speech perception. *NeuroImage*, 33(1):316–325, 2006.

Wisneski, K. J., Anderson, N., Schalk, G., Smyth, M., Moran, D., and Leuthardt, E. C. Unique cortical physiology associated with ipsilateral hand movements and neuroprosthetic implications. *Stroke*, 39(12):3351–3359, 2008.

Wolpaw, J. R., and McFarland, D. J. Control of a two-dimensional movement signal by a noninvasive brain–computer interface in humans. *Proc Natl Acad Sci USA*, 101(51):17849–17854, 2004.

Yamawaki, N., Wilke, C., Liu, Z., and He, B. An enhanced time-frequencyspatial approach for motor imagery classification. *IEEE Trans Neural Syst Rehabil Eng*, 14(2):250–254, 2006.

Yin, E., Zhou, Z., Jiang, J., Chen, F., Liu, Y., and Hu, D. A novel hybrid BCI speller based on the incorporation of SSVEP into the P300 paradigm. *J Neural Eng*, 10(2):026012, 2013.

Yin, E., Zhou, Z., Jiang, J., Chen, F., Liu, Y., and Hu, D. A speedy hybrid BCI spelling approach combining P300 and SSVEP. *IEEE Trans Biomed*, 61(2):473–483, 2014.

Zhao, J., Li, W., Mao, X., and Li, M. SSVEP-based experimental procedure for brain–robot interaction with humanoid robots. *JoVE (J Vis Exp)*, (105), 2015.

Zickler, C., Halder, S., Kleih, S. C., Herbert, C., and Kübler, A. Brain painting: Usability testing according to the user-centered design in end users with severe motor paralysis. *Artif Intell Med*, 59(2):99–110, 2013.

# Part III

Signal Processing, Feature Extraction, and Classification in BCI

# 18 Gentle Introduction to Signal Processing and Classification for Single-Trial EEG Analysis

*Benjamin Blankertz*

## CONTENTS

18.1 Univariate Features and the Amplitude Threshold Criterion .............................................. 344
18.2 From Uni- to Multivariate Features ............................................................................... 346
18.3 Multivariate Approach to Classification of Single-Trial EEG .......................................... 347
18.4 Introduction to Discriminative Features of Brain Activity—Signal and Noise ................. 349
    18.4.1 Modulations of ERPs ........................................................................................ 350
    18.4.2 Amplitude Modulations of Brain Rhythms ....................................................... 351
18.5 Introduction to Linear Classification ............................................................................. 353
    18.5.1 Motivation—Nearest Centroid Classifier .......................................................... 353
    18.5.2 Linear Discriminant Analysis ........................................................................... 355
    18.5.3 Interlude: Gaussian Distributions and Related Transformations ........................ 356
    18.5.4 Relation of LDA to NCC, Whitening, and Mahalanobis Distance ..................... 359
    18.5.5 Remark on the Assumptions of LDA ................................................................ 359
    18.5.6 LDA with Shrinkage of the Covariance Matrix ................................................. 361
    18.5.7 Other Classification Methods ........................................................................... 362
18.6 Feature Extraction ...................................................................................................... 362
    18.6.1 Guideline for Transient Activity: ERP and LRP ............................................... 362
    18.6.2 Guideline for Oscillatory Brain Activity ........................................................... 362
    18.6.3 Feature Extraction: CSP Analysis .................................................................... 363
    18.6.4 Feature Extraction: CCA ................................................................................. 366
18.7 Appendix: Formalization of CSP as a Two-Step Procedure ............................................ 366
References ........................................................................................................................... 367

## Abstract

This introduction presents basic concepts for the analysis of single-trial electroenchephalogram (EEG) data. This is done in a way that is accessible to readers whose main experience rather lies in other fields. While attempting to be as illustrative as possible, our exposition contains the mathematically precise formalism of the methods discussed. Readers not familiar with basic mathematical notions such as vectors and matrices should nevertheless not be discouraged, as they hopefully benefit from reading this tutorial even when skipping the technical parts. For the classification of event-related potentials, spatiotemporal features and classification with regularized linear discriminant analysis is discussed. Modulations of oscillatory brain activity are detected with common spatial pattern analysis and log(arithmized) band-power features. All of those methods are well comprehensible and easy to implement and show nevertheless competitive performance. The first two sections motivate the transition from univariate features, such as signal amplitude in a certain channel and at a certain latency toward multivariate features. Readers familiar with the benefits of multivariate analyses are encouraged to step very quickly over those two sections and to start with Section 18.3.

## 18.1 UNIVARIATE FEATURES AND THE AMPLITUDE THRESHOLD CRITERION

A good starting point for discussing single-trial classification is the amplitude threshold criterion, which is a simple classification rule for a single quantity derived from measured data, which we will refer to as a univariate* *feature*. We will notice that this univariate setting is ideal for studying the basic concept of classification, which can be extended easily to multidimensional (multivariate) features and more complex classification rules. We here consider electroenchephalogram (EEG) data acquired in a so-called *oddball* experiment. In this experiment, six different visual stimuli were presented to the participant in random order at a presentation rate of 5 Hz. The participants were instructed to pay attention to one kind of stimulus (i.e., 16.66 %) and to mentally count the number of their occurrences. Attended stimuli (called *targets* or "oddballs") elicit a so-called *P300 component* (Key et al. 2005) in the EEG, which is a positive voltage deflection observable at central EEG channels. Targets are thus characterized by larger amplitudes in these channels than the stimuli that were to be ignored (the *nontargets*). The P300 can be related to brain processes evaluating the relevance of the given stimulus for the task (see also Ref. Wenzel et al. 2017). Since it is locked to the time of the stimulus onset, the P300 belongs to the class of so-called *event-related potentials* (ERPs).

A typical problem occurring in *brain–computer interface* (BCI) research is to determine the attended stimulus from the acquired brain signals. In order to investigate how well this task can be achieved, it is helpful to acquire the so-called *calibration data*, for which the *ground truth* is known. This is achieved by instructing the participant to pay attention to a specified stimulus when recording the calibration measurement. Thus, we can divide the presented stimuli into the two groups: targets (attended) and nontargets (nonattended). Figure 18.1 shows exemplarily five *single-trial* ERP time courses for both of the two groups (thin lines), as well as the groupwise *averages* calculated over all recorded trials (thick lines) in the time interval ranging from −200 to 800 ms at electrode location Cz.[†]

The most simple criterion that can be used to predict whether a given stimulus was attended or not is an amplitude threshold criterion that aims at the detection of the P300 component. For measuring the P300 amplitude, we consider to assess only the measured activity at channel Cz (which is expected to show the strongest P300 amplitude) and time point 220 ms (at which the P300 peak is observed in this particular data; see the maximum of the thick orange line in Figure 18.1). Those values are marked by filled circles in Figure 18.1. To fix a detection threshold, we calculate the mean of the two average ERPs, which amounts to 4.86 µV in this example. Now, a trial would be classified as a *target* if its amplitude (at 220 ms and Cz) exceeds that threshold. In our example, three *target* trials are correctly detected by this rule, while one *nontarget* is misclassified as target. On the other hand, four *nontargets* are correctly labeled as such, but there are also two *target* trials, which are erroneously classified as *nontargets*. In machine learning terminology, these are three *hits* (or true positives), one *false alarm* (or false positive), four *correct rejections* (or true negatives), and two *misses* (or false negatives). In statistics, false alarms are sometimes also called type I errors, while misses are called type II errors.

---

* *Univariate* data refer to a single scalar (i.e., one-dimensional) variable.
[†] For the convention of denoting electrode positions, refer to Figure 18.2.

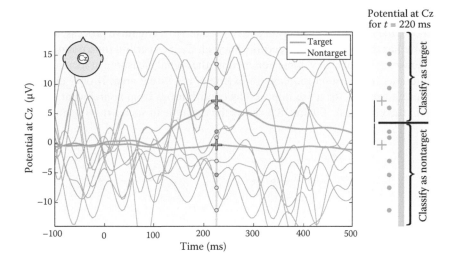

**FIGURE 18.1**    Illustration of the amplitude threshold criterion. The plot shows signals of five randomly picked single trials as well as the ERP (classwise average across trials) of each class. The gray shaded line indicates the time point at which the amplitude is taken. It is selected as the peak amplitude in the *target* ERP. The panel on the right shows the amplitude values of the single trials in relation to a simple classification rule: the threshold is selected as being in the middle between the average amplitudes of the two classes (indicated by crosses here).

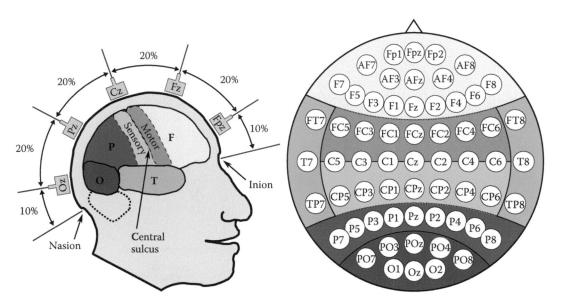

**FIGURE 18.2**    Labels of electrode position according to the international 10–20 system. A widely used method to specify EEG electrode positions is the *international 10–20 system* (cf. Ref. Klem et al. 1999) Those labels are composed of letters and a number. The letters correspond to anatomical structures, the **F**rontal lobe, the **P**arietal lobe, the **O**ccipital lobe, the **T**emporal lobe, and the **C**entral sulcus. The "rows" of electrodes centrally over those structures are denoted with the corresponding single letter. These principal electrode rows are positions that are specified as percentages of the distance between the *nasion* and the *inion* as illustrated in the figure. Rows between those principal rows have two-letter labels, the first one being the one from the row that is more frontal, for example, "FC" between the "F" and the "C" rows. The rows anterior to the "F" row are denoted by "AF" (anterior frontal) and "Fp" (fronto-polar). The position in the left-right direction is specified by numbers, the odd ones going from the vertex down the left hemisphere, the even ones going from the vertex down the right hemisphere, and the vertex itself indicated by the letter "z" for the number 0 (zero).

## 18.2 FROM UNI- TO MULTIVARIATE FEATURES

In the case above, the task is to detect brain activity related to a cognitive process, with the approach of checking whether the amplitude in a certain channel, Cz, at a certain time point, 220 ms, exceeds a threshold. However, because of volume conduction, the signal measured at location Cz can include strong contributions from distant sources, for example, the visual area. If only channel Cz is considered (univariate feature), the noise imposed by contributions from nonrelevant areas can impede classification in the given task. Figure 18.3 shows the example of such a mixing and a case in which

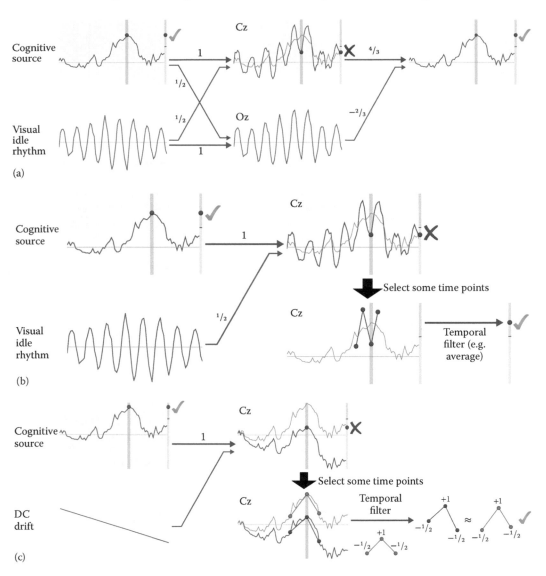

**FIGURE 18.3** The virtue of multivariate features. These illustrations motivate why multivariate features are required for robust classification. Classification on a univariate feature (here amplitude at channel Cz at the time point of the P300 peak) would work well, if the signal from the (here cognitive) source was available. However, in the presence of volume conduction and drifts, including information from distant channels or other time points (multivariate feature) will improve classification. (a) For a given classification task (here cognitive), including channels from distant locations (here visual area) can improve classification as it may help reducing noise by spatial filtering. (b) Also considering several time points may help classification as it allows temporal filtering. (c) Temporal filtering also allows making the classfication more robust against the influence of drifts.

the phase of the oscillation of the visual idle rhythm is at a trough at the relevant time point, such that the mixed signal at Cz misses the threshold. Employing a multivariate classification method that also uses information from the channel Oz opens the possibility to filter out the disturbing influence and to reconstruct the signal of the source of interest. This is not possible with the univariate approach that looks only at one channel and one time point. The calculation of the weighted average of the values at channel Cz and Oz is called *spatial filtering*. Saving the classification is also possible by temporal filtering (see Figure 18.3b). Temporal filtering is also useful for counterbalancing the effect of drifts (see Figure 18.3c).

This illustration should motivate the following fact. Even if channel Cz and time point 220 ms shows the difference between the classes *target* and *nontarget* most pronounced, it can (and in almost all case will) be beneficial to include further features (measurements from different channels and/or time points) into the decision. Note that this applies not (only) to channels in the proximity of the source (here Cz) but can also include distant channels (here Oz). This corresponds to the fact that spatial filters can have substantial weights over areas that do not directly contribute to the information of interest. For a more thorough discussion on this issue, refer to Refs. (Blankertz et al. 2011; Haufe et al. 2014).

## 18.3  MULTIVARIATE APPROACH TO CLASSIFICATION OF SINGLE-TRIAL EEG

While the original approach to brain–computer interfacing using operand conditioning involved feedback of simple features of brain activity, more complex methods from the field machine learning form nowadays an essential part in most BCI approaches, as ERP-based spellers (Farwell and Donchin 1988; Hong et al. 2009; Krusienski et al. 2006; Schreuder et al. 2010; Treder and Blankertz 2010), motor imagery–driven BCIs (Blankertz et al. 2006a; Guger et al. 2000; Vidaurre et al. 2011c), BCIs based on steady-state visual evoked potentials (SSVEPs) (Bin et al. 2009; Lin et al. 2006), and shifting visual attention (Treder et al. 2011). Recently, machine learning is even used in the conditioning approach (van der Heiden et al. 2010). One reason why the machine learning approach is successful in BCIs is that the adaptation of the system to the specific brain signals of each user from a calibration is essential to account for the huge interpersonal variability in the brain signals (Blankertz et al. 2006b).

Before going into the details, we give an overview of the data processing procedure. At the core of a BCI system is a classifier that assigns the incoming brain signals to a certain mental state, for example, the last visual stimuli was an *attended target* versus it was *unattended*; or motor imagery of the *left hand* versus *right hand* versus *foot*; or visual attention was shifted toward the "2 o'clock direction." If the output of the classifier does not correspond to a predefined set of mental states, but is rather a continuous value (e.g., for cursor control), one should more precisely call it regressor or controller. But the basic principle is the same in all cases, so we do not make this distinction here.

The processing, from the raw brain signals to the control signal, can roughly be divided into the following steps: segmentation, preprocessing, classification, and translation into a control signal: From the continuous signals, short-term windows (called *epochs*) are extracted for further processing. Such an epoch is the input to the preprocessing (or feature extraction), and the output is a vector of real numbers, which is called *feature vector*. This feature vector is the input for the classifier and its output can be given in various forms, for example, as probabilities that reflect the likelihood of the input sample belonging to the different mental states (e.g., last stimulus was *attended*). The output can also be one real-valued number that interpolates between the states *left hand motor imagery* (ideally output −1) and *right hand motor imagery* (ideally output +1), which could be used, for example, to control a cursor. This basic case of a processing chain is depicted in Figure 18.4. The final step of translating the classifier outputs into a control signal depends very much on the actual application that is controlled by the BCI, which is out of the scope of this chapter. For ERP-based spellers, for example, consecutive classifier outputs are averaged for each type of stimuli across

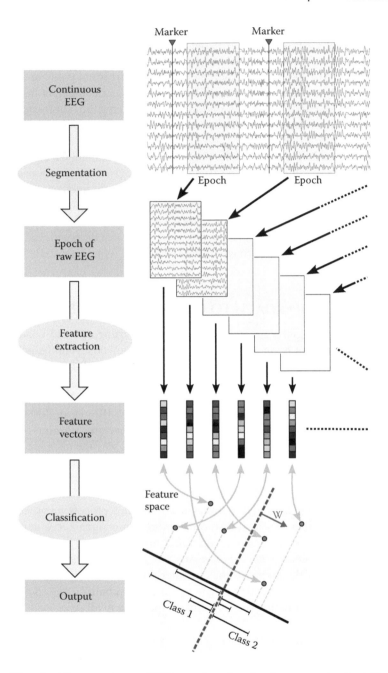

**FIGURE 18.4** Flowchart from continuous EEG neuroimaging signals to control output. From the continuous signals, short windows (epochs) are cut out. The time interval is often related to markers that indicate, for example, the occurrence of a cue. For continuous online control like cursor movement, the epoch may be, for example, the most recently acquired window of 500 ms. From these epochs of raw data, the so-called features vectors are calculated, which often include several preprocessing steps. These features are either used to train a classifier (calibration phase) or fed into a classifier in order to obtain a control signal as output (feedback phase). For more information on calibration and feedback phase, see Figure 18.5 and the corresponding text.

repeated presentations to generate a control signal that corresponds to that type of stimulus that has the highest accumulated evidence.

The classifier could be just a fixed formula with no free parameters, which determines the output in the very same way for each user. In this case, the processing is tuned to the "average brain" or to the neurophysiology that is deduced from analyzing the grand average of a larger database. One example for such a classification scheme was given in Section 18.1, the amplitude threshold criterium. Similarly, for the operand conditioning of slow cortical potentials (Elbert et al. 1980), for example, the classifier output is roughly the potential at electrode Cz averaged across 500 ms. This value is used for a continuous feedback signal. Some more degrees of freedom are used in the approach of Wolpaw et al. (1991), which is based on the modulation of mu/beta rhythms. Band-power values are translated into cursor movement by a linear regression based on two- to three-dimensional features. Furthermore, two free parameters of the regression (slope and intercept) are adapted online.

The huge interpersonal variability with respect to the patterns of brain activity can be better accounted for, when spatial filters are adapted to the individual. The optimization of spatial filters is instrumental in the machine learning approach. Early examples of individually adapted spatial filters are (Farwell and Donchin 1988) for ERP-based BCIs (implicitly by training a linear classifier on spatiotemporal filters) and the common spatial pattern (CSP) analysis for BCIs based on motor imagery (Ramoser et al. 2000) (see Section 18.6.3).

In the machine learning approach, the flexibility to adapt the system to the specific brain signal of each user is increased with the aim to minimize the time required for user training and to increase the performance of the system. This is typically accomplished by a so-called calibration. In this phase, the participant follows cues that indicate what mental activity they should perform. Therefore, the epochs of EEG data related to the cues can be endowed with the labels of the corresponding mental states. These labels carry over to the extracted feature vectors, which form the training data. Accordingly, the training data are groups of samples, each group (or class) being defined by the label, that is, corresponding to one particular mental state. In the training procedure, values for the free parameters of the classifier are determined in order to maximize classification performance. Figure 18.5 shows the concept of machine learning–based BCIs [69,70].

Note that this figure shows only the basic case. The calibration can be implemented as a coadaptive procedure during a feedback application (Sannelli et al. 2012; Vidaurre et al. 2011c; Wang et al. 2007). Still, the concept shown in Figure 18.5 applies in that mental activity is cued. Furthermore, the classifier might be adapted during online operation even without information about the true mental state ("unsupervised adaptation" Vidaurre et al. 2011a,b,c).

The higher power of multivariate methods like machine learning–based classifiers for BCI comes at a risk. The increased flexibility is related to the higher degree of freedom or, speaking in terms of the feature vectors, the higher dimensionality. In high-dimensional data, a lot of accidental correlations of certain features with the labels exist, which might mislead the optimization. Such a classifier would perform well on the training data, but not on "new data." In BCI context, the new data are the brain signals that are acquired during the actual application (e.g., freespelling with a mental typewriter). This failure of generalization is called "overfitting." Therefore, it is crucial to be able to estimate the "generalization performance" from the given training data. This issue is discussed in detail in Ref. (Lemm et al. 2011).

## 18.4  INTRODUCTION TO DISCRIMINATIVE FEATURES OF BRAIN ACTIVITY—SIGNAL AND NOISE

To follow the introduction to classification better, we start by giving an overview of the typical features that are used in a BCI context because these are the input to the classification procedure. In view of classification, it is important to have an intuition of how the feature vectors are distributed—what is the signal, what is the noise, and how are they related. To discuss that, we take a look at two

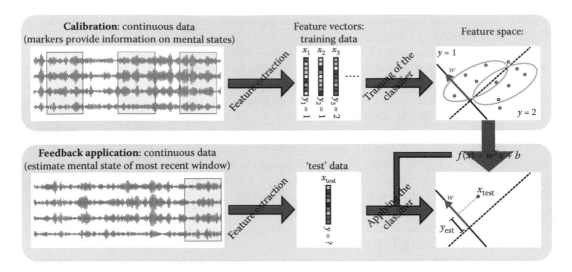

**FIGURE 18.5** Concept of machine learning–based BCIs. In the machine learning approach, a classification model is adapted to training data. To this, the so-called calibration data are recorded at the beginning of a session, in which the user is cued to perform certain tasks. High-dimensional feature vectors that are extracted from the corresponding trials of EEG signals are the input to this machine training. After estimating the parameters of the classification model, the system is ready to be used. In the feedback application, recent EEG trials (which might be aligned to external stimuli like in the ERP-based speller or continuously acquire as in cursor control) are translated into feature vectors and then fed into the classifier. The output of the classifier might be further processed to obtain a control signal for the BCI application, for example, the selection of a letter in a speller, or the movement of an orthosis contingent on environmental data (shared control) (From R. Leeb et al., *Artificial Intelligence in Medicine*, 59(2):121–132, 2013; G. Vanacker et al., *Computational Intelligence and Neuroscience*, 2007:3–3, 2007.)

components of brain activity that are widely used in BCI research, since they can be voluntarily modulated.

### 18.4.1 Modulations of ERPs

A basic feature vector for an ERP component is the vector of amplitudes of each channel at the peak latency (see Section 18.6.1 and Ref. Blankertz et al. 2011 for more complex features). For illustrative purposes, we use just two channels (Cz and Oz). Figure 18.6 (left plots) displays the ERPs for the conditions *target* (attended stimulus) and *nontarget* (unattended stimulus) of an oddball paradigm. The thick line is the average (ERP) while the lighter thin lines are the single-trial epochs. The gray shaded line marks the time point, which is used to calculate the respective feature vector. The values marked by crosses are the ERP amplitudes, for both conditions and channels.

The respective values of the single trials (marked by little dots) show a considerable variation around the average value. This is mainly due to the ongoing background activity, which is different in each trial. The voltage changes of the ERP are "phase-locked" to the stimulus and are therefore represented by the mean, which is the target "signal" in this case. The background activity is non–phase-locked to the stimulus and represents noise. The amplitude of this noise is reduced by the factor $1/\sqrt{N}$, when averaging across $N$ trials (according to a rule of thumb that holds under the assumption that the phase-locked activity is the same in each trial and that the noise has a Gaussian distribution). Accordingly, with a sufficient number of trials, the non–phase-locked background activity should only have a negligible impact and the across-trial average is a reasonable approximation of the underlying ERP. A further (but much weaker) source of variation may be the trial-to-trial variability of the ERPs (e.g., caused by variable states of attention, vigilance, and task engagement).

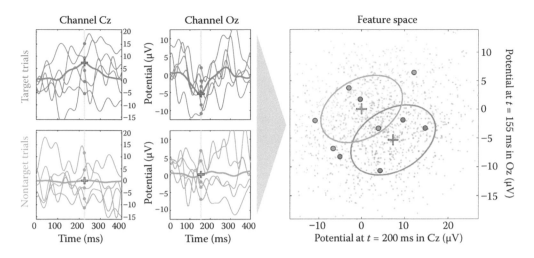

**FIGURE 18.6** ERP features and their distribution. A basic feature for an ERP component is the vector of amplitudes in all channels at the peak latency (spatial feature). For illustration purposes, we just use two channels here. *Left plots:* Signals of five randomly picked single trials of each class as well as the ERP (classwise average across trials) are shown for the two channels Cz and Oz. A time is shaded where the amplitude is taken as a value of the feature vector. *Right plot:* The scatterplot shows the distribution of the two classes. The larger dots show the features taken from the selected single trials shown on the left. Ellipses are determined from the covariance matrices and indicate the fit of a Gaussian distribution.

When aiming at classification, the classwise distributions of the feature vectors are crucial. In our example, we take simple two-dimensional features composed of the amplitudes in channels Cz and Oz at certain latencies. The corresponding distributions (for the conditions *targets* and *nontargets*) can be visualized in a so-called scatterplot: For each single trial, the amplitude at $t = 220$ ms in channel Cz is plotted on the $x$ axis and the amplitude at $t = 155$ ms in channel Oz is plotted on the $y$ axis. This gives one data point per trial in Figure 18.6.

An approximation of the distributions as Gaussians are indicated by the ellipsoids (this way of visualization is explained below; see Section 18.5.3). The mean amplitudes in Figure 18.6 (left plots), which are marked by crosses, correspond to the means of the distributions in subplot (right plot). Accordingly, the *signal* of the ERP features is reflected by the mean (or centroid) of the distribution, while the *noise* corresponds to the dispersion of the data points around the mean (represented by the ellipsoid and mathematically by the covariance matrix; see Section 18.5.3).

## 18.4.2  AMPLITUDE MODULATIONS OF BRAIN RHYTHMS

The amplitude of some spontaneous brain rhythms is modulated by the mental state, for example, the attenuation of the sensorimotor rhythms during motor imagery (Kalcher and Pfurtscheller 1995). In this case, the modulation of the amplitude is time-locked to the change of the mental state (event-related modulation). However, the oscillation of the brain rhythm is not phase-locked to the event. This is a crucially different situation that for ERPs, and when simply averaging oscillatory signals, the result will be a flat line and the modulations just vanish.* Accordingly, a different method is required to investigate the event-related amplitude modulations of brain rhythms than for ERPs. A simple way to visualize the time course of amplitude modulations of brain rhythms is to band-pass filter the signals to the frequency range of interest, rectify the signals (that is taking the absolute value), and then average across epochs (Pfurtscheller and Lopes da Silva 1999). Slightly

---

* There may be a residual low frequency shift, since the oscillations of some brain rhythms are not symmetric (Nikulin et al. 2010).

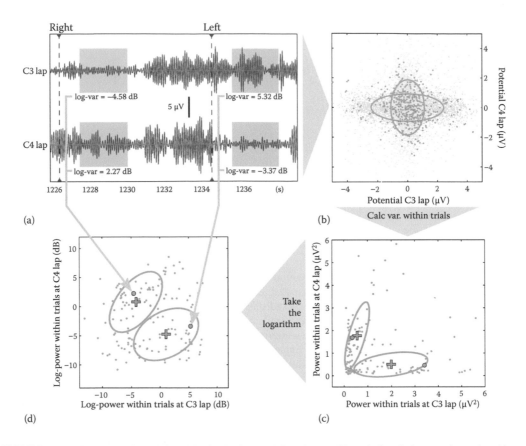

**FIGURE 18.7** Features of modulated brain rhythms. (a) Band-pass–filtered signals in two channels with one phase of right and another of left hand motor imagery, shaded in blue and orange, respectively. (b) Scatterplot of the signals shown in (a). Each point here corresponds to one time point in the signals (of all trials, not only the two shown left). (c) After calculating the variance within each trial, we obtain a scatterplot in which each point corresponds to one trial. (d) In order to make the distributions more Gaussian, the logarithm is applied. Note that the orthogonality of the distributions shown in (b) is not typical for EEG, as the channels are highly correlated because of volume conduction. This ideal case is taken here for illustration purposes. Realistic distributions are shown in Figure 18.15a with the rest of the figure showing how orthogonal distributions can be obtained.

better results might be obtained by employing the Hilbert transform to determine the amplitude hull curve of single-trials and averaging (see Ref. Burgess and Gruzelier 1996).

Here, we will focus more on the aspect of classification. To that end, it is important to consider how the *features* corresponding to the modulations of brain rhythms look like. Again, we consider only two channels for illustration purposes and take the two conditions of *left* and *right hand motor imagery* and assume that the signals are already band-pass filtered to the frequency band of the respective rhythm. In contrast to the ERP case, the whole time interval of motor imagery displays the condition-specific modulation (see Figure 18.7a).

In the first step of visualizing the brain signals in a feature space, we plot the C3 and the C4 amplitude value* for *each time point* as a dot in a scatterplot (see subplot b). (Remember that, in the ERP case [Figure 18.6], each dot represented one trial.) As the signals were band-pass filtered, the mean of the class-specific distributions is at the origin (0,0). The oscillations display here as variation around the center. Again, each distribution is approximated by a Gaussian and visualized by an ellipsoid (see Section 18.5.3 for an explanation). This is just an intermediate step, as the feature

---

* Laplace-filtered, see "the need for spatial filtering" in Ref. Blankertz et al. 2008b.

vectors for classification are not calculated from a single time point, but from one epoch of motor imagery (for continuous control, these epochs may be as short as 250 ms; see Ref. Blankertz et al. 2008b). To that end, the variance within such epochs is calculated, and the resulting feature vectors are visualized in Figure 18.7c. The variance of band-pass–filtered signals coincides with the band-power. Note that the distributions of these band-power features are far from looking like Gaussians. Therefore, the logarithm is often applied. Then, the unit of the features is decibels, and the distributions are more like Gaussians (see subplot d). These log band-power features can typically be well classified by linear methods (the link between Gaussian distributions and linear separability will be discussed in Section 18.5.2).

## 18.5    INTRODUCTION TO LINEAR CLASSIFICATION

With this intuition of how the features of discriminative brain activity are typically distributed in the feature space, we proceed to introduce linear classification. It starts with a simple setting that naturally relates to the classification method called nearest centroid classifier (NCC), which will be intuitively clear to everyone. Then, we advance to the more complex linear discriminant analysis (LDA) and show that it is equivalent to the simple NCC plus accounting for the structure of the noise.

We use boldface letters in lowercase to denote (column) vectors, while scalars (i.e., real numbers) are typeset in normal font weight. Hence, a sample is formally written as $\mathbf{x} = [x^1,\ldots, x^k]^T$, where each $x^i$ is a scalar and T denotes transposition of a matrix or a vector. Matrices are denoted by uppercase letters in boldface.

### 18.5.1    MOTIVATION—NEAREST CENTROID CLASSIFIER

Let us assume we have data given from two conditions. In the context of classification, one typically uses the term *classes* rather than *conditions*. Each observation is derived from one epoch (or trial) of neuroimaging data and represented as a vector of real numbers, which is also called a *sample* or *feature vector* (see Section 18.3). These values can either be the raw data itself, or the result of applying some processing steps to the raw data, as sketched above and explained in more detail in Section 18.4. This procedure of preprocessing is also called feature extraction, as the goal is to extract features that more explicitly reflect the information of interest, which is latent in the raw signals. Feature extraction is discussed in more detail in Section 18.6.

Suppose that our task is to decide from a given sample to which of two classes it belongs. If we know only the means of the two classes $\mu_1$ and $\mu_2$ (also called centroids in this context), then the best strategy is to assign the given sample $\mathbf{x}$ to that class, whose centroid is closest to $\mathbf{x}$ (see Figure 18.8a). This assignment corresponds to a linear separation of the plane with the separation line perpendicularly crossing the line from $\mu_2$ to $\mu_1$ in the middle (see Figure 18.8b): all samples on one side of the separation line (half-plane) are assigned to class 1 and samples on the other half-plane are assigned to class 2.

Let us put this into the mathematical framework, which can be used to generalize to more complex cases. Generally, binary classification is formalized by a decision function $f: \mathbb{R}^k \rightarrow \{-1,+1\}$ that assigns an observation $\mathbf{x}$ to the numbers $-1$ or $+1$, which are used as labels for the two classes. In the case of linear classification, the separation can be defined by a hyperplane (which is a "flat" subspace of $k-1$ dimensions in the $k$-dimensional space; special cases are a line in 2D and a plane in 3D space). In this case, $f$ is typically parameterized by its normal vector $\mathbf{w}$ and a bias term $b$. The predicted class label $y$ is given by

$$f : \mathbf{x} \rightarrow y := \text{sign}(\mathbf{w}^\top \mathbf{x} - b). \tag{18.1}$$

The set of points $\mathbf{x}$ that satisfy $\mathbf{w}^\top \mathbf{x} - b = 0$ is the *separating hyperplane*. The normal vector $\mathbf{w}$ is the crucial parameter of the classifier; it defines the orientation of the separating hyperplane. Changing the bias $b$ corresponds to a parallel translation of the separating hyperplane (see Figure 18.8c). In terms

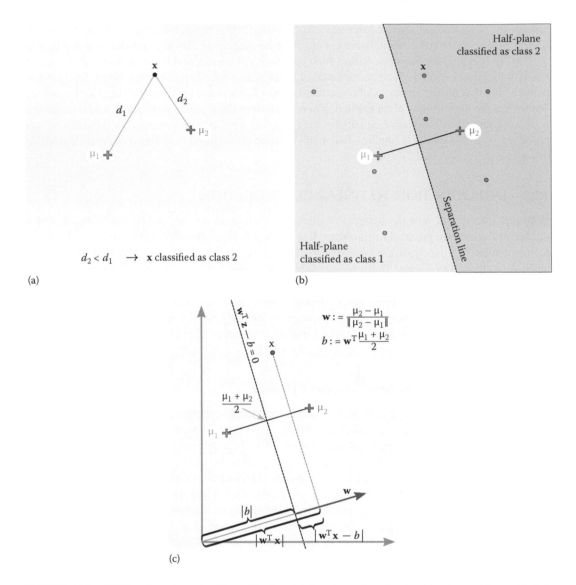

**FIGURE 18.8** NCC and mathematical formalization. (a) Simple setting of a classification problem with little information. Only the means (or centroids) $\mu_1$ and $\mu_2$ of the two distributions are known. In this situation, the natural strategy to classify a sample x is to assign it to that class, whose centroid is nearer. (b) This leads to a linear separation of the space with the separation line (or hyperplane in higher dimensions) cross perpendicular to the line connecting the centroids in the middle. (c) Putting this into a mathematical formalism, a line separation is described by a normal vector $\mathbf{w}$ and a bias term $b$. For the nearest centroid classification, $\mathbf{w}$ is defined as the difference of the centroids $\mu_2 - \mu_1$. For the visualization, we normalize $\mathbf{w}$. Bias $b$ is length of the projection of the middle between the centroids $(\mu_1 + \mu)/2$ onto the normal vector $\mathbf{w}$. The term $|\mathbf{w}^T\mathbf{x}|$ corresponds to the projection of the sample point $\mathbf{x}$ onto $\mathbf{w}$.

of classification, it can impose a bias toward one or the other class. In our simple example, $\mathbf{w}$ could be defined as $\mu_2 - \mu_1$ and $b$ as $\mathbf{w}^T(\mu_1 + \mu_2)/2$, that is, the length of the projection of the middle between the class means onto the normal vector (see Figure 18.8c). Note that the scaling of $\mathbf{w}$ and $b$ does not matter in this formalization—multiplying $\mathbf{w}$ and $b$ by a common factor would not alter the decision function. In Figure 18.8c, $\mathbf{w}$ was scaled to have length 1 for demonstration purposes. (Otherwise, the formulas for the length of the projections onto the normal vector would require scaling.)

## 18.5.2    LINEAR DISCRIMINANT ANALYSIS

While this is a reasonable classification strategy in the case, that we do not have any further information about the classes than their means would not perform well in most applications involving noisy observations. The idea in machine learning (Bishop 2006; Duda et al. 2001; Hastie et al. 2008) is to have a set of observations (training set), for which the true class affiliation is known. This labeled sequence $(\mathbf{x}_1, y_1),\ldots,(\mathbf{x}_n, y_n)$ of feature vectors $\mathbf{x}_i$ and corresponding labels $y_i$ can then be used to estimate further properties of the two class distributions of samples in order to derive a more specific classification function. Choosing a certain method of classification means (at least implicitly) assuming certain models for the class distributions. In the following, we take LDA as an example. Its assumptions are discussed in Section 18.5.5. Later, in Section 18.5.6, we present a simple extension to LDA that makes it a powerful classification technique, which is performing competitively in most BCI classification tasks, when suitable features are used (Blankertz et al. 2011; Krusienski et al. 2006).

First, we assume that the samples of both classes obey Gaussian (=normal) distributions. A multivariate (i.e., observations are vectors, rather than numbers) Gaussian distribution is characterized by its mean (vector) $\mu$ and its covariance matrix $\Sigma$. Given these distribution parameters, one can determine for a specific test sample $\mathbf{x}$ and a class $c$ what the expected loss of classifying $\mathbf{x}$ as $c$ is (the loss being 0 in case of correct classification and being 1 otherwise). In this sense, the optimal classifier (which has minimum risk of misclassification) is the one that decides for that class $c$, which has the minimal expected loss. Assuming that both distributions have the same covariance matrix $\Sigma$, the normal vector $\mathbf{w}$ of the optimal separating hyperplane can be determined as $\mathbf{w} = \Sigma^{-1}(\mu_2 - \mu_1)$ and the bias $b = \mathbf{w}^{\top}(\mu_2 + \mu_1)/2$ (see Ref. Duda et al. 2001). This yields the decision function of LDA (see Figure 18.9)

$$\mathbf{x} \mapsto \mathrm{sign}\left(\mathbf{x}^{\top} \Sigma^{-1}(\mu_2 - \mu_1) - b\right). \tag{18.2}$$

The same separating hyperplane is obtained by different approaches, for example, Fisher's discriminant or least squares regression (Duda et al. 2001). Without the assumption that both covariance matrices are equal, the optimal solution is given by quadratic discriminant analysis, but this method is much more sensible to violations of the basic assumptions and requires considerably more training data (Wald and Kronmal 1977). Note that the NCC corresponds to LDA with the identity matrix as covariance ($\Sigma = \mathbf{I}$ in Equation 18.2). Therefore, NCC is the canonical classifier when Gaussian distributions are assumed, but no estimate or assumption about the noise exists.

Since the "true" distributions are unknown, one has to approximate the actual mean and covariance matrix for both classes on the basis of training data. In statistics, it is shown that the empirical mean and empirical covariance matrix are the best unbiased estimators (unbiased means that the expected value of the estimator is the true value). These estimators are also called sample mean and sample covariance and are defined for class $c$ as

$$\hat{\mu}_c = \frac{1}{n_c} \sum \left\{ \mathbf{x}_i \,\middle|\, i \text{ such that } y_i = c \right\} \text{ and}$$

$$\hat{\Sigma}_c = \frac{1}{n_c - 1} \sum \left\{ (\mathbf{x}_i - \hat{\mu}_c)(\mathbf{x}_i - \hat{\mu}_c)^{\top} \,\middle|\, i \text{ such that } y_i = c \right\},$$

with $n_c$ being the number of samples of class $c$. Using these estimates and setting $\hat{\Sigma} = \left(\hat{\Sigma}_1 + \hat{\Sigma}_2\right)/2$, the separation imposed by LDA is determined* from the calibration data, and one can assign test samples to one of the classes via Equation 18.2.

---

\* The same separation is obtained (for equally sized classes) by using the pooled covariance matrix $\hat{\Sigma} = \frac{1}{n-1}\sum\left\{(\mathbf{x}_i - \hat{\mu})(\mathbf{x}_i - \hat{\mu})^{\top}\,\middle|\,\text{for all } i\right\}.$

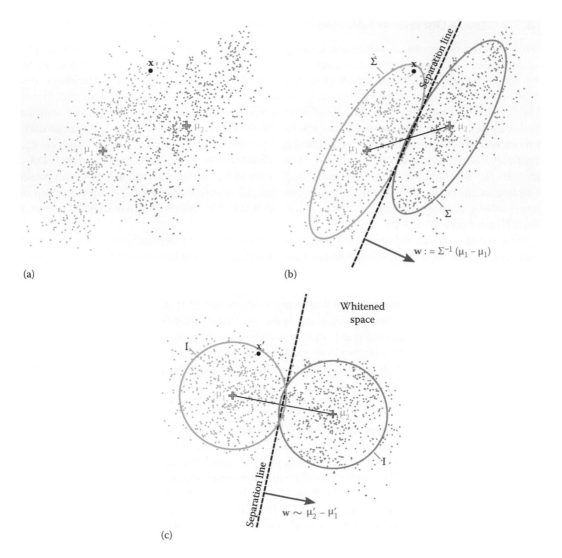

**FIGURE 18.9** Linear discriminent analysis. (a) The setting of the classification problem here is the same as in Figure 18.8a, but here distributions of (training) data points for both classes are known. Note that the means $\mu_1$, $\mu_2$ and the sample point **x** are exactly the same as in Figure 18.8. (b) In LDA, a common covariance matrix for both classes is estimated, which describes the (class-independent) noise. Based on probability theory, the optimal classifier for two Gaussian distributions $\mathcal{N}(\mu_1,\Sigma)$ and $\mathcal{N}(\mu_2,\Sigma)$ can be determined to have the normal vector $\mathbf{w} = \Sigma^{-1}(\mu_2 - \mu_1)$. Note that this leads to a different separation (and opposite classification of the illustrated test sample x) compared to Figure 18.8, although the *signal*, that is, the means $\mu_1$ and $\mu_2$ are the same, "just" the *noise*, that is, covariance $\Sigma$ is different. In other words, NCC is LDA under the assumption that the noise is white. (c) LDA is equivalent to whitening the whole space (including the test sample) and performing nearest centroid classification as in Figure 18.8.

In order to illustrate the principle of LDA from another perspective, we first give an introduction to Gaussian distributions and related linear transformations.

### 18.5.3  INTERLUDE: GAUSSIAN DISTRIBUTIONS AND RELATED TRANSFORMATIONS

In order to provide a better understanding of the functioning of LDA, we provide an intuitive exposé on Gaussian distributions and involved transformations. Gaussian distributions can be well characterized by an eigenvalue decomposition (EVD). Let us investigate the distribution $\mathcal{N}(\mu, \Sigma)$, that is, a Gaussian distribution with mean $\mu$ and covariance matrix $\Sigma$. Covariance matrices are symmetric and positive-semidefinite, which implies that there exists a so-called EVD

$$\Sigma = \mathbf{VDV}^\top, \tag{18.3}$$

with orthonormal matrix $\mathbf{V}$ (i.e., $\mathbf{V}^\top\mathbf{V} = \mathbf{I}$, the identity matrix) and diagonal matrix $\mathbf{D}$. The columns $\mathbf{v}_i$ of $\mathbf{V}$ are called eigenvectors and the corresponding diagonal elements $d_i$ of $\mathbf{D}$ are the eigenvalues. When $\Sigma$ is the empirical covariance matrix of samples $\mathbf{X} = [\mathbf{x}_1,...,\mathbf{x}_n]$, then the eigenvalue $d_i$ is the variance of the samples in the direction of the Eigenvector $\mathbf{v}_i$ and

$$\text{std}\left(\mathbf{v}_i^\top\mathbf{X}\right) = \sqrt{\text{var}\left(\mathbf{v}_i^\top\mathbf{X}\right)} = \sqrt{\frac{1}{n}\mathbf{v}_i^\top\mathbf{X}\left(\mathbf{v}_i^\top\mathbf{X}\right)^\top} = \sqrt{\frac{1}{n}\mathbf{v}_i^\top\mathbf{X}\mathbf{X}^\top\mathbf{v}_i} = \sqrt{\mathbf{v}_i\Sigma\mathbf{v}_i} = \sqrt{d_i} \text{ since } \mathbf{V}^\top\Sigma\mathbf{V} = \mathbf{D}.$$

For this exposé, the involved math does not matter. Rather, we will give a geometric interpretation of eigenvectors and eigenvalues of a covariance that is simple. Here, it is just important to note that multiplication of a vector with an orthonormal matrix (like $\mathbf{V}$) is a rotation (may also involve mirroring), and multiplication with a diagonal matrix (like $\mathbf{D}$) corresponds to scaling along the coordinate axes.

For visualization, distributions can be represented by the equidensity contour lines. For Gaussian distributions, all equidensity lines are ellipsoids centered around the mean $\mu$ (see Figure 18.10a). The principal axes of those ellipsoids are given by the eigenvectors of $\Sigma$ and their radii are proportional to the square root of the corresponding eigenvalues. Figure 18.10b visualizes a Gaussian distribution by one equidensity contour. Here, that contour line is chosen, for which the radii are the standard deviation in the direction of the corresponding principal axes.

As a first step, we show what kind of transformation to the space is implied by the multiplication with a positive-semidefinite matrix (such as a covariance). Using the EVD of Equation 18.3, the process can be decomposed into three steps of multiplications with matrices $\mathbf{V}^\top$, $\mathbf{D}$, and $\mathbf{V}$, which correspond to simple transformations (see Figure 18.11).

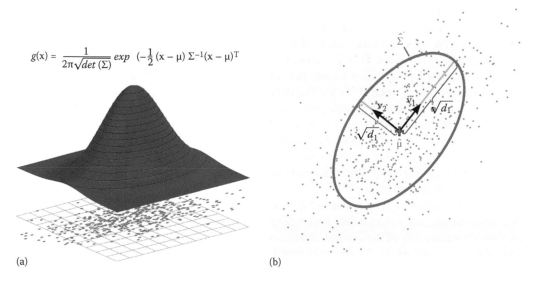

$$g(x) = \frac{1}{2\pi\sqrt{\det(\Sigma)}} exp \left(-\frac{1}{2}(x - \mu)\,\Sigma^{-1}(x - \mu)^\mathrm{T}\right)$$

(a)

(b)

**FIGURE 18.10** Visualization of a 2D Gaussian distribution. (a) Surface plot of the density function of a two-dimensional Gaussian distribution. Contours are equidensity lines, which are for Gaussians all concentric ellipsoids with the same ratio of radii. (b) To visualize a Gaussian distribution in the plane, an ellipsoid representing one equidensity line is drawn. The direction of the axes and then lengths of the corresponding radii can be determined by an EVD.

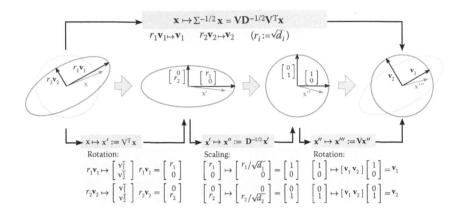

**FIGURE 18.11** Illustration of the multiplication of a covariance matrix and a vector. The process of the multiplication is split into three steps by using the Eingevalue decomposition. This figure shows that the multiplication is a transformation of the space that maps the unit sphere to an ellipsoid, which is defined by the covariance matrix. But note that the radii here are defined by the eigenvalues, not by the square root of the eigenvalues as in Figure 18.10; compare also Figure 18.12. In other words, it is a scaling along the principal axes of the ellipsoid defined by $\Sigma$. *Step 1.* The multiplication of a vector with the orthonormal matrix $\mathbf{V}^{\mathsf{T}}$ is a rotation. The calculation shows that the rotation is defined by mapping the eigenvectors $\mathbf{v}_i$ to the coordinate axes. *Step 2.* The multiplication of a vector with the diagonal matrix $\mathbf{D}$ is a scaling along the coordinate axes. *Step 3.* The multiplication with $\mathbf{V}$ is the inverse rotation to the multiplication with $\mathbf{V}^{\mathsf{T}}$ (due to orthonormality). This means the coordinate axes are maps "back" to the eigenvectors.

In this illustration, the point $\mathbf{x}$ is transformed by the multiplication with $\Sigma$. The gray arrow represents $\mathbf{x}$ as position vector (i.e., a vector pointing from the origin to $\mathbf{x}$). In the first panel, the unit circle is shown for reference (solid line). Furthermore, an ellipsoid is indicated by a dashed line. The principal axes are the eigenvectors $\mathbf{v}_1$ and $\mathbf{v}_2$, the columns of $\mathbf{V}$. The first step is the multiplication with the orthonormal vector $\mathbf{V}^{\mathsf{T}}$, which is a rotation (it could also involve a mirroring, but that can be neglected here). Since $\mathbf{V}^{\mathsf{T}}\mathbf{V} = \mathbf{I}$ (orthonormality) implies $\mathbf{v}_1^{\mathsf{T}}\mathbf{v}_1 = \mathbf{v}_2^{\mathsf{T}}\mathbf{v}_2 = 1$ and $\mathbf{v}_1^{\mathsf{T}}\mathbf{v}_2 = \mathbf{v}_2^{\mathsf{T}}\mathbf{v}_1 = 0$, the rotation is defined by mapping the eigenvectors $\mathbf{v}_i$ to the coordinate axes: $\mathbf{V}^{\mathsf{T}}\mathbf{v}_1 = [1\ 0]^{\mathsf{T}}$ and $\mathbf{V}^{\mathsf{T}}\mathbf{v}_2 = [0\ 1]^{\mathsf{T}}$. Vector $\mathbf{x}$ is rotated accordingly, with the result denoted by $\mathbf{x}'$. The second step is a multiplication with $\mathbf{D}$. Since $\mathbf{D}$ is diagonal, this transformation is a scaling along the coordinate axes, the horizontal one by factor $d_1$, and the vertical one by factor $d_2$. The final step is the inverse rotation to the first step, since $\mathbf{V}^{-1} = \mathbf{V}^{\mathsf{T}}$. The coordinate axes are rotated back to the direction of the eigenvectors. To emphasize the whole process, the unit circle, which was used as reference for $\mathbf{x}$ in the first panel, is drawn in the last panel by a dashed line. The new reference for $\mathbf{x}$ is the ellipsoid in solid line. Viewing the total transformation, the original space is squeezed (or extended) along the principal axes $\mathbf{v}_1$, $\mathbf{v}_2$ such that the unit sphere becomes the shown ellipsoid. Note that this ellipsoid does not exactly coincide with the equidensity contour of $\Sigma$. Here, the radii are the eigenvalues, not the square root of the eigenvalues.

The transformation in LDA is somewhat different. It involves the multiplication with the inverse covariance matrix. For a reason that becomes apparent later, we will consider here the multiplication with the square root of the inverse covariance matrix. Using the EVD (Equation 18.3) and basic linear algebra, we obtain the decomposition of $\Sigma^{-1/2}$ as

$$\Sigma^{-1/2} = \mathbf{V}\mathbf{D}^{-1/2}\mathbf{V}^{\top}. \tag{18.4}$$

Note that $\mathbf{D}^{-1/2}$ is the diagonal matrix with elements $1/\sqrt{d_i}$. Again, $\mathbf{v}_1$ and $\mathbf{v}_2$ denote the column vectors of $\mathbf{V}$ (i.e., eigenvectors of $\Sigma$). Drawn in the first panel of Figure 18.12 is the ellipsoid corresponding to $\Sigma$ with its principal axes $\mathbf{v}_1$ and $\mathbf{v}_2$, and the vector $\mathbf{x}$, which will be transformed to $\Sigma^{-1/2}\mathbf{x}$.

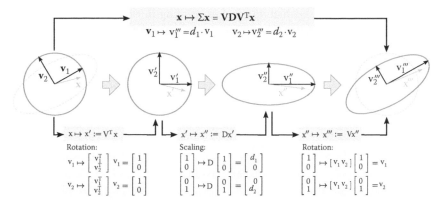

**FIGURE 18.12**   Illustration of whitening. The transformation performed by the multiplication with the inverse square root of the covariance matrix is called whitening. It maps the space such that a Gaussian distribution with the given covariance matrix becomes a standard normal distribution, that is, the variance in all directions is 1. This transformation maps the ellipsoid given by the standard isodensity line of the Gaussian distribution to the unit sphere. The three-step process illustrated here is kind of the inverse way of Figure 18.11. But as we took the square root of the covariance matrix here, the scaling relates to the square root of the eigenvalues.

As before, the first transformation rotates the principal axes of the ellipsoid to the coordinate axes. In the second step, the multiplication with the diagonal matrix $\mathbf{D}^{-1/2}$ scales along the coordinate axes with the factors $1/\sqrt{d_1}$ for the horizontal and $1/\sqrt{d_2}$ for the vertical axis. Since $\sqrt{d_1}$ and $\sqrt{d_2}$ are the radii of the ellipsoid, this step transforms the ellipsoid into a unit circle. The final transformation step is the inverse of the first one; that is, it rotates the coordinate axes back into the directions of the original eigenvectors. Viewing the total transformation, the original space is squeezed (or extended) along the principal axes such that the ellipsoid defined by $\Sigma$ becomes a unit sphere.

Applying this transformation to a whole set of samples (i.e., multiplying all samples with $\Sigma^{-1/2}$, where $\Sigma$ is the sample covariance matrix) is called whitening. In the whitened samples, variance in all directions is 1; that is, the sample covariance matrix is the identity matrix.

### 18.5.4   RELATION OF LDA TO NCC, WHITENING, AND MAHALANOBIS DISTANCE

Writing the essential term of Equation 18.3 slightly differently as $(\Sigma^{-1/2}\mathbf{x})^{\top}\Sigma^{-1/2}(\mu_2 - \mu_1)$, we can see that the general case given (nonspherical) covariance matrices can be reduced to our simple example above. The multiplication with $\Sigma^{-1/2}$ is a whitening (see Section 18.5.3), which transforms the space into a new coordinate system in which the distribution has variance 1 in all directions. In other words, in the transformed space, the classes have spherical distributions. In the transformed spaces, an observation $\mathbf{x}$ (which is $\Sigma^{-1/2}\mathbf{x}$ there) is assigned to that class $c$ whose transformed mean $\Sigma^{-1/2}\mu_c$ is closer to $\mathbf{x}$ (see Figure 18.9c). Taking this view, LDA classification is equivalent to NCC (introduced in Section 18.5.1) in the space that is whitened with respect to the common covariance matrix.

For the reader familiar with the Mahalanobis distance (Mahalanobis 1936), we remark that this can be rephrased as LDA being equivalent to using Mahalanobis metric (corresponding to the common covariance matrix) in calculating the distance to the centroids in the NCC.

### 18.5.5   REMARK ON THE ASSUMPTIONS OF LDA

Here, we discuss the assumptions underlying the optimality criterion of LDA (see Section 18.5.2). It is clear that such ideal conditions are never met in practice, but the better the fit, the better performance can be expected. Therefore, a good understanding of this issue might help in tuning feature extraction procedures for good classifiability and in deciding in which situations it is worthwhile to try nonlinear classification methods.

LDA is derived by minimizing the risk of misclassification based on the following three assumptions (see Section 18.5.2):

- Classes obey Gaussian distributions.
- The covariance matrices of all classes are equal.
- The parameters (mean, covariance) of true class distributions are known.

Obviously, these assumptions impose severe constraints on the applicability (or the power) of LDA. There are many sophisticated nonlinear classification methods that allow much more flexibility in the assumed distributions. However, it turned out that in the single-trial classification of brain signals, linear classification is widely successful. One basic argument may be that linear classification is more robust than nonlinear classification, which is a big advantage in case of strong background noise and a relatively low number of samples, which is the typical scenario in BCI. (Classifiers that allow more complex separations require more parameters, and the estimation of those parameters may suffer from overfitting to noise, or be hampered by outliers.) For the classification of single-trial EEG data, it turned out that the features often fulfill the assumptions of LDA about the distributions quite well (ERPs), or that the features can be transformed to accomplish them (e.g., by taking the logarithm of band-power features; see Section 18.6.3). Here, we discuss the case of ERP features. For a more detailed examination and code of practice to visually investigate the distributions, see Ref. (Blankertz et al. 2011).

In ERP data, the (simplified) assumption is that the underlying ERP component is constant in every trial; that is, the signals of each trial $i$ can be formalized as

$$\mathbf{x}_i(t) = \mathbf{p}(t) + \mathbf{n}_i(t), \qquad (18.5)$$

where $\mathbf{p}(t)$ is the ERP (phase-locked activity) and $\mathbf{n}_i(t)$ is the noise term that models (non–task-related) background activity (non–phase-locked). The noise is assumed to be independent in each trial $i$ and Gaussian distributed according to $\mathcal{N}(0, \Sigma)$. Given a specific time point $t_0$, the distribution of $\langle \mathbf{x}_i(t_0) \rangle_i$ for all trials is Gaussian with $\mathcal{N}(\mu, \Sigma)$. Here, $\mu$ is the average of $\mathbf{x}_i(t_0)$ across all trials, which is $\mathbf{p}(t_0)$, that is, the amplitude of the ERP component in all channels at time $t$ (see Figure 18.6). Furthermore, the covariance matrix of $\mathbf{x}_i(t)$ is the covariance of the noise $\mathbf{n}_i$, which corresponds to the dispersion of the background activity.

Modeling the non–phase-locked activity in ERP data as Gaussians fits reasonably well with our experience. The assumption implicit in Equation 18.5 that the ERP is the same in every trial is a simplification. There are trial-to-trial variations in amplitude and latency, for example, related to attention, vigilance, and so on, but in most experimental settings, they can be assumed to be negligible in comparison to the background activity.

The assumption of equal covariance matrices boils down to the question whether the background activity is the same in both conditions. This question cannot be answered in general, because it depends on the experimental paradigm. While the experimental design is typically such that the background activity is the same in all conditions, this is not necessarily the case. If ERP responses to tones are compared under the two conditions eyes open and eyes closed, there is a much stronger visual alpha rhythm in the eyes closed condition that would dominate the ongoing activity. This example is not a typical paradigm, in particular not for BCI research, but it should make clear what kind of considerations are indicated when choosing a classification method. Blankertz et al. (2011) proposes a method for verifying the assumption of equal covariance matrices in a given data set by visualization using a principal component analysis.

However, most condition-specific components are phase-locked to the stimulus and are therefore captured in the mean of distributions and not in the covariance matrix. Last but not least, LDA is not overly sensitive with respect to differences in the covariance matrices and may even in that case still outperform more complex methods that estimate the covariance matrices individually for each class.

Concerning the third assumption that class distributions are known, see Section 18.5.6.

### 18.5.6    LDA WITH SHRINKAGE OF THE COVARIANCE MATRIX

The discussion of the third requirement for the optimality criterion of LDA was left open in Section 18.5.5. It is the assumption that the true distributions are known, which is, in real applications, of course, never the case. Accordingly, for applying LDA, empirical estimates of the distribution parameters (obtained from some calibration data) are taken as approximation. This works well if the number of training samples is high compared to the dimensionality of the samples. (Unfortunately, this statement cannot easily be made more precise, because the required ratio depends also on the data, not only on the number of samples and dimensions.) Otherwise, the approximation of the true covariance matrix by the empirical estimate is imprecise, and classification with LDA can break down completely (overfitting).

Luckily, the estimation error in the empirical covariance matrix $\hat{\Sigma}$ typically has a systematic bias, and there is a method for counteracting. The so-called shrinkage (Friedman 1989; Stein 1956) is a linear morphing (by parameter $\gamma$ in [0, 1]) between $\Sigma$ ($\gamma = 0$: LDA) and a matrix representing a spherical distribution ($\gamma = 1$: NCC). Selecting the shrinkage parameter used to be somewhat cumbersome and time consuming, until recently an analytical formula for the optimal $\gamma^*$ has been found (Ledoit and Wolf 2004; Schäfer and Strimmer 2005; Vidaurre et al. 2009). It results from minimizing the difference between the (unknown) true covariance matrix and $\tilde{\Sigma}(\gamma)$. While this does not necessarily imply optimality for classification, the choice was empirically found to be a good one; that is, for the optimal shrinkage parameter $\gamma^*$, the shrunk covariance matrix $\tilde{\Sigma}(\gamma^*)$ provides classification competitive with the result of an exhaustive search for the best $\gamma$ with cross-validation. The formula for $\gamma^*$ is comparably simple and easy to implement. It is based on the sample-to-sample variations of the correlation coefficient. Figure 18.13 illustrates linear classification with shrinkage.

Note that the choice of the shrinkage parameter $\gamma$ reflects the belief in the estimation of the noise. If the training set is large enough for a reliable estimation of the noise, one should make full use of it ($\gamma = 0$: LDA). In the other extreme, if the estimation of the noise is so unreliable that the information cannot be used at all without risking overfitting, classification is based on the distribution means only, leading to NCC ($\gamma = 1$: NCC), as discussed in Section 18.5.1.

The first application of the automatic parameter selection for Shrinkage-LDA to BCI data was reported in Ref. (Vidaurre et al. 2009). A more detailed presentation of Shrinkage-LDA is given elsewhere (Blankertz et al. 2011).

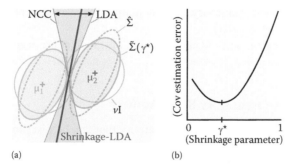

(a)                                                    (b)

**FIGURE 18.13**    Classification with shrinkage of the covariance matrix. Shrinkage of the estimated covariance is used to counteract the estimation bias in small sample settings. (a) The distributions of two classes are illustrated with difference covariance matrices. Dashed lines correspond to the empirical covariance matrix while the gray circles correspond to a spherical covariance matrix. The solid colored ellipsoids are obtained from shrinkage with the optimal shrinkage parameter $\gamma^*$. (b) For classification, the parameter with the minimum expected error is desired.

### 18.5.7 Other Classification Methods

For a more advanced and highly promising classification method in BCI context, see Refs. (Barachant et al. 2013; Congedo et al. 2013, 2015). A very good overview is given in Ref. (Lotte et al. 2007). Concerning nonlinear classifiers and a discussion of linear versus nonlinear methods, see Ref. (Müller et al. 2003) and the introduction to the methods in Ref. (Lemm et al. 2011), as well as the references therein.

## 18.6 FEATURE EXTRACTION

There are many different ways to process and classify brain signals (Dornhege et al. 2007; Lotte et al. 2007; McFarland et al. 2006). Which methods are good candidates for given data depend on which types of components of brain activity are discriminative for the task at hand. Although a lot of experience is required for choosing (presumably) optimal methods and tuning their parameters, some basic guidelines can be given. After that, we review some popular feature extraction methods that are validated by being used in several online BCI systems and being the basis for many methods that did well in the BCI competitions (Blankertz et al. 2004, 2006c).

### 18.6.1 Guideline for Transient Activity: ERP and LRP

Transient components like ERPs and the (lateralized) readiness potential (RP, LRP; see Refs. Kornhuber and Deecke 1965; Schultze-Kraft et al. 2016) are phase-locked modulations of the electrical brain potentials. If two conditions are different with respect to such components, the corresponding sample distributions have different means (see Section 18.4.1). Such data can, in principle, directly be fed into a classifier. As the arguments in Section 18.5.5 apply to all kinds of transient activity, employing LDA can be assumed to yield good results.

Even if it is possible to feed the raw single trials of EEG data into a classifier, it is advisable to do some preprocessing of the data in order to reduce the dimensionality. But this is a trade-off that is subject to experience. In principle, if a huge amount of training samples was available, applying a classifier to the raw data would be optimal (with respect to classification performance, computational load would be a different issue). But this is not the case in BCI applications, and extraction of lower-dimensional features improves classification performance. Since the transient activity resides in relatively low frequencies, a common strategy for dimensional reduction in this type of data is subsampling in time. This can be done for a fixed subsampling frequency (Krusienski et al. 2008) or by selecting discriminative time intervals of ERP components in which the difference pattern between the two conditions is stationary and calculating the average within those subject-specific time intervals (Blankertz et al. 2011).

A tutorial on feature extraction and classification of transient brain activity is provided in Ref. (Blankertz et al. 2011).

### 18.6.2 Guideline for Oscillatory Brain Activity

There are several features of oscillatory brain activity that can be discriminative for specific mental states. Note that oscillatory brain activity ideally has zero mean. Accordingly in this case, the means of the respective distributions of raw data are not separated, implying that linear classification applied to raw data would not be successful. In principle, a general nonlinear classifier could be applied to the raw data, but this has rarely been reported to yield competitive results (but see Refs. Congedo et al. 2017; Tomioka and Müller 2010). Rather, the predominantly reported experience is that it is most effective to apply (nonlinear) preprocessing to the data, to obtain features that can be linearly separated (Müller et al. 2003).

In the BCI context, the most commonly exploited neurophysiological feature of oscillatory brain activity is the amplitude modulation of brain rhythms (event-related desynchronization [ERD] and event-related synchronization [ERS] Pfurtscheller and Lopes da Silva 1999). Brain rhythms are oscillations of a certain frequency (or in a narrow frequency band) generated in a certain area of the brain. The amplitude of a brain rhythm can be quantified as band-power, determined, for example, by Fourier analysis or by calculating the variance of band-pass–filtered signals (strictly speaking, the amplitude is the square root of band-power). Because of volume conduction, calculating such features from raw channels often leads to an unfavorable signal-to-noise ratio. Therefore, it is advisable to apply spatial filters (corresponding to the sources that generate the rhythms). Apart from fixed filters like common average reference and Laplacians (McFarland et al. 1997), data-driven methods can be used to optimize spatial filters toward given properties. For discriminating motor imagery conditions, the CSP analysis is widely used (see Section 18.6.3).

In contrast to those internally initiated modulations, in the case of externally induced oscillations, for example, the SSVEPs elicited by periodic visual stimulation, the exact frequency of the oscillatory signals is known. This opens up the floor for methods that explicitly exploit this additional information, like canonical correlation analysis (CCA) (see Section 18.6.4).

### 18.6.3   Feature Extraction: CSP Analysis

The CSP technique (Fukunaga 1990; Koles 1991) allows one to determine spatial filters that maximize the variance of signals of one condition and at the same time minimize the variance of signals of another condition. Since variance of band-pass–filtered signals is equal to band-power, CSP filters are well suited to detect amplitude modulations of sensorimotor rhythms and consequently to discriminate mental states that are characterized by ERD/ERS effects. As such, it has been well used online in BCI systems (Blankertz et al. 2008a; Ramoser et al. 2000) where CSP filters are calculated individually for each participant on initially recorded calibration data. Note that, unlike unsupervised decomposition techniques like PCA and ICA, CSP makes explicit use of the label information to optimize the discriminative aspect of oscillatory processes. It is of paramount importance to take this into account in the validation of CSP-based classification procedures (see Figure 18.14). For example, when performing cross-validation, the CSP filters have to be determined within the cross-validation, on the respective training data only, and then applied to the test data (see Ref. Lemm et al. 2011).

CSP analysis decomposes multichannel EEG signals in the sensor space. The number of spatial filters that are obtained equals the number of channels of the original data. The CSP filter

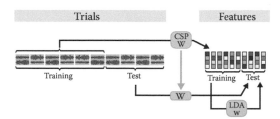

**FIGURE 18.14**   Validation of a classification on features that are based on CSP analysis. Cross-validation is commonly used to estimate the performance of classifiers. When the feature extraction is data dependent, like the optimization of spatial filters with CSP, the feature extraction process also has to be taken into account into the validation procedure. It would be invalid to determine CSP features on a whole data set and to perform cross-validation only for the classification. In contrast, for a correct validation, trials are split into training and test data, and model parameters of the feature extraction (like the weights of CSP filters) and of the classifier are estimated on training data only and transferred to extract features of test data and to classify them. For cross-validation, this whole process has to be done within the loop of cross-validation.

matrix can be calculated in one step as the solution of the following generalized Eigenvalue problem (Blankertz et al. 2008b):

$$\mathbf{W}^\top \Sigma_1 \mathbf{W} = \mathbf{D} \text{ and } \mathbf{W}^\top \left(\Sigma_1 + \Sigma_2\right) \mathbf{W} = \mathbf{I}. \tag{18.6}$$

The CSP filters are the columns of $\mathbf{W}$. Before we investigate the properties of the CSP filters mathematically, we illustrate the process. It can be better understood when it is broken down into two steps. First, the data are whitened (see Section 18.5.3) with respect to the covariance sum $\Sigma_1 + \Sigma_2$ (which is equal to the pooled covariance matrix, if $\mathbf{X}_1$ and $\mathbf{X}_2$ have the same number to time points). Then, a rotation is performed that aligns the principal axes of the individual covariance matrices with the coordinate axes. This procedure is illustrated with two-dimensional data in Figure 18.15. The mathematics describing those two transforms are shown in Section 18.7.

To show the effect of CSP mathematically, let $\mathbf{X}_1$ and $\mathbf{X}_2$ be data matrices of band-pass–filtered signals from two conditions. The dimensionality of those matrices is number of channels times number of time points. In the time dimension, they may be concatenated from all available trials. We define $\Sigma_i = 1 T_i \mathbf{X}_i \mathbf{X}_i^\top$ to be the class conditional covariance matrices (with $T_i$ being the number of samples in $\mathbf{X}_i$). Since the signals are band-pass filtered, we may assume that the mean across time is zero. Furthermore, let $\mathbf{w}_i$ denote the columns of $\mathbf{W}$, that is, the CSP filters, and $d_i$ indicate the elements of the diagonal matrix $\mathbf{D}$. The dimensionality of the CSP filters $\mathbf{w}_i$ is the number of channels. These spatial filters are applied to data matrices by multiplication: $\mathbf{w}_i^\top \mathbf{X}$. This maps the multichannel time series $\mathbf{X}$ to one single time series. The effect of CSP can be readily shown using the first identity of Equation 18.6

$$\text{var}\left(\mathbf{w}_i^\top \mathbf{X}_1\right) = \frac{1}{T_i} \mathbf{w}_i^\top \mathbf{X}_1 \left(\mathbf{w}_i^\top \mathbf{X}_1\right)^\top = \frac{1}{T_i} \mathbf{w}_i^\top \mathbf{X}_1 \mathbf{X}_1^\top \mathbf{w}_i = \mathbf{w}_i^\top \Sigma \mathbf{w}_i = d_i$$

and analog, but also using the second identity of Equation 18.6, it follows that

$$\text{var}\left(\mathbf{w}_i^\top \mathbf{X}_2\right) = 1 - d_i.$$

Accordingly, the variances of both signals, after applying the spatial filter $\mathbf{w}_i$, have values between 0 and 1 and sum up to 1. Furthermore, also the generalized eigenvalues $d_i$ are between 0 and 1. Now comes the clue. By choosing a spatial filter $\mathbf{w}_i$ that corresponds to a large $d_i$, that is, a value near 1, we know the following property concerning a signal that has been filtered with $\mathbf{w}_i$: a large variance (near 1) indicates that the signal belongs to class 1, and a small variance (near 0) indicates that the

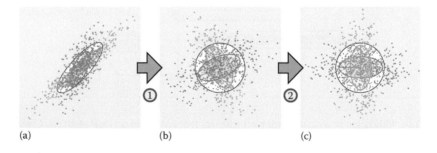

(a)                              (b)                              (c)

**FIGURE 18.15** Essential steps of CSP analysis. The blue and orange ellipsoids refer to the two-class conditional covariance matrices along with the principal axes, while the covariance sum is depicted in white. (a) Original data distributions. (b) Data distributions after whitening with respect to the covariance sum (white distribution becomes unit shpere). (c) After a final rotation, the variance along the horizontal direction is maximal for the orange class, while it is minimal for the blue class and vice versa along the vertical direction.

signal belongs to class 2. For example, an eigenvalue of 0.9 for class 1 means an average ratio of 9:1 of variances during conditions 1 and 2. For spatial filters with a small $d_i$, the opposite is true. That means, if "extreme" generalized eigenvalues (near 0 or near 1) in Equation 18.6 are obtained, the classification problem is more or less solved. The variance of the filtered test signal reveals to which class it belongs.

If both conditions do not differ with respect to the spatial distribution of band-power, all $d_i$ values will be approximately 0.5, and no discriminative spatial filter can be determined.

In a typical application, only few filters will be discriminative, while the rest corresponds to eigenvalues near 0.5.

Note that while CSP filters *can* be visualized as scalp maps, their interpretation is problematic (which is generally the case with spatial filters). Rather, such filters should be transformed into the corresponding spatial patterns that are suitable for neurophysiological interpretation (see Ref. Haufe et al. 2014).

Endowed with the technique of CSP analysis, we can describe the whole process of a CSP-based BCI (taking the case of continuous control in the application). This process is depicted as a flowchart in Figure 18.16.

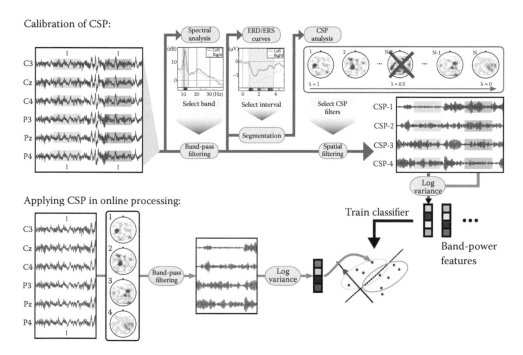

**FIGURE 18.16** Flowchart of CSP analysis and application. (*Calibration*) CSP analysis is used to optimize spatial filters based on calibration data. Input signals have periods that belong to two experimental conditions that are characterized by differently modulated brain rhythms (here "left" and "right" hand motor imagery, coded by blue and orange color). Segments of both conditions are subjected to a spectral analysis in order to find a frequency band that best shows the difference in band-power between the two conditions. Furthermore, the time interval that shows the most pronounced difference between the conditions is selected. The concatenated segments (epochs) of band-pass–filtered brain signals for the two conditions are the input to the CSP analysis. The result is a sequence of spatial filters (generalized eigenvectors) and corresponding eigenvalues. Based on those eigenvalues (or alternative measures), suitable filters for the discrimination task are selected. Those filters are applied to the continuous, band-pass–filtered signals. Finally, features such as log variance are calculated and used to train a classifier. (*Application*) After the calibration, incoming signals can be classified in a straightforward way. First, the CSP filters are applied and the resulting signals are band-pass filtered. From these segments, features are calculated and fed into the classifier. This process can be applied continuously, at each step taking the most recent, say 750 ms of data; see text for details.

**Calibration:** The complete training process for CSP-based classification includes the following steps: Selection of a frequency band and a time interval that best show the difference between the two conditions. Then, the input signals are band-pass filtered to the selected frequency band and epochs according to the selected time interval are extracted from the continuous signals and concatenated. This results in the data matrices $\mathbf{X}_1$ and $\mathbf{X}_2$ that are fed into the CSP analysis. Discriminative CSP filters are selected based on their eigenvalues (as discussed above) and stored. Those spatial filters are applied to the band-pass–filtered epochs and the log variance is calculated within each epoch. This results in a feature vector, whose dimensionality coincides with the number of selected filters. Finally, an LDA classifier is trained on the set of feature vectors. Because of the low dimensionality, shrinkage is typically not required, but may help in cases of scarce calibration data.

**Application:** The most recently acquired signals are spatially filtered by applying the chosen CSP filters and then band-pass filtered. Calculating the log variance within time intervals of a certain length (see remark below) results in the feature vector that is fed to the LDA classifier. This gives the output signal that is transmitted to the feedback application, for example, cursor control (Blankertz et al. 2007; Guger et al. 2000).

**Remark:** The (expected value of the) variance of a stationary signal is independent of its length. Hence, the length of the segment from which the feedback signal is calculated can be changed. The value has an impact on the dynamics of the output control signal. A short length (like 250 ms) gives a responsive but more turbulent control. A long one (like 1000 ms) results in smooth control at the cost of higher inertia.

An interesting aspect about CSP is that this technique can also be applied for optimizing spatial filters absent of any discrimination task. For example, CSP can be used to enhance the signal-to-noise ratio in (single-condition) event-related modulations of brain rhythms by optimizing the contrast between pre- and post-stimulus band-power (see Ref. Blankertz et al. 2008b). More recently, a CSP-based method called spatio-spectral decomposition (SSD) was published (Nikulin et al. 2011). SSD allows the extraction of components that have maximal band-power at a specified frequency, while minimizing the power at surrounding frequencies.

For details about the technique of CSP analysis and its extensions, we refer to Refs. (Ang et al. 2009; Blankertz et al. 2008b; Grosse-Wentrup et al. 2009; Lemm et al. 2005; Lotte and Guan 2011).

### 18.6.4 Feature Extraction: CCA

When the target signals are sinusoidal signals (possibly with harmonics) of different frequencies, and additionally the phase of the oscillations is the same in each epoch, a good alternative to CSP is the CCA. This method is very successfully applied to SSVEP-based BCIs, where that premise is fulfilled (Bin et al. 2008, 2009; Yan et al. 2009). More recent techniques exploit the possibility to differentiate neural responses to SSVEP stimulation based on the phase differences (additional to frequency) (see Refs. Chen et al. 2015; Jia et al. 2011).

## 18.7 APPENDIX: FORMALIZATION OF CSP AS A TWO-STEP PROCEDURE

Effectively, the filters provided by the CSP analysis $\mathbf{W}$ are determined by a generalized EVDs of the matrices $\Sigma_1$ and $\Sigma_1 + \Sigma_2$. Mainly for illustration purposes, the CSP transformation matrix $\mathbf{W}$ can be decomposed in two steps: first, a whitening with respect to $\Sigma_1 + \Sigma_2$, and then a rotation of the principal components of $\Sigma_1$ and (at the same time) $\Sigma_2$ onto the coordinate axes (see Figure 18.15). Here is the corresponding math:

Let (the columns of) $\mathbf{X}_1$ and $\mathbf{X}_2$ be the samples of the two classes. Assuming zero mean for samples $\mathbf{X}_1$ and $\mathbf{X}_2$, the covariance matrices are given by $\Sigma_{\mathbf{X}_1} = \dfrac{1}{T_1 - 1} \mathbf{X}_1 \mathbf{X}_1^\top$ and $\Sigma_{\mathbf{X}_2} = \dfrac{1}{T_2 - 1} \mathbf{X}_2 \mathbf{X}_2^\top$.

Taking the EVD of $\Sigma_{X_1} + \Sigma_{X_2} = \mathbf{V}\Lambda\mathbf{V}^\top$ with $\mathbf{V}\mathbf{V}^\top = \mathbf{I}$ and diagonal $\Lambda = \text{diag}(\lambda_1,\ldots,\lambda_k)$, we define $\mathbf{P} = \mathbf{V}\Lambda^{-\frac{1}{2}}\mathbf{V}^\top$.

1. The transformation ① from the original space to the whitened space is $\mathbf{z} \mapsto \mathbf{P}^\top \mathbf{z}$. For the projected distributions, we obtain $(I = 1,2)$

$$\Sigma_{\mathbf{P}^\top \mathbf{X}_I} = \mathbf{P}^\top \Sigma_{\mathbf{X}_I} \mathbf{P}. \tag{18.7}$$

2. We define the transform ② by diagonalizing the distribution $\mathbf{P}^\top \mathbf{X}_1$, that is, a rotation that maps the eigenvectors of $\Sigma_{\mathbf{P}^\top \mathbf{X}_1}$ on the coordinate axes. We take the EVD of $\Sigma_{\mathbf{P}^\top \mathbf{X}_1} = \mathbf{R}\mathbf{D}\mathbf{R}^\top$ with $\mathbf{R}\mathbf{R}^\top = \mathbf{I}$ and diagonal $\mathbf{D}$. The transformation is then given by $\mathbf{z} \mapsto \mathbf{R}^\top \mathbf{z}$ and has the desired property:

$$\Sigma_{\mathbf{P}^\top \mathbf{X}_1} \mapsto \Sigma_{\mathbf{R}^\top \mathbf{P}^\top \mathbf{X}_1} = \mathbf{R}^\top \Sigma_{\mathbf{P}^\top \mathbf{X}_1} \mathbf{R} = \mathbf{D}. \tag{18.8}$$

This shows that the transform does the right thing for the first distribution $\mathbf{P}^\top \mathbf{X}_1$. We have to check that it also diagonalizes the second distribution, that is, maps the eigenvectors of $\Sigma_{\mathbf{P}^\top \mathbf{X}_2}$ to the coordinate axes.

Since $\mathbf{P}$ is the whitening for $\Sigma_1 + \Sigma_2$, we obtain

$$\mathbf{P}^\top \Sigma_{\mathbf{X}_2} \mathbf{P} = \mathbf{I} - \mathbf{P}^\top \Sigma_{\mathbf{X}_1} \mathbf{P}. \tag{18.9}$$

Using this identity, we find the transform of the second distribution as

$$
\begin{aligned}
\Sigma_{\mathbf{P}^\top \mathbf{X}_2} &\to \mathbf{R}^\top \Sigma_{\mathbf{P}^\top \mathbf{X}_2} \mathbf{R} \\
&= \mathbf{R}^\top \mathbf{P}^\top \Sigma_{\mathbf{X}_2} \mathbf{P}\mathbf{R} \\
&\overset{(18.9)}{=} \mathbf{R}^\top (\mathbf{I} - \mathbf{P}^\top \Sigma_{\mathbf{X}_1} \mathbf{P})\mathbf{R} \\
&= \mathbf{R}^\top \mathbf{I}\mathbf{R} - \mathbf{R}^\top \mathbf{P}^\top \Sigma_{\mathbf{X}_1} \mathbf{P}\mathbf{R} \\
&\overset{(18.8)}{=} \mathbf{I} - \mathbf{D}
\end{aligned} \tag{18.10}
$$

Since $\mathbf{I}-\mathbf{D}$ is a diagonal matrix, this proves that the second distribution is also diagonalized by the defined transform. Moreover, it shows that the eigenvalues of the transformed distributions for $\Sigma_1$ and $\Sigma_2$ sum up to 1. If one distribution has high variance along one axis (transformed eigenvalue $d_i \approx 1$), the other distribution has low variance along that axis (transformed eigenvalue $1 - d_i \approx 0$).

## REFERENCES

Ang, K. K., Chin, Z. Y., Zhang, H., and Guan, C. Robust filter bank common spatial pattern (RFBCSP) in motor-imagery-based brain–computer interface. *Conf Proc IEEE Eng Med Biol Soc*, 2009:578–581, 2009.

Barachant, A., Bonnet, S., Congedo, M., and Jutten, C. Classification of covariance matrices using a riemannian-based kernel for BCI applications. *Neurocomputing*, 112:172–178, 2013.

Diu, G., Gao, X., Yan, Z., Hong, B., and Gao, S. An online multi-channel SSVEP-based brain–computer interface using a canonical correlation analysis method. *J Neural Eng*, 6:046002, Aug 2009.

Bin, G., Lin, Z., Gao, X., Hong, B., and Gao, S. The SSVEP topographic scalp maps by canonical correlation analysis. *Conf Proc IEEE Eng Med Biol Soc*, 2008:3759–3762, 2008.

Bishop, C. M. *Pattern Recognition and Machine Learning*. Springer, 2006.

Blankertz, B., Dornhege, G., Krauledat, M., Müller, K.-R., and Curio, G. The non-invasive Berlin Brain–Computer Interface: Fast acquisition of effective performance in untrained subjects. *NeuroImage*, 37(2):539–550, 2007.

Blankertz, B., Dornhege, G., Krauledat, M., Müller, K.-R., Kunzmann, V., Losch, F., and Curio, G. The Berlin Brain–Computer Interface: EEG-based communication without subject training. *IEEE Trans Neural Syst Rehabil Eng*, 14(2):147–152, 2006a.

Blankertz, B., Dornhege, G., Lemm, S., Krauledat, M., Curio, G., and Müller, K.-R. The Berlin Brain–Computer Interface: Machine learning based detection of user specific brain states. *J Universal Computer Sci*, 12(6):581–607, 2006b.

Blankertz, B., Lemm, S., Treder, M. S., Haufe, S., and Müller, K.-R. Single-trial analysis and classification of ERP components—A tutorial. *NeuroImage*, 56:814–825, 2011.

Blankertz, B., Losch, F., Krauledat, M., Dornhege, G., Curio, G., and Müller, K.-R. The Berlin Brain–Computer Interface: Accurate performance from first-session in BCI-naive subjects. *IEEE Trans Biomed Eng*, 55(10):2452–2462, 2008a.

Blankertz, B., Müller, K.-R., Curio, G., Vaughan, T. M., Schalk, G., Wolpaw, J. R., Schlögl, A., Neuper, C., Pfurtscheller, G., Hinterberger, T., Schröder, M., and Birbaumer, N. The BCI competition 2003: Progress and perspectives in detection and discrimination of EEG single trials. *IEEE Trans Biomed Eng*, 51(6):1044–1051, 2004.

Blankertz, B., Müller, K.-R., Krusienski, D., Schalk, G., Wolpaw, J. R., Schlögl, A., Pfurtscheller, G., Millán, J. del R., Schröder, M., and Birbaumer, N. The BCI competition III: Validating alternative approaches to actual BCI problems. *IEEE Trans Neural Syst Rehabil Eng*, 14(2):153–159, 2006c.

Blankertz, B., Tomioka, R., Lemm, S., Kawanabe, M., and Müller, K.-R. Optimizing spatial filters for robust EEG single-trial analysis. *IEEE Signal Process Mag*, 25(1):41–56, 2008b.

Burgess, A. P., and Gruzelier, J. H. The reliability of event-related desynchronisation: A generalisability study analysis. *Int J Psychophysiol*, 23(3):163–169, 1996.

Chen, X., Wang, Y., Nakanishi, M., Gao, X., Jung, T.-P., and Gao, S. High-speed spelling with a noninvasive brain–computer interface. *Proc Natl Acad Sci U S A*, 112(44):E6058–E6067, 2015.

Congedo, M., Afsari, B., Barachant, A., and Moakher, M. Approximate joint diagonalization and geometric mean of symmetric positive definite matrices. *PLoS ONE*, 10(4):1–25, 04 2015.

Congedo, M., Barachant, A., and Andreev, A. A new generation of brain–computer interface based on riemannian geometry. *arXiv preprint arXiv:1310.8115*, 2013.

Congedo, M., Barachant, A., and Bhatia, R. Riemannian geometry for eeg-based brain–computer interfaces; a primer and a review. *Brain–Computer Interfaces*, 1–20, 2017.

Dornhege, G., Millán, J. del R., Hinterberger, T., McFarland, D., and Müller, K.-R. editors. *Toward Brain–Computer Interfacing*. MIT Press, Cambridge, MA, 2007.

Duda, R. O., Hart, P. E., and Stork, D. G. *Pattern Classification*. Wiley & Sons, 2nd edition, 2001.

Elbert, T., Rockstroh, B., Lutzenberger, W., and Birbaumer, N. Biofeedback of slow cortical potentials. I. *Electroencephalogr Clin Neurophysiol*, 48:293–301, 1980.

Farwell, L. A., and Donchin, E. Talking off the top of your head: Toward a mental prosthesis utilizing event-related brain potentials. *Electroencephalogr Clin Neurophysiol*, 70:510–523, 1988.

Friedman, J. H. Regularized discriminant analysis. *J Amer Statist Assoc*, 84(405):165–175, 1989.

Fukunaga, K. *Introduction to Statistical Pattern Recognition*. Academic Press, Boston, 2nd edition, 1990.

Grosse-Wentrup, M., Liefhold, C., Gramann, K., and Buss, M. Beamforming in noninvasive brain–computer interfaces. *IEEE Trans Biomed Eng*, 56:1209–1219, Apr 2009.

Guger, C., Ramoser, H., and Pfurtscheller, G. Real-time EEG analysis with subject-specific spatial patterns for a brain computer interface (BCI). *IEEE Trans Neural Syst Rehabil Eng*, 8(4):447–456, 2000.

Hastie, T., Tibshirani, R., and Friedman, J. *The Elements of Statistical Learning*. Springer, 2008.

Haufe, S., Meinecke, F., Görgen, K., Dähne, S., Haynes, J.-D., Blankertz, B., and Bießmann, F. On the interpretation of weight vectors of linear models in multivariate neuroimaging. *NeuroImage*, 87:96–110, 2014. Neuroimage single best paper of 2014 Award.

Hong, B., Guo, F., Liu, T., Gao, X., and Gao, S. N200-speller using motion-onset visual response. *Clin Neurophysiol*, 120:1658–1666, Sep 2009.

Jia, C., Gao, X., Hong, B., and Gao, S. Frequency and phase mixed coding in SSVEP-based brain–computer interface. *IEEE Trans Biomed Eng*, 58:200–206, Jan 2011.

Kalcher, J., and Pfurtscheller, G. Discrimination between phase-locked and non-phase-locked eventrelated EEG activity. *Electroencephalogr Clin Neurophysiol*, 94:381–384, 1995.

Key, A. P., Dove, G. O., and Maguire, M. J. Linking brainwaves to the brain: An ERP primer. *Dev Neuropsychol*, 27:183–215, 2005.

Klem, G. H., Lüders, H. O., Jasper, H. H., Elger, C. et al. The ten–twenty electrode system of the international federation. *Electroencephalogr Clin Neurophysiol*, 52(3):3–6, 1999.

Koles, Z. J. The quantitative extraction and topographic mapping of the abnormal components in the clinical EEG. *Electroencephalogr Clin Neurophysiol*, 79(6):440–447, 1991.

Kornhuber, H. H., and Deecke, L. Hirnpotentialänderungen bei Willkürbewegungen und passive Bewegungen des Menschen: Bereitschaftspotential und reafferente Potentiale. *Pflugers Arch*, 284:1–17, 1965.

Krusienski, D. J., Sellers, E. W., Cabestaing, F., Bayoudh, S., McFarland, D. J., Vaughan, T. M., and Wolpaw, J. R. A comparison of classification techniques for the P300 speller. *J Neural Eng*, 3(4):299–305, Dec 2006.

Krusienski, D. J., Sellers, E. W., McFarland, D. J., Vaughan, T. M., and Wolpaw, J. R. Toward enhanced P300 speller performance. *J Neurosci Methods*, 167:15–21, Jan 2008.

Ledoit, O., and Wolf, M. A well-conditioned estimator for large-dimensional covariance matrices. *J Multivar Anal*, 88:365–411, 2004.

Leeb, R., Perdikis, S., Tonin, L., Biasiucci, A., Tavella, M., Creatura, M., Molina, A., Al-Khodairy, A., Carlson, T., and Millán, J. del R. Transferring brain–computer interfaces beyond the laboratory: Successful application control for motor-disabled users. *Artificial Intelligence in Medicine*, 59(2):121–132, 2013.

Lemm, S., Blankertz, B., Curio, G., and Müller, K.-R. Spatio-spectral filters for improving classification of single trial EEG. *IEEE Trans Biomed Eng*, 52(9):1541–1548, 2005.

Lemm, S., Blankertz, B., Dickhaus, T., and Müller, K.-R. Introduction to machine learning for brain imaging. *NeuroImage*, 56:387–399, 2011.

Lin, Z., Zhang, C., Wu, W., and Gao, X. Frequency recognition based on canonical correlation analysis for SSVEP-based BCIs. *IEEE Trans Biomed Eng*, 53:2610–2614, Dec 2006.

Lotte, F., and Guan, C. Regularizing common spatial patterns to improve BCI designs: Unified theory and new algorithms. *IEEE Trans Biomed Eng*, 58:355–362, Feb 2011.

Lotte, F., Congedo, M., Lécuyer, A., Lamarche, F., and Arnaldi, B. A review of classification algorithms for EEG-based brain–computer interfaces. *J Neural Eng*, 4:R1–R13, Jun 2007.

Mahalanobis, P. C. On the generalised distance in statistics. *Proc Natl Inst Sci India*, 2:49–55, 1936.

McFarland, D. J., Anderson, C. W., Müller, K. R., Schlögl, A., and Krusienski, D. J. BCI Meeting 2005—Workshop on BCI signal processing: Feature extraction and translation. *IEEE Trans Neural Syst Rehabil Eng*, 14:135–138, Jun 2006.

McFarland, D. J., McCane, L. M., David, S. V., and Wolpaw, J. R. Spatial filter selection for EEG-based communication. *Electroencephalogr Clin Neurophysiol*, 103:386–394, 1997.

Müller, K.-R., Anderson, C. W., and Birch, G. E. Linear and non-linear methods for brain–computer interfaces. *IEEE Trans Neural Syst Rehabil Eng*, 11(2):165–169, 2003.

Nikulin, V. V., Linkenkaer-Hansen, K., Nolte, G., and Curio, G. Non-zero mean and asymmetry of neuronal oscillations have different implications for evoked responses. *Clin Neurophysiol*, 121(2):186–93, 2010.

Nikulin, V. V., Nolte, G., and Curio, G. A novel method for reliable and fast extraction of neuronal EEG/MEG oscillations on the basis of spatio-spectral decomposition. *NeuroImage*, 55:1528–1535, Apr 2011.

Pfurtscheller, G., and Lopes da Silva, F. H. Event-related EEG/MEG synchronization and desynchronization: Basic principles. *Clin Neurophysiol*, 110(11):1842–1857, Nov 1999.

Ramoser, H., Müller-Gerking, J., and Pfurtscheller, G. Optimal spatial filtering of single trial EEG during imagined hand movement. *IEEE Trans Rehabil Eng*, 8(4):441–446, 2000.

Sannelli, C., Vidaurre, C., Müller, K.-R., and Blankertz, B. Common spatial pattern patches: Online evaluation on naive users. In *Conf Proc IEEE Eng Med Biol Soc*, 2012, 2012.

Schäfer, J., and Strimmer, K. A shrinkage approach to large-scale covariance matrix estimation and implications for functional genomics. *Stat Appl Genet Mol Biol*, 4:Article32, 2005.

Schreuder, M., Blankertz, B., and Tangermann, M. A new auditory multi-class brain–computer interface paradigm: Spatial hearing as an informative cue. *PLoS ONE*, 5(4):e9813, 2010. Open Access.

Schultze-Kraft, M., Birman, D., Rusconi, M., Allefeld, C., Görgen, K., Dähne, S., Blankertz, B., and Haynes, J.-D. The point of no return in vetoing self-initiated movements. *Proc Natl Acad Sci U S A*, 113(4):1080–1085, 2016. Open Access.

Stein, C. Inadmissibility of the usual estimator for the mean of a multivariate normal distribution. In *Proc. 3rd Berkeley Sympos. Math. Statist. Probability*, 1:197–206, 1956.

Tomioka, R., and Müller, K. R. A regularized discriminative framework for EEG analysis with application to brain–computer interface. *NeuroImage*, 49:415–432, 2010.

Treder, M. S., and Blankertz, B. (C)overt attention and visual speller design in an ERP-based brain–computer interface. *Behav Brain Funct*, 6:28, May 2010. Open Access.

Treder, M. S., Bahramisharif, A., Schmidt, N. M., van Gerven, M., and Blankertz, B. Brain–computer interfacing using modulations of alpha activity induced by covert shifts of attention. *J Neuroeng Rehabil*, 8:24, 2011.

van der Heiden, L., Furdea, A., Matuz, T., Ruf, C., De Massari, D., Halder, S., Jaskowski, P., and Birbaumer, N. Conditioning of cortical responses to the trueness and falseness of word pairs: A new paradigm for basic communication by means of BCI. In *4th International BCI Meeting*, 2010.

Vanacker, G., Millán, J. del R., Lew, E., Ferrez, P. W., Moles, F. G., Philips, J., Van Brussel, H., and Nuttin, M. Context-based filtering for assisted brain-actuated wheelchair driving. *Computational Intelligence and Neuroscience*, 2007:3–3, 2007.

Vidaurre, C., Krämer, N., Blankertz, B., and Schlögl, A. Time domain parameters as a feature for EEGbased brain computer interfaces. *Neural Networks*, 22:1313–1319, 2009.

Vidaurre, C., Kawanabe, M., von Bünau, P., Blankertz, B., and Müller, K.-R. Toward unsupervised adaptation of LDA for brain–computer interfaces. *IEEE Trans Biomed Eng*, 58(3):587–597, 2011a.

Vidaurre, C., Sannelli, C., Müller, K.-R., and Blankertz, B. Co-adaptive calibration to improve BCI efficiency. *J Neural Eng*, 8(2):025009 (8 pp), 2011b.

Vidaurre, C., Sannelli, C., Müller, K.-R., and Blankertz, B. Machine-learning based co-adaptive calibration. *Neural Comput*, 23(3):791–816, 2011c.

Wald, P., and Kronmal, R. Discriminant functions when covariance are unequal and sample sizes are moderate. *Biometrics*, 33:479–484, 1977.

Wang, Y., Hong, B., Gao, X., and Gao, S. Implementation of a brain–computer interface based on three states of motor imagery. *Engineering in Medicine and Biology Society, 2007 EMBS 2007 29th Annual International Conference of the IEEE*, 14:234–240, Aug 2007.

Wenzel, M. A., Bogojeski, M., and Blankertz, B. Real-time inference of word relevance from electroencephalogram and eye gaze. *J Neural Eng*, 2017. Open Access.

Wolpaw, J. R., McFarland, D. J., Neat, G. W., and Forneris, C. A. An EEG-based brain–computer interface for cursor control. *Electroencephalogr Clin Neurophysiol*, 78:252–259, 1991.

Yan, Z., Gao, X., Bin, G., Hong, B., and Gao, S. A half-field stimulation pattern for SSVEP-based brain–computer interface. *Conf Proc IEEE Eng Med Biol Soc*, 2009:6461–6464, 2009.

# 19 Riemannian Classification for SSVEP-Based BCI

## Offline versus Online Implementations

*Sylvain Chevallier, Emmanuel K. Kalunga,*
*Quentin Barthélemy, and Florian Yger*

## CONTENTS

19.1 Introduction ...................................................................................................... 372
19.2 A Review of SSVEP-Based BCI ...................................................................... 373
    19.2.1 Steady-State Visually Evoked Potentials ............................................ 373
    19.2.2 Online and Offline Implementations for BCI ...................................... 373
19.3 Classifying SSVEP Signals .............................................................................. 374
    19.3.1 Notations .............................................................................................. 374
    19.3.2 Classification Using Canonical Correlation ........................................ 374
    19.3.3 Classification Using Riemannian Geometry ........................................ 377
19.4 Riemannian Geometry ...................................................................................... 378
    19.4.1 Geometry of Covariance Matrices ...................................................... 378
    19.4.2 Estimators of Covariance Matrices ...................................................... 380
    19.4.3 Distances and Means ............................................................................ 382
    19.4.4 Minimum Distance to Mean Classifier ................................................ 384
    19.4.5 MDM for SSVEP .................................................................................. 386
    19.4.6 Online MDM ........................................................................................ 386
19.5 Experimental Evaluation on SSVEP Data Set .................................................. 390
    19.5.1 SSVEP Data Set Description ................................................................ 390
    19.5.2 Evaluation of the Covariance Estimators ............................................ 390
    19.5.3 Offline Classification of SSVEP .......................................................... 392
    19.5.4 Online Classification of SSVEP .......................................................... 392
19.6 Conclusions ...................................................................................................... 394
References ................................................................................................................ 394

## Abstract

This chapter focuses on the different implementations of brain–computer interface (BCI) based on steady-state visually evoked potentials (SSVEPs). In offline BCI, feature extraction and classification are performed at the end of the session, when all trials are available, whereas in online settings, they are performed several times during each trial, usually for each available epoch recorded by the electroencephalogram (EEG) device, enabling real-time and asynchronous BCI. A recent successful approach in feature extraction and signal processing for BCI is Riemannian geometry, which deals with covariance matrices. They capture the degree of correlation between several random variables, that is, how the brain signals change relatively to each other. These techniques have demonstrated their benefit on several occasions, leading to winning algorithms in international competitions and to state-of-the-art results on renowned BCI benchmarks. After reviewing some of the most robust approaches in feature extraction for SSVEP, this chapter will introduce newer tools based on Riemannian geometry. With an application to SSVEP, this article shows through a comparison how Riemannian geometry allows one to easily define offline and online implementations that have better accuracies than state of the art.

## 19.1   INTRODUCTION

This chapter presents the feature extraction and classification techniques applied for signals of a particular paradigm of brain–computer interface (BCI). The most successful approaches, that is, those providing the highest transfer rates and the most robust representations, share one common ground: they are all estimating the covariance from the signal to build or to derive their feature. The covariance captures the degree of linear dependence between several random variables, that is, how the brain signals change relatively to each other. If two signals show the same variations, increasing and decreasing at the same time, they are dependent. The notion of covariance is central in several fields of science, such as mathematical finance, meteorology, oceanography, and, of course, signal processing. A correct covariance estimation requires to take into account a noticeable part of the time signal history. This fact has a strong impact when setting up a BCI system, as it introduces a delay to allow a correct processing and interpretation of the brain signal. Special attention is thus needed when dealing with covariance-based approaches in online systems, to aim for a robust system without impeding the interactions with a high latency.

After reviewing some of the most robust approaches in features extraction for steady-state visually evoked potentials (SSVEPs), this chapter will present recently introduced tools for signal processing based on a non-Euclidean geometry, namely, the Riemannian geometry. These techniques have demonstrated their benefit on several occasions, leading to winning algorithms in international competitions and to state-of-the-art results on renowned BCI benchmarks. Most of these achievements are built on the theoretical advances of a very active community working on Information Geometry and its applications to signal processing, for example, in radar imagery, computer vision, or finance. A thorough review of the existing Riemannian approaches for BCI is proposed, with its application to SSVEP.

Regarding the implementation in offline BCI, feature extraction and classification are performed at the end of the session, when all trials are available. Based on such a setting, it is difficult to design algorithms for real-time BCI. On the contrary, in online implementation, feature extraction and classification are performed several times during each trial, usually for each available epoch recorded by the electroencephalogram (EEG) device. This setting being more realistic, it enables the development of real-time and asynchronous BCI. Applied to SSVEP, this chapter will compare on real data how Riemannian geometry allows one to easily design offline and online implementations for BCI with a better accuracy than state of the art. Moreover, using covariance matrices as feature allows one to define a resting-state class, which is a crucial point in BCI design.

Section 19.2 gives an overall view of the SSVEP-based BCI and the state-of-the-art approaches. The implication of designing online algorithms are explained and highlighted. Section 19.3 provides a detailed description of the mathematical and theoretical principles involved in the feature extraction step. The importance of the covariance matrices is shown and the link with Riemannian geometry is explained. In Section 19.4, an overview of the Riemannian tools and their application to covariance matrices are proposed. The existing approaches to estimate covariance matrices are explained before this section covers the known distances, the mean estimation, and the classification in the space of covariance matrices. Offline and online implementations are described. Section 19.5 explains how these Riemannian approaches are applied to EEG signal. The existing algorithms are evaluated on an SSVEP data set and the results are analyzed in terms of quality of prediction and computing load. Section 19.6 concludes this chapter and opens on questions on the future of Riemannian-based BCI.

## 19.2 A REVIEW OF SSVEP-BASED BCI

This section quickly reviews some points about SSVEP and then details its application in BCI. As the notion of offline analysis and online algorithms is at the center of this chapter, this section explains the differences between those approaches.

### 19.2.1 STEADY-STATE VISUALLY EVOKED POTENTIALS

Dealing with sensory evoked potentials, it is a common view to oppose event-related potential and steady-state response (SSR) (Regan 1982), including their visual counterpart, SSVEP. This distinction originates from the idea that the SSR may be generated by neural oscillations elicited by the repeated stimulations (Takahashi 2004, pp. 241–262) whereas the ERP is the transient response to an event occurring at a sufficiently long time interval to allow the system to return to its initial state (Niedermeyer and Lopes da Silva 2004).

The SSVEP-based BCI is often employed as a dependent BCI (Wolpaw et al. 2002); that is, some residual muscular capabilities are required to move the eye toward the blinking stimulus as opposed to independent BCI, such as motor imagery (MI), where the communication does not rely on any motor capability. It has been shown that SSVEP could be used as an independent BCI (Morgan et al. 1996; Müller et al. 2006) as the neural oscillations are strongly related to the focus of attention. Using covert attention, that is, shifting the focus of attention without moving the eyes, subjects can generate different SSVEP responses.

Visual stimulus plays a crucial role, affecting the SSVEP-based BCI performance, and should be designed carefully. An in-depth review of the literature (Zhu et al. 2010) shows that LED stimuli provide better results than those obtained on a computer screen. Any stimulation between 2 and 50 Hz induces visible oscillations in the visual cortex (Herrmann 2001), with a peak in signal-to-noise ratio visible around 15 Hz (Pastor et al. 2003). Common values employed in SSVEP studies are between 12 and 25 Hz, as they induce oscillations with higher amplitudes (Zhu et al. 2010). One should note that safety considerations should be taken into account as some frequency ranges of the stimulation train may trigger epileptic seizures (Fisher et al. 2005).

Review articles (Liu et al. 2014; Stawicki et al. 2017; Vialatte et al. 2010; Zhu et al. 2010) provide more details on SSVEP: properties of the visual stimuli (influence of the number of visual stimulation frequencies to accommodate an increasing number of BCI commands), stimulation paradigm (multiple frequencies sequential coding and frequency shift keying), and electrophysiological response. For more details about SSVEP, one should refer to the Chapter 8 of this book ("Affective Brain–Computer Interfacing and Methods for Affective State Detection" by Ian Daly).

### 19.2.2 ONLINE AND OFFLINE IMPLEMENTATIONS FOR BCI

It is important to define some of the terminologies used in the chapter and in the literature. A first important notion is to differentiate between synchronous and asynchronous BCI. In synchronous setting, the system provides temporal cues for the subject, asking to perform specific action at a specific time. This is not the case in asynchronous BCI, where the subject could act or elicit an action from the system at any time. In SSVEP, both settings could be found, even if the synchronous setting is very common in the literature, as it is simpler to obtain meaningful and reproducible results.

Implementations of feature extraction and classification could be online or offline. Distinguishing between those two implementations requires one to define some necessary notions. We call samples the values acquired by the system at each time step. A group of successive samples of a predetermined size is called an epoch; it is used to simplify the feature extraction. We define a trial as the sequence in the experimental plan where the user is asked to perform a specific task. A session is defined here as a group of trial performed successively by the subject. The classification results are generally obtained by averaging performances across all trials.

We can thus distinguish the different implementations:

- In offline settings, feature extraction and classification are performed at the end of the session; thus, all trials are available. It is not possible to design a real-time BCI system with such implementation.
- In block-online settings, classification is performed at the end of each trial; the trials are available one after the other. This is the common setting for synchronous interactions.
- In online settings, feature extraction and classification are performed several times during each trial, usually for each available epoch recorded by the EEG device, sometimes for each sample if the computation time is compatible with the real-time constraints. With this implementation, it is possible to set up an asynchronous BCI.

Note that using or not using a preliminary calibration on a training set does not change these distinctions.

One of the most crucial problems in BCI is the difference between these offline and online implementations. Offline analyses represent the major part of the scientific publications, but they cannot serve, as they are, in practical implementations of a BCI, which are necessarily online or block-online. Offline implementations often use noncausal processing (e.g., bilateral filtering), normalizations, or whitening that requires one to know the whole data distribution of the session. But these computations are not possible in online settings; hence, converting an offline implementation to an online one is not trivial and can generate a loss of performances, in terms of classification accuracy.

## 19.3 CLASSIFYING SSVEP SIGNALS

This section presents the common techniques to classify SSVEP signals, that is, finding the frequencies of brainwaves in the visual cortex that correspond to the target stimulus.

### 19.3.1 NOTATIONS

In the following, $C$ denotes the number of electrodes recorded by the EEG system. Depending on the sampling rate of the EEG system, a certain number of samples are recorded each second. Each sample contains $C$ values indicating the potential difference, usually expressed in microvolts, measured at each electrode site. The potential differences are represented in a vector of $C$ lines, denoted $x_n$, where $n = 1,\ldots,N$. This is illustrated in the upper part of Figure 19.1. A recording is represented as a matrix $X = [x_1,\ldots,x_n]$, $X \in \mathbb{R}^{C \times N}$, which is the concatenation of all samples, as shown in the bottom of Figure 19.1. We will make the hypothesis that all $N$ samples $x_n$ are randomly drawn from a distribution. It follows that $x$ is a variable of random vectors and its expected vector is $\omega = E(x)$ (Fukunaga 1990). The covariance matrix of the random vector $x$ is defined by $\Sigma = E\{(x - \omega)(x - \omega)^T\}$.

### 19.3.2 CLASSIFICATION USING CANONICAL CORRELATION

To classify SSVEP signal, one should find the frequencies of brainwaves in the visual cortex corresponding to the target stimulus. Several methods have been proposed, using power spectral density

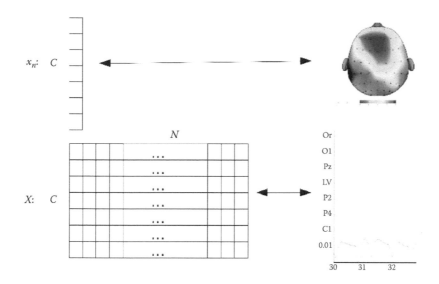

**FIGURE 19.1** Potential differences measured on the scalp are gathered in vector $x_n$ (top). A complete recording is represented as a matrix $X$ of $C$ lines, corresponding to the number of electrodes, and $N$ columns, corresponding to the number of samples (bottom).

or other decomposition methods (Liu et al. 2014). The most robust approaches are based on either canonical correlation or Riemannian geometry.

Until recently, methods relying on canonical correlation analysis (CCA) originating from Hotelling (1936) were achieving the highest classification performances, but implementation is offline (Lin et al. 2006). Given two sets of signals, CCA aims at finding the projection space that maximizes their cross-covariance while jointly minimizing their covariance.

For SSVEP, the CCA aims to find a new subspace such that the two sets of variables have maximal correlation when projected on this subspace. The main idea is to use $X \in \mathbb{R}^{C \times N}$ as a first set of variables and $2N_h$ reference signals $Y_f \in \mathbb{R}^{2N_h \times N}$ as the second set. A common way of generating the representation of the simulation signal at frequency $f$ is

$$
Y_f = \begin{bmatrix} \sin(2\pi f n) \\ \cos(2\pi f n) \\ \vdots \\ \sin(2\pi N_h f n) \\ \cos(2\pi N_h f n) \end{bmatrix}, \; n = \frac{1}{T_S}, \frac{2}{T_S}, \dots, \frac{N}{T_S}, \tag{19.1}
$$

where $T_S$ is the EEG sampling frequency, $N_h$ is the number of harmonics, and $N$ is the number of samples. $N_h$ is a parameter that can be defined by cross validation.

The CCA seeks two projection directions $w_X$ and $w_{Y_f}$ such that $w_X^T X$ and $w_{Y_f} Y_f$ have maximal correlation. $w_X$ and $w_{Y_f}$ maximize the correlation function $\rho\left(w_X, w_{Y_f}\right)$:

$$
\rho\left(w_X, w_{Y_f}\right) = \mathrm{corr}\left(w_X^T X, w_{Y_f} Y_f\right)
$$

$$
= \frac{w_X^T \Sigma_{XY_f} w_{Yf}}{\sqrt{w_X^T \Sigma_X w_X w_{Y_f}^T \Sigma_{Y_f} w_{Y_f}}}, \tag{19.2}
$$

where $\Sigma_{XY_f}$ is the between-set covariance matrix; $\Sigma_X$ and $\Sigma_{Y_f}$ are the within-set covariance matrices. CCA can be solved as in Hardoon et al. (2004):

$$\text{maximize}_{w_X, w_{Y_f}} \qquad w_X^T \Sigma_{XY_f} w_{Y_f}$$

$$\text{subject to} \qquad \begin{aligned} w_X^T \Sigma_X w_X &= 1 \\ w_{Y_f}^T \Sigma_{Y_f} w_{Y_f} &= 1. \end{aligned}$$

The CCA objective is to maximize the correlation $\rho$ between $w_X^T X$ and $Y_f^T w_{Y_f}$ as follows:

$$\rho_f = \max_{w_X, w_{Y_f}} \frac{w_X^T X Y_f^T w_{Y_f}}{\sqrt{w_X^T X X^T w_X w_{Y_f}^T Y_f Y_f^T w_{Y_f}}}. \tag{19.3}$$

Note that when more than one couple of directions $w_X$ and $w_{Y_f}$ are needed, a deflation step can be applied and then another problem of CCA is solved. To determine the target frequency $\hat{f}$, the values of $\rho_f$ are used for classification as (Lin et al. 2006)

$$\hat{f} = \text{argmax}_f \{\rho_f\}. \tag{19.4}$$

A different approach considers CCA only to obtain a spatial filter, using a support vector machine (SVM) to process the spectral features of the filtered signal (Kalunga et al. 2013). This approach is referred to as CCA+SVM in this work.

Several aspects regarding the CCA are still debated and not clearly established, especially concerning the harmonics. The number of harmonics to choose and its impact on the classification accuracy are unclear. Chen et al. (2015) introduce the filter bank canonical correlation analysis (FBCCA), which is an online algorithm. The EEG signal is filtered into $n = 1 \ldots N_b$ sub-bands covering multiple harmonic frequency bands. As described above, CCA allows one to obtain a correlation coefficient $\rho_f^n$ for each sub-band $n$. The correlation coefficients are combined as

$$\bar{\rho}_f = \sum_{n=1}^{N_b} w_n \left( \rho_f^n \right)^2, \tag{19.5}$$

where $N_b$ is the number of sub-bands and $n_b$ and $w_n$ are the index and the weight of a sub-band, respectively. The weights are defined as

$$w_n = n^{-a} + b, \ n \in \left[ 1, \ldots, N_b \right], \tag{19.6}$$

where $a$ and $b$ are constants that maximize the classification performance. Hyperparameters $a$, $b$, and $N_b$ are determined in practice with a grid search conducted on an offline analysis. Once all $\bar{\rho}_f$ are determined, the classification is done with Equation 19.4. FBCCA significantly improves the performance of standard CCA (Chen et al. 2015).

Recent studies conducted by Nakanishi et al. (2014) and Chen et al. (2015) made a breakthrough in high-speed SSVEP-based speller, used in online settings. The objective of these experiments is to successively select letters for a spelling task; SSVEP achieves the highest information transfer rate

(ITR) reported in EEG-based BCI. Nakanishi et al. brought the ITR to an average of 166.91 bits/min (Nakanishi et al. 2014), and later, Chen et al. raised it to an average of 270 bits/min (Chen et al. 2015). Nakanishi et al. (2014) achieved high classification performances, mainly relying on methodological improvement of the stimulation protocol (phase modulation and combination of frequencies) and stimulus presentation (the proposed letters follow a similar scheme to SMS writing). However, there are two strong limitations to these works.

First, these studies do not consider a resting-state class (or a reject class), where the user does not gaze at any specific stimulus, meaning that the system continuously outputs a selected letter without any pause. Allowing users to act at their own pace is utterly important in human–machine interface (HMI) and hence in BCI. Moreover, taking into account the case where the user does not gaze at any stimulus is a challenging issue as traces of stimulation frequencies are still observable in the EEG. Second, the stimulation protocol is complex: a successful classification requires a synchronization between the stimulation and EEG acquisition devices to ensure a proper time reference for the phase measurements. This is not guaranteed in many experimental settings and it is a limitation for the potential applications.

### 19.3.3 CLASSIFICATION USING RIEMANNIAN GEOMETRY

The covariance is central in state-of-the-art CCA approaches as it allows one to estimate spatial filters that are projections of the original sensor space into a surrogate sensor space that enhances the signal of interest. Spatial filters are user-specific signal processing techniques yielding a robust representation, with strong discrimination properties, allowing good accuracy in classification. Spatial filters are very efficient on clean data sets obtained from strongly constrained environment, but they are sensitive to artifacts and outliers (Lotte 2011; Tomioka et al. 2007). But working directly on covariance matrices is advantageous: it simplifies the whole BCI system (Yger 2013), avoiding the alignment of two learning steps (spatial filters and classifiers) that might lead to overfitting. The covariance matrices, being symmetric and positive-definite (SPD), are best handled by tools provided by Riemannian geometry (Bhatia 2009). Classification in the space of SPD matrices eliminates the need of spatial filters and improves the system robustness (Barachant et al. 2012; Congedo et al. 2013; Yger 2013). Riemannian-based approaches have demonstrated their efficiency by outranking all other existing techniques on real competitive problems: DecMeg 2014 challenge,* BCI Challenge—NER 2015,[†] and Grasp-and-Lift EEG Detection 2015.[‡]

To detail how Riemannian geometry can improve machine learning algorithms, one can argue that it takes explicitly into consideration the underlying structure of the data. Different approaches in the literature use the geometry of data in machine learning (for complete reviews, see Congedo et al. 2017; Yger et al. 2017). A first possibility is to rely on the mapping of the Riemannian manifold onto a Euclidean vector space, where common algorithm could be applied. One such mapping, called logarithmic mapping, exists between the manifold and its tangent space, which is a Euclidean space, and has been used in classification task for BCI (Barachant et al. 2013b). Some kernels have been applied successfully to this end: Stein kernel, Log-Euclidean kernels, as well as their normalized versions (Yger 2013). The family of kernels defined on the Riemannian manifold allows the implementation of extensions of all kernel-based methods, such as SVM, kernel-PCA, or kernel $k$-means (Jayasumana et al. 2013). Apart from the kernel approaches, once the data are mapped onto a vector space, any machine learning algorithm working in Euclidean space, such as LDA, could be applied (Barachant et al. 2012).

Another possibility is to develop new algorithms directly for Riemannian manifolds. The minimum distance to Riemannian mean (MDRM) relies on a Riemannian metric to implement

---

\* https://www.kaggle.com/c/decoding-the-human-brain
[†] https://www.kaggle.com/c/inria-bci-challenge
[‡] https://www.kaggle.com/c/grasp-and-lift-eeg-detection

a multiclass classifier and have been applied on EEG. New EEG trials are assigned to the class whose average covariance matrix is the closest to the trial covariance matrix (Barachant et al. 2012). The MDRM classification can be preceded by a spatial filtering of covariance matrices, like in Barachant et al. (2010), where covariance matrices are filtered with LDA components in the tangent space, and then brought back to the Riemannian space for classification with MDRM. Another example is the Riemannian Potato (Barachant et al. 2013a), an unsupervised and adaptive artifact detection method, providing an online EEG outlier removal. Incoming epochs are rejected if their covariance matrix lies beyond a predefined $z$-score.

To apply Riemannian geometry to SSVEP, the sample covariance matrices can be defined from a rearrangement of the recorded data. The rearrangement is done such that the temporal or frequency information is captured (Congedo 2013; Congedo et al. 2013). With similar motivations, Li et al. (2012) and Li and Wong (2013) defined a new Riemannian distance between SPD matrices filtered in different frequency bands: an optimized spatial weighting matrix is commonly applied on covariance matrices of each frequency band. They use this new distance as a dissimilarity between weighted matrices of power spectral density to classify EEG into different sleep states by $k$-nearest neighbors.

## 19.4  RIEMANNIAN GEOMETRY

This section starts with a presentation of the tools and characteristics of the geometry of SPD matrices. A simple classification algorithm is then described, which works directly in the space of covariance matrices. This simple yet efficient classifier allows one to achieve near state-of-the-art results. It relies on two key aspects, the estimation of covariance matrices, which should be as accurate as possible, and the choice of a metric to estimate the center of mass of a set of covariance matrices. These aspects, covariance estimation and existing metrics, are presented in this section. Finally, MDRM classifier is presented for offline and online implementations.

### 19.4.1  GEOMETRY OF COVARIANCE MATRICES

Covariance matrices are SPD and are thus constrained to lie strictly inside a convex cone, as shown in Figure 19.2. This special topological space is a Riemannian manifold. A manifold could be described as a collection of small flat structures, "glued" together. For each of these small structures, the neighborhood of an element could be considered as flat, which is similar to a tangent space. The bijection between the neighborhood of a manifold element and $\mathbb{R}^m$ is called a chart. A smooth differentiable atlas is a collection of charts verifying that the elements overlap smoothly (Absil et al. 2009). When the manifold is equipped with a complete, smooth differentiable atlas and with an inner product defined on the tangent space of each element, it is called a Riemannian manifold.

As illustrated by Yger et al. (2017), we can draw the parallel with the situation that occurs on Earth. Indeed, the surface of Earth is a smooth lower-dimensional subspace. At every point of the surface, we can approximate the surface as a map (a locally accurate flat approximation). Then, the shortest path between two points on the surface is a curved called a geodesic.

The covariance matrices are elements of $\mathcal{M}_C$, a manifold of $C \times C$ symmetric positive-definite matrices,

$$\mathcal{M}_C = \left\{ \Sigma \in \mathbb{R}^{C \times C} \middle| \Sigma = \Sigma^T \text{ and } x^T \Sigma x > 0, \ \forall x \in \mathbb{R}^C \backslash 0 \right\}.$$

SPD matrices verify the properties listed in Table 19.1.

The tangent space $T_\Sigma \mathcal{M}_C$, which is a local linear approximation of the manifold at the point $\Sigma$, is identified to the Euclidean space of symmetric matrices:

$$\mathcal{S}_C = \left\{ \Theta \in \mathbb{R}^{C \times C} : \Theta = \Theta^T \right\}.$$

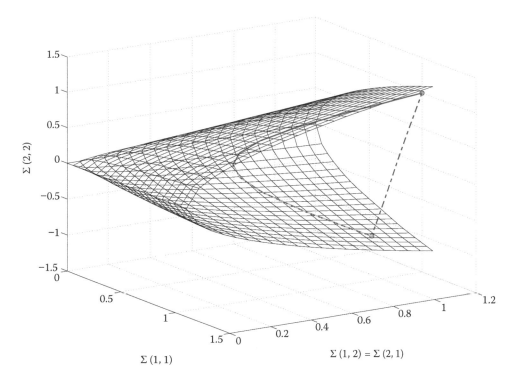

**FIGURE 19.2** Visualization of the covariance matrices $\Sigma \in \mathbb{R}^{2 \times 2}$. The Euclidean distance (dashed red line) does not consider the curvature of the space and define chordal distance between elements. Riemannian distances (AIR in plain blue and Log-Euclidean in dashed-dotted green) follow a geodesic and thus take into account the shape of the space where covariance matrices lie.

**TABLE 19.1**

**Properties of the SPD Matrices**

| | |
|---|---|
| Symmetry | $\Sigma = \Sigma^T$ |
| Positive definiteness | $x^T \Sigma x > 0, \ \forall x \in \mathbb{R}^C \setminus 0$ |
| Strict positivity of diagonal elements | $\Sigma(i,j) > 0 \big| i = j, \ \forall i, j \in \{1, \dots, C\}$, i.e., positive variance |
| Cauchy–Schwarz inequalities | $\left| \Sigma(i,j) \right| \leq \left( \Sigma(i,i) \, \Sigma(j,j) \right)^{\frac{1}{2}}, \ \forall i, j \in \{1, \dots, C\}$ |

The dimension of the manifold $\mathcal{M}_C$, and its tangent space $T_\Sigma \mathcal{M}_C$, is $m = \dfrac{C(C+1)}{2}$.

The mapping from a point $\Theta_i$ of the tangent space to the manifold is called the exponential mapping $\mathrm{Exp}_\Sigma (\Theta_i)$: $T_\Sigma \mathcal{M}_C \rightarrow \mathcal{M}_C$ and is defined as

$$\mathrm{Exp}_\Sigma (\Theta_i) = \Sigma^{\frac{1}{2}} \mathrm{Exp}\left( \Sigma^{-\frac{1}{2}} \Theta_i \Sigma^{-\frac{1}{2}} \right) \Sigma^{\frac{1}{2}}. \tag{19.7}$$

Its inverse mapping, from the manifold to the tangent space, is called the logarithmic mapping $\mathrm{Log}_\Sigma \left( \Sigma_i \right)$: $\mathcal{M}_C \rightarrow T_\Sigma \mathcal{M}_C$ and is defined as

$$\mathrm{Log}_\Sigma (\Sigma_i) = \Sigma^{\frac{1}{2}} \mathrm{Log}\left( \Sigma^{-\frac{1}{2}} \Sigma_i \Sigma^{-\frac{1}{2}} \right) \Sigma^{\frac{1}{2}}. \tag{19.8}$$

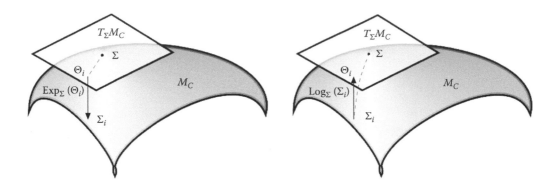

**FIGURE 19.3**   Left: the exponential mapping of $\Theta_i$, an element of the tangent space $T_\Sigma \mathcal{M}_C$ at point $\Sigma$, on the manifold $\mathcal{M}_C$ is $\Sigma_i$. Right: the logarithmic mapping of $\Sigma_i$ at point $\Sigma$ is $\Theta_i$ on the tangent space $T_\Sigma \mathcal{M}_C$.

Exp ($\cdot$) and Log ($\cdot$) are the matrix exponential and matrix logarithm, respectively. These two mappings are illustrated in Figure 19.3. The computation of these operators is straightforward for SPD matrices of $\mathcal{M}_C$. They are obtained from their eigenvalue decomposition:

$$\Sigma = U\mathrm{diag}(\lambda_1, \ldots, \lambda_C)U^T,$$
$$\mathrm{Exp}(\Sigma) = U\mathrm{diag}\big(\exp(\lambda_1), \ldots, \exp(\lambda_C)\big)U^T,$$
$$\mathrm{Log}(\Sigma) = U\mathrm{diag}\big(\log(\lambda_1), \ldots, \log(\lambda_C)\big)U^T,$$

where $\lambda_1, \ldots, \lambda_C$ are the eigenvalues and $U$ is the matrix of eigenvectors of $\Sigma$. As any SPD matrix can be diagonalized with strictly positive eigenvalues, Log ($\cdot$) is always defined. Similarly the square root $\Sigma^{\frac{1}{2}}$ is obtained as

$$\Sigma = U\mathrm{diag}\left(\lambda_1^{\frac{1}{2}}, \ldots, \lambda_C^{\frac{1}{2}}\right)U^T,$$

and is unique. The same goes for $\Sigma^{-\frac{1}{2}}$.

### 19.4.2 ESTIMATORS OF COVARIANCE MATRICES

Estimation of covariance matrices is a critical step required to design a working and efficient BCI system. The covariance matrix is defined as $\Sigma = E\{(x - \omega)(x - \omega)^T\}$ and is unknown. Only an estimate $\hat{\Sigma}$ could be computed from the observations. The first step is to choose an appropriate estimator. It is crucial to verify that the obtained covariance matrices fulfill the following properties: they should be accurate, symmetric, positive-definite, and well conditioned. The second step is to remove the outliers properly, that is, the samples that are contaminated either by exogenous or endogenous noise, to avoid bias when estimating the mean of a class or when processing newly recorded EEG signals.

Regarding the first step, that is, the covariance estimation, an important property is matrix conditioning. It requires that the ratio between the maximum and minimum eigenvalue is not too large. Moreover, to ensure the computational stability of the algorithm, the estimator should provide full-rank matrices, and its inversion should not amplify estimation errors.

This section describes three different classes of estimators: the sample, the shrinkage, and the fixed-point estimators. These classes of estimators are evaluated on a real EEG data set to assess their accuracy in terms of classification and the condition of the obtained matrices. The most common estimator is the maximum likelihood estimator (MLE) under a multivariate Gaussian assumption. It is called the empirical *sample covariance matrix* (SCM), defined as

$$\hat{\Sigma}_{\text{scm}} = \frac{1}{N-1} \sum_{n=1}^{N} (x_n - \bar{x})(x_n - \bar{x})^T$$
$$= \frac{1}{N-1} X \left( I_N - \frac{1}{N} 1_N 1_N^T \right) X^T, \tag{19.9}$$

where $\bar{x} \in \mathbb{R}^C$ is the sample mean vector $\bar{x} = \frac{1}{N} \sum_{n=1}^{N} x_n$. In the matrix notation, $I_N$ is the $N \times N$ identity matrix and $1_N$ is the vector $[1,...,1]$. The SCM is often normalized (Fukunaga 1990) as

$$\hat{\Sigma}_{\text{nscm}} = \frac{C}{N} \sum_{n=1}^{N} \frac{(x_n - \bar{x})(x_n - \bar{x})^T}{\sigma_{x_n}^2}, \tag{19.10}$$

with the interchannel variance at time $n$ defined as $\sigma_{x_n}^2 = (x_n - \bar{x})^T (x_n - \bar{x})$. Other normalization techniques could be used. This estimation is fast and computationally simple. However, when $C \approx N$, the SCM is not a good estimator of the true covariance. In the case $C > N$, the SCM is not even full rank.

To overcome the shortcomings of SCM, the shrinkage estimators have been developed as a weighted combination of the SCM and a target covariance matrix, which is often chosen to be close to the identity matrix, that is, resulting from almost independent variables of unit variance:

$$\hat{\Sigma}_{\text{shrink}} = \kappa \Gamma + (1 - \kappa) \hat{\Sigma}_{\text{scm}}, \tag{19.11}$$

where $0 \leq \kappa < 1$. This estimator provides a regularized covariance that outperforms the empirical $\hat{\Sigma}_{\text{scm}}$ for small sample size, that is, $C \approx N$. The shrinkage estimator has the same eigenvectors as the SCM, but the extreme eigenvalues are modified, that is, the estimator is shrunk or elongated toward the average. The different shrinkage estimators differ in their definition of the target covariance matrix $\Gamma$. Ledoit and Wolf (2004) ($\hat{\Sigma}_{\text{shrink\_ledoit}}$) have proposed $\Gamma = \nu I_C$, with $\nu = \text{Tr}(\hat{\Sigma}_{\text{scm}})$. Blankertz et al. (2011) ($\hat{\Sigma}_{\text{shrink\_blank}}$) define $\Gamma$ also as $\nu I_C$ but with $\nu = \frac{\text{Tr}(\hat{\Sigma}_{\text{scm}})}{C}$. Schäfer ($\hat{\Sigma}_{\text{shrink\_schaf}}$) proposes several ways of defining $\Gamma$ depending on the observed $\hat{\Sigma}_{\text{scm}}$ (Schäfer and Strimmer 2005).

The fixed-point covariance matrix (Pascal et al. 2005) is based on an M-estimator, which generalizes the MLE, and is a solution to the following equation:

$$\hat{\Sigma}_{\text{fp}} = \hat{\ell} = \frac{C}{N} \sum_{n=1}^{N} \frac{(x_n - \bar{x})(x_n - \bar{x})^T}{(x_n - \bar{x})^T \hat{\ell}^{-1} (x_n - \bar{x})}, \tag{19.12}$$

As there is no closed form expression to Equation 19.12, it can be written as a function of $\hat{\ell}$. $g(\hat{\ell}) = \hat{\Sigma}_{\text{fp}}$. $g$ admits a single *fixed point* $\hat{\ell}*$, where $g(\hat{\ell}*) = \hat{\ell}*$, which is a solution to Equation 19.12. Using $\hat{\ell}_0 := \hat{\Sigma}_{\text{nscm}}$ as the initial value of $\hat{\ell}$, it is solved recursively as $\hat{\ell}_t \xrightarrow[t \to \infty]{} \hat{\ell}*$.

**TABLE 19.2**

**Properties of a Distance**

| | |
|---|---|
| (i) Non-negativity | $d(\Sigma_1 = \Sigma_2) \geq 0$ |
| (ii) Identity | $d(\Sigma_1 = \Sigma_2) = 0$ iff $\Sigma_1 = \Sigma_2$ |
| (iii) Symmetry | $d(\Sigma_1, \Sigma_2) = d(\Sigma_2, \Sigma_1)$ |
| (iv) Triangular inequality | $d(\Sigma_1, \Sigma_3) \leq d(\Sigma_1, \Sigma_2) + d(\Sigma_2, \Sigma_3)$ |

### 19.4.3 DISTANCES AND MEANS

From the definition of Riemannian manifolds, we have seen that they are defined by their atlas and by the choice of an inner product defined on the tangent space. In the case of covariance matrices, there exist several candidate inner products that lead to different distances and, thus, to different geometries of Riemannian manifolds. A distance function $d = \mathcal{M}_C \times \mathcal{M}_C \rightarrow \mathbb{R}^+$ has the properties listed in Table 19.2 for all $\Sigma_1, \Sigma_2, \Sigma_3 \in \mathcal{M}_C$.

Divergences are very similar to distances, with the difference that properties (iii) and (iv) do not have to be satisfied. In the context of SPD matrices, divergences and distances are carefully chosen to induce a Riemannian metric. Divergences offer interesting properties but do not lead to qualitatively different results. For the sake of clarity, this chapter focuses only on distances; an in-depth review of the existing divergence and the analysis of their results are available in Kalunga et al. (2015).

As we will see in Section 19.4.4, the notion of mean, or center of mass, of a set of SPD matrices is tightly linked with the task of classification in machine learning approaches. Given a set of covariance matrices $\{\Sigma_i\}_{i=1,\ldots,I}$, the mean $\bar{\Sigma}$ of those SPD matrices is a covariance matrix that minimizes the dispersion of matrices $\Sigma_i$:

$$\bar{\Sigma} = \mu\left(\left\{\Sigma_1, \ldots, \Sigma_I\right\}\right) = \operatorname{argmin}_{\Sigma \in \mathcal{M}_C} \sum_{i=1}^{I} d^2(\Sigma_i, \Sigma), \tag{19.13}$$

where $d(\cdot, \cdot)$ is a distance between two matrices. In the literature, $\bar{\Sigma}$ could be referred to as the geometric mean, the *Cartan mean*, the *Frechet mean*, or the *Karcher mean** (Ando et al. 2004; Lim and Pálfia 2012). Depending on the distance used, several means can be defined from Equation 19.13. Hereafter, some of the existing distances are briefly presented, along with their associated mean, and they are summarized in Table 19.3.

A trivial choice is the Euclidean distance, which is not a Riemannian distance, and is derived from the Frobenius inner product:

$$d_E(\Sigma_1, \Sigma_2) = \left\|\Sigma_1 - \Sigma_2\right\|_F, \tag{19.14}$$

Euclidean distance yields the arithmetic mean:

$$\bar{\Sigma}_E = \frac{1}{I} \sum_{i=1}^{I} \Sigma_i. \tag{19.15}$$

---

* This appellation has been recently criticized by Karcher (2014) himself.

**TABLE 19.3**

**Some of the Distances and Means Considered in This Chapter**

| | Distance | Mean | Reference |
|---|---|---|---|
| Euclidean | $d_E = \|\Sigma_1 - \Sigma_2\|_F$ | $\bar{\Sigma}_E = \dfrac{1}{I}\displaystyle\sum_{i=1}^{I}\Sigma_i$ | |
| Log-Euclidean | $d_{LE} = \|\mathrm{Log}(\Sigma_1) - \mathrm{Log}(\Sigma_2)\|_F$ | $\bar{\Sigma}_{LE} = \mathrm{Exp}\left(\dfrac{1}{I}\displaystyle\sum_{i=1}^{I}\log(\Sigma_i)\right)$ | Arsigny et al. 2007 |
| Affine-invariant | $d_{AIR} = \left\|\mathrm{Log}\left(\Sigma_1^{-1}\,\Sigma_2\right)\right\|_F$ | Algorithm 3 in Fletcher et al. 2004 | Moakher 2005 |

Averaging covariance matrices with this arithmetic mean is not adequate in the space of SPD matrices for two main reasons: first, the Euclidean distance and averaging do not guarantee invariance under inversion: a matrix and its inverse are supposed to be at the same distance from the identity matrix. Second, the Euclidean averaging of covariance SPD leads to a *swelling effect*: the determinant of the arithmetic mean of SPD matrices can be larger than the determinant of its individual components, as illustrated in Figure 19.4. Since the determinant of a covariance matrix is a direct measure of the dispersion of the multivariate variable, the swelling effect introduces a large distortion on the dispersion of data (Arsigny et al. 2007). For these reasons, other means that adapt to the convex cone of SPD matrices are more adequate than this arithmetic mean.

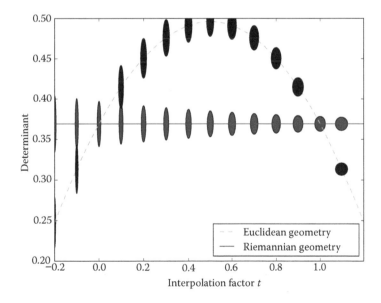

**FIGURE 19.4** Evolution of the determinant of a matrix along a geodesic. Both matrices being interpolated have the same determinant (for $t = 0$ and $t = 1$), and along a Riemannian geodesic (in gray), the determinant remains the same, but along a Euclidean geodesic (in black), the determinant rises. This latter phenomenon is called the swelling effect.

To avoid these problems, a natural approach is to consider a distance built on curves from the manifold, called geodesics; Pennec and Ayache (1998) give a method to generate invariant distance on the manifold. The tangent vector of the geodesic $\gamma(t)$ between $\Sigma_1$ and $\Sigma_2$, where $\gamma(0) = \Sigma_1$ and $\gamma(1) = \Sigma_2$, is defined as $v = \overrightarrow{\Sigma_1 \Sigma_2} = \text{Log}_{\Sigma_1}(\Sigma_2)$. A natural distance between $\Sigma_1$ and $\Sigma_2$ can thus be defined as (Moakher 2005)

$$d_{\text{AIR}}\left(\Sigma_1, \Sigma_2\right) = \left\| \text{Log}\left(\Sigma_1^{-\frac{1}{2}} \Sigma_2 \Sigma_1^{-\frac{1}{2}}\right) \right\|_F = \left(\sum_{c=1}^{C} \log^2 \lambda_c\right)^{\frac{1}{2}}, \tag{19.16}$$

where $\lambda_c$, $c = 1,\ldots,C$, are the eigenvalues of $\Sigma_1^{-\frac{1}{2}}\Sigma_2\Sigma_1^{-\frac{1}{2}}$. This distance is known as the *affine-invariant Riemannian* (AIR) distance. Inserting Equation 19.16 in Equation 19.13 yields the mean $\bar{\Sigma}_{\text{AIR}}$ associated to the affine-invariant Riemannian metric:

$$\sum_{i=1}^{I} \text{Log}\left(\Sigma_{\text{AIR}}^{-\frac{1}{2}} \Sigma_i \Sigma_{\text{AIR}}^{-\frac{1}{2}}\right) = 0. \tag{19.17}$$

It has no closed form solution and can be solved iteratively through a gradient descent algorithm (Fletcher et al. 2004). This AIR distance has many properties (Bhatia 2009), and the most interesting one is the invariance under congruent transformation:

$$d_{\text{AIR}}(\Sigma_1, \Sigma_2) = d_{\text{AIR}}(W^T \Sigma_1 W, \ W^T \Sigma_2 W), \tag{19.18}$$

for any invertible matrix $W \in \mathbb{R}^{C \times C}$. This property is crucial, since it shows that a full-rank spatial filter has no influence on Riemannian distance. Using Riemannian geometry, calculus is already performed on the optimal feature space.

Another distance is the Log-Euclidean, which was introduced to alleviate the complexity involved in the computation of the affine-invariant Riemannian distance and its related mean (Arsigny et al. 2007). The mean associated to the Log-Euclidean distance corresponds to an arithmetic mean in the domain of matrix algorithm. The distance between two SPD matrices is expressed as

$$d_{\text{LE}}(\Sigma_1, \Sigma_2) = \left\| \text{Log}(\Sigma_1) - \text{Log}(\Sigma_2) \right\|_F, \tag{19.19}$$

and its associated mean is defined explicitly:

$$\bar{\Sigma}_{\text{LE}} = \text{Exp}\left(\frac{1}{I}\sum_{i=1}^{I} \log(\Sigma_i)\right). \tag{19.20}$$

Note that $d_{\text{LE}}$ can be interpreted as the Euclidean distance computed on the tangent plane at the identity matrix. Hence, this distance can be generalized as in Yger and Sugiyama (2015) to other reference points.

The distances presented above are summed up in Table 19.3.

### 19.4.4 Minimum Distance to Mean Classifier

The distances seen in Section 19.4.3 allow one to take into account the curvature of the space of SPD matrices. Nonetheless, to be able to exploit those Riemannian metric in the context of BCI, one needs to design an algorithm to discriminate between the different patterns in brain signals. One of the most simple classification algorithms consists in assigning a previously unseen signal to

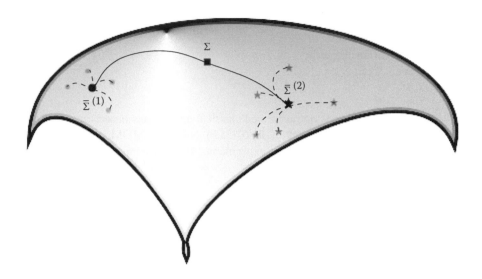

**FIGURE 19.5** Illustration of a two-class classification in the space of SPD matrices with the MDM algorithm.

the class with the closest mean. This implies a computation of means of classes and a measure of distances from the means.

The classifier *minimum distance to mean* (MDM), introduced in Barachant et al. (2010, 2012), is presented for multiclass classification.* It is a simple Bayesian classifier, under the hypotheses that classes have identical dispersions and that it is operating on a manageable space. The covariance matrices of EEG trials are classified based on their distance to the $k = 1,...,K$ centers of the classes $\overline{\Sigma}^{(k)}$, that is, means, medians, or centroids, as illustrated in Figure 19.5. The predicted class $k^*$ of the current matrix $\Sigma$ is defined as

$$k^* = \operatorname{argmin}_k \ d(\Sigma, \overline{\Sigma}^{(k)}). \tag{19.21}$$

As described in Algorithm 2, from $I$ labeled training trials $\left\{X_i\right\}_{i=1}^{I}$ recorded per subject, $K$ centers of classes $\overline{\Sigma}^{(k)}$ are estimated (step 3, detailed in Algorithm 1). A new unlabeled test trial $Z$ is predicted to belong to the class whose mean $\overline{\Sigma}^{(k)}$ is the closest to the trial covariance matrix, with respect to one of the distances from Table 19.3 (step 2).

**Algorithm 1: Offline Estimation of Riemannian Centers of Classes**

Inputs: $X_i \in \mathbb{R}^{C \times N}$, for $i = 1,...,I$, a set of labeled trials.
Inputs: $\mathcal{I}(k)$, a set of indices of trials belonging to class $k$.
Output: $\overline{\Sigma}^{(k)}, k = 1,...,K$, centers of classes.
   1: Compute covariance matrices $\Sigma_i$ of $X_i$
   2: **for** $k = 1$ **to** $K$ **do**
   3:      $\overline{\Sigma}^{(k)} = \mu\left(\left\{\Sigma_i \big| i \in \mathcal{I}(k)\right\}\right)$ (Equation 19.13)
   4: **end**
   5: **return** $\overline{\Sigma}^{(k)}$

---

* A sample code is available at https://git.io/vDVRB.

**Algorithm 2: Minimum Distance to Mean**

Inputs: $\overline{\Sigma}^{(k)}$, $K$ centers of classes from Algorithm 1.
Input: $Z \in \mathbb{R}^{C \times N}$, an unlabeled test trial.
Output: $k^*$, the predicted label of $Z$.
  1: Compute covariance matrix $\Sigma$ of $Z$
  2: $k^* = \text{argmin}_k \, d\left(\Sigma, \overline{\Sigma}^{(k)}\right)$
  3: **return** $k^*$

This very simple classifier has outperformed classical approaches based on spatial filtering and machine learning classifiers (Barachant et al. 2013a,b). Note that MDM is a classifier that can be applied offline or block-online (thus, in the experiments, these two cases will be grouped), but not online.

## 19.4.5 MDM FOR SSVEP

The MDM has been extended in Congedo (2013) and Congedo et al. (2013) for possible offline applications on SSVEP signals. For SSVEP classification, $K = F + 1$ classes are considered: one class for each target frequency, and one for the resting state.

To embed frequency information of SSVEP in the covariance matrices, we use a construction of matrices proposed in Congedo et al. (2013). Let $X \in \mathbb{R}^{C \times N}$ be an EEG trial measured on $C$ channels and $N$ samples in an SSVEP experiment with $F$ stimulus blinking at different frequencies. The covariance matrices are estimated* from a modified version of the input signal $X$:

$$X \in \mathbb{R}^{C \times N} \rightarrow \begin{bmatrix} X_{\text{freq}_1} \\ \vdots \\ X_{\text{freq}_F} \end{bmatrix} \in \mathbb{R}^{FC \times N}, \tag{19.22}$$

where $X_{\text{freq}_f}$ is the input signal $X$ band-pass filtered around frequency $\text{freq}_f$, $f = 1,\dots,F$. Henceforth, all EEG signals will be considered as filtered and modified by Equation 19.22, as shown in Figure 19.6. The associated covariance matrix $\Sigma \in \mathcal{M}_{FC}$ (i.e., a manifold of dimension $m = FC(FC + 1)/2$) is estimated using the Schäfer shrinkage estimator (Schäfer and Strimmer 2005), which was experimentally found to be the most adequate for the set of data used (Kalunga et al. 2016). These matrices are shown in Figure 19.7.

## 19.4.6 ONLINE MDM

The MDM algorithm as described above is suitable for offline and block-online BCI settings. Covariance matrices were computed from a reference time given by the cue onsets used to locate SSVEP occurrences. However, in an online and asynchronous setup, there is no cue onset, and EEG epochs are thus classified on the fly. In this section, we present an MDM online algorithm suitable for asynchronous BCI (Kalunga et al. 2016).

The algorithm identifies a period (i.e., time interval) in the online EEG $\mathcal{X} \in \mathbb{R}^{FC \times \mathcal{N}}$, where $\mathcal{N}$ is the number of recorded samples, associated with a high probability (above threshold) of observing an SSVEP at a specific frequency, as illustrated in Algorithm 3.

---

* A code example is available at https://git.io/vDVRI.

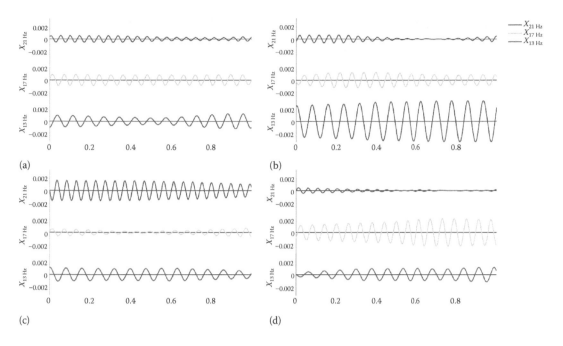

**FIGURE 19.6** Samples of EEG trials from Equation 19.22. For each sub-band $X_{\text{freq}_f}$, only channel $O_z$ is shown. Each subplot shows the first seconds of a trial from classes: (a) resting state, (b) 13 Hz, (c) 21 Hz, and (d) 17 Hz.

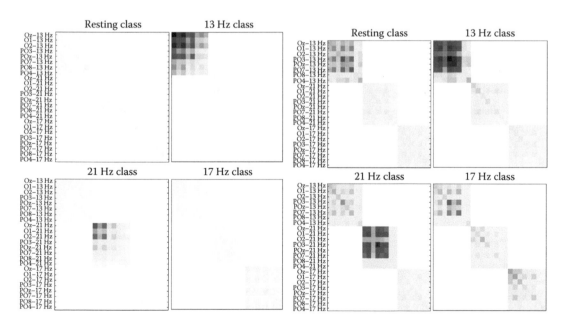

**FIGURE 19.7** Representations of covariance matrices: each image is the covariance matrix mean $\overline{\Sigma}^{(k)}$ of the class $k$, for one session of the recording. The diagonal blocks show the covariance in different frequency bands, that is, 13 Hz in the upper-left block, 21 Hz in the middle block, and 17 Hz in the bottom-right block. Subjects with the highest (left) and lowest (right) BCI performance.

**Algorithm 3: Online MDM**

Inputs: hyperparameters $w$, $\Delta n$, $D$, $\vartheta$.
Inputs: $\overline{\Sigma}^{(k)}$, $k = 1,\ldots,K$, centers of classes from Algorithm 2 (offline training).
Inputs: Online EEG recording $\mathcal{X}(n)$.
Output: $\tilde{k}(n)$, online predicted class.
    1: $d = 1$
    2: **for** $n = w$ **to** $\mathcal{N}$ **step** $\Delta n$
    3:      Epoch $X_d$ (Equation 19.23) and classify it with Algorithm 2
    4:      **if** $d \geq D$
    5:          Find the most recurrent class in $\mathcal{K} = k^*_{j \in \mathcal{J}(d)} \big| \overline{k} = \mathrm{argmax}_k \, \rho(k)$ (Equation 19.24)
    6:          **if** $\rho(\overline{k}) > \vartheta$
    7:              Compute $\tilde{\delta}_{\overline{k}}$ (Equation 19.25)
    8:              **if** $\tilde{\delta}_{\overline{k}} < 0$
    9:                 **return** $\tilde{k} = \overline{k}$
    10:          **end**
    11:      **end**
    12:    **end**
    13:    $d = d + 1$
    14: **end**

To locate this interval, we focus on the last $D$ recorded EEG overlapping epochs $\left\{ X_j \in \mathbb{R}^{FC \times \omega} \right\}_{j \in \mathcal{J}(d)}$, with the set of indices $\mathcal{J}(d) = d - D + 1,\ldots,d - 1, d$, where $d$ is the index of the current epoch $X_d$ in the online recording $\mathcal{X}(n)$. Epochs have size $w$, and the interval between two consecutive epochs is $\Delta n$, with $w > \Delta n$:

$$X_d = \mathcal{X}(n - w, \ldots, n). \tag{19.23}$$

To obtain the first $D$ epochs $X_{j \in \mathcal{J}(d)}$, at least $w + (D - 1)\Delta n$ samples of $\mathcal{X}$ should be recorded (step 4).

The classification outputs $k^*_{j \in \mathcal{J}(d)}$ obtained in step 3 by applying Algorithm 2 on $X_{j \in \mathcal{J}(d)}$ are stored in a vector $\mathcal{K}$, which always contains the latest $D$ classification outputs. The class that occurs the most in $\mathcal{K}$ (step 5), with an occurrence probability $\rho(k)$ above a defined threshold $\vartheta$, is considered to be the class, denoted $\overline{k}$, of the ongoing EEG recording $\mathcal{X}(n)$. The vector $\rho$ is defined as

$$\rho(k) = \frac{\#\left\{ k^*_{j \in \mathcal{J}(d)} = k \right\}}{D}, \text{ for } k = 1, \ldots, K, \tag{19.24}$$

with $k^* = \mathrm{argmax}_k \, \rho(k)$; then, $\rho(\overline{k})$ is compared to the threshold $\vartheta$. If $\vartheta$ is not reached within the last $D$ epochs, the classification output is held back, and the sliding process continues until $\vartheta$ is reached. In the last $D$ epochs, once a class $\overline{k}$ has been identified, a curve direction criterion is introduced to enforce the robustness of the result. For class $\overline{k}$ to be validated, this criterion requires that the direction taken by the displacement of covariance matrices $\Sigma_{j \in \mathcal{J}(d)}$ be toward the center of class $\overline{\Sigma}^{(\overline{k})}$. Hence, $\tilde{\delta}_{\overline{k}}$, the sum of gradients (i.e., differentials) of the curve made by distances from $\Sigma_{j \in \mathcal{J}(d)}$ to $\overline{\Sigma}^{(\overline{k})}$, should be negative (step 8):

$$\tilde{\delta}_{\bar{k}} = \sum_{j \in \mathcal{J}(d)} \frac{\Delta \delta_{\bar{k}}(j)}{\Delta j} = \sum_{j=d-D+2}^{d} \delta_{\bar{k}}(j) - \delta_{\bar{k}}(j-1) < 0$$

$$\text{with } \delta_{\bar{k}}(j) = \frac{\delta\left(\Sigma_j, \overline{\Sigma}^{(\bar{k})}\right)}{\sum_{k=1}^{K} \delta\left(\Sigma_j, \overline{\Sigma}^{(k)}\right)}. \tag{19.25}$$

The occurrence criterion is inspired by the dynamic stopping of Verschore et al. (2012); there is no fixed trial length for classification. The occurrence criterion ensures that the detected user intention is unaffected by any short time disturbances attributed to noise or subject inattention, as presented in Algorithm 3. This approach offers a good trade-off to obtain robust results within a short and flexible time.

The curve direction criterion solves both the problem of latency in the EEG synchronization and the problem of the delays inserted by the EEG epochs processing. Indeed, some EEG epochs gather signals from different classes, that is, intermediary states, and might be wrongly classified if the decision is solely based on the distance with the center of the class. This situation and the effect of the curve direction criterion are shown in Figure 19.8. The colors in the figure show the classification result before the curve direction criteria. Ensuring that the covariance matrices are displaced toward the center of the detected class provides a guarantee that it matches the current EEG state. Inversely, if the direction of the curve is moving away from the center of the detected class, it might indicate that there has been a change in the EEG state that has not been detected.

Algorithm 3 has four hyperparameters: $w$, $\Delta n$, $D$, $\vartheta$. For the results of online classification presented in Table 19.5, they are set through cross validation to $D = 5$, $\vartheta = 0.7$, $w = 2.6$, $\Delta n = 0.2$.

Although a large window size $w$ is expected to increase the classification accuracy, it increases the response time, thus reducing the time resolution, and extends the overlap between different EEG states. The step size $\Delta n$ should be set to a minimum value to allow a maximum number of overlapping epochs ($D$) within a short time. However, it should be large enough to avoid too many calculations within a time interval with small or inexistent changes in EEG states. If the number of epochs $D$ is too small, the classification will be sensitive to nonintentional and abrupt changes in

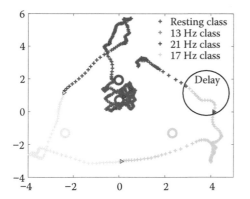 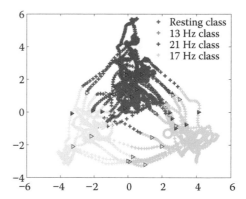

**FIGURE 19.8** Covariance matrices trajectory during a four-class SSVEP online recording. The circles represent class centers. The triangles mark the beginning of a new trial in the experiment, whose true class is indicated by the triangle's color. The colors of the crosses show the class identified by MDM before the curve direction criterion is applied. The plot on the left shows the first seven trials. The first three trials are from the resting class, the remaining are class 13, 17, and 21 Hz, respectively. The plot on the right shows the entire recording. Data are taken from the subject with the highest BCI performance.

the EEG. A very large $D$ will increase the momentum and reinforce the influence of the past EEG signals. It should also be mentioned that both the occurrence and the curve direction criteria cannot have a significant impact if the value of $D$ is too small. The probability threshold parameter $\vartheta$ acts like a rejection parameter: high $\vartheta$ values correspond to a high rejection rate.

## 19.5 EXPERIMENTAL EVALUATION ON SSVEP DATA SET

### 19.5.1 SSVEP DATA SET DESCRIPTION

To assess the covariance estimators, a benchmark is proposed on real SSVEP data set; this data set is freely available.* The signals are recorded from 12 subjects during an SSVEP experiment. EEG is measured on $C = 8$ channels: $O_Z$, $O_1$, $O_2$, $PO_Z$, $PO_3$, $PO_4$, $PO_7$, and $PO_8$. The ground and the reference electrodes were placed on $F_Z$ and the right hear mastoid, respectively. The acquisition rate is $T_s = 256$ Hz on a gTec MobiLab Amp (gTec, Graz, Austria). The subjects are presented with $F = 3$ visual target stimuli blinking respectively at freq = 13, 17, and 21 Hz. It is a $K = 4$ classes BCI setup made of the $F = 3$ stimulus classes and one resting class (no-SSVEP). In a session, which lasts 5 min, 32 trials are recorded: 8 for each visual stimulus and 8 for the resting class. The number of sessions recorded per subject varies from 2 to 5. Thus, the longest EEG recorded for a single subject is 25 min or 160 trials. The trial length is 6 s, that is, $N = 6 \times T_s = 1536$ samples. For each subject, a test set is made of 32 trials, whereas the remaining trials (which might vary from 32 to 128) make up the training set.

### 19.5.2 EVALUATION OF THE COVARIANCE ESTIMATORS

The effectiveness of covariance matrix estimators is evaluated for SSVEP signals. The evaluation is done in terms of classification accuracy, and the conditioning of covariance matrices is also investigated. A bootstrapping with 1000 replications is performed to assess the performances of each estimator. Estimators are compared on 10 trial lengths $t \in \{0.5, 1.0, \ldots 5.0\}$ s, as these are known to affect the estimators' performance. Here, $N \in \{128, 256, \ldots, 1280\}$ is computed as $N = t \times T_s$.

Figure 19.9 shows the classification accuracy of each estimator computed across all subjects. Even if the error bars show an important intersubject variability, the increase in the accuracy can be attributed to the fact that the relevant patterns in EEG accumulate with the trial length, producing better estimation of the covariance matrices. This is known to be particularly true for the SCM estimator, and it could be seen in Figure 19.9. It appears that shrinkage estimators (especially Ledoit and Schäfer) are less affected by the reduction of epoch sizes than the other estimators. This is a direct consequence of the regularization between the sample covariance matrices and the targeted (expected) covariance matrix of independent variables.

For computational purposes, it is important to look at the matrix conditioning. Figure 19.10 shows the ratio $\mathcal{C}$ between the largest and smallest eigenvalues: in well-conditioned matrices, $\mathcal{C}$ is small. Shrinkage estimators offer better conditioned matrices whereas the SCM, NSCM, and fixed-point matrices are ill-conditioned below 2 s of trial length and may result in singular matrices.

It appears in Figures 19.9 and 19.10 that the shrinkage estimator, especially the Ledoit–Wolfe and the Schäfer ones, are a good choice to obtain robust and accurate results, even if the covariance matrices are estimated on a small number of samples. This is an important aspect, as the processing time induces a delay in the processing and should thus be reduced to provide responsive HMI.

---

* Data could be freely downloaded from https://github.com/sylvchev/dataset-ssvep-exoskeleton.

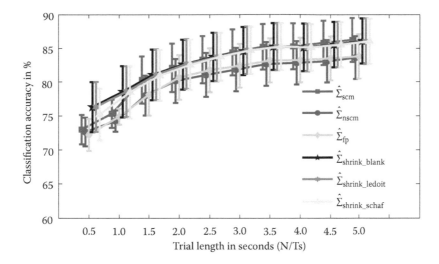

**FIGURE 19.9** Comparison of covariance estimators in terms of classification accuracy obtained with offline MDRM with increasing EEG trial length. For each trial length, the accuracy mean ± SD across all subjects and across all replications is shown.

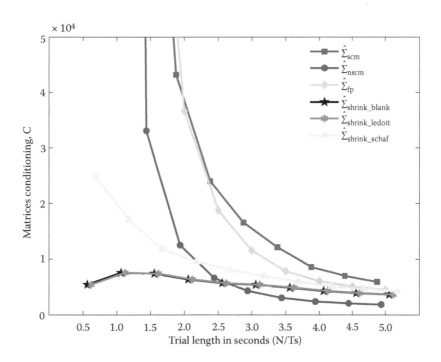

**FIGURE 19.10** Covariance matrices condition expressed as the ratio $\mathcal{C}$ between the largest and smallest eigenvalues for the different covariance estimators. The comparison is made with increasing EEG trial length.

**TABLE 19.4**
**Offline Algorithms for SSVEP Classification**

| | CCA | | | | MDM | | | | | |
| | Lin et al. | | Nakanishi et al. | | Euclidean | | Log-Euclidean | | Affine-Invariant | |
| | Acc (%) | ITR (bpm) | Acc (%) | ITR (bpm) | Acc (%) | ITR (bpm) | Acc (%) | ITR (bpm) | Acc (%) | ITR (bpm) |
|---|---|---|---|---|---|---|---|---|---|---|
| S1 | 91.7 | 16.3 | 67.6 | 3.5 | 71.6 | 6.6 | 86.2 | 13.1 | 84.7 | 12.22 |
| S2 | 45.8 | 0.7 | 66.0 | 3.2 | 46.7 | 0.8 | 77.4 | 8.8 | 79.4 | 9.79 |
| S3 | 100.0 | 23.8 | 90.2 | 10.3 | 83.6 | 11.6 | 99.2 | 22.7 | 99.3 | 22.7 |
| S4 | 97.9 | 21.3 | 78.3 | 6.1 | 66.2 | 4.9 | 89.7 | 15.0 | 89.7 | 15.05 |
| S5 | 83.3 | 11.5 | 76.0 | 5.5 | 46.5 | 0.8 | 85.7 | 12.7 | 89.5 | 14.94 |
| S6 | 77.1 | 8.7 | 72.2 | 4.5 | 46.64 | 0.8 | 84.5 | 12.1 | 87.2 | 13.63 |
| S8 | 97.9 | 21.3 | 90.4 | 10.3 | 80.5 | 10.2 | 98.9 | 22.3 | 99.7 | 23.2 |
| S9 | 91.7 | 16.3 | 64.0 | 2.8 | 68.2 | 5.5 | 83.3 | 11.5 | 85.8 | 12.8 |
| S10 | 80.2 | 10.0 | 79.2 | 6.4 | 53.9 | 1.9 | 90.9 | 15.8 | 93.1 | 17.3 |
| S11 | 89.6 | 15.0 | 54.8 | 1.4 | 56.2 | 2.4 | 77.4 | 8.8 | 78.2 | 9.2 |
| S12 | 95.8 | 19.4 | 82.3 | 7.4 | 82.9 | 11.2 | 97.8 | 21.2 | 98.6 | 22.0 |
| Mean | 87.5 ± 15.1 | 15.5 ± 6.8 | 81.2 ± 14.1 | 11.8 ± 6.0 | 65.1 ± 9.5 | 5.5 ± 4.2 | 89.2 ± 4.9 | 15.5 ± 5.2 | 90.4 ± 7.8 | 16.3 ± 5.3 |

*Note:* Offline performance in terms of accuracy and ITR of five methods are compared: (1) CCA approach introduced by Lin et al. (2006), (2) CCA approach introduced by Nakanishi et al. (2014), (3) MDM approach with Euclidean mean and distance, (4) MDM with Log-Euclidean mean and distance, and (5) MDM with affine-invariant distance and mean as described in Algorithm 2.

### 19.5.3 OFFLINE CLASSIFICATION OF SSVEP

Table 19.4 shows the offline classification accuracy for each subject obtained by the application of the MDM described in Section 19.4.4. The distances and mean listed in Table 19.3 are used: Euclidean, Log-Euclidean, and affine-invariant Riemannian. The performance of MDM approaches is compared to two CCA-based state-of-the-art methods proposed by Lin et al. (2006) and Nakanishi et al. (2014). In the implementation of these methods, the epochs are taken from $\tau_0 + 2$ s, where $\tau_0$ is the start time of the trial.

The MDM approach with Riemannian distances outperforms both CCA-based methods with an average classification accuracy of 89.2% ± 4.9% and an ITR of 15.52 ± 5.2 bits/min for the Log-Euclidean, and 90.4% ± 7.8% and 16.3 ± 5.3 bits/min for the AIR. The method by Lin et al. ranks third with 87.5% ± 15.1% and 15.5 ± 6.8 bits/min. The method proposed by Nakanishi et al., which could be expected to achieve better results as reported in Nakanishi et al. (2014), only ranks fourth. This is mainly due to the fact that this method requires information on the phase of the stimuli. In fact, Nakanishi et al. use the average of all training trials belonging to a unique class as a reference signal in the CCA. When SSVEP trials belonging to a unique trial are not in-phase, which is the case in the current work, averaging them will cancel the signal. The MDM approach with Euclidean distance has the lowest performance. This shows how inappropriate it is to use Euclidean geometry on covariance matrices as they lie on a curved space.

### 19.5.4 ONLINE CLASSIFICATION OF SSVEP

For online implementation, the different algorithms are compared in terms of classification accuracy. The performances achieved using online MDM with the distances mentioned in Table 19.3

are compared to the two state-of-the-art methods, CCA+SVM and FBCCA, both described in Section 19.3.2. For these methods, the number of harmonics is set to $N_h = 6$. This value maximizes the classification accuracy of standard CCA in an offline analysis on training data. In CCA+SVM, the EEG is filtered between 13 and 126 Hz to accommodate all six harmonics. In FBCCA, the $N_b$ sub-bands are constructed such that the $n$th sub-band starts from $n \times 8$ Hz and ends at 93 Hz, that is, 10 times the stimuli frequency range of 8 Hz (i.e., 13 to 21 Hz). Parameters $a$, $b$ and $N_b$ from Equations 19.6 and 19.5 were set to 2, 0, and 3, respectively, through a grid search where their values were respectively limited to $a = 0.25 \times i_a$, with $i_a = 0, 1, ..., 40$, $b = 0.25 \times i_b$, with $i_b = 0, 1, ..., 4$, and $N_b = i_N$, with $i_N = 1, ..., 7$.

Table 19.5 summarizes results obtained for each subject and each method. Using AIR distance significantly improves classification performances (81.27%), in comparison with the state-of-the-art CCA-based methods that have an average performance across subjects of 70.45% and 72.56% for CCA+SVM and FBCCA, respectively, and in comparison to the MDM with Euclidean distance that has an average performance across subjects of 52.83%. Relying on CCA coefficients for classification, as in the classic CCA method (Lin et al. 2006) or as in FBCCA (Chen et al. 2015), has a strong limitation as it could not account for the reject class. As the reject class does not have a specific reference signal, it is not possible to determine the correlation coefficients associated with this class. This limitation disqualifies the FBCCA for any real implementation of BCI and avoids confronting the most challenging case (identifying when the user does not look at any stimulus) from a machine learning perspective. Nonetheless, to propose a thorough comparison with the existing approaches, we provide the results obtained with FBCCA without including the resting-state (no-SSVEP) class.

This experiment on real EEG data shows that it is crucial to process covariance matrices with dedicated Riemannian tools, affecting the efficiency of the classification. The obtained results show that the simple MDM classification scheme used within the Riemannian framework outperforms CCA-based state-of-the-art methods for SSVEP classification. With only four classes (three SSVEP stimulation frequencies and a reject class), this experiment does not aim at improving the ITR of the BCI system.

**TABLE 19.5**
**Online Algorithms for SSVEP Classification**

| Sub. | CCA+SVM Kalunga et al. Acc (%) | FBCCA Chen et al. Acc (%) | Online MDM Euclidean Acc (%) | Online MDM Log-Euclidean Acc (%) | Online MDM Affine-Invariant Acc (%) |
|---|---|---|---|---|---|
| 1 | 54.68 | 75.00 | 53.12 | 71.88 | 73.44 |
| 2 | 37.50 | 41.67 | 43.75 | 78.13 | 79.69 |
| 3 | 89.06 | 85.42 | 67.19 | 85.94 | 85.93 |
| 4 | 79.69 | 97.92 | 54.68 | 84.38 | 87.50 |
| 5 | 50.00 | 64.58 | 37.50 | 62.50 | 68.75 |
| 6 | 87.50 | 75.00 | 34.37 | 84.38 | 85.94 |
| 7 | 77.08 | 80.56 | 60.42 | 87.50 | 88.54 |
| 8 | 73.44 | 72.92 | 67.19 | 90.63 | 92.19 |
| 9 | 60.94 | 66.67 | 57.81 | 70.31 | 70.31 |
| 10 | 67.97 | 65.62 | 38.28 | 75.00 | 80.47 |
| 11 | 71.88 | 64.58 | 48.44 | 60.94 | 65.63 |
| 12 | 95.63 | 80.83 | 71.25 | 96.25 | 96.69 |
| Mean | 70.45 ± 16.5 | 72.56 ± 13.3 | 52.83 ± 12.0 | 78.98 ± 10.6 | 81.27 ± 9.5 |

*Note:* Subject classification accuracies [Acc (%)] elapsed for the classification of a single trial. Classification is performed with MDM using either Euclidean or Riemannian means (see Table 19.3).

## 19.6 CONCLUSIONS

In this chapter, we have reviewed the different algorithms and implementations for feature extraction in SSVEP-based BCI. The spatial covariance, which describes the relative changes observed between the electrodes, plays a key role in the success of the state-of-the-art approaches. This observation also applies for several EEG-based BCIs, such as systems relying on ERP or MI. SSVEP offers promising results, as it is suggested by the fact that the highest ITR reported in the literature is using SSRs. It is thus important to use the appropriate tools and algorithms when building up such a BCI system, to ensure that all the signal processing chain could work in online or block-online settings.

To estimate correctly the covariance from the data, a trade-off should be sought between accuracy and temporal precision: using some large time windows to estimate covariance allows one to compute accurate and well-conditioned matrices at the expense of time resolution. Using an adequate estimator, it is possible to use smaller time windows (on the order of 1 or 2 s) for estimating covariance, while avoiding ill-conditioned matrices. One should keep in mind that this trade-off has a direct impact on the system reactivity and on the precision for online settings. The delay introduced by the covariance estimation lowers the ITR: this has a strong incidence on the HMI aspect and it should be taken into account when designing experiments.

In the BCI literature, most of the studies propose offline analyses, which are of interest for a better understanding of the neurological phenomena. But offline implementations are not suitable to design a BCI as they need information from the whole session to extract features and to provide classification decisions. Converting offline algorithms to online ones is not an easy task, and it systematically has a negative impact on the classification accuracy.

A common approach is to rely on spatial filters that are carefully tuned during a calibration session. The system could then work online, applying the learned spatial filters on the acquired signal. The main disadvantage of these filters is that they are user specific and session specific. Moreover, these filters are best exploited when dealing with a clean signal, without artifacts, constraining the experiments to be conducted in a strongly controlled environment. Riemannian approaches offer different methods that are efficient and more robust to noise. The algorithms could be relatively simple, such as the MDRM classifiers. Note that the online MDM introduced here for SSVEP data could be applied identically to MI-based BCI.

Future work on this topic could range from very practical works and theoretical advances. For example, it is possible to improve the MDM classifier, taking into account various information about the subject. Another possibility is to investigate the distribution of covariance matrices on the manifold, as suggested in the work of Zanini et al. (2016) or Gayraud et al. (2016). From a machine learning point of view, there are still many open questions on the possibilities to include transfer learning to cope with session-to-session or intersubject variability (Waytowich et al. 2016).

## REFERENCES

Absil, P.-A., R. Mahony, and R. Sepulchre. 2009. *Optimization Algorithms on Matrix Manifolds*. Princeton University Press.

Ando, T., C.-K. Li, and R. Mathias. 2004. Geometric means. *Linear Algebra and Its Applications* 385: 305–334.

Arsigny, V., P. Fillard, X. Pennec, and N. Ayache. 2007. Geometric means in a novel vector space structure on symmetric positive-definite matrices. *SIAM Journal on Matrix Analysis and Applications* 29(1): 328–347.

Barachant, A., A. Andreev, and M. Congedo. 2013a. The Riemannian Potato: An automatic and adaptive artifact detection method for online experiments using Riemannian geometry. In *Proceedings of TOBI Workshop IV*, 19–20.

Barachant, A., S. Bonnet, M. Congedo, and C. Jutten. 2010. Riemannian geometry applied to BCI classification. In *Latent Variable Analysis and Signal Separation*, 629–636. Springer.

Barachant, A., S. Bonnet, M. Congedo, and C. Jutten. 2012. Multiclass brain–computer interface classification by Riemannian geometry. *Biomedical Engineering, IEEE Transactions on* 59(4): 920–928.

Barachant, A., S. Bonnet, M. Congedo, and C. Jutten. 2013b. Classification of covariance matrices using a Riemannian-based kernel for BCI applications. *Neurocomputing* 112: 172–178.

Bhatia, R. 2009. *Positive Definite Matrices*. Princeton University Press.

Blankertz, B., S. Lemm, M. Treder, S. Haufe, and K.-R. Müller. 2011. Single-trial analysis and classification of ERP components: A tutorial. *NeuroImage* 56(2): 814–825.

Chen, X., Y. Wang, S. Gao, T.-P. Jung, and X. Gao. 2015. Filter bank canonical correlation analysis for implementing a high-speed SSVEP-based brain–computer interface. *Journal of Neural Engineering* 12(4): 46008.

Congedo, M. 2013. EEG source analysis. Habilitation à diriger des recherches, Université de Grenoble.

Congedo, M., A. Barachant, and A. Andreev. 2013. A new generation of brain–computer interface based on Riemannian geometry. *arXiv Preprint arXiv:1310.8115*.

Congedo, M., A. Barachant, and R. Bathia. 2017. Riemannian geometry for EEG-based brain–computer interfaces: A primer and a review. *Brain–Computer Interfaces*, 1–20. doi:10.1080/2326263X.2017.1297192.

Fisher, R.S., G. Harding, G. Erba, G.L. Barkley, A. Wilkins, and Epilepsy Foundation of America Working Group. 2005. Photic- and pattern-induced seizures: A review for the Epilepsy Foundation of America Working Group. *Epilepsia* 46(9): 1426–1441. doi:10.1111/j.1528-1167.2005.31405.x.

Fletcher, P.T., C. Lu, S.M. Pizer, and S. Joshi. 2004. Principal geodesic analysis for the study of nonlinear statistics of shape. *Medical Imaging, IEEE Transactions on* 23(8): 995–1005.

Fukunaga, K. 1990. *Introduction to Statistical Pattern Recognition*. Academic Press.

Gayraud, N., N. Foy, and M. Clerc. 2016. A separability marker based on high-dimensional statistics for classification confidence assessment. In *IEEE International Conference on Systems, Man, and Cybernetics*.

Hardoon, D.R., S. Szedmak, and J. Shaw-Taylor. 2004. Canonical correlation analysis: An overview with application to learning methods. *Neural Computation* 16: 2639–2664.

Herrmann, C.S. 2001. Human EEG responses to 1–100 Hz flicker: Resonance phenomena in visual cortex and their potential correlation to cognitive phenomena. *Experimental Brain Research* 137: 346–353.

Hotelling, H. 1936. Relations between two sets of variates. *Biometrika* 28 (3/4): 321–377. doi:10.2307/2333955.

Jayasumana, S., R. Hartley, M. Salzmann, H. Li, and M. Harandi. 2013. Kernel methods on the Riemannian manifold of symmetric positive definite matrices. In *Computer Vision and Pattern Recognition (CVPR), 2013 IEEE Conference on*, 73–80. IEEE.

Kalunga, E.K., S. Chevallier, Q. Barthélemy, K. Djouani, Y. Hamam, and E. Monacelli. 2015. From Euclidean to Riemannian means: Information geometry for SSVEP classification. In *Geometric Science of Information*, edited by F. Nielsen and F. Barbaresco, 595–604. Springer International Publishing.

Kalunga, E.K., S. Chevallier, Q. Barthélemy, K. Djouani, E. Monacelli, and Y. Hamam. 2016. Online SSVEP-based BCI using Riemannian geometry. *Neurocomputing* 191: 55–68.

Kalunga, E.K., K. Djouani, Y. Hamam, S. Chevallier, and E. Monacelli. 2013. SSVEP enhancement based on canonical correlation analysis to improve BCI performances. In *AFRICON, 2013*, 1–5. doi:10.1109/AFRCON.2013.6757776.

Karcher, H. 2014. Riemannian center of mass and so called Karcher mean. *arXiv Preprint arXiv:1407.2087*. http://arxiv.org/abs/1407.2087.

Ledoit, O., and M. Wolf. 2004. A well-conditioned estimator for large-dimensional covariance matrices. *Journal of Multivariate Analysis* 88(2): 365–411.

Li, Y., and K.M. Wong. 2013. Riemannian distances for signal classification by power spectral density. *IEEE Journal of Selected Topics in Signal Processing* 7(4): 655–669.

Li, Y., K.M. Wong, and H. De Bruin. 2012. Electroencephalogram signals classification for sleepstate decision: A Riemannian geometry approach. *Signal Processing, IET* 6(4): 288–299.

Lim, Y., and M. Pálfia. 2012. Matrix power means and the Karcher mean. *Journal of Functional Analysis* 262(4): 1498–1514.

Lin, Z., C. Zhang, W. Wu, and X. Gao. 2006. Frequency recognition based on canonical correlation analysis for SSVEP-based BCIs. *Biomedical Engineering, IEEE Transactions on* 53(12): 2610–2614.

Liu, Q., K. Chen, Q. Ai, and S.Q. Xie. 2014. Review: Recent development of signal processing algorithms for SSVEP-based brain computer interfaces. *Journal of Medical and Biological Engineering* 34: 299–309.

Lotte, F. 2011. Generating artificial EEG signals to reduce BCI calibration time. In *5th International Brain–Computer Interface Workshop*, 176–179.

Moakher, M. 2005. A differential geometric approach to the geometric mean of symmetric positive-definite matrices. *SIAM Journal on Matrix Analysis and Applications* 26(3): 735–747.

Morgan, S.T., J.C. Hansen, and S.A. Hillyard. 1996. Selective attention to stimulus location modulates the steady-state visual evoked potential. *Proceedings of the National Academy of Sciences* 93(10): 4770–4774.

Müller, M.M., S. Andersen, N.J. Trujillo, P. Valdés-Sosa, P. Malinowski, and S.A. Hillyard. 2006. Feature-selective attention enhances color signals in early visual areas of the human brain. *Proceedings of the National Academy of Sciences* 103(38): 14250–14254.

Nakanishi, M., Y. Wang, Y.-T. Wang, Y. Mitsukura, and T.-P. Jung. 2014. A high-speed brain speller using steady-state visual evoked potentials. *International Journal of Neural Systems* 24(6): 1450019.

Niedermeyer, E., and F. Lopes da Silva. 2004. *Electroencephalography: Basic Principles, Clinical Applications, and Related Fields*. 5th ed. Lippincott Williams & Wilkins.

Pascal, F., P. Forster, J.-P. Ovarlez, and P. Arzabal. 2005. Theoretical analysis of an improved covariance matrix estimator in non-Gaussian noise. In *IEEE International Conference on Acoustics, Speech, and Signal Processing (ICASSP)*. Vol. 4.

Pastor, M.A., J. Artieda, J. Arbizu, M. Valencia, and J.C. Masdeu. 2003. Human cerebral activation during steady-state visual-evoked responses. *The Journal of Neuroscience* 23(37): 11621–11627.

Pennec, X., and N. Ayache. 1998. Uniform distribution, distance and expectation problems for geometric features processing. *Journal of Mathematical Imaging and Vision* 9(1): 49–67.

Regan, D. 1982. Comparison of transient and steady-state methods. *Annals of the New York Academy of Sciences* 388(1): 45–71.

Schäfer, J., and K. Strimmer. 2005. A shrinkage approach to large-scale covariance matrix estimation and implications for functional genomics. *Statistical Applications in Genetics and Molecular Biology* 4(1).

Stawicki, P., F. Gembler, and I. Volosyak. 2017. *Brain Computer Interfaces Handbook: Technological and Theoretical Advances*, edited by Lotte, Nam, and Nijholt. CRC Press.

Takahashi, T. 2004. *Electroencephalography: Basic Principles, Clinical Applications, and Related Fields*. 5th ed., 241–262. Lippincott Williams & Wilkins.

Tomioka, R., K. Aihara, and K.-R. Müller. 2007. Logistic regression for single trial EEG classification. In *Advances in Neural Information Processing Systems (NIPS)*, 19: 1377–1384.

Verschore, H., P.-J. Kindermans, D. Verstraeten, and B. Schrauwen. 2012. Dynamic stopping improves the speed and accuracy of a P300 speller. In *Artificial Neural Networks and Machine Learning—ICANN 2012*, 661–668. Springer.

Vialatte, F.-B., M. Maurice, J. Dauwels, and A. Cichocki. 2010. Steady-state visually evoked potentials: Focus on essential paradigms and future perspectives. *Progress in Neurobiology* 90(4): 418–438.

Waytowich, N.R., V.J. Lawhern, A.W. Bohannon, K.R. Ball, and B.J. Lance. 2016. Spectral transfer learning using information geometry for a user-independent brain–computer interface. *Frontiers in Neuroscience* 10.

Wolpaw, J., N. Birbaumer, D.J. McFarland, G. Pfurtscheller, and T.M. Vaughan. 2002. Brain–computer interfaces for communication and control. *Clinical Neurophysiology* 113(6): 767–791. doi:10.1016/S1388-2457(02)00057-3.

Yger, F. 2013. A review of kernels on covariance matrices for BCI applications. In *Machine Learning for Signal Processing (MLSP), 2013 IEEE International Workshop on*, 1–6. IEEE.

Yger, F., M. Berar, and F. Lotte. 2017. Riemannian approaches in brain–computer interfaces: A review. *IEEE Transactions on Neural Systems and Rehabilitation Engineering* (to appear).

Yger, F., and M. Sugiyama. 2015. Supervised LogEuclidean Metric Learning for Symmetric Positive Definite Matrices. *arXiv Preprint arXiv:1502.03505*.

Zanini, P., M. Congedo, C. Jutten, S. Said, and Y. Berthoumieu. 2016. Parameters estimate of Riemannian Gaussian distribution in the manifold of covariance matrices. In *IEEE Sensor Array and Multichannel Signal Processing Workshop*.

Zhu, D., J. Bieger, G.G. Molina, and R.M. Aarts. 2010. A survey of stimulation methods used in SSVEP-based BCIs. *Computational Intelligence and Neuroscience* 2010: 1–12.

# 20 The Fundamentals of Signal Processing for Evoked Potential BCIs: *A Guided Tutorial*

*Garett D. Johnson and Dean J. Krusienski*

## CONTENTS

20.1 Introduction ..................................................................................................398
20.2 Four-Class P300 Oddball .............................................................................398
    20.2.1 Data Collection ................................................................................398
    20.2.2 Data Preprocessing .........................................................................398
    20.2.3 Data Segmentation and Feature Extraction ....................................399
    20.2.4 Classifier Training ...........................................................................401
    20.2.5 Classification....................................................................................401
    20.2.6 Considerations .................................................................................402
20.3 $n$-Class SSVEP ...........................................................................................402
    20.3.1 Data Collection ................................................................................403
    20.3.2 Data Preprocessing .........................................................................404
    20.3.3 Data Segmentation and Classification ............................................404
    20.3.4 Considerations .................................................................................405
Acknowledgments....................................................................................................405
References.................................................................................................................405

**Abstract**

This chapter presents the implementation of several electroencephalogram (EEG)-based brain–computer interface (BCI) signal processing approaches for evoked potentials. Sample code is provided for two well-established BCI paradigms: (1) P300 Oddball and (2) Steady-State Visual Evoked Potentials (SSVEP). These examples can be straightforwardly extended to more sophisticated designs employing evoked potentials.

1. Transient Evoked Potentials: Four-class P300 Oddball BCI (synchronous operation with discrete selections)
2. Steady-state evoked potentials: $n$-class SSVEP (steady-state visually evoked potential) BCI (asynchronous operation with discrete selections)

## 20.1 INTRODUCTION

This chapter provides an introductory tutorial on how to implement several fundamental electro-encephalogram (EEG)-based brain–computer interface (BCI) processing approaches for evoked potentials using MATLAB®. The examples are intended to provide a simplified, hands-on frame-work for better understanding the basic structure and parameters used for BCI processing appli-cations. Two examples will be presented, which are representative of common BCI processing scenarios and can be straightforwardly extended to more specific and complex scenarios:

1. Transient Evoked Potentials: Four-class P300 Oddball BCI (synchronous operation with discrete selections)
2. Steady-state evoked potentials: $n$-class steady-state visually evoked potential (SSVEP) BCI (asynchronous operation with discrete selections)

## 20.2 FOUR-CLASS P300 ODDBALL

This scenario is based on the classical P300 oddball where stimuli (visual, auditory, or tactile) are presented sequentially and one of the stimuli is to be selected as the target (Farwell & Donchin 1988). In this case, four stimuli are repeatedly presented in block-wise random order. The target stimuli elicit a charac-teristic P300 response, whereas the nontarget stimuli should not elicit the same neural behavior. A classi-fier can then be trained in order to distinguish between the target and nontarget stimuli. A segment of the data, denoted as a response, is collected after every stimulus. Multiple responses are collected for a given stimulus and averaged to increase the reliability of response detection. The averaged response for each stimulus is input into a classifier to determine which stimulus was a target, that is, elicited a characteristic P300 response. Classifier calibration is typically required before online operation. When collecting the calibration data, the user is instructed which stimulus to focus on. This is done so that the responses can be properly labeled in order to train the classifier to a given user. The following basic scenario can be generalized to the P300 speller and other variants. Next, the typical scenario during operation is detailed.

### 20.2.1 DATA COLLECTION

The characteristic P300 event-related potential (ERP) response is typically found to be strongest over the parietal lobe. Additional relevant neural information can also be found in areas over the occipital lobe, especially when the stimuli are presented visually. The typical setup for a P300 visual oddball BCI includes electrode coverage over Fz, Cz, Pz, P3, P4, PO7, PO8, and Oz. EEG data from these channels are collected synchronously using stimulus presentation software that time locks the stimulus events to the EEG, for example, BCI2000 and Psychtoolbox. The sampling rate should be kept above roughly 100 Hz in order to accurately reflect the time progression of the P300 waveform. Here, we assume the data to be loaded into MATLAB in a matrix format of $k$ samples × $n$ channels. We also assume that there is a vector of length $k$ denoting the start of each stimulus, with zeros everywhere excepting "1" through "4" where a stimulus starts. An additional vector of length $k$ is also necessary to record during the collection of calibration data, where a "1" represents the presentation of a target oddball stimulus, and zeros everywhere else.

### 20.2.2 DATA PREPROCESSING

The data can be band-pass filtered between 0.1 Hz and approximately 20 to 30 Hz, and then deci-mated. Care must be taken to accordingly downsample the label vectors to match the rate of the signal. This frequency range was chosen as it still allows for an accurate representation of the dynamics of the EEG ERPs while limiting the number of temporal data points that will ultimately be used as features in our classifier. This smoothing of the data often helps to prevent overfitting of classifiers. Additionally, there is a computational advantage to starting with a smaller feature space, but with modern computing capabilities, this is becoming less of an issue. Once the data have been preprocessed, the next step is to extract the useful features from the EEG data.

### 20.2.3 Data Segmentation and Feature Extraction

Below is a sample MATLAB function that takes a labeled EEG signal matrix (EEGsignal) and outputs a MATLAB structure containing a matrix of ERPs corresponding to each stimulus label (StimulusCode). Section 1 determines the sample index corresponding to the onset of each stimulus, in this case the transition of StimulusCode from 0 to any label 1–4. The ERPwindow input argument defines the number of samples before and after each stimulus that contains the desired ERP window (this can be converted to milliseconds based on the sampling rate if desired). The ERP windows will be positioned at each stimulus transition. For example, assuming a sampling rate of 100 Hz and a P300 paradigm, a reasonable window would be −100 to 800 ms in order to capture the entire temporal dynamics of the ERP. In this case, an ERPwindow = [−10 80] would collect 10 samples before and 80 samples after each stimulus onset for a total of 91 samples representing each ERP (counting the zeroth sample). Samples collected before the stimulus onset can be used to correct for baseline signal shifts before the stimuli. The final two lines of the function extract the stimulus and type labels for each ERP in the resulting matrix for use in classifier training and validation. It should be noted that the functions in this chapter do not include any error or exception checking. It is left to the user to ensure that the input arguments and variables are properly constructed and configured for specific application scenarios (e.g., window positions should not exceed the length of the signal, etc.). Refer to Figure 20.1 for a graphical depiction of the variables.

```
function [ERPs]=GetERPs(EEGsignal,StimulusCode,StimulusType,ERPwindow)

%%%%%%%%%%%%%%%%%%%%%%%%%%%%%%%%%%%%%%%%%%%%%%%%%%%%%%%%%%%%%%%%%%%%%%%%%%%
%
% This function extracts time-locked EEG responses (ERPs) from
% a single trial of a P300 Oddball paradigm.
%
% input arguments:
%       EEGsignal:    Preprocessed EEG signal matrix    [time samples X
%                     channels]
%       StimulusCode: Values 0-4.  0 for all samples when no stimulus is
%                     presented, 1-4 for all samples associates when
%                     respective stimulus 1-4 is presented. Same number of
%                     samples as signal.
%       StimulusType: 1 for all samples for which a target stimulus is
%                     presented.  0 for all samples for which a non-target
%                     stimulus is presented.  Same number of samples as
%                     signal.
%       ERPwindow:    ERP window start and end time samples with respect
%                     to stimulus onset of 0 samples [begin end]
%
% output arguments:
%       ERPs:       Structure containing the following:
%             ERPs:  Array of collected responses [stimuli X response window
%                    X channels]
%             ERPCode: Vector containing the StimulusCode of each ERP
%                    [stimuli X 1]
%             ERPType: Vector containing the StimulusType of each ERP
%                    [stimuli X 1]
%%%%%%%%%%%%%%%%%%%%%%%%%%%%%%%%%%%%%%%%%%%%%%%%%%%%%%%%%%%%%%%%%%%%%%%%%%%%
```

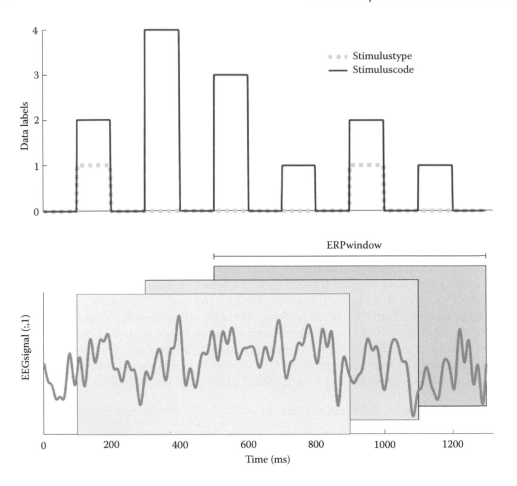

**FIGURE 20.1** Graphical depiction of the variables for the P300 oddball paradigm. The figure shows the alignment of one sample EEG channel, *EEGsignal (:,1)*, with the data labels. The consecutive *ERPwindows* are aligned with the transition of *StimulusCode* from zero to nonzero values (i.e., when the next stimulus is presented). *StimulusType* represents whether the stimulus is a target ("1") or nontarget ("0").

```
%%%%%%%%%%%%%%%%%%%%%%%%%%%%%%%%%%%%%%%%%%%%%%%%%%%%%%%%%%%%%%%%%%%%%%%%%%
%%%% Section 1: Identify the onset of the stimuli
%%%%%%%%%%%%%%%%%%%%%%%%%%%%%%%%%%%%%%%%%%%%%%%%%%%%%%%%%%%%%%%%%%%%%%%%%%
[NumberSamples,NumberChannels]=size(EEGsignal);
StimulusIndex=find(StimulusCode(1:NumberSamples-1)==0 & ...
    StimulusCode(2:NumberSamples)~=0)+1;  % find indices of stim onset
NumberStimuli=length(StimulusIndex);        % number of stimuli in trial


%%%%%%%%%%%%%%%%%%%%%%%%%%%%%%%%%%%%%%%%%%%%%%%%%%%%%%%%%%%%%%%%%%%%%%%%%%
%%%% Section 2: Extract the ERPs from the EEG signal
%%%%%%%%%%%%%%%%%%%%%%%%%%%%%%%%%%%%%%%%%%%%%%%%%%%%%%%%%%%%%%%%%%%%%%%%%%
ERPs.ERPs=zeros(xx,ERPwindow(2)-ERPwindow(1),NumberChannels);
for cnt=1:NumberStimuli                        % gather the ERPs
   ERPs.ERPs(cnt,:,:)=EEGsignal(ind(kk)+ERPwindow(1)-1: ...
                          ind(kk)+ERPwindow(2)-2,:);
end

ERPs.Code=StimulusCode(StimulusIndex); % extract stimulus code for each ERP
ERPs.Type=StimulusType(StimulusIndex); % extract stimulus type for each ERP
```

## 20.2.4 CLASSIFIER TRAINING

The output of the function from the Section 20.2.3 contains an array of ERPs with dimensions (stimulus, samples, channels) along with the associated stimulus labels Code and Type, both vectors of dimension (1, stimulus). All or a subset of the ERPs in the array can be used to train a classifier to determine whether a single trial or averaged ERP is the result of a target or nontarget stimulus (as defined by vector Type). Below is a sample MATLAB function for creating a simple binary classifier based on linear discriminant analysis (LDA) (Fisher 1936) to classify the ERPs as targets or nontargets. Note that this is one of the most simplistic classifiers, which is selected primarily for pedagogical purposes. However, LDA classifiers can be very effective in certain contexts. Alternative classifiers such as support vector machines, artificial neural networks, and so on can also be implemented by replacing the regress() function call with one for another classifier with comparable input/output arguments (Krusienski et al. 2006). The input argument TrainERPs is the same form as the ERP structure from the Section 20.2.3, but renamed for the case that the ERPs were separated for training and testing. The first line of code reshapes the spatiotemporal ERPs as (samples*channels, stimuli) to create a single feature vector corresponding to each stimulus, as required by the regress() classification function. The regress() function assumes a linear combination of each of the samples*channels feature in the input vector. The function finds a weight for each feature that minimizes the mean squared error between the equation output and the Type variable representing the targets and nontargets. These weights can be applied to independent ERPs to estimate if they are a target or nontarget. Essentially, the EEG measurement at each spatial location (channel) and time point with respect to the stimulus is being weighted to form a version of a "spatiotemporal detection template." For example, by taking an independent stimulus observation feature vector (samples*channels) and vector multiplying it by FeatureWeights, the result will be a single scalar value used for classification.

```
function [FeatureWeights]=TrainERPClassifier(TrainERPs,ERPwindow)

%%%%%%%%%%%%%%%%%%%%%%%%%%%%%%%%%%%%%%%%%%%%%%%%%%%%%%%%%%%%%%%%%%%%%%%%%%%%%%
%
%  This function is used to generate feature weights for a linear
classifier from a set of labeled responses.
%
%  input arguments:
%      TrainERPs:   Structure containing collected ERPs and stimulus
%                   code/type labels
%      windowlen:   Begin and end time samples after stimuli of
%                   collected responses   [begin end]
%
%  output arguments:
%      FeatureWeights: Vector containing the weights to multiply to each
%                      spatiotemporal feature for classification
%%%%%%%%%%%%%%%%%%%%%%%%%%%%%%%%%%%%%%%%%%%%%%%%%%%%%%%%%%%%%%%%%%%%%%%%%%%%%%

FeatureVectors=reshape(TestERPs.ERPs,NumberERPs,NumberChannels*WindowLen);

FeatureWeights=regress(ERPs.Type,[FeatureVectors,...
                       ones(1,size(FeatureVectors,1))']);
FeatureWeights=FeatureWeights(1:end-1); % exclude the bias term
```

## 20.2.5 CLASSIFICATION

At this point, classification to identify which stimulus evoked the oddball response can be performed. For Type labels of 0 and 1, the decision threshold will be 0.5 for deciding if an ERP represents a target or nontarget response. That is, if this scalar is <0.5, the ERP can be classified as a nontarget, and if this scalar is >0.5, the ERP can be classified as a target. If it is known that only one class contains a target, selecting the highest scalar output is a sensible approach and is implemented in the following `TestClassifier()`function. Keep in mind that ERPs are generally formed by averaging multiple single-trial responses. However, this same detection approach can be applied to the averaged feature vectors.

```
function
[PredictedStimulus]=TestClassifier(TestERPs,FeatureWeights,ERPwindow);

%%%%%%%%%%%%%%%%%%%%%%%%%%%%%%%%%%%%%%%%%%%%%%%%%%%%%%%%%%%%%%%%%%%%%%%%%%%
%
%  This function tests the performance of a linear classifier generated
using %  TrainClassifier.m
%
%  input arguments:
%      TestERPs:      Structure containing collected responses and labels
%      FeatureWeights: Vector containing the weights to multiply to each
%                      spatiotemporal feature for classification
%      ERPwindow:     ERP window start and end time samples with respect
%                      to stimulus onset of 0 samples [begin end]
%
%  output arguments:
%      PredictedStimulus:  Predicted target stimulus for a given trial
%%%%%%%%%%%%%%%%%%%%%%%%%%%%%%%%%%%%%%%%%%%%%%%%%%%%%%%%%%%%%%%%%%%%%%%%%%%

%%%%%%%%%%%%%%%%%%%%%%%%%%%%%%%%%%%%%%%%%%%%%%%%%%%%%%%%%%%%%%%%%%%%%%%%%
%%%% Section 1: Put test data through the classifier
%%%%%%%%%%%%%%%%%%%%%%%%%%%%%%%%%%%%%%%%%%%%%%%%%%%%%%%%%%%%%%%%%%%%%%%%%
WindowLen= ERPwindow(2)-ERPwindow(1);
[NumberERPs,NumberChannels]=size(TrainERPs.ERPs);

FeatureVectors=reshape(TrainERPs.ERPs,NumberERPs,NumberChannels*Window
Len);
scores=FeatureVectors*FeatureWeights;

%%%%%%%%%%%%%%%%%%%%%%%%%%%%%%%%%%%%%%%%%%%%%%%%%%%%%%%%%%%%%%%%%%%%%%%%%
%%%% Section 2: Select the predicted 'Target' stimulus
%%%%%%%%%%%%%%%%%%%%%%%%%%%%%%%%%%%%%%%%%%%%%%%%%%%%%%%%%%%%%%%%%%%%%%%%%
for stimuli=1:4
      AvgScore(stimuli)=mean(scores(TestERPs.Code==stimuli));
end
[~,PredictedStimulus]=max(AvgScore);
```

### 20.2.6 CONSIDERATIONS

The structure of the classification function presented assumes that a decision will be made after a fixed number of presentations of each of the four stimuli have occurred. However, this may be sub-optimal in terms of information transfer rate, and a method for dynamic stopping after a variable number of stimuli could also be implemented (Throckmorton et al. 2013).

### 20.3  N-CLASS SSVEP

This scenario is based on an SSVEP interface with arbitrary number $n$ possible classes (Sutter 1992). The $n$ targets are spatially distinct symbols, that is, icons, that each flash at distinct constant

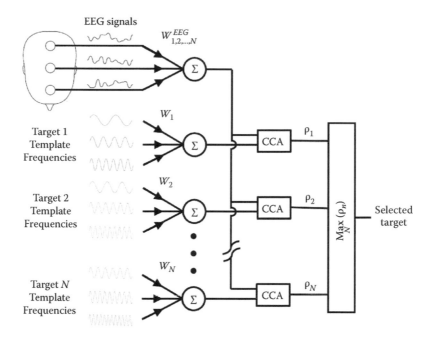

**FIGURE 20.2** Graphical depiction of CCA for an $n$-class SSVEP paradigm. For each $N$ target, a weighted sum of EEG channels is correlated to a weighted sum of sinusoidal templates at the harmonic frequencies (3 in this case) of the respective target stimulus. The optimal weights are computed separately for each target via CCA, which produces a maximized Pearson's correlation coefficient. The resulting correlation coefficients are compared across targets. The target that produced the maximum correlation is output as the current selection. Note that distinct EEG signal weights are generated for each target, corresponding to the subscript of the weight matrix.

frequency on a computer monitor or LED display. As the user shifts visual attention to one of the targets, the EEG over the visual cortex exhibits stronger oscillatory components at the target frequency and its harmonics. For this case, the canonical correlation analysis (CCA) algorithm generates an EEG spatial filter for each target that maximizes the correlation between a set of sinusoidal templates at each target frequency and its harmonic frequencies (Bin et al. 2009). The spatial filter associated with one of the target frequencies that produces the highest correlation for a given data window designates the current target of the user's visual attention. The idea is that the sinusoidal templates corresponding to the target frequency should better match the EEG than the templates at the other frequencies. See Figure 20.2 for a graphical depiction of CCA. This approach has an advantage over standard spectral analysis, for example, techniques based on the Fourier transform, in that it simultaneously combines spatial and spectral information in the classification decision and tends to provide more reliable performance. This approach does not require calibration or training before online operation and allows for continuous, asynchronous operation.

## 20.3.1 Data Collection

The SSVEP response is strongest over the occipital lobe, with typical electrode coverage over O1, O2, Oz, PO7, and PO8. In contrast to the P300 paradigm, it is not necessary to synchronize the EEG data with the flashing stimuli for this approach, although it may be necessary for more sophisticated approaches or offline analyses. The sampling rate should be set above at least twice the frequency of the highest harmonic of interest in order to satisfy the Nyquist–Shannon sampling theorem. Here, we assume that the data to be analyzed are loaded into MATLAB in a matrix format of $k$ samples × $m$ channels.

### 20.3.2 DATA PREPROCESSING

The data can be band-pass filtered between 0.1 Hz and just above the frequency of the maximum stimulus harmonic of interest. This filter is primarily to eliminate noise outside of the frequency range of interest, which can improve the performance of CCA. Other studies have shown that the performance can be improved by further isolating each harmonic using individual sub-band or comb filters (Chen et al. 2015).

### 20.3.3 DATA SEGMENTATION AND CLASSIFICATION

Below is a sample MATLAB function that takes a segment of EEG data (`EEGsignal`) as an input and outputs a classification decision for that data segment. Additionally, the function outputs the correlation coefficients for each of the classes presented. The CCA reference templates at each stimulus frequency are first created. They consist of sine and cosine segments at the fundamental frequency and `numHarm` harmonics, creating waveforms consisting of $k$ samples (matching the temporal length of the EEG segment) for each target frequency listed in the vector `stimF`. Both sine and cosine templates are used because a linear combination of the two can represent a single sinusoid with arbitrary phase, matching the characteristics of the EEG observation. Typically, only two or three harmonics are needed for an accurate classification, but the number of harmonics can be easily reconfigured to meet the performance needs. For each EEG data segment, CCA is performed for the template corresponding to each target frequency. CCA returns a set of optimized spatial weights for the EEG channels and the CCA sinusoidal templates that maximize the resulting correlation, as well as returning the value of this correlation. The provided function then selects the target frequency corresponding to the CCA template that produced the largest correlation for the given data segment. This process is repeated for each subsequent EEG data segment. The data segments can overlap, and the function can be called using varying durations of collected EEG data. For instance, a classification decision could be made every second while using a sliding buffer of the previous 1.5 s worth of EEG data.

```
function [class,rCoeff] = CCA_Classification(EEGsignal,Fs,stimF,numHarm)

%%%%%%%%%%%%%%%%%%%%%%%%%%%%%%%%%%%%%%%%%%%%%%%%%%%%%%%%%%%%%%%%%%%%%%%%%%%%
%  This function performs CCA classification for a block of data
%
%  input arguments:
%      EEGSignal:    EEG data, of dimension [time x mChannels]
%      Fs:           Sampling rate of EEG data
%      stimF:        Vector of stimulation frequencies in Hz e.g. [6, 7,
%                    8, 9]
%      numHarm:      Number of harmonic frequencies to include in the CCA
%
%  output arguments:
%      class:        Predicted class (class label with highest correlation)
%      rCoeff:       Vector of correlation coefficients for each freq. in
stimF
%%%%%%%%%%%%%%%%%%%%%%%%%%%%%%%%%%%%%%%%%%%%%%%%%%%%%%%%%%%%%%%%%%%%%%%%%%%%

%%%%%%%%%%%%%%%%%%%%%%%%%%%%%%%%%%%%%%%%%%%%%%%%%%%%%%%%%%%%%%%%%%%%%%%%%
%%%% Section 1: Create reference signals of sines and cosines
%%%%%%%%%%%%%%%%%%%%%%%%%%%%%%%%%%%%%%%%%%%%%%%%%%%%%%%%%%%%%%%%%%%%%%%%%
refSigs = zeros(size(EEGsignal,1),numHarm*2,length(stimF));
t = (1/Fs:1/Fs:size(EEGSignal)/Fs)';   % vector of time points
for i = 1:length(stimF)                % for each stimulus frequency
    for j = 1:numHarm                  % and for each harmonic
```

```
        refSigs(:,(2*j-1):(2*j),i) = … % create a sine and cosine
            [sin(2*pi*j*stimF(i)*t) cos(2*pi*j*stimF(i)*t)];
    end
end

%%%%%%%%%%%%%%%%%%%%%%%%%%%%%%%%%%%%%%%%%%%%%%%%%%%%%%%%%%%%%%%%%%%%%%
%%%% Section 2: Compute the correlations for each stimulus frequency
%%%%%%%%%%%%%%%%%%%%%%%%%%%%%%%%%%%%%%%%%%%%%%%%%%%%%%%%%%%%%%%%%%%%%%
rCoeff = zeros(length(stimF),1);
for j = 1:length(stimF)            % compute the CCA for each stimulus freq
    [~,~,r]=canoncorr(EEGsignal,squeeze(refSigs(:,:,j)));
    rCoeff(j)=r(1);
end
[~,class]=max(rCoeff);            % the largest coefficient is chosen
```

### 20.3.4 CONSIDERATIONS

The processing time for performing CCA can be limiting. For this reason, it would be beneficial to pass in the reference templates to the CCA _ Classification() function as an additional input argument. Generating the sine and cosine templates each time CCA _ Classification() is called is unnecessary when using a constant data window length for each classification. A classification decision based simply on the largest correlation coefficient is also not necessarily optimal. For instance, a classification decision can be postponed (and more data collected) until the highest correlation coefficient in rCoeff reaches a threshold, or until rCoeff from one class distinguishes itself significantly from the other classes. It is also possible to achieve improved performance by including user-specific EEG reference templates in addition to the sinusoidal reference templates (Chen et al. 2015); however, this results in an additional calibration phase to collect the EEG reference templates. These considerations exemplify the speed versus accuracy and calibration time trade-offs in the design of an online BCI.

Sample four-class P300 and SSVEP data are available upon e-mail request from the authors.

## ACKNOWLEDGMENTS

Dean J. Krusienski was supported in part by the National Science Foundation (NSF) under Grants IIS-1608140, IIS-1421948 and IIS-1451028. Any opinions, findings, and conclusions or recommendations expressed in this material are those of the authors and do not necessarily reflect the views of the NSF.

## REFERENCES

Bin, G., Gao, X., Yan, Z., Hong, B., & Gao, S., An online multi-channel SSVEP-based brain–computer interface using a canonical correlation analysis method, *Journal of Neural Engineering*, 6(4), 2009.

Chen, X., Wang, Y., Nakanishi, M., Gao, X., Jung, T.P., & Gao, S., High-speed spelling with a noninvasive brain–computer interface, *Proceedings of the National Academy of Sciences*, 112(44), 2015.

Farwell, L. & Donchin, E., Talking off the top of your head: Toward a mental prosthesis utilizing event-related brain potentials, *Electroencephalography and Clinical Neurophysiology*, 70, 510–523, 1988.

Fisher, R.A., The use of multiple measurements in taxonomic problems, *Ann. Eugenics*, 7, 179–188, 1936.

Krusienski, D.J., Sellers, E.W., Cabestaing, F., Bayoudh, S., McFarland, D.J., Vaughan, T.M., & Wolpaw, J.R., A comparison of classification techniques for the P300 Speller, *Journal of Neural Engineering*, 3, 299–305, 2006.

Sutter, E.E., The brain response interface: Communication through visually-induced electrical brain response, *J Microcomput Appl*, 15, 31–45, 1992.

Throckmorton, C.S., Colwell, K.A., Ryan, D.D., Sellers, E.W., & Collins, L.M., Bayesian approach to dynamically controlling data collection in P300 spellers. *IEEE Transactions on Neural Systems and Rehabilitation Engineering*, 21(3), 508–517, 2013.

# 21 Bayesian Learning for EEG Analysis

*Yu Zhang*

## CONTENTS

21.1 Introduction ...........................................................................................................408
21.2 Equivalence between LDA and LSR ................................................................... 410
21.3 Maximum Likelihood and Regularized Least Squares....................................... 411
21.4 Bayesian Learning .............................................................................................. 413
    21.4.1 Bayesian Discriminant Analysis............................................................ 413
    21.4.2 Sparse Bayesian Learning ...................................................................... 414
21.5 Experimental Study ............................................................................................ 415
    21.5.1 ERP Data Set .......................................................................................... 415
        21.5.1.1 Data Description ..................................................................... 415
        21.5.1.2 Performance Evaluation.......................................................... 416
        21.5.1.3 Results...................................................................................... 416
    21.5.2 SMR Data Set ......................................................................................... 418
        21.5.2.1 Data Description ..................................................................... 418
        21.5.2.2 Performance Evaluation.......................................................... 418
        21.5.2.3 Results...................................................................................... 419
21.6 Discussion............................................................................................................ 419
21.7 Conclusions.........................................................................................................420
References.......................................................................................................................421

## Abstract

As a noninvasive neuroimaging technique, electroencephalogram (EEG) has been most popularly applied to brain–computer interface (BCI) development. Informative feature extraction and accurate classification of EEG patterns are considerably challenging because of the poor signal-to-noise ratio caused by volume conduction effects, interferences from various noises, and intrinsic signal nonstationarity. In this chapter, we provide a tutorial of applying Bayesian learning-based algorithms to EEG feature optimization and classification in BCI applications. The algorithm principles of Bayesian learning are detailedly explained in the aspects of prior designing, posterior inference, and hyperparameter estimation. With two representative examples based on event-related potential and sensorimotor rhythm BCI paradigms, we further introduce the usage of Bayesian learning-based algorithms for EEG analysis. Extensive experimental comparisons are carried out among different competing algorithms to validate the effectiveness of Bayesian learning in BCI applications. A discussion is provided on various extensions of Bayesian learning for exploring more complex but potentially important properties of EEG, toward improved performance of BCI systems.

## 21.1 INTRODUCTION

Brain–computer interface (BCI) is a new communication technique that aims at establishing a nonmuscular connection between a human brain and a computer (Chaudhary et al. 2016). A BCI system is developed to translate the intent of a user into computer commands by recognizing a task-related brain activity typically measured using electroencephalography (EEG), for operating external devices, such as wheelchair navigation, character spelling, prosthesis controlling, Internet browsing, and so on (Carlson and Millan 2013; Zhang et al. 2012, 2014a; Chen et al. 2014; Mugler et al. 2010; Yu et al. 2012; Jin et al. 2012). With the help of BCIs, severely disabled patients (e.g., spinal cord injuries, amyotrophic lateral sclerosis, etc.) can potentially recover their environmental control abilities and hence improve their living quality (Leeb et al. 2015; Li and Nam 2016; Klein and Nam 2016).

By far, one of the most popularly adopted EEG activities for BCI development is event-related potential (ERP), a time- and phase-locked brain response to stimulus events of interest. Typical ERP components P300, N170, and N200 have been successfully applied to the design of BCIs. P300 is a positive deflection in EEG occurring at approximately 300 ms after a rare but task-related stimulus (i.e., oddball paradigm) (Krusienski et al. 2008), while N170 and N200 are the two negative deflections at about 170 and 200 ms, respectively. Through classifying the ERP components corresponding to controlled stimuli, an ERP-based BCI can be developed to detect the desired commands from a user. The ERP-based BCI has proven its promising potential for spelling application with a relatively robust performance for target character detection and also no requirement for subject training (Sellers and Donchin 2006; Jin et al. 2015). Another frequently adopted EEG activity for BCI development is sensorimotor rhythm (SMR), characterized as a bandpower change of particular EEG frequency band, appearing at the contralateral sensorimotor area during imagination of unilateral band movement (i.e., so-called motor imagery) (Pfurtscheller et al. 2006; Blankertz et al. 2010). Accordingly, an SMR-based BCI can be designed by recognizing the spatial pattern difference of EEG between different motor imagery tasks, typically including imagining left and right hand, foot, or tongue movements. In recent years, SMR-based BCI has shown its application value in both wheelchair control and stroke rehabilitation (Ang et al. 2011; Huang et al. 2012).

Accurate classification of EEG patterns is considerably challenging because of their poor signal-to-noise ratio caused by volume conduction effects, interferences from various noises, and intrinsic signal nonstationarity (Krusienski et al. 2011). One of the main issues likely to deteriorate EEG classification in BCI applications is the so-called curse of dimensionality. The curse of dimensionality is caused by the fact that samples (i.e., feature vectors) for EEG classification in BCI applications are generally extracted from the multichannel-based complex representation in a feature subspace and hence have typically high dimensionality. That is, the feature dimensionality is relatively larger than the number training sample that is limitedly available when taking into account the practicability of the BCI system. As a result, the bias–variance trade-off restricts the generalization capability in a small sample size scenario since a limited training set would most probably result in overfitting (i.e., high variance but low bias) of the model to outliers in noisy EEG signals. Thus, a good classification performance of EEG usually requires sufficient data recordings for effective calibration of a classification model. For example, although linear discriminant analysis (LDA), also known as Fisher's linear discriminant analysis (FDA), has proven its powerful strength in EEG classification, its effective calibration usually requires 5 to 10 times as many training samples per class as the feature dimensionality (Lotte et al. 2007). Recording such a relatively large number of data will inevitably take a long calibration time, thereby most probably depressing system practicability and causing a user to be reluctant to use BCI. On the other hand, extracting discriminative features can be considerably challenging because of the nonstationary nature of EEG signals (Zhang et al. 2013a). Characterized by the variations of signal properties over time, the nonstationarities of EEG are probably caused by various sources, including muscular activity, increased fatigue, and electrode artifacts (Samek et al. 2012). All these variations will result in a time-varying feature distribution and hence bring negative effects on the feature extraction and classification performance in BCI applications. Accordingly, developing a powerful machine learning-based framework for robust feature extraction and classification of EEG, especially in a small sample setting, is quite crucial to promote the development of improved BCIs (Lotte 2015; Zhang et al. 2014b).

Until now, regularization techniques have been mostly applied to prevent overfitting in EEG classification. Typically, support vector machine (SVM) adopts a regularization item to control the prediction error in training for enhancing the generalization capability for testing data. A good SVM performance has been confirmed by many studies on EEG classification (Siuly and Li 2012; Rakotomamonjy and Guigue 2008; Koo et al. 2015). By imposing the $l_2$-norm constraint on the discriminant vector to be learned, Müller et al. (2004) proposed regularized Fisher's discriminant analysis (RFDA) for BCI applications. RFDA effectively prevented the influence of outliers and performed better than FDA on motor-imagery EEG classification. Instead of using the $l_2$-norm, Blankertz et al. (2002) introduced a sparse variant of FDA by exploiting the $l_1$-norm regularization for finger movement-related EEG classification, which yields a lower classification error than both FDA and SVM. Zhang et al. (2014b) introduced a sparse FDA under the least-squares regression (LSR) framework for ERP classification in BCI applications. Sparse FDA automatically implements feature selection for dimensionality reduction to alleviate the curse of dimensionality and hence yielded a better performance than the standard FDA. Another regularized version of FDA is stepwise linear discriminant analysis (SWLDA), which improves classification performance by iteratively selecting useful features. SWLDA was originally introduced to EEG classification by Farwell and Donchin (1988) in a P300 speller BCI paradigm and has been widely applied to BCIs and referred to as the state-of-the-art P300 classification algorithm with superiority over various algorithms including linear SVM and Gaussian kernel-based SVM (Krusienski et al. 2006). Another more recently applied algorithm is called shrinkage LDA (SKLDA), which has proven to be effective for ERP classification in small sample settings (Blankertz et al. 2011). The inverse of sample covariance matrix can hardly be accurately estimated using limited training samples, thereby reducing the generalization capability of LDA. By exploiting a shrinkage covariance estimator (Schäfer and Strimmer 2005), SKLDA remedies the ill-conditioned covariance matrix toward the real one so that the trained classifier can achieve relatively high generalization capability even when using insufficient training samples.

Although the aforementioned regularization technique-based classification algorithms have achieved promising improvement in EEG classification accuracy, their performances highly depend on the selection of corresponding regularization parameters. These regularization parameters are typically determined manually by experience or based on cross-validation (CV) procedure. However, the empirically selected parameters could hardly provide the best classification accuracy since the optimal parameters are usually subject specific. Although CV is able to determine the subject-specific parameters, it requires a large amount of training data to construct an additional validation set with expensive computation for classifier calibration. Such limitation of CV will dramatically reduce the BCI system's practicability. Instead of the time-consuming CV procedure, Bayesian learning provides an elegant approach to automatically and quickly estimate model parameters under the so-called evidence framework. Without the need of additional validation set, all available training data can be used for calibrating the probabilistic model-based classifier. On the other hand, instead of outputting a "hard" classification decision, Bayesian learning is able to capture the uncertainty in the prediction by estimating the posterior probability with an appropriately specified prior distribution (Tipping 2001).

Through a Bayesian treatment of linear regression, Hoffmann (2007) and Hoffmann et al. (2008) introduced Bayesian linear discriminant analysis (BLDA) for ERP classification in BCI applications. BLDA is basically a Bayesian version of RFDA and can efficiently determine the degree of regularization by exploiting a standard zero-mean Gaussian prior without the need for the time-consuming CV procedure. The good performance of BLDA has been confirmed by many studies on BCI development for both healthy and disabled subjects (Xu et al. 2011; Manyakov et al. 2011). It should be noted that the standard Gaussian prior does not result in a sparse discriminative vector but a relatively smooth one. Since EEG sources generally present relatively sparse distribution in the spatial, temporal, spectral, or time–frequency domain (Li et al. 2014), sparse learning has been increasingly suggested for BCI applications (Zhang et al. 2014; Tomioka and Müller 2010; Arvaneh et al. 2011). Accordingly, accurate estimation of the sparse discriminative vector under a Bayesian learning framework becomes more promising for EEG feature optimization and classification. Through an elegant Bayesian treatment, sparse Bayesian learning (SBL) was originally developed by Tipping (2001) to achieve a probabilistic realization of the sparse penalized linear regression problem. Different from BLDA, SBL exploits a separate Gaussian prior to effectively control the sparsity of the estimated discriminant vector so that the crucial features can be automatically selected by excluding those nonsignificant ones. In the past few years, SBL has attracted increasing interests of researchers in various fields, including compressive sensing (Babacan et al. 2010), source reconstruction (Zhang and Rao 2011), and visual tracking (Williams et al. 2005). More recently, SBL has been successfully applied to simultaneous feature selection and classification in ERP-based BCI (Zhang et al. 2016b) and subband feature optimization for SMR classification in motor imagery-based BCI (Zhang et al. 2017a).

In this chapter, we present a tutorial for applying Bayesian learning-based algorithms to EEG feature optimization and classification in BCI applications. Some basic concepts on the regularization technique in classification algorithm are given. The algorithm principles of BLDA and SBL are described in detail. With EEG data sets of ERP and SMR paradigms, we further explain the usage of BLDA and SBL for EEG analysis. Extensive experimental comparisons are carried out among different competing algorithms to validate the effectiveness of Bayesian learning on EEG analysis. A discussion is provided on some promising extensions based on Bayesian learning algorithms for more effective EEG analysis, followed by conclusions.

## 21.2 EQUIVALENCE BETWEEN LDA AND LSR

LDA is known as a benchmark method to find the optimal combination of features separating two classes. Since LDA requires relatively low computational cost and usually provides good classification results, it has been widely used for EEG classification in BCI applications. Assume $\mathbf{X} = [\mathbf{x}_1, \mathbf{x}_2, \ldots, \mathbf{x}_N]^T \in \mathbb{R}^{N \times D}$ is an EEG data matrix consisting of $N$ samples (i.e., feature vectors) with a feature dimensionality of $D$ and $\mathbf{y} = [y_1, y_2, \ldots, y_N]^T \in \mathbb{R}^N$ denotes a vector containing the class labels with $y_i \in \{1, -1\}$. The mean feature vectors of the two classes are computed by

$$\boldsymbol{\mu}_c = \frac{1}{N_c} \sum_{i \in \mathcal{I}_c} \mathbf{x}_i, \quad c = 1, 2, \tag{21.1}$$

where $\mathcal{I}_c$ and $N_c$ are the index and the number of samples in class $c$, respectively. The common covariance matrix is estimated as

$$\boldsymbol{\Sigma} = \frac{1}{N} \sum_{c=1}^{2} \sum_{i \in \mathcal{I}_c} (\mathbf{x}_i - \boldsymbol{\mu}_c)(\mathbf{x}_i - \boldsymbol{\mu}_c)^T. \tag{21.2}$$

Then, the discriminant vector of the LDA is given by

$$\mathbf{w} = \boldsymbol{\Sigma}^{-1}(\boldsymbol{\mu}_1 - \boldsymbol{\mu}_2). \tag{21.3}$$

Note that the LDA is equivalent to FDA since the class covariances are assumed to be identical and equal to $\Sigma$. The LDA can be actually derived from a special case of LSR for a binary classification problem (Bishop 2006). Let us consider the following LSR problem:

$$\mathbf{w} = \arg \min_{\mathbf{w}} \frac{1}{2} \|\mathbf{y} - \mathbf{X}\mathbf{w}\|_2^2, \tag{21.4}$$

where $\| \cdot \|_2$ denotes the $l_2$-norm. Suppose the class labels $y_i$ have been specified to $\frac{N}{N_1}$ for samples from class 1 and to $-\frac{N}{N_2}$ for samples from class $-1$. By setting the derivate of Equation 21.4 with respect to $\mathbf{w}$ to zero, the solution is formulated as $\mathbf{w} = (\mathbf{X}^T\mathbf{X})^{-1} \mathbf{X}^T\mathbf{y}$. Without loss of generality, let us assume all samples in $\mathbf{X}$ have been de-meaned. We can then derive $\mathbf{X}^T\mathbf{X} = N\Sigma$ and $\mathbf{X}^T\mathbf{y} = \frac{N_1 N_2}{N}(\boldsymbol{\mu}_1 - \boldsymbol{\mu}_2)$. That is, the solution of LSR can be reformulated as $\mathbf{w} = \frac{N_1 N_2}{N^2}\Sigma^{-1}(\boldsymbol{\mu}_1 - \boldsymbol{\mu}_2)$, which holds the same form as that of LDA in Equation 21.3 since the irrelevant scale factor $\frac{N_1 N_2}{N^2}$ could be ignored for the discriminant vector.

## 21.3 MAXIMUM LIKELIHOOD AND REGULARIZED LEAST SQUARES

Let us define a probabilistic model for LSR in Equation 21.4 by considering an error term with zero mean and variance $\sigma^2$. The likelihood function for weight is written as

$$p(\mathbf{y} \mid \mathbf{w}, \sigma^2) = \left( \frac{1}{2\pi\sigma^2} \right)^{\frac{N}{2}} \exp\left( -\frac{1}{2\sigma^2} \|\mathbf{y} - \mathbf{Xw}\|_2^2 \right). \tag{21.5}$$

Taking the logarithm of the likelihood function yields

$$\ln p(\mathbf{y} \mid \mathbf{w}, \sigma^2) = -\frac{N}{2}\ln(2\pi\sigma^2) - \frac{1}{2\sigma^2}\|\mathbf{y} - \mathbf{Xw}\|_2^2. \tag{21.6}$$

Thus, the maximum likelihood estimation for $\mathbf{w}$ is equivalent to minimizing the squared error $\|\mathbf{y} - \mathbf{Xw}\|_2^2$, which gives a solution $\mathbf{w} = (\mathbf{X}^T\mathbf{X})^{-1} \mathbf{X}^T\mathbf{y}$, the same as that of LSR. A potential issue of LSR and maximum likelihood estimation is that they are likely to suffer from an overfitting problem, especially when the number of samples is small relative to the dimensionality of the feature space (Tipping 2004). Figure 21.1 illustrates the overfitting problem when fitting to 16 samples artificially generated according to the sine function characterized by the red curve with an added Gaussian noise of variance of 0.25. The polynomial fit with a relatively high model complexity (i.e., with order $L = 14$) estimates a model that exactly interpolates the data but largely deviates from the true model because of serious overfitting.

In order to alleviate the overfitting problem, the regularization technique has been most popularly used since it provides a potentially useful prior to control the model complexity. Typically, an $l_2$-norm regularized LSR can be formulated as

$$\mathbf{w} = \arg\min_{\mathbf{w}} \frac{1}{2}\|\mathbf{y} - \mathbf{Xw}\|_2^2 + \lambda\|\mathbf{w}\|_2. \tag{21.7}$$

By setting the derivate of Equation 21.7 with respect to $\mathbf{w}$ to zero, this regularized LSR gives a solution $\mathbf{w} (\mathbf{X}^T\mathbf{X} + \lambda\mathbf{I})^{-1} \mathbf{X}^T\mathbf{y}$. The hyperparameter $\lambda$ plays an important role in balancing the trade-off between minimization of squared error and smoothness of $\mathbf{w}$. An appropriately selected $\lambda$ could assist in adjusting the model toward the real one and hence mitigate overfitting to the limited samples.

By replacing the $l_2$-norm with the $l_1$-norm, a sparse regularized LSR (also known as Lasso Tibshirani 1996) is formulated as

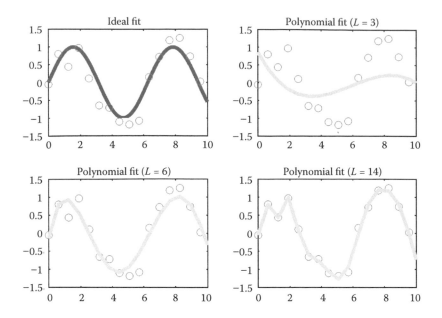

**FIGURE 21.1** Illustration of overfitting problem when fitting to 16 samples artificially generated according to the sine function characterized by the red curve with an added Gaussian noise of variance of 0.25. These subfigures show the ideal fit and polynomial fit with various orders $L = 3, 6$, and 14, respectively.

$$\mathbf{w} = \arg \min_{\mathbf{w}} \frac{1}{2} \left\| \mathbf{y} - \mathbf{X}\mathbf{w} \right\|_2^2 + \lambda \left\| \mathbf{w} \right\|_1 , \qquad (21.8)$$

where the hyperparameter $\lambda$ controls the sparsity of $\mathbf{w}$. Since the EEG sources are believed to be sparsely distributed in a spatial, time, or time–frequency domain (Li et al. 2014), sparse learning based on $l_1$-norm regularization provides a promising approach to EEG feature optimization.

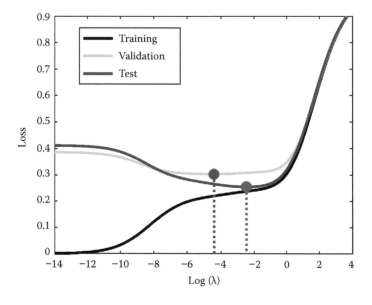

**FIGURE 21.2** Illustration of training, validation and, test loss at different values of hyperparameter $\lambda$. The lowest validation and test losses are marked by blue and pink circles, respectively.

As mentioned above, the optimal selection of the hyperparameter $\lambda$ plays a key role in regularization techniques. So far, most studies involving regularization have generally determined the hyperparameter by experience or by using a CV procedure. However, manual selection can hardly give the optimal parameter value that is typically subject specific. Although CV provides an accurate estimate for $\lambda$ when using enough training samples for constructing training and validation sets (as shown in Figure 21.2), it usually requires expensive computations and is hardly applicable to small sample size scenarios (Zhang et al. 2014b). As a result, these limitations substantially depress the system's practicability and even probably cause a subject to be reluctant to use BCI.

## 21.4 BAYESIAN LEARNING

### 21.4.1 BAYESIAN DISCRIMINANT ANALYSIS

Bayesian inference provides an effective approach for automatic and relatively quick estimation of the regularization parameter using only the training set (MacKay 1992). This allows all available samples to be used for training without the need of a validation set for CV (Bishop 2006). With Bayesian linear regression, Hoffmann et al. (2008) introduced BLDA to EEG classification for P300-based BCIs. Instead of the regularization term in Equation 21.7, a zero-mean Gaussian prior in a probabilistic model is defined to express the penalty:

$$p(\mathbf{w} \mid \alpha) = \prod_{d=1}^{D} \mathcal{N}(w_d \mid 0, \alpha^{-1}) = \left(\frac{\alpha}{2\pi}\right)^{\frac{D}{2}} \exp\left(-\frac{\alpha}{2}\|\mathbf{w}\|_2^2\right), \tag{21.9}$$

where $\alpha$ is a shared inverse variance hyperparameter similar to the regularization parameter $\lambda$ in Equation 21.7. However, different from the selection of $\lambda$, $\alpha$ will be automatically estimated based on the evidence method instead of the time-consuming CV procedure. Given the likelihood function in Equation 21.5, the posterior distribution can be computed according to the Bayesian rule:

$$p(\mathbf{w} \mid \alpha, \sigma^2, \mathbf{y}) = \frac{p(\mathbf{y} \mid \mathbf{w}, \sigma^2)p(\mathbf{w} \mid \alpha)}{p(\mathbf{y} \mid \alpha, \sigma^2)}. \tag{21.10}$$

As a result of combining a Gaussian prior and a Gaussian likelihood function, the posterior distribution is also Gaussian, with covariance and mean being

$$\boldsymbol{\Sigma} = (\sigma^{-2}\mathbf{X}^T\mathbf{X} + \alpha\mathbf{I})^{-1}, \quad \boldsymbol{\mu} = \sigma^{-2}\boldsymbol{\Sigma}\mathbf{X}^T\mathbf{y}. \tag{21.11}$$

To estimate the optimal hyperparameters $\alpha$ and $\sigma$, the evidence method (Bishop 2006; MacKay 1992) has been popularly adopted, which maximizes the marginal likelihood $p(\mathbf{y} \mid \alpha, \sigma^2)$. By integrating out the weights, the marginal likelihood is given by

$$\begin{aligned} p(\mathbf{y} \mid \alpha, \sigma^2) &= \int p(\mathbf{y} \mid \mathbf{w}, \sigma^2)p(\mathbf{w} \mid \alpha)\, d\mathbf{w} \\ &= \left(\frac{\alpha}{2\pi}\right)^{\frac{D}{2}} \left(\frac{1}{2\pi\sigma^2}\right)^{\frac{N}{2}} |\boldsymbol{\Sigma}^{-1}|^{-\frac{1}{2}} \exp\left(-\frac{\|\mathbf{y} - \mathbf{X}\boldsymbol{\mu}\|_2^2}{2\sigma^2} - \frac{\alpha}{2}\boldsymbol{\mu}^T\boldsymbol{\mu}\right). \end{aligned} \tag{21.12}$$

By setting the derivate of $\log p(\mathbf{y} \mid \alpha, \sigma^2)$ with respect to $\alpha$ and $\sigma^2$ to zero, the two hyperparameters can be automatically and iteratively estimated as follows:

$$\alpha \leftarrow \frac{\gamma}{\mu^T \mu}, \quad \sigma^2 \leftarrow \frac{\|y - X\mu\|_2^2}{N - \gamma}, \tag{21.13}$$

where $\gamma = \sum_{d=1}^{D} \eta_d / (\alpha + \eta_d)$, and $\eta_d$ is the $d$th eigenvalue of matrix $X^T X / \sigma^2$. For a new test sample $\hat{x}$, the predictive distribution can be computed as

$$p(\hat{y} \mid \alpha, \sigma^2, \hat{x}, y) = \int p(\hat{y} \mid w, \sigma^2, \hat{x}) p(w \mid \alpha, \sigma^2, y) \, dw, \tag{21.14}$$

which is again Gaussian with mean and variance

$$\hat{\mu} = \mu^T \hat{x}, \hat{\sigma}^2 = \sigma^2 + \hat{x}^T \Sigma \hat{x}. \tag{21.15}$$

A larger predictive mean more strongly represents the characteristics of EEG patterns as defined by the training set.

### 21.4.2 Sparse Bayesian Learning

The standard Gaussian prior in Equation 21.9 used by BLDA is similar to the effect of $l_2$-norm regularization in Equation 21.7, which does not result in a sparse solution. However, a sparse projection vector has been suggested to be promising for automatic feature reduction and hence to improve the classification of EEG (Zhang et al. 2014b). SBL, also known as relevance vector machine (Tipping 2001), provides an elegant way to obtain a sparse solution under the probabilistic framework by defining the following separate Gaussian prior:

$$p(w \mid \alpha) = \prod_{d=1}^{D} \mathcal{N}\left(w_d \mid 0, \alpha_d^{-1}\right) = \prod_{d=1}^{D} \left(\frac{\alpha_d}{2\pi}\right)^{\frac{1}{2}} \exp\left(-\frac{1}{2}\alpha_d w_d^2\right). \tag{21.16}$$

Instead of a shared hyperparameter $\alpha$ as in BLDA, Equation 21.16 adopts $D$ automatic relevance determination hyperparameters $\alpha = [\alpha_1, \alpha_2, \ldots, \alpha_D]$ to separately control the inverse variances of weights $w_1, w_2, \ldots, w_D$. Following the Bayesian rule with the likelihood function given in Equation 21.5, we can estimate the covariance and mean of the posterior $p(w \mid \alpha, \sigma^2, y)$ by

$$\Sigma = (\sigma^{-2} X^T X + \Lambda)^{-1}, \quad \mu = \sigma^{-2} \Sigma X^T y, \tag{21.17}$$

where $\Lambda = \text{diag}([\alpha_1, \alpha_2, \ldots, \alpha_D])$. Again, we adopt the evidence-based marginal likelihood maximization (MacKay 1992) to estimate hyperparameters $\alpha$ and $\sigma^2$. The marginal likelihood $p(y \mid \alpha, \sigma^2)$ is derived by integrating out the weights as

$$p(y \mid \alpha, \sigma^2) = \int p(y \mid w, \sigma^2) p(w \mid \alpha) \, dw = \left(\frac{1}{2\pi}\right)^{\frac{N}{2}} |C|^{-\frac{1}{2}} \exp\left(-\frac{1}{2} y^T C^{-1} y\right), \tag{21.18}$$

where $C = \sigma^2 I + X \Lambda^{-1} X^T$. By maximizing the logarithm of the marginal likelihood with respect to $\alpha$ and $\sigma^2$, we obtain the following iterative estimation formulas for hyperparameter optimization:

$$\alpha_d \leftarrow \frac{\gamma_d}{\mu_c^2}, \quad \sigma^2 \leftarrow \frac{\|y - X\mu\|_2^2}{N - \sum_{d=1}^{D} \gamma_d}, \tag{21.19}$$

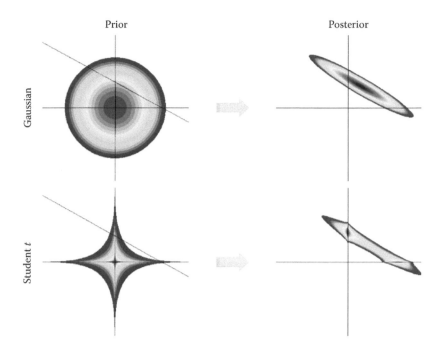

**FIGURE 21.3** Contour plots of the Gaussian prior, Student $t$ prior and the corresponding posterior distributions in two dimensions. The Student $t$ prior is derived by integrating out the hyperparameter $\alpha$ for the separate Gaussian prior.

where $\mu_d$ is the $d$th posterior mean computed by Equation 21.17, and $\gamma_d = 1 - \alpha_d \Sigma_{dd}$ with $\Sigma_{dd}$ being the $d$th diagonal entry of the posterior covariance computed in with the current values.

Figure 21.3 depicts the differences between the Bayesian linear regression and SBL in terms of priors and posteriors. Compared with the standard Gaussian prior, the separate Gaussian prior heavily shrinks the posterior probability mass toward the axes, which encourages sparse solutions.

## 21.5 EXPERIMENTAL STUDY

In this section, we introduce the usage of Bayesian learning-based algorithms for analyses of two types of EEG patterns, that is, ERP and SMR for BCI applications. Extensive experimental comparisons are carried out among different competing methods to validate the effectiveness of Bayesian learning for EEG feature optimization and classification.

### 21.5.1 ERP DATA SET

#### 21.5.1.1 Data Description

The EEG data were recorded from seven healthy subjects (S1–S7, from 24 to 49 years of age). The subjects were seated in a comfortable chair 60 cm from a 17-inch LCD monitor. In the experimental layout, eight arrow commands were presented to simulate a navigation control. Randomly specified objects were used as the visual stimuli to elicit ERPs. Each subject performed 16 experimental runs. In each run, a randomly cued target arrow was first presented in the middle of the screen for 1 s followed by a black screen period of 1 s. A block-randomized sequence of object presentations was subsequently presented. The presentation block was repeated five times. In each block, an object was presented on one arrow position once with a duration of 100 ms and an interstimulus interval of 80 ms. During the experiment, the subjects were asked to gaze at the cued arrow positions and silently count the number of times the object stimuli appeared. EEG signals were recorded using the g.USBamp amplifier (g.tec, Austria) at a 256-Hz sampling rate followed by band pass filtering between 0.1 and 30 Hz. Sixteen electrodes were used for signal recording and analysis—F3, Fz, F4, T7, C3, Cz, C4, T8, P7, P3, Pz, P4, P8, PO7, PO8, and Oz—referenced to the average of two mastoids and grounded to the electrode Fpz. More details about the experimental settings and data recordings can be found in the literature (Zhang et al. 2012). A data segment of 700 ms was extracted from each object stimulus presentation and downsampled by a 12-point moving average. A sample (i.e., feature vector) with a dimensionality of 240 was then formed by concatenating 15 temporal points from each of the 16 channels. A total of 640 samples consisting of 80 targets and 560 nontargets were derived from each subject, where every 40 samples (5 targets and 35 nontargets) correspond to one command selection.

### 21.5.1.2  Performance Evaluation

To validate the effectiveness of Bayesian learning algorithms on ERP classification, we carry out an extensive experimental comparison among SVM, SWLDA, BLDA, and SBL. A linear kernel was adopted for SVM training. The parameter settings of SWLDA are those in the literature (i.e., $p$ value < 0.1 for adding feature; $p$ value > 0.15 for removing feature; the maximal number of features is 60). No parameter tuning is required for both BLDA and SBL algorithms. Four, six, and eight command selections were used for classifier training while the remaining half was used for performance evaluation. The program was repeated 100 times and the average classification accuracies were then calculated. It should be noted that the number of available training samples is relatively small compared with the feature dimensionality. Theoretically, higher classification accuracy can be achieved using more training data for classifier training or a larger number of trial averages for command detection. However, more training data take longer time for recording EEG signals while a larger number of trial averages require a longer time for deciding a command. Thus, an effective classification algorithm for ERP-based BCI should be able to obtain high classification accuracy with fewest possible training data and the smallest number of averaged trials.

### 21.5.1.3  Results

Figure 21.4 depicts the classification accuracies derived by the four methods, averaged over all seven subjects, for different numbers of training data. The results indicate that the SBL method achieved a more obvious superiority over the other competing methods as the number of training data decreased. More specifically, with training data from six runs ($N = 240$) or eight runs ($N = 320$),

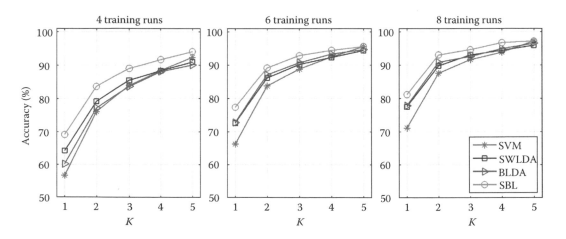

**FIGURE 21.4**  Classification accuracies derived by SVM, SWLDA, BLDA, and SBL algorithms, averaged for different numbers of training data. Four training runs: $N = 160$. Six training runs: $N = 240$. Eight training runs: $N = 320$. $K$ denotes the number of trials' average.

BLDA and SWLDA achieved comparable accuracy, performing better than SVM but worse than SBL. When decreasing the number of training data to $N = 120$ (i.e., using four training runs), SBL still yielded the best performance among all methods while BLDA performed worse than SWLDA and comparable to SVM. Through the feature reduction based on sparse learning, SBL effectively alleviated the overfitting in a small sample size scenario, especially when the number of training samples is smaller than the feature dimensionality.

As shown in Figure 21.5, the most discriminative features are found to mainly result from the ERP components across 200–600 ms and are indeed relatively sparse in the spatial–temporal distribution. Figure 21.6 further shows the discriminant vectors (presented in the form of channels × temporal points) learned by SWLDA, BLDA, and SBL, respectively. Compared with BLDA, SBL captured the most discriminative features more accurately and excluded those redundant ones by exploiting the separate Gaussian prior for enforcing sparsity of the learned discriminative vector. Although SWLDA also obtained a sparse discriminative vector because of its feature selection procedure, it failed to capture the significant features located in P3 at the fifth and seventh temporal points but put a large weight on the nonsignificant features located in C3 at the fourth temporal point.

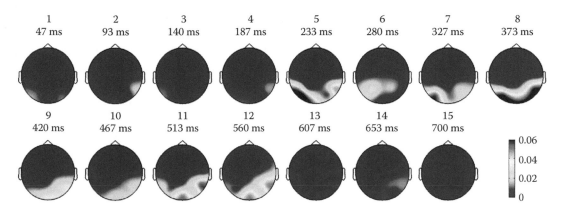

**FIGURE 21.5** Scalp topographies of the discriminative information ($r^2$ values) at different temporal points for a typical subject.

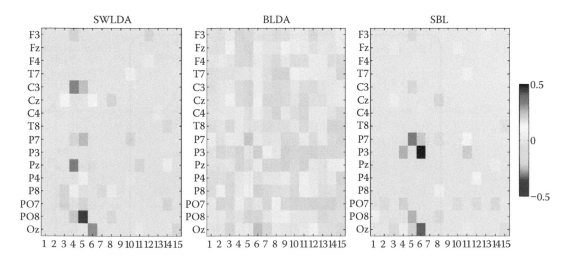

**FIGURE 21.6** Discriminative vectors derived by the SWLDA, BLDA, and SBL methods for a typical subject, which are presented in the form of channels × temporal points.

### 21.5.2 SMR Data Set

#### 21.5.2.1 Data Description

The public BCI Competition IV data set IIb is used to validate the effectiveness of the SBL method for the two-class problem of SMR classification. This data set was recorded from nine subjects at three electrodes C3, Cz and C4 with a sampling rate of 250 Hz, during right/left hand motor imagery tasks. The data were band pass filtered between 0.5 and 100 Hz with a notch filter at 50 Hz. Only the third training sessions of the data set were used for our experimental study. For each subject, a total of 160 trials of EEG data are available (half for each class of motor imagery tasks). In each trial, the subject was instructed by a visual cue to perform a motor imagery task for 4.5 s. More details about the data set can be found at http://www.bbci.de/competition/iv/. Following the segment way in (Ang et al. 2012), an EEG sample is extracted from each trial, starting from 0.5 to 2.5 s after the visual cue, which consists of three-channel data with 500 temporal points in each channel.

#### 21.5.2.2 Performance Evaluation

Common spatial pattern (CSP) has been one of the most popular methods for SMR feature extraction in motor imagery-based BCI applications (Blankertz et al. 2008). The effectiveness of CSP generally depends on the filter band selection to a large degree. Since the most proper band can be typically subject specific, the subband optimization has been suggested to enhance the classification accuracy of SMR (Ang et al. 2012; Zhang et al. 2015; Higashi and Tanaka 2013). SBL provides a promising way to simultaneously implement subband feature selection and classification of SMR. Figure 21.7 illustrates the SBL-based algorithm for SMR classification in MI-based BCI (Zhang et al. 2017a). Specifically, instead of using a wide filter band, we perform band pass filtering on raw EEG data using a set of overlapping subbands that are chosen f rom the frequency range 4–40 Hz with 4 Hz bandwidth and 2 Hz overlapping rate. CSP is implemented on the filtered signals at each subband to extract the SMR features. With SBL, a sparse discriminant vector is automatically estimated for simultaneous feature selection and classification.

To validate the effectiveness of the SBL method, we carry out an extensive experimental comparison among different competing methods including (1) CSP+SVM, (2) filter bank CSP (FBCSP)+SVM (Ang et al. 2008), and (3) CSP+SBL. A 10 × 10-fold CV is carried out to evaluate the classification performance. Specifically, the available data are equally divided into 10 subsets in 10 different orders. In each order, a procedure, in which nine subsets are used for feature extraction and classifier training and the left one subset for accuracy testing, is repeated 10 times so that each subset serves once for testing. The classification accuracy is then averaged on all the 10 orders.

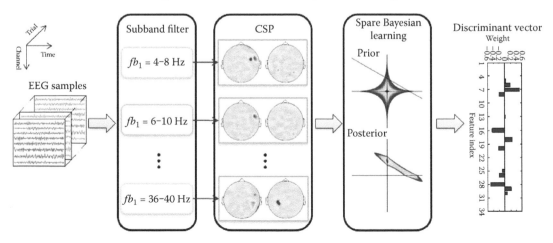

**FIGURE 21.7** Illustration of the sparse Bayesian learning-based algorithm for EEG classification in motor-imagery BCI.

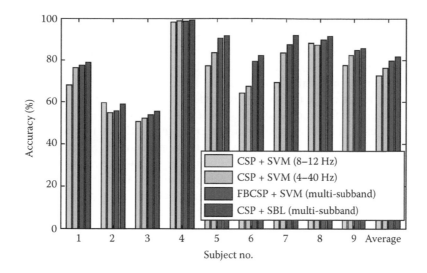

**FIGURE 21.8** Classification accuracies (%) derived from different algorithms for the nine subjects in BCI Competition IV data set IIb, respectively.

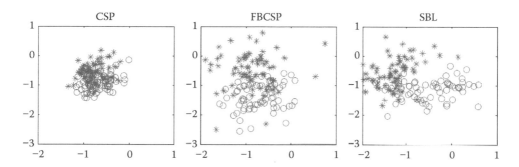

**FIGURE 21.9** Distribution of the two most significant features obtained by CSP, FBCSP, and SBL, respectively, for a typical subject.

### 21.5.2.3 Results

Figure 21.8 depicts the SMR classification accuracies obtained by the four methods for all nine subjects, respectively. Though optimizing the subband features, both the FBCSP+SVM and the CSP+SBL methods performed better than the CSP+SVM with the alpha band (8–12 Hz) only or a wide band (4–40 Hz). More importantly, CSP+SBL further improved the classification accuracy in comparison with FBCSP+SVM. Under the probabilistic framework with a sparsity-inducing prior, SBL implemented simultaneous feature selection and classification. As a result, the selected features naturally provide good discriminant information toward higher separability between different motor imagery tasks. The results shown in Figure 21.9 indicate that the SBL method obtained more separable feature distribution than those of CSP and FBCSP.

## 21.6 DISCUSSION

In our experimental study, we mainly investigated the effectiveness of Bayesian learning based algorithms for the simultaneous feature optimization and classification of EEG in BCI applications. In fact, Bayesian learning-based methods have gained widespread successes in various problems of brain signal analysis, including spatial filtering (Zhang et al. 2013a), automatic source estimation (Zhang et al. 2017b; Wipf et al. 2010), channel selection (Yu et al. 2015), data reconstruction (Zhang et al. 2014c), and so on. By extending the automatic relevance determination to a group version, Yu et al. (2015) proposed a group SBL algorithm for channel optimization in P300-based BCI. With the marginal likelihood maximization technique, hyperparameters are automatically estimated from training data to determine the sparsity of model for significant channel selection. By exploiting variational algorithm for groupwise SBL, Wu et al. (2015) established a probabilistic model of CSP for a reliable estimation of the spatiotemporal pattern of EEG in a Stroop color naming task, which effectively alleviates the overfitting issue of the conventional CSP algorithm. Suk and Lee (2012) designed a Bayesian framework by formulating the spatio-spectral filter optimization as the estimation of a posterior probability density function. The EEG features with significant discriminative powers were then effectively extracted based on a particle-based probabilistic approximation algorithm, which effectively improved EEG classification accuracy for BCI applications.

The prior knowledge plays a key role in Bayesian learning since it characterizes what hypothesis or constraint we expect to impose on the data-driven model. BLDA adopted a standard Gaussian prior for $l_2$-norm regularization while SBL exploited a separate Gaussian prior for sparse learning. In addition to these two priors, several other types of priors may also be adopted for developing effective Bayesian learning algorithms. For instance, the Laplace prior provides a unimodal posterior with log-concavity to avoid the possible local minima of inference (Zhang et al. 2016b; Figueiredo 2003). On the other hand, the spike-and-slab prior provides a mixture of narrow and wide Gaussian to effectively implement sparse variable selection (Ishwaran et al. 2010).

More recently, an increasing number of advanced algorithms based on Bayesian learning have arisen, which were mostly developed based on the so-called tensor decomposition (Cichocki et al. 2015). Collaboratively multiway optimization has been suggested to be more effective than the conventional one-way optimization for EEG data analysis because of the potential multidimensional structure (i.e., space, time–frequency, trial, condition, etc.) of neurological signals (Cichockie et al. 2008; Zhang et al. 2013b,c; Zhou et al. 2016). Thus, multiway Bayesian learning holds great promise for exploring discriminative features from the multidimensional structure of EEG by exploiting well-designed priors in different dimensions. By combining Bayesian learning and tensor decomposition, a multiway extension of Bayesian learning has been proposed for tensor completion using probabilistic inference-based automatic rank determination (Zhao et al. 2015). With a constructed EEG tensor data, a fully Bayesian tensor factorization-based method was successfully developed to implement accurate EEG completion for artifact removal in ERP-based BCI (Zhang et al. 2016a). A variational scheme-based Bayesian tensor modeling method has also proven its strength on ERP component estimation from multicondition and multichannel EEG (Wu et al. 2014). More studies on developing sophisticated Bayesian learning algorithms are ongoing, which would provide more promising performance for outlier detection and artifact removal, feature optimization, and robust classification for various BCI applications.

## 21.7 CONCLUSIONS

In this chapter, we presented a tutorial that introduced how to implement Bayesian learning, including BLDA and SBL in EEG feature optimization and classification for BCI applications. Preceded by describing the relationships among discriminant analysis, LSR, maximum likelihood estimation, and regularization, the algorithmic principles and features of BLDA and SBL are detailedly explained in the aspects of prior designing, posterior inference, and hyperparameter estimation. Two examples were provided to explicitly explain the usage of BLDA and SBL for EEG analysis on two data sets recorded from ERP and SMR BCI paradigms, respectively. Extensive experimental comparisons were carried out among the Bayesian learning algorithms and other state-of-the-art methods. The experimental results confirmed the superiority of Bayesian learning on discriminative feature extraction and robust classifier calibration for improving BCI performance. A discussion was provided on the more widespread applications of Bayesian learning in brain signal analysis and some potential extensions for exploring more complex but important information from EEG for further performance improvement of BCI systems.

## REFERENCES

Ang, K. K., Chin, Z. Y., Wang, C., Guan, C., and Zhang, H. Filter bank common spatial pattern algorithm on BCI competition IV datasets 2a and 2b. *Frontiers in Neuroscience*, 2012, 6: 39.

Ang, K. K., Chin, Z. Y., Zhang, H., and Guan, C. Filter bank common spatial pattern (FBCSP) in brain–computer interface. In: *IEEE International Joint Conference on Neural Networks (IJCNN 2008)*, 2008: 2390–2397.

Ang, K. K., Guan, C., Chua, K. S. G., Ang, B. T., Kuah, C. W. K., Wang, C., Phua, K. S., Chin, Z. Y., and Zhang, H. A large clinical study on the ability of stroke patients to use an EEG-based motor imagery brain–computer interface. *Clinical EEG and Neuroscience*, 2011, 42(4): 253–258.

Arvaneh, M., Guan, C., Ang, K. K., and Quek, C. Optimizing the channel selection and classification accuracy in EEG-based BCI. *IEEE Transactions on Biomedical Engineering*, 2011, 58(6): 1865–1873.

Babacan, S. D., Molina, R., and Katsaggelos, A. K. Bayesian compressive sensing using Laplace priors. *IEEE Transactions on Image Processing*, 2010, 19(1): 53–63.

Bishop, C. M. Pattern recognition and machine learning. New York: Springer, 2006.

Blankertz, B., Curio, G., and Müller, K. R. Classifying single trial EEG: Towards brain computer interfacing. In: *Advances in Neural Information Processing Systems (NIPS)*, 2002, 14: 157–164.

Blankertz, B., Lemm, S., Treder, M., Haufe, S., and Müller, K. R. Single-trial analysis and classification of ERP components—A tutorial. *NeuroImage*, 2011, 56(2): 814–825.

Blankertz, B., Sannelli, C., Halder, S., Hammer, E. M., Kübler, A., Müller, K.-R., Curio, G., and Dickhaus, T. Neurophysiological predictor of SMR-based BCI performance. *NeuroImage*, 2010, 51(4): 1303–1309.

Blankertz, B., Tomioka, R., Lemm, S., Kawanabe, M., and Müller, K. R. Optimizing spatial filters for robust EEG single-trial analysis. *IEEE Signal Processing Magazine*, 2008, 25(1): 41–56.

Carlson, T., and Millan, J. d. R. Brain-controlled wheelchairs: A robotic architecture. *IEEE Robotics & Automation Magazine*, 2013, 20(1): 65–73.

Chaudhary, U., Birbaumer, N., and Ramos-Murguialday, A. Brain–computer interfaces for communication and rehabilitation. *Nature Reviews Neurology*, 2016, 12: 513–525.

Chen, X., Chen, Z., Gao, S., and Gao, X. A high-ITR SSVEP-based BCI speller. *Brain–Computer Interfaces*, 2014, 1(3–4): 181–191.

Cichocki, A., Mandic, D., Lathauwer, L., Zhou, G., Zhao, Q., Caiafa, C., and Phan, H. A. Tensor decompositions for signal processing applications: From two-way to multiway component analysis. *IEEE Signal Processing Magazine*, 2015, 32(2): 145–163.

Cichocki, A., Washizawa, Y., Rutkowski, T., Bakardjian, H., Phan, A.-H., Choi, S., Lee, H., Zhao, Q., Zhang, L., and Li, Y. Noninvasive BCIs: Multiway signal-processing array decompositions. *IEEE Computer*, 2008, 41(10): 34–42.

Farwell, L. A., and Donchin, E. Talking off the top of your head: Toward a mental prosthesis utilizing event-related brain potentials. *Electroencephalography and Clinical Neurophysiology*, 1988, 70(6): 510–523.

Figueiredo, M. A. Adaptive sparseness for supervised learning. *IEEE Transactions on Pattern Analysis and Machine Intelligence*, 2003, 25(9): 1150–1159.

Higashi, H., and Tanaka, T. Simultaneous design of FIR filter banks and spatial patterns for EEG signal classification. *IEEE Transactions on Biomedical Engineering*, 2013, 60(4): 1100–1110.

Hoffmann, U. Bayesian machine learning applied in a brain–computer interface for disabled users. PhD thesis, 2007.

Hoffmann, U., Vesin, J. M., Ebrahimi, T., and Diserens, K. An efficient P300-based brain–computer interface for disabled subjects. *Journal of Neuroscience Methods*, 2008, 167(1): 115–125.

Huang, D., Qian, K., Fei, D.-Y., Jia, W., Chen, X., and Bai, O. Electroencephalography (EEG)-based brain–computer interface (BCI): A 2-D virtual wheelchair control based on event-related desynchronization/synchronization and state control. *IEEE Transactions on Neural Systems and Rehabilitation Engineering*, 2012, 20(3): 379–388.

Ishwaran, H., Rao, J., and Kogalur, U. Spikeslab: Prediction and variable selection using spike and slab regression. *The R Journal*, 2010, 2(2): 68–73.

Jin, J., Allison, B. Z., Kaufmann, T., Kübler, A., Zhang, Y., Wang, X., and Cichocki, A. The changing face of P300 BCIs: A comparison of stimulus changes in a P300 BCI involving faces, emotion, and movement. *PLoS One*, 2012, 7(11): e49688.

422                                                                                                    Brain–Computer Interfaces Handbook

Jin, J., Sellers, E. W., Zhou, S., Zhang, Y., Wang, X., and Cichocki, A. A P300 brain–computer interface based on a modification of the mismatch negativity paradigm. *International Journal of Neural Systems*, 2015, 25(3): 1550011.

Klein, E., and Nam, C. Neuroethics and brain–computer interfaces (BCIs). *Brain–Computer Interfaces*, 2016, 3(3): 123–125.

Koo, B., Lee, H.-G., Nam, Y., Kang, H., Koh, C. S., Shin, H.-C., and Choi, S. A hybrid NIRS-EEG system for self-paced brain computer interface with online motor imagery. *Journal of Neuroscience Methods*, 2015, 244: 26–32.

Krusienski, D. J., Grosse-Wentrup, M., Galan, F., Coyle, D., Miller, K. J., Forney, E., and Anderson, C. W. Critical issues in state-of-the-art brain–computer interface signal processing. *Journal of Neural Engineering*, 2011, 8(2): 025002.

Krusienski, D. J., Sellers, E. W., Cabestaing, F., Bayoudh, S., McFarland, D. J., Vaughan, T. M., and Wolpaw, J. R. A comparison of classification techniques for the P300 Speller. *Journal of Neural Engineering*, 2006, 3(4): 299–305.

Krusienski, D. J., Sellers, E. W., McFarland, D. J., Vaughan, T. M., and Wolpaw, J. R. Toward enhanced P300 speller performance. *Journal of Neuroscience Methods*, 2008, 167(1): 15–21.

Leeb, R., Tonin, L., Rohm, M., Desideri, L., Carlson, T., and Millán, J. d. R. Towards independence: A BCI telepresence robot for people with severe motor disabilities. *Proceedings of the IEEE*, 2015, 103(6): 969–982.

Li, Y., and Nam, C. S. Collaborative brain–computer interface for people with motor disabilities. *IEEE Computational Intelligence Magazine*, 2016, 11(3): 56–66.

Li, Y., Yu, Z., Bi, N., Xu, Y., Gu, Z., and Amari, S. I. Sparse representation for brain signal processing: A tutorial on methods and applications. *IEEE Signal Processing Magazine*, 2014, 31(3): 96–106.

Lotte, F., Congedo, M., Lecuyer, A., Lamarche, F., and Arnaldi, B. A review of classification algorithms for EEG-based brain–computer interfaces. *Journal of Neural Engineering*, 2007, 4(2): R1–R13.

Lotte, F. Signal processing approaches to minimize or suppress calibration time in oscillatory activity based brain–computer interfaces. *Proceedings of the IEEE*, 2015, 103(6): 871–890.

MacKay, D. J. Bayesian interpolation. *Natural Computing*, 1992, 4(3): 415–447.

Manyakov, N. V., Chumerin, N., Combaz, A., and Van Hulle, M. M. Comparison of classification methods for P300 brain–computer interface on disabled subjects. *Computational Intelligence and Neuroscience*, 2011, 2011(2): Article ID 519868.

Mugler, E. M., Ruf, C. A., Halder, S., Bensch, M., and Kubler, A. Design and implementation of a P300-based brain–computer interface for controlling an internet browser. *IEEE Transactions on Neural Systems and Rehabilitation Engineering*, 2010, 18(6): 599–609.

Müller, K. R., Krauledat, M., Dornhege, G., Curio, G., and Blankertz, B. Machine learning techniques for brain–computer interfaces. *Biomedizinische Technik/Biomedical Engineering*, 2004, 49(1): 11–12.

Pfurtscheller, G., Brunner, C., Schlögl, A., and Lopes, S. F. H. Mu rhythm (de)synchronization and EEG single-trial classification of different motor imagery tasks. *NeuroImage*, 2006, 31(1): 153–159.

Rakotomamonjy, A., and Guigue, V. BCI Competition III: Dataset II—Ensemble of SVMs for BCI P300 Speller. *IEEE Transactions on Biomedical Engineering*, 2008, 55(3): 1147–1154.

Samek, W., Vidaurre, C., Muller, K. R., and Kawanabe, M. Stationary common spatial patterns for brain–computer interfacing. *Journal of Neural Engineering*, 2012, 9(2): 026013.

Schäfer, J., and Strimmer, K. A shrinkage approach to large-scale covariance matrix estimation and implications for functional genomics. *Statistical Applications in Genetics and Molecular Biology*, 2005, 4(1): Article32.

Sellers, E. W., and Donchin, E. A P300-based brain–computer interface: Initial tests by ALS patients. *Clinical Neurophysiology*, 2006, 117(3): 538–548.

Siuly, S., and Li, Y. Improving the separability of motor imagery EEG signals using a cross correlation based least square support vector machine for brain–computer interface. *IEEE Transactions on Neural Systems and Rehabilitation Engineering*, 2012, 20(4): 526–538.

Suk, H. I., and Lee, S. W. A novel Bayesian framework for discriminative feature extraction in brain–computer interfaces. *IEEE Transactions on Pattern Analysis and Machine Intelligence*, 2012, 35(2): 286–299.

Tibshirani, R. Regression shrinkage and selection via the Lasso. *Journal of the Royal Statistical Society Series B—Methodological*, 1996, 58(1): 267–288.

Tipping, M. E. Bayesian inference: An introduction to principles and practice in machine learning. In: *Advanced Lectures on Machine Learning, Lecture Notes in Computer Science (LNCS)*, Springer, 2004, 3176: 41–62.

Tipping, M. E. Sparse Bayesian learning and the relevance vector machine. *Journal of Machine Learning Research*, 2001, 1(1): 211–244.

Tomioka, R., and Müller, K. R. A regularized discriminative framework for EEG analysis with application to brain–computer interface. *NeuroImage*, 2010, 49(1): 415–432.

Williams, O., Blake, A., and Cipolla, R. Sparse bayesian learning for efficient visual tracking. *IEEE Transactions on Pattern Analysis and Machine Intelligence*, 2005, 27(8): 1292–1304.

Wipf, D. P., Owen, J. P., Attias, H. T., Sekihara, K., and Nagarajan, S. S. Robust Bayesian estimation of the location, orientation, and time course of multiple correlated neural sources using MEG. *NeuroImage*, 2010, 49(1): 641–655.

Wu, W., Chen, Z., Gao, X., Li, Y., Brown, E., and Gao, S. Probabilistic common spatial patterns for multichannel EEG analysis. *IEEE Transactions on Pattern Analysis and Machine Intelligence*, 2015, 37(3): 639–653.

Wu, W., Wu, C., Gao, S., Liu, B., Li, Y. and Gao, X. Bayesian estimation of ERP components from multicondition and multichannel EEG. *NeuroImage*, 2014, 88: 319–339.

Xu, P., Yang, P., Lei, X., and Yao, D. Z. An enhanced probabilistic LDA for multi-class brain computer interface. *PLoS One*, 2011, 6(1): e14634.

Yu, T., Li, Y., Long, J., and Gu, Z. Surfing the internet with a BCI mouse. *Journal of Neural Engineering*, 2012, 9(3): 036012.

Yu, T., Yu, Z., Gu, Z., and Li, Y. Grouped automatic relevance determination and its application in channel selection for P300 BCIs. *IEEE Transactions on Neural Systems and Rehabilitation Engineering*, 2015, 23(6): 1068–1077.

Zhang, H., Yang, H., and Guan, C. Bayesian learning for spatial filtering in an EEG-based brain–computer interface. *IEEE Transactions on Neural Networks and Learning Systems*, 2013a, 24(7): 1049–1060.

Zhang, Y., Wang, Y., Jin, J., and Wang, X. Sparse Bayesian learning for obtaining sparsity of EEG frequency bands based feature vectors in motor imagery classification. *International Journal of Neural Systems*, 2017a, 27(2): 1–13.

Zhang, Y., Zhao, Q., Jin, J., Wang, X., and Cichocki, A. A novel BCI based on ERP components sensitive to configural processing of human faces. *Journal of Neural Engineering*, 2012, 9(2): 026018.

Zhang, Y., Zhao, Q., Zhou, G., Jin, J., Wang, X., and Cichocki, A. Removal of EEG artifacts for BCI applications using fully Bayesian tensor completion. In: *2016 Acoustics, Speech and Signal Processing (ICASSP)*, 2016a: 819–823.

Zhang, Y., Zhou, G., Jin, J., Wang, M., Wang, X., and Cichocki, A. L1-regularized multiway canonical correlation analysis for SSVEP-based BCI. *IEEE Transactions on Neural System and Rehabilitation Engineering*, 2013b, 21(6): 887–896.

Zhang, Y., Zhou, G., Jin, J., Wang, X., and Cichocki, A. Frequency recognition in SSVEP-based BCI using multiset canonical correlation analysis. *International Journal of Neural Systems*, 2014a, 24(2): 1450013 (14 pages).

Zhang, Y., Zhou, G., Jin, J., Wang, X., and Cichocki, A. Optimizing spatial patterns with sparse filter bands for motor-imagery based brain–computer interface. *Journal of Neuroscience Methods*, 2015, 255: 85–91.

Zhang, Y., Zhou, G., Jin, J., Zhang, Y., Wang, X., and Cichocki, A. Sparse Bayesian multiway canonical correlation analysis for EEG pattern recognition. *Neurocomputing*, 2017b, 225: 103–110.

Zhang, Y., Zhou, G., Jin, J., Zhao, Q., Wang, X., and Cichocki, A. Aggregation of sparse linear discriminant analysis for event-related potential classification in brain–computer interface. *International Journal of Neural Systems*, 2014b, 24(1): 1450003 (15 pages).

Zhang, Y., Zhou, G., Jin, J., Zhao, Q., Wang, X., and Cichocki, A. Sparse Bayesian classification of EEG for brain–computer interface. *IEEE Transactions on Neural Networks and Learning Systems*, 2016b, 27(11): 2256–2267.

Zhang, Y., Zhou, G., Zhao, Q., Jin, J., Wang, X., and Cichocki, A. Spatial–temporal discriminant analysis for ERP-based brain–computer interface. *IEEE Transactions on Neural Systems and Rehabilitation Engineering*, 2013c, 21(2): 233–243.

Zhang, Z., and Rao, B. D. Sparse signal recovery with temporally correlated source vectors using sparse Bayesian learning. *IEEE Journal of Selected Topics in Signal Processing*, 2011, 5(5): 912–926.

Zhang, Z., Jung, T.-P., Makeig, S., Pi, Z., and Rao, B. D. Spatiotemporal sparse Bayesian learning with applications to compressed sensing of multichannel physiological signals. *IEEE Transactions on Neural Systems and Rehabilitation Engineering*, 2014c, 22(6): 1186–1197.

Zhao, Q., Zhang, L., and Cichocki, A. Bayesian CP factorization of incomplete tensors with automatic rank determination. *IEEE Transactions on Pattern Analysis and Machine Intelligence*, 2015, 37(9): 1751–1763.

Zhou, G., Zhao, Q., Zhang, Y., Adali, T., Xie, S., and Cichocki, A. Linked component analysis from matrices to high-order tensors: Applications to biomedical data. *Proceedings of the IEEE*, 2016, 1104(2): 310–331.

# 22 Transfer Learning for BCIs

*Vinay Jayaram, Karl-Heinz Fiebig, Jan Peters,*
*and Moritz Grosse-Wentrup*

## CONTENTS

22.1 Introduction: Why Do We Need to Worry about Session Transfer? ...................................426
    22.1.1 Transfer Learning ..........................................................................................426
    22.1.2 Mathematical Notation ..................................................................................427
22.2 Approaches in the Feature Space ..............................................................................427
    22.2.1 Nonlinear Representations...............................................................................428
    22.2.2 Riemannian Classification in BCIs....................................................................428
    22.2.3 Regularized Common Spatial Patterns ...............................................................429
22.3 Model Space Learning: A Statistical Learning Framework.............................................431
    22.3.1 MTL in Regression Problems...........................................................................434
    22.3.2 MTL in Classification Problems........................................................................435
    22.3.3 Calibration-Free Decoding and Model Adaptation................................................437
    22.3.4 Dimensionality Reduction in EEG: Feature Decomposition....................................437
    22.3.5 Which Approach Should I Use?........................................................................439
22.4 Conclusions...........................................................................................................440
References.....................................................................................................................440

**Abstract**

Classification and regression in brain–computer interfaces (BCIs) suffer from performance variations across subjects as well as across sessions within individual subjects due to various technical and biological reasons. Such variations limit the amount of data that can be used to train machine learning models, rendering BCIs highly subject specific and requiring tedious calibration and retraining before each usage in order to achieve optimal performance. This chapter presents state-of-the-art approaches to calibration-free and improved decoding through transfer learning techniques from multiple subjects and sessions. Within the feature space, a generalized framework for the popular common spatial patterns is described in terms of covariance regularization with multiple subjects. Recent methods using Riemannian features offer invariance to spatial characteristics between subjects and sessions. Finally, a probabilistic Bayesian multitask learning framework is presented that works on top of feature spaces and learns prior distribution over decision rules of different subjects and sessions. The mathematical details are left in for more technically inclined readers, but intuitions and (when applicable) code bases are referenced for the more pragmatic developer.

## 22.1  INTRODUCTION: WHY DO WE NEED TO WORRY ABOUT SESSION TRANSFER?

Whether due to fatigue, hunger, or a drying out of sensor gel, the signal that comes out of current noninvasive brain measurement techniques changes with time. Worse, while human brains share a generic pattern of functionality, individuals vary significantly. Both of these issues mean that it is impossible to use a brain–computer interface (BCI) like a plug-and-play keyboard for the brain. Rather, continuous BCI usage requires a painstaking process of attaching sensors in precise locations, calibrating them (whether by using training data or some other method), and then being able to use the device (often unreliably) until recalibration is required. In large part, it is not unreasonable to say that this issue is one of the major reasons BCIs are not more widely used today. Humans deal well with complicated devices and even highly unintuitive devices (e.g., consider the QWERTY keyboard layout)—but what they deal very poorly with is inconsistent devices. The combination of the imperfect decoding of human intent from BCI signals and the calibration necessary every time the device is used results in very poor usability for both healthy and disabled users. Happily, over time, the field has come up with many strategies to fight this limitation—and while they have not yet been used in combination with each other, there is no reason that cannot be done in the future.

The oldest, most reliable strategy to deal with session-to-session variation is training (cf. Birbaumer et al. 1999; Wolpaw et al. 1991, 1994)—in essence, teaching the human to boost the signal strength. The human brain can be induced, with much time and effort, to generate effects so strong that they are visible despite the various degradations in the signal. It is the reason that it was possible 20 years ago, using purely noninvasive signals, to have one-dimensional control of a cursor (cf. Wolpaw et al. 1991). Though, in addition to the obvious drawback of time, the other issue with this approach is that it cannot be generalized to new users without their undergoing the same sort of training.

Marginally better than long months of training, we can simply recalibrate the BCI for each new usage. While somewhat tiresome for the subject, it is still better than months of operant conditioning and can require as little as 10 min. The procedure is quite simple: For each new subject or session, simply record some trials in which the subject is told what to do and use these labeled trials to train a session-specific classifier. Throw away all previous data.

The drawback is that, even a linear classifier or regression model usually requires, as a rule of thumb, 10 times more data than it has dimensions to be reliable, forcing the algorithm to use a low-dimensional space of features. Given the noise inherent to BCIs, choosing only very few features is difficult as the information is usually quite widely dispersed within the signal.

### 22.1.1  TRANSFER LEARNING

All machine learning algorithms require some sort of assumptions on the data to learn successfully. The basic idea behind the transfer learning approach presented in the following sections is to replace the generic, uninformed assumptions one might make about an isolated data set with knowledge obtained from different related tasks. Instead of forcing the user to generate strong activity patterns or retraining decoders before each session, one creates decoders that are able to deal with and exploit the changing properties of the signal, also called nonstationarities, by leveraging information from other users and tasks. Transfer learning is the field of crafting algorithms that manage to take information from many related tasks in order to better adapt to a new task. In the realm of BCIs, the related tasks can correspond to past sessions from many previous subjects or days, and the current task can be considered the session of interest. Though well-studied within other classes of machine learning problems, it is only recently coming into focus as an active avenue of research and improvement for BCIs. Following the approach in Jayaram et al. (2016), we divide the transfer learning in BCIs into two subgroups: Feature space learning and model space learning. Both approaches are illustrated in Figure 22.1.

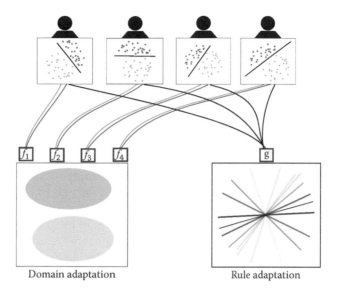

Domain adaptation                    Rule adaptation

**FIGURE 22.1** Schematic of the difference between feature space and model space approaches to transfer learning. Transfer learning is useful in situations in which a single classification rule is incapable of good classification on all the data. Feature space approaches (left) attempt to compute a function that, when applied to the data, brings it to a space in which a single classification boundary suffices for all the tasks. New tasks need to compute a function that brings the data into this space, instead of a full classifier. Model space approaches (right) use the class-specific classification boundaries to learn which decision rules are more likely than other ones, and use this to regularize new tasks.

### 22.1.2 MATHEMATICAL NOTATION

Much of this chapter is written to impart algorithms that can be followed and intuition behind why certain ideas work, but we also include mathematical notation for certain sections to help more technically inclined readers follow along. Formulas throughout this chapter are mostly presented in vectorized form using matrix multiplications. Sets and matrices are denoted with capital letters (e.g., $X$ or $\Sigma$ for EEG time series or covariance matrices, respectively, and $D$ for data sets). Vectors are denoted with bold lowercase letters (e.g., $\mathbf{w}$ for weight vectors and $\mathbf{x}$ for feature vectors or model inputs). Scalar parameters take the form of Greek lowercase letters (they usually describe variable hyperparameters of a model, e.g., $\lambda$, $\alpha$, and $\beta$) and constants with lowercase Latin letters (e.g., $c$ to describe constant terms or factors, $i$ and $j$ for indexing, and $m$, $n$, $d$, and $k$ to indicate dimensionalities).

In general, we denote EEG signals from a session or subject with $X \in \mathbb{R}^{k \times n}$, which means that the $n$ signal samples (number of time points) were recorded at $k$ channels (electrodes).

## 22.2 APPROACHES IN THE FEATURE SPACE

The generic idea behind feature space approaches to transfer learning is that there exists either a single transform or a session-dependent transform that can move all the data into a space in which a single machine learning algorithm can be used for regression or classification. The space of possible transforms is, unsurprisingly, unreasonable to mention anywhere. In the interests of salience and conciseness, we will mention—with intuition, if not derivation—some methods here, giving precedence to methods that have available code in any language or constitute very general techniques that are applicable in a wide range of BCI problems.

### 22.2.1 Nonlinear Representations

First, we might consider the simplest transform: The identity transform. We might assume that there exists a classification function that can, regardless of when the device is put on or who does so, accurately decode intention. But, as mentioned in the beginning, this means that the function must be able to deal with not only differences in signal qualities but also anatomical or functional differences in the various humans who might want to use the BCI. That means that the function would have to be quite complicated in order to infer so much context about each data point it is presented with, which is a problem in itself: The more complicated a function, the more data it needs to be trained with to avoid overfitting and generalize well to new data.

When it comes to learning highly complex functions that are very accurate, the reader may think of neural networks. As a parametrization of a very rich function class, they have become more and more common and powerful; unfortunately, they are also very data hungry. While this is not a problem for neural networks trained on databases of millions of images, this poses a problem for networks intended for human use, as we quickly become fatigued when asked to provide thousands of examples to train such networks. However, some work in the area of deep learning still shows promising success when large data sets are used (cf. Hennrich et al. 2015; Lu et al. 2016). Outside of noninvasive interfaces, we refer to the approach by Sussillo et al. (2016) that has also been shown to be very powerful in invasive BCI technology.

### 22.2.2 Riemannian Classification in BCIs

Looking at the neural network, it is interesting to note that the output class really only appears at the end. The network spends most of its energy trying to figure out some sort of feature representation that allows it to accurately decode the classes, but the decoding itself only happens in the last layer. If we want to try and match the performance in a transfer learning setting, but we do not have very much data, we may try to find features that are interesting and robust ourselves, instead of giving the classifier the raw time series. Feature engineering has been a focus of BCI research for decades, with the most recent advances in the field due to approaches in Riemannian geometry.

We know that many voluntary actions are related to the oscillations of activity of neurons in the brain (such as the sensorimotor rhythm). Conveniently, these oscillations are related to the variance of a measured time series—a fact that has been used to develop many popular methods. However, what was recently realized is that instead of looking purely at variance, one can look at covariance instead. By computing the covariance matrix over space for a given trial (preprocessed into the appropriate frequency range), one can generate an object that is surprisingly powerful in decoding intentions from brain signals. The trick is to not think of each entry in this covariance matrix as a separate feature, but rather to imagine the whole as a single mathematical object on a manifold and then train a classifier that respects the underlying geometry.

The idea of manifolds is intuitively quite simple. Much as humans, though existing in three dimensions, are only found on the surface of the earth, which is two-dimensional, mathematical constructs often live in spaces that are smaller and less obvious than the ones they are found in. Riemannian geometry means taking that into account when computing distances; for example, when determining the distance between America and China, one does not compute the line that goes through the earth's core, but rather a path that an airplane would take. Similarly for objects on Riemannian manifolds, it is often far more useful not to look at the linear distance between their embeddings but something else. Specifically in the case of BCIs, the mathematical construct in question is the covariance matrix, which is always symmetric with positive diagonal elements. Given $k$ channels, the covariance matrix can be unrolled into a $k(k + 1)/2$-dimensional vector (once you eliminate duplicate entries); however, simply looking at the standard, Euclidean distance between two such vectors is often unhelpful. Barachant et al. (2012) realized that there are two ways of dealing with this issue, in light of the underlying structure: Either to use methods that are based on this true, manifold structure, or mapping these points onto a space where the Euclidean distance is a more reasonable measure. In his 2012 paper, he proposes methods for both: the mean distance to the Riemannian mean (MDRM) method for objects on the manifold and the idea of tangent space approximation.

Mathematically, the Euclidean distance between two covariance matrices is noted as $d_{Fr}(X,Y) = X - Y_2 = \sqrt{\text{Tr}((X-Y)^T(X-Y))}$. This is equivalent to taking the squared difference between every entry of the matrices, summing them, and taking the root—it in effect assumes each dimension is unrelated to the other ones (e.g., if we were to shuffle indices of the elements of both matrices, the distance would remain unchanged). The distance measure that Barachant proposed is called the affine-invariant distance, written $d_{AI}(X, Y) = \|\log(X^{-1}Y)\|_2$. This measure cannot be used for all matrices—it requires the matrix log of an inverse, both of which are whole-matrix operations. Further, it is called the affine-invariant measure because the distance does not change if we multiply both matrices by any invertible matrix on the left:

$$d_{AI}(MX, MY) = \left\|\log((MX)^{-1}MY)\right\|_2 = \left\|\log(X^{-1}M^{-1}MY)\right\|_2 = d_{AI}(X,Y) \tag{22.1}$$

One example of how this distinction can be very helpful is in the case of electrode shift. If, during use or between sessions, the positions of the electrodes are shifted (or if there is an error and electrode indices are permuted), the Frobenius distance between the pre- and post-shift matrices will reflect the displacements. The affine invariant distance, since both of these changes are invertible, is unaffected, thereby removing some sources of nonstationarity from the classification task.

MDRM can be thought of as clustering on a manifold when all the labels are known. For each class in a multiclass task, the labeled points are used to compute a class mean. New points are classified based on which mean they are closest to, according to a Riemannian distance. This clustering approach can be used as a transfer learning technique by simply pooling data from many previous sessions.

Tangent space approximation refers to projecting data onto a space tangent to the manifold at a certain point, such that the projected data are well-described by Euclidean distances. This allows classifiers that are normally used with Euclidean spaces—LDA, SVM, logistic regression—to be used. However, it requires computing a point from which to determine the tangent space, which may be problematic if the new task is far enough away on the manifold for the assumptions of this method to break down.

Both the previous algorithms can be used with ERP paradigms as well (Barachant and Congedo 2014) and the code to do these transforms can be found in Python at https://github.com/alexandrebarachant.

### 22.2.3 REGULARIZED COMMON SPATIAL PATTERNS

While the previous methods are powerful ways of using both spatial and power-based features, they have an issue of dimensionality. Given $k$ channels, one has a mathematical object that is of a size nearing $k^2/2$. Even small amounts of noise become very problematic in these high-dimensional spaces and require more data to average over. To deal with this problem, we might consider dimensionality reduction measures—which in BCIs has historically been delegated to spatial filtering.

The most widely used supervised spatial filtering method in BCIs is common spatial patterns (CSPs). It is discussed in more detail elsewhere in the book, but we will briefly review the fundamentals here. For a two-class problem, a covariance matrix of the time-series data is computed per class. These two matrices are used to find directions that maximize the difference between classes—some number of these (heuristically 6) are used to project the data down to a more manageable and task-specific space. Unfortunately, this method is highly sensitive to nonstationarities, and therefore the recovered directions tend to preserve very little of the signal of interest when applied to other subjects or other sessions. Lotte and Guan (2011) unified two main approaches to increase the robustness of CSP filters: Either the estimation of the class covariance matrices can be regularized, or the estimation of the directions can be regularized. Both can be done in single task and transfer learning settings, but here we will focus on the ways regularization can be applied as a method for transfer learning.

Mathematically, we want to find a set of filters $W$ that we can multiply to our trial data matrix by, such that the filtered signal $S = WX$ only contains only specific information and is more useful for decoding. CSP computes a spatial filter $w$ by maximizing the ratio between interclass signal variances. The CSP objective is very simple: Assume that $X_1$ and $X_2$ are the signals each corresponding to one of two brain states (we can get these by, for example, concatenating the trials corresponding to each class). The CSP filter is then obtained by optimizing for

$$\max_{\mathbf{w}} \frac{\mathbf{w}^T \Sigma_1 \mathbf{w}}{\mathbf{w}^T \Sigma_2 \mathbf{w}}, \tag{22.2}$$

where $\Sigma_1$ is the spatial covariance matrix of $X_1$ and $\Sigma_2$ is the covariance of $X_2$. If the DC offset of the signal is removed, the estimates amount to $\Sigma_1 \propto X_1^T X_1$ and $\Sigma_2 \propto X_2^T X_2$. Hence, Equation 22.2 is maximized by maximizing the band-power of signals originating from one state while at the same time minimizing the band-power within the other state, resulting in filtered signals that can be further processed into discriminative features. A solution of Equation 22.2 is an eigendecomposition of $\Sigma_2^{-1} \Sigma_1$ where the eigenvectors with the largest and smallest eigenvalues constitute spatial filters in CSP.

Finding robust filters that work well across sessions or even subjects is an active research area and many methods have been proposed so far to overcome these difficulties (cf. Devlaminck et al. 2011; Lotte and Guan 2011; Samek et al. 2014, and references therein). In this chapter, we present the framework to regularize CSP filters proposed by Lotte and Guan (2011). This framework unifies regularization on the level of the covariance estimates for CSP as well as on the objective and incorporates many regularization techniques including session and subject transfer approaches.

Instead of using the empirical covariance matrix computed from some brain state, we use a regularized covariance estimate

$$\mathrm{rcov}(\Sigma; \alpha, \beta, c, G) = (1 - \alpha)((1 - \beta)c\Sigma + \beta G) + \alpha I, \tag{22.3}$$

where $\beta \in [0,1]$ is a hyperparameter that shrinks the original covariance estimate toward a generic a priori covariance matrix $G$, $\alpha \in [0,1]$ further shrinks the estimate toward the identity matrix $I$, and $c \in \mathbb{R}$ is some constant scaling factor. The shrinkage toward the identity matrix is also known as diagonal loading and is used to increase the numerical stability of the estimated covariance. The a priori covariance matrix $G$ on the other hand encodes prior knowledge of the corresponding brain state and is therefore subject to transfer learning techniques. This means that $G$ may be obtained in a data-driven manner from recordings of other subjects or sessions. For an exhaustive list of approaches, please consult Lotte and Guan (2011), Samek et al. (2014), and Devlaminck et al. (2011). The simplest way to compute $G$ with transfer knowledge is to average (either in the Euclidean or Riemannian sense) over the covariance estimates of other subjects and past sessions.

The next regularization within this framework occurs directly at the objective in Equation 22.2. The idea takes the form of penalizing deviations from some prior belief of the CSP filter. Assume that we computed appropriate regularized class-wise covariances $\hat{\Sigma}_1 = \mathrm{rcov}(\Sigma_1; \alpha, \beta, c, G_1)$ and

$\hat{\Sigma}_2 = \mathrm{rcov}(\Sigma_2; \alpha, \beta, c, G_2)$ from the original covariance estimates. Regularization on the solutions for the spatial filters is then performed by optimizing for

$$\max_{\mathbf{w}} \frac{\mathbf{w}^T \hat{\Sigma}_1 \mathbf{w}}{\mathbf{w}^T \hat{\Sigma}_2 \mathbf{w} + \lambda r(\mathbf{w})} \quad \text{and} \quad \max_{\mathbf{w}} \frac{\mathbf{w}^T \hat{\Sigma}_2 \mathbf{w}}{\mathbf{w}^T \hat{\Sigma}_1 \mathbf{w} + \lambda r(\mathbf{w})}, \tag{22.4}$$

where $r(\mathbf{w})$ is the regularization function that encodes the prior belief in the filter (i.e., higher values correspond to higher deviations of the given $w$ from the prior belief) and $\lambda \in \mathbb{R}$ is the regularization factor to control the amount of penalization. The final regularized CSP framework in Equation 22.4 has two objectives: one corresponds to maximizing the variances of class 1 while minimizing the constraints, while the other consists of the same for class 2. This framework has a lot of hyperparameters but captures many robust CSP methods in special cases of parameter settings. For instance, $\beta = 0$ and $c = 1$ is equivalent to a covariance estimate with diagonal loading. A simple choice for the filter penalty is to use a Tikhonov regularizer $r(\mathbf{w}) = \mathbf{w}^T K \mathbf{w}$ where $K$ encodes the prior for the filter and induces L2 regularization in the objective. In this case, the solution for Equation 22.4 corresponds to taking the eigenvectors with the largest eigenvalues of $(\hat{\Sigma}_2 + \lambda K)^{-1} \hat{\Sigma}_1$ and $(\hat{\Sigma}_1 + \lambda K)^{-1} \hat{\Sigma}_2$.

The empirical evaluation of the regularized CSP framework showed that indeed subject transfer at different levels seems to outperform regular CSP. The authors found that for subjects that perform well from the start, such regularizations do not seem to be necessary. However, for subjects that do not perform well, training spatial filters with data from other subjects is preferable (cf. Lotte and Guan 2011 and their results for CCSP, GLRCSP, and SSRCSP). We can also assume that these results hold for the case where only few samples for training are available, as the RCSP optimization process will pull spatial filters toward the generic structure employed by the corresponding regularization component.

## 22.3 MODEL SPACE LEARNING: A STATISTICAL LEARNING FRAMEWORK

In contrast to approaches that attempt to find a consistent feature representation for all our data from various users and sessions, there is the idea of regularizing in the model space. In essence, it is the assumption that the classifier from user A is related in some way to user B. This idea has been used far less in the literature than feature space learning, being mostly limited to work by Alamgir et al. (2010) and Kang and Choi (2014). However, Alamgir et al. (2010) and the improvement added in Jayaram et al. (2016) presented convenient generic approaches that can be adapted to fit many situations, and so we will go through the derivation in more detail here.

The primary goal of any prediction model in machine learning is not to fit the data one already has, but to reliably fit data in the future. In order to find the true underlying model for a given task (assuming such a model exists), statistics and learning theory tell us that with more data to use, we get closer to finding it. However, acquiring data in BCIs is a tedious process and the amount of available data for training is limited. In order to deal with the instabilities arising from small data sets, strong assumptions must be made. As seen in Section 22.2, these assumptions have historically been made about the most appropriate feature space to use: with very predictive features, even a few samples are enough to learn the rule. However, we can also turn this around and ask ourselves whether there are useful assumptions we can make about the model space.

Assumptions on the model space are often incorporated via regularization. Common versions of this are, for example, penalties that penalize how far away a regression vector is from zero and force the model to be simpler. By restricting the space of acceptable solutions to be much smaller than the actual space of possibilities, more reliable predictions can be made. However, the crucial idea behind this form of transfer learning is that there is no reason to assume that the difference from zero is the best thing to penalize. It simply represents one form of prior belief on the form of the regression vector. While this is reasonable in a single task setting, if we have multiple tasks, then we might consider learning the most appropriate form of penalization at the same time as we learn the models themselves. For example, in the most simple way, we might choose the appropriate coefficient for ridge regression not with cross-validation on a single task, but by using the other data sets as validation sets and seeing which one works best across all of them.

The basic idea behind the transfer learning approach presented in the following sections is to replace the generic, uninformed prior assumptions with informed priors obtained from different related tasks. In the context of BCIs, a task is the decoding of brain activity from a subject or session. The goal is to find commonalities in the decoding task between subjects and sessions and use this information as prior belief to regularize training of new decoders. This process is also known as multitask learning (MTL) and we will look at the details of a Bayesian framework for MTL in the following. A major advantage of this framework is the ability to perform calibration-free decoding (i.e., no session-specific data are required and decoding can be done out-of-the-box in new sessions) as well as adapt to new sessions when data become available. In what follows, things might get more mathematical than some readers may find comfortable. The reason is that the presented MTL technique is based on a theoretical setting that allows for the derivations of MTL versions of many learning algorithms by establishing appropriate probabilistic links. In keeping with published literature, MTL versions of two very popular models for regression and classification, namely, linear and logistic regression, are derived in the subsections. These serve as applications of the framework to particular settings, such that the practical user can already use the final algorithms for regression or classification tasks in BCIs. The theoretical practitioner may use the details of the framework presented in the following to derive MTL versions of their own learning algorithms that are able to perform transfer learning. For a more thorough introduction, we suggest to read Jayaram et al. (2016).

Assume that data for a certain paradigm from $m$ subjects or sessions are available. Such data sets may be, for instance, motor imagery of limbs or visually evoked potentials obtained from training sessions with subjects. We will formally denote the set of all task data with

$$T = \left\{ D^{(t)} \right\}_{t=1}^{m}, \text{ where } D^{(t)} = \left\{ \left( \mathbf{x}_i^{(t)}, y_i^{(t)} \right) \right\}_{i=1}^{n_t} \subset \mathbb{R}^d \times C. \tag{22.5}$$

Hence, each of the $m$ data sets contains $n_t$ data points that consist of $d$-dimensional feature vectors $\mathbf{x}_i^{(t)}$ representing brain activity of interest and have a corresponding target label $y_i^{(t)}$ from a set $C$ associated that is to be decoded. For instance, the feature vectors may be trials of band-power values obtained from the sensorimotor rhythms of a subject performing an EEG session and the target labels represent the motor-imagery brain state at which the trial was recorded.

In general, the MTL framework introduced by Alamgir et al. (2010) and Jayaram et al. (2016) is based on a model $f^{(t)} : \mathbb{R}^d \to C$ for the decoding task of each subject individually. An MTL algorithm is then derived in two steps. First, a probabilistic relationship between the target labels and the observations is established through the corresponding task model

$$y_i^{(t)} \sim p\left( y_i^{(t)} \mid f^{(t)}\left( \mathbf{x}_i^{(t)} \right) \right). \tag{22.6}$$

This relationship of observing the true label given the model prediction is also known as the *data likelihood*. In a second step, a *prior distribution* over the task models is introduced

$$f^{(t)} \sim p(f^{(t)}). \tag{22.7}$$

The goal of the prior distribution is to encode commonalities within the models that are found across the decoding tasks of each subject. Bayes' rule then links the data likelihood with the prior belief in the models: assuming that the data and task models are drawn independently, the *posterior distribution* is given by $p(F|T) = p(T|F)\, p(F)\, p(T)^{-1}$ and reads

$$p(F \mid T) = \prod_{t=1}^{m} \prod_{i=1}^{n_t} p\left(y_i^{(t)} \mid f^{(t)}\left(\mathbf{x}_i^{(t)}\right)\right) \prod_{t=1}^{m} p(f^{(t)}) p(T)^{-1}, \qquad (22.8)$$

where $F$ denotes the set of task models. As the *evidence* $p(T)$ does not depend on the model, a maximum a posteriori (MAP) estimate of the parameters in Equation 22.8 is obtained by optimizing for the objective

$$\min_{f^{(t)}, p(f^{(t)})} \sum_{t=1}^{m} \sum_{i=1}^{n_t} \ln p\left(y_i^{(t)} \mid f^{(t)}\left(\mathbf{x}_i^{(t)}\right)\right) + \sum_{t=1}^{m} \ln p(f^{(t)}). \qquad (22.9)$$

The first term in Equation 22.9 can be seen as minimizing a loss function on the task-specific data sets, while the second term regularizes the solution toward the shared structure. The task that is to be performed (e.g., regression or classification) is determined by the likelihood that induces the loss function, while the type of regularization depends on the chosen prior assumption. The procedure of this approach is shown in Figure 22.2. In the following two sections, we present MTL versions of two very common models that may be used to perform transfer learning for regression or classification tasks.

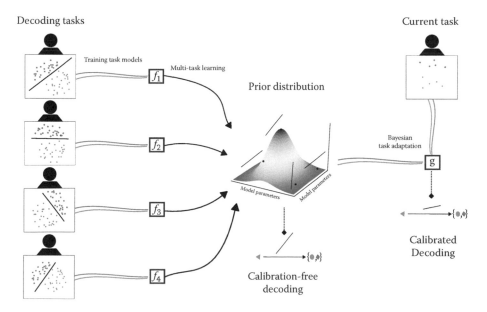

**FIGURE 22.2** Flow of using the MTL approach. Past sessions are used to learn a distribution over classification rule parameters in order to better solve future tasks. The mean (or mode, or median) of this distribution can be used out-of-the-box to classify new points, and with some task-specific data, the distribution can be used to regularize the classifier so a task-specific classifier can be obtained more quickly.

## 22.3.1 MTL in Regression Problems

BCIs sometimes have to deal with problems in which the brain activity has to be decoded into some continuous quantity. For instance, such problems are encountered in response speed estimation (e.g., Wu et al. 2017), determining a subject's attention level (e.g., Kim et al. 2013) or determining the capabilities of subjects to operate a BCI from neurophysiological predictors (e.g., Blankertz et al. 2010 or Grosse-Wentrup and Schölkopf 2012). Another very popular use case for BCIs is also the correction of artifacts using linear regression methods (e.g., Wallstrom et al. 2004). The goal of regression tasks is to create a model that is able to predict a continuous outcome from observations. Hence, the data set represented by Equation 22.5 contains real numbered target variables $C = \mathbb{R}$.

One of the most prominent regression algorithms, because of its simplicity of understanding and closed-form solution, is known under the general term of linear regression. The linear model states a simple weighted sum of the features $f(\mathbf{x}) = \mathbf{w}^T \mathbf{x} + b$, where $\mathbf{w} \in \mathbb{R}^d$ is the weight vector of the model and $b \in \mathbb{R}$ is a bias term. In the following, we will assume that the bias term is subsumed into the weight vector by padding an artificial 1 to the feature vector $\mathbf{x}$ (i.e., the features include the bias term). In the first step of the MTL framework, we have to establish a probabilistic relationship between the observed target variables and model prediction according to Equation 22.6. A common assumption in linear regression is to assume that the observed targets originate from the model's prediction but are distorted by Gaussian noise through factors that have not been explicitly accounted for. Hence, the observed targets are drawn from a normal distribution

$$y_i^{(t)} \sim N\left(y_i^{(t)} \mid f^{(t)}\left(\mathbf{x}_i^{(t)}\right), \sigma^2\right) \tag{22.10}$$

centered at the model prediction with some variance $\sigma^2 \in \mathbb{R}$. This distribution constitutes the data likelihood for the posterior objective that is stated in short. The second step is to find an appropriate prior distribution over the models according to Equation 22.7. In fact, it turns out that assuming a zero mean Gaussian prior over the model parameters with scalar covariance is equivalent to L2 regularization and results in ridge regression. Hence, a suggestive prior assumption is the generalization to a multivariate Gaussian

$$\mathbf{w}^{(t)} \sim N(\mathbf{w}^{(t)} \mid \boldsymbol{\mu}, \boldsymbol{\Sigma}), \tag{22.11}$$

where we want to learn a parameter mean $\boldsymbol{\mu} \in \mathbb{R}^d$ and covariance matrix $\boldsymbol{\Sigma} \in \mathbb{R}^{d \times d}$ that encodes transfer knowledge in an MTL fashion. We can now plug the density functions for the likelihood in Equation 22.10 and prior (Equation 22.11) into the MAP objective from Equation 22.9 and optimize for the prior parameters. It turns out that the optimal parameter estimates for the prior are just the standard sample estimates of the Gaussian distribution obtained from the individual optimal task weights. However, while the MAP estimates for the optimal task weights have a closed-form solution, they need the prior parameters for regularization. Hence, an iterative update procedure has to be applied between updating the model and learning the prior distribution. The MTL algorithm for linear regression with the corresponding update rules is presented in Algorithm 1.

**Algorithm 1: Multitask Linear Regression**

**Input:** Task data sets $T$ as described in Equation 22.5
**Output:** Gaussian prior $N(\boldsymbol{\mu}, \boldsymbol{\Sigma})$, over model weights

1. For each task $t = 1, 2, \ldots, m$ do:
   1.1. Compute the feature matrix $X^{(t)} \in \mathbb{R}^{n_t \times d}$ containing the row-wise stored features;
   1.2. Compute the label vector $\mathbf{y}^{(t)} \in \mathbb{R}^{n_t}$;

2. Initialize $\mu := 0$ and $\Sigma := I$;
3. While $\mu$ and $\Sigma$ are not converged do:
   3.1. Perform a MAP estimate for each task model $t = 1, 2, \ldots, m$ with

$$\mathbf{w}^{(t)} := \left( \frac{1}{\sigma^2} \Sigma X^{(t)T} X^{(t)} + I \right)^{-1} \left( \frac{1}{\sigma^2} \Sigma X^{(t)T} \mathbf{y}^{(t)} + \mu \right)$$

   3.2. Update the prior parameters from the current optimal task weights with

$$\mu := \frac{1}{m} \sum_{t=1}^{m} \mathbf{w}^{(t)} \quad \Sigma := \frac{1}{m-1} \sum_{t=1}^{m} (\mathbf{w}^{(t)} - \mu)(\mathbf{w}^{(t)} - \mu)^T$$

4. Return $\mu$ and $\Sigma$;                                                                                      ■

Using a particular labeling scheme, it is possible to also use this regression-based method for classification; indeed, it can be shown that linear discriminant analysis, a popular linear classifier, is a special case of linear regression as shown above. In this classification setting, the ideas above have been used in the case of the P300 response by Kindermans et al. (2012).

In their work, they also assume a Gaussian prior over the weights and use it to regularize the model for new subjects. However, they assume that the covariance of their prior distribution is a multiple of the identity matrix, unlike in our framework where the full distribution is learned in a maximum likelihood procedure. Whether this is more or less useful is a question that can only be answered empirically; in their experiments as well as later work, Kindermans et al. (2014) show their restriction to give quite robust results. Still, as more and more data from more and more subjects are gathered, the maximum likelihood approach converges to the true covariance of the distribution and is thus more flexible. Moreover, analysis of the trained covariances revealed that they encode task-specific properties and act as an implicit feature selection method based on the presented data.

Also worth pointing out for the work in Kindermans et al. (2014) is that it is not necessary to only look at likelihood as a function of only the EEG data. In the case of spelling paradigms, one can make use of the fact that words and sentences are highly structured to learn language models either within or across patients and use this relation as another form of transfer learning. The details of how to combine these two can be seen in Kindermans et al. (2012) and Kindermans et al. (2014).

### 22.3.2 MTL in Classification Problems

While regression tasks frequently occur in BCI applications, decoding brain activity into distinct mental states representing the subjects' intention is the main application of BCIs. This kind of task belongs to the regime of classification problems in which the goal of the model is to predict a certain class to which the observations belong. For instance, one could operate a switch, or say yes or no, via imagining right or left hand movement. In classification problems, the dependent variable is discrete and the linear Gaussian model previously used for regression is not appropriate anymore. Fiebig et al. (2016) altered the model and derived an MTL version of logistic regression, a popular probabilistic classification method.

In case of binary classification, the data sets described by Equation 22.5 contain target variables of the form $C = \{c_1, c_2\}$, where $c_1$ and $c_2$ represent one of two mental states that we want to decode from brain activity (e.g., right hand or left hand movement imagination). A common interpretation for such a classification problem is to assign conditional probabilities to each class. In particular, if we observe some feature vector $\mathbf{x} \in \mathbb{R}^d$, we are interested in the probability $p(c_1|\mathbf{x})$ of observing brain state $c_1$ given that we observed the brain activity $\mathbf{x}$. In binary classification, the probability $p(c_2|\mathbf{x})$ of observing $c_2$ under $\mathbf{x}$ is then given by the complementary event $1 - p(c_1|\mathbf{x})$. Such a distribution can be modeled with the function $f(\mathbf{x}) = \varphi(\mathbf{w}^T \mathbf{x} + b)$, where $\mathbf{w} \in \mathbb{R}^d$ is the weight vector of the model, $b \in \mathbb{R}$ is a bias term, and $\varphi(s) = (1 + e^{-s})^{-1}$ is called the *logistic sigmoid* function. Again, we will assume that the bias term is represented as an additional artificial feature and pulled into the weight vector. Notice that this model is essentially the same linear regression that was described above, but uses the logistic sigmoid activation to map the output into a probabilistic range (0, 1). Hence, we can model the conditional class probabilities with $p(c_1|\mathbf{x}) = f(\mathbf{x})$ and $p(c_2|\mathbf{x}) = 1 - f(\mathbf{x})$. By regarding the observed labels in the data sets as certain and uncertain events (we know to which class they belong when observing a feature vector), we can represent the classes with $C = \{1, 0\}$ and label features for class $c_1$ with 1 and for class $c_2$ with 0. We are now able to perform the first step from Equation 22.6 of the MTL framework and link the observed target variables to the logistic model prediction through a Bernoulli distribution

$$y_i^{(t)} \sim \mathrm{Ber}\left(y_i^{(t)} \mid f^{(t)}\left(\mathbf{x}_i^{(t)}\right)\right), \tag{22.12}$$

where $\mathrm{Ber}(y \mid p = p^y (1 - p)^{1-y}$. With Equation 22.12, we have the data likelihood at hand and need an appropriate prior distribution over the logistic model to complete the second step from Equation 22.7 in the MTL framework. One may resort to the conjugate prior of the Bernoulli distribution, which is the Beta distribution. However, the similarities to the linear regression model and the properties of the Gaussian prior there (e.g., implicit feature selection through the covariance matrix) led to the decision of using a general multivariate Gaussian prior over the weights. Hence, the prior over logistic models is the same as the prior over the weights in Equation 22.11, which again captures similarities across decoding tasks in a mean $\boldsymbol{\mu} \in \mathbb{R}^d$ and covariance matrix $\Sigma \in R^{d \times d}$. Putting the likelihood in Equation 22.12 together with the prior assumption (Equation 22.11) into the MAP objective in Equation 22.9 and going through a little bit of math yields the optimization problem

$$\min_{\mathbf{w}^{(t)}, \boldsymbol{\mu}, \Sigma} \sum_{t=1}^{m} \sum_{i=1}^{n_t} -y_i^{(t)} \ln f\left(\mathbf{x}_i^{(t)}\right) - \left(1 - y_i^{(t)}\right) \ln\left(1 - f\left(\mathbf{x}_i^{(t)}\right)\right) + \frac{m}{2} \ln |\Sigma| + \frac{1}{2} \sum_{t=1}^{m} (\mathbf{w}^{(t)} - \boldsymbol{\mu})^T \Sigma^{-1} (\mathbf{w}^{(t)} - \boldsymbol{\mu}),$$

$$\tag{22.13}$$

where the first term constitutes a cross-entropy error function fitting the task-specific data set while the second term regularizes the solution toward the commonalities encoded in the shared prior. Again, the optimal prior parameters that minimize Equation 22.13 can be obtained by standard sample estimates of the multivariate Gaussian distribution from the optimal task-specific weights. Unfortunately, the MAP estimates of the data set–specific weights do not only depend on the prior mean and covariance, but further do not have a closed-form solution as in the linear regression case. However, an analytic gradient for Equation 22.13 with respect to a task-specific weight vector $w^{(t)}$ is given by

$$\sum_{i=1}^{n_t} \left(f\left(\mathbf{x}_i^{(t)}\right) - y_i^{(t)}\right) \mathbf{x}_i^{(t)} + \Sigma^{-1}(\mathbf{w}^{(t)} - \boldsymbol{\mu}). \tag{22.14}$$

The MAP weights can be efficiently obtained using Equation 22.14 with any highly optimized gradient-based numerical optimization library. The iterative algorithm to learn a logistic regression prior distribution using MTL can be found in Algorithm 2.

**Algorithm 2: Multitask Logistic Regression**

**Input:** Task data sets $T$ as defined in Equation 22.5
**Output:** Gaussian prior $N(\mu, \Sigma)$, over model weights

1. Initialize $\mu := 0$ and $\Sigma := I$;
2. While $\mu$ and $\Sigma$ are not converged, do:
   2.1. Compute $\mathbf{w}^{(t)}$ for all tasks $t = 1, 2,\ldots, m$ by optimizing the loss function in Equation 22.13 using the gradient from Equation 22.14.
   2.2. Update the prior parameters from the current optimal task weights with

$$2.2.1.\ \mu := \frac{1}{m}\sum_{t=1}^{m}\mathbf{w}^{(t)} \quad \Sigma := \frac{1}{m-1}\sum_{t=1}^{m}(\mathbf{w}^{(t)} - \mu)(\mathbf{w}^{(t)} - \mu)^{T}$$

3. Return $\mu$ and $\Sigma$; ∎

### 22.3.3 CALIBRATION-FREE DECODING AND MODEL ADAPTATION

The advantages of the presented MTL approach are twofold. Once the Gaussian prior parameters are trained, they can be used immediately for decoding with new subjects or sessions by parameterizing the corresponding model for regression or classification with the mean. Hence, we obtain a calibration-free decoder that works based on the commonalities found across the decoding tasks for the subjects.

The second benefit to this hierarchical approach is that it allows for model adaptation on-the-fly. As new data come in, each point can be used to adapt the classifier to the current time or subject. What this means in practice is that one can start with a middling classifier (the prior mean) and then update it successively such that it quickly becomes a well-optimized, session-specific classifier. In fact, empirical evaluation of this approach with a sensorimotor rhythm paradigm shows very promising results. All MTL approaches started out with a calibration-free performance above chance and increase accuracy with more and more session-specific data. Figure 22.3 indicates that especially with few samples to train on, MTL clearly outperforms the standard classification method by making effective use of the shared prior distribution trained from other subjects.

### 22.3.4 DIMENSIONALITY REDUCTION IN EEG: FEATURE DECOMPOSITION

The approach so far gives the training data as a matrix, per task, of features from each trial. However, in the light of approaches like CSP, which takes explicit advantage of the spatial pattern of sensors, this may strike one as somewhat odd. Let us imagine that we compute, for a given trial, the band-power in the various canonical functional frequency bands—delta, theta, alpha, beta, and gamma—at each channel. So, given a matrix $X \in \mathbb{R}^{k \times d}$, it would consist of $d$ features computed from $k$ channels. Why should we unroll this richly structured matrix of features into a single vector? Instead, let us consider a model that takes advantage of this spatial and spectral decomposition inherent in our feature matrix:

$$f(X) = \mathbf{a}^{T} X\mathbf{w} + b. \tag{22.15}$$

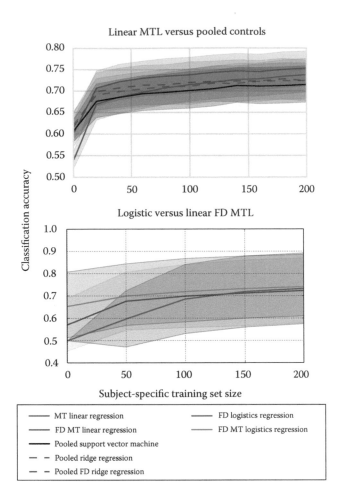

**FIGURE 22.3**   Performance of MTL models compared to standard control models on a real-world EEG data set of a sensorimotor rhythm paradigm. The experiment was conducted on 10 subjects with 300 trials each and the task was to classify if subjects were performing left or right hand haptic motor imagery. Details on the experimental setup can be obtained from Jayaram et al. (2016) or Fiebig et al. (2016). Both plots show how the accuracy evolves over an increasing amount of subject-specific training data provided for calibration. The MTL models are prefixed by MT and feature decomposition is suffixed with FD. The top plot was taken from Jayaram et al. (2016) and shows how a support vector machine (SVM) and ridge regression (RR) where the data of all subjects were pooled perform against the MTL models for linear regression. The bottom plot was taken from Fiebig et al. (2016) and shows how the MTL version of logistic regression performs against a standard logistic regression control and the MTL linear regression (all using the feature decomposition because of the high number of channels).

From this, we can see that we now only need to compute one feature weighting and one channel weighting, which is far smaller than the previous necessity for a weight corresponding to every individual feature. With less weights to compute, less training trials are needed overall. For example, imagine we have a 16-channel setup and take the band-power in 12 2-Hz bands from 6 to 30 Hz from each channel to have 12 band-power features per channel. If we were to unroll the feature matrix, we would have $16 \times 12 = 192$ features, requiring almost 2000 trials for reliable training with linear models. However, using the method suggested above, we would have $16 + 12 = 28$ features, cutting that number by a factor of nearly 100.

The need for less training data can be beneficial for another reason as well: it allows for more exploration in the space of possible paradigms for users. Until now, the paradigm has always dictated the feature space of the classifier. For example, using the ERP features corresponding to trial onset for a motor imagery paradigm would be entirely useless, as would using the appropriate log-band-power features from channels too far from the anatomical motor cortex. Adding relevant features to both paradigms, however, forces the participant to generate an unreasonable amount of data before a good classifier can be determined. This approach allows one to specify a large range of features per channel—say many different frequency windows—and lets the algorithm figure out which features are most relevant. Or, given a set of previously known spatial filters, the decomposition can be used to determine algorithmically how to best combine them for robust classification over many subjects.

The optimization required to extend the model for spatial decomposition is, happily, quite easy. It is not convex, however, meaning that whenever a solution is found, there is no way to guarantee that it is the best solution. In practice, the nonconvexity does not seem to be an issue. The crucial idea behind the updated formula is to consider that when we hold either $\mathbf{a}$ or $\mathbf{w}$ constant, the problem reduces to a standard linear regression problem as we have seen many times before.

$$\mathbf{a}^T X \mathbf{w} = (\mathbf{a}^T X)\mathbf{w} \quad \text{and} \quad \mathbf{a}^T X \mathbf{w} = \mathbf{a}^T (X\mathbf{w}). \tag{22.16}$$

Given either $\mathbf{a}$ or $\mathbf{w}$, we can reshape this bilinear form into a standard linear regression problem and solve it as usual. Assuming the priors on the two vectors are independent, we arrive at coupled linear regression tasks that can be solved sequentially to arrive at a local minimum of the loss function. Figure 22.3 shows that, indeed, the employed dimensionality reduction increases calibration-free and adaptation performance.

Code for the bilinear as well as the linear and logistic approaches can be found in MATLAB under https://github.com/bibliolytic/MTlearning and a scikit compatible version in Python at https://github.com/bibliolytic/pyMTL.

## 22.3.5 Which Approach Should I Use?

Perhaps the greatest drawback for transfer learning in BCIs is that there has yet to be a systemic comparison of the various techniques across various setups. As such, the question of which approach to use is one that each laboratory has dealt with independently; below is a table of suggestions from personal experience for beginners in the field, but it should be noted that there is no official evaluation of them yet.

- Regularized CSP: Has a focus on ERD-based paradigms (e.g., motor imagery). Most effective if the data quality is bad or the EEG setup has many channels (32–256).
- Riemannian features: Has been shown to have large success in motor imagery paradigms, but employs a very high feature dimensionality. Hence, should be used with less than ~32 channels.
- Language model priors according to Kindermans et al.: Showed success with ERP-based paradigms and is reliably applicable with noisy data sets for less than ~32 channels.
- Neural network approaches: Showed convincing success where larger data sets are available. This is not the case for most ERD-based paradigms, but ERP approaches may have enough data in some situations.
- MTL: Best applicable when data from multiple subjects are available. In case of few channels, we suggest to use standard MTL linear or logistic regression. With a high number of channels, MTL feature decomposition should be applied additionally. MTL is also eligible for cases where the paradigm is to be studied in a data-driven manner or features are unknown.

It is also possible to use hybrid techniques and combine approaches on the feature and model space. For instance, Riemannian features can be extracted from a regularized CSP filter bank and combined using MTL. Whether such a combination does yield better performance will likely depend on the situation and is open for investigation.

## 22.4 CONCLUSIONS

The last decades of research have led to hundreds of methods for dealing with the problem of inconsistent signals in BCIs, which can be generalized into the categories explained in this section. We have introduced multiple families of techniques that can be used to effect transfer learning in the particular case of brain–machine interfacing. However, none of the families mentioned here is complete—there is still far more space to improve and develop an algorithm that is robust enough to allow for an out-of-the-box BCI that is good enough for anyone to use.

## REFERENCES

Alamgir, Morteza, Moritz Grosse-Wentrup, and Yasemin Altun. Multitask learning for brain–computer interfaces. AISTATS. Vol. 10. 2010.

Barachant, Alexandre et al. Multiclass brain–computer interface classification by Riemannian geometry. *IEEE Transactions on Biomedical Engineering* 59.4 (2012): 920–928.

Barachant, Alexandre, and Marco Congedo. A plug&play P300 BCI using information geometry. arXiv preprint arXiv:1409.0107 (2014).

Birbaumer, Niels et al. A spelling device for the paralysed. *Nature* 398.6725 (1999): 297–298.

Blankertz, Benjamin et al. Neurophysiological predictor of SMR-based BCI performance. *Neuroimage* 51.4 (2010): 1303–1309.

Devlaminck, Dieter et al. Multisubject learning for common spatial patterns in motor-imagery BCI. *Computational Intelligence and Neuroscience* 2011 (2011): 8.

Fiebig, Karl-Heinz et al. Multi-task logistic regression in brain-computer interfaces. *2016 IEEE International Conference on Systems, Man, and Cybernetics (SMC)*. IEEE, 2016.

Grosse-Wentrup, Moritz, and Bernhard Schölkopf. High gamma-power predicts performance in sensorimotor-rhythm brain–computer interfaces. *Journal of Neural Engineering* 9.4 (2012): 046001.

Hennrich, Johannes et al. Investigating deep learning for fNIRS based BCI. *Engineering in Medicine and Biology Society (EMBC), 2015, 37th Annual International Conference of the IEEE* (2015).

Jayaram, Vinay et al. Transfer learning in brain–computer interfaces. *IEEE Computational Intelligence Magazine* 11.1 (2016): 20–31.

Kang, Hyohyeong, and Seungjin Choi. Bayesian common spatial patterns for multi-subject EEG classification. *Neural Networks* 57 (2014): 39–50.

Kim, Min-Ki et al. A review on the computational methods for emotional state estimation from the human EEG. *Computational and Mathematical Methods in Medicine* (2013).

Kindermans, Pieter-Jan et al. Integrating dynamic stopping, transfer learning and language models in an adaptive zero-training ERP speller. *Journal of Neural Engineering* 11.3 (2014): 035005.

Kindermans, Pieter-Jan et al. A P300 BCI for the masses: Prior information enables instant unsupervised spelling. *Advances in Neural Information Processing Systems* (2012).

Lotte, Fabien, and Cuntai Guan. Regularizing common spatial patterns to improve BCI designs: Unified theory and new algorithms. *IEEE Transactions on Biomedical Engineering* 58.2 (2011): 355–362.

Lu, Na et al. A deep learning scheme for motor imagery classification based on restricted Boltzmann machines. *IEEE Transactions on Neural Systems and Rehabilitation Engineering* (2016).

Samek, Wojciech, Motoaki Kawanabe, and Klaus-Robert Muller. Divergence-based framework for common spatial patterns algorithms. *IEEE Reviews in Biomedical Engineering* 7 (2014): 50–72.

Sussillo, David et al. Making brain–machine interfaces robust to future neural variability. *Nature Communications* 7 (2016).

Wallstrom, Garrick L. et al. Fox. Automatic correction of ocular artifacts in the EEG: A comparison of regression-based and component-based methods. *International Journal of Psychophysiology* 53.2 (2004): 105–119.

Wolpaw, Jonathan R. et al. An EEG-based brain–computer interface for cursor control. *Electroence-phalography and Clinical Neurophysiology* 78.3 (1991): 252–259.

Wolpaw, Jonathan R., and Dennis J. McFarland. Multichannel EEG-based brain–computer communication. *Electroencephalography and Clinical Neurophysiology* 90.6 (1994): 444–449.

Wu, Dongrui et al. Spatial filtering for EEG-based regression problems in brain–computer interface (BCI). *IEEE Transactions on Fuzzy Systems* (2017).

# Part IV

---

*Brain–Computer Interface Paradigms*

# 23 A Step-by-Step Tutorial for a Motor Imagery–Based BCI

*Hohyun Cho, Minkyu Ahn, Moonyoung Kwon, and Sung Chan Jun*

## CONTENTS

23.1 Introduction: Motor Imagery–Based BCI....................................................................446
23.2 Training Session .........................................................................................................446
    23.2.1 Recording MI Data...........................................................................................446
        23.2.1.1 Recording Device and Software ........................................................446
        23.2.1.2 Subjects..............................................................................................447
        23.2.1.3 Environment.......................................................................................447
        23.2.1.4 Experimental Paradigm .....................................................................447
        23.2.1.5 MI Instructions ..................................................................................449
        23.2.1.6 Questionnaire .....................................................................................449
        23.2.1.7 Discussions.........................................................................................449
    23.2.2 Training Algorithms and Offline Analysis........................................................451
        23.2.2.1 Preprocessing.....................................................................................451
        23.2.2.3 Feature Extraction ............................................................................453
        23.2.2.4 Classification......................................................................................454
        23.2.2.5 Discussion ..........................................................................................456
23.3 Testing Session...........................................................................................................456
    23.3.1 Online Experiment ...........................................................................................456
    23.3.2 Discussion .........................................................................................................457
23.4 Summary .....................................................................................................................458
Acknowledgments....................................................................................................................458
References.................................................................................................................................458

**Abstract**

Motor imagery (MI)–based brain–computer interface (BCI) is one of the standard concepts of BCI, in that the user can generate induced activity from motor cortex by imagining motor movements without any limb movement or external stimulus. In this chapter, we present a step-by-step tutorial on MI BCI and discuss the issues involved in each step. We describe detailed examples of our MI experiment with a general procedure from training session to testing session. In training session, we introduce and discuss recording devices and software, experimental settings, collecting MI data and questionnaires, offline analysis for inhibition of somatosensory rhythm, and training simple machine learning algorithms, including common spatial patterns and Fisher's linear discriminant analysis. Next, we introduce basic procedures used in the testing session and discuss important issues including session variabilities of electroencephalogram signal and information transfer rate. Last, we summarize the tutorial and list the challenging issues that remain in MI BCI.

## 23.1  INTRODUCTION: MOTOR IMAGERY–BASED BCI

Motor imagery (MI) brain–computer interface (BCI) employs the user's endogenous brain activity in the absence of any external stimuli (Pfurtscheller and Da Silva 1999; Ramoser et al. 2000; Schalk et al. 2004; Wolpaw and Wolpaw 2012; Wolpaw et al. 1991). A standard concept in BCI is the translation of the user's intention via mental imagination of motor movement, which serves an interface through which to communicate the user's intention without limb movement. The most representative application of MI BCI is for neurorehabilitation, and researchers have reported that repetitive MI can have positive effects in such rehabilitation (Mattia et al. 2016; Pichiorri et al. 2015). Thus, MI BCI remains a fascinating topic, although it already has been investigated for approximately 20 years.

Similar to other BCI paradigms, the MI BCI paradigm entails training and testing sessions. In the training session, the experimenter collects each user's MI data, does feature extraction with them, and makes classification algorithms through the data collected. Thus, it is very important to collect highly informative MI data, as they may provide an easier way to train algorithms. If the data contain many artifacts, then they may require preprocessing techniques that are more complex to remove or reduce any unwanted effects of the artifacts. During the testing session, algorithms already trained are applied to new MI data for classification on a real-time basis. Minimizing the psychological and environmental differences between training and testing sessions is also of significant importance, as trained algorithms do not work properly in the testing session because of session-to-session variability in electroencephalograms (EEGs).

In this chapter, we present a step-by-step tutorial on MI BCI. We describe a detailed MI experiment conducted in the BioComputing laboratory and then discuss the issues involved in each step. This tutorial is composed primarily of two sections: training and testing sessions. First, we introduce the way in which to collect high-quality, informative MI data, as well as several feature extraction and classification algorithms, including the common spatial pattern (CSP) and Fisher's linear discriminant analysis (FLDA). Next, we introduce basic procedures used in the testing session and review briefly existing techniques used to overcome variability between training and testing sessions. Last, we summarize the tutorial and list the challenging issues that remain in MI BCI.

## 23.2  TRAINING SESSION

### 23.2.1  RECORDING MI DATA

Here, we introduce the procedures involved in an MI experiment in the BioComputing laboratory (https://biocomput.gist.ac.kr) at Gwangju Institute of Science and Technology (GIST), South Korea. Public access to our data set will be available soon in GigaDB (Cho et al. 2017). At the end of this section, we discuss possible research topics related to recording techniques, subjects, experimental environments, experimental paradigms, MI instruction for subjects, and metadata (questionnaire).

#### 23.2.1.1  Recording Device and Software

As Figure 23.1 shows, we used a 64-channel montage based on the international 10–10 system to record EEG signals at 512-Hz sampling rates. Each subject wore an EEG cap. The EEG device used in this experiment was the Biosemi ActiveTwo system (Amsterdam, Netherlands), which uses a direct current (DC) battery as the power source. The BCI2000 system 3.0.2 (Schalk et al. 2004) was used to collect EEG data and present instructions (left-hand or right-hand MI). Furthermore, we recorded electromyography (EMG) and EEG simultaneously to check actual hand movements. Four EMG electrodes were attached to the flexor digitorum profundus and extensor digitorum on both forearms.

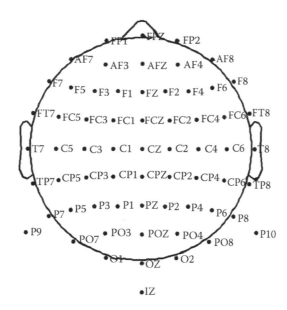

**FIGURE 23.1** EEG channel labeling. (Adapted from Cho, H., Ahn, M., Ahn, S., Kwon, M., and Jun, S.C., 2017. EEG datasets for motor imagery brain computer interface. *GigaScience*. DOI: https://doi.org/10.1093/gigascience/gix034. Copyright 2017 by GigaScience.)

### 23.2.1.2 Subjects

We conducted an MI experiment of the left and right hands with 52 subjects (19 females, mean age ± SD = 24.8 ± 3.86); the Institutional Review Board of GIST (2013-2) approved the experiment. First, we posted a notice on the GIST website. Graduate and undergraduate students, employees, and staff on campus participated in this experiment. All subjects gave informed consent for the researchers to collect information on brain signals and were paid 30,000 Korean Won (approximately $27) after they participated in the experiment. If a subject's MI data were discriminable—or, if the classification accuracy of left- and right-hand MI was higher than 80%—we paid him or her twice the reward to encourage each subject's concentration.

### 23.2.1.3 Environment

All experiments were conducted in our laboratory during one of four time slots: T1 (9:30–12:00), T2 (12:30–15:00), T3 (15:30–18:00), or T4 (19:00–21:30), as we were interested to know whether BCI performance varied with time. The background noise level was 37–39 decibels because of an air conditioner. The experiments began in August 2011 and ended in September 2011.

### 23.2.1.4 Experimental Paradigm

For each subject, we recorded data for non–task-related and (MI) task-related states, as follows:

> **Six types of non–task-related data.** We recorded six types of noise data (eye blinking, eyeball movement up/down, eyeball movement left/right, head movement, jaw clenching, and resting state) for the 52 subjects. Each type of noise was collected twice for 5 s, except for the resting state, which was recorded for 60 s.
>
> **MI experiment.** The experimental design was nearly the same as the Graz MI experiment (Ramoser et al. 2000). Subjects sat in a chair with armrests and watched a monitor. At the beginning of each trial, the monitor showed a black screen with a fixation cross for 2 s; the subject was then prepared to imagine hand movements, and the screen gave a ready signal to the subject. As Figure 23.2 shows, one of two instructions ("left hand" or "right hand")

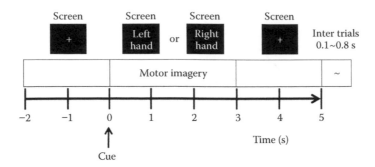

**FIGURE 23.2** Experimental paradigm. One trial of the MI experiment. (Adapted from Cho, H., Ahn, M., Ahn, S., Kwon, M., and Jun, S.C., 2017. EEG datasets for motor imagery brain computer interface. *GigaScience.* DOI: https://doi.org/10.1093/gigascience/gix034. Copyright 2017 by GigaScience.)

appeared randomly on the screen for 3 s, and subjects were asked to imagine the hand movement depending on the instruction given. After imagination, when the blank screen appeared, the subject was given a random break of 4.1 to 4.8 s. These processes were repeated 20 times for one class (one run), and five runs were performed. After each run, we calculated the classification accuracy over one run and gave the subject feedback to increase his or her motivation. Between each run, the subjects received a maximum 4-m break depending on their wishes. If interested in a more detailed description of the procedures used to set parameters and configuration, we recommend a mu rhythm BCI tutorial in BCI2000 wiki.

The entire experimental procedure is presented in Table 23.1.

### TABLE 23.1
### Experimental Procedure

| Number | Task | Duration (min) |
|--------|------|----------------|
| 1 | Filling out consent form and questionnaire | 10 |
| 2 | EEG electrode placement | 20 |
| 3 | Acquisition of the six types of non–task-related data | 2 |
| 4 | Practicing actual finger movements | 3 |
| 5 | RUN 1 | 6 |
| 6 | Filling out questionnaire | 4 |
| 7 | RUN 2 | 6 |
| 8 | Filling out questionnaire | 4 |
| 9 | RUN 3 | 6 |
| 10 | Filling out questionnaire | 4 |
| 11 | RUN 4 | 6 |
| 12 | Filling out questionnaire | 4 |
| 13 | RUN 5 | 6 |
| 14 | Filling out questionnaire | 4 |
| 15 | Online experiment | 6 |
| 16 | Digitizing 3D coordinates of EEG electrodes | 15 |
| 17 | Removing electrodes and cleaning laboratory | 20 |
| | Sum | 126 |

*Source:*  Adapted from Cho, H., Ahn, M., Ahn, S., Kwon, M., and Jun, S.C., 2017. EEG datasets for motor imagery brain computer interface. *GigaScience.* DOI: https://doi.org/10.1093/gigascience/gix034. Copyright 2017 by GigaScience.

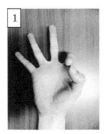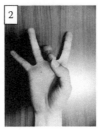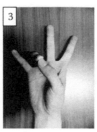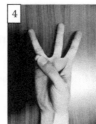

**FIGURE 23.3** Motor imagery instruction. We asked subjects to imagine four actual finger movements: touching each index, middle, ring, and little finger with the thumb within 3 s. Before the MI experiment began, subjects practiced executing the four movements within that time. (Adapted from Cho, H., Ahn, M., Ahn, S., Kwon, M., and Jun, S.C., 2017. EEG datasets for motor imagery brain computer interface. *GigaScience*. DOI: https://doi.org/10.1093/gigascience/gix034. Copyright 2017 by GigaScience.)

### 23.2.1.5 MI Instructions

Before the MI experiment began, we asked each subject to move his or her fingers, beginning with the index finger and proceeding to the little finger (depicted in Figure 23.3) within 3 s after onset. Each subject practiced these actual finger movements before performing the MI experiment. When imagining the movement, we asked subjects to imagine the kinesthetic, rather than the visual experience.

### 23.2.1.6 Questionnaire

We asked subjects to fill out a questionnaire during the MI experiment, as shown in Table 23.2. Before the MI experiment began, subjects answered 15 questions (questions 101 to 115). After every run, they answered another 10 questions (questions 210 to 219, 220 to 229, etc.). After the MI experiment, we asked the subjects to answer a final set of questions (questions 301 to 304). All numerical responses to the questions were stored in a Microsoft Excel file (Cho et al. 2017).

### 23.2.1.7 Discussions

In this section, we discuss several points that must be considered in MI BCI experiments, each of which may be an interesting topic for future research.

#### 23.2.1.7.1 Recording Software and Device

It is important to consider the line noise when recording EEG data. A signal power of 50–60 Hz line noise (220 or 110 V, respectively) is much higher than neural oscillation. Although software solutions exist to remove the line noise (e.g., notch filtering), data acquisition hardware that uses DC can reduce the line noise much more than can systems that use alternating current, for example, battery-based hardware. Therefore, we recommend a DC system. Hardware engineers in the BCI field are interested in developing wireless, dry electrode, tripolar concentric electrode, or multimodal EEG to study more accurate and convenient uses of BCI (Ahn et al. 2016; Besio et al. 2006; Cincotti et al. 2006; Nguyen et al. 2016). We believe that the most important issue in software engineering is saving data with correct trigger information and using EEG to study accurate, single-trial–based, and real-time experiments. The literature (Wolpaw and Wolpaw 2012) includes representative types of software for MI experiments: BCI2000 (Schalk et al. 2004), OpenVibe (Renard et al. 2010), and BCILAB (Kothe and Makeig 2013).

#### 23.2.1.7.2 Subjects

The initial goal of research on MI BCIs was to provide a new communication channel for people who are paralyzed completely. For these patients, it is very helpful even to answer "yes" or "no" using left- and right-hand MI. Researchers today tend to study MI for neurorehabilitation of stroke

**TABLE 23.2**

**Questionnaire for Motor Imagery Experiment**

Questionnaire

| Number | Individual Information | | | Subject ID: | |
|--------|----------------------|---|---|---|---|
| 101 | Time slot (1 = 9:30; 2 = 12:30; 3 = 15:30; 4 = 19:00) | | | | |
| 102 | Handedness (0 = left; 1 = right; 2 = both) | | | | |
| 103 | Age (number) | | | | |
| 104 | Sex (0 = female; 1 = male) | | | | |
| 105 | BCI experience (0 = no; number = how many times) | | | | |
| 106 | Biofeedback experience (0 = no; number = how many times) | | | | |
| | **Before motor imagery experiment** | | | | |
| 107. | 3. How long did you sleep? (1 = less than 4 h; 2 = 5–6 h; 3 = 6–7 h; 4 = 7–8 h; 5 = more than 8 h) | | | | |
| 108. | 4. Did you drink coffee within the past 24 h? (0 = no; number = hours before) | | | | |
| 109. | 5. Did you drink alcohol within the past 24 h (0 = no; number = hours before) | | | | |
| 110. | 6. Did you smoke within the past 24 h (0 = no; number = hours before) | | | | |
| 111. | 7. How do you feel? | Relaxed | 1 2 3 4 5 | Anxious | |
| 112. | | Excited | 1 2 3 4 5 | Bored | |
| 113. | Physical state | Very good | 1 2 3 4 5 | Very bad or tired | |
| 114. | Mental state | Very good | 1 2 3 4 5 | Very bad or tired | |
| 115. | 8. BCI performance (accuracy) expected? (%) | | | | |
| | **During motor imagery experiment** | | | | |
| | Run 1 (after the first run) | | | | |
| 210. | 1. Can you continue to the next run? (0 = No; 1 = Yes) | | | | |
| 211. | 2. How do you feel? | Relaxed | 1 2 3 4 5 | Anxious | |
| 212. | | Excited | 1 2 3 4 5 | Bored | |
| 213. | Attention level | High | 1 2 3 4 5 | Low | |
| 214. | Physical state | Very good | 1 2 3 4 5 | Very bad or tired | |
| 215. | Mental state | Very good | 1 2 3 4 5 | Very bad or tired | |
| 216. | 3. Have you nodded off (slept awhile) during this run? (0 = no; number = how many times) | | | | |
| 217. | 4. Was it easy to imagine finger movements? | | Easy 1 2 3 4 5 Difficult | | |
| 218. | 5. How many trials did you miss? (0 = none; number = how many times) | | | | |
| 219. | 6. Was your BCI performance (accuracy) for this run as you expected? (%) | | | | |
| | Run 2 (after the second run) | | | | |
| 220–229 | | ... | | | |
| | Run 3 (after the third run) | | | | |
| 230–239 | | ... | | | |
| | Run 4 (after the fourth run) | | | | |
| 240–249 | | ... | | | |
| | Run 5 (after the fifth run) | | | | |
| 250–259 | | ... | | | |
| | **After the motor imagery experiment** | | | | |
| 301. | 1. How was this experiment? | Duration | Short 1 2 3 4 5 Long | | |
| 302. | | Procedure | Good 1 2 3 4 5 Bad | | |
| 303. | | Environment | Comfortable 1 2 3 4 5 Uncomfortable | | |
| 304. | 2. Was your overall BCI performance (accuracy) as you expected? (%) | | | | |

*Source:* Adapted from Cho, H., Ahn, M., Ahn, S., Kwon, M., and Jun, S.C., 2017. EEG datasets for motor imagery brain computer interface. *GigaScience*. DOI: https://doi.org/10.1093/gigascience/gix034. Copyright 2017 by GigaScience.

patients. Clinicians have reported that MI neurofeedback is effective in reestablishing their motor movements immediately after a stroke (Mattia et al. 2016; Pichiorri et al. 2015). For normal subjects, BCI researchers have been interested in performance variation and subject-to-subject transfer to provide subject-independent algorithms (Blankertz et al. 2006; Fazli et al. 2009; Lotte et al. 2009; Reuderink et al. 2011; Samek et al. 2013; Tu and Sun 2012). There is a fraction of BCI-illiterate users in whom it is difficult to detect the mu rhythms from their somatosensory cortex. Identifying and understanding the neurophysiological and psychological characteristics that distinguish high and low performers in MI BCI are also very challenging (Ahn et al. 2013; Ahn and Jun 2015; Blankertz et al. 2010).

### 23.2.1.7.3 Environment

BCI experiments conducted in real time and outside the laboratory are receiving more attention. Most such studies, including this experiment, have been performed in a relatively silent laboratory (37–39 decibels). Ideally, however, we should be able to conduct BCI anywhere. Thus, movement and environmental issues are quite important.

### 23.2.1.7.4 Experimental Paradigm

The classic MI BCI paradigm introduced in this section is simple to follow. To obtain more informative MI data, the co-adaptive framework (Vidaurre et al. 2011), instructive framework (Jeunet et al. 2016), and merging steady-state somatosensory evoked potential and MI (Ahn et al. 2014) have been proposed, using the same stimulus timing as in online experimentation as much as possible (Cho et al. 2015).

### 23.2.1.7.5 MI Instructions

Interestingly, optimal MI instruction remains unknown. Here, we adopted the imagination of complex finger movements, as shown in Figure 23.3, based on a mu rhythm tutorial in a BCI2000 workshop held in 2011 that proposed kinesthetic and visual MI (Guillot et al. 2009; Neuper et al. 2005; Stinear et al. 2006). Stinear et al. (2006) reported that kinesthetic MI modulates corticomotor excitability more than visual MI does. Furthermore, the speed of the imagined clenching has been demonstrated (Yuan et al. 2010), and recently, an instructive framework of MI has been proposed (Jeunet et al. 2016).

### 23.2.1.7.6 Questionnaire

Although we have indicated already that BCI illiteracy, performance variation, and subject-to-subject transfer are complex issues, understanding subjects' metadata is also challenging, including examples such as "woman versus man," "younger versus older," size of head, individual personality, and so on.

## 23.2.2 TRAINING ALGORITHMS AND OFFLINE ANALYSIS

Here, we introduce the procedures for preprocessing, training the spatial filter, and selecting a classifier in BioComputing. At the end of this section, we discuss research topics with respect to preprocessing, the training feature extraction filter, and classification.

### 23.2.2.1 Preprocessing

After recording MI data, we had five files (*.dat) from the BCI2000 system because we recorded five runs, as shown in Table 23.1. BCI2000 provides a MATLAB® code, "BCI2000import.m," to convert each *.dat file to the EEGlab format of MATLAB. EEGlab is a well-known EEG signal processing toolbox (Delorme and Makeig 2004). In the EEGlab data structure, an "event" variable contains trigger information. The data length of each "event" variable is the same with respect to the number of stimuli. The "event" variable includes three variables: latency, position, and type.

The "latency" variable contains the time point value of a triggered stimulus within the run data. The "position" variable indicates the position of the stimulus array of the configuration in BCI2000. This value can be considered a class label, because the first and second values in our MI experiment are left- and right-hand MI instructions, as shown in Figure 23.2. Last, the "type" variable indicates the type of stimulus code. In an online experiment, there are many types of stimulus codes in BCI2000, for example, the stimulus, target, and feedback codes, and so on; then, we have raw EEG and trigger information, including latency and stimulus labels. We can extract each trial data from five runs of data. Depending on the latency of each stimulus (onset), the data frame extracted was between −2000 and 5000 ms. We carried out the same procedure for non–task-related data as well.

### 23.2.2.1.1 Offline Analysis

We checked the event-related desynchronization/synchronization (ERD/ERS) of somatosensory rhythm (SMR) for each subject (Pfurtscheller and Da Silva 1999). To calculate ERD/ERS for each channel, we followed the same procedure as did those authors using the following steps:

- Band-pass filtering of all trials at 8–30 Hz.
- Hilbert transformation of all trials.
- Taking absolute magnitude for each complex value of all trials.
- Averaging the magnitude of Hilbert transformed samples across all trials.
- We performed baseline correction for each trial to obtain percentage values for ERD/ERS

  using the formula $\text{ERD}\% = \dfrac{A - R}{R} \times 100$ , where $A$ is each time sample and $R$ is the mean

  value of the baseline period, which was between −500 and 0 ms.

Figure 23.4 illustrates the ERD/ERS results and shows the grand averaged ERD/ERS% over 38 subjects who had better classification rates than random chance. We plotted the topography and a bar graph of the intensive ERD period (500–2500 ms), as shown in Figure 23.4b and c. The

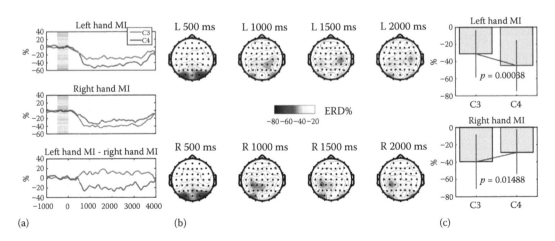

**FIGURE 23.4**  ERD of SMR (8–14 Hz) from discriminative subjects (38 subjects). (a) The first and second rows show ERD of the C3 and C4 channels in left- and right-hand MI, respectively, and the last row shows the difference in ERDs between the two. The gray shaded region is the baseline period. Cyan vertical lines represent time points, such as 500, 1000, 1500, and 2000 ms. (b) Topographies of ERDs at the cyan-colored time points in (a). Initials "L" and "R" indicate left and right MI movements, respectively. (c) Comparison of ERD at C3 and C4 channels within 500–2500 ms. *p* values were estimated by paired *t* test. (Adapted from Cho, H., Ahn, M., Ahn, S., Kwon, M., and Jun, S.C., 2017. EEG datasets for motor imagery brain computer interface. *GigaScience*. DOI: https://doi.org/10.1093/gigascience/gix034. Copyright 2017 by GigaScience.)

topographies showed that central, parietal, and occipital areas are involved in the MI task. Bar graphs of left-hand MI show that the contralateral ERD (C4 channel) was stronger than was the ipsilateral ERD (C3 channel).

### 23.2.2.3 Feature Extraction

For the training algorithm, each trial was band-pass filtered with an 8- to 30-Hz filter and extracted temporally 500–2500 ms after the stimulus onset. The range 8–30 Hz is a well-known frequency band of the SMR or alpha and beta rhythms (Pfurtscheller and Da Silva 1999). Researchers have reported that there are individual frequency bands of SMR. It is possible to improve classification accuracy by applying individual frequency bands of SMR to train algorithms (Ang et al. 2008; Cho et al. 2012, 2015; Dornhege et al. 2006; Lemm et al. 2005; Nikulin et al. 2011; Tomioka et al. 2006). Here, we simply filtered the data spectrally with a broad band of SMR. In the temporal behavior of SMR, inhibition begins at 500 ms and is quite general for most subjects (Pfurtscheller and Da Silva 1999). Similar to the individual differences found in SMR, individual featured time windows also exist and knowing these can improve classification accuracy. However, for the simplicity of our step-by-step tutorial, we applied the same temporal window to each participant.

In the field of EEG-based MI BCI, the CSP algorithm is a very well-known and efficient method used to extract discriminative features from two different conditioned brain signals—generally, left-/right-hand MI (Blankertz et al. 2008; Fukunaga 1972; Koles 1991; Ramoser et al. 2000). The CSP algorithm finds vectors that maximize the variance for one class while simultaneously minimizing the variance for the other. The vectors are common spatial filters focused on channels that are highly effective in differentiating between the two classes. This is expressed by the following optimization problem:

$$\max_{w} \left( \frac{\mathbf{w}^T C_1 \mathbf{w}}{\mathbf{w}^T C_2 \mathbf{w}} \right), \tag{23.1}$$

where $T$ denotes transpose, $C_i$ is the spatial covariance matrix of $X_i$ from class $i$, and $X_i$ are the raw data for class $i$ (matrix of size # of channels × # of the time samples), assuming a zero mean for the EEG signals. This assumption is generally met when the EEG signals are band-pass filtered. The optimization problem is equivalent to this form:

$$C_1 \mathbf{w} = \lambda C_2 \mathbf{w}. \tag{23.2}$$

We obtained a generalized eigenvalue problem. By solving this problem, we were able to identify the filters, or the eigenvectors corresponding to the largest eigenvalues. We referred to the eigenvectors $W$ spatial filters and $(W^{-1})^T$ spatial patterns. Meanwhile, we are able to call filter $W$ the de-mixing (backward model) matrix and $(W^{-1})^T$ the mixing matrix (forward model) for time points (Blankertz et al. 2008; Parra et al. 2005). For example, if $X$ equals the data observed (mixed data), then $Z$ $(=W^T X)$ is the data projected (de-mixed data or source data). Thus, $X$ $(=(W^{-1})^T Z)$ are mixed data with different sources in $Z$, and the values in the spatial filters explain which channels are important in extracting the source feature, while the values in spatial patterns explain which sources are important in generating mixed data $X$. When we used CSP for feature extraction, the EEG signal was projected onto the $w$ filters. Next, we took the logarithm to the projected EEG signal variance.

As Figure 23.5 shows, $w_1$ and $w_2$ are the eigenvectors corresponding to the largest eigenvalue and the smallest eigenvalue obtained by solving Equation 23.2. $w_1$ is for class 1 or left-hand MI, while $w_2$ is for class 2 or right-hand MI. By using the "eig()" function in MATLAB, we can obtain the CSP filters easily. Here, $w_1$ is a 64 × 1-dimensional vector because of the number of channels, as shown in Figure 23.1. $X^{(k)}$ is the trial data in a 64 × 1024 (= sampling rate × 2 s of extracted window) matrix.

Spatial feature
extraction

Classification

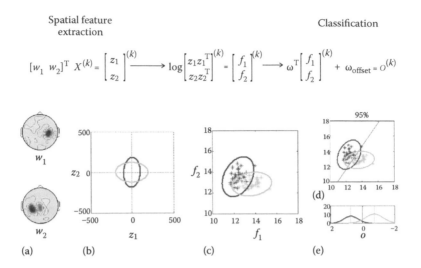

$$[w_1 \ w_2]^T \ X^{(k)} = \begin{bmatrix} z_1 \\ z_2 \end{bmatrix}^{(k)} \longrightarrow \log \begin{bmatrix} z_1 z_1^T \\ z_2 z_2^T \end{bmatrix}^{(k)} = \begin{bmatrix} f_1 \\ f_2 \end{bmatrix}^{(k)} \longrightarrow \omega^T \begin{bmatrix} f_1 \\ f_2 \end{bmatrix}^{(k)} + \omega_{\text{offset}} = O^{(k)}$$

**FIGURE 23.5** Conventional CSP and FLDA model: (a) CSP filters; (b) projected signal variance: green indicates left-hand MI and red indicates right-hand MI; (c) log variance of projected feature; (d) FLDA's discrimination line; and (e) distributions of classifier outputs for two classes. (Adapted from Cho, H., Ahn, M., Kim, K., and Jun, S.C., 2015. Increasing session-to-session transfer in a brain–computer interface with on-site background noise acquisition. *Journal of Neural Engineering*, 12 (6), 66009. Copyright 2015 by the *Journal of Neural Engineering*.)

Figure 23.5a shows that the topographies of $w_1$ and $w_2$. $z_1 (= w_1^T \cdot X^{(k)})$ and $z_2 (= w_2^T \cdot X^{(k)})$ are projected data. Figure 23.5b shows the distribution along the $z_1$ and $z_2$ axes. Each point in Figure 23.5b is $(z_1(t),$ $z_2(t))$, where $t$ is the time index among the 1024 time points. Figure 23.5b shows two distributions of a left MI trial and right MI data. The green distribution indicates the projected left MI $X_1^{(k)}$, and the red distribution indicates the projected right MI $X_2^{(k)}$. Each distribution was maximized to the corresponding axis. $f_1$ and $f_2$ are scalar values. Because the projected data are squared, the distribution of the squared values is not Gaussian. If we take the logarithm of the squared data, then the variation in large values can be reduced to obtain a Gaussian distribution. This log-variance also helps satisfy the basic assumption for FLDA, which is that two-class data have a Gaussian distribution. Therefore, the number of red stars in Figure 23.5c is equal to the number of training trials. Figure 23.5c shows the distributions of trials for left and right MI data. Finally, we can obtain the $F_i$ matrix (2 × trials) for class $i$, where $F = [F_i^{(1)}, F_i^{(2)}, ..., F_i^{(N)}]$ and $F_i^{(k)} = [f_1 f_2]^{T(k)}$.

### 23.2.2.4 Classification

As Figure 23.5c shows, the training data $F_i$ are prepared for classification. FLDA is a simple classifier used frequently in the BCI field and assumes that the two distributions are Gaussian. Interestingly, the objective functions of FLDA also use a Rayleigh quotient similar to the objective function of CSP, as shown in Equation 23.1. The formula of FLDA is expressed as

$$\max_{\omega} \left( \frac{\omega^T S_B \omega}{\omega^T S_w \omega} \right), \tag{23.3}$$

where $S_B$ is $(\mu_1 - \mu_2) \cdot (\mu_1 - \mu_2)^T$, $\mu_i$ is a mean vector of data of $F_i$ from class $i$, and $S_w$ is the sum of two covariance matrices of $F_1$ and $F_2$. This equation maximizes the difference between mean vectors while minimizing both covariances of the two-class data. The optimization problem can be solved as

$$S_B \omega = \lambda S_w \omega. \tag{23.4}$$

Here, we encounter a generalized eigenvalue problem again. By solving this problem, we can obtain an eigenvector $\omega$ corresponding to the largest eigenvalue. The eigenvector $\omega$ is the normal to the discriminant hyperplane. The $\omega_{offset}$ can be calculated by $\omega^T \cdot 0.5 \cdot (\mu_1 + \mu_2)$. Finally, we can classify a trial data set by ensuring that $\omega^T \cdot F^{(k)} + \omega_{offset} > 0$. In Figure 23.5d, if $\omega^T \cdot F^{(k)} + \omega_{offset} > 0$, then the trial can be classified as right MI data.

Last, we conducted cross-validation to calculate the performance of our MI data. For each class, we divided the 100 trials of MI data into 10 subsets of 10 trials each. Seven subsets were chosen randomly and used to train CSP and FLDA, and the three subsets remaining were used to test them. This procedure was repeated 120 times by choosing 3 among the 10 subsets randomly. Finally, we estimated and averaged 120 classification accuracies.

The mean accuracy of the BCI performance over the 50 subjects, excluding bad subjects, was 67.46% (±13.17%) in our data sets. In the BCI2000 MI data set (EEG Motor Movement/Imagery Dataset 2016; Goldberger et al. 2000; Schalk et al. 2004), the average accuracy was 60.42% (±11.68%) over 109 subjects using CSP and FLDA. In our data sets, 14 subjects (26.92% of 52 subjects) showed low BCI performance (below chance, which is the upper confidence limit of chance with $\alpha = 5\%$), as shown in Figure 23.6. This is greater than a report on 99 subjects (Guger et al. 2003) and showed that 6.7% of the subjects had accuracies lower than 60% (here, the average accuracy over the 99 subjects was not reported). Compared with the EEG Motor Movement/Imagery Dataset (2016), our data sets included more trials, although we rejected bad trials and excluded them from the results. The EEG Motor Movement/Imagery Dataset (2016) includes MI data for 109 subjects, but the number of total trials for each subject is approximately 20 trials, which has a random chance level of 65% ($\alpha = 5\%$).

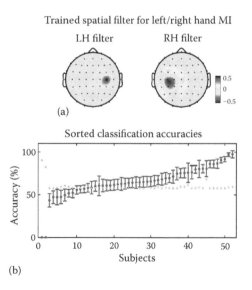

(a)

(b)

**FIGURE 23.6** Trained CSP filters for left and right hand motor imagery data and sorted cross-validated classification results. (a) To demonstrate the discriminative feature of our data set, CSP filters were trained by averaged covariance matrix of thirty-eight subjects who have high BCI performance (>random chance). (b) Sorted cross-validated classification results. Sorted accuracies are depicted in increasing order. Fourteen subjects showed low BCI performance (<chance marked with yellow diamond). Because of sorting, the number on the $x$ axis does not correspond to subject numbers "s01" to "s52." (Adapted from Cho, H., Ahn, M., Ahn, S., Kwon, M., and Jun, S.C., 2017. EEG datasets for motor imagery brain computer interface. *GigaScience*. DOI: https://doi.org/10.1093/gigascience/gix034. Copyright 2017 by GigaScience.)

### 23.2.2.5 Discussion

#### 23.2.2.5.1 Preprocessing

In any trial, various artifacts—movement-related noise, eye blinking, eye movement, heart-related noise, and so on—can contaminate the data. In this tutorial, we simply used an 8- to 30-Hz band-pass filter to remove eye-related noise above the 8-Hz earmark. To remove eye blinking or heart-related noise, an independent component analysis is a better solution than is band-pass filtering. Here, we recommend using the EEGlab MATLAB toolbox (Delorme and Makeig 2004; Wang et al. 2012). To extract reliable and stationary EEG, stationary subspace analysis (von Bünau et al. 2009) and spatio-spectral decomposition (Nikulin et al. 2011) have been proposed.

#### 23.2.2.5.2 Offline Analysis

Understanding the SMR of MI can improve hyperparameter selection for training feature extraction and classification algorithms. The $r$-squared analysis is a well-known method used to identify individual frequency bands (Schalk et al. 2004). In their appendix, Blankertz et al. (2008) introduced simple algorithms to identify discriminant time windows and frequency bands. To select the best frequency band, the algorithm calculates correlations between each point in a channel using a frequency matrix of MI trials and class labels. Similar to frequency band selection, the algorithm used to locate the best time window of MI calculates correlations between each point in a channel using a time matrix of absolute Hilbert transformed trial and class labels. Therefore, BCI performance can be improved using the results of offline analysis to identify individual frequency bands and time windows. In addition, the well-known offline analysis MATLAB toolboxes EEGlab (Delorme and Makeig 2004) and Fieldtrip (Oostenveld et al. 2010) can be used.

#### 23.2.2.5.3 Feature Extraction

Because of the spatial properties of left and right MI, CSP is a very powerful method. As shown in Figure 23.4, the spatial features of left MI can be observed in the right sensorimotor area, while the spatial features of right MI can be observed in the left sensorimotor area. Since CSP was first proposed approximately a decade ago, many variants of CSP algorithms have been developed, and numerous CSP ideas have been proposed to overcome session and subject variation. Representatively, regularized CSP theory adopts two approaches to regularize the CSP algorithm: regularizing covariance matrix and the objective function of CSP (Lotte and Guan 2011). Furthermore, expanding the spatio-spectral feature space also can improve BCI performance with respect to session and subject variation.

#### 23.2.2.5.4 Classification

A review of classification methods for BCI (Lotte et al. 2007) showed that a support vector machine (SVM) was the best classifier among the existing algorithms. Compared with FLDA, SVM is a successful system to classify outliers and therefore is a more universal classifier than is FLDA. Previously, there were few studies that addressed the deep neural network (Sakhavi et al. 2015; Walker et al. 2015). However, a recent study of this topic showed compelling results. DNN accomplishes both feature extraction and classification in one structure. To achieve improved BCI performance, the DNN approach requires more investigation of its hyperparameters (optimal number of layers, activation functions, etc.) and weights analysis. After the training DNN, what is the meaning of weights in the layers with respect to signal processing?

## 23.3 TESTING SESSION

### 23.3.1 ONLINE EXPERIMENT

In any testing session, the method used to classify new data largely is the same as that used in training sessions. New data were processed every 2 s in our testing sessions. A trial of the online experimental paradigm implemented by the BCI2000 system is shown in Figure 23.7. We used the

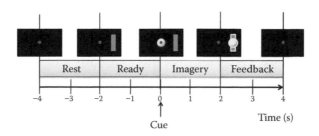

**FIGURE 23.7**   Online experimental paradigm. The yellow ball is controlled by the data collected from 0 to 2 s after the cue (blue). The red point on the screen was the fixation point. (Adapted from Cho, H., Ahn, M., Kim, K., and Jun, S.C., 2015. Increasing session-to-session transfer in a brain–computer interface with on-site background noise acquisition. *Journal of Neural Engineering*, 12 (6), 66009. Copyright 2015 by the *Journal of Neural Engineering*.)

Biosemi acquisition module for signal acquisition and adopted the MATLAB signal processing module to load trained weights of CSP and FDLA and to classify the new data in real time. The application module was a cursor task application with a 2-s sliding window. After the 2-s rest, 2 s of MI instruction were shown as a gray bar. Following this instruction, the subject conducted left- or right-hand MI. If a gray bar appeared on the right side, then the subject was supposed to imagine right-hand finger movements. This 2-s period was classified by trained CSP and FLDA in the MATLAB signal processing module, and the classified result was transmitted to the cursor task application. Finally, after the 2-s imagination period, the cursor was moved according to the classified result, as shown in Figure 23.7. These new data were band-pass filtered at 8–30 Hz, filtered spatially by CSP, and the feature extracted was classified by FLDA, as shown in Figure 23.5. Here, the size of the sliding window was 2 s because it was the period used in the training session.

### 23.3.2   DISCUSSION

Representatively, BCI2000 (Schalk et al. 2004) and OpenVibe (Renard et al. 2010) are recommended for online BCI feedback. For BCI beginners, OpenVibe is easy to use because it supports graphical language. However, based on our experience, because of the graphical language, OpenVibe requires relatively large memory spaces. Thus, the BCI2000 system is lighter than is OpenVibe.

A limitation of our online experiment was a mismatch between the time windows featured. While the training session time window was 500–2500 ms after onset, the time window of the classified new data was 0–2000 ms. To overcome this mismatch problem, we applied an online experimental paradigm used in training sessions in other work (Cho et al. 2015). For MI data classification, it is very important to extract the most discriminative time window for offline data in training algorithms. The online experimental paradigm in this chapter was included in synchronous BCI, which has trial and stimulus cues. For asynchronous BCI, which has no instruction onset or cue, recognizing the user's self-cues is also challenging, for example, classifying the resting and task states.

To minimize the gap between training and testing sessions, BCI researchers have proposed adaptive and co-adaptive approaches (Baldwin and Penaranda 2012; Satti et al. 2010; Shenoy et al. 2006; Shin et al. 2015; Sun and Zhang 2006; Vidaurre et al. 2011). Here, "adaptive" means "let the machine learn in real time" and "co-adaptive" means "let both the user and machine learn." In the adaptive approach, either CSP or FLDA was updated with new data after each online trial. Controlling the learning rate or gradient was challenging. The co-adaptive approach showed improved BCI performance and a possible solution to BCI illiteracy. Furthermore, there are additional reasons for the gap between training and testing sessions, including psychological and environmental differences, among others. Thus, minimizing the gap between training and testing sessions remains a difficult issue to resolve.

A particular missing point in the training session section was the information transfer rate (ITR), which provides a general assessment of BCI performance. Actually, ITR is a critical feature of MI

BCI with respect to human–computer interaction. At the beginning of BCI research, many people were interested in BCI because it can provide a new communication channel without any limb movement; however, the ITR in BCI is much lower than that in other input interfaces, including keyboard, mouse, and joystick. Very few studies (Bin et al. 2011; Wang et al. 2008) have shown an ITR that exceeds 100 bits/min (not based on MI). For comparison, the ITRs using a keyboard or mouse are 900 bits/min and a few hundred bits per minute, respectively (Clerc et al. 2016). If a BCI could somehow demonstrate a rate similar to that of keyboard use, that would be highly innovative.

## 23.4 SUMMARY

In this chapter, we provided a step-by-step tutorial for MI BCI and discussed research topics related to each step. In the training sessions, we detailed recording data issues, including software, device, environment, experimental paradigm, MI instruction, and questionnaire, offline analysis, and training algorithms. In the testing session, we introduced a simple procedure of cursor task application and discussed time window and synchronous/asynchronous issues.

We not only provided a step-by-step tutorial but also discussed possible ways to improve the data quality and MI BCI performance. We selected the most promising, yet challenging issues, as follows: recording device, experimental paradigm or MI instruction, metadata analysis for subject/session variation or BCI illiteracy, DNN, asynchronous MI BCI, and ITR. BCI researchers have made tremendous efforts to resolve these challenging issues. Thus, it is our hope that more innovative and easy-to-use BCI will be developed in the near future.

## ACKNOWLEDGMENTS

This work was supported by Institute for Information and Communications Technology Promotion (IITP) grant funded by the Korean government (No. 2017-0-00451) and Ministry of Culture, Sports and Tourism (MCST) and Korea Creative Content Agency (KOCCA) in the Culture Technology (CT) Research and Development Program 2017.

## REFERENCES

Ahn, M., Cho, H., Ahn, S., and Jun, S.C., 2013. High theta and low alpha powers may be indicative of BCI-illiteracy in motor imagery. *PloS one*, 8 (11), e80886.

Ahn, M. and Jun, S.C., 2015. Performance variation in motor imagery brain–computer interface: A brief review. *Journal of Neuroscience Methods*, 243, 103–110.

Ahn, S., Ahn, M., Cho, H., and Jun, S.C., 2014. Achieving a hybrid brain–computer interface with tactile selective attention and motor imagery. *Journal of Neural Engineering*, 11 (6), 66004.

Ahn, S., Nguyen, T., Jang, H., Kim, J.G., and Jun, S.C., 2016. Exploring neuro-physiological correlates of drivers' mental fatigue caused by sleep deprivation using simultaneous EEG, ECG, and fNIRS data. *Frontiers in Human Neuroscience*, 10.

Ang, K.K., Chin, Z.Y., Zhang, H., and Guan, C., 2008. Filter bank common spatial pattern (FBCSP) in brain–computer interface. In: *Neural Networks, 2008. IJCNN 2008 (IEEE World Congress on Computational Intelligence). IEEE International Joint Conference on*. IEEE, 2390–2397.

Baldwin, C.L. and Penaranda, B.N., 2012. Adaptive training using an artificial neural network and EEG metrics for within-and cross-task workload classification. *NeuroImage*, 59 (1), 48–56.

Besio, G., Koka, K., Aakula, R., and Dai, W., 2006. Tri-polar concentric ring electrode development for Laplacian electroencephalography. *IEEE Transactions on Biomedical Engineering*, 53 (5), 926–933.

Bin, G., Gao, X., Wang, Y., Li, Y., Hong, B., and Gao, S., 2011. A high-speed BCI based on code modulation VEP. *Journal of Neural Engineering*, 8 (2), 25015.

Blankertz, B., Dornhege, G., Krauledat, M., Muller, K.-R., Kunzmann, V., Losch, F., and Curio, G., 2006. The Berlin Brain–Computer Interface: EEG-based communication without subject training. *IEEE Transactions on Neural Systems and Rehabilitation Engineering*, 14 (2), 147–152.

Blankertz, B., Sannelli, C., Halder, S., Hammer, E.M., Kübler, A., Müller, K.-R., Curio, G., and Dickhaus, T., 2010. Neurophysiological predictor of SMR-based BCI performance. *Neuroimage*, 51 (4), 1303–1309.

Blankertz, B., Tomioka, R., Lemm, S., Kawanabe, M., and Muller, K.-R., 2008. Optimizing spatial filters for robust EEG single-trial analysis. *IEEE Signal Processing Magazine*, 25 (1), 41–56.

von Bünau, P., Meinecke, F.C., and Müller, K.-R., 2009. Stationary subspace analysis. In: *International Conference on Independent Component Analysis and Signal Separation*. Springer, 1–8.

Cho, H., Ahn, M., Ahn, S., and Jun, S.C., 2012. Invariant common spatio-spectral patterns. In: *Proc. of TOBI 3rd Workshop*. 31–32.

Cho, H., Ahn, M., Ahn, S., Kwon, M., and Jun, S.C., 2017. EEG datasets for motor imagery brain computer interface. *GigaScience*. DOI: https://doi.org/10.1093/gigascience/gix034

Cho, H., Ahn, M., Kim, K., and Jun, S.C., 2015. Increasing session-to-session transfer in a brain–computer interface with on-site background noise acquisition. *Journal of Neural Engineering*, 12 (6), 66009.

Cincotti, F., Bianchi, L., Birch, G., Guger, C., Mellinger, J., Scherer, R., Schmidt, R.N., Suárez, O.Y., and Schalk, G., 2006. BCI Meeting 2005—Workshop on technology: Hardware and software. *IEEE Transactions on Neural Systems and Rehabilitation Engineering*, 14 (2), 128–131.

Clerc, M., Bougrain, L., and Lotte, F., 2016. *Brain–Computer Interfaces 1: Methods and Perspectives*. John Wiley & Sons.

Delorme, A. and Makeig, S., 2004. EEGLAB: An open source toolbox for analysis of single-trial EEG dynamics including independent component analysis. *Journal of Neuroscience Methods*, 134 (1), 9–21.

Dornhege, G., Blankertz, B., Krauledat, M., Losch, F., Curio, G., and Muller, K.-R., 2006. Combined optimization of spatial and temporal filters for improving brain-computer interfacing. *IEEE Transactions on Biomedical Engineering*, 53 (11), 2274–2281.

EEG Motor Movement/Imagery Dataset [online], 2016. Available from: https://physionet.org/pn4/eegmmidb /[Accessed 20 Dec 2016].

Fazli, S., Popescu, F., Danóczy, M., Blankertz, B., Müller, K.-R., and Grozea, C., 2009. Subject-independent mental state classification in single trials. *Neural Networks*, 22 (9), 1305–1312.

Fukunaga, K., 1972. *Introduction to Statistical Pattern Recognition*. Academic Press.

Goldberger, A.L., Amaral, L.A.N., Glass, L., Hausdorff, J.M., Ivanov, P.C., Mark, R.G., Mietus, J.E., Moody, G.B., Peng, C.-K., and Stanley, H.E., 2000. PhysioBank, PhysioToolkit, and PhysioNet. *Circulation*, 101 (23), e215–e220.

Guger, C., Edlinger, G., Harkam, W., Niedermayer, I., and Pfurtscheller, G., 2003. How many people are able to operate an EEG-based brain–computer interface (BCI)? *IEEE Transactions on Neural Systems and Rehabilitation Engineering*, 11 (2), 145–147.

Guillot, A., Collet, C., Nguyen, V.A., Malouin, F., Richards, C., and Doyon, J., 2009. Brain activity during visual versus kinesthetic imagery: An fMRI study. *Human Brain Mapping*, 30 (7), 2157–2172.

Jeunet, C., Jahanpour, E., and Lotte, F., 2016. Why standard brain–computer interface (BCI) training protocols should be changed: An experimental study. *Journal of Neural Engineering*, 13 (3), 36024.

Koles, Z.J., 1991. The quantitative extraction and topographic mapping of the abnormal components in the clinical EEG. *Electroencephalography and Clinical Neurophysiology*, 79 (6), 440–447.

Kothe, C.A. and Makeig, S., 2013. BCILAB: A platform for brain–computer interface development. *Journal of Neural Engineering*, 10 (5), 56014.

Lemm, S., Blankertz, B., Curio, G., and Muller, K.-R., 2005. Spatio-spectral filters for improving the classification of single trial EEG. *IEEE Transactions on Biomedical Engineering*, 52 (9), 1541–1548.

Lotte, F., Congedo, M., Lécuyer, A., Lamarche, F., and Arnaldi, B., 2007. A review of classification algorithms for EEG-based brain–computer interfaces. *Journal of Neural Engineering*, 4 (2), R1.

Lotte, F., Guan, C., and Ang, K.K., 2009. Comparison of designs towards a subject-independent brain–computer interface based on motor imagery. In: *2009 Annual International Conference of the IEEE Engineering in Medicine and Biology Society*. IEEE, 4543–4546.

Lotte, F. and Guan, C., 2011. Regularizing common spatial patterns to improve BCI designs: unified theory and new algorithms. IEEE Transactions on biomedical Engineering, 58 (2), 355–362.

Mattia, D., Astolfi, L., Toppi, J., Petti, M., Pichiorri, F., and Cincotti, F., 2016. Interfacing brain and computer in neurorehabilitation. In: *Brain–Computer Interface (BCI), 2016 4th International Winter Conference on*. IEEE, 1–2.

Neuper, C., Scherer, R., Reiner, M., and Pfurtscheller, G., 2005. Imagery of motor actions: Differential effects of kinesthetic and visual–motor mode of imagery in single-trial EEG. *Cognitive Brain Research*, 25 (3), 668–677.

Nguyen, T., Ahn, S., Jang, H., Jun, S.C., and Kim, J.G., 2016. Applying support vector machine on hybrid fNIRS/EEG signal to classify driver's conditions (Conference Presentation). In: *SPIE BiOS*. International Society for Optics and Photonics, 969003–969003.

Nikulin, V.V., Nolte, G., and Curio, G., 2011. A novel method for reliable and fast extraction of neuronal EEG/MEG oscillations on the basis of spatio-spectral decomposition. *NeuroImage*, 55 (4), 1528–1535.

Oostenveld, R., Fries, P., Maris, E., and Schoffelen, J.-M., 2010. FieldTrip: Open Source Software for Advanced Analysis of MEG, EEG, and Invasive Electrophysiological Data. *Computational Intelligence and Neuroscience*, 2011, e156869.

Parra, L.C., Spence, C.D., Gerson, A.D., and Sajda, P., 2005. Recipes for the linear analysis of EEG. *Neuroimage*, 28 (2), 326–341.

Pfurtscheller, G. and Da Silva, F.L., 1999. Event-related EEG/MEG synchronization and desynchronization: basic principles. *Clinical Neurophysiology*, 110 (11), 1842–1857.

Pichiorri, F., Morone, G., Petti, M., Toppi, J., Pisotta, I., Molinari, M., Paolucci, S., Inghilleri, M., Astolfi, L., Cincotti, F., and others, 2015. Brain–computer interface boosts motor imagery practice during stroke recovery. *Annals of Neurology*, 77 (5), 851–865.

Ramoser, H., Muller-Gerking, J., and Pfurtscheller, G., 2000. Optimal spatial filtering of single trial EEG during imagined hand movement. *IEEE Transactions on Rehabilitation Engineering*, 8 (4), 441–446.

Renard, Y., Lotte, F., Gibert, G., Congedo, M., Maby, E., Delannoy, V., Bertrand, O., and Lécuyer, A., 2010. Openvibe: An open-source software platform to design, test, and use brain–computer interfaces in real and virtual environments. *Presence: Teleoperators and Virtual Environments*, 19 (1), 35–53.

Reuderink, B., Farquhar, J., Poel, M., and Nijholt, A., 2011. A subject-independent brain–computer interface based on smoothed, second-order baselining. In: *2011 Annual International Conference of the IEEE Engineering in Medicine and Biology Society*. IEEE, 4600–4604.

Sakhavi, S., Guan, C., and Yan, S., 2015. Parallel convolutional-linear neural network for motor imagery classification. In: *Signal Processing Conference (EUSIPCO), 2015 23rd European*. IEEE, 2736–2740.

Samek, W., Meinecke, F.C., and Müller, K.R., 2013. Transferring subspaces between subjects in brain–computer interfacing. *IEEE Transactions on Biomedical Engineering*, 60 (8), 2289–2298.

Satti, A., Guan, C., Coyle, D., and Prasad, G., 2010. A covariate shift minimisation method to alleviate non-stationarity effects for an adaptive brain–computer interface. In: *Pattern Recognition (ICPR), 2010 20th International Conference on*. IEEE, 105–108.

Schalk, G., McFarland, D.J., Hinterberger, T., Birbaumer, N., and Wolpaw, J.R., 2004. BCI2000: A general-purpose brain–computer interface (BCI) system. *IEEE Transactions on Biomedical Engineering*, 51 (6), 1034–1043.

Shenoy, P., Krauledat, M., Blankertz, B., Rao, R.P.N., and Müller, K.-R., 2006. Towards adaptive classification for BCI. *Journal of Neural Engineering*, 3 (1), R13.

Shin, Y., Lee, S., Ahn, M., Cho, H., Jun, S.C., and Lee, H.-N., 2015. Simple adaptive sparse representation based classification schemes for EEG based brain–computer interface applications. *Computers in Biology and Medicine*, 66, 29–38.

Stinear, C.M., Byblow, W.D., Steyvers, M., Levin, O., and Swinnen, S.P., 2006. Kinesthetic, but not visual, motor imagery modulates corticomotor excitability. *Experimental Brain Research*, 168 (1–2), 157–164.

Sun, S. and Zhang, C., 2006. Adaptive feature extraction for EEG signal classification. *Medical and Biological Engineering and Computing*, 44 (10), 931–935.

Tomioka, R., Dornhege, G., Nolte, G., Blankertz, B., Aihara, K., and Müller, K.-R., 2006. Spectrally weighted common spatial pattern algorithm for single trial EEG classification. *Dept. Math. Eng., Univ. Tokyo, Tokyo, Japan, Tech. Rep*, 40.

Tu, W. and Sun, S., 2012. A subject transfer framework for EEG classification. *Neurocomputing*, 82, 109–116.

Vidaurre, C., Sannelli, C., Müller, K.-R., and Blankertz, B., 2011. Co-adaptive calibration to improve BCI efficiency. *Journal of Neural Engineering*, 8 (2), 25009.

Walker, I., Deisenroth, M., and Faisal, A., 2015. Deep convolutional neural networks for brain computer interface using motor imagery. *Imperial College of Science, Technology and Medicine Department of Computing*.

Wang, Y., Gao, X., Hong, B., Jia, C., and Gao, S., 2008. Brain–computer interfaces based on visual evoked potentials. *IEEE Engineering in Medicine and Biology Magazine*, 27 (5).

Wang, Y., Wang, Y.-T., and Jung, T.-P., 2012. Translation of EEG spatial filters from resting to motor imagery using independent component analysis. *PloS one*, 7 (5), e37665.

Wolpaw, J. and Wolpaw, E.W., 2012. *Brain–Computer Interfaces: Principles and Practice*. OUP USA.

Wolpaw, J.R., McFarland, D.J., Neat, G.W., and Forneris, C.A., 1991. An EEG-based brain–computer interface for cursor control. *Electroencephalography and Clinical Neurophysiology*, 78 (3), 252–259.

Yuan, H., Perdoni, C., and He, B., 2010. Relationship between speed and EEG activity during imagined and executed hand movements. *Journal of Neural Engineering*, 7 (2), 26001.

# 24 Eye Gaze Collaboration with Brain–Computer Interfaces
## Using Both Modalities for More Robust Interaction

*Gaye Lightbody, Chris P. Brennan, Paul J. McCullagh, and Leo Galway*

## CONTENTS

24.1 Introduction ...................................................................................................... 461
24.2 Overview of Current SSVEP and ET Advances ............................................... 464
    24.2.1 SSVEP .................................................................................................... 465
    24.2.2 *h*BCI with Eye Gaze ............................................................................. 466
24.3 Eye Gaze and SSVEP *h*BCI............................................................................. 469
    24.3.1 Concepts for the Inclusion of ET into the *h*BCI ................................. 469
    24.3.2 Visual Interface Application Design ..................................................... 470
    24.3.3 The ET Component................................................................................ 470
    24.3.4 The SSVEP BCI Component................................................................. 472
    24.3.5 The *h*BCI Architecture ........................................................................ 472
    24.3.6 Experimental Protocol.......................................................................... 475
    24.3.7 Postprocessing ...................................................................................... 476
24.4 Discussion and Conclusions............................................................................. 478
References............................................................................................................... 479

### Abstract

In this chapter, we discuss the motivation for the hybrid brain–computer interface (BCI) and review progress toward more robust user interaction from existing studies. In addition, we discuss the design and development of a *hybrid* brain–computer interface (*h*BCI) example that combines two symbiotic modalities: steady-state visual evoked potential and eye gaze technology. By adopting a modular design, we show that it has been possible to implement such hybridization by integrating mostly existing software components and, indeed, facilitate future updates to the system that will be necessary as hardware, software, and interfaces continue to evolve.

## 24.1 INTRODUCTION

Brain–computer interfaces (BCIs) have offered the hope of more autonomous communication and control for those with the most severe forms of muscular and neurological disability (Sellers et al. 2010). BCIs are also emerging as a supplemental technology for human–computer interaction (HCI) (Allison 2011; Allison et al. 2012b; Brunner et al. 2015). Interaction with computing systems and embedded smart devices is typically achieved through a set of tailored BCI paradigms that in some way instigate an intended and measurable activity within the electroencephalogram (EEG).

Historically, BCI paradigms fall into two categories. The first category is motor imagery (MI), in which the user thinks of moving a limb, a hand, or foot for example, and in doing so initiates an identifiable pattern over the sensorimotor region of the cortex (Pfurtscheller and Neuper 2001). The second category relies on an external stimulus to evoke a response within the EEG. Although auditory (Kim et al. 2012) and somatosensory (Rutkowski et al. 2012) stimuli produce discernable event-related responses (ERPs), it has been prevalent for BCI paradigms to use visual stimuli in the form of flashing light-emitting diodes (LEDs) or flickering icons on a screen. The resultant evoked cortical activity, known as steady-state visual evoked potential (SSVEP), is dependent on the frequency of stimulation. This typically tends to be in the region of 6–20 Hz (Müller-Putz et al. 2005), although higher-frequency variations, which are deemed as less annoying, have also been proposed and investigated (Durka et al. 2009). Higher-frequency stimuli mitigate photo-sensitivity effects (e.g., people with epilepsy) but produce smaller components in the EEG. Where the stimulation occurs unpredictably, for example, a *target* stimulus that can be distinguished from a more frequent stimulus, a positivity occurs in the EEG approximately 300 ms after the stimulus; this is the well-known P300 waveform. This component has been successfully harnessed for user interaction (Farwell and Donchin 1988; Guger et al. 2009; Sellers et al. 2010), as it is reliably detected in most people, reduces the processing time for feature extraction, and hence expedites classification. Other paradigms such as the slow cortical potential have received attention from the research community but are not widely used (Hinterberger et al. 2004).

Each paradigm (MI, SSVEP, and P300) has its strength and weakness (Allison et al. 2013). MI requires training, which is time consuming and requires significant subject compliance; it can be difficult to achieve greater than a reliable two-way classification consistently and over long durations. For example, in order to achieve a three-way communication channel, classification algorithms need to differentiate between individual imagined hand movement (left, right) and feet (the latter is often undertaken as combined imagined movement to strengthen the response). Other possibilities can be chosen specifically tailored to the most promising brain activity components of the user. For example, imagined tongue movement has also been used as a possible input (Morash et al. 2008), as it can be discriminated from hands because of its location of activation on the motor cortex. Unfortunately, in some individuals, it is difficult to differentiate the EEG MI activity to a suitable level for robust and usable BCI operation (Ahn and Jun 2015).

The P300 paradigm has the advantage that a significant number of stimuli [usually in the form of icons, and more recently faces (Jin et al. 2014), which tend to produce a robust response] can be placed on screen at one time. A good example of this is with the P300 speller (Cecotti 2011; Farwell and Donchin 1988; Vaughan et al. 2006). A typical configuration contains a grid of 6 by 6 icons flashing sequentially by row and column, although variations of less or more icons have been used (Sellers et al. 2006). A balance is needed between having enough icons to create a "random" enough stimulus but not so many as to make it too slow to determine the target icon. Depending on the subject and experimental parameters, it can take from one (single trial) to multiple (up to 16) repeat flashes of the target icon to enhance the P300 response from the background EEG. The number of repetitions of the stimulus is dependent on both the P300 screen setup and the user and, in turn, has an impact on the performance in terms of robustness (determined by sensitivity and lack of errors) and information transfer rate (ITR), which equates to speed and interactivity for the user.

With SSVEP, there is also a trade-off in these performance metrics. The choice of discriminable frequencies for the icons is important and is often dependent on the user. Furthermore, the greater the number of distinct icons flashing on the screen, the greater the challenge in differentiating between frequency characteristics of the EEG. Furthermore, improved discrimination could depend on tuning an algorithm to tailor the threshold power values in the EEG for each frequency associated with each user. Such choices have an impact on the duration of recording before a decision can be made with a certain degree of confidence. Ware et al. (2010) reported a gap in what was considered an acceptable accuracy by some users (77%–81%) and what they were able to achieve using SSVEP (16%–95%). This highlights the importance of a minimum viable accuracy before such systems can be deemed usable. To be accepted by users, BCI systems need to have a high enough accuracy to be robust in terms of errors, and with a suitable speed and performance to alleviate frustration. Consequently, accuracy and ITR have been applied as metrics to indicate this overall system performance of a BCI. Performance metrics are further addressed in Section 24.3 and described in more detail in Chapter 7 of this book.

Conventional BCI systems have been impeded by an extensive list of constraints (such as intersubject performance variability, robustness, and comfortable EEG acquisition) that prevent ubiquitous distribution and widespread adoption (Abdulkader et al. 2015; Brunner et al. 2015). Consequently, *hybrid* brain–computer interface (*h*BCI) (Allison et al. 2012b; Vilimek and Zander 2009) is an emerging research area that has the potential to address many of the limitations and associated hindrances by combining two or more BCI paradigms within a single system (e.g., MI and sensory stimulation) or by combining a BCI system with other input/output modalities. Allison et al. (2012a) provide definitions of different classes of *h*BCIs. Based on these definitions Figure 24.1 illustrates examples of the different types of *h*BCI.

There are many reasons why additional inputs could provide a more robust and usable system. In combining the different mechanisms, Pfurtscheller et al. (2010a) discuss how systems can be combined to enhance the quality of the decision making (*simultaneous processing*), as also highlighted by Millán et al. (2010); or so that one component can act as a "*switch*" to initiate the control while the other is used to determine the ongoing action (*sequential processing*). For further details on *h*BCI control mechanisms, please see Henshaw et al. (2014). In their work, they provide a review of *h*BCI since 2011, putting the example of *h*BCI into the categories of *simultaneous* and *sequential* processing, and highlighting in their overview the key benefits that the combinations provide over pure BCI systems. In addition, they reported associated improvements, such as an increase in accuracy (Allison et al. 2014), specificity (Spüler et al. 2012), performance (Yin et al. 2014), and function (Choi and Jo 2013).

Such examples demonstrate how multiple BCI systems can be combined to provide a purely EEG-reliant interaction. These fall into the traditional concept of a BCI (Pfurtscheller et al. 2010a) in which there must be an element of determined patterns detectable in the EEG in response to the user's goal-directed behavior. Zander and Kothe provide an alternative argument through studying BCI technology as a passive input for human–machine interfaces (Zander and Kothe 2011). Other

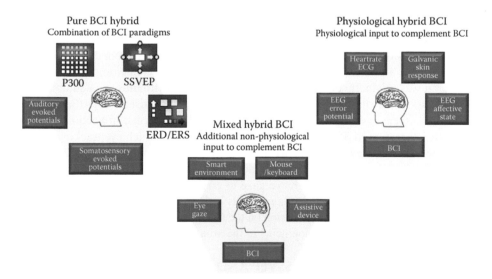

**FIGURE 24.1** Hybrid BCI approaches: Pure BCI hybrid, which combines a number of existing BCI paradigms, Mixed hybrid BCI, which employs nonphysiological sensors as an additional input modality to the BCI system; Physiological hybrid BCI, which combines physiological-based sensor input with a BCI system.

examples combine physiological inputs with EEG components to provide a level of classification reinforcement (Leeb et al. 2011; Shahid et al. 2011) or to extend the number of classification targets (Lin et al. 2016). Passive BCIs (Zander and Kothe 2011) utilize the modulating EEG, for example, due to the affective state of the subject, to reinforce the active BCI.

Millán et al. (2010) discuss the combining of all the individual decisions from each component of the hBCI in such a way as to assign a confidence or certainty on the classifications. The result would be a "weighted" fusion of the incoming information and classifications. Consideration is given to a number of factors: from the reliability of the systems and channels through to the inclusion of supervision signals such as mental states (e.g., fatigue and error potentials [ErrPs], which may occur when a subject realizes that an incorrect classification occurred) and physiological parameters (e.g., muscular fatigue). Ongoing performance monitoring could also play a beneficial role. Incorporating evidence of error occurrence from the EEG using ErrPs has also been applied to hBCI design (Buttfield et al. 2006), with Schmidt et al. (2012) showing that including automatic error detection enhanced the writing speed of their BCI speller.

The future of BCI has been envisioned in a roadmap (Brunner et al. 2015). The roadmap categorizes BCI from the most extreme cases, whereby using EEG within the BCI offers the only route for communication and control, through to the inclusion of a BCI modality to supplement and guide an activity, or to be used for rehabilitation or neuroscience research. Blankertz et al. (2016) provide a review of examples of BCI deployment covering a range of applications, for example, monitoring alertness in safety critical situations. Another interesting example discusses combining ET technologies with BCI for implicit monitoring of the use of computing applications to enable augmentation of the HCI to the user needs. Indeed, the vision for BCI has extended beyond an assistive technology to the extent that EEG monitoring is envisaged to become a ubiquitous activity for a very wide group of users (Blankertz et al. 2010, 2016; Nijboer et al. 2011; Van Erp et al. 2012; Zander and Kothe 2011).

By broadening the scope of BCI with the addition of complementary modalities within hybrid systems, it may be possible to produce stronger, more usable systems, thereby promoting greater adoption. Furthermore, as developments in wearable devices and BCI technology continue to progress, application areas will certainly extend beyond disabled user groups. This is a plausible concept, albeit the technology is still in the "Innovation Trigger" phase of the Gartner 2016 Hype Cycle (Gartner 2016). The report envisages that "technology will continue to become more human-centric to the point where it will introduce transparency between people, businesses and things." As part of this vision, they highlight BCI, human augmentation, affective computing, and connected home (among others) to be key driving technologies.

This potential increase in widespread user acceptance and interest from commercial developers should in turn have a positive impact on the availability of BCI technology as an assistive device for those that it was originally designed for. Indeed, this market stimulus can additionally reinforce further BCI research into hardware, algorithms, and synergies with user groups (Saproo et al. 2016).

This chapter's focus is on combining eye gaze with BCI paradigms. In Section 24.2, we review the current BCI literature in SSVEP, and in BCI mechanisms in which eye tracking (ET) has been used in a complementary way to enhance performance and usability. Section 24.3 provides an overview of the challenges and techniques in developing an hBCI. This is demonstrated through an example that combines SSVEP with eye gaze to create more robust navigation through a user interface for control over a virtual smart home. This includes an experimental protocol and evaluation. Section 24.4 concludes with a discussion on the subtleties in operation of the hybrid design and provides commentary on future developments in the area.

## 24.2 OVERVIEW OF CURRENT SSVEP AND ET ADVANCES

This section provides an overview of the state of the art in SSVEP systems, which will set the background for the algorithm used in the hybrid example in Section 24.3. We also investigate the application of ET metrics into EEG and BCI systems.

## 24.2.1 SSVEP

The visual evoked potential (VEP) can be detected in the EEG in response to external visual stimuli. The stimuli can be pattern reversal (e.g., a checkerboard on computer screen), flashing icons on a computer screen, or externally modulated flashing lights, usually LEDs (Zhu et al. 2010). The VEP component is prominent in the visual region of the occipital cortex (Regan 1988). If the visual stimulus is presented at a rate greater than 6 Hz, an oscillatory response is evoked. This response is termed steady-state visual evoked potential (SSVEP). If users pay attention to one or more stimuli that oscillate between 6 and 50 Hz, corresponding frequencies may be measured over visual areas of the brain. Users can thus communicate by focusing on one stimulus while ignoring others. Different frequencies elicit different SSVEP activity across different subjects (Gao et al. 2003; Kelly et al. 2005) Allison et al. (2008) showed that SSVEP sufficient for BCI control may be elicited by selective attention to one of two overlapping stimuli. Thus, some SSVEP-based BCI approaches may not depend on gaze control and could function in severely disabled users (Allison et al. 2010; Pfurtscheller et al. 2010b; Volosyak et al. 2011).

Hwang et al. (2013) surveyed the percentages of each BCI paradigm used in EEG-based BCI articles published between 2007 and 2011. For a review of these paradigms, please refer to Amiri et al. (2013). In 2011, SSVEP comprised 10% and hBCI comprised 4% of these articles. The main paradigms were MI (56%) and Visual P300 (18%).

The SSVEP component is maximum for 10 Hz stimulation. The EEG activity has peaks at the fundamental frequency and its harmonics; thus, 10 Hz stimulation enhances activity in the EEG at 10 Hz, 20 Hz, 30 Hz, and so on. These components of the EEG are best measured in the frequency domain using signal processing techniques, typically by analyzing the power spectrum of the EEG (Friman et al. 2007; Gao et al. 2003; Lalor et al. 2005). In order to operate as a BCI, the user focuses his or her attention on a target stimulus (possibly attending to one of many stimuli).

Most SSVEP-based BCIs use stimulation frequencies in the 6–30 Hz range (classified as "low-frequency" stimulation up to 12 Hz and "medium-frequency" stimulation up to 30 Hz). The SSVEPs elicited by frequencies in this range have high amplitude but can induce visual fatigue and may not be suitable BCI devices for people who are photosensitive, for example, people with epilepsy (Fisher et al. 2005). Although SSVEP systems may allow excellent control without training, the flickering stimuli typically produces a degree of annoyance and fatigue. Presenting stimuli above 30 Hz (to approximately 50 Hz) can provide a better user experience as it is prone to less flicker and, therefore, annoyance (Volosyak et al. 2011) but with a lower signal-to-noise ratio (Pastor et al. 2003) for the SSVEP components, thus requiring improved signal processing tools. One of the continuing challenges is finding the best stimulation frequencies for a user. Gembler et al. (2015a) proposed a wizard-based approach to address this. If this could be reliably deployed in practice, it would be a big advance.

For detection, spatial filters may be used to enhance the response (Garcia-Molina and Mihajlovic 2010). Principal component analysis (PCA) seeks uncorrelated components with maximal variance, while independent component analysis (ICA) decomposes signals into statistically independent components. ICA, PCA, and combinations of both methods have been applied to BCIs based on SSVEP (Allison et al. 2008; Friman et al. 2007). However, canonical correlation analysis (Hardoon et al. 2004) has become a key algorithm choice for SSVEP (Lin et al. 2007; Zhang et al. 2014). See Chapter 7 for an overview of other spatial filters.

Various techniques have been proposed to enhance the stimulation paradigm. The approaches are similar to the techniques adopted in communication modems to enhance effective bit rate. Multiple stimulation frequencies can be combined into one time-locked stimulus (Cheng et al. 2001; Mukesh et al. 2006), evoking more SSVEP component power for detection (assuming that the signal processing can decode these components). Another approach adopted is to use the same stimulating frequency but with different phases (Kluge and Hartmann 2007; Wang et al. 2008). The SSVEP response is phase-locked with the stimulus facilitating target identification. If the Fourier transform is used to produce a spectrum, the epoch length for analysis should be a multiple of the stimulus period. This reduces the communication throughput (Wilson and Palaniappan 2009). Garcia-Molina et al. (2010) used the Hilbert transform to detect phase, after narrow band filtering of the EEG. The difference between the instantaneous phase of SSVEP and the stimulation-signal reference phase was calculated in order to identify the stimulus. Such phase difference is dependent on the user's SSVEP response to the frequency. Phase synchrony analysis can extract the phase difference between the SSVEP and the reference light signal. The difference between these two values deviates slightly from the expected value, but the difference is sufficient for detection. Bit rates greater than 70 bits/min were reported.

More recent performance results demonstrate a higher ITR in the range of 100 bits/min (Volosyak 2011). Cited improvements in the signal processing and feedback modules constituted the basis for achieving this accuracy. In their study, five out of seven subjects spelled all copy spelling words without errors. SSVEP has also been used for assistive technology application. Gollee et al. (2010) developed a LED panel system that allows the control of a functional electrical stimulation–based neuroprosthesis. The system is robust, achieving accuracies of typically more than 90%. Volosyak et al. (2017) explored the effects of age on SSVEP usability. The mean ITR of the young age group was 27.36 (6.50) bits/min while the older age group achieved a significantly lower ITR of 16.10 (5.90) bits/min, showing that the subject age must be taken into account during the development of SSVEP-based applications.

### 24.2.2 *H*BCI with Eye Gaze

This section provides a review of BCI hybrids in which the BCI is combined with an additional input modality coming from eye gaze metrics. Consideration is given to how eye gaze can be combined with BCI methods to enhance the robustness of the BCI decision making (*explicit use*) or to infer (*implicit use*) information about user engagement with computer-based applications through associating gaze location onscreen to EEG responses. Figure 24.2 illustrates eye gaze combined with BCI for both explicit and implicit interaction. In (a), the Eye Tracker signal is employed for search activity with subsequent use of BCI signal to provide command decisions; in (b), classification employs explicit use of BCI signal and Eye Tracker signal as feature vectors in a combined classifier in which each input reinforces the output classification; in (c), the Eye Tracker signal is implicitly used to identify onscreen components of interest. By analyzing the epochs of the BCI signal that correspond temporally to the spatial onscreen component of interest, then some output decision can be made.

One of the benefits with BCI systems relying solely on EEG is that they require no peripheral movement by the user, in particular, eye movement. Although the extent to which this is true for VEPs is under some debate Brunner et al. (2010) and Treder and Blankertz (2010) observed a drop in performance within ERP-based BCI when attention was not overt, that is, with a user unable to shift their gaze to the object of interest. For a review on eye gaze–independent auditory and tactile BCI, please refer to Riccio et al. (2012).

In contrast, ET is an assistive technology relying on gaze direction and is widely accepted by users up to the point when gaze control has been lost (Pasqualotto et al. 2015). Combining active eye gaze technology with BCI can bridge the gap between the two systems. In particular, eye trackers used to navigate onscreen commands can meet challenges when a decision or action needs to be confirmed. *Dwell time** is an example technique used to activate a command. Here, a subject gazes at an object for an intended length of time, notably longer than natural gaze behavior and thus indicating a desired action. However, this interaction can lead to unintended selection if the duration of the dwell time is too short. Alternatively, BCIs could lend themselves to performing this

---

\* Dwell time is the time that a user focuses on a screen object, with gaze set stationary.

"switch" (Amiri et al. 2013; Zander et al. 2010) operation to perform the selection, thereby providing a greater level of intentional control to the user (Figure 24.2a).

Early EEG responses referred to as eye fixation-related potentials (EFRPs) have been investigated as a method to provide insight on "the cognitive processes that occur during a single eye fixation" (Baccino and Manunta 2005). The combination of analyzing ET with EEG is of great interest in the research of lexical processing with ERP components (P1, N1, and P2, between 100 and 200 ms post-stimulus), offering potential understanding of the cognitive processes (Sereno and Rayner 2003). Such insight can subsequently be utilized to automatically augment the HCI in response to ET and EEG patterns to enhance usability and personalization to the needs of the user.

Implicit selection of relevant onscreen content was demonstrated by Eugster et al. (2016) through their development of a natural interface for reading onscreen text and inferring the user's interest in the content that their eyes were focused on. Their system used a combination of eye gaze and "semantic" ERPs to classify if the particular words onscreen had relevance to the reader. By gathering this information from user's interaction with online material, they developed a participant-specific single-trial prediction model based on word relevance. This model was then used to search for more relevant online content and provide recommendations to the user. For all their participants, they found it possible to distinguish between two classes of relevant versus irrelevant words by looking at the grand average–based ERP between 300 and 600 ms. This extends beyond the initial window for EFRPs (Rama and Baccino 2010).

One of the challenges that face the combination of ET and ERPs is that user recognition of an onscreen target can occur in the foveal or peripheral vision. Wenzel et al. (2016) investigated this variability of the latency between the recognition of the visual target object and the corresponding evoked response. They performed a gaze search task in which there were targets and distractors. EEG epochs were captured over 800 ms after fixation onset. They found that despite such variability, ET data can be effectively correlated with brain activity to provide "appearance aligned EEG features" to determine user interest of visual online material.

Hild et al. (2014) show the use of ET and EEG to allow spatiotemporal event selection. Their system (Putze et al. 2016) combined eye gaze with BCI to enable the implicit selection of onscreen objects from nontarget objects within a graphical user interface without the need for manual user intervention. By using eye gaze to determine where on the screen the user is looking

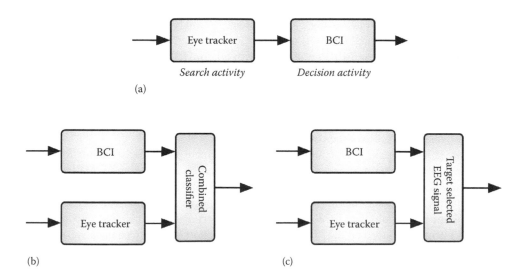

**FIGURE 24.2** Explicit and implicit use of eye tracking and BCI: (a) sequential mixed *h*BCI; (b) combined classification; (c) collaborative target selection.

and combining this with ERP changes in brain activity, they found it possible to determine the onscreen object of interest to the user and hence the user's selection. They did not suggest their method as a sole selection mechanism for a user interface but instead for it to be part of a combined approach (Putze et al. 2015).

The concept of "cortically coupled computing" presented by Gerson et al. (2006) uses the ability of the human brain to rapidly analyze a visual scene at a glance for the purpose of triaging images. Through EEG analysis during *rapid serial visual presentation* of a series of images, they can determine those images of greatest relevance. A more recent review of cortically coupled computing is provided by Saproo et al. (2016). They make the distinction between BCI systems in which the user actively performs a task that leads to a decision classification and the implicit or explicit monitoring of brain states to infer the decision through machine learning without a priori information. They provide the example of cortically coupled computer vision in which eye gaze is used to determine the object that the user is viewing while their associated brain state information is being analyzed to determine or infer some condition, for example, a target image selection. Their goal for this process is to allow the images to be automatically "tagged" through the response from the EEG. By collating large amounts of data, machine learning approaches can be employed using supervised learning to tag patterns in unknown data.

From these examples, it can be determined that ET can be effective in associating temporal EEG, and hence user brain state information, with spatial objects such as images or onscreen text. Achieving this is not without challenges but offers a promising input modality (Nikolaev et al. 2016; Ušćumlić and Blankertz 2016). The main challenge, as always, is decoding and understanding the EEG given the high levels of competing sensory, motor, and cognitive processes. The human and software form a closed loop, and the software may have to adapt to continue to extract information. The EEG activity is nonstationary and may change over time, due to attention, tiredness, familiarization and habituation effect, and the use of alternative interaction strategies.

Eye gaze is a natural interaction method for an onscreen application; however, users have free eye movement and may unintentionally fixate on undesired areas, thus implementing unwanted actions. This is referred to as the "Midas Touch" problem in which free eye movement can cause unintentional selection. Methods such as setting a certain dwell time on a fixation point or using intended eye blinks have been used to help make the selection with ET-based interfaces (Holmqvist et al. 2011). Combining ET with another form for making the decision can help resolve unintentional actions. This is demonstrated by Shishkin et al. (2016) in which they combined ET with EFRPs to enable control over a game solely using eye movement. By analyzing the EEG, they were able to differentiate between intentional fixations and spontaneous fixations. Finke et al. (2016) also demonstrate the possibility of using EFRPs combined with ET for HCI.

Combining ET with more explicit BCI decision mechanisms, namely, SSVEP (or MI and P300), can also help make a more robust system. Huang et al. (2013) present an *h*BCI with ET to perform a continuous cursor control task. Here, the user is asked to navigate a cursor around onscreen obstacles toward a target position. They use MI to decide if the cursor movement is an intended action, thus providing more control over the cursor movement.

Yong et al. (2011) propose an ET and BCI hybrid that incorporate on/off states for intentional control. When on, BCI operation is active and selection can be made using an MI task. If off, no BCI interaction is used. This is done to restrict possible false positives when operating the BCI in a self-paced manner. The system demonstrated is for a speller operation in which the ET points to the letter or word; the user would then fixate on this item for a certain dwell time and activate a selection through BCI interaction based on the MI paradigm. They report a lower true negative/false positive ratio with their system as compared to similar systems, highlighting the additional computational load and the importance of choosing a suitable dwell time so as not to impact speed performance.

A combination of SSVEP with ET is presented by Hwang et al. (2012) for a spelling application. This example incorporated a web camera for ET with a custom-made QWERTY keyboard in which each letter displayed an associated LED key with a unique frequency. The SSVEP speller in this example is not screen based, but through a combination of the ET and SSVEP, classification between each of the characters is obtainable, reporting a mean accuracy over five subjects of 87.58% and a mean ITR of 40.72 bits/min.

In general, the search and select combination of ET and BCI offers a promising solution to the difficulty in robust selection through ET alone. Naturally, as the previous examples demonstrate, ET is used to locate an object of interest on the screen. A BCI paradigm such as MI can then be used to activate the command (Zander et al. 2010). There are examples, however, where the eye gaze is used to determine spatial locations within an environment in order to select a device that the user will then communicate with via the BCI (Valbuena et al. 2011). This is an example of how the environment in which the user is situated can provide context to the decisions available to the user. Comparably, a simultaneous BCI combining MI with ET has been proposed by Meena et al. (2015) with the goal to increase the number of available command choices. As with Valbuena et al. (2011), the eye gaze is used to detect (*search*) the spatially located device, while the BCI (MI) is used to perform selection.

## 24.3 EYE GAZE AND SSVEP *H*BCI

The versatility and usability of ET as an input metric to complement EEG and BCI systems have been demonstrated in Section 24.2. The example presented in this section details the method in which ET is employed to navigate (*search*) a computer screen for a target object, while the BCI, which in this case is SSVEP, is then used to instigate a command (*selection*). In this specific example, the ET has been used to provide the onscreen selection of directional arrows for navigation through a user interface to control domestic appliances (Galway et al. 2015). The SSVEP then performs the switch operation in order to activate the desired movement through the user interface or to activate a command on an external device.

This allows us to understand the interplay between eye gaze and SSVEP components in the decision process for a task-based user interface comprising four possible onscreen selections. The following sections provide an overview of the design of the hybrid architecture. It includes the combination of an existing SSVEP solution with a commercial ET collaborating through a custom-designed user interface, displaying both navigational options and visual stimulus (Galway et al. 2015; Volosyak 2011). An example experimental protocol is provided, and a study to measure ITR, accuracy, and efficiency was carried out on healthy volunteers (Brennan et al. 2017). The evaluation aims to highlight the intricacies of combining the two modalities into a usable system.

### 24.3.1 CONCEPTS FOR THE INCLUSION OF ET INTO THE *H*BCI

Because of collaborative decision making, an *h*BCI may be endowed with slower information throughput in comparison to a single modality BCI; however, we hypothesize that it will provide more robust HCI by enhancing accuracy, and we can reduce the number of incorrect decisions and hence improve efficiency.

Typically, it is considered that an increase in accuracy can lead to a slower speed of operation, thus a reduction in efficiency while increasing effectiveness. However, by making a more robust system with a higher accuracy, we hypothesize that there will be a reduction in incorrect decisions and hence an overall reduction in total decision classifications needed to perform a set of tasks. Thus, this can offer a reduction in the overall duration for these tasks. This aligns with the ISO 9241 (ISO 1998) definition of efficiency, which relates to the resources expended with regard to the accuracy and completeness of the goals achieved. The full extent of this improvement depends on any increase duration of an individual classification versus the duration needed to correct failed decisions within a set of tasks.

Our *h*BCI architecture, described herein, comprises two complementary modalities: (1) SSVEP-based BCI and (2) ET using a low-cost eye tracker (EyeTribe). The BCI software component, similar to Volosyak (2011), was employed for onscreen frequency-modulated stimulation and signal processing.

The introduction of ET as a complementary technology removes the need for the precise tuning of EEG parameters, in addition to potentially overcoming the Midas Touch problem that would occur with the use of ET alone, as the *h*BCI will only make a selection when the gaze-fixation point corresponds with the SSVEP decision. Consequently, this permits SSVEP parameters that would normally lead to usage instability with an SSVEP-only BCI to be used successfully. Furthermore, the command classification decision is now a collaborative one. Of course, the eye tracker should also be calibrated; however, this is a more straightforward and generally more stable process.

The tasks facilitated by the *h*BCI system require a four-way command choice (*left*, *right*, *up*, *down*) that influences a menu system, which is utilized in order to actuate events in a "smart environment." This environment comprises a number of rooms, fitted with appliances that can be controlled by computer actuation. Metrics traditionally used to define performance are as follows: *Accuracy* (*Acc.*), *Efficiency* (*Eff.*), and *ITR*. There exists a degree of interplay between these measures; for example, in some cases, SSVEP-BCI *ITR* can be improved at the expense of *Acc.* and *Eff.*, but this leads to frustration for the user as task errors may have to be corrected. Correspondingly, the operator of the BCI system can tune the operation of the SSVEP by adapting the frequencies and thresholds that are used to classify commands. To add complexity to the process, these variables are typically subject specific and may also change over time because of habituation and tiredness during a long session (i.e., in excess of 1 h). Because of the amount of operator intervention, it may then be difficult to compare performance across subjects or subject groups.

### 24.3.2 VISUAL INTERFACE APPLICATION DESIGN

The first component to be discussed is the design of the user interface application, which facilitates user interaction and provides feedback and assessment of both system and user performance. In this *h*BCI architecture, we focused on the design of an interface that allows interaction and actuation of local events within a domestic smart environment. The example application was originally developed to address the needs of a brain-injured user group with motor impairment. It followed on from investigations as part of the BRAIN project (BRAIN Project 2011).

The user interface design followed HCI recommendations (Nielsen 1995) and a user evaluation from the brain-injured user group (BRAIN Project 2011; Ware et al. 2014). A screenshot of the developed user interface is shown in Figure 24.3. The visual interface was structured hierarchically and allowed the user to navigate Left, Right, Up, or Down in order to traverse through nested menu levels to select items. Users operate devices (e.g., control home lighting or the kitchen extractor fan), interact with multimedia applications, or communicate via predefined iconography and auditory feedback. The interface was additionally designed to be controlled using standard computer input peripherals and through receipt of packets across a network.

### 24.3.3 THE ET COMPONENT

The second component of the *h*BCI architecture is the design of an algorithmic process to facilitate ET-based control, which should be structured around the number and location of selectable icons. In our example, there are four active icons located to the left (Left, L), right (Right, R), top (Up, U), and bottom (Down, D) of the interface. Each icon is selectable via dwell time (Holmqvist et al. 2011), thereby allowing the selection of items based on gaze-fixation time. The approach employed divided the visual display of the interface into quadrants (Figure 24.4). The metrics from the eye tracker provided onscreen coordinates for the user's gaze, and thus, which quadrant the fixation point fell within and for what period of time during operation. Figure 24.4 illustrates the ET selection zones utilized by the ET control algorithm.

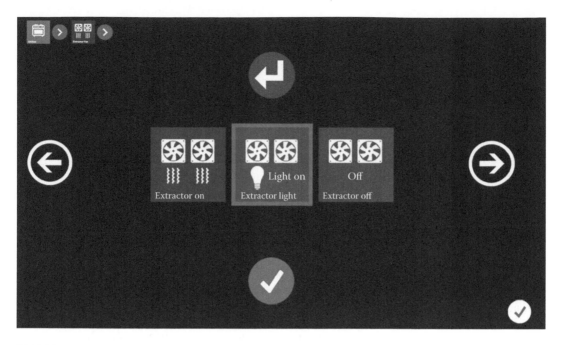

**FIGURE 24.3** The visual interface comprising four choices: Left, Right, Up, and Down. For example, at this point, the user is controlling a fan within the kitchen.

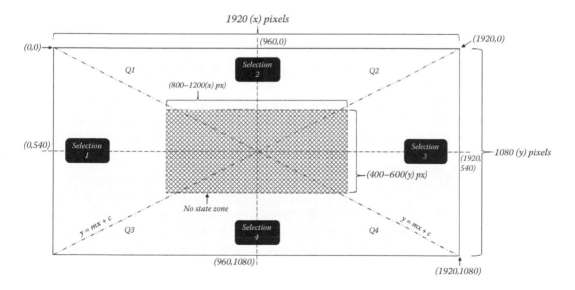

**FIGURE 24.4** Eye tracking zones.

As may be observed in Figure 24.4, the screen resolution of a "full HD" monitor (1920px*1080px) used for the hBCI was divided into four quadrants, each measuring 540px in width and 960px in height, along with a "No-State Zone," measuring 200px in width and 400px in height, which was designated centrally. If the gaze-fixation point was situated within the no-state zone, then no decisions could occur. Such a structure allowed menu icons to be located in this area, so that a user could freely observe the changes they were affecting without accidentally triggering false-positive commands. Each quadrant was then further divided diagonally based on a simple linear equation and therefore a selection could be determined based on the portion of the quadrant that the user was fixating upon.

### 24.3.4 The SSVEP BCI Component

The design of the BCI component needs to consider the intended hardware that will be used to capture the EEG recordings. If utilizing a low-cost commercially available EEG acquisition device, there may be a trade-off between cost and performance. In one of our early iterations, we employed the Emotiv EPOC as our method of EEG acquisition but were unable to achieve acceptable performance for SSVEP paradigms because of the restrictions on electrode placement and the low signal-to-noise ratio.

Since the design of the BCI component centered on the use of the SSVEP paradigm, acquisition of EEG was handled by the g.USBamp, g.GAMMAcap, and g.LADYbird passive electrodes (www.gtec.com), which provided flexibility regarding electrode montages and a much higher signal-to-noise ratio. As the SSVEP response emanates most prominently from the visual cortex, positioning of the electrodes over the occipital region of the cerebral cortex was required. Utilizing the International 10–20 system, the recommended positioning for SSVEP recordings was employed: $AF_Z$ (Ground), $C_Z$ (Ref), $P_Z$, $PO_3$, $PO_4$, $O_1$, $O_Z$, $O_2$, $O_9$, and $O_{10}$. In a passive electrode setup, it is particularly important to prepare and gently agitate the skin with an abrasive solution to reduce impedance below 5 kΩ (although 10 kΩ probably suffices in practice). Values for electrode impedance can be returned using acquisition tools, such as those available in OpenViBE (http://openvibe.inria.fr/), which was utilized within the work carried out herein.

SSVEP signal detection and classification utilized the minimum energy combination (MEC) (Volosyak 2011) method to create a spatial filter and enhance the SSVEP response while reducing ambient signals and other interference. The system automatically determined the best spatial filter for each subject at each frequency. Each stimulating frequency in the EEG was detected by spatial filtering, power estimation, and a probabilistic method, which enhanced the signal at each electrode location. If classification of the input signal was not possible using the initial, shortest time frame for the input vector, a longer time frame was subsequently used. The adaptive windowing technique automatically extended the time frame of the input vector in order to facilitate data processing (a maximum of four potential epochs resulting in a "window" of approximately 4 s) based on the work by Durka et al. (2009).

The hBCI uses SSVEP stimulation frequencies that are a division of the display refresh rate (100 Hz) to ensure that they are reasonably constant. Verification of screen-based stimulation frequency used an external Arduino-based photodiode tool to independently measure flicker rates. Indeed, high accuracy is not necessarily a requirement here, as long as (i) the stimulation frequencies induce a feature that can be reliably detected using spatial filter/MEC approach and (ii) the components are sufficiently different so that a four-way decision can be enacted. The modulation used is rectangular (i.e., on/off) and only a subset of frequencies can be used so that division does not produce the same component. Manyakov et al. (2013) have demonstrated that more sophisticated modulation techniques allow finer-grained frequency coverage that is independent of refresh rate; this could allow many more stimuli for other applications or indeed reduce the need for a hierarchical menu structure. Gembler et al. (2015b) conducted an experiment with seven subjects and showed that six could reliably detect 28 individual SSVEP targets (22–120 bits/min) and two could control a screen comprising 60 modulated targets (24–73 bits/min) (Gembler et al. 2015a). Clearly, these advances could influence the design of the interaction (beyond four-way) and facilitate easier interaction.

### 24.3.5 The hBCI Architecture

The final aspect of the hBCI design was to create an architecture that combines the ET and BCI components and to implement a decision-making algorithm. The ET component was implemented within the visual interface application. Consequently, the visual interface had to wait until a corresponding vote from the BCI component is received before a selection could be made. The dataflow and overarching architecture of the hBCI is presented in Figure 24.5.

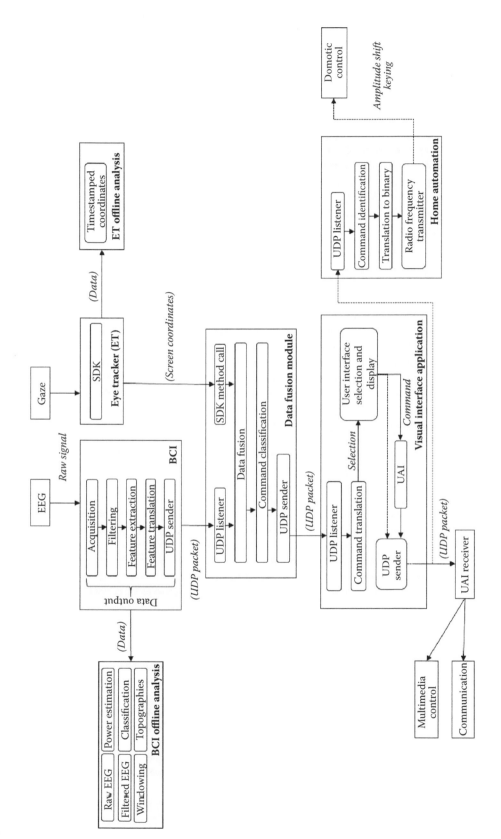

**FIGURE 24.5** The *h*BCI system architecture and corresponding dataflow.

As may be observed in Figure 24.5, utilizing functionality within the associated SDK, the Eye Tracker component repeatedly acquires screen coordinates at 128 samples per second for each eye gaze event, which are also time stamped for subsequent offline analysis. Simultaneously, the BCI component acquires and processes the raw EEG signal, resulting in a command decision, which is then encapsulated in a User Datagram Protocol (UDP) packet and transmitted to the Data Fusion Module. The EEG data can be used for further offline analysis. Once the Data Fusion Module has received the coordinates from the Eye Tracker component and the command derived from the BCI component, it performs further processing and comparative analysis in order to determine whether or not there has been a unanimous agreement in the choice of command.

Based on screen coordinates the ET component generates a vote for a screen zone. The ET vote for each command increments/decrements based on the fixation point until they exceed the dwell time threshold. The ET vote for each command increments/decrements based on the fixation point until they exceed the dwell time threshold. When this is the case, an ET command is transmitted to the Data Fusion Module. SSVEP votes are based on the power estimation of detected frequencies, which classifies the SSVEP response and also transmits the SSVEP command to the Data Fusion Module. When both votes are in agreement, a collaborative selection is performed. This is to reduce the chance of a false classification.

If agreement occurs, a collaborative command is subsequently issued by the Data Fusion Module, encapsulated within a UDP packet, and transmitted to the Visual Interface Application in order to execute the relevant command. Depending on the menu item selected within the visual interface by the agreed upon command, the UDP packet containing the command may be additionally transmitted to an external receiver in order to perform an action on an external peripheral, for example, switching on/off a light via a home automation system. Table 24.1 provides further details.

By contrast, if no agreement occurs, no command is issued by the Data Fusion Module, and the voting levels are reset, which subsequently results in a delay occurring before the next command may be potentially issued. Consequently, a more sophisticated fusion of the SSVEP and

## TABLE 24.1
## Component of the *h*BCI: SSVEP and Eye Tracker

| Module | Activity | Attributes | Comment |
|---|---|---|---|
| EEG | BCI acquisition | Acquisition, filtering, feature extraction, feature translation | Standard acquisition using gTec USB amp |
| EEG | BCI offline analysis | Spatial filtering, power estimation | Signal analysis using minimum energy combination (Volosyak 2011) |
| Gaze | SDK | Screen coordinated, time stamp | Screen coordinates extracted and sector determined, time stamp added for synchronization with SSVEP-BCI component |
| Data fusion | Software component that listens to interface (UDP listener) | Which command? SSVEP and ET | Combines BCI and eye gaze parameters to make a "hard" decision |
| Visual interface | See Figure 24.3 | Four-way choice (R, L, U, D) | Interaction between user (BCI + ET) and environment used to navigate and select |
| Home automation | UAI, user application interface | Radio-frequency Amplitude shift keying, can be interchanged with raspberry PI server | Interact with environment to provide domotic control, e.g., play a video, switch on a light |
| Communication protocol | UDP | UDP sender, UDP listener | Asynchronous activity at visual interface |

ET components is needed to further enhance the overall operation of the system. Furthermore, through observation of the recorded EEG sessions, there is evidence that the ET or SSVEP should be allowed to dominate the classification at a particular time, dependent on the current operation. In other words, if one of the components is failing, then a mechanism needs to be in place to allow the operational component to lead the classification or to allow the voting level to be reduced to activate the classification earlier.

### 24.3.6 EXPERIMENTAL PROTOCOL

Evaluation of the *h*BCI system was performed by creating an experimental protocol and conducting user trials. With such an *h*BCI, we recommend using a dual-monitor setup, with the experimenter operating on monitor 1 and the participant interacting with monitor 2.

The experimenter initializes the BCI acquisition and ET software and launches the user interface. This displays command data, data logs containing internal values from the SSVEP algorithm and ET co-ordinates, and EEG and eye signal visualization. Monitor 1 is also used on the BCI setup of the EEG electrodes on the user's scalp to ensure that impedances have been suitably reduced. Additionally, the experimenter launches the ET calibration tool and displays this on monitor 2 for user interaction. The participant focuses on monitor 2; they are asked to follow the instructions to fixate on certain areas on the screen. The experimenter monitors the calibration from screen 1, establishing if a suitable level of accuracy has been achieved. If not, the ET calibration process is repeated. Distance from the screen, environmental light condition, and the use of spectacle are all consideration for this calibration.

Once the BCI and ET have been set up, the experimental protocol may begin. As with the setup, the participant should only focus on monitor 2, which is employed to display the visual interface. For the set of tasks defined within the protocol, the experimenter should provide the participant with instructions on the command to issue; however, in one of the predefined tasks (Task 4), the participant is given free control of the system in order to complete a preset goal. Participants are instructed to complete the following set of tasks:

1. Task 1—Lights (Total = 13)
   Navigate to Dining Room, turn on the Lamp, and return to Back Garden. The sequence of commands is R-R-R-R-D-R-R-D-U-L- L-L-L.
2. Task 2—Media player (Total = 25)
   a. Navigate to Living Room, select Home Media menu, select Home Cinema, select the "Exoskeleton BCI" video, return to Home Media menu, select Controls, and play video. The sequence of commands is L-L-L-D-L-D-R-R-D-R-R-R-D (video).
   b. Stop the video and return to high level menu: U-L-L-D-R-D (stop) U-U-U-R-R-R (back to garden).
3. Task 3—Feelings (Total = 7)
   Navigate to Talk icon, indicate you want to Eat, and return to high level menu. The sequence of commands is L-D-L-L-D (eat) U-R (garden).
4. Task 4—Free control
   Freely navigate around the GUI to turn off the extractor fan in the kitchen and return to the starting point (back garden icon).

Each of the tasks should be assessed in terms of *Acc.*, *Eff.*, and ITR. Accuracy is calculated as follows:

$$\text{Accuracy} = \frac{P_{\text{total}}}{P_{\text{max}}} * 100,$$

where $P_{total}$ is the total number of correct commands and $P_{max}$ is the maximum number of detected commands. Efficiency as defined by Volosyak et al. (2009) is calculated as follows:

$$\text{Efficiency} = \frac{C_{min}}{C_{total}} * 100,$$

where $C_{min}$ is the minimum number of compulsory commands (13 for Task 1 in our visual interface layout) and $C_{total}$ is the total number of detected commands. Finally, within the BCI community, ITR is the most widely used metric for performance evaluation (Gao et al. 2014) and was first defined by Wolpaw et al. in 1998 (Wolpaw et al. 1998). ITR is calculated as follows:

$$\text{ITR} = \left( \log_2 M + P\log_2 P + (1 - P)\log_2 \left[ \frac{1 - P}{M - 1} \right] \right) * \left( \frac{60}{T} \right),$$

where $M$ is the number of choices, $P$ is the accuracy of target detections, and $T$ (in seconds/selection) is the average time for a selection.

### 24.3.7 POSTPROCESSING

The EEG and command data can be analyzed offline to further assess performance and visualize information. Plotting the ET data can provide useful information regarding performance. The graph in Figure 24.6, for example, shows the ET vote for each selection during Task 1. A threshold has been set at a predefined value, and until the vote reaches this level of confidence, a selection cannot be made. In an ET-only system, the selection could be made as soon as the vote reaches this level; however, in a collaborative system, the decision for a selection cannot be made until the BCI is in agreement. If a user's gaze-fixation point moves from within the area associated with the desired command, then the voting confidence begins to decline and could stall operation. From Figure 24.6, it can be seen that the user began by trying to select the *right* command, but for the first 5 s, no selection was made, as it was waiting for agreement from the BCI component. Then, the second *right* command

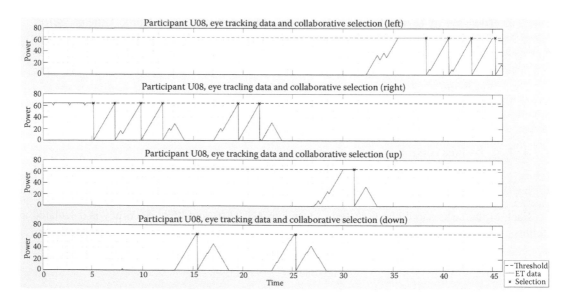

**FIGURE 24.6**  Eye tracking–based vote and collaborative selections for Task 1.

was made within the next 2 s, as soon as the ET vote met its threshold, suggesting that the BCI vote for the second selection came in before the ET had made its decision. This is particularly important as it indicates that the ET threshold may be set too high; hence, a reduction of this threshold could potentially improve the time per selection, thereby the overall ITR. More statistical approaches to combining the modalities could lead to a more robust system with enhanced interaction (Dong et al. 2015).

It is equally as important to analyze the BCI command detection. In Figure 24.7, the signal power of each frequency, left (7.5 Hz), right (8.57 Hz), up (12 Hz), and down (6.67 Hz), is displayed. The circles denote a BCI-based command, which can only be triggered once the value of the signal power reaches a preset threshold for the BCI decision. Like the ET component, this alone cannot make a selection and must wait for a corresponding decision. This information allows us to establish if the thresholds for BCI-based decisions are too low and classification is made based on noise level rather than the elicited SSVEP response.

To analyze the data from the *h*BCI, it is possible to utilize tools such as MATLAB® in order to overlay the ET vote and collaborative selections onto the signal-to-noise ratio values and BCI-based decisions, as shown in Figure 24.8. Doing so provides detailed information on the experiment and allows future recommendations to be made with a degree of certainty. Figure 24.8 shows that the participant took approximately 46 s to complete Task 1 and executed a total of 13 selections, which is 100% accurate and 100% efficient and resulted in an ITR of 34.67 bits/min. Further analysis of each individual selection conveys that for 10 of the total 13 selections, the BCI made a decision first; hence, the performance was limited by the ET component. The average difference between the BCI and ET decision can then be calculated in order to determine the optimal values for each threshold, and therefore, in this case, performance and ITR can be improved by reducing the threshold for the ET decision.

In summary, Figure 24.6 shows the simultaneous eye movement data for left, right, up, and down channels and Figure 24.7 isolates the EEG components for 7.5 Hz (left), 8.57 Hz (right), 12 Hz (up), and 6.67 Hz (down). Command classification is based on threshold imposed on these isolated components. In some cases, as illustrated in Figure 24.8, the EEG makes a classification (denoted by circles) before the eye tracker (red line reaching the threshold appropriate to that zone). Agreed classification (selection) is denoted by crosses. There is, of course, still the potential for false positives and false negatives to occur.

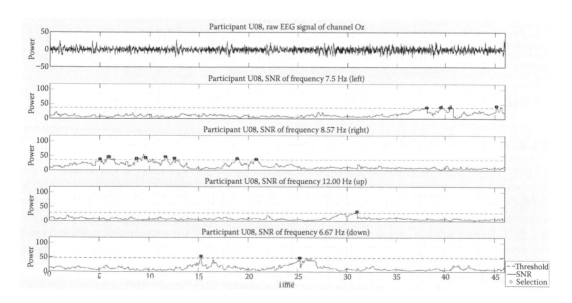

**FIGURE 24.7** Signal power values and BCI-based decisions for each stimulating frequency for Task 1.

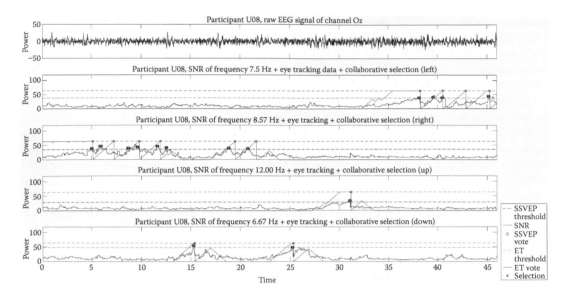

**FIGURE 24.8**   BCI and ET data for a representative participant completing Task 1.

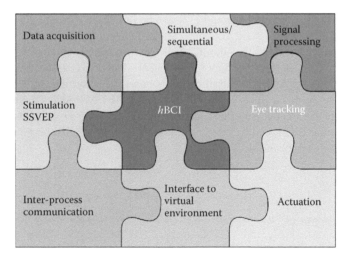

**FIGURE 24.9**   Components of an *h*BCI system.

## 24.4   DISCUSSION AND CONCLUSIONS

In general, *h*BCI development and different modalities (MI, SSVEP, P300, ET) and approaches (simultaneous/sequential, implicit/explicit) provide us with many possibilities for enhancing performance and for testing acceptance and usability. Figures 24.6 through 24.8 serve as an illustrative example, to indicate the data that can be made available to aid the decision process. In some cases, the BCI decides first; in others, the ET predominates. Currently, the experimenter can influence the decision-making process by tuning thresholds. An automated process to combine these inputs appropriate to the participant and temporal changes with more sophisticated decision-making algorithms would enhance the systems, potentially improving performance metrics.

Figure 24.9 illustrates the interplay of some of the constituent components. Each component can utilize tools that have been developed by the BCI community such as BCI2000, OpenVibe, or more general signal processing and classification tools such as MATLAB and Weka. Brunner et al. (2012) provides a classification of some of these components.

Component-based modular systems allow the swapping in and out of different components for data acquisition, stimulation, and analysis and allow us to test various applications. Standardization and the use of well-defined APIs are key to expediting development. Low-cost (hundreds rather than thousands of pounds/Euros) data acquisition components have become available for recording both EEG and ET. Both are in a fast period of evolution.

Although we have utilized SSVEP and ET, other permutations are of course available. Examples may be found in Amiri et al. (2012) and Henshaw et al. (2014). Amiri et al. (2012) discuss the advantages and disadvantages of different EEG paradigm combinations forming *h*BCIs. They highlight that the decision to combine different BCI mechanisms influences the practicality of the data acquisition and how the control signals are isolated from the EEG. Signal processing and classification methods for the BCI mechanisms could conflict with each other. Hence, effort is needed to determine analysis and classification strategies that are tuned for each BCI component of the hybrid system.

When we adopt more than one modality, we need fusion of the decision-making process. If based on agreement to reinforce the decision, as is in the case presented here, failure to agree can cause a noticeable delay, which will be obvious to the user, and the command will eventually fail (time out). The experimenter may be able to pinpoint whether this was due to SSVEP or ET performance. Parameters can then be modified intuitively, for example, reduce threshold for SSVEP "up" command activation. This will of course be manifest in reduced ITR and diminish usability. Indeed, there is an obvious need for a more sophisticated approach to scoring classified commands rather than our existing approach that requires both systems to "agree" within close epochs of operation.

The interaction between an MI BCI and onscreen ET has been refined by Dong et al. (2015). In their hybrid system, they reinforce the decision-making process by combining a four-class MI BCI with the eye trajectories coming from the eye tracker using a probabilistic Bayesian approach. The goal with their system is to facilitate more natural interaction rather than explicit eye gaze. The paper provides a good example of how refinement of the combined systems can lead to a more elegant and robust solution.

Overall, our experience and initial results indicate that the *h*BCI provides increased reliability when compared to SSVEP or ET alone (for healthy subject volunteers). Vilimek and Zander (2009) reported that this reliability came as a cost to the ITR; however, our study has shown that this may not be the case. The reason being that even though the time per individual selection may have increased, there is a reduction in the number of commands required to complete each task due to the improvement in accuracy. This, in turn, is a factor in the calculation of the ITR.

Volosyak (2011) has reported a peak SSVEP ITR of 124 bits/min, which shows that development in BCI alone has further to go. Indeed, adding more "intelligence" to the environmental devices has been demonstrated to enhance BCI function and improve self-calibration (Cavrini et al. 2014; Faller et al. 2012; Jarosiewicz et al. 2015; Schettini et al. 2014). In some applications, this reliability may be key to acceptance by users; in others, such as gaming for example, ITR and robust operation will predominate.

## REFERENCES

Abdulkader, S. N., Atia, A. and Mostafa, M. S. M. (2015) Brain computer interfacing: Applications and challenges, *Egyptian Informatics Journal*, pp. 213–230. doi: 10.1016/j.eij.2015.06.002.

Ahn, M. and Jun, S. C. (2015) Performance variation in motor imagery brain–computer interface: A brief review, *Journal of Neuroscience Methods*, 243, pp. 103–110. doi: 10.1016/j.jneumeth.2015.01.033.

Allison, B. (2011) Trends in BCI research, *XRDS: Crossroads, The ACM Magazine for Students*, 18(1), p. 18. doi: 10.1145/2000775.2000784.

Allison, B., Dunne, S., Leeb, R., Mill, R. and Nijholt, A. (2013) *Towards Practical Brain–Computer Interfaces*. Edited by B. Z. Allison, S. Dunne, R. Leeb, J. Del R. Millán, and A. Nijholt. Berlin, Heidelberg: Springer Berlin Heidelberg (Biological and Medical Physics, Biomedical Engineering), pp. 1–13. doi: 10.1007/978-3-642-29746-5.

Allison, B., Jin, J., Zhang, Y. and Wang, X. (2014) A four-choice hybrid P300/SSVEP BCI for improved accuracy, *Brain–Computer Interfaces*, 1(1), pp. 17–26. doi: 10.1080/2326263X.2013.869003.

Allison, B., Leeb, R., Brunner, C., Müller-Putz, G., Bauernfeind, G., Kelly, J. W. and Neuper, C. (2012a) Toward smarter BCIs: Extending BCIs through hybridization and intelligent control, *Journal of Neural Engineering*, 9(1), p. 13001. doi: 10.1088/1741-2560/9/1/013001.

Allison, B., Luth, T., Valbuena, D., Teymourian, A., Volosyak, I. and Graser, A. (2010) BCI demographics: How many (and what kinds of) people can use an SSVEP BCI?, *IEEE Transactions on Neural Systems and Rehabilitation Engineering*, 18(2), pp. 107–116. doi: 10.1109/TNSRE.2009.2039495.

Allison, B., McFarland, D. J., Schalk, G., Zheng, S. D., Jackson, M. M. and Wolpaw, J. R. (2008) Towards an independent brain–computer interface using steady state visual evoked potentials, *Clinical Neurophysiology*, 119(2), pp. 399–408. doi: 10.1016/j.clinph.2007.09.121.

Allison, B., Millan, J. del R., Nijholt, A., Dunne, S., Leeb, R., Whitmer, D., Poel, M. and Neuper, C. (2012b) *Future BNCI: A Roadmap for Future Direction in Brain/Neuronal Computer Interaction Research, Future Directions in Brain/Neuronal Computer Interaction (Future BNCI)*. doi: 10.1080/2326263X.2015.1008956.

Amiri, S., Fazel-Rezai, R. and Asadpour, V. (2012) A review of hybrid brain–computer interface systems, *Advances in Human–Computer Interaction*, 2013, pp. 1–8. doi: 10.1155/2013/187024.

Amiri, S., Rabbi, A., Azinfar, L. and Fazel-Rezai, R. (2013) A review of P300, SSVEP, and hybrid P300/SSVEP brain–computer interface systems, *Brain–Computer Interface Systems—Recent Progress and Future Prospects*, 2013, pp. 1–8. doi: 10.5772/56135.

Baccino, T. and Manunta, Y. (2005) Eye-fixation-related potentials: Insight into parafoveal processing, *Journal of Psychophysiology*, 19(3), pp. 204–215. doi: 10.1027/0269-8803.19.3.204.

Blankertz, B., Acqualagna, L., Dähne, S., Haufe, S., Schultze-Kraft, M., Sturm, I., Uščumlić, M., Wenzel, M., Curio, G., Mueller, K. R., Cumlí C, M. U. and Müller, K.-R. (2016) The Berlin Brain–Computer Interface: Progress beyond communication and control, *Front. Neurosci*, 10(November). doi: 10.3389/fnins.2016.00530.

Blankertz, B., Tangermann, M., Vidaurre, C., Fazli, S., Sannelli, C., Haufe, S., Maeder, C., Ramsey, L., Sturm, I., Curio, G. and Müller, K.-R. (2010) The Berlin Brain–Computer Interface: Non-medical uses of BCI technology, *Frontiers in Neuroscience*. Frontiers, 4, p. 198. doi: 10.3389/fnins.2010.00198.

BRAIN Project (2011) *EU Project BRAIN (ICT-2007-224156), Project Web Site*. Available at: http://www.brain-project.org/(Accessed: 5 April 2017).

Brennan, C., McCullagh, P., Lightbody, G. and Galway, L. (2017) Evaluation of an SSVEP and eye gaze hybrid BCI, in *7th Graz Brain-Computer Interface Conference*. Graz.

Brunner, C., Andreoni, G., Bianchi, L., Blankertz, B., Breitwieser, C., Kanoh, S., Kothe, C. A., Lécuyer, A., Makeig, S., Mellinger, J., Perego, P., Renard, Y., Schalk, G., Susila, I. P., Venthur, B. and Müller-Putz, G. R. (2012) *BCI Software Platforms*, Springer Berlin Heidelberg, pp. 303–331. doi: 10.1007/978-3-642-29746-5_16.

Brunner, C., Birbaumer, N., Blankertz, B., Guger, C., Kübler, A., Mattia, D., Millán, J. del R., Miralles, F., Nijholt, A., Opisso, E., Ramsey, N., Salomon, P. and Müller-Putz, G. R. (2015) BNCI Horizon 2020: Towards a roadmap for the BCI community, *Brain–Computer Interfaces*, 2(1), pp. 1–10. doi: 10.1080/2326263X.2015.1008956.

Brunner, P., Joshi, S., Briskin, S., Wolpaw, J. R., Bischof, H. and Schalk, G. (2010) Does the "P300" speller depend on eye gaze?, *Journal of Neural Engineering*, 7(5), p. 56013. doi: 10.1088/1741-2560/7/5/056013.

Buttfield, A., Ferrez, P. W. and Del R. Millan, J. (2006) Towards a Robust BCI: Error Potentials and Online Learning, *IEEE Transactions on Neural Systems and Rehabilitation Engineering*, 14(2), pp. 164–168. doi: 10.1109/TNSRE.2006.875555.

Cavrini, F., Quitadamo, L. R., Bianchi, L. and Saggio, G. (2014) Combination of classifiers using the fuzzy integral for uncertainty identification and subject specific optimization—Application to brain–computer interface, in *Proceedings of the International Conference on Fuzzy Computation Theory and Applications*. SCITEPRESS—Science and and Technology Publications, pp. 14–24. doi: 10.5220/0005035900140024.

Cecotti, H. (2011) Spelling with non-invasive brain–computer interfaces—Current and future trends, *Journal of Physiology, Paris*. Elsevier Ltd, 105(1–3), pp. 106–114. doi: 10.1016/j.jphysparis.2011.08.003.

Cheng, M., Gao, X., Gao, S. and Xu, D. (2001) Multiple color stimulus induced steady state visual evoked potentials, in *2001 Conference Proceedings of the 23rd Annual International Conference of the IEEE Engineering in Medicine and Biology Society*. IEEE, pp. 1012–1014. doi: 10.1109/IEMBS.2001.1020359.

Choi, B. and Jo, S. (2013) A low-cost EEG system-based hybrid brain–computer interface for humanoid robot navigation and recognition, *PLoS ONE*, 8(9). doi: 10.1371/journal.pone.0074583.

Dong, X., Wang, H., Chen, Z. and Shi, B. E. (2015) Hybrid brain computer interface via Bayesian integration of EEG and eye gaze, *7th Annual International IEEE EMBS Conference on Neural Engineering*, 1, pp. 22–24. doi: 10.1109/NER.2015.7146582.

Durka, P., Kus, R. and Zygierewicz, J. (2009) High-frequency SSVEP responses parametrized by multichannel matching pursuit, ... *Abstract: 2nd INCF* .... doi: 10.3389/conf.neuro.11.2009.08.055.

Eugster, M. J. A., Ruotsalo, T., Spapé, M. M., Barral, O., Ravaja, N., Jacucci, G. and Kaski, S. (2016) Natural brain-information interfaces: Recommending information by relevance inferred from human brain signals, *Scientific Reports*. Nature Publishing Group, 6(arXiv:1607.03502), p. 38580. doi: 10.1038/srep38580.

Faller, J., Torrellas, S., Miralles, F., Holzner, C., Kapeller, C., Guger, C., Bund, J., Muller-Putz, G. R. and Scherer, R. (2012) Prototype of an auto-calibrating, context-aware, hybrid brain–computer interface, *Proceedings of the Annual International Conference of the IEEE Engineering in Medicine and Biology Society, EMBS*, pp. 1827–1830. doi: 10.1109/EMBC.2012.6346306.

Farwell, L. A. and Donchin, E. (1988) Talking off the top of your head: Toward a mental prosthesis utilizing event-related brain potentials, *Electroencephalography and Clinical Neurophysiology*, 70, pp. 510–523. doi: 10.1016/0013-4694(88)90149-6.

Finke, A., Essig, K., Marchioro, G. and Ritter, H. (2016) Toward FRP-based brain–machine interfaces single-trial classification of fixation-related potentials, *PLoS ONE*, 11(1), p. e0146848. doi: 10.1371/journal.pone.0146848.

Fisher, R. S., Harding, G., Erba, G., Barkley, G. L. and Wilkins, A. (2005) Photic- and pattern-induced seizures: A review for the epilepsy foundation of america working group, *Epilepsia*. Blackwell Science Inc, pp. 1426–1441. doi: 10.1111/j.1528-1167.2005.31405.x.

Friman, O., Luth, T., Volosyak, I. and Graser, A. (2007) Spelling with steady-state visual evoked potentials, in *Proceedings of International IEEE EMBS Conference on Neural Engineering*. IEEE, pp. 354–357. doi: 10.1109/CNE.2007.369683.

Galway, L., Brennan, C., McCullagh, P. and Lightbody, G. (2015) BCI and eye gaze: Collaboration at the interface, in *Lecture Notes in Computer Science (including subseries Lecture Notes in Artificial Intelligence and Lecture Notes in Bioinformatics)*. Springer, Cham, pp. 199–210. doi: 10.1007/978-3-319-20816-9_20.

Gao, S., Wang, Y., Gao, X. and Hong, B. (2014) Visual and auditory brain–computer interfaces, *IEEE Transactions on Biomedical Engineering*, 61(5), pp. 1436–1447. doi: 10.1109/TBME.2014.2300164.

Gao, X., Xu, D., Cheng, M. and Gao, S. (2003) A BCI-based environmental controller for the motion-disabled, *IEEE Transactions on Neural Systems and Rehabilitation Engineering*, 11(2), pp. 137–140. doi: 10.1109/TNSRE.2003.814449.

Garcia-Molina, G. and Mihajlovic, V. (2010) Spatial filters to detect steady-state visual evoked potentials elicited by high frequency stimulation: BCI application, *Biomedizinische Technik/Biomedical Engineering*, 55(3), pp. 173–182. doi: 10.1515/bmt.2010.013.

Garcia-Molina, G., Zhu, D. and Abtahi, S. (2010) Phase detection in a visual-evoked-potential based brain–computer interface, in *18th European Signal Processing Conference (EUSIPCO)*, pp. 949–953.

Gartner (2016) *Gartner's 2016 Hype Cycle for Emerging Technologies*. Available at: http://www.gartner.com/newsroom/id/3412017 (Accessed: 5 April 2017).

Gembler, F., Stawicki, P. and Volosyak, I. (2015a) Autonomous parameter adjustment for SSVEP-based BCIs with a novel BCI wizard, *Frontiers in Neuroscience*. Frontiers, 9(DEC), p. 474. doi: 10.3389/fnins.2015.00474.

Gembler, F., Stawicki, P. and Volosyak, I. (2015b) How many targets can be used in a SSVEP-based BCI-system, in Volosyak, I. (ed.) *EBCI 2015 Workshop*. Aachan: Shakler-Verlag, pp. 53–62.

Gerson, A. D., Parra, L. C. and Sajda, P. (2006) Cortically coupled computer vision for rapid image search, *IEEE Transactions on Neural Systems and Rehabilitation Engineering*, 14(2), pp. 174–179. doi: 10.1109/TNSRE.2006.875550.

Gollee, H., Volosyak, I., McLachlan, A. J., Hunt, K. J. and Graser, A. (2010) An SSVEP-based brain–computer interface for the control of functional electrical stimulation, *IEEE Transactions on Biomedical Engineering*, 57(8), pp. 1847–1855. doi: 10.1109/TBME.2010.2043432.

Guger, C., Daban, S., Sellers, E., Holzner, C., Krausz, G., Carabalona, R., Gramatica, F. and Edlinger, G. (2009) How many people are able to control a P300-based brain–computer interface (BCI)?, *Neuroscience Letters*, 462(1), pp. 94–98. doi: 10.1016/j.neulet.2009.06.045.

Hardoon, D. R., Szedmak, S. and Shawe-Taylor, J. (2004) Canonical correlation analysis: An overview with application to learning methods, *Neural Computation*. MIT Press 238 Main St., Suite 500, Cambridge, MA 02142-1046 USA journals-info@mit.edu, 16(12), pp. 2639–2664. doi: 10.1162/0899766042321814.

Henshaw, J., Liu, W. and Romano, D. (2014) Problem solving using hybrid brain–computer interface methods: A review, in *2014 5th IEEE Conference on Cognitive Infocommunications (CogInfoCom)*. IEEE, pp. 215–219. doi: 10.1109/CogInfoCom.2014.7020448.

Hild, J., Putze, F., Kaufman, D., Kühnle, C., Schultz, T. and Beyerer, J. (2014) Spatio-temporal event selection in basic surveillance tasks using eye tracking and EEG, *Proceedings of the 2014 Workshop on Eye Gaze in Intelligent Human Machine Interaction*, pp. 3–8. doi: 10.1145/2666642.2666645.

Hinterberger, T., Schmidt, S., Neumann, N., Mellinger, J., Blankertz, B., Curio, G. and Birbaumer, N. (2004) Brain–computer communication and slow cortical potentials, *IEEE Transactions on Biomedical Engineering*, 51(6), pp. 1011–1018. doi: 10.1109/TBME.2004.827067.

Holmqvist, K., Nyström, M., Andersson, R., Dewhurst, R., Jarodzka, H. and Van de Weijer, J. (2011) *Eye Tracking: A Comprehensive Guide to Methods and Measures*. 1st Edition. OUP Oxford.

Huang, B., Lo, A. H. P. and Shi, B. E. (2013) Integrating EEG information improves performance of gaze based cursor control, *International IEEE/EMBS Conference on Neural Engineering, NER*, pp. 415–418. doi: 10.1109/NER.2013.6695960.

Hwang, H. J., Kim, S., Choi, S. and Im, C. H. (2013) EEG-based brain–computer interfaces: A thorough literature survey, *International Journal of Human–Computer Interaction*. Taylor & Francis, 29(12), pp. 814–826. doi: 10.1080/10447318.2013.780869.

Hwang, H. J., Lim, J. H., Jung, Y. J., Choi, H., Lee, S. W. and Im, C. H. (2012) Development of an SSVEP-based BCI spelling system adopting a QWERTY-style LED keyboard, *Journal of Neuroscience Methods*, 208(1), pp. 59–65. doi: 10.1016/j.jneumeth.2012.04.011.

ISO (1998) *ISO 9241-11:1998(en), Ergonomic requirements for office work with visual display terminals (VDTs)—Part 11: Guidance on usability*. Available at: https://www.iso.org/obp/ui/#iso:std:iso:9241:-11:ed-1:v1:en (Accessed: 15 June 2017).

Jarosiewicz, B., Masse, N., Bacher, D. and Sarma, A. (2015) Context-Aware Self-Calibration, US Patent 20,150,370,325.

Jin, J., Allison, B., Zhang, Y., Wang, X. and Cichocki, A. (2014) An ERP-based BCI using an oddball paradigm with different faces and reduced errors in critical functions, *International Journal of Neural Systems*, 24(8), p. 1450027. doi: 10.1142/S0129065714500270.

Kelly, S. P., Lalor, E. C., Finucane, C., McDarby, G. and Reilly, R. B. (2005) Visual spatial attention control in an independent brain–computer interface, *IEEE Transactions on Bio-medical Engineering*, 52(9), pp. 1588–1596. doi: 10.1109/TBME.2005.851510.

Kim, D.-W., Lee, J.-C., Park, Y.-M., Kim, I.-Y. and Im, C.-H. (2012) Auditory brain–computer interfaces (BCIs) and their practical applications, *Biomedical Engineering Letters*, 2(1), pp. 13–17. doi: 10.1007/s13534-012-0051-1.

Kluge, T. and Hartmann, M. (2007) Phase coherent detection of steady-state evoked potentials: Experimental results and application to brain–computer interfaces, in *2007 3rd International IEEE/EMBS Conference on Neural Engineering*. IEEE, pp. 425–429. doi: 10.1109/CNE.2007.369700.

Lalor, E. C., Kelly, S. P., Finucane, C., Burke, R., Smith, R., Reilly, R. B. and Mcdarby, G. (2005) Steady-state VEP-based brain–computer interface control in an immersive 3D gaming environment, *EURASIP Journal on Applied Signal Processing*, 19, pp. 3156–3164.

Leeb, R., Sagha, H., Chavarriaga, R. and Millán, J. del R. (2011) A hybrid brain–computer interface based on the fusion of electroencephalographic and electromyographic activities, *Journal of Neural Engineering*. IOP Publishing, 8(2), p. 25011. doi: 10.1088/1741-2560/8/2/025011.

Lin, K., Cinetto, A., Wang, Y., Chen, X., Gao, S. and Gao, X. (2016) An online hybrid BCI system based on SSVEP and EMG, *Journal of Neural Engineering*. IOP Publishing, 13(2), p. 26020. doi: 10.1088/1741-2560/13/2/026020.

Lin, Z., Zhang, C., Wu, W. and Gao, X. (2007) Frequency recognition based on canonical correlation analysis for SSVEP-based BCIs, *IEEE Transactions on Biomedical Engineering*, 54(6), pp. 1172–1176. doi: 10.1109/TBME.2006.889197.

Manyakov, N. V, Chumerin, N., Robben, A., Combaz, A., van Vliet, M. and Van Hulle, M. M. (2013) Sampled sinusoidal stimulation profile and multichannel fuzzy logic classification for monitor-based phase-coded SSVEP brain–computer interfacing, *Journal of Neural Engineering*, 10(3), p. 36011. doi: 10.1088/1741-2560/10/3/036011.

Meena, Y. K., Cecotti, H., Wong-Lin, K. and Prasad, G. (2015) Towards increasing the number of commands in a hybrid brain–computer interface with combination of gaze and motor imagery, *Proceedings of the Annual International Conference of the IEEE Engineering in Medicine and Biology Society, EMBS*, 2015–Novem, pp. 506–509. doi: 10.1109/EMBC.2015.7318410.

Millán, J. D. R., Rupp, R., Müller-Putz, G. R., Murray-Smith, R., Giugliemma, C., Tangermann, M., Vidaurre, C., Cincotti, F., Kübler, A., Leeb, R., Neuper, C., Müller, K. R. and Mattia, D. (2010) Combining brain–computer interfaces and assistive technologies: State-of-the-art and challenges, *Frontiers in Neuroscience*, 4(SEP), pp. 1–15. doi: 10.3389/fnins.2010.00161.

Morash, V., Bai, O., Furlani, S., Lin, P. and Hallett, M. (2008) Classifying EEG signals preceding right hand, left hand, tongue, and right foot movements and motor imageries, *Clinical Neurophysiology*. International Federation of Clinical Neurophysiology, 119(11), pp. 2570–2578. doi: 10.1016/j.clinph.2008.08.013.

Mukesh, T. M. S., Jaganathan, V. and Reddy, M. R. (2006) A novel multiple frequency stimulation method for steady state VEP based brain computer interfaces, *Physiological Measurement*. IOP Publishing, 27(1), pp. 61–71. doi: 10.1088/0967-3334/27/1/006.

Müller-Putz, G. R., Scherer, R., Brauneis, C. and Pfurtscheller, G. (2005) Steady-state visual evoked potential (SSVEP)-based communication: Impact of harmonic frequency components, *Journal of Neural Engineering*, 2(4), pp. 123–130. doi: 10.1088/1741-2560/2/4/008.

Nielsen, J. (1995) 10 Usability heuristics for user interface design, *Conference Companion on Human Factors in Computing Systems CHI 94*. Nielsen Norman Group, pp. 152–158. doi: 10.1145/191666.191729.

Nijboer, F., Allison, B., Dunne, S., Bos, D., Nijholt, A. and Haselager, P. (2011) A preliminary survey on the perception of marketability of Brain–Computer Interfaces (BCI) and initial development of a repository of BCI companies, *5th International Brain-Computer Interface Conference, BCI 2011*, pp. 344–347.

Nikolaev, A. R., Meghanathan, R. N. and van Leeuwen, C. (2016) Combining EEG and eye movement recording in free viewing: Pitfalls and possibilities, *Brain and Cognition*, 107, pp. 55–83. doi: 10.1016/j.bandc.2016.06.004.

Pasqualotto, E., Matuz, T., Federici, S., Ruf, C. A., Bartl, M., Olivetti Belardinelli, M., Birbaumer, N. and Halder, S. (2015) Usability and workload of access technology for people with severe motor impairment: A comparison of brain–computer interfacing and eye tracking, *Neurorehabilitation and Neural Repair*, 29(10), pp. 950–7. doi: 10.1177/1545968315575611.

Pastor, M. A., Artieda, J., Arbizu, J., Valencia, M. and Masdeu, J. C. (2003) Human cerebral activation during steady-state visual-evoked responses, *The Journal of Neuroscience: The Official Journal of the Society for Neuroscience*, 23(37), pp. 11621–7. doi: 23/37/11621 [pii].

Pfurtscheller, G., Allison, B., Brunner, C., Bauernfeind, G., Solis-Escalante, T., Scherer, R., Zander, T. O., Mueller-Putz, G., Neuper, C. and Birbaumer, N. (2010a) The hybrid BCI, *Frontiers in Neuroscience*, 4(April), p. 30. doi: 10.3389/fnpro.2010.00003.

Pfurtscheller, G. and Neuper, C. (2001) Motor imagery and direct brain-computer communication, *Proceedings of the IEEE*, 89(7), pp. 1123–1134. doi: 10.1109/5.939829.

Pfurtscheller, G., Solis-Escalante, T., Member, S., Ortner, R., Linortner, P. and Müller-Putz, G. R. (2010b) Self-paced operation of an SSVEP-based orthosis with and without an imagery-based "Brain Switch": A feasibility study towards a hybrid BCI, *IEEE Transactions on Neural Systems and Rehabilitation Engineering*, 18(4), pp. 409–414.

Putze, F., Amma, C. and Schultz, T. (2015) Design and evaluation of a self-correcting gesture interface based on error potentials from EEG, in *Proceedings of the 33rd Annual ACM Conference on Human Factors in Computing Systems—CHI '15*. New York, USA: ACM Press, pp. 3375–3384. doi: 10.1145/2702123.2702184.

Putze, F., Popp, J., Hild, J., Beyerer, J. and Schultz, T. (2016) Intervention-free selection using EEG and eye tracking, in *Proceedings of the 18th ACM International Conference on Multimodal Interaction—ICMI 2016*. New York, USA: ACM Press, pp. 153–160. doi: 10.1145/2993148.2993199.

Rama, P. and Baccino, T. (2010) Eye fixation–related potentials (EFRPs) during object identification, *Visual Neuroscience*, 27(5–6), pp. 187–192. doi: 10.1017/S0952523810000283.

Regan, D. (1988) Human visual evoked potentials, in *Handbook of Electroencephalography and Clinical Neurophysiology*. Vol. 3 ed T. Elsevier, pp. 159–244.

Riccio, A., Mattia, D., Simione, L., Olivetti, M. and Cincotti, F. (2012) Eye-gaze independent EEG-based brain–computer interfaces for communication, *Journal of Neural Engineering*, 9(4), p. 45001. doi: 10.1088/1741-2560/9/4/045001.

Rutkowski, T. M., Mori, H., Matsumoto, Y., Cai, Z., Chang, M., Nishikawa, N., Makino, S. and Mori, K. (2012) Haptic BCI paradigm based on somatosensory evoked potential. *arXiv:1207.5720*, pp. 1–2.

Saproo, S., Faller, J., Shih, V., Sajda, P., Waytowich, N. R., Bohannon, A., Lawhern, V. J., Lance, B. J. and Jangraw, D. (2016) Cortically coupled computing: A new paradigm for synergistic human–machine interaction, *Computer*, 49(9), pp. 60–68. doi: 10.1109/MC.2016.294.

Schettini, F., Aloise, F., Aricò, P., Salinari, S., Mattia, D. and Cincotti, F. (2014) Self-calibration algorithm in an asynchronous P300-based brain–computer interface, *Journal of Neural Engineering*. IOP Publishing, 11(3), p. 35004. doi: 10.1088/1741-2560/11/3/035004.

Schmidt, N. M., Blankertz, B. and Treder, M. S. (2012) Online detection of error-related potentials boosts the performance of mental typewriters, *BMC Neuroscience*, 13(1), p. 19. doi: 10.1186/1471-2202-13-19.

Sellers, E. W., Krusienski, D. J., McFarland, D. J., Vaughan, T. M. and Wolpaw, J. R. (2006) A P300 event-related potential brain–computer interface (BCI): The effects of matrix size and inter stimulus interval on performance, *Biological Psychology*, 73(3), pp. 242–252. doi: 10.1016/j .biopsycho.2006.04.007.

Sellers, E. W., Vaughan, T. M. and Wolpaw, J. R. (2010) A brain–computer interface for long-term independent home use, *Amyotrophic Lateral Sclerosis: Official Publication of the World Federation of Neurology Research Group on Motor Neuron Diseases*, 11(5), pp. 449–55. doi: 10.3109/17482961003777470.

Sereno, S. and Rayner, K. (2003) Measuring word recognition in reading: Eye movements and event-related potentials, *Trends in Cognitive Sciences*, 7(11), pp. 489–493. doi: 10.1016/j.tics.2003.09.010.

Shahid, S., Prasad, G. and Sinha, R. K. (2011) On fusion of heart and brain signals for hybrid BCI, in *2011 5th International IEEE/EMBS Conference on Neural Engineering*. IEEE, pp. 48–52. doi: 10.1109 /NER.2011.5910486.

Shishkin, S. L., Nuzhdin, Y. O., Svirin, E. P., Trofimov, A. G., Fedorova, A. A., Kozyrskiy, B. L. and Velichkovsky, B. M. (2016) EEG negativity in fixations used for gaze-based control: Toward converting intentions into actions with an eye–brain–computer interface, *Frontiers in Neuroscience*, 10(November). doi: 10.3389/fnins.2016.00528.

Spüler, M., Bensch, M., Kleih, S., Rosenstiel, W., Bogdan, M. and Kübler, A. (2012) Online use of error-related potentials in healthy users and people with severe motor impairment increases performance of a P300-BCI, *Clinical Neurophysiology: Official Journal of the International Federation of Clinical Neurophysiology*, 123(7), pp. 1328–37. doi: 10.1016/j.clinph.2011.11.082.

Treder, M. S. and Blankertz, B. (2010) (C)overt attention and visual speller design in an ERP-based brain–computer interface, *Behavioral and Brain Functions: BBF*, 6, p. 28. doi: 10.1186/1744-9081-6-28.

Ušćumlić, M. and Blankertz, B. (2016) Active visual search in non-stationary scenes: Coping with temporal variability and uncertainty, *Journal of Neural Engineering*. IOP Publishing, 13(1), p. 16015. doi: 10.1088/1741-2560/13/1/016015.

Valbuena, D., Volosyak, I., Malechka, T. and Gräser, A. (2011) A novel EEG acquisition system for brain computer interfaces, *Journal of Bioelectromagnetism*, 13(2), pp. 74–75.

Van Erp, J. B. F., Lotte, F. and Tangermann, M. (2012) Brain–computer interfaces: Beyond medical applications, *Computer*, 45(4), pp. 26–34. doi: 10.1109/MC.2012.107.

Vaughan, T. M., McFarland, D. J., Schalk, G., Sarnacki, W. A., Krusienski, D. J., Sellers, E. W. and Wolpaw, J. R. (2006) The Wadsworth BCI Research and Development Program: At home with BCI, *IEEE Transactions on Neural Systems and Rehabilitation Engineering: A Publication of the IEEE Engineering in Medicine and Biology Society*, 14(2), pp. 229–33. doi: 10.1109/TNSRE.2006.875577.

Vilimek, R. and Zander, T. O. (2009) BC(eye): Combining eye-gaze input with brain–computer interaction, Springer Berlin Heidelberg, pp. 593–602. doi: 10.1007/978-3-642-02710-9_66.

Volosyak, I. (2011) SSVEP-based Bremen-BCI interface—Boosting information transfer rates, *Journal of Neural Engineering*, 8(3), p. 36020. doi: 10.1088/1741-2560/8/3/036020.

Volosyak, I., Cecotti, H., Valbuena, D. and Graser, A. (2009) Evaluation of the Bremen SSVEP based BCI in real world conditions, in *2009 IEEE International Conference on Rehabilitation Robotics*. IEEE, pp. 322–331. doi: 10.1109/ICORR.2009.5209543.

Volosyak, I., Gembler, F. and Stawicki, P. (2017) Age-related differences in SSVEP-based BCI performance, *Neurocomputing*. doi: 10.1016/j.neucom.2016.08.121.

Volosyak, I., Valbuena, D., Lüth, T., Malechka, T. and Gräser, A. (2011) BCI demographics II: How many (and what kinds of) people can use a high-frequency SSVEP BCI?, *IEEE Transactions on Neural Systems and Rehabilitation Engineering: A Publication of the IEEE Engineering in Medicine and Biology Society*, 19(3), pp. 232–9. doi: 10.1109/TNSRE.2011.2121919.

Wang, Y., Gao, X., Hong, B., Jia, C. and Gao, S. (2008) Brain–computer interfaces based on visual evoked potentials: Feasibility of practical system designs, *IEEE Engineering in Medicine and Biology Magazine*, pp. 64–71. doi: 10.1109/MEMB.2008.923958.

Ware, M. P., Lightbody, G., McCullagh, P. J., Mulvenna, M. D., Martin, S. and Thomson, E. (2014) A method for assessing the usability of an on screen display for a brain-computer interface, *International Journal of Computers in Healthcare*, 2(1), p. 43. doi: 10.1504/IJCIH.2014.065811.

Ware, M. P., McCullagh, P. J., McRoberts, A., Lightbody, G., Nugent, C., McAllister, G., Mulvenna, M. D., Thomson, E. and Martin, S. (2010) Contrasting levels of accuracy in command interaction sequences for a domestic brain–computer interface using SSVEP, *2010 5th Cairo International Biomedical Engineering Conference*. IEEE, pp. 150–153.

Wenzel, M. A., Golenia, J.-E. and Blankertz, B. (2016) Classification of eye fixation related potentials for variable stimulus saliency, *Frontiers in Neuroscience*, 10(FEB), pp. 1–14. doi: 10.3389/fnins.2016.00023.

Wilson, J. J. and Palaniappan, R. (2009) Augmenting a SSVEP BCI through single cycle analysis and phase weighting, in *2009 4th International IEEE/EMBS Conference on Neural Engineering*. IEEE, pp. 371–374. doi: 10.1109/NER.2009.5109310.

Wolpaw, J. R., Ramoser, H., McFarland, D. J. and Pfurtscheller, G. (1998) EEG-based communication: Improved accuracy by response verification, *IEEE Transactions on Rehabilitation Engineering*, 6(3), pp. 326–333. doi: 10.1109/86.712231.

Yin, E., Zhou, Z., Jiang, J., Chen, F., Liu, Y. and Hu, D. (2014) A speedy hybrid BCI spelling approach combining P300 and SSVEP, *IEEE Transactions on Biomedical Engineering*, 61(2), pp. 473–483. doi: 10.1109/TBME.2013.2281976.

Yong, X., Fatourechi, M., Ward, R. K. and Birch, G. E. (2011) The design of a point-and-click system by integrating a self-paced brain–computer interface with an eye-tracker, *IEEE Journal on Emerging and Selected Topics in Circuits and Systems*, 1(4), pp. 590–602. doi: 10.1109/JETCAS.2011.2175589.

Zander, T., Gaertner, M., Kothe, C. and Vilimek, R. (2010) Combining eye gaze input with a brain–computer interface for touchless human–computer interaction, *International Journal of Human–Computer Interaction*, 27(1), pp. 38–51. doi: 10.1080/10447318.2011.535752.

Zander, T. O. and Kothe, C. (2011) Towards passive brain–computer interfaces: Applying brain–computer interface technology to human–machine systems in general, *Journal of Neural Engineering*, 8(2), p. 25005. doi: 10.1088/1741-2560/8/2/025005.

Zhang, Y. U., Zhou, G., Jin, J., Wang, X. and Cichocki., A. (2014) Frequency recognition in SSVEP-based BCI using multiset canonical correlation analysis, *International Journal of Neural Systems*. World Scientific Publishing Company, 24(4), p. 1450013. doi: 10.1142/S0129065714500130.

Zhu, D., Bieger, J., Garcia Molina, G. and Aarts, R. M. (2010) A survey of stimulation methods used in SSVEP-based BCIs, *Computational Intelligence and Neuroscience*. Hindawi Publishing Corp., 2010, pp. 1–12. doi: 10.1155/2010/702357.

# 25 Designing a BCI Stimulus Presentation Paradigm Using a Performance-Based Approach

*Boyla O. Mainsah, Leslie M. Collins,
and Chandra S. Throckmorton*

## CONTENTS

25.1 Introduction ..................................................................................................488
25.2 The Performance-Based Paradigm................................................................490
    25.2.1 Bayesian DS Algorithm ......................................................................490
    25.2.2 Performance-Based Parameters............................................................491
    25.2.3 Codebook Development........................................................................493
25.3 Methods ........................................................................................................494
    25.3.1 BCI Implementation ............................................................................494
    25.3.2 P300 Speller Task ................................................................................495
25.4 Results............................................................................................................495
25.5 Discussion and Future Work..........................................................................498
Acknowledgments....................................................................................................498
List of Abbreviations...............................................................................................498
References................................................................................................................499

**Abstract**

Stimulus-driven brain–computer interfaces (BCIs), such as the P300 speller, rely on eliciting and detecting event-related potentials (ERPs) that are embedded in noisy electroencephalography data. However, these BCIs are currently limited by their relatively slow spelling speeds due to repetitive data measurements to increase the signal-to-noise ratios of the elicited ERPs for improved selection accuracy. In addition, psycho-physiological factors such as refractory effects limit the ability to elicit a strong ERP response with every target stimulus event presentation. The stimulus presentation pattern encodes information about an intended message a user wishes to communicate. The role of the BCI is to translate the user's attention-modulated responses to the stimulus events into a selection that conveys the user's intent. Consequently, a BCI can be approached from an information-theoretic perspective in order to determine how best to reliably encode information to be robust to noisy channel transmission errors. In this chapter, we present a principled approach to design the stimulus presentation paradigm for the P300 speller that exploits an information-theoretic approach to maximize the information content that is presented to the user. We use a probabilistic performance prediction method to evaluate and compare the performances of different stimulus presentation configurations during the design optimization process. We select a final configuration that maximizes BCI performance while minimizing refractory effects. We present results with online BCI use, which demonstrate significant performance improvements with our performance-based stimulus presentation paradigm compared to the conventional method of stimulus presentation.

## 25.1  INTRODUCTION

The P300-based BCI (Farwell and Donchin 1988) relies predominantly on detecting event-related potentials (ERPs) within noisy electroencephalography (EEG) data. These ERPs are elicited in response to a user attending to specific stimuli during an oddball recognition task (Sutton et al. 1965). In a typical P300 speller with a visual interface, a user is presented with a set of choices, such as the grid shown in Figure 25.1a. To select a character, the user focuses on that character while groups of characters are randomly flashed on the screen. In this scenario, the user's intended character is present in a few of the flash groups, representing the *oddball* or *target* stimulus events, which, ideally, should elicit a P300 ERP when presented. The BCI system analyzes the EEG responses to the stimulus events to determine the user's intended character. However, because of the low signal-to-noise ratios (SNRs) of the elicited ERPs, data are collected from multiple presentations of a

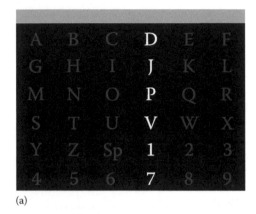

(a)

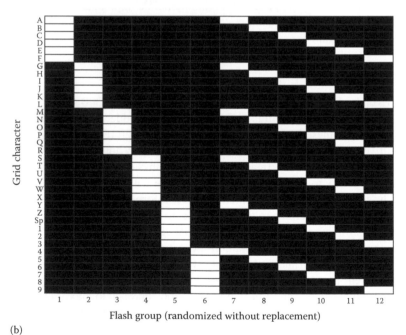

(b)

**FIGURE 25.1**  (a) BCI speller interface with a 6 × 6 grid layout. In this example, the fourth column is flashed. (b) Corresponding codebook for the RCP. Each column represents a flash group, with presented characters highlighted in white. For example, the fourth column in the 6 × 6 grid in (a) is represented by flash group 10 in (b). Each row represents a character's presentation pattern or codeword.

potential target character to increase the SNR for improved selection accuracy. These repetitive data measurements contribute to the slow spelling speeds of ERP-based BCIs.

The stimulus presentation paradigm defines the manner in which the stimulus events are presented, which includes the flash group elements and the order of presentation of the flash groups. While some P300 spellers are designed to present a single character in a stimulus event (e.g., Ref. Orhan et al. 2012), typically, a group of characters is presented in the same stimulus event in order to increase the character presentation rate. For example, the row–column paradigm (RCP) (Farwell and Donchin 1988) is the most commonly used method of stimulus presentation (Mak et al. 2011), where the flash groups consist of the rows and columns of characters arranged in a grid layout. However, grouping characters together in a single stimulus event increases the likelihood of selection errors for characters with similar presentation patterns owing to the added correlation in the EEG responses associated with each character's presentation. For example, in the RCP, erroneous character selections are usually in the same row or column as the target character (Fazel-Rezai 2007; Townsend et al. 2010).

Other parameters of the stimulus presentation paradigm that can also affect performance are the order and timing of stimulus events. In particular, the time interval between target stimulus events, or the target-to-target interval (TTI), affects the ability to elicit a strong ERP response due to *refractory effects* (Martens et al. 2009). Several studies have shown that the ERP SNR and detection rate increase with longer TTIs (Citi et al. 2009; Jin et al. 2012; Lu et al. 2013; Martens et al. 2009). Because of the randomized order of presentation of the row and column flash groups in the RCP, there is the possibility of two consecutive presentations of the target character, for example, the target row followed by the target column. Further, anecdotal evidence suggests that users experience visual fatigue with the RCP (Townsend et al. 2010).

Several stimulus paradigms have been designed to address some of the shortcomings of the RCP. Some paradigms have focused on changing cosmetic aspects of the visual interface to minimize visual distractions, such as presenting groups of characters sequentially in the center of the interface (Gavett et al. 2012), or arranging flash groups in spatially distinct clusters (Trender et al. 2011). Other approaches have incorporated salient elements in the visual interface during stimulus presentation to increase user focus or elicit additional ERPs that can improve performance, for example, using color or familiar faces (Kaufmann et al. 2011; Li et al. 2015). Other stimulus paradigms have been designed to reduce the proportion of short TTIs by imposing a minimum TTI to mitigate refractory effects (Jin et al. 2012; Polprasert et al. 2013; Townsend et al. 2010).

However, in all these previous approaches, the generation and presentation of subsets of characters are randomized without consideration of the potential benefit to performance of actively designing the composition of character subsets and their presentation order. The role of a BCI is to accurately convey a user's intent based on extracting and decoding relevant information from a user's brain responses to stimulus events. Consequently, the P300 speller can be approached from an information-theoretic perspective by exploiting *coding theory*, which is the study of how best to encode information for noisy channel transmission to minimize errors in the decoding process (Cover and Tomas 2012; Mackay 2003).

In the P300 speller, a character is encoded via its presentation pattern, which can be represented as a binary codeword, $X_1^T = [x_1, x_2, \ldots x_T]$, where $x_t \in \{0,1\}$ denotes the absence or presence, respectively, of a character in a flash group, $\mathscr{F}_t$. A stimulus presentation paradigm is represented by a collection of codewords, or a codebook $\mathfrak{C} \in [0,1]^{M \times T}$, where $\mathfrak{C}(m, 1{:}T)$ corresponds to the codeword for character $C_m$. For the speller grid shown in Figure 25.1a, Figure 25.1b shows the base codebook for the RCP, with a mapping of each character to its codeword. Some studies have used an information-theoretic approach to design codebooks for the stimulus presentation paradigm (e.g., Refs. Geuze et al. 2012; Hill et al. 2009; Martens et al. 2011; Verhoeven et al. 2015). However, the proposed codebooks ultimately performed similarly to or worse than the RCP when tested in healthy participants. These previous approaches likely underestimated the negative impact of refractory effects on performance, thereby negating any potential benefit to performance despite an optimized codebook design process.

We hypothesize that obtaining the benefits of using an information-theoretic approach relies on adequately characterizing the dynamics of the noisy communication channel. We present a new approach to designing the stimulus presentation paradigm for the P300 speller using a codebook design process that explicitly considers the physiological limitations of ERP elicitation. We denote the stimulus presentation paradigm developed with our new method as the *performance-based paradigm* (PBP). We provide empirical evidence of the utility of the PBP, with results from an online BCI study that show statistically significant performance improvements over the RCP.

## 25.2 THE PERFORMANCE-BASED PARADIGM

Our design approach is to construct a codebook of $M$ $l$-bit codewords, or an $(M,l)$-code, that maximizes a user's performance with a given BCI algorithm. The main performance criteria we consider are as follows: improving selection accuracy by facilitating the distinction of characters via their respective flash patterns and, within the context of a dynamic stopping (DS) algorithm, increasing the spelling speed by reducing the amount of stimulus event presentations before character selection.

Given a BCI algorithm, we define a combinatorial problem with the following objective function:

$$\underset{\mathfrak{C}\in[0,1]^{M\times l}}{\text{minimize}}\ \text{EST}(\alpha_{\mathfrak{C}}),\ \text{subject to } A(\alpha_{\mathfrak{C}}) \geq A_{\min}, \tag{25.1}$$

where EST is the expected stopping time, which we define as the mean number of stimulus event presentations before character selection; $A$ is the selection accuracy; $A_{\min}$ is the minimum accuracy desired; and $\alpha_{\mathfrak{C}}$ is a generic parameter that we define to quantify a user's performance level with a given codebook, $\mathfrak{C}$. A user's performance level is determined by the BCI system's ability to distinguish between EEG responses following nontarget and target stimulus event presentations.

### 25.2.1 BAYESIAN DS ALGORITHM

In this work, we consider the Bayesian DS algorithm (Throckmorton et al. 2013), where the amount of data collection before character selection is based on attaining a certain level of confidence in correctly selecting the target character. A probability distribution, $\left\{ P_m(t) \right\}_{m=1}^{M}$, is maintained over the character choices, where each character's probability, $P_m(t)$, represents the probability that it is the target character at time index $t$.

Following each stimulus event presentation, $\mathscr{F}_t$, the resulting classifier score after processing the EEG response, $y_t$, is used to update the probability model using Bayesian inference:

$$P_m(t) = \frac{p_m(t)P_m(t-1)}{\sum_{j=1}^{M} p_j(t)P_j(t-1)}, \tag{25.2}$$

$$p_m(t) = \begin{cases} p\left(y_t \middle| H_0\right), & \text{if } C_m \notin \mathscr{F}_t \\ p\left(y_t \middle| H_1\right), & \text{if } C_m \in \mathscr{F}_t \end{cases}, \tag{25.3}$$

where $P_m(t-1)$ and $P_m(t)$ are the prior and posterior probabilities, respectively, for character $C_m$; $p_m(t)$ is the likelihood of the classifier score, $y_t$, for character $C_m$, assigned based on whether $C_m$ is present in the current flash group, $\mathscr{F}_t$; and $p\left(y_t \middle| H_0\right)$ and $p\left(y_t \middle| H_1\right)$ are the classifier likelihood probability density functions (pdfs) for the nontarget and the target classifier scores, respectively. Data collection is stopped when the maximum character probability achieves a threshold value, $P_{th}$, or a data collection limit is reached. After data collection, the character with the maximum probability is selected as the user's intended character.

Under a normality assumption, a user's performance level with the Bayesian DS algorithm can be parameterized by the *detectability index* based on the parameters of the class conditional pdfs (Mainsah et al. 2016). Because of the low probability of occurrence of target flash groups, the classifier is usually trained with a larger proportion of nontarget feature observations compared to target feature observations. Consequently, the target classifier scores may exhibit higher variance. To account for unequal variances, we use the formula proposed in Ref. (Simpson and Fitter 1973):

$$d = \frac{\mu_1 - \mu_0}{\sqrt{0.5\left(\sigma_1^2 + \sigma_0^2\right)}},$$
(25.4)

where $d$ is the detectability index and $\left(\mu_0, \sigma_0^2\right)$ and $\left(\mu_1, \sigma_1^2\right)$ are the means and variances of the nontarget and target classifier pdfs, respectively.

### 25.2.2 PERFORMANCE-BASED PARAMETERS

The search space of $l$-bit codewords is an exponentially large space from which a subset of $2^l-1$ possible codewords can be selected to design a codebook. To reduce the search time, we restrict the search space based on parameters that are tuned to positively affect performance (Jin et al. 2012; MacKay 2003; Martens et al. 2009), which include the minimum Hamming distance, the minimum TTI, and the codeword density.

For most BCI algorithms, the character with the maximum cumulative EEG response after data collection is selected as the user's intended character. As the correlation between the EEG responses associated with each character's presentation decreases, the discriminability between the character choices during the decoding process increases. The correlation between the EEG responses associated with each character can be minimized by having many dissimilarities between the presentation patterns or codewords for the characters.

A measure to quantify the dissimilarity between two codewords of equal-sized lengths is the Hamming distance (Hamming 1950), denoted as $d^H(c_i,c_j)$, which is the number of differences between the two codewords, $c_i$ and $c_j$. For example, $d^H(0100,1101) = 2$, as the two codewords differ at position 1 and 4. For binary codes, the minimum Hamming distance of a codebook defines its *error-correcting capacity* (MacKay 2003),

$$e_b = \left\lfloor \frac{d_{\min}^H(\mathfrak{C}) - 1}{2} \right\rfloor,$$
(25.5)

where $d_{\min}^H(\mathfrak{C})$ is minimum Hamming distance of a codebook, $\mathfrak{C}$; and $e_b$ is the maximum error-correcting capacity number of bit errors that are guaranteed to be corrected during the decoding process.

It is hypothesized that a codebook with a higher error-correcting capacity results in better performance during the decoding process (MacKay 2003). Previous approaches to codebook design for the P300 speller focused on maximizing error-correcting capacity (e.g., Geuze et al. 2012; Hill et al. 2009; Martens et al. 2011; Verhoeven et al. 2015). However, a consequence of maximizing Hamming distances is the selection of codewords with a relatively high proportion of short TTIs, especially those with long streams of repetitive character presentations (Geuze et al. 2012; Hill et al. 2009; Martens et al. 2011). We impose a minimum interval between a character's presentation, $TTI_{\min}$, to increase the likelihood of generating ERPs with higher SNRs.

The codeword Hamming weight, $w(c)$, is the proportion of 1's in a binary codeword and determines the number of times a character gets presented. Presenting the target character more often increases the likelihood of generating high classifier scores and the possibility of the target character having the maximum cumulative response in order to be selected by the BCI as the user's intended character. However, there is a direct relationship between codeword density and TTI: the denser a codeword, the shorter the time interval between target character presentations. It has been shown that classification performance improves with increasing TTI; because of refractory effects, lower classification scores usually result from target character presentations with shorter TTIs (Jin et al. 2012; Martens et al. 2009).

Let a TTI of 1 be represented by the presentation pattern [...11...] and a TTI of 3 by [...1001...], where "1" denotes the target stimulus event under consideration. The relationship between classification performance and TTI is illustrated in Figure 25.2a, which shows the pdfs of a trained classifier and the pdfs of the target classifier scores, segregated by TTI, obtained during testing of the classifier. At the extremes are the nontarget pdf $\left(H_0^{\text{train}}\right)$ and the target pdf $\left(H_1^{\text{train}}\right)$ of the classifier. The other pdfs represent those of test classifier scores segregated by TTI for specific values, TTI1, TTI2, and TTI3. The means of the

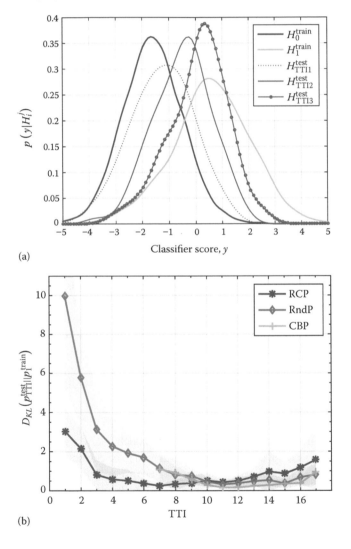

**FIGURE 25.2** (a) Illustration of the relationship between the classifier likelihoods for nontarget $\left(H_0^{\text{train}}\right)$ and target $\left(H_1^{\text{train}}\right)$ classifier scores estimated during training, and the likelihood of the target classifier scores grouped by TTI $\left(H_{\text{TTI}}^{\text{test}}\right)$, estimated during testing of the trained classifier. (b) Kullback–Leibler divergence, $D_{\text{KL}}\left(p_{\text{TTI}}^{\text{test}}\middle\|p_1^{\text{train}}\right)$, between the TTI-segregated $\left(p_{\text{TTI}}^{\text{test}}\right)$ and target classifier likelihoods, $\left(p_1^{\text{train}}\right)$, for row–column (RCP), random (RndP), and checkerboard (CBP) paradigms, averaged across participants. The means (solid lines) and standard deviations (shaded regions) across participants ($n = 13$) are shown.

TTI-grouped classifier score pdfs increases as the TTI increases. For example, the pdf for test classifier scores with a TTI of 1 is more similar to the nontarget classifier pdf. Hence, for a target character presented twice in succession, the BCI system is more likely to infer the second presentation as a nontarget stimulus event, which can lead to an erroneous character selection. The pdf for classifier scores with a TTI of 3 is more similar to the target classifier pdf, which is desirable for more accurate character selection.

An appropriate $TTI_{min}$ can be selected that not only minimizes refractory effects but also minimizes the EST. We analyzed participant EEG data from Ref. (Throckmorton et al. 2010) to quantify refractory effects in three stimulus paradigms, RCP, checkerboard (CBP) (Townsend et al. 2010), and random paradigms (RndP), to generate pdfs like those in Figure 25.2a. In the RndP, the character subsets are randomly generated, with the condition that within a codebook instantiation, a character can only be presented again after all of the other characters have been presented. The CBP is a special case of the random paradigm where a minimum TTI is imposed and spatial restrictions, with respect to a grid layout, are placed on the composition of the flash groups. For each participant, 10-fold cross-validation was performed to train and test the P300 classifier.

The Kullback–Leibler divergence (KLD) (Kullback and Leibler 1951) between the target pdf obtained from the training data and the TTI-segregated pdfs of the test data was calculated for multiple TTIs in order to determine the similarity between the pdfs, thereby providing an indication of acceptable TTIs. Figure 25.2b shows the results for the KLD as a function of TTI, averaged across participants. The TTI-segregated pdfs of shorter TTIs for the RndP are noticeably dissimilar from the target classifier pdf. These dissimilarities are minimized in the CBP where a $TTI_{min}$ (of 7 in this case) is imposed. For the RCP, the pdfs of shorter TTIs also have the most dissimilarity with the target pdf, although to a lesser degree than the RndP: from a TTI of 3 or greater, the TTI-segregated pdfs more or less converge to that of the target pdf.

Given the stimulus timing parameters, we select a minimum TTI to achieve a balance between minimizing refractory effects, maximizing target classifier scores, and minimizing the EST. Based on this analysis, we estimated that a TTI of 3 appears to be a suitable selection that achieves all three aims.

### 25.2.3 CODEBOOK DEVELOPMENT

Several approaches can be used to solve the combinatorial problem of selecting an $(M,l)$-code from a search space. In this study, we use a greedy search to iteratively build a codebook, by adding a new codeword to a partially filled codebook such that the objective function is minimized with respect to the other codewords. To solve the minimization problem defined in Equation 25.1, it is necessary to estimate how a user's performance level, $\alpha(\mathfrak{C})$, changes with a given codebook configuration, especially due to refractory effects.

Based on the studies in Refs. (Hill et al. 2009; Martens et al. 2011), we hypothesize that the TTI characteristics of a codebook, particularly the relative proportions of short TTIs, determines the relative degree with which refractory effects negatively affect performance. Changes in a user's performance level can significantly affect the amount of data collection or the EST required to achieve a certain accuracy level (Mainsah et al. 2016). However, it is difficult to estimate how a user's performance level varies across different codebook configurations, as empirical data collection is impractical: for a binary codebook with $M$ codewords of length $l$, there are $\binom{2^l - 1}{M}$ possible codebook configurations. In addition, a large user pool is needed to characterize codebook performance across a wide range of user performance levels.

Instead of empirical data collection, we use the performance prediction method we developed in Ref. (Mainsah et al. 2016) to estimate performance with a given codebook analytically. To simplify our analysis, we make the assumption that if a user's performance level is fixed, minimizing the EST with a DS algorithm using an $(M,l)$-code is equivalent to maximizing accuracy with a static stopping algorithm, given the same data collection limit for both algorithms. We believe that this assumption is reasonable because we consider a codebook space where refractory effects are minimized via the imposition of a minimum TTI. Consequently, we assume that changes to a user's performance level within this restricted search space are minimal. In the case of the Bayesian DS algorithm, we assume that the detectability index is fixed when predicting performance. Algorithm 1 outlines the pseudo-code we used to develop a codebook for the PBP, with a given set of performance-based parameters.

**Algorithm 1: Pseudo-code for performance-based codebook design**

**Input:** $M$ = codebook size, $l$ = codeword length, $\omega$ = codeword density, $d_{min}^H$ = minimum Hamming distance, $TTI_{min}$ = minimum target-to-target interval

**Output:** $\mathfrak{C}_{new}$ = New codebook of size $M \times l$

Definition — $X \left\{ \overset{add}{\leftarrow} / \overset{remove}{\rightarrow} \right\} x$ : add/remove codeword $x$ to/from codebook $X$

1: **function** BUILDPBPCODEBOOK($M$, $l$, $\omega$, $d_{min}^H$, $TTI_{min}$)

2:      $\mathfrak{C}^{2^l \times l}$ = Space of all $2^l$ $l$-bit codewords

3:      $\mathfrak{C}_{old} = \mathfrak{C}^{2^l \times l} \overset{remove}{\rightarrow} c_i \in \{w(c_i) \notin \omega, TTI(c_i) < TTI_{min} \text{ and } d^H(c_i, c_j) < d_{min}^H \}$

4:      $\mathfrak{C}_{new} = \underset{remove\ c_i}{\arg\max} \sum_{j=1}^{|\mathfrak{C}_{old}|-1} d^H(c_i, c_j), c_i \neq c_j, c_i, c_j \in \mathfrak{C}_{old}$

5:      $\mathfrak{C}_{old} \rightarrow \mathfrak{C}_{new}$

6:      **while** $|\mathfrak{C}_{new}| < M$ **do**

7:          **for** $i = 1$: $|\mathfrak{C}_{old}|$ **do**

8:              $c_i = \mathfrak{C}_{old}(i, 1:l)$

9:              $\mathfrak{C}_{temp} = \mathfrak{C}_{new} \overset{add}{\leftarrow} c_i$

10:              $A_{temp}(i) = \text{predictedAccuracy}\left(\mathfrak{C}_{temp}\right)$      $\triangleright$ (see [Mainsah et al. 2016])

11:          **end for**

12:          $a = \arg\max \left\{ A_{temp}(i) \right\}_{i=1}^{|\mathfrak{C}_{old}|}$

13:          $c_{new} = \mathfrak{C}_{old}^j(a, 1:l)$

14:          $\mathfrak{C}_{new} = \mathfrak{C}_{new} \overset{add}{\leftarrow} c_{new}$

15:          $\mathfrak{C}_{old} = \mathfrak{C}_{old} \overset{remove}{\rightarrow} c_{new}$

16:      **end while**

17:      **return** $\mathfrak{C}_{new}$

18: **end function**

## 25.3 METHODS

We performed an online study to compare user performances with the RCP and a codebook configuration of the PBP. The study protocol was approved by the Duke Institutional Review Board. Twenty healthy participants from the student and work population at Duke University were recruited. All participants gave informed consent before participating in the study. The participants were numbered in the order that they were recruited.

### 25.3.1 BCI IMPLEMENTATION

The open source BCI2000 software (Schalk et al. 2004) was used to implement the P300 speller with the Bayesian DS algorithm (Throckmorton et al. 2013). EEG signals were acquired using a

32-channel wet electrode cap (Electro-Cap) and relayed to a computer via g.USBamp biosignal amplifiers (Guger Technologies). The left and right mastoids were used as ground and reference electrodes, respectively. Electrode impedance values were adjusted until ≤40 kΩ.

Electrode channel selection is usually employed in BCIs to minimize computational complexity during signal processing and to reduce setup time (Colwell et al. 2014; Krusienski et al. 2008). Data collected from electrodes [Fz, Cz, P3, Pz, P4, PO7, PO8, Oz] were used for signal processing. We typically use this set of electrodes in our P300 speller studies as they have been shown to generalize well across participants (Krusienski et al. 2006, 2008). EEG signals were sampled at 256 samples/s and filtered between 0.5 and 30 Hz before feature extraction. A stepwise linear discriminant analysis classifier was trained to distinguish between features extracted from EEG data following target and nontarget stimulus event presentations. The signal processing methods used for feature extraction, classifier weight vector training, and classifier likelihood estimation are detailed in Ref. (Throckmorton et al. 2013).

The codebooks for the stimulus paradigm to be tested online, RCP and PBP, were developed based on the 6 × 6 speller grid shown in Figure 25.1a. For both stimulus paradigms, the flash duration, interstimulus interval, and time pause between character selections were set to 62.5 ms, 62.5 ms, and 3.5 s, respectively, and the online data collection limit was set to 72 stimulus presentations. We performed a grid search over parameter values to select a (36,24)-code for the PBP using algorithm 1. The codeword length was increased with respect to the base codebook of a 6 × 6 RCP (see Figure 25.1b) to allow for a wider degree of freedom in selecting codewords. Consequently, the codeword length for the RCP was increased to match the PBP codebook resulting in a (36,24)-code with $d_{\min}^H = 4$, $w(c) = 1/6$, and $\mathrm{TTI}_{\min} = 1$ for the base RCP codebook. For the PBP, a uniform distribution over characters was assumed and an iterative search was performed over parameter values, $d_{\min}^H > 4$, $w(c) > 1/6$, and $\mathrm{TTI}_{\min} = 3$, with multiple codebook configurations compared. A final codebook configuration of the PBP that minimized the performance ratio $\dfrac{\mathrm{EST}}{A}$ with respect to other codebook configurations was selected to be tested online.

### 25.3.2  P300 Speller Task

During a BCI session, a participant performed word copy-spelling tasks with the P300 speller, where the user was instructed on which characters to focus on by the BCI. A BCI session had two blocks, with each block consisting of a calibration run and a test run for a stimulus presentation paradigm condition. The block order was randomized across participants. The calibration run involved copy-spelling without character selection or BCI feedback. Data collected in the calibration run were used to train user-specific classifier parameters. In the test run, using the trained classifier parameters, the user performed copy-spelling using the Bayesian DS algorithm ($P_{th} = 0.9$), with feedback presentation and no error correction.

### 25.4  RESULTS

Participant performance measures were estimated from the P300 speller outcomes from the test run. Based on offline predictions, it was hypothesized that the PBP would result in noticeable improvements in accuracy at low-range $d$ values and reduced EST at mid-range $d$ values. Figure 25.3 compares the online results for both codebooks, as well as their predicted performances, as a function of participant detectability index. The online results exhibit a higher degree of variability as the performance measures were estimated from a low number of samples (30 or 48 characters). Nonetheless, the performance trends of the current results are consistent with the performance predictions, where the PBP performs with increased accuracies for lower-level performers and reduced ESTs for mid-level performers.

Statistical significance was tested using the Wilcoxon signed-rank test, ($p < 0.05$). The average results are summarized in Table 25.1. Participant-specific results are shown in Figure 25.4.

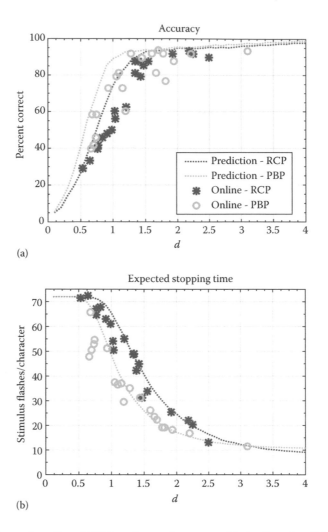

**FIGURE 25.3** Online and predicted P300 speller performance with the Bayesian DS algorithm, (a) accuracy, and (b) expected stopping time, as a function of participant detectability index, d. Each scatter point represents a participant, with the performance level quantified by the detectability index. The dashed lines represent predicted performances.

**TABLE 25.1**

**Summary of Mean Online Results**

| Performance Measure | RCP | PBP | p Value |
|---|---|---|---|
| Character selection time (s) | 9.97 ± 2.06 | 8.45 ± 1.78 | $<10^{-4}$ |
| Accuracy (%) | 67.08 ± 22.51 | 74.96 ± 18.15 | $<10^{-2}$ |
| Bit rate (bits/min) | 18.94 ± 12.90 | 24.93 ± 12.50 | $<10^{-3}$ |

Statistically significant performance improvements were obtained with the PBP. Figure 25.4a shows participant accuracies. A significant increase in accuracy was observed with the PBP ($p < 10^{-2}$), particularly those who performed with low accuracy levels using the RCP. The mean character selection time is estimated from the EST and takes into account the interstimulus interval, the flash duration, and the time pause between character selections. The mean character selection time was

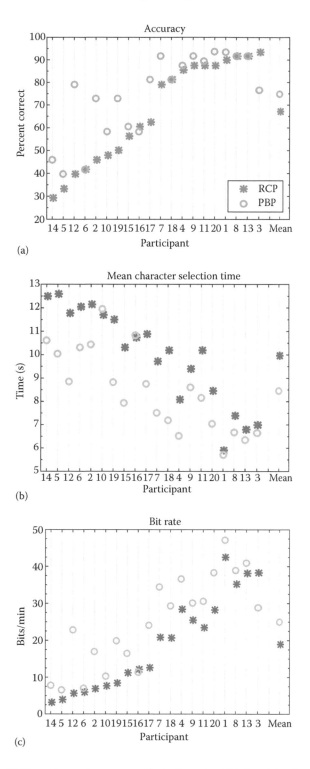

**FIGURE 25.4** Online P300 speller performance with the Bayesian DS algorithm, for the RCP and the PBP: (a) accuracy, (b) mean character selection time, which includes a 3.5-s pause between character selections, and (c) bit rate. Participant results are ordered by increasing RCP accuracy, with participants numbered in the order that they were recruited. The mean participant results for each stimulus presentation paradigm are also displayed on the far right of each plot.

significantly reduced with the PBP ($p < 10^{-4}$), as shown in Figure 25.4b. Figure 25.4c shows participant bit rates. The improvements in accuracy and reductions in the mean character selection time resulted in a significant increase in participant bit rates ($p < 10^{-3}$).

## 25.5 DISCUSSION AND FUTURE WORK

Previous approaches to design the stimulus presentation paradigm for the P300 speller that focused predominantly on error-correcting codes (Geuze et al. 2012; Martens et al. 2011; Verhoeven et al. 2015) did not obtain the expected performance improvements, possibly due to underestimating the significant negative impact that refractory effects can have on performance. Refractory effects can be mitigated by imposing a minimum time interval between target character presentations to increase the SNR of elicited ERPs. Some stimulus paradigms adopt this approach by specifying a long minimum TTI to mitigate refractory effects (Jin et al. 2012; Polprasert et al. 2013; Townsend et al. 2010). However, the imposition of a long minimum TTI can decrease the BCI's spelling rate, especially within the context of a DS algorithm, as it takes a longer time for the BCI algorithm to converge to a decision threshold.

We have developed a stimulus presentation paradigm that achieves a balance between improved error-correcting capacity and minimizing refractory effects, by tuning stimulus parameters to positively affect performance. Based on empirical analysis, a shorter minimum TTI was chosen to achieve a compromise between improving spelling rate and minimizing refractory effects. With online BCI use, significant performance improvements, in both accuracy and spelling speed, were obtained with our PBP compared to the conventional RCP. Users with low performance levels (low $d$ values) are able to significantly improve their accuracy levels. A significant decrease in the EST was observed across a wide range of users, without a detriment to accuracy. By using a principled method in the codebook design process, we obtained statistically significant improvements in communication rates in healthy users, across a wide range of user performance levels.

Our approach to stimulus presentation design requires validation in a target BCI end-user population. Performance improvements in a healthy user population may not always translate to a population with severe neuromuscular limitations, especially due to the differences in psychophysiological responses to stimuli. For example, we typically use slower stimulus presentation rates in our target end user BCI studies (Mainsah et al. 2015). Additional consideration in the selection of stimulus presentation parameters is required for users with severe neuromuscular limitations.

Another area of future work is using the performance predictive method for adaptive codebook design. In this work, we developed an optimized static codebook where the flash groups and their order of presentation are fixed and only the character-to-codeword assignments can be randomized with each codebook instantiation. Similar to a DS algorithm, an alternative approach is to design flash groups dynamically based on previous user responses. This approach provides the flexibility to include additional information, such as from a statistical language model, in order to present the most likely characters based on the BCI system's current belief of the user's intended character.

## ACKNOWLEDGMENTS

This research project was funded by the NIH/NIDCD under grant number R33 DC010470 and the Kristina M. Johnson Fellowship.

## LIST OF ABBREVIATIONS

**CBP**     Checkerboard paradigm
**DS**     Dynamic stopping
**EEG**     Electroencephalography
**ERP**     Event-related potential

| **EST** | Expected stopping time |
|---|---|
| **KLD** | Kullback–Leibler divergence |
| **PBP** | Performance-based paradigm |
| **PDF** | Probability density function |
| **RCP** | Row–column paradigm |
| **RndP** | Random paradigm |
| **SNR** | Signal-to-noise ratio |
| **TTI** | Target-to-target interval |

## REFERENCES

Citi, L., Poli, R., and Cinel, C. Exploiting P300 amplitude variations can improve classification accuracy in Donchin's BCI speller. In *4th International IEEE/EMBS Conference on Neural Engineering*, pages 478–481, 2009.

Colwell, K. A., Ryan, D. B., Throckmorton, C. S., Sellers, E. W., and Collins, L. M. Channel selection methods for the P300 speller. *Journal of Neuroscience Methods*, 232:6–15, 2014.

Cover, T. M., and Thomas, J. A. *Elements of Information Theory*. John Wiley & Sons, 2012.

Farwell, L. A., and Donchin, E. Talking off the top of your head: Toward a mental prosthesis utilizing event-related brain potentials. *Electroencephalography and Clinical Neurophysiology*, 70(6):510–523, 1988.

Fazel-Rezai, R. Human error in P300 speller paradigm for brain–computer interface. *29th Annual International Conference of the IEEE Engineering in Medicine and Biology Society*, 2007:2516–2519, 2007.

Gavett, S., Wygant, Z., Amiri, S., and Fazel-Rezai, R. Reducing human error in P300 speller paradigm for brain–computer interface. In *Annual International Conference of the IEEE Engineering in Medicine and Biology Society*, pages 2869–2872, 2012.

Geuze, J., Farquhar, J. D. R., and Desain, P. Dense codes at high speeds: Varying stimulus properties to improve visual speller performance. *Journal of Neural Engineering*, 9(1):016009, 2012.

Hamming, R. W. Error detecting and error correcting codes. *The Bell System Technical Journal*, 29(2): 147–160, 1950.

Hill, J., Farquhar, J., Martens, S., Biessmann, F., and Schölkopf, B. Effects of stimulus type and of error-correcting code design on BCI speller performance. In *Advances in Neural Information Processing Systems*, pages 665–672. 2009.

Jin, J., Sellers, E. W., and Wang, X. Targeting an efficient target-to-target interval for P300 speller brain–computer interfaces. *Medical & Biological Engineering & Computing*, 50(3):289–296, 2012.

Kaufmann, T., Schulz, S. M., Grünzinger, C., and Kübler, A. Flashing characters with famous faces improves ERP-based brain–computer interface performance. *Journal of Neural Engineering*, 8(5):056016, 2011.

Krusienski, D. J., Sellers, E. W., Cabestaing, F., Bayoudh, S., McFarland, D. J., Vaughan, T. M., and Wolpaw, J. R. A comparison of classification techniques for the P300 speller. *Journal of Neural Engineering*, 3(4):299, 2006.

Krusienski, D. J., Sellers, E. W., McFarland, D. J., Vaughan, T. M., and Wolpaw, J. R. Toward enhanced P300 speller performance. *Journal Neuroscience Methods*, 167(1):15–21, 2008.

Kullback, S., and Leibler, R. A. On information and sufficiency. *The Annals of Mathematical Statistics*, 22(1):79–86, 1951.

Li, Q., Liu, S., Li, J., and Bai, O. Use of a green familiar faces paradigm improves P300-speller brain–computer interface performance. *PloS one*, 10(6):e0130325, 2015.

Lu, J., Speier, W., Hu, X., and Pouratian, N. The effects of stimulus timing features on P300 speller performance. *Clinical Neurophysiology*, 124(2):306–314, 2013.

MacKay, D. J. *Information Theory, Inference and Learning Algorithms*. Cambridge University Press, 2003.

Mainsah, B. O., Collins, L. M., and Throckmorton, C. S. Using the detectability index to predict P300 speller performance. *Journal of Neural Engineering*, 13(6):066007, 2016.

Mainsah, B. O., Collins, L. M., Colwell, K. A., Sellers, E. W., Ryan, D. B., Caves, K., and Throckmorton, C. S. Increasing BCI communication rates with dynamic stopping towards more practical use: An ALS study. *Journal of Neural Engineering*, 12(1):016013, 2015.

Mak, J. N., Arbel, Y., Minett, J. W., McCane, L. M., Yuksel, B., Ryan, D., Thompson, D., Bianchi, L., and Erdogmus, D. Optimizing the P300-based brain–computer interface: Current status, limitations and future directions. *Journal of Neural Engineering*, 8(2):025003, 2011.

Martens, S. M. M., Hill, N. J., Farquhar, J., and Schölkopf, B. Overlap and refractory effects in a brain-computer interface speller based on the visual P300 event-related potential. *Journal of Neural Engineering*, 6(2), 2009.

Martens, S. M. M., Mooij, J. M., Hill, J. N., Farquhar, J., and Schölkopf, B. A graphical model framework for decoding in the visual ERP-based BCI speller. *Neural Computation*, 23(1):160–182, 2011.

Orhan, U., Hild, K.E., Erdogmus, D., Roark, B., Oken, B., and Fried-Oken, M. Rsvp keyboard: An EEG based typing interface. In *IEEE International Conference on Acoustics, Speech and Signal Processing (ICASSP)*, pages 645–648, 2012.

Polprasert, C., Kukieattikool, P., Demeechai, T., Ritcey, J. A., and Siwamogsatham, S. New stimulation pattern design to improve P300-based matrix speller performance at high flash rate. *Journal of Neural Engineering*, 10(3):036012, 2013.

Schalk, G., McFarland, D. J., Hinterberger, T., Birbaumer, N., and Wolpaw, J. R. BCI2000: A general purpose brain–computer interface (BCI) system. *IEEE Transactions on Biomedical Engineering*, 51(6):1034–1043, 2004.

Simpson, A. J., and Fitter, M. J. What is the best index of detectability? *Psychology Bulletin*, 80(6):481–488, 1973.

Sutton, S., Braren, M., Zubin, J., and John, E. R. Evoked-potential correlates of stimulus uncertainty. *Science*, 150(3700):1187–1188, 1965.

Throckmorton, C. S., Colwell, K. A., Ryan, D. B., Sellers, E. W., and Collins, L. M. Bayesian approach to dynamically controlling data collection in P300 spellers. *IEEE Transaction on Neural Systems and Rehabilitation Engineering*, 21(3):508–517, 2013.

Throckmorton, C. S., Ryan, D. B., Hamner, B., Caves, K., Colwell, K. A., Sellers, E. W., and Collins, L. M. Towards clinically acceptable BCI spellers: Preliminary results for different stimulus-selection patterns and pattern-recognition techniques. In *Fourth International BCI Meeting, Asilomar, CA*, 2010.

Townsend, G., LaPallo, B. K., Boulay, C. B., Krusienski, D. J., Frye, G. E., Hauser, C. K., Schwartz, N. E., Vaughan, T. M., Wolpaw, J. R., and Sellers, E. W. A novel P300-based brain–computer interface stimulus presentation paradigm: Moving beyond rows and columns. *Clinical Neurophysiology*, 121(7):1109–1120, 2010.

Treder, M. S., Schmidt, N. M., and Blankertz, B. Gaze-independent brain–computer interfaces based on covert attention and feature attention. *Journal of Neural Engineering*, 8(6), 2011.

Verhoeven, T., Buteneers, P., Wiersema, J. R., Dambre, J., and Kindermans, P. J. Towards a symbiotic brain–computer interface: Exploring the application-decoder interaction. *Journal of Neural Engineering*, 12(6):066027, 2015.

# 26 Issues and Challenges in Designing P300 and SSVEP Paradigms

*Ali Haider and Reza Fazel-Rezai*

## CONTENTS

26.1 Introduction .................................................................................................................. 502
26.2 Overview of Visual Paradigms ..................................................................................... 502
26.3 P300 Paradigms ............................................................................................................ 503
26.4 SSVEP Paradigms ........................................................................................................ 507
26.5 P300 and SSVEP Detection .......................................................................................... 508
26.6 Challenges in Paradigm Design .................................................................................... 509
    26.6.1 Crowding Effect ................................................................................................ 509
    26.6.2 Adjacency Problem ........................................................................................... 509
    26.6.3 Repetition Blindness ......................................................................................... 511
    26.6.4 Fatigue .............................................................................................................. 511
    26.6.5 User Comfortability .......................................................................................... 512
    26.6.6 User Training ..................................................................................................... 512
    26.6.7 Hardware Capacity ........................................................................................... 512
26.7 Paradigm and Efficiency ............................................................................................... 512
26.8 Paradigm Dependence of BCI Applications ................................................................. 513
26.9 Hybrid SSVEP–P300 Paradigm .................................................................................... 513
26.10 Evolvement of New BCI Applications ......................................................................... 516
26.11 Conclusion .................................................................................................................... 517
References ............................................................................................................................... 517

**Abstract**

One of the key components of brain–computer interface (BCI) design is the interfacing paradigm. Progress in BCI research and applications significantly depends on a successful paradigm implementation. BCI paradigm requires simple interpretation and ease of use for end users so that electroencephalogram (EEG) data can be mapped to an application, for example, to drive a prosthetic arm or to send a command to operate an external device. Another remarkable use of the BCI system is to set up a communication network with exterior environment. Such actions necessitate the user to disburse voluntary or involuntary mental or control task without making the subject fatigued or tired. To ensure these criteria, the paradigm design should be leveraged to deliver optimal performance. P300 and SSVEP are two paradigms that have gathered large attentions from BCI communities. Over the last decade, advancement of BCI research has experienced successful design of various hybrid BCI systems. This chapter focuses on the issues and challenges involved during the development of BCI paradigm to harness the advantages associated with recently developed BCI paradigms. In addition, importance of paradigms will be highlighted to open up novel BCI applications for future use, which, in turn, might have a great potential to increase the BCI users to a large extent.

## 26.1  INTRODUCTION

An interface paradigm is the first connection point of a user to a brain–computer interface (BCI) system. Despite the recent important ongoing advancement in the BCI field, issues and challenges related with the BCI paradigm design still need to be addressed and resolved in more detail. As such, a comprehensive study of the relative advantages and disadvantages of different BCI paradigms is needed. As the goal of BCI is to gather as much information as possible from the brain and computer interaction, the context of user experience with particular user interface is important in designing a BCI system.

In fact, BCI paradigms play an important role in letting the user decide how effectively he or she can use the brain activity to issue a command or control an application. The voluntarily executed mental efforts or control tasks can take many different forms such as imaginary or bodily movement, visualization of objects, relaxing thoughts, humming or counting, focused attention or reading, each of which can result in an exogenous change in brain signals.

In this chapter, the BCI systems with visual stimuli are considered for discussion. Adhering to the objective of this book, this chapter begins with an initial assessment of graphical user interface design of two common BCIs, namely, P300 peak of event-related potentials (ERP) and steady-state visually evoked potentials (SSVEPs). Here, we review the state-of-the-art BCI paradigms from the perspective of signal enhancement and user-friendly control interface, based on electroencephalogram (EEG)-based noninvasive P300 and SSVEP. We survey a few paradigms as reported in the scientific literatures and findings and discuss the associated advantages and drawbacks. First, the review examines the paradigms used during the signal acquisition step under SSVEP and P300 BCI modalities. The second part of the review discusses different techniques employed in the design of paradigms to control the brain stimulation in order to enhance the electrophysiological control signals and the system accuracy. Finally, it provides an overview of the latest development in the BCI paradigms and recent available tools and techniques to address the design issues that might open the avenues for many more BCI applications and thereby increase the number of BCI users. Depending on the health status of the user, the user's intended function, activities and needs, and sensitivity of the BCI outcome, BCI paradigms should be modified to satisfy the underlying preferences of the users.

## 26.2  OVERVIEW OF VISUAL PARADIGMS

A visual paradigm is a key part of a usable BCI that the user can observe during BCI interaction. In other words, a BCI paradigm is a control interface that allows the users to perform mental tasks and obtain feedback through a display representing the users' intentions. Therefore, the design and organization of a BCI paradigm are very important to satisfy the BCI goals. In order to design an interface, it is valuable to recognize the user experience of the interface. As the main purpose of the interface is to allow explicit control of computer or computer-controlled devices, understanding the cognitive state and activities of the user helps improve the quality of the BCI. Human brain activity can be controlled by the user's activities and desires, which, in turn, can be used to control the application, employing a BCI interface.

The importance of a paradigm is underscored by the following functions, which are necessary to develop a BCI system: (a) representing visual control functions to the user, (b) providing the state of the BCI and feedback to the user, and (c) displaying the user's neural signals.

Eventually, the purpose of the P300 and SSVEP interfaces is to establish an environment, which can modulate the neural signals as an indication of the user's interest or action. As such computer interfaces allow avoiding the need for motor movements, BCI technology can be utilized by patients with severe motor disabilities, both for communication and for controlling devices by brain signals (McFarland and Wolpaw 2011). In these systems, the users do not need to manipulate their brain activity. Instead, the computer interface stimulates the brain signal depending on the users' attention to some specific physical phenomena in the form of implicit inputs such as flashing characters or flickering images. Ease of performing mental tasks with P300 and SSVEP to select an object is comparable to a touch screen (Fazel-Rezai and Ahmad 2011). One of the important aspects of the BCI research is to improve the lifestyles of patients who have minimal to zero control of their physical body parts, such as people suffering from amyotrophic lateral sclerosis (ALS). As most of the time such patients have their own cognitive abilities intact, they can control their brain signals by utilizing the BCI interface, and thereby their cognitive abilities can be employed to improve their lifestyle.

## 26.3 P300 PARADIGMS

It is mentioned earlier that activation of P300 response requires that the user is focusing on a particular stimulus (a target object or character) of a visual paradigm, presenting a set of stimuli (objects or characters). In fact, the positive electrical peak in P300 BCI appears in the EEG after 300 ms of the irregular visual stimulation. The row–column matrix speller paradigm uses an alphanumerical square matrix interface to produce P300 in EEG (Farwell and Donchin 1988) as shown in Figure 26.1. Rows and columns of this 6 × 6 matrix are flashed randomly and the subject is asked to mentally count the number of times that the attended character is flashed. During the brain signal measurement in the parietal area, the detectable P300 in EEG appears as evoked response 300 ms after the stimulation of the row and column, which contain the target character. The nonflashing rows and columns do not generate P300. Because of the nature of the stimulation mechanism and to the increase in the accuracy of detection, the P300 system requires multiple trials to reach acceptable accuracy (Gavett and Fazel-Rezai 2012). The computational device can determine the target row and column after averaging several P300 responses.

Researchers have explored many possible paradigms to optimize the stimulus presentation as well as to reduce the trials to make smaller selection time (Salvaris and Sepulveda 2009). For instance, a Hex-o-Spell orientation obtained seven characters per minute to spell from a very small group of six characters (Blankertz et al. 2006). Apart from this, use of predictive speller and single trial detection of targets can further increase the efficacy of the system (Li et al. 2009).

A single-character paradigm (SCP) is a simple speller (Fazel-Rezai et al. 2012). This paradigm also uses an alphanumeric matrix with six rows and six columns like RCP. However, unlike the RCP, only a single character is flashed in SCP instead of a row or column (Figure 26.2). It was reported that RCP takes less time than SCP to flash all the characters at least once (Guger et al. 2009). Nevertheless, in it was noticed that if the number of flashes is constant, the SCP speller produces stronger P300 ERP than the RCP speller (Fazel-Rezai et al. 2011b; Hoffmann et al. 2008b).

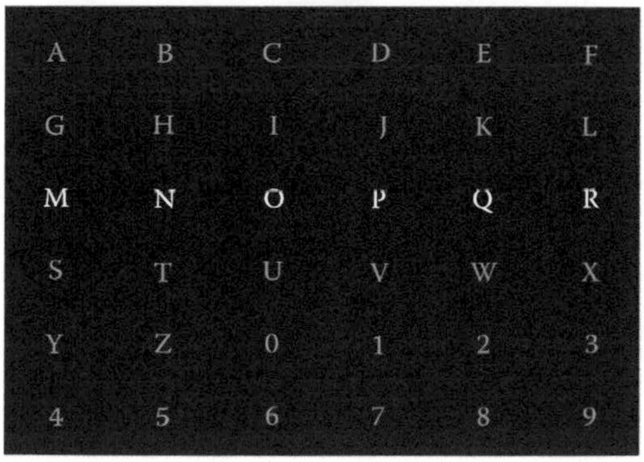

**FIGURE 26.1** The row–column paradigm (RCP) for the 6 × 6 matrix with the third row flashed. (From Farwell, Lawrence Ashley, and Emanuel Donchin. 1988. Talking off the top of your head: Toward a mental prosthesis utilizing event-related brain potentials. *Electroencephalography and Clinical Neurophysiology* 70 (6): 510–23.)

| A | B | C | D | E | F |
|---|---|---|---|---|---|
| G | H | I | J | K | L |
| M | N | O | P | Q | R |
| S | T | U | V | W | X |
| Y | Z | 1 | 2 | 3 | 4 |
| 5 | 6 | 7 | 8 | 9 | _ |

**FIGURE 26.2** Single-character paradigm (SCP): where only a single character is flashed. Here, M is flashing at this moment. (From Fazel-Rezai, Reza, Brendan Z. Allison, Christoph Guger, Eric W. Sellers, Sonja C. Kleih, and Andrea Kübler. 2012. P300 brain computer interface: Current challenges and emerging trends. *Frontiers in Neuroengineering* 5 (July): 14.)

Another paradigm for a P300 BCI is the region-based paradigm (RBP), where the choice of an object is split in dual selection levels (Fazel-Rezai and Abhari 2009). In this paradigm, visual space is divided into seven regions. The desired characters are split into seven groups, and each group is placed into a single region as shown in Figure 26.3. Depending on the level of interface, each group can contain either seven characters or a single character as in first level and second level, respectively. For any given spelling task, the user has a few seconds to focus on the characters before the action of each level. Instead of the rows and columns as in the Farwell and Donchin (1988) paradigm, regions are flashed in a random order by changing its color between black and white. Choice of color was justified for better contrast in each color transition. Both levels are needed to detect a single character. In short, first level is used to select a group of characters in a region, which

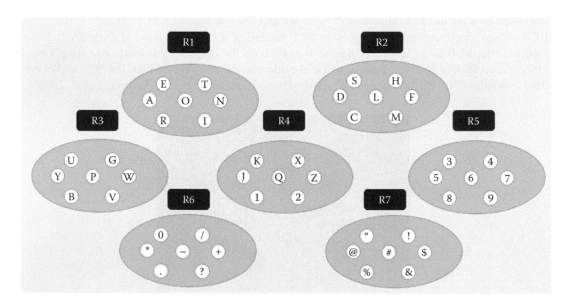

**FIGURE 26.3** A region-based paradigm with the locations of seven regions. Here, "Rn" represents region n and each region contains seven characters. (From Fazel-Rezai, Reza, and Kamyar Abhari. 2009. A region-based P300 speller for brain–computer interface. *Canadian Journal of Electrical and Computer Engineering* 34 (3): 81–5.)

contains the target character while the second level is used to select the single target character from the chosen region. Following the similar procedure of two levels for each character, all characters are detected one after another in a given spelling task. Each time a target is flashed, a strong P300 potential is expected in the EEG wave.

Although the Farwell and Donchin (1988) paradigm contains 36 characters, the use of the seven-region paradigm allows one to allocate 49 characters. In addition, this arrangement allows one to distribute the characters spatially on the screen considering their probability of linguistics use in a word. As paralyzed people need to spell the desired word with minimum movement, the arrangement of the letters can be adjusted accordingly to optimize the performance (Fazel-Rezai et al. 2012).

As mentioned earlier, the probability of characters' usage (Koblitz et al. 2001) was considered in distributing them into all seven regions and characters with close frequency of usage were placed in one region. After successful selection of a region in the first level, characters in the selected region are again subdivided into seven regions in the second level where each region consists of only one character (Haider et al. 2016).

In a checkerboard paradigm (CBP) (Townsend et al. 2010), the row–column paradigm was modified to eliminate the error caused by an adjacency problem, discussed by Fazel-Rezai (2007) as human error in P300 BCI. In order to increase the time between successive flashes of a target character, modification to the row–column paradigm was implemented in a CBP. Although a CBP is a matrix containing 72 characters in a standard 9 × 8 matrix, the characters are distributed in two virtual levels, where each level is a virtual checkerboard (Figure 26.4). Each virtual checkerboard contains a matrix of 6 × 6 in size, and a white and black checkerboard contains the items in white and black cells in the standard matrix, respectively (Figure 26.5).

In order to reduce the adjacency errors, the items in white and black matrices are randomized before a sequence of flashes. Virtual matrices are kept hidden from the users, and this action keeps the spatially adjacent items apart in flashing domain. It is interesting to see that the standard matrix does not change, but the randomized 12 virtual rows (6 white rows and 6 black rows) with 12 virtual columns (6 white columns and 6 black columns) make a distinct flashing pattern in each sequence of flashes (Figure 26.6).

| A | B | C | D | E | F | G | H |
|---|---|---|---|---|---|---|---|
| I | J | K | L | M | N | O | P |
| Q | R | S | T | U | V | W | X |
| Y | Z | Sp | 1 | 2 | 3 | 4 | 5 |
| 6 | 7 | 8 | 9 | 0 | . | Ret | Bs |
| ? | , | ; | \ | / | + | − | Alt |
| Ctrl | = | Del | Home | UpAw | End | PgUp | Shift |
| Save | ' | F2 | LfAw | DnAw | RtAw | PgDn | Pause |
| Caps | F5 | Tab | EC | Esc | email | ! | Sleep |

**FIGURE 26.4** Standard CBP with 9 rows and 8 columns. (Adapted from Townsend, George, Brandon K. LaPallo, Chadwick B. Boulay, Dean J. Krusienski, G. E. Frye, Christopher K. Hauser, Nicholas Edward Schwartz, Theresa M. Vaughan, Jonathan R. Wolpaw, and Eric W. Sellers. 2010. A novel P300-based brain–computer interface stimulus presentation paradigm: Moving beyond rows and columns. *Clinical Neurophysiology* 121 (7). NIH Public Access: 1109–20.)

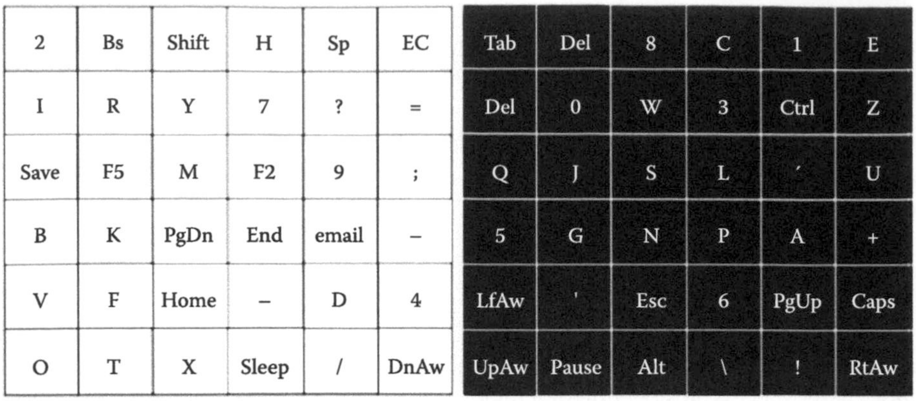

| 2 | Bs | Shift | H | Sp | EC |
|---|----|-------|---|----|----|
| I | R | Y | 7 | ? | = |
| Save | F5 | M | F2 | 9 | ; |
| B | K | PgDn | End | email | – |
| V | F | Home | – | D | 4 |
| O | T | X | Sleep | / | DnAw |

| Tab | Del | 8 | C | 1 | E |
|-----|-----|---|---|---|---|
| Del | 0 | W | 3 | Ctrl | Z |
| Q | J | S | L | ' | U |
| 5 | G | N | P | A | + |
| LfAw | ' | Esc | 6 | PgUp | Caps |
| UpAw | Pause | Alt | \ | ! | RtAw |

**FIGURE 26.5** Two virtual CBP, each with 6 × 6 matrix, originated from the standard CBP. (Adapted from Townsend, George, Brandon K. LaPallo, Chadwick B. Boulay, Dean J. Krusienski, G. E. Frye, Christopher K. Hauser, Nicholas Edward Schwartz, Theresa M. Vaughan, Jonathan R. Wolpaw, and Eric W. Sellers. 2010. A novel P300-based brain–computer interface stimulus presentation paradigm: Moving beyond rows and columns. *Clinical Neurophysiology* 121 (7). NIH Public Access: 1109–20.)

| A | B | C | D | E | F | G | H |
|---|---|---|---|---|---|---|---|
| I | J | K | L | M | N | O | P |
| Q | R | S | T | U | V | W | X |
| Y | Z | Sp | 1 | 2 | 3 | 4 | 5 |
| 6 | 7 | 8 | 9 | 0 | . | Ret | Bs |
| ? | , | ; | \ | / | + | – | Alt |
| Ctrl | = | Del | Home | UpAw | End | PgUp | Shft |
| Save | ' | F2 | LfAw | DnAw | RtAw | PgDn | Pause |
| Caps | F5 | Tab | EC | Esc | email | F11 | Sleep |

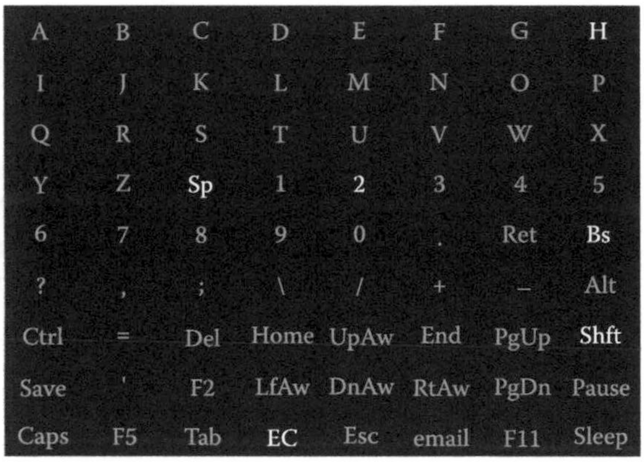

**FIGURE 26.6** Top row of the white virtual matrix is flashing, which includes the following items: 2, Bs, Shift, H, Sp, and EC. Adapted from Townsend, George, Brandon K. LaPallo, Chadwick B. Boulay, Dean J. Krusienski, G. E. Frye, Christopher K. Hauser, Nicholas Edward Schwartz, Theresa M. Vaughan, Jonathan R. Wolpaw, and Eric W. Sellers. 2010. A novel P300-based brain–computer interface stimulus presentation paradigm: Moving beyond rows and columns. *Clinical Neurophysiology* 121 (7). NIH Public Access: 1109–20.)

It was reported that RBP and CBP paradigms have decreased the adjacency problem significantly (Fazel-Rezai et al. 2012). These studies showed new directions in BCI speller paradigms apart from RCP.

In addition to those discussed above, there is another type of paradigm that is based on rapid serial visual presentation (RSVP) where symbols or characters are presented successively at a single location. Subjects' attention on a single symbol of this visual presentation can elicit P300 ERP (Acqualagna et al. 2010; Acqualagna and Blankertz 2011). However, the RSVP-based BCI speller requires a high number of sequential trials to obtain a reliable output. Though the RSVP paradigm does not require eye movements as the subject focuses on a single place, the information transfer rate (ITR) is less owing to the longer time it takes for stimulus presentation. Nevertheless, absence of eye movement makes RSVP a suitable paradigm for patients with impaired oculomotor control (Acqualagna and Blankertz 2013).

## 26.4 SSVEP PARADIGMS

SSVEP-based BCI is another type of system where EEG signals are measured over the visual cortex area. It can be realized by making the stimulus flash at a steady pace. SSVEP appears as an oscillation in the EEG signals with a steady flashing frequency that can be detected by the application of a suitable signal processing algorithm. Studies have found that SSVEP interfaces benefit from more brain states than P300 owing to the use of multiple frequencies each representing a degree of freedom on a control paradigm (Moore Jackson and Mappus 2010). Similar to the P300 paradigm, SSVEP needs to select the object within a time frame. Whereas P300 is detected in the time domain, SSVEP appears as a peak on the frequency spectrum close or equal to the frequency of the repetition of stimulus in which the subject focuses. Detected SSVEP can be translated either to a character to spell a word or to a control signal to drive a device for a BCI system. SSVEP BCIs are not entirely dependent on muscle-based gaze control. However, the flickering stimulus is annoying to some users and produces fatigue to the eyes. At higher frequencies, the annoying effect of the flickering stimuli reduces, making it more comfortable, but the SSVEP magnitude attenuates to such a level, which makes the SSVEP harder to detect. Usually, the SSVEP-based BCI system benefits from higher accuracy and less or no training time, and fewer numbers of EEG channels (Amiri et al. 2013b).

A relationship study between SSVEP amplitude and the corresponding frequency found that SSVEP peak rises after 5 Hz and continues to increase until 15 Hz (Figure 26.7). After reaching the highest point, it starts decreasing following an irregular pattern as the frequency inclines further with almost insignificant SSVEP evoked about 50 Hz (Pastor et al. 2003). Although it is evident that SSVEP is more pronounced at low-frequency stimulation, this lower band suffers from two major difficulties: human eyes become more tired at this frequency range and risk of prompting epileptic seizure for SSVEP is in the 15- to 25-Hz range (Pastor et al. 2003).

Many conventional SSVEP-based BCI systems use light-emitting diodes (LEDs) for flickering at a specific frequency. Use of LED allows one to distribute the flickering frequencies within a very narrow range and all stimuli are detectable with an interstimulus difference of just 0.2 Hz (Gao et al. 2003). Other than LED, a cathode ray tube or a liquid crystal display can also be employed to

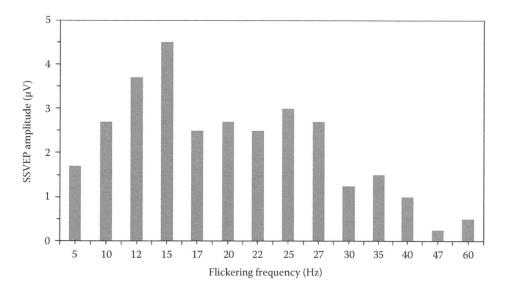

**FIGURE 26.7** SSVEP amplitudes with different flickering frequencies. (Adapted from Pastor, Maria A., Julio Artieda, Javier Arbizu, Miguel Valencia, and Jose C. Masdeu. 2003. Human cerebral activation during steady-state visual-evoked responses. *The Journal of Neuroscience: The Official Journal of the Society for Neuroscience* 23 (37): 11621–7.)

generate SSVEP. Studies are still investigating the SSVEP differences that result from these different stimulating interfaces to find the most useful flickering interface to improve the accuracy of SSVEP-based BCI (Chen et al. 2015b). SSVEP has an advantage over P300: it allows the user to have small eye movement (Bakardjian et al. 2010).

## 26.5 P300 AND SSVEP DETECTION

Both the P300 and SSVEP paradigms require the users to select a target by means of their eye gaze. In case of the P300, the brain responds to the external stimulus by showing the positive (P) or negative (N) deflections in the EEG. Eventually, users' focus on the paradigms will modulate the EEG signal. However, the stimulation mechanism is different in these two paradigms. An SSVEP signal is elicited over occipital areas in reaction to visual stimuli flickering at a frequency higher than 6 Hz (Nicolas-Alonso and Gomez-Gil 2012), whereas P300 evoked potential is elicited as positive EEG peaks in reaction to infrequent or irregular appearance of visual stimuli. Distinctive cognitive functions are formulated by several patterns of brain activity. With the help of EEG, brain activity in the neocortex is measured as voltage differences over the scalp. An appropriate signal processing strategy is critical in revealing the complexity and difficulty issues as well as the possibilities, which lies in the fact that optimization of accuracy and speed heavily depends on a suitable signal processing scheme (Mirghasemi et al. 2006b). In general, any signal processing is composed of two major steps. In the first stage, different feature extraction algorithms are applied to optimize the number of suitable features. Afterward, classification algorithms are employed for translating the extracted features to a corresponding target class. However, both stages are designed to meet one common goal: reduce the computing complexity and, thereby, decrease the task completion period. The first stage is employed to reveal the brain signal features that can be modulated by a BCI user. Various methods can be applied to the digitized EEG signal such as spatial and spectral analysis and measurements of voltage distribution. This stage is immediately followed by a translation procedure. All signal features are mapped to some classes representative of device commands by employing either a linear or a nonlinear method. These device-independent signal features can be applied to build a functional or communicative relationship between the user and the device under operation. In order to satisfy the criteria of an application, the BCI system needs an effective translational algorithm, which requires adaptation to the specific signal features that can be either controlled or learned by the user to improve individual performance. In summary, the effective interaction between the user and the BCI system necessitates incorporation of a better signal processing method (Alamdari et al. 2016; Mirghasemi et al. 2006a).

Before stepping into the details of the signal processing methods, key descriptors to categorize and describe the complex brain activity have been briefly highlighted in Table 26.1 (Fazel-Rezai and Peters 2005). EEG recording for BCI research needs a large number of descriptors, which are commonly used with cognitive research (Fazel-Rezai and Ramanna 2005; Nuwer 1997). Though behavioral and functional aspects are a major concern in BCI, many other aspects of EEG activity such as spatial distribution, frequency, amplitude, morphology, and periodicity are identically worthwhile (Lange et al. 1997).

Both P300 and SSVEP signals can easily be contaminated by other biosignals or environmental noise as nuisance signals. Generally, band-pass and notch filters are used to discard unwanted signal and limit the processing within a certain frequency range. For example, SSVEP stimulation frequencies can be divided into three groups: low (1–12 Hz), medium (12–30 Hz), and high (30–60 Hz) (Wang et al. 2008). Although low stimulating frequency evokes higher-amplitude SSVEPs, it may lead to visual fatigue and epileptic seizures (Fisher et al. 2005). In a variety of occasions, it was suggested to use higher stimulation frequencies, if possible. The most frequently used P300 and SSVEP signal processing methods have also been listed in Table 26.2 with the reference their relevant studies.

**TABLE 26.1**
**Key Factors of EEG Signal**

| EEG Signal Features | Description | Comments |
|---|---|---|
| Morphology | Wave shape | Brain activities form wave shapes that are the identifier of some events or characteristics |
| Repetition | Defines the recurrence of waveform types | Rhythmical repetitive waveforms. Also may gradually increase and then decrease in amplitude |
| Frequency | Number of repetitions of similar waveforms in a single unit of time | – |
| Amplitude | Microvolts ($\mu$V); peak to peak or from the calibrated zero reference | Typical range: 10–100 $\mu$V |
| Distribution | Electrodes record electrical activity, which are spatially oriented over different parts of the head | Spatial orientation is described using electrode names, not by head regions or brain areas |
| Phase relation | Change in troughs and peaks of the wave components over time considering single or multiple channels | Phase refers to the temporal relationship between different components of a rhythm |
| Timing | Relative occurrence of activity in time at different channels | – |
| Reactivity | Changes that can be introduced by one or multiple features as mentioned above due to various maneuvers or functions; appears as some normal and abnormal patterns | Used to train or evaluate the subject's condition; study of drug addiction |

## 26.6 CHALLENGES IN PARADIGM DESIGN

To transform a system under test to a usable one, it should satisfy several criteria. From a user point of view, the system should be easy to learn, efficient and effective, and able to handle error (Nielsen 1993). Both P300 and SSVEP paradigms are synchronous or system-initiated, so these two interfaces do not need a lengthy cumbersome training phase as required in a motor imagery–based BCI (McFarland and Wolpaw 2005). However, during the design of the BCI interface, the designer should consider that human factors can play an important role to achieve a useful BCI meeting the needs of users. In the context of BCI, users' psychological state in terms of attention, workload, or emotion depends on the following paradigm factors, to a greater extent.

### 26.6.1 CROWDING EFFECT

P300 and SSVEP BCIs rely heavily on sensory load through visual channel. In a multitasking approach, the paradigm may encompass overcrowded objects as stimulators, causing too much busy views for the sensory organs (Fazel-Rezai 2007). Such a crowded interface may risk sensory overload.

### 26.6.2 ADJACENCY PROBLEM

In an interface paradigm, the stimulating characters are distributed over the whole visual space and the user looks on the entire paradigm but focuses only on the target. Hence, the characters or objects adjacent to the target also send scattered stimulation to the visual organ. The user has no control to

## TABLE 26.2
## Summary of Signal Processing Methods

| Neuro-mechanism | Methods | System Performance |
|---|---|---|
| P300 | 6 × 6 targets on the menu; 36 feature vectors; feature vectors were continually ranked and either a correlation/threshold was used to select a cell. | 7.8 characters/min and 80% accuracy; accuracy >90% for 5 subjects (Donchin et al. 2000). 2.3 characters/min (Farwell and Donchin 1988). |
| | GA (genetic algorithm); high resource consumption; possible premature convergence. | Variable accuracy, 34%–90% (Dal Seno et al. 2010). |
| | Bayesian analysis, BLDA (Bayesian linear discriminant analysis); feature vector is labeled to the class to which it has the highest probability. | Transfer rate of 7 commands/min with 95% false-positive classification accuracy (Pires et al. 2008). Average accuracy 98% and ITR 25.1 bits/min (Jin et al. 2015). |
| | LDA (linear discriminant analysis); simple, low computation. | Accuracy for the able-bodied subjects was on average close to 100% and the best classification accuracy for disabled subjects was on average 100%. 15.9 bits/min for the disabled subjects and 29.3 bits/min for the able-bodied subjects. Accuracy varies with electrodes 4–32 (Hoffmann et al. 2008a). |
| | SVM (support vector machine); linear and non-linear (Gaussian) modalities, faster processing | 96.5% accuracy (Rakotomamonjy and Guigue 2008). Accuracies are 66%, 69%, and 72%, for LDA, neural networks, and SVM, respectively (Garrett et al. 2003); accuracy 84.5% and information transfer rate (ITR) up to 84.7 bits/min (Kaper et al. 2004). |
| | ML (maximum likelihood); feature detection using a priori knowledge, uses thresholds for a set of classes. | Accuracy is 90% with a communication rate of 4.19 symbols/min (Serby et al. 2005). |
| | ANPCA (adaptive nonlinear principal component analysis) and NN (neural network); four-stage operation: pre-separation, whitening, separation, and estimation. | Optimum interstimulus interval (ISI) is 350 ms. Average accuracy, about 89% (Turnip et al. 2011). |
| | CNN (convolutional neural network); 7 classifier models based on the CNN; employed single classifiers and multiclassifiers. | Maximum accuracy, 95.5%; ITR, 8.25 bits/min (Cecotti and Graser 2011). |
| | ANNC (adaptive neural network classifier); features extracted using autoregressive (AR) model | Average accuracy about 100%. Maximum ITRs of 35 bits/min and 47 bits/min for disabled and healthy subjects, respectively (Turnip and Hong 2012). |
| | SWDA (stepwise linear discriminant analysis). | Participants were with and without acquired brain injury (ABI). Average accuracy, 78% and 55% for healthy control group and end users with ABI, respectively (Daly et al. 2015). |
| SSVEP | MCC (maximum contrast combination); maximizes SNR; object function is used for computing filter. | Average accuracy is 95.5% and average bit rate is 34 bits/min (Zhu et al. 2011). |
| | PCA (principal component analysis); decomposes signals; reduces the dimension of original data. | Average accuracy range 76.4%–91.8% for 8 experiments per subject (Pouryazdian and Erfanian 2010). |

*(Continued)*

**TABLE 26.2 (CONTINUED)**
**Summary of Signal Processing Methods**

| Neuro-mechanism | Methods | System Performance |
|---|---|---|
| | ACSP (analytic common spatial pattern); common spatial pattern method; reflects both amplitude and phase information. | Classification accuracy of 84%, 93%, and 94% for number of harmonics = 1, 2, and 3, respectively (Falzon et al. 2012). |
| | EMD (empirical mode decomposition); compute the instantaneous frequency; reduces noise. | Average ITR, 36.99 bits/min; accuracy, 84.63% (Wu et al. 2011). |
| | Hilbert transform computes phases after spatial filtering; needs a shorter data length than that for the Fourier method. | Phase detection accuracy ranges from 70% to 94% (Zhu et al. 2011); phase detection accuracy 99% (Zhu et al. 2010). |
| | Wiener filtering together with a stepwise discriminant procedure to reduce feature vector dimensionality; Bayesian classifier; use covariance information. | Accuracy, 80% (Vidal 1977). |
| | MEC (minimum energy combination), 5 LEDs flickering at 13, 14, 15, 16, and 17 Hz, respectively. Low-pass filter cut-off at 32 Hz. Cancel nuisance signals as much as possible. | Average ITR, 29 bpm; 97.5% accuracy (Friman et al. 2007). |
| | CCA (canonical correlation analysis); uses harmonics, considers user variation, interrelates two multi-variable data sets as a linear combinations of original data. | Average accuracy, 95.3%; ITR, 58 bits/min (Bin et al. 2009). |
| | Relative amplitude, phase and a combination of both to create the feature matrix; threshold and amplitude ratio criteria were used to select stimuli. | Average, 92% correct selections; average selection time, 2.1 s (Middendorf et al. 2000). |
| | FBCCA (filter bank canonical correlation analysis); frequency range: 8–15.8 Hz, frequency interval: 0.2 Hz | 40 targets, multiple harmonic frequency bands get best performance, average and maximum accuracy is 92% and 99%, respectively. Average and maximum ITR of 151.18 bits/min and 172 bits/min, respectively (Chen et al. 2015a). |

restrict those stimulations, and until today, there is no convenient device to filter out the unwanted energy (Fazel-Rezai et al. 2011b).

### 26.6.3 REPETITION BLINDNESS

Repetition blindness is a cognitive phenomenon that presents the difficulty in repeated words or items (Cinel et al. 2004). This interesting property is incorporated with the event where a rapid presentation of target object following the presentation of the same object results in the reduced probability of detection. It greatly depends on the age of the user; older people are more prone to repetition blindness than younger ones. However, designing the paradigm with the less crowding effect can reduce the possibility of repetition blindness.

### 26.6.4 FATIGUE

Prolonged on screen look can cause uncomfortable response from the visual tool, resulting in visual fatigue. Experiment shows the presence of significant interaction between display resolution and fixation duration, causing stronger fatigue in the low-resolution display condition (62 dots per inch [dpi]) as compared with the high-resolution condition (89 dpi) (Ziefle 1998). Visual fatigue also correlates with eye movement parameters. Earlier research recommends that visual performance can be optimized by engaging high-resolution displays (90 dpi and greater).

### 26.6.5  USER COMFORTABILITY

Due to the constant staring on paradigm, P300 BCI may result in unpleasant feelings in the user engaged in lengthy training sessions. For this or other reasons, such paradigm outcomes varying success among subjects or patients (Rabbi et al. 2009). On the other hand, SSVEP paradigm requires the user to attend for a shorter time than P300 on a constantly flickering object, resulting in stress on the eyes. However, both P300 and SSVEP benefit from synchronous interfaces, which take less amount of time and show less false-positive errors. These benefits are not always obtainable from an asynchronous system (Scherer et al. 2007, 2008).

All of the basic tasks involved with graphical interfaces require the user to focus his attention on a specific stimulus. P300 paradigms require to have the user focus on the interface for a sufficient time to generate a discernible ERP (Polich 2007). If the user finds it difficult to stare at the interface, then it might result in errors. These facts also limit the group of users who can use these BCI systems. Both systems assume that the users can pay attention within an angle not larger than 3° so that robust SSVEP can be elicited (Thurlings et al. 2010). However, some users may find difficulties in adjusting the gaze because of their inability to control their muscles.

### 26.6.6  USER TRAINING

It is evident that training is necessary to make the user familiar with the interface system and to make the interface responsive to the user's intent by supervising the learning machine. However, it is not always feasible to obtain the knowledge of what type and amount of training would optimize the system performance. For example, a subject may need a long training session to increase BCI accuracy, which might cause exhaustion for the same individual, adding the potential risk of producing unreliable results (Pastor et al. 2003; Rabbi et al. 2012a,b).

### 26.6.7  HARDWARE CAPACITY

Timing accuracy is of great importance for stimulus presentation and stimulating visual organ. EEG measurements have a very good temporal resolution with small delays of tens of milliseconds, which makes EEG a predominant technology in BCI research. To accommodate the different hardware components of a BCI system, a regular update of the software is necessary. As data collection and analysis can be accomplished by different personnel in different locations, the BCI system should be developed while making room for potentially different hardware. In comparison to invasive BCI, both healthy and disabled users find EEG-based BCI to be portable, safe, cheaper, and simple to use (Machado et al. 2010).

## 26.7  PARADIGM AND EFFICIENCY

Almost in all cases, BCI throughput highly depends on the control interface (van Gerven et al. 2009). Depending on the specific task, the regulated steps to increase the efficiency may vary. For instance, spell checking and auto-completion can be incorporated to the interface to raise the accuracy. Similarly, proper design of target areas and adjacency can be critical to elevate BCI performance. Some works have attempted to create an adaptive BCI interface to maintain a high level of performance accuracy (Vidaurre et al. 2006). However, this approach is limited by two unresolved issues: it needs a multiple calibration process for the same user and it requires perfect measurement of the user's intent. As BCI is a highly interdisciplinary field of neurotechnology, it is of no surprise that concepts of software and machine learning can be utilized to increase the efficiency of the paradigm. It saves the time by avoiding cumbersome training sessions, which sometimes may be as long as several hours, by letting the machine learn to decode the different brain states of an individual BCI user. The calibration phase also plays an important role in designing a better BCI paradigm. Calibration is necessary to allow room for system correction before running the experiment. Certain brain states are needed to be produced during the training session. Indeed, a BCI system needs to be calibrated when a paradigm is changed or modified, when the BCI user is changed, or when the same subject is going to use BCI in another session. During the calibration period, the machine learning algorithms take care of the above events by estimating the statistical parameters, which allows the machine to separate learned brain states into their correct categories.

## 26.8 PARADIGM DEPENDENCE OF BCI APPLICATIONS

BCIs have unfathomable potentials as the ultimate hands-free control and communication interface for conventional applications. Ironically, the BCI interface cannot be optimized for all types of users. Over the last few decades, the BCI community has seen significant progress in BCI research, targeting the people who are mainly in need of assistive technology (Sellers and Donchin 2006). Yet, the underlying BCI mechanism has been challenging, with its relative slow speed, low accuracy, sensitivity to error, and complex working principles. Although the modern computing and sensing technologies have been incorporated with the BCI system to gradually overcome those limitations, the BCI paradigm also needs to be considered during the system deign to extend BCI for mainstream applications. The importance of paradigm for the expansion of BCI applications comes from the fact that addressing the above problems is not solvable in a piecewise manner; rather, all issues and related drawbacks should be encountered in a compound manner. For example, users with BCI illiteracy need to have a paradigm with a larger P300 by increasing the number of flashes needed to identify the target character, which, in turn, reduces the ITR. There are multiple of areas of BCI applications that have been gradually flourishing such as assistive, recreation, and rehabilitation. Whether it is binary (limited only to "yes" or "no") or multiarray communication, the paradigm needs to be designed so that the environment and other parameters are not affected much by the human factors. Maintaining an ambient environment while pacifying all the human factors is not an easy task. Interestingly, some of the human issues have been identified and addressed in many spellers so that character selection pace and accuracy increase (Hiley et al. 2006).

Other than spelling, the web browsing ability of a disabled person can have a phenomenal impact in life. Such an opportunity can open up several other communicative ways leading to online education, access of online benefits that can encompass managing economics, and running a business and working at home, among others (Karim et al. 2006).

## 26.9 HYBRID SSVEP–P300 PARADIGM

Although both P300 and SSVEP BCIs are good candidates to form a hybrid BCI, it is challenging to process the resulting hybrid signals to simultaneously extract both SSVEP and P300 features. Traditional signal processing theory is not efficient enough to meet the general goal and performance expectation of a physical hybrid BCI (Thompson et al. 2014). The main goal of a hybrid BCI is to overcome the existing limitations and disadvantages of conventional BCI systems. In a similar reason, in the last few years, the hybrid BCI field has drawn the focus and attention of researchers toward combining multiple BCI systems. Based on the Scopus search engine, and the title–abstract–keyword (("hybrid" AND ("BCI" OR "brain computer interface"))) and ("SSVEP" AND "P300"), limited to "Engineering," "Neuroscience," and "Computer Science" subject areas, it is evident that the number of hybrid BCI publications is fast increasing (Figure 26.8). With this in mind, the design objectives of a hybrid (P300 and SSVEP) BCI paradigm should be incorporated

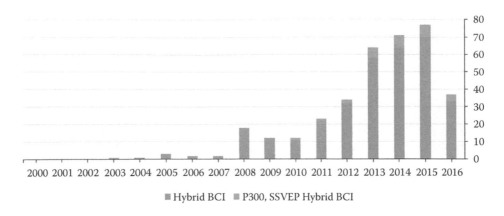

**FIGURE 26.8**   The increasing number of hybrid BCI research published over the recent years.

with the development of necessary signal processing algorithms to improve accuracy and ITR. To accomplish these objectives, the interface should be composed of random flashings and periodic flickers spatially distributed on an electronic display paradigm that would be easy and comfortable for the subjects to gaze at. Implementation of real-time hybrid system requires a computationally efficient system that ensures the least amount of signal processing time to identify the target characters. In order to optimize the estimation, the classifier should be trained for each individual subject. Depending on the health status of the user, the user's intended function, activities and needs, and sensitivity of the BCI outcome, the classifiers, weights, and other parameters would be adjusted to satisfy the underlying preferences of the users. In general, the hybrid BCI signal processing step is not merely a trivial function that employs just a simple signal processing algorithm similar to what is used in a single P300 or SSVEP BCI. A signal of interest could be a product of multiple brain signals that overlap in time and space. To overcome this limitation, computational cost and feature selection process from the brain signals should carefully be considered.

In fact, the resulting hybrid BCI will open up the possibilities for extracting temporal and spectral information at the same time. Interestingly, although both the P300 and SSVEP are good candidates to form a hybrid BCI as they are well documented by different research groups, little attention has been given so far to combining the SSVEP and P300 features. For instance, a hybrid speller is promising for achieving a better ITR and more stable system performance compared with any other BCI speller. It has also been reported in the literature that the hybrid BCI is expected to compensate for a weak response of an individual to a stimulating paradigm by supplementing the weakness of any specific feature (Müller-Putz 2011). However, it is challenging to process the resulting hybrid signals to simultaneously extract both SSVEP and P300 features (Amiri et al. 2013a). To emphasize, combining P300 and SSVEP BCI systems is a novel approach in several ways.

As hybrid P300/SSVEP BCI is composed of two reactive BCIs, this system should provide an indirect voluntary control and communication. Similarly, as the hybrid P300/SSVEP BCI is synchronous, it is supposed to be a successful solution to the long hauling "Midas Touch" problem.

The basic architecture of a BCI system can be divided into two different main categories: (1) sequential hybrid BCI where the individual BCI systems work in series and (2) simultaneous hybrid BCI where the individual BCI systems work in parallel to each other (Pfurtscheller et al. 2010). The conceptual block diagram of the two hybrid BCI systems is presented in Figure 26.9. In the design of a hybrid BCI system, it is necessary to assess the key factors including system complexity, cost, and user workload. In addition, it is of great importance to identify the optimal combination of BCI signals to accomplish desired goals, or in other words, to satisfy the user's need. Understanding of the relationship among the tasks at hand is required to combine several BCI systems.

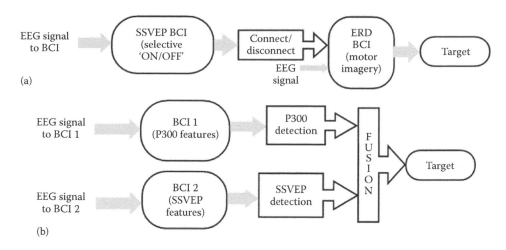

**FIGURE 26.9** (a) Sequential and (b) simultaneous hybrid BCI systems. Hybrid system in (a) uses SSVEP BCI as a selector to activate the next stage, ERD BCI. (From Pfurtscheller, Gert, Brendan Z. Allison, Clemens Brunner, Gunther Bauernfeind, Teodoro Solis-Escalante, Reinhold Scherer, Thorsten O. Zander, Gernot Mueller-Putz, Christa Neuper, and Niels Birbaumer. 2010. The hybrid BCI. *Frontiers in Neuroscience* 4: 30.) Hybrid BCI in (b) fuses both P300 and SSVEP BCI systems to select the target. (Adapted from Erwei, Yin, Timothy Zeyl, Rami Saab, Tom Chau, Hu Dewen, and Zhou Zongtan. 2015. A hybrid brain–computer interface based on the fusion of P300 and SSVEP scores. *Neural Systems and Rehabilitation Engineering, IEEE Transactions on* 23 (4): 693–701.)

So far, hybrid BCI has enhanced the chance that the user's response can be more effectively obtained through utilizing the BCI type that is more appropriate for him or her. Additional benefits lie in the fact that the user can have the option to reduce fatigue by shifting the attention for some time to alternative BCI systems. Such advantages are appreciated by the increase in accuracy when a conventional BCI is replaced by a hybrid BCI (Fazli et al. 2012). In fact, a hybrid BCI is designed to go beyond the traditional BCI system to achieve a specific goal set by a particular BCI application. For instance, two or more brain patterns (e.g., SSVEP and P300, MI and SSVEP) can be combined to improve the system performance of a brain "on/off" switch (Figure 26.9a) or a speller paradigm (Figure 26.9b). In fact, the SSVEP response is usually detected quicker than P300. As a result, many researchers deploy the SSVEP system as a switch to control the second BCI dealing with P300 response (Panicker et al. 2011). A hybrid BCI user may exhibit as less as 50% false positives encountered while using the SSVEP BCI alone (Pfurtscheller et al. 2010).

Panicker et al. (2011) introduced an asynchronous hybrid BCI using both P300 and SSVEP. They have implemented the pattern in a single screen combining P300 and SSVEP. The flashes of this paradigm for generating the P300 were developed by the standard 6 × 6 speller matrix based on the original P300 RCP introduced by Farwell and Donchin (1988). As SSVEP was used just as a switch by identifying the intended control state (CS), only one frequency was sufficient for the SSVEP paradigm. Screen background was alternating between black and white at a rate of 18 Hz. During the classification, a band-pass filter facilitates the SSVEP detection by separating it from P300. It was one of the simplest hybrid BCIs where the SSVEP is utilized to detect the user gaze on the screen as a CS, and it was assumed that the user intends to send a command by gazing at the screen. This hybrid BCI system simultaneously detects P300 for target selection and SSVEP for CS.

Another group of researchers used the P300 and SSVEP combination to control a smart home environment (Edlinger and Guger 2012). SSVEP was employed as a switch to recognize the P300 BCI operation, but the P300-based BCI was used for controlling the virtual smart home environment (Panicker et al. 2011). In general, SSVEP is suitable for continuous control signals as it is detected much quicker than P300, and for the same reason, P300 is suitable for discrete control commands. Research efforts of the BCI community is heading toward the new direction of developing BCI systems that will use new approaches in stimulating brain patterns, as echoed by efforts set forth with the new trend in studying more hybrid BCIs to keep the system complexity low and user acceptability high. Another group combined P300 and SSVEP to control a wheelchair in real time (Li et al. 2013). Simultaneous detection of the P300 and SSVEP was used to separate control and idle states, a key to the satisfactory performance of an asynchronous BCI system. It is important to note that in the case of device control operation, detection accuracy and response time are very critical in terms of system operation.

In addition to the kinds of hybrid BCIs described above, there are several other hybrid systems designed with other modalities such as multimodal signal-based hybrid BCI. For example, two or more combinations of EEG, MEG (magneto-encephalography), fMRI (functional magnetic resonance imaging), fNIRS (functional near-infrared spectroscopy), EMG (electromyography), and EOG (electrooculography) signals can be used for greater system accuracy (Li et al. 2016). However, these modalities limit the applications of a hybrid BCI since they cannot be used outside the laboratory. A hybrid system can also be constituted by combining a conventional BCI with another system to develop a smart, reliable, effective, and user-friendly BCI. For example, an autonomous navigation system had been capitalized to share the destination's info and reroute a smart wheelchair. A P300-based BCI was then employed to select a destination and help route the autonomous system to the desired location (Iturrate et al. 2009).

## 26.10   EVOLVEMENT OF NEW BCI APPLICATIONS

An understanding of the cognitive response to exogenous stimulation has been captured in the literature in form of various mathematical representations, or models, at different levels, leading to the new use of visual evoked potentials, for instance, controlling devices such as television, thermostat, and video devices (Kübler et al. 2006). Moreover, remote controlling of various electronic devices and robots has been implemented on a wheelchair-mounted device (Carlson and Del R. Millan 2013; Rajangam et al. 2015; Sanders 2016). The fine selection capability of the SSVEP control interface makes it a good candidate for making a phone call by dialing the numbers (Cheng et al. 2002). With the ability of BCI to control frequently used devices, BCI continuously evolves to encompass mainstream applications such as recreational activities, training, arts, and music, among others (Eaton and Miranda 2016; Eskandari and Erfanian 2008; Zickler et al. 2013).

To unravel further applications of other modalities, the underlying physiological mechanisms and brain responses in each application need to be carefully investigated. For example, a study to unfold more insights into the cognitive process showed that neurofeedback can be applied to augment the cognitive diagnosis (Schmorrow and Fidopiastis 2015). The cognitive augmentation opened up the possibility of real-time evaluation of cognitive workload during a mental task so that the user's mental capacity is not overloaded (Lee et al. 2013; Rabbi et al. 2012a). Visual image classification (Kapoor et al. 2008), attention monitoring (Nijholt and Tan 2008), and neural rehabilitation are some other BCI applications that drew interests of researchers from various disciplines. BCI rehabilitation can rewire the brain by manipulating the neural plasticity of paralyzed stroke patients (Daly and Wolpaw 2008). An audiovisual BCI system combined visual (P100, N200, and P300 ERP) and audio stimuli (saying numbers) to detect the awareness of disorders of consciousness (DOC) patients (Wang et al. 2015). Interestingly, another study used a combination of P300 and SSVEP to detect potential awareness in patients suffering from DOC (Pan et al. 2014). Depending on the patients' health, classification accuracy varied from 46% to 100%. However, this visual hybrid BCI was able to detect the command following ability of some patients. As the traditional awareness measurement tool heavily depends on behavioral observations and DOC patients suffer from limited behavioral response, the hybrid BCI has potential application as a supportive awareness detection tool.

In addition, recent BCI studies have made extensive progress to develop other attractive applications such as painting artworks, controlling a smart home, designing games, and furnishing Internet tasks (Fazel-Rezai et al. 2011a, 2012). Recent BCI studies have expressed considerable interest in virtual reality–based smart homes. Such a research group allowed the users to execute a group of modest controlling commands such as running a coffee maker, operating a television set, switching the light on and off, or controlling the doors and windows (Kosmyna et al. 2016). Surprisingly, disabled subjects (81%) outperformed healthy subjects (77%) considering the controlling accuracy. A P300 BCI system was used to execute the Internet tasks of ALS patients by browsing the websites. It provided a solution for paralyzed subjects who can surf through web pages and select the desired links to browse different sites or read the news (Mugler et al. 2010). Such freedom and unrestricted access are keys to communication with the outside world. Studies found that performing natural tasks brings happiness and increases the quality of life of ALS patients (Münßinger et al. 2010; Zickler et al. 2013). Another BCI application known as "Brain Painting" allows the user to express their creativity by painting pictures (Hintermüller et al. 2015). This also improves patients' mood by offering a medium of entertainment. BCI systems have been used to design a paradigm to control simple games that do not require strong time constraints such as playing chess (Ahn et al. 2014; Andreev et al. 2016; Boland et al. 2011). Other popular games are MindGame (Finke et al. 2009), Bacteria Hunt (Mühl et al. 2010), and Brain Invaders (Congedo et al. 2011; Korczowski et al. 2016). As no training is required to start playing simple BCI games as mentioned here, it can be useful to familiarize individuals to the BCI tools. Note that BCI-based games have been designed to treat ADHD (attention-deficit/hyperactivity disorder) by incorporating simultaneous training and entertainment (Kim and Bae 2014). Apart from clinical, entertaining, and routine applications, the BCI system can be used to train users in a skilled profession such as learning to control an aircraft in a flight simulator (Kryger et al. 2016).

## 26.11 CONCLUSION

Although there exist many obstacles for BCI researchers such as low accuracy and slow response time, BCI works beyond laboratory experiments have increased over the last decade with the help of modern high-speed computational and sensor technologies to develop an alternative to traditional assistive and mainstream technologies. Reasons for this growth range from the potential improvement of lifestyle to the financial benefits of these applications. In fact, fundamental research on hardware, signal processing, machine learning, and neurophysiology is the main criteria for designing an interaction paradigm. Although every design is accomplished for keeping a specific application in mind, opportunities are revived with the potential space to accommodate other supplementary applications. In order to promote BCI research just from the exploratory field to a profitable level with better acceptance, further insightful study and research need to be directed toward exploring other usability areas that are not yet exposed. This chapter has covered only one particular objective of BCI research, modulating brain activity applying external stimulation. Visual stimulation forms two types of modulated brain activities, P300 and SSVEP. The interfacing paradigm can be designed to capture these evoked potentials in a manner such that many human factors are properly taken care of to diminish their overall impact. Many new applications can develop with efficient design of the control interface. It is evident that P300 and SSVEP can be fused together to form a hybrid BCI with much more interesting features.

## REFERENCES

Acqualagna, Laura, and Benjamin Blankertz. 2011. A gaze independent spelling based on rapid serial visual presentation. In *2011 Annual International Conference of the IEEE Engineering in Medicine and Biology Society, 2011:* 4560–63.

Acqualagna, Laura, and Benjamin Blankertz. 2013. Gaze-independent BCI-spelling using rapid serial visual presentation (RSVP). *Clinical Neurophysiology* 124 (5): 901–8.

Acqualagna, Laura, Matthias Sebastian Treder, Martijn Schreuder, and Benjamin Blankertz. 2010. A novel brain–computer interface based on the rapid serial visual presentation paradigm. In *Engineering in Medicine and Biology Society (EMBC), 2010 Annual International Conference of the IEEE*, 2686–9.

Ahn, Minkyu, Mijin Lee, Jinyoung Choi, and Sung Jun. 2014. A review of brain–computer interface games and an opinion survey from researchers, developers and users. *Sensors* 14 (8): 14601–33.

Alamdari, Nasim, Ali Haider, Riadh Arefin, Ajay K. Verma, Kouhyar Tavakolian, and Reza Fazel-Rezai. 2016. A review of methods and applications of brain computer interface systems. In *2016 IEEE International Conference on Electro Information Technology (EIT)*, 0345–50.

Amiri, Setare, Reza Fazel-Rezai, and Vahid Asadpour. 2013a. A review of hybrid brain–computer interface systems. *Advances in Human–Computer Interaction* 2013: 1–8.

Amiri, Setare, Ahmed Rabbi, Leila Azinfar, and Reza Fazel-Rezai. 2013b. A review of P300, SSVEP, and hybrid P300/SSVEP brain–computer interface systems. In *Brain–Computer Interface Systems—Recent Progress and Future Prospects*, 2013: 1–8. InTech.

Andreev, Anton, Alexandre Barachant, Fabien Lotte, and Marco Congedo. 2016. Recreational applications of OpenViBE: Brain invaders and use-the-force. In *Brain–Computer Interfaces 2: Technology and Applications*, edited by Maureen Clerc, Laurent Bougrain, and Fabien Lotte, chap. 14: 241–57. John Wiley.

Bakardjian, Hovagim, Toshihisa Tanaka, and Andrzej Cichocki. 2010. Optimization of SSVEP brain responses with application to eight-command brain–computer interface. *Neuroscience Letters* 469 (1): 34–38.

Bin, Guangyu, Xiaorong Gao, Zheng Yan, Bo Hong, and Shangkai Gao. 2009. An online multi-channel SSVEP-based brain–computer interface using a canonical correlation analysis method. *Journal of Neural Engineering* 6 (4): 46002.

Blankertz, Benjamin, Guido Dornhege, Matthias Krauledat, Michael Schroeder, John Williamson, Roderick Murray-Smith, and Klaus-Robert Müller. 2006. The Berlin brain–computer interface presents the novel mental typewriter Hex-O-Spell. *3rd International BCI Workshop and Training Course, Graz, 2006, Graz, Austria (2006)*, 2–3.

Boland, Daniel, Melissa Quek, Michael Tangermann, John Williamson, and Roderick Murray-Smith. 2011. Using simulated input into brain–computer interfaces for user-centred design. *International Journal of Bioelectromagnetism* 13 (2): 86–7.

Carlson, Tom, and Jose Del R. Millan. 2013. Brain-controlled wheelchairs: A robotic architecture. *IEEE Robotics and Automation Magazine* 20 (1): 65–73.

Cecotti, Hubert, and A. Graser. 2011. Convolutional neural networks for P300 detection with application to brain–computer interfaces. *IEEE Transactions on Pattern Analysis and Machine Intelligence* 33 (3): 433–45.

Chen, Xiaogang, Yijun Wang, Shangkai Gao, Tzyy-Ping Jung, and Xiaorong Gao. 2015a. Filter bank canonical correlation analysis for implementing a high-speed SSVEP-based brain–computer interface. *Journal of Neural Engineering* 12 (4): 46008.

Chen, Xiaogang, Yijun Wang, Masaki Nakanishi, Xiaorong Gao, Tzyy-Ping Jung, and Shangkai Gao. 2015b. High-speed spelling with a noninvasive brain–computer interface. *Proceedings of the National Academy of Sciences* 112 (44): 1–10.

Cheng, Ming, Xiaorong Gao, Shangkai Gao, and Dingfeng Xu. 2002. Design and implementation of a brain–computer interface with high transfer rates. *IEEE Transactions on Biomedical Engineering* 49 (10): 1181–6.

Cinel, Caterina, Riccardo Poli, and Luca Citi. 2004. Possible sources of perceptual errors in P300-based speller paradigm. In *Biomedizinische Technik, 2nd International BCI Workshop and Training Course*, 49: 39–40.

Congedo, Marco, Matthieu Goyat, Nicolas Tarrin, Gelu Ionescu, Léo Varnet, Bertrand Rivet, Ronald Phlypo, Nisrine Jrad, Michael Acquadro, and Christian Jutten. 2011. "Brain Invaders": A prototype of an open-source P300-based video game working with the OpenViBE platform. In *5th International BCI Conference, Graz, Austria, 280–283*, 2011: 1–6.

Dal Seno, Bernardo, Matteo Matteucci, and Luca Mainardi. 2010. Online detection of P300 and error potentials in a BCI speller. *Computational Intelligence and Neuroscience* 2010: 1–5.

Daly, Janis J., and Jonathan R. Wolpaw. 2008. Brain–computer interfaces in neurological rehabilitation. *The Lancet Neurology* 7 (11): 1032–43.

Daly, Jean, Elaine Armstrong, Eileen Thomson, Pinegger Andreas, Muller-Putz Gernot, and Suzanne Martin. 2015. P300 brain computer interface control after an acquired brain injury. *International Journal on Recent and Innovation Trends in Computing and Communication* 3 (1): 318–25.

Donchin, Emanuel, Kevin M. Spencer, and R. Wijesinghe. 2000. The mental prosthesis: Assessing the speed of a P300-based brain–computer interface. *IEEE Transactions on Rehabilitation Engineering* 8 (2): 174–9.

Eaton, Joel, and Eduardo R. Miranda. 2016. The hybrid brain computer music interface—Integrating brain-wave detection methods for extended control in musical performance systems. In *Lecture Notes in Computer Science (Including Subseries Lecture Notes in Artificial Intelligence and Lecture Notes in Bioinformatics)*, 9617 LNCS: 132–45. Springer, Cham.

Edlinger, Gunter, and Christoph Guger. 2012. A hybrid brain–computer interface for improving the usability of a smart home control. In *2012 ICME International Conference on Complex Medical Engineering (CME)*, 182–5.

Erwei, Yin, Timothy Zeyl, Rami Saab, Tom Chau, Hu Dewen, and Zhou Zongtan. 2015. A hybrid brain–computer interface based on the fusion of P300 and SSVEP scores. *Neural Systems and Rehabilitation Engineering, IEEE Transactions on* 23 (4): 693–701.

Eskandari, Parvaneh, and Abbas Erfanian. 2008. Improving the performance of brain–computer interface through meditation practicing" In *2008 30th Annual International Conference of the IEEE Engineering in Medicine and Biology Society*, 662–5.

Falzon, Owen, Kenneth Camilleri, and Joseph Muscat. 2012. Complex-valued spatial filters for SSVEP-based BCIs with phase coding. *IEEE Transactions on Biomedical Engineering* 59 (9): 2486–95.

Farwell, Lawrence Ashley, and Emanuel Donchin. 1988. Talking off the top of your head: Toward a mental prosthesis utilizing event-related brain potentials. *Electroencephalography and Clinical Neurophysiology* 70 (6): 510–23.

Fazel-Rezai, Reza. 2007. Human error in P300 speller paradigm for brain–computer interface. In *2007 29th Annual International Conference of the IEEE Engineering in Medicine and Biology Society*, 2516–9.

Fazel-Rezai, Reza, and Kamyar Abhari. 2009. A region-based P300 speller for brain–computer interface. *Canadian Journal of Electrical and Computer Engineering* 34 (3): 81–5.

Fazel-Rezai, Reza, Waqas Ahmad, Christoph Guger, Günter Edlinger, and Gunther Krausz. 2011a. *Recent Advances in Brain–Computer Interface Systems*. Edited by Reza Fazel. Rijeka, Croatia: InTech.

Fazel-Rezai, Reza, Brendan Z. Allison, Christoph Guger, Eric W. Sellers, Sonja C. Kleih, and Andrea Kübler. 2012. P300 brain computer interface: Current challenges and emerging trends. *Frontiers in Neuroengineering* 5 (July): 14.

Fazel-Rezai, Reza, Scott Gavett, Waqas Ahmad, Ahmed Rabbi, and Eric Schneider. 2011b. A comparison among several P300 brain–computer interface speller paradigms. *Clinical EEG and Neuroscience* 42 (4): 209–13.

Fazel-Rezai, Reza, and John F. Peters. 2005. P300 wave feature extraction: Preliminary results. In *Electrical and Computer Engineering, 2005. Canadian Conference on*, 390–3.

Fazel-Rezai, Reza, and Sheela Ramanna. 2005. Brain signals: Feature extraction and classification using rough set methods. *Brain*, 709–18.

Fazli, Siamac, Jan Mehnert, Jens Steinbrink, Gabriel Curio, Arno Villringer, Klaus-Robert Müller, and Benjamin Blankertz. 2012. Enhanced performance by a hybrid NIRS–EEG brain computer interface. *NeuroImage* 59 (1): 519–29.

Finke, Andrea, Alexander Lenhardt, and Helge Ritter. 2009. The MindGame: A P300-based brain–computer interface game. *Neural Networks* 22 (9): 1329–33.

Fisher, Robert S., Graham Harding, Giuseppe Erba, Gregory L. Barkley, and Arnold Wilkins. 2005. Photic- and pattern-induced seizures: A review for the Epilepsy Foundation of America Working Group. *Epilepsia*. Blackwell Science Inc.

Friman, Ola, Ivan Volosyak, and Axel Graser. 2007. Multiple channel detection of steady-state visual evoked potentials for brain–computer interfaces. *IEEE Transactions on Biomedical Engineering* 54 (4): 742–50.

Gao, Xiaorong, Dingfeng Xu, Ming Cheng, and Shangkai Gao. 2003. A BCI-based environmental controller for the motion-disabled. *IEEE Transactions on Neural Systems and Rehabilitation Engineering* 11 (2): 137–40.

Garrett, Deon, David A. Peterson, Charles W. Anderson, and Michael H. Thaut. 2003. Comparison of linear, nonlinear, and feature selection methods for EEG signal classification. *IEEE Transactions on Neural Systems and Rehabilitation Engineering* 11 (2): 141–4.

Gavett, Scott, and Reza Fazel-Rezai. 2012. P-300 based brain–computer interface virtual keyboard with predictive spelling. *Journal of Medical Devices* 6 (1): 17597.

Guger, Christoph, Shahab Daban, Eric Sellers, Clemens Holzner, Gunther Krausz, Roberta Carabalona, Furio Gramatica, and Guenter Edlinger. 2009. How many people are able to control a P300-based brain–computer interface (BCI)? *Neuroscience Letters* 462 (1): 94–8.

Haider, Ali, Ben Cosatto, M.N. Alam, Kouhyar Tavakolian, and Reza Fazel-Rezai. 2016. A new region-based BCI speller design using steady state visual evoked potentials. In *6th International Brain–Computer Interface Meeting*, 1. Pacific Grove, CA.

Hiley, Jonathon B., Andrew H. Redekopp, and Reza Fazel-Rezai. 2006. A low cost human computer interface based on eye tracking. In *2006 International Conference of the IEEE Engineering in Medicine and Biology Society*, 1:3226–9.

Hintermüller, Christoph, Eloisa Vargiu, Sebastian Halder, Jean Daly, Felip Miralles, Hannah Lowish, Nick Anderson, Suzanne Martin, and Günter Edlinger. 2015. Brain neural computer interface for everyday home usage. In *Universal Access in Human–Computer Interaction. Access to Interaction*, 9176: 437–46. Springer, Cham.

Hoffmann, Ulrich, Jean-Marc Vesin, Touradj Ebrahimi, and Karin Diserens. 2008a. An efficient P300-based brain–computer interface for disabled subjects. *Journal of Neuroscience Methods* 167 (1): 115–25.

Hoffmann, Ulrich, Ashkan Yazdani, Jean Marc Vesin, and Touradj Ebrahimi. 2008b. Bayesian feature selection applied in a P300 brain–computer interface. In *European Signal Processing Conference*, 1–5.

Iturrate, Iñaki, Jevier M. Antelis, Andrea Kübler, and Javier Minguez. 2009. A noninvasive brain-actuated wheelchair based on a P300 neurophysiological protocol and automated navigation. *IEEE Transactions on Robotics* 25 (3): 614–27.

Jin, Jing, Eric W. Sellers, Sijie Zhou, Yu Zhang, Xingyu Wang, and Andrzej Cichocki. 2015. A P300 brain–computer interface based on a modification of the mismatch negativity paradigm. *International Journal of Neural Systems* 25 (3): 1550011.

Kaper, Matthias, Peter Meinicke, Ulf Grossekathoefer, Thomas Lingner, and Helge Ritter. 2004. BCI Competition 2003—Data Set IIb: Support vector machines for the P300 speller paradigm. *IEEE Transactions on Biomedical Engineering* 51 (6): 1073–6.

Kapoor, Ashish, Pradeep Shenoy, and Desney Tan. 2008. Combining brain computer interfaces with vision for object categorization. In *2008 IEEE Conference on Computer Vision and Pattern Recognition*, 1–8.

Karim, Ahmed A., Thilo Hinterberger, Jürgen Richter, Jürgen Mellinger, Nicola Neumann, Herta Flor, Andrea Kübler, and Niels Birbaumer. 2006. Neural Internet: Web surfing with brain potentials for the completely paralyzed. *Neurorehabilitation and Neural Repair* 20 (4): 508–15.

Kim, Ji Yun, and Jae Hwan Bae. 2014. A study on serious game technology based on BCI for ADHD treatment. In *Advanced Science and Technology Letters*, 46: 208–11.

Koblitz, Neal, Johannes A. Buchmann, Joseph Kirtland, and Robert Edward Lewand. 2001. Introduction to cryptography. *The American Mathematical Monthly* 108 (10): 983.

Korczowski, Louis, Alexandre Barachant, Anton Andreev, Christian Jutten, and Marco Congedo. 2016. "Brain Invaders 2': An open source plug & play multi-user BCI videogame. In *6th International Brain-Computer Interface Meeting*, 224.

Kosmyna, Nataliya, Franck Tarpin-Bernard, Nicolas Bonnefond, and Bertrand Rivet. 2016. Feasibility of BCI control in a realistic smart home environment. *Frontiers in Human Neuroscience* 10 (August). Frontiers Media SA: 1–10.

Kryger, Michael, Brock Wester, Eric A. Pohlmeyer, Matthew Rich, Brendan John, James Beaty, Michael McLoughlin, Michael Boninger, and Elizabeth C. Tyler-Kabara. 2016. Flight simulation using a brain–computer interface: A pilot, pilot study. *Experimental Neurology* 287: 473–8.

Kübler, Andrea, Vivian K. Mushahwar, Leigh R. Hochberg, and John P. Donoghue. 2006. BCI Meeting 2005—Workshop on clinical issues and applications. In *IEEE Transactions on Neural Systems and Rehabilitation Engineering*, 14: 131–4.

Lange, Daniel H., Hillel Pratt, and Gideon F. Inbar. 1997. Modeling and estimation of single evoked brain potential components. *IEEE Transactions on Biomedical Engineering* 44 (9): 791–9.

Lee, Seungchan, Younghak Shin, Soogil Woo, Kiseon Kim, Heung-No Lee, and Reza Fazel-Rezai. 2013. Review of wireless brain–computer interface systems. In *Brain–Computer Interface Systems—Recent Progress and Future Prospects*, 215–38.

Li, Kun, Ravi Sankar, Yael Arbel, and Emanuel Donchin. 2009. P300 based single trial independent component analysis on EEG signal. In *Foundations of Augmented Cognition. Neuroergonomics and Operational Neuroscience*, 5638: 404–10.

Li, Yuanqing, Jiahui Pan, Fei Wang, and Zhuliang Yu. 2013. A hybrid BCI system combining P300 and SSVEP and its application to wheelchair control. *IEEE Transactions on Biomedical Engineering* 60 (11): 3156–66.

Li, Yuanqing, Jiahui Pan, Jinyi Long, Tianyou Yu, Fei Wang, Zhuliang Yu, and Wei Wu. 2016. Multimodal BCIs: Target detection, multidimensional control, and awareness evaluation in patients with disorder of consciousness. *Proceedings of the IEEE* 104 (2): 332–52.

Machado, Sergio, Fernanda Araújo, Flávia Paes, Bruna Velasques, Mario Cunha, Henning Budde, Luis F. Basile et al. 2010. EEG-based brain–computer interfaces: An overview of basic concepts and clinical applications in neurorehabilitation. *Reviews in the Neurosciences* 21 (6): 451–68.

McFarland, Dennis J., and Jonathan R. Wolpaw. 2005. Sensorimotor rhythm-based brain–computer interface (BCI): Feature selection by regression improves performance. *IEEE Transactions on Neural Systems and Rehabilitation Engineering* 13 (3): 372–9.

McFarland, Dennis J, and Jonathan R Wolpaw. 2011. Brain–computer interfaces for communication and control. *Communications of the ACM* 54 (5): 60–6.

Middendorf, Matthew, Grant McMillan, Gloria Calhoun, and Keith S. Jones. 2000. Brain–computer interfaces based on the steady-state visual-evoked response. *IEEE Transactions on Rehabilitation Engineering* 8 (2): 211–4.

Mirghasemi, Hamed, Reza Fazel-Rezai, and Mohammad B. Shamsollahi. 2006a. Analysis of P300 classifiers in brain computer interface speller. In *Annual International Conference of the IEEE Engineering in Medicine and Biology—Proceedings*, 6205–8. IEEE.

Mirghasemi, Hamed, Mohammad B. Shamsollahi, and Reza Fazel-Rezai. 2006b. Assessment of preprocessing on classifiers used in the P300 speller paradigm. In *Annual International Conference of the IEEE Engineering in Medicine and Biology—Proceedings*, 1319–22.

Moore Jackson, Melody, and Rudolph Mappus. 2010. Applications for brain–computer interfaces. In *Brain–Computer Interfaces*, 89–103.

Mugler, Emily M., Carolin A. Ruf, Sebastian Halder, Michael Bensch, and Andrea Kübler. 2010. Design and Implementation of a P300-based brain–computer interface for controlling an Internet browser. *IEEE Transactions on Neural Systems and Rehabilitation Engineering* 18 (6): 599–609.

Mühl, Christian, Hayrettin Gürkök, Danny Plass-Oude Bos, Marieke E. Thurlings, Lasse Scherffig, Matthieu Duvinage, Alexandra A. A. Elbakyan, SungWook Kang, Mannes Poel, and Dirk Heylen. 2010. Bacteria hunt. *Journal on Multimodal User Interfaces* 4 (1): 11–25.

Müller-Putz, Gernot R. 2011. Tools for brain–computer interaction: A general concept for a hybrid BCI. *Frontiers in Neuroinformatics* 5: 30.

Münßinger, Jana I., Sebastian Halder, Sonja C. Kleih, Adrian Furdea, Valerio Raco, Adi Hösle, and Andrea Kübler. 2010. Brain painting: First evaluation of a new brain–computer interface application with ALS-patients and healthy volunteers. *Frontiers in Neuroscience* 4: 182.

Nicolas-Alonso, Luis Fernando, and Jaime Gomez-Gil. 2012. Brain computer interfaces, a review. *Sensors*.

Nielsen, Jakob. 1993. *Usability Engineering. Usability Engineering.* Vol. 44.

Nijholt, Anton, and Desney Tan. 2008. Brain–computer interfacing for intelligent systems. *IEEE Intelligent Systems* 23 (3): 72–9.

Nuwer, Marc. 1997. Assessment of digital EEG, quantitative EEG, and EEG brain mapping: Report of the American Academy of Neurology and the American Clinical Neurophysiology Society. *Neurology* 49 (1): 277–92.

Pan, Jiahui, Qiuyou Xie, Yanbin He, Fei Wang, Haibo Di, Steven Laureys, Ronghao Yu, and Yuanqing Li. 2014. Detecting awareness in patients with disorders of consciousness using a hybrid brain–computer interface. *Journal of Neural Engineering* 11 (5). IOP Publishing: 56007.

Panicker, Rajesh C., Sadasivan Puthusserypady, and Ying Sun. 2011. An asynchronous P300 BCI with SSVEP-based control state detection. *IEEE Transactions on Biomedical Engineering* 58 (6): 1781–8.

Pastor, Maria A., Julio Artieda, Javier Arbizu, Miguel Valencia, and Jose C. Masdeu. 2003. Human cerebral activation during steady-state visual-evoked responses. *The Journal of Neuroscience: The Official Journal of the Society for Neuroscience* 23 (37): 11621–7.

Pfurtscheller, Gert, Brendan Z. Allison, Clemens Brunner, Gunther Bauernfeind, Teodoro Solis-Escalante, Reinhold Scherer, Thorsten O. Zander, Gernot Mueller-Putz, Christa Neuper, and Niels Birbaumer. 2010. The hybrid BCI. *Frontiers in Neuroscience* 4: 30.

Pires, Gabriel, Miguel Castelo-Branco, and Urbano Nunes. 2008. Visual P300-based BCI to steer a wheelchair: A Bayesian approach. In *2008 30th Annual International Conference of the IEEE Engineering in Medicine and Biology Society*, 658–61.

Polich, John. 2007. Updating P300: An integrative theory of P3a and P3b. *Clinical Neurophysiology* 118 (10): 2128–48.

Pouryazdian, Saeed, and Abbas Erfanian. 2010. Detection of steady-state visual evoked potentials for brain–computer interfaces using PCA and high-order statistics. In *World Congress on Medical Physics and Biomedical Engineering 2009*, edited by Olaf Dössel and Wolfgang C. Schlegel, 25: 480–3. IFMBE Proceedings. Berlin, Heidelberg: Springer Berlin Heidelberg.

Rabbi, Ahmed F., Kevin Ivanca, Ashley V. Putnam, Ahmed Musa, Courtney B. Thaden, and Reza Fazel-Rezai. 2009. Human performance evaluation based on EEG signal analysis: A prospective review. In *2009 Annual International Conference of the IEEE Engineering in Medicine and Biology Society*, 2009: 1879–82.

Rabbi, Ahmed F., Abongwa Zony, Pablo de Leon, and Reza Fazel-Rezai. 2012a. Mental workload and task engagement evaluation based on changes in electroencephalogram. *Biomedical Engineering Letters* 2 (3): 139–46.

Rabbi, Ahmed F., Abongwa N. Zony, P. de Leon, and Reza Fazel-Rezai. 2012b. Preliminary results of mental workload and task engagement assessment using electroencephalogram in a space suit. In *2012 Annual International Conference of the IEEE Engineering in Medicine and Biology Society*, 3549–52.

Rajangam, Sankaranarayani, Po-He Tseng, Allen Yin, Mikhail A. Lebedev, and Miguel A. L. Nicolelis. 2015. Direct cortical control of primate whole-body navigation in a mobile robotic wheelchair, *arXiv:1504.02496*.

Rakotomamonjy, Alain, and Vincent Guigue. 2008. BCI Competition III: Dataset II—Ensemble of SVMs for BCI P300 speller. *IEEE Transactions on Biomedical Engineering* 55 (3): 1147–54.

Salvaris, Mathew, and Francisco Sepulveda. 2009. Visual modifications on the P300 speller BCI paradigm. *Journal of Neural Engineering* 6 (4): 46011.

Sanders, David Adrian. 2016. Using self-reliance factors to decide how to share control between human powered wheelchair drivers and ultrasonic sensors. *IEEE Transactions on Neural Systems and Rehabilitation Engineering*, 1–1.

Scherer, Reinhold, Felix Lee, A. Schlogl, Robert Leeb, Horst Bischof, and Gert Pfurtscheller. 2008. Toward self-paced brain computer communication: Navigation through virtual worlds. *IEEE Transactions on Biomedical Engineering* 55 (2): 675–82.

Scherer, Reinhold, Alois Schloegl, Felix Lee, Horst Bischof, Janez Janša, and Gert Pfurtscheller. 2007. The self-paced Graz brain–computer interface: Methods and applications. *Computational Intelligence and Neuroscience* 2007: 1–9.

Schmorrow, Dylan D., and Cali M. Fidopiastis. 2015. *Foundations of Augmented Cognition*. Edited by Dylan D. Schmorrow and Cali M. Fidopiastis. *Lecture Notes in Computer Science (Including Subseries Lecture Notes in Artificial Intelligence and Lecture Notes in Bioinformatics)*. Vol. 9183. Lecture Notes in Computer Science. Cham: Springer International Publishing.

Sellers, Eric W., and Emanuel Donchin. 2006. A P300-based brain–computer interface: Initial tests by ALS patients. *Clinical Neurophysiology* 117 (3): 538–48.

Serby, Hilit, Elad Yom-Tov, and Gideon F. Inbar. 2005. An improved P300-based brain-computer interface. *IEEE Transactions on Neural Systems and Rehabilitation Engineering* 13 (1): 89–98.

Thompson, David E., Lucia R. Quitadamo, Luca Mainardi, Khalil ur Rehman Laghari, Shangkai Gao, Pieterjan Kindermans, John D. Simeral et al. 2014. Performance measurement for brain–computer or brain–machine interfaces: A tutorial. *Journal of Neural Engineering* 11 (3): 35001.

Thurlings, Marieke E., Jan B. F. van Erp, Anne-Marie Brouwer, and Peter J Werkhoven. 2010. EEG-based navigation from a human factors perspective. In *Brain–Computer Interfaces*, 0: 71–86.

Townsend, George, Brandon K. LaPallo, Chadwick B. Boulay, Dean J. Krusienski, G. E. Frye, Christopher K. Hauser, Nicholas Edward Schwartz, Theresa M. Vaughan, Jonathan R. Wolpaw, and Eric W. Sellers. 2010. A novel P300-based brain–computer interface stimulus presentation paradigm: Moving beyond rows and columns. *Clinical Neurophysiology* 121 (7). NIH Public Access: 1109–20.

Turnip, Arjon, Keum-Shik Hong, and Myung-Yung Jeong. 2011. Real-time feature extraction of P300 component using adaptive nonlinear principal component analysis. *Biomedical Engineering Online* 10 (1): 83.

Turnip, Arjon, and Keum Shik Hong. 2012. Classifying mental activities from EEG-P300 signals using adaptive neural networks. *International Journal of Innovative Computing, Information and Control* 8 (9): 6429–43.

van Gerven, Marcel, Jason Farquhar, Rebecca Schaefer, Rutger Vlek, Jeroen Geuze, Anton Nijholt, Nick Ramsey et al. 2009. The brain–computer interface cycle. *Journal of Neural Engineering* 6 (4): 41001.

Vidal, Jacques J. 1977. Real-time detection of brain events in EEG. *Proceedings of the IEEE* 65 (5): 633–41.

Vidaurre, Carmen, Alexander Schlöogl, Rafael Cabeza, Reinhold Scherer, and Gert Pfurtscheller. 2006. A fully on-line adaptive BCI. *IEEE Transactions on Biomedical Engineering* 53 (6): 1214–19.

Wang, Fei, Yanbin He, Jiahui Pan, Qiuyou Xie, Ronghao Yu, Rui Zhang, and Yuanqing Li. 2015. A novel audiovisual brain–computer interface and its application in awareness detection. *Scientific Reports* 5 (October 2014). Nature Publishing Group: 9962.

Wang, Yijun, Xiaorong Gao, Bo Hong, Chuan Jia, and Shangkai Gao. 2008. Brain–computer interfaces based on visual evoked potentials. *IEEE Engineering in Medicine and Biology Magazine* 27 (5): 64–71.

Wu, Chi Hsun, Hsiang Chih Chang, Po Lei Lee, Kuen Shing Li, Jyun Jie Sie, Chia Wei Sun, Chia Yen Yang, Po Hung Li, Hua Ting Deng, and Kuo Kai Shyu. 2011. Frequency recognition in an SSVEP-based brain computer interface using empirical mode decomposition and refined generalized zero-crossing. *Journal of Neuroscience Methods* 196 (1): 170–81.

Zhu, Danhua, Jordi Bieger, Gary Garcia Molina, and Ronald M. Aarts. 2010. A survey of stimulation methods used in SSVEP-based BCIs. *Computational Intelligence and Neuroscience.* Hindawi Publishing Corp.

Zhu, Danhua, Gary Garcia-Molina, Vojkan Mihajlović, and Ronald M Aarts. 2011. Online BCI implementation of high-frequency phase modulated visual stimuli. In *Universal Access in Human–Computer Interaction. Users Diversity: 6th International Conference, UAHCI 2011, Held as Part of HCI International 2011, Orlando, FL, USA, July 9–14, 2011, Proceedings, Part II,* edited by Constantine Stephanidis, 645–54. Berlin, Heidelberg: Springer Berlin Heidelberg.

Zickler, Claudia, Sebastian Halder, Sonja C. Kleih, Cornelia Herbert, and Andrea Kübler. 2013. Brain painting: Usability testing according to the user-centered design in end users with severe motor paralysis. *Artificial Intelligence in Medicine* 59 (2): 99–110.

Ziefle, Martina. 1998. Effects of display resolution on visual performance. *Human Factors* 40 (4): 554–68.

# 27 Hybrid Brain–Computer Interfaces and Their Applications

*Jiahui Pan and Yuanqing Li*

## CONTENTS

27.1 Introduction .................................................................................................................. 526
27.2 Hybrid BCIs Based on Multibrain Patterns ............................................................. 528
    27.2.1 P300-and-SSVEP–Based BCIs ...................................................................... 528
        27.2.1.1 P300-and-SSVEP–Based BCI Spellers ......................................... 528
        27.2.1.2 P300-and-SSVEP–Based Brain Switch ......................................... 529
    27.2.2 MI-and-SSVEP–Based BCIs ........................................................................... 531
        27.2.2.1 MI-and-SSVEP–Based Orthosis Control ...................................... 531
        27.2.2.2 MI-and-SSVEP–Based MI Training .............................................. 531
    27.2.3 MI-and-P300–Based BCIs ............................................................................... 532
        27.2.3.1 An MI-and-P300–Based BCI Mouse ............................................. 532
        27.2.3.2 MI-and-P300–Based Wheelchair Control ..................................... 534
27.3 Multisensory Hybrid BCIs ......................................................................................... 535
    27.3.1 Audio-Visual P300 BCIs ................................................................................. 535
    27.3.2 Audio-Tactile P300 BCIs ................................................................................ 537
27.4 Hybrid BCIs Based on Multiple Signals ................................................................... 538
    27.4.1 EEG-and-EMG–Based BCIs ........................................................................... 539
    27.4.2 EEG-and-EOG–Based BCIs ............................................................................ 539
27.5 Hybrid BCIs Based on Multiple Intelligent Techniques .......................................... 541
    27.5.1 An Intelligent Wheelchair Based on a BCI and an Autonomous Navigation System .... 541
    27.5.2 A Rehabilitative System Based on a BCI and an Intelligent Robot ........................ 542
27.6 Discussions and Conclusion ....................................................................................... 543
Acknowledgments .............................................................................................................. 544
References ........................................................................................................................... 544

## Abstract

In the past decade, big progresses have been made in BCI studies. However, there have been a lot of challenges, including a low information transfer rate, multidimension/function control, man–machine adaptability, long-term robustness, and stability. In this chapter, we review the recent progress in hybrid brain–computer interface (BCIs; also called multimodal BCIs), which may provide potential solutions for addressing these challenges. In particular, four main classes of hybrid BCIs are introduced, including hybrid BCIs based on multibrain patterns, multisensory hybrid BCIs, hybrid BCIs based on multiple signals, and hybrid BCIs based on multiple intelligent techniques. We review state-of-the-art hybrid BCI systems by analyzing their general principles, paradigm, experimental results, advantages, and applications. We conclude that hybrid BCI techniques can be utilized to improve the target detection performance of BCIs and to perform multidimensional object control.

## 27.1   INTRODUCTION

Brain–computer interface (BCI) systems provide communication channels that allow brain messages to be conveyed to the periphery independent of the brain's normal output pathway (Wolpaw et al. 2002). There are several techniques for measuring brain activities, which include near-infrared spectroscopy (NIRS), functional magnetic resonance imaging (fMRI), magnetoencephalography (MEG), electrocorticography (ECoG), and electroencephalography (EEG). EEG is one of the most commonly used modalities in BCIs because of its relatively low cost, its ability to capture near real-time responses, and its technical ease of acquiring signals. In this study, we primarily focus on EEG-based BCIs. The brain patterns used in EEG-based BCIs mainly include P300 potentials (Farwell and Donchin 1988), steady-state evoked potentials such as steady-state visual evoked potentials (SSVEPs) (Muller-Putz et al. 2006), and event-related desynchronization/synchronization (ERD/ERS) produced by motor imagery (MI) (Pfurtscheller and Lopes Da Silva 1999).

Conventional "simple" EEG-based BCIs generally rely on a single signal input (i.e., EEG) and a single brain pattern, such as P300 potentials, which are produced by stimuli applied to a single sensory modality (e.g., visual stimuli), while no other intelligent/automation techniques are incorporated into the system. The general architecture of a BCI system is shown in Figure 27.1, which includes four stages of brain signal processing: data acquisition, preprocessing, feature extraction, and translation algorithms. In the data acquisition, brain signals are first acquired using sensors. For example, the EEG measures signals acquired from electrodes placed on the scalp, as shown in Figure 27.1. In BCI signal processing, many signal components are noisy. Preprocessing methods such as spatial filtering and temporal filtering can improve signal quality by greatly reducing noise and artifacts. Then, useful signal features reflecting the user's intent are then extracted from the preprocessed brain signals. For EEG-based BCIs, the selection of feature extraction methods depends on the brain patterns such as event-related potentials (ERPs), ERD, and ERS reflected by mu and beta rhythms. After the features that reflect the intentions of the user are extracted, the next step is to translate these features into device control commands, using a classification method, such as the Fisher linear discriminant (FLD), support vector machine (SVM), and Bayesian model (Li et al. 2009). Major progress has been made in the paradigm designs, brain signal processing algorithms, and control systems of such simple BCIs. However, these BCI systems are faced with several challenges, including a low information transfer rate (ITR), multidimension/function control, man–machine adaptability, long-term robustness, and stability.

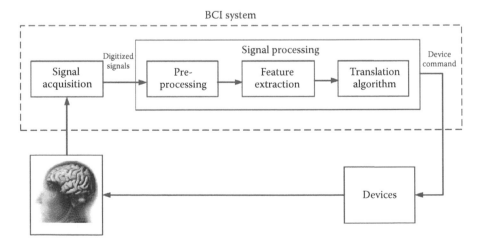

**FIGURE 27.1**   Basic design and operation of a BCI system. (Modified from Li, Y., K. K. Ang, and C. Guan. 2009. *Digital Signal Processing and Machine Learning.*)

A potential solution to the above challenges is the use of a recently developed type of BCI, namely, hybrid BCIs. As described in Allison (2010), Allison et al. (2007), and Pfurtscheller et al. (2010a), a hybrid BCI is composed of a BCI system and an additional system, which might be a second BCI system, and is designed to perform specific goals better than conventional BCIs. Compared to a conventional BCI system (as shown in Figure 27.1), the signal flow of a hybrid BCI system can be described as follows. (1) In the signal acquisition, the signal input can be from multiple signals (e.g., EEG and NIRS), or multibrain patterns (e.g., P300 and SSVEP), which are evoked by multisensory stimuli (e.g., audio-visual stimuli). (2) In the signal processing, a hybrid BCI system can provide only a single output/control signal or multiple outputs/control signals. In the former case, when multiple brain patterns or multiple signals are involved, data fusion is generally required at the feature or decision level. In the latter case, the multiple control signals may be separately manipulated by the different brain patterns probed by the system, and the fusion of these brain patterns is generally not necessary. (3) In the BCI application, a BCI system can be combined with an intelligent device (e.g., an intelligent robot) to achieve shared control.

"Hybrid BCIs" and "multimodal BCIs" are two highly related concepts. In the literature (Li et al. 2016), researchers reported that "hybrid BCIs" and "multimodal BCIs" are interchangeable terms referring to the same definitions of BCIs. In the literature (Gürkök and Nijholt 2012), researchers described that multimodal BCI appeared mostly in the human–computer interaction and could be categorized as BCIs based on multimodal stimuli (also called BCIs in multimodal interaction) and BCIs based on multimodal signals (only refer to brain signals). Here, we further expand upon the definition of hybrid BCIs (Pfurtscheller et al. 2010a) or multimodal BCIs (Gürkök and Nijholt 2012). As shown in Figure 27.2, there are four main classes of hybrid BCIs.

1. Hybrid BCIs based on multibrain patterns, in which at least two brain patterns (e.g., P300 and SSVEP or MI and P300) are used. In this type of hybrid BCI, multiple brain patterns are evoked by single sensory stimulus.
2. Multisensory hybrid BCIs, in which brain patterns are evoked simultaneously by multisensory stimuli, such as audio-visual stimuli. In this class of hybrid BCIs, one or more brain patterns are evoked by multiple sensory stimuli.

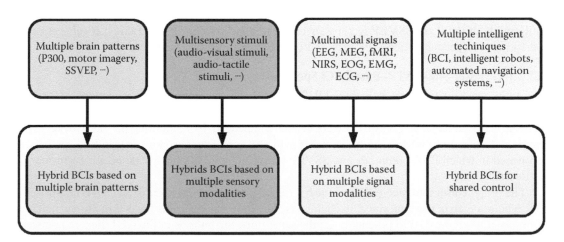

**FIGURE 27.2** Four classes of hybrid BCIs. (Modified from Li, Y., J. Pan, J. Long, T. Yu, F. Wang, Z. Yu, and W. Wu. 2016. Multimodal BCIs: Target detection, multidimensional control, and awareness evaluation in patients with disorder of consciousness. *Proceedings of the IEEE* no. 104 (2):332–352.)

3. Hybrid BCIs based on multiple signals, in which two or more input signals, such as EEG, MEG, fMRI, NRIS, electro-oculogram (EOG), or electromyogram (EMG), are combined in a hybrid BCI system.

4. Hybrid BCIs based on multiple intelligent techniques, in which the BCI is combined with another intelligent system to achieve shared control. Such combinations may lead to more reliable, flexible, usable, and powerful BCI systems by allowing subjects to focus their attention on a final target and to ignore low-level details related to the execution of an action (Brouwer et al. 2010).

The aim of this chapter is to introduce hybrid BCIs. The various classes of hybrid BCIs are explained in the following sections, beginning with general principles and designs and leading to their applications. Finally, concluding remarks and future perspectives are presented.

## 27.2 HYBRID BCIs BASED ON MULTIBRAIN PATTERNS

Hybrid BCIs combining multiple brain patterns, such as P300, SSVEP, and MI-based ERD/ERS, have been designed for various applications, such as spelling (Panicker et al. 2011; Xu et al. 2013; Yin et al. 2013, 2014), idle state detection (Li et al. 2013), orthosis (Horki et al. 2011; Pfurtscheller et al. 2010b), wheelchair navigation, and control of computer components, such as a two-dimensional (2D) cursor (Allison 2010; Li et al. 2010), mouse (Li et al. 2010; Long et al. 2012b), browser (Yu et al. 2012), explorer (Bai et al. 2015), or mail client (Yu et al. 2013). In the following section, we describe several P300-and-SSVEP–based BCIs, MI-and-SSVEP–based BCIs, and MI-and-P300–based BCIs.

### 27.2.1 P300-AND-SSVEP–BASED BCIs

Several P300-and-SSVEP–based BCIs have been proposed, such as for spelling (Panicker et al. 2011; Xu et al. 2013; Yin et al. 2013, 2014) and for toggling an on/off switch (Li et al. 2013). In these systems, SSVEP is a suitable candidate for incorporation into the P300 paradigm for two reasons. First, both P300 potentials and SSVEPs can be elicited by visual stimuli, allowing the subjects to simultaneously produce both brain patterns by simply performing a visual attention task without exerting extra mental load. Second, the P300 and SSVEP features are located in different domains (time domain vs. frequency domain), and the two brain patterns have significant independence. By utilizing both P300 and SSVEP features, hybrid P300-and-SSVEP–based BCIs can achieve better performance than conventional P300 or SSVEP BCIs, as described below.

#### 27.2.1.1 P300-and-SSVEP–Based BCI Spellers

Recently, several studies have combined P300 and SSVEP to improve the conventional 6 × 6 BCI speller (Panicker et al. 2011; Xu et al. 2013; Yin et al. 2013, 2014). Generally, in these hybrid spellers, the P300 potential and SSVEP are elicited simultaneously by combining periodic flickers with random flashes. In a previous study (Panicker et al. 2011), an asynchronous hybrid BCI speller was proposed in which P300 potentials and SSVEP were combined to improve detection performance, as described below.

The graphic user interface (GUI) of the hybrid BCI speller in Panicker et al. (2011) comprised a 6 × 6 button matrix that contained 36 characters. The rows and columns flashed in orange in a random order to produce P300 potentials. At the same time, the buttons in the GUI flickered between white and black at 17.7 Hz to produce SSVEPs when the subject is focusing on one particular character. In this system, detection of the control state was performed through SSVEP detection, and recognition of the target button was carried out through P300 detection.

Detection of the P300 potentials and SSVEPs was performed separately (see the details in Panicker et al. 2011). For each round of intensifications for the rows and columns, SSVEP detection was performed. Specifically, the mean power values in a narrow and wide band were utilized to calculate a power ratio; the previously reported central frequency was 17.7 Hz, and the bandwidths were 0.6 and 4 Hz, respectively. When the power ratio exceeded a predefined threshold (i.e., 0.5 in Panicker et al. 2011), a control state was detected for this round; otherwise, an idle state was determined. If the control state was detected for at least three of five adjacent rounds, the subjects were expected to input a character, and P300 detection was performed, which included band-pass filtering, P300 feature extraction, and Bayes linear discriminant analysis (BLDA) or Fischer's linear discriminant analysis (FLDA) classification. The target character was then determined according to the result of P300 detection.

In the online experiment, 10 healthy subjects underwent three experimental sessions that included 18 characters in each session. A character was identified and displayed on the screen once per presentation of five rounds, and the character was determined to be null if the control state was not detected. The experimental results demonstrated the effectiveness of this hybrid system, with an average control state detection accuracy of approximately 88%, an average P300 classification accuracy in the control state of 94.44%, and an average ITR of 19.05 bits/min.

### 27.2.1.2 P300-and-SSVEP–Based Brain Switch

In asynchronous brain switches, an important task is to distinguish the control and idle states based on the ongoing brain signals. Many studies have addressed the issue of asynchronous brain switches based on single brain pattern, such as SSVEP or MI. When designing the visual paradigm and the detection algorithm, we need to improve the accuracy of the control state detection (true-positive rate [TPR]) and reduce the false alarm rate (false-positive rate [FPR]) when the user is in the idle state.

In a study (Li et al. 2013), a hybrid BCI-based brain switch was proposed, in which P300 and SSVEP were combined to improve the performance of idle/control state detection. As shown in Figure 27.3, four groups of buttons are displayed on the GUI, and each group contains one large button in the center and eight small buttons surrounding it. All buttons in each of the four groups flicker at a four different frequencies of 6.0, 6.67, 7.5, and 8.57 Hz, respectively, to evoke SSVEP. At the same time, the large buttons of the four groups are intensified in a random order through changing their shape and color to evoke P300 potentials. One group of buttons, for example, at the top, is set as a target for "on/off" command, and the other buttons are set as pseudo keys that do not activate any commands (the usefulness of pseudo keys were explained in detail in Pan et al. 2013). In the control state, the user can switch between "on" and "off" states of the system by focusing on the target and counting its flashes, whereas in the idle state, no particular button is attended to. The system detects the control/idle state by determining whether both P300 and SSVEP occur at the target.

The P300 and SSVEP detections were performed separately. In the asynchronous algorithm, the detection of P300, including low-pass filtering, P300 feature extraction, and SVM classification, was accomplished every 800 ms corresponding to one round of button flashes, and four SVM scores were obtained for the four button groups. The SSVEP detection, including band-pass filtering and power feature extraction, was performed every 200 ms, and four power ratios were computed for the four groups' flickering frequencies. The decision was made every 200 ms. Specifically, summing the normalized P300 SVM scores and the normalized SSVEP power ratios, a detection index was obtained to discriminate the control and idle states. The detection of the control state was performed by judging whether any of two conditions was satisfied: (i) the difference of the detection index between target group and the other groups (pseudo keys) exceeds a predefined threshold; (ii) the target is recognized simultaneously by both P300 and SSVEP detection for a predefined number of consecutive times, for example, three times in Li et al. (2013). Two experiments involving eight subjects were conducted to validate the hybrid approach and system. For the purpose of comparison, three sessions were conducted in the first experiment for the hybrid P300-and-SSVEP–based BCI, a P300-based BCI, and an SSVEP-based BCI, respectively. It was shown that the performance of asynchronous control was better for a combined hybrid BCI than for the corresponding P300-only– or SSVEP-only–based brain switch. This improvement could be explained by the fusion of the

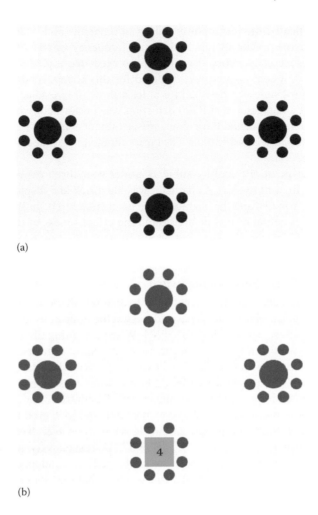

(a)

(b)

**FIGURE 27.3** GUI of the hybrid brain switch combining the P300 and SSVEPs. (a) Each group of buttons flickers at a fixed frequency (6.0, 6.67, 7.5, or 8.57 Hz) by changing color between black and red. (b) Large buttons of the four groups are intensified with green squares in a random order, with each intensification lasting 100 ms with a 100-ms interval between two consecutive intensifications.

time–frequency features of the P300 and SSVEPs, which might provide additional information to facilitate the classification of the control state versus the idle state. In the second experiment, an online asynchronous experiment was conducted. The system sent a correct control command in an average of 4.30 s, and achieved an average ITR of 22.11 bits/min. Furthermore, it was found that this hybrid paradigm not only simultaneously evoked P300 and SSVEP but also elicited a strong N200, which could further enhance the discrimination between the control state and the idle state and improved the classification accuracy.

As an application, this hybrid brain switch was used to produce a "go/stop" command in real-time wheelchair control, where "go" and "stop" commands were always sent at the static and the in-motion conditions, respectively. A wheelchair control experiment involving five subjects was conducted. The subjects could send a "go" command in the static condition with an average response time (RT) of 4.21 s and an average false activation rate (FAR) of 0.48 events/min. In the in-motion condition, the subjects could send a "stop" command in an average RT of 5.50 s with an average FAR of 0.52 events/min.

### 27.2.2 MI-AND-SSVEP–BASED BCIs

Several MI-and-SSVEP–based BCIs have been proposed for various applications, such as orthosis/artificial limb control (Horki et al. 2011; Pfurtscheller et al. 2010b) or MI training (Yu et al. 2015). In these systems, MI and SSVEP were combined such that MI induced the ERS/ERD and visual attention modulated the SSVEPs.

#### 27.2.2.1 MI-and-SSVEP–Based Orthosis Control

MI- and SSVEP-based BCIs can be combined sequentially to reduce false activations during non-intentional control. Pfurtscheller et al. (2010b) proposed a hybrid MI-and-SSVEP BCI in which an MI-based brain switch was used to turn on/off an SSVEP-controlled orthosis. In this system, an SSVEP-based BCI was utilized to open the orthosis by gazing at an 8-Hz light-emitting diode (LED) and close the system by gazing at a 13-Hz LED. An MI-based brain switch was used to activate the SSVEP-based BCI only when orthosis control was needed and to deactivate the LEDs mounted on the orthosis during resting periods.

For the SSVEP-based BCI, the power density spectrum of the past 1-s EEG segment recorded from one bipolar channel was calculated every 250 ms based on a discrete Fourier transform. A weighted sum of each stimulation frequency and its second and third harmonics yielded the harmonic sum decision (HSD). The flickering light source with the highest HSD was selected if it was consecutively detected several times (see the details in Pfurtscheller et al. 2010b). For the MI-based brain switch, foot MI was detected from the "Cz" Laplacian EEG channel in a moving window of 1 s. From the training data (30 trials during MI and 30 trials during resting periods), the frequency bands with the most pronounced beta ERS were used to set up the FLDA classifier. The training of the FLDA classifier was performed based on a $10 \times 10$ cross-validation, and the classifier with the highest classification accuracy was used for online classification.

Six subjects participated in the experiment to control an electrical hand orthosis (see the details in Pfurtscheller et al. 2010b). For comparison, the orthosis was also operated using the SSVEP-based modality alone, without incorporation of the MI-based brain switch. Four of the six subjects succeeded in operating the asynchronous hybrid BCI with good performance (positive prediction value > 70%). The combination of these two BCI modalities, which are operated using different mental strategies, achieved much lower FPR during resting periods or breaks than the BCI based on SSVEP alone (FP = $1.46 \pm 1.18$ vs. $5.40 \pm 0.90$).

#### 27.2.2.2 MI-and-SSVEP–Based MI Training

MI-induced ERD/ERS has been widely used in EEG-based BCIs. However, the differences in EEG between two MIs, such as left and hand MIs, are generally not sufficient to provide reliable control, especially for naïve subjects. It is believed that positive neuro-feedback can help subjects learn how to perform MIs to achieve effective BCI control. In one study (Yu et al. 2015), SSVEPs were combined with MI to provide positive feedback to facilitate MI training. SSVEPs are generally chosen as a supplementary tool for calculating feedback because (i) SSVEP- and MI-related brain patterns can be produced simultaneously; (ii) SSVEP is a type of evoked potential that can be stably detected in naïve subjects who have undergone little training; and (iii) SSVEPs can be detected based on a single trial of EEG data. This detection does not require an averaging procedure, as in ERP calculations. Therefore, the speed of detection of SSVEPs is comparable to that of MI, which is useful for providing real-time feedback.

The GUI contained a horizontal feedback bar in the center of the GUI, two SSVEP stimulus buttons (the two red arrows) presented on the left and right sides of the bar, and a cue arrow above the feedback bar that indicated the current task type. The flicker frequencies of these two buttons were 7.5 Hz (left) and 6.0 Hz (right). During training, the subjects were instructed to focus on the left or right flickering button to evoke SSVEPs as they performed left- or right-hand MI, respectively.

The algorithm of the hybrid BCI was based on hybrid features consisting of MI- and SSVEP-related brain signals. First, a common spatial pattern (CSP) algorithm is applied for MI discrimination, whereas a canonical correlation analysis (CCA) is employed for SSVEP detection. Then, the hybrid features are constructed by concatenating the CSP features and canonical correlation coefficients, which are then fed into an SVM classifier. Before training, a calibration data set is collected to update the classifier. The length of the feedback bar is determined according to the online classification results and is updated every 200 ms.

At the beginning of training, SSVEPs are more likely to dominate the feedback because (i) SSVEPs can be effectively evoked without requiring much training, and therefore, the SSVEP features are more discriminative than the MI features; and (ii) the classifier tends to automatically assign large weights to more discriminative features. Therefore, relatively accurate feedback is available at the beginning of training. However, as the training progresses, the subjects become more skilled in performing MI and, thus, gradually shift their attention to MI. In this case, the MI features become more discriminative and are automatically assigned higher weights in the SVM classification, whereas the SSVEP features deteriorate and become less dominant than at the beginning of training. Therefore, effective feedback is still available, where MI plays a more dominant role, and thus, MI training may be facilitated.

Twenty-four naïve subjects were randomly divided into two groups: one group participated in MI training based on hybrid feedback, and the other group, corresponding to a control group, participated in MI training based on the normal feedback of the MI features. The experimental results demonstrated that the subjects generated distinguishable brain patterns based on hand MI after only five hybrid feedback training sessions lasting approximately 1.5 h each. The subjects who received hybrid feedback significantly outperformed the subjects of the control group who received normal feedback. Moreover, as training proceeded, a shift of the corresponding classifier weights from SSVEP to MI features was observed. It was thus validated that the hybrid BCI system can be used to enhance MI training.

### 27.2.3 MI-and-P300–Based BCIs

An important aspect of EEG-based BCI systems is multidimensional control, which involves multiple independent control signals. These control signals may be obtained from multiple brain patterns, such as MI and P300 potentials. On one hand, P300 potentials represent a reliable type of brain pattern for generating discrete control output commands. On the other hand, MI-based ERD/ERS of BCIs is more efficient for producing continuous control commands. Recently, several studies have discussed multidimensional control based on MI-and-P300–based BCIs (Jennett and Plum 1972; Li et al. 2010; Long et al. 2012a,b; Rebsamen et al. 2008; Wang et al. 2014; Yu et al. 2013).

#### 27.2.3.1 An MI-and-P300–Based BCI Mouse

When using a BCI mouse, the user must sequentially perform two tasks. First, the user must move the cursor to a target on a monitor (termed 2D cursor control), and second, the user must click the target of interest (termed target selection). In this case, multiple control signals that can be generated by multiple brain patterns are essential.

Li and colleagues proposed a hybrid BCI combining MI brain patterns and P300 potentials for 2D cursor control (Li et al. 2010) and target selection (Long et al. 2012b). The GUI is shown in Figure 27.4, in which the circle and square represent the cursor and target, respectively, where the initial position of the cursor and the initial position and color (gray or dark gray) of the target are randomly provided. The three "up" buttons, three "down" buttons, and two "stop" buttons flash in a random order to evoke P300 potentials. The task of the subject is to move the cursor to the target and to then select or reject the gray/dark gray target. The control strategy of the user is described below. The user can move the cursor to the left or right by imagining his or her own left or right hand movement, respectively, and the user can move the cursor up or down by focusing on one of

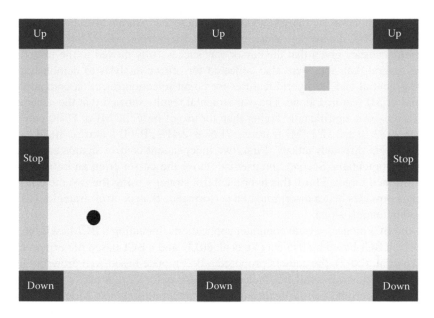

**FIGURE 27.4** GUI of the hybrid BCI combining MI and P300 potentials for 2D cursor control and target selection in which a cursor (black circle), target (gray square), and eight flashing buttons (three "up," three "down," and two "stop" buttons) are included. (From Long, J., Y. Li, H. Wang, T. Yu, J. Pan, and F. Li. 2012. A hybrid brain computer interface to control the direction and speed of a simulated or real wheelchair. *IEEE Transactions on Neural Systems & Rehabilitation Engineering* no. 20 (5):720–729; Li, Y., J. Long, T. Yu, Z. Yu, C. Wang, H. Zhang, and C. Guan. 2010. An EEG-based BCI system for 2-D cursor control by combining Mu/Beta rhythm and P300 potential. *Biomedical Engineering, IEEE Transactions on* no. 57 (10):2495–2505.)

the three flashing "up" or "down" buttons to evoke P300 potentials. If the user does not intend to move the cursor in the vertical direction, then the user can focus on either of the two "stop" buttons.

To further implement a BCI mouse, target selection and rejection functions are required. Specifically, once the cursor hits the target of interest (gray square), the user can select the target by focusing attention on a flashing "stop" button and simultaneously maintaining an idle state of MI. If the target is not of interest (dark gray square), the user can reject it by continuing to imagine left or right hand movement without focusing on any flashing buttons.

The algorithm for the 2D cursor control includes two parts: P300 detection for vertical movement control and MI detection for horizontal movement control, with the details presented in Li (2010). The signal processing procedure for P300 detection consists of three stages: low-pass filtering, P300 feature extraction, and SVM classification. For MI detection, the signal processing stages include common average reference (CAR) spatial filtering, band-pass filtering of the specific mu rhythm band (8–13 Hz), feature extraction based on a CSP algorithm, and SVM classification.

The algorithm for target selection or rejection was based on the hybrid features of P300 potentials and MI, with the details presented in Long et al. (2012b). After extracting the features of the P300 potentials and MI using the same algorithms described above, a hybrid feature vector for each trial is constructed by concatenating the feature vector of the MI with the feature vector of the P300 potentials, which is then fed into the SVM for classification.

Eleven healthy subjects attended the online experiment, which included one session of 80 trials for each subject. Each trial included two sequential tasks. During the first task, subjects were instructed to move the cursor to a target that was presented at a randomized position on the screen. After the cursor hit the target, the subject was instructed to perform the second task of selecting or rejecting the target according to the color of the target (gray for selection and dark gray for rejection). The time interval for the second task was set to 2 s. Among all subjects, the average time for one trial was 18.96 s, the average accuracy for successful trials was 92.84%, and the average for target selection accuracy given that the cursor was successfully moved to the target was 93.99%. Additionally, several data sets were also collected for offline analysis to demonstrate the advantage of P300 potential and MI hybrid features for target selection/rejection compared with use of P300 potential or MI features alone. The experimental results showed that the accuracy for use of the hybrid features was significantly higher than for use of only the MI or P300 potential features (hybrid features: 83.10 ± 2.12%; MI features: 71.68 ± 2.41%; P300 features: 80.44 ± 1.82%). This hybrid system offers three advantages. First, two independent control signals are generated based on MI and P300 potentials. Second, the user can move the cursor from an arbitrary position to a randomly positioned target. Third, this hybrid control strategy using the two modalities of MI and P300 potentials provides better discrimination performance than control strategies based on the use of MI or P300 potentials alone.

Based on the BCI mouse, several computer applications, including a BCI-based Internet browser (Yu et al. 2012), a BCI-based mail client (Yu et al. 2013), and a BCI-based file explorer, were implemented. In Yu et al. (2012), the authors proposed a BCI mouse-based web browser, in which common navigation functions are available, including traversing forward or backward through browsing history, selecting hyperlinks, scrolling through pages, and inputting text. Moreover, Yu et al. (2013) also proposed a hybrid BCI–based mail client that implemented electronic mail communication. Using this BCI mail client, the users are able to receive, read, write, and attach files to e-mails. Bai et al. (2015) proposed a hybrid BCI combining P300 and MI to operate an explorer. Using this system, users can access a computer and manipulate (open, close, copy, paste, and delete) files, such as documents, pictures, music, movies, and so on.

### 27.2.3.2 MI-and-P300–Based Wheelchair Control

Multiple control signals are also essential for the multidimensional control of a wheelchair. In a study, Long et al. (2012a) proposed a hybrid BCI paradigm based on MI and P300 potentials to provide directional (left or right) and speed control (acceleration and deceleration) commands to operate a real wheelchair.

The GUI is similar to that shown in Figure 27.4 for 2D cursor control except that no cursor or target is presented. In this hybrid BCI system, the user can control the left and right directions of the wheelchair via left- and right-hand imagery. For speed control, a hybrid paradigm is applied. For deceleration, the user must imagine a third motor event (e.g., movement of the foot) without paying attention to any of the flashing buttons. For acceleration, the user must pay attention to a specific flashing button without imagining any movement. Furthermore, the user can remain in an idle state to prevent activation of any commands.

The algorithm for wheelchair control includes two parts: the detection of directional control signals and the detection of speed control signals, and the details are presented in Long et al. (2012a). The algorithm first detects left or right MI for directional control. The direction detection module includes CAR spatial filtering, band-pass filtering, feature extraction based on a CSP algorithm, and linear discriminant analysis (LDA) classification. If no left or right MI is detected, no direction control is applied. Then, the algorithm performs speed control by discriminating among three states: foot imagery without P300 potentials (low speed), P300 potentials without foot imagery (high speed), and an idle state (no speed control). The speed detection module includes MI pattern extraction, P300 pattern extraction, and LDA classification.

To test the effectiveness of the control mechanism, two subjects were required to control a real wheelchair to follow a predefined route. In the experiment, each subject performed five trials. For each trial, the subjects were required to drive the wheelchair from the starting point to the end of the route (i.e., PL5) and then perform a "U" turn and drive the wheelchair back to the starting point. For the two subjects, the average distances driven while in low-speed and high-speed mode (path length) were 5.43 and 5.21 m, respectively. The average time for which the subjects operated the wheelchair in the low- and high-speed modes were 45.38 and 20.14 s, respectively, of which the subjects incorrectly operated the wheelchair at high and low speeds in areas of the route that were designated as low- and high-speed areas for 4.54 and 4.1 s, respectively. In addition, no collisions occurred. These experimental results thus demonstrated that the two subjects could successfully control the wheelchair's direction and velocity over the predefined route using the proposed hybrid BCI.

In this section, we described several hybrid BCIs based on multibrain patterns and presented several application systems. In fact, hybrid BCIs based on multiple brain patterns may be beneficial not only for normal subjects but also for BCI-illiterate subjects. Approximately 13% of healthy users are unable to effectively control simple BCIs based on P300 potential (Guger et al. 2009) or SSVEP (Allison et al. 2010b) brain patterns. Hybrid BCIs involving two or more brain patterns offer a possible solution for decreasing the number of users who are BCI-illiterate. For instance, a hybrid BCI combining MI and SSVEPs improved BCI performance in Allison et al. (2010a). The experimental results of 14 healthy subjects showed that the average accuracy of performing a task using the hybrid system was improved by approximately 6% compared to using conventional MI-only or SSVEP-only methods. Furthermore, there were no users who were unable to use the hybrid BCI, whereas there were five users who were unable to use the MI-only or SSVEP-only BCIs. This improvement in performance for hybrid systems may be due to the addition of a second task that provides more information to the classifier (Allison 2010).

Other hybrid BCIs based on multibrain patterns have also been reported. For instance, Allison et al. (2012) presented a new type of hybrid BCI based on MI and SSVEPs for continuous 2D cursor control. In this system, the users controlled the vertical movement of a virtual ball based on left- and right-hand MI while simultaneously controlling horizontal movement via SSVEP activity. The authors also developed a P300- and SSVEP-based hybrid BCI with a four-choice paradigm (Allison et al. 2014). The experimental results showed that the hybrid system led to improved detection performance compared to the SSVEP-only system, although the performance was not improved compared to the P300-only condition.

## 27.3 MULTISENSORY HYBRID BCIs

Humans possess multiple sensory pathways for processing information from the real world. This integration of multisensory stimuli is known to give rise to modulated ERPs, possibly through the strengthening of top-down attention (Stein and Stanford 2008). These enhanced effects of multisensory integration may be useful for improving the performance of BCI systems. Based on this consideration, several studies based on audio-visual (An et al. 2014; Belitski et al. 2011; Wang et al. 2015), audio-tactile (Rutkowski and Mori 2015; Yin et al. 2015), and visual-tactile BCIs (Brouwer et al. 2010; Thurlings et al. 2012) have been reported, in which bimodal stimuli are employed for improving system performance.

### 27.3.1 AUDIO-VISUAL P300 BCIs

Recently, several studies based on audio-visual BCIs have been reported. An offline audio-visual P300-speller and the corresponding data analysis results were presented in Belitski et al. (2011), which showed that the strength of the P300 response was higher in audio-visual conditions than in visual-only or auditory-only conditions. An et al. explored a parallel speller for gaze-independent BCI in which the auditory and visual domains are independent from one another (An et al. 2014). Their results showed that 15 users could spell online with a mean accuracy of 87.7%. These existing results have shown that audio-visual integration could be a potential method to enhance brain patterns and to further improve BCI performance.

Wang et al. proposed a novel audio-visual BCI system in which spatially, temporally, and semantically congruent audio-visual stimuli based on numbers were employed (Wang et al. 2015). In the

GUI of this audio-visual BCI, there are two number buttons corresponding to two numbers randomly selected from 0 to 9 that are located on the left and right sides of the GUI, and two speakers are placed laterally to the monitor. The two buttons flash in an alternating manner. When a number button is visually intensified, the corresponding spoken number is presented from the ipsilateral speaker. In this way, the user is presented with temporally, spatially, and semantically congruent audio-visual stimuli that last for 300 ms, where the interstimulus interval (ISI) is randomized from 700 to 1500 ms.

Ten healthy subjects participated in the experiment, which consisted of three sessions that were administered in a random order. The sessions corresponded to the visual-only, auditory-only, and audio-visual conditions. In each session, the subject first performed a training run of 10 trials, followed by a test run of 30 trials. The online average accuracies across all healthy subjects were 95.67%, 86.33% and 62.33% for the audio-visual, visual-only and auditory-only sessions, respectively. The audio-visual BCI significantly outperformed the visual-only and auditory-only BCIs. As shown in Figure 27.5, the ERP waveforms at the "Pz" electrode indicated that for the target stimuli, there were stronger P100, N200, and P300 responses in the audio-visual condition than in the visual-only and auditory-only conditions. As shown in Figure 27.6, there were more discriminative features for the audio-visual condition than for the visual-only and auditory-only conditions. The enhanced ERP components associated with the audio-visual stimuli, such as P100, N200, and P300, improved the performance of the audio-visual BCI system.

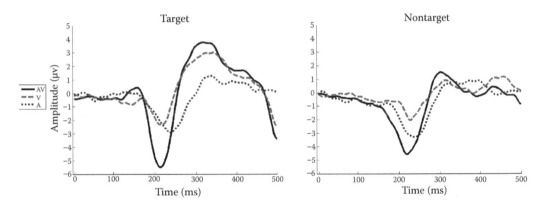

**FIGURE 27.5**  Average ERP waveforms from the "Pz" electrode for each stimulus condition among all subjects.

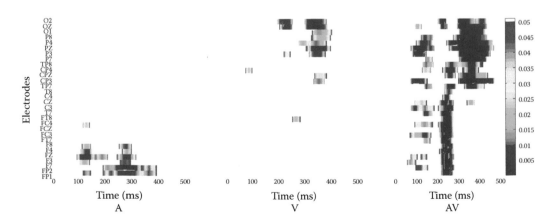

**FIGURE 27.6**  Point-wise running *t* tests were used to compare the target responses with the nontarget responses for the multisensory and unisensory stimulus conditions across all subjects for the 30 electrodes. Significant differences were plotted when data points met an alpha criterion of 0.05.

This audio-visual BCI system was applied to detect the awareness of patients with a disorder of consciousness (DOC). Currently, clinical diagnosis and awareness evaluations of patients with a DOC, such as patients in a vegetative state (VS) or a minimally conscious state (MCS), rely mainly on behavioral observation scales, such as the Coma Recovery Scale–Revised. There exists a high misdiagnosis rate (ranging from 37% to 43%) because these patients cannot provide sufficient behavioral responses. Detecting awareness in these patients is extremely challenging. Recently, the potential applications of BCIs in awareness detection and online communication for DOC patients have been explored in several studies (Coyle et al. 2012; Lulé et al. 2012). However, DOC patients with severe brain injuries have a much lower ability to use BCIs than healthy individuals. One possible solution is to apply the aforementioned audio-visual BCI to improve sensitivity in awareness detection. Seven patients with DOC performed a calibration run of 10 trials and a test run of 50 trials. Specifically, the test run contained five blocks, each of which was composed of 10 trials and was conducted on separate days because the patients became easily fatigued. Among the seven patients, the online accuracies for five patients (one VS and four MCS) were significantly higher than the chance level. For each of the five patients, the ERP waveforms measured at the "Fz" and "Oz" electrodes showed robust P300 responses elicited by the target stimuli. The results demonstrated the presence of command following and residual number recognition in the five DOC patients.

## 27.3.2 Audio-Tactile P300 BCIs

The aforementioned bimodal BCIs require visual interactions in terms of attending to stimuli and feedback, which limits their applicability to users with good visual acuity and intact gaze control. Because users require no visual interaction when operating auditory or tactile BCIs, auditory/tactile-based bimodal stimulus approaches may allow for visual saccade-independent BCIs. In a previous study, Yin et al. proposed a direction-congruent bimodal P300 BCI using the simultaneous presentation of auditory and tactile stimuli from the same spatial direction (Yin et al. 2015).

As shown in Figure 27.7, four selectable items were set up in the BCI system. The speakers and motors were placed at corresponding locations around the user such that the auditory-tactile stimuli from each speaker–motor pair represented one selectable item associated with a distinct spatial direction. Specifically, auditory stimuli were randomly delivered from one of four speakers, which played a short digital message in a female or male voice. Tactile stimuli were delivered in each target direction by two motors, oscillating between low- and high-power states to maximize tactile sensitivity. The bimodal stimulus duration was 200 ms, with an ISI of 200 ms. The users were

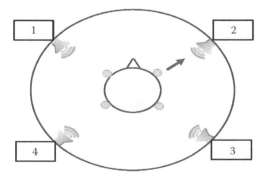

**FIGURE 27.7** Schematic of the audio-tactile BCI. The auditory and tactile stimuli were simultaneously presented from a random direction. Each shaded circle represents a pair of motors mounted at waist level. The arrow represents the stimulus direction to which the participant is focusing attention (front-right in this case). The boxed numbers represent the auditory stimuli. (Modified from Yin, E., T. Zeyl, R. Saab, D. Hu, Z. Zhou, and T. Chau. 2015. An auditory-tactile visual saccade-independent P300 brain–computer interface. *International Journal of Neural Systems* no. 26 (1):1650001.)

instructed to simultaneously focus their attention on the target stimulus according to the pre-trial auditory prompt while ignoring the stimuli from the other directions (nontargets).

Twelve healthy subjects participated in the experiments. Each subject took part in three sessions corresponding to bimodal auditory-tactile, auditory-only, and tactile-only conditions. Each session consisted of 15 runs, comprising a training phase and an online selection phase, with 150 selections in total. The experimental results showed that the bimodal approach achieved a higher average accuracy of 88.67% than the auditory (79.17%) and tactile (80.50%) approaches. Furthermore, the average ITR of the bimodal approach (10.77 bits/min) improved by 45.43% ($p < 0.05$) compared to the auditory approach (7.41 bits/min) and by 51.05% ($p < 0.001$) compared to the tactile approach (7.13 bits/min). These findings suggest that the proposed bimodal system is a promising practical visual saccade-independent P300 potential BCI.

Audio-tactile BCI study is still at the initial stages of research and development. For instance, Rutkowski and Mori reported a tactile and bone-conduction auditory BCI for vision- and hearing-impaired users (Rutkowski and Mori 2015). These existing results revealed several advantages of audio-tactile BCIs. First, the audio-tactile bimodal BCI yielded better overall system performance than both the auditory or tactile unimodal P300 BCIs. Second, audio-tactile BCIs offer the attractive possibility of targeting sensory domains that do not rely on visual stimuli to elicit potentials during visual computer applications, although the performances achieved using such systems are lower than the performances of gaze shift–dependent BCI systems. Third, audio-tactile BCIs represent an alternative type of BCI for users suffering from impaired vision.

In this section, we reviewed several promising multisensory hybrid BCIs, including audio-visual P300 BCIs and audio-tactile P300 BCIs. Initial results regarding visual-tactile BCIs have also been reported (Brouwer et al. 2010; Thurlings et al. 2012). For instance, Thurlings et al. investigated the effects of bimodal visual-tactile stimuli presentation on ERP components and discovered enhanced early components (N1) that may improve BCI performance (Thurlings et al. 2012).

## 27.4 HYBRID BCIs BASED ON MULTIPLE SIGNALS

To establish a hybrid BCI system, multiple signals can be used, including EEG, MEG, fMRI, EOG, NRIS, and EMG, as reported in Fazli et al. (2012), Kauhanen et al. (2006), Khan et al. (2014), Koo et al. (2015), Leeb et al. (2011), Lin et al. (2016), Ma et al. (2014), Punsawad et al. (2010), Soekadar et al. (2015), and Wang et al. (2014).

The variety of brain signals has different signal characteristics (shown in Table 27.1) and can be used therefore for distinct functions. For instance, brain signals can be categorized according to the manner of deployment as being invasive or noninvasive. On one hand, invasive methods are implemented by placing electrodes on the surface of the cortex (i.e., ECoG) and thus provide good signal quality with high temporal and spatial resolution. However, they require surgery for deployment and

**TABLE 27.1**
**Properties of Different Brain Signal Acquisition Modalities**

|  | EEG | MEG | fMRI | NIRS | ECoG |
|---|---|---|---|---|---|
| Deployment | Noninvasive | Noninvasive | Noninvasive | Noninvasive | Invasive |
| Temporal resolution | Good | Good | Low | Low | High |
| Spatial resolution | Low | Low | Good | Low | High |
| Cost | Low | High | High | Low | High |
| Portability | High | Low | Low | High | High |

*Note:* EEG, electroencephalography; MEG, magnetoencephalography; fMRI, functional magnetic resonance imaging; NIRS, near-infrared spectroscopy; ECoG, electrocorticography.

extreme care for stability and against possible infections. On the other hand, noninvasive methods measure the activity from the scalp and hence do not carry the same risks as invasive methods. Thus, they are used more frequently in human research.

Among noninvasive methods, EEG and NIRS are portable, easily deployable, and relatively inexpensive devices. Their wireless implementations are also feasible, making them even more convenient to use. In this respect, MEG and fMRI are immobile machines and require good shielding from the environment, so they are bound to controlled laboratory environments. The EEG and MEG measurements have high temporal resolution, whereas fMRI and NIRS measure the blood oxygenation in the brain, which is a much slower correlate of the brain activity (i.e., lower temporal resolution). Noninvasive methods provide lower spatial resolution in comparison to invasive ones. Among noninvasive methods, fMRI has relatively higher spatial resolution, as it can sample the activity of deep brain structures. In the following, we present several EEG-and-EMG–based BCIs and EEG-and-EOG–based BCIs.

## 27.4.1 EEG-and-EMG–Based BCIs

Practical BCIs for disabled persons should allow the best available remaining functionalities to be exploited. Sometimes, these users have residual activity of their muscles, and therefore, EEG and EMG signals can be combined in a BCI system. Such a combination allows for very reliable control and smooth handover, even though subjects may become fatigued or exhausted during the day (Leeb et al. 2011; Lin et al. 2016).

Leeb et al. proposed a hybrid BCI combining EEG and EMG (Leeb et al. 2011). Twelve healthy subjects participated in a synchronous experiment, which included four runs composed of 30 trials each. In each trial, the subject was instructed to perform repetitive movements with the left or right hand (i.e., clutching the hand in a fist) for a period of 5 s depending on a visual cue (an arrow pointing to the left or right).

The EEG and EMG signals were separately processed and classified and then fused. The EEG signals were recorded over the motor cortex using 16 electrodes. Using a Laplacian filter, the power spectral density of the EEG was estimated in the band of 4–48 Hz. A canonical variate analysis was used to select the subject-specific features that maximized the separability between the different tasks, and the stable features determined according to cross-validation with the training data were used to train a Gaussian classifier. EMG signals were recorded from four channels over the flexor and extensor muscles of the right and left forearms. The prehensile EMG signals were rectified and averaged (0.3 s) to extract the envelopes. The resulting features thresholded in a subject-specific manner, normalized, and classified based on the maximum distance. Finally, the two classifier probabilities were fused using a native Bayesian approach to generate one control signal (see the details in Leeb et al. 2011).

The accuracy was 73% for EEG activity alone and 87% for EMG activity alone. However, the accuracy was improved to 91% in the hybrid BCI. Furthermore, to simulate fatigue of exhausted muscles, the amplitudes of the EMG channels were degraded over the run time (attenuation from 10% up to 100%), such that the EEG activity became increasingly more important in the fusion data as the EMG muscles became more fatigued. The results showed that increased muscle fatigue led to a moderate and graceful degradation of performance. The subjects could achieve good control of their hybrid BCI independent of their level of muscle fatigue. This represents a distinct advantage of EEG-and-EMG–based BCI systems.

## 27.4.2 EEG-and-EOG–Based BCIs

Because many disabled persons retain control of their eye movements, for many users, EOG signals are an appropriate option as an input signal for BCI systems. Recently, several studies have combined EEG and EOG to construct hybrid BCIs (Ma et al. 2014; Punsawad et al. 2010; Soekadar et al. 2015; Wang et al. 2014).

In Ma et al. (2014), EOG and EEG signals were combined to control a multifunctional robot. The GUI of the ERP paradigm used in Ma et al. (2014) included eight arrow icons placed in eight directions on the screen (N, W, S, E, NW, NE, SW, SE), where each icon represented one ERP command. For one trial, stimuli (invert facial images) were displayed upon each arrow icon once in a random order. Each stimulus was presented for 100 ms with a 100-ms ISI. When the user focuses on one target icon, the stimulus that flashed on that icon evokes ERPs, including P300 potentials, vertex positive potentials (VPPs), and N170 potentials. In the EOG paradigm, the EOG signals, including vertical EOGs and horizontal EOGs, were used to detect four types of eye movements: blink, frown, wink, and gaze. More specifically, the system detected double blinks, triple blinks, and frowns based on the vertical EOG and detected winks (left/right) and gazes (toward left/right) based on the horizontal EOG.

This hybrid BCI functioned in two modes, an EOG mode and an EEG mode. The two subsystems had separate functions: the EOG-based subsystem was employed for fast-response tasks, and the EEG (ERP)-based subsystem was used for menu-selection tasks. In EOG mode, the system was asynchronous, which indicates that the system continually detects eye movements and that users can send commands using EOG at any time. In EEG mode, the system was synchronous, indicating that there must be an external command to enable/disable the system and that the subject must follow the system's predefined pace. Here, a frown detected via the eye movement paradigm was used to switch between the EOG and EEG modes.

The EOG and EEG signals were processed separately. For EOG processing, a simple multi-threshold algorithm was proposed for all four types of eye movements, and the details are presented in Ma et al. (2014). The speed, amplitude, and duration of EOGs were used as features to determine an eye movement event. The threshold values were determined by a calibration process before each experiment. For EEG processing, a 700-ms data segment was extracted from the beginning of each flash stimulus and baseline-corrected based on a 100-ms prestimulus interval. A total of 320 such data segments consisting of 40 targets and 280 nontargets were obtained for each subject. Each segment was down-sampled to obtain a data vector with a length of 15. The training samples (i.e., feature vectors) were then formed by the concatenation of 15 temporal points of data segments from eight channels. The extracted feature vectors were used to train an LDA classifier for subsequent online classification.

Two online experiments that included 13 subjects were carried out to verify the proposed system. One experiment was conducted to control a multifunctional humanoid robot, and the other was conducted to control multiple mobile robots. EOG commands were used to control the robots' movements, and ERP commands were used to activate the robots' preprogrammed behaviors or to select the control target for multiple robots. The first experiment stimulated a scenario in which the user controlled a humanoid robot to engage in simple communication with other people. The second experiment simulated a scenario in which the user controlled multiple robots to move around and gather information. In each experiment, most of the subjects achieved satisfactory performance, and a few subjects were even able to complete tasks with performances that were comparable to hand operations. The experimental results suggested that there is a complementary effect between eye movements and ERP paradigms and also suggested that this hybrid interface is promising for various BCI applications. Combining eye movements and ERPs can potentially make full use of the advantages of both systems. Using eye movements, the system can achieve a very high ITR, which compensates for the greatest weakness of ERP interfaces. A GUI incorporating ERPs can allow for many commands to be easily integrated and supported.

In this section, we described several promising hybrid BCIs based on multiple signals, including EEG-and-EMG–based BCIs and EEG-and-EOG–based BCIs, and we highlighted their advantages based on the various signal characteristics. Other types of hybrid BCIs based on multiple signals have also been reported, such as EEG-and-fMRI–based BCIs (Krebs and Hogan 2006; Leeb et al. 2011), EEG-and-fNIRS–based BCIs (Fazli et al. 2012), EEG-and-MEG–based BCIs (Kauhanen et al. 2006), and NIRS-and-fMRI–based BCIs (Cui et al. 2011; Hoge et al. 2005; Mehagnoul-Schipper et al. 2002; Strangman et al. 2002).

## 27.5　HYBRID BCIs BASED ON MULTIPLE INTELLIGENT TECHNIQUES

In recent years, several BCIs that are combined with other intelligent systems have been developed to achieve shared control. These shared control techniques incorporate the strengths of both the user and the assistive device by allowing each user to control different aspects of the system in situations that require contributions from both the user and the assistive device, that is, shared control. In a shared controller, each task incorporates simultaneous contributions from both the assistive device and the human operator, meaning that the tasks are not controlled in a mutually exclusive manner concerning user and machine command signals. In this section, we introduce these shared control systems and discuss several intelligent wheelchairs that are based on BCIs and autonomous navigation systems, in addition to several rehabilitative systems based on BCIs and intelligent robots.

### 27.5.1　An Intelligent Wheelchair Based on a BCI and an Autonomous Navigation System

To control a wheelchair, multi-objective control commands, including start and stop controls, directional control, and speed control, are needed. The task of producing numerous control signals is challenging for an EEG-based BCI. Although multiple control signals can also be obtained using the aforementioned hybrid BCIs (Long et al. 2012a), producing an accurate control command is time-consuming. Furthermore, the continuous control of a wheelchair based on a BCI may induce a heavy mental burden for the user, especially for disabled patients. One feasible solution is to integrate a BCI with automated navigation techniques and to implement shared control.

In a previous study, Zhang et al. develop an intelligent wheelchair that combines an MI- or P300-based BCI and an autonomous navigation system (Zhang et al. 2016). As shown in Figure 27.8, the wheelchair is equipped with a laser range finder (LRF), two encoders, and an array of three ultrasonic sensors. Specifically, an LRF and two encoders are employed to track the position of the wheelchair in real time. An array of three ultrasonic sensors fixed in the front of the wheelchair is used to prevent collisions when new dynamic obstacles, such as pedestrians or pets, appear near the wheelchair. The users first select one of the candidate destinations using the MI- or P300 potential-based BCI system. According to the determined destination and the current location of

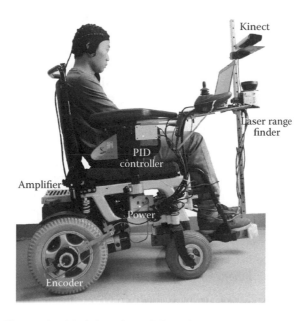

**FIGURE 27.8**　An intelligent wheelchair based on a BCI and an autonomous navigation system.

the wheelchair, the autonomous navigation system plans a path and then navigates the wheelchair to the destination.

To validate the effectiveness of this intelligent wheelchair, two experiments, an experiment based on MI and an experiment based on P300 potentials, were conducted. The experimental results demonstrated the effectiveness of this system and the several advantages of the system, as follows: (i) The candidate destinations and paths are automatically generated based on the current environment, as detected by two webcams, allowing the system to adapt to changes in the environment. (ii) Once the user selects a destination with the BCI, the wheelchair automatically navigates to the destination, and the user does not need to issue additional mental commands. Thus, the user's required workload is significantly decreased. (iii) While the wheelchair is in motion, the user can issue a stop command via the BCI.

## 27.5.2 A REHABILITATIVE SYSTEM BASED ON A BCI AND AN INTELLIGENT ROBOT

Hybrid BCIs based on multiple intelligent techniques can also be designed by combining a BCI system and an intelligent robot or a prosthesis. Motor recovery after stroke is known to be influenced by enhanced activity of the ipsilesional primary motor cortex induced by motor training. On one hand, studies have shown that effective movement therapy can be delivered by robots (Krebs and Hogan 2006). When a patient is unable to move, the robot provides guidance and assistance to the patient by performing movements with the stroke-affected limb. On the other hand, MI shares many cognitive aspects of movement without including movement execution and thus provides a substitute for movement execution as a means to activate the primary motor cortex. By reestablishing contingency between cortical activity related to MI and robotic feedback, BCIs that incorporate robot-assisted movement feedback might strengthen the sensorimotor loop and foster neuroplasticity that could facilitate motor recovery. Using this hybrid approach, several rehabilitative systems have been designed that employ an MI-BCI–controlled robot to provide motor feedback to the patient.

Ang et al. combined an MI-based BCI and a haptic knob (HK) robot for arm rehabilitation of stroke patients (Ang et al. 2014). The system setup comprised an EEG cap, EMG electrodes, an EEG amplifier, and an HK robot. During training with the HK robot, the subjects were comfortably seated and instructed to imagine opening and closing their stroke-impaired hand while voluntary movements were restrained by static resistance from the HK robot. Specifically, instructions and feedback were provided via a computer screen to indicate the progress of the HK robot–assisted physical therapy in the form of a picture manipulation task in which a solid frame represented the current position and a dotted frame represented the target position. The EEG-based BCI was used to detect MI while the HK robot provided movement feedback to the subjects.

Twenty-one chronic hemiplegic stroke patients (Fugl-Meyer Motor Assessment [FMMA] score 10–50) were randomly allocated to BCI-HK, HK, or standard arm therapy (SAT) groups. All groups received 18 sessions of intervention for 6 weeks comprising 3 sessions per week and 90 min per session (see the details in Ang et al. 2014). The experimental results showed that the FMMA scores improved in all groups, although no intergroup differences were found at any time points. Significantly larger motor gains were observed in the BCI-HK group than in the SAT group at weeks 3, 12, and 24, but the motor gains of the HK group did not differ from the SAT group at any time point. In conclusion, BCI-HK is effective, is safe, and may have the potential to enhance the motor recovery of chronic stroke patients when combined with therapist-assisted arm mobilization. Similar benefits were observed in another study that investigated chronic stroke patients who utilized an MI-BCI system that included hand and arm orthoses feedback versus those who received random orthoses feedback not linked to the BCI (Ramos-Murguialday et al. 2013), suggesting a possible advantage of the use of robot-assisted BCIs in rehabilitation following stroke.

Other hybrid BCIs for shared control have also been reported. For instance, a previous study (Iturrate et al. 2009) reported shared control of a wheelchair based on multi-stages. At each stage, a 3D environmental map, which presented a set of distributed candidate destinations to the user, was constructed using an LRF. After the user selected a destination using a P300 potential-based BCI, the wheelchair autonomously moved to the selected destination based on the navigation system. Through a series of destination selections and navigations, the final destination could be reached. In another previous study (Ang et al. 2011), a rehabilitative system in which an MI-based BCI was combined with the Inmotion[2] MIT-Manus planar shoulder and elbow robotic arm was proposed for stroke patients. The BCI was used to detect MI while the MIT-Manus robot provided movement feedback to the subjects. In summary, hybrid BCIs combined with other intelligent systems may be more reliable, usable, and powerful than traditional "simple" BCI systems.

## 27.6 DISCUSSIONS AND CONCLUSION

This chapter reviewed the state-of-the-art hybrid BCI techniques. We first described four classes of hybrid BCIs: hybrid BCIs based on multibrain patterns, multisensory hybrid BCIs, hybrid BCIs based on multiple signals, and hybrid BCIs based on multiple intelligent techniques. However, this categorization is not strict because different classes of hybrid BCIs may overlap. For instance, a multisensory hybrid BCI may elicit two or more brain patterns. Next, we briefly analyzed these four classes of hybrid BCI systems, including discussions of their principles, paradigms, experimental results, advantages, and applications. In the following section, we provide several concluding remarks and future studies.

Considering the four classes of hybrid BCIs and their respective applications, we may summarize two fundamental advantages of hybrid BCIs (Li et al. 2016).

1. Improving target detection performance. Hybrid BCIs have been shown to improve target detection performance, as outlined in the aforementioned sections. The two major strategies that lead to these improvements are as follows: (1) The combination of multiple brain patterns, for example, MI-based ERD/ERS, P300 potentials, and SSVEPs, or multiple signals, such as EEG, EMG, EOG, or NIRS. The fusion of multiple brain patterns or multiple signals can be performed at the feature level (e.g., Horki et al. 2011) or at the output level (e.g., Krebs and Hogan 2006; Leeb et al. 2011; Li et al. 2013); (2) The enhancement of brain patterns through the presentation of multisensory stimuli, such as audio-visual stimuli (Wang et al. 2015).
2. Multidimensional/function control. Herein, the implementation of multidimensional or function control based on hybrid BCIs and several application systems have been presented. Three main methods can be used: (1) combining multiple brain patterns to obtain multiple independent control signals, for example, MI-and-P300–based 2D cursor control (Li et al. 2010) and MI-and-SSVEP–based orthosis control (Pfurtscheller et al. 2010b); (2) employing different signal characteristics to perform distinct functions, for example, EEG-and-EOG–based robot control (Ma et al. 2014); and (3) incorporating BCIs with other intelligent systems to achieve shared control, for example, an intelligent wheelchair based on a BCI and an autonomous navigation system (Zhang et al. 2016).

Here, we consider several challenges for further study, and the details are presented in Li et al. (2016). A hybrid BCI system may involve multibrain patterns, multisensory modalities, multiple signal inputs, or multiple intelligent systems. To ensure the effective coordination of these components in a hybrid BCI system, investigations into the related brain mechanisms are needed. However, there have been few brain mechanism studies for hybrid BCIs until now.

Moreover, noninvasive brain stimulation by means of repetitive transcranial magnetic stimulation (rTMS) or transcranial direct current stimulation (tDCS) has driven important discoveries in the field of human memory functions. In recent studies (Capotosto et al. 2015; Roy et al. 2014;

Sparing and Mottaghy 2008), researchers have combined rTMS/tDCS with EEG or fNIRS to assess issues such as location and timing of brain activity, connectivity and plasticity of neural circuits, and functional relevance of a circumscribed brain area to a given cognitive task. Further studies should extend the use of these hybrid approaches from research tools in neuroscience to the treatment of neurological and psychiatric patients.

Furthermore, future studies should focus on the design and implementation of hybrid BCIs. When designing a hybrid BCI based on multibrain patterns, one challenge is identifying the best combination of brain patterns, which will likely differ considerably across users, to accomplish the desired goals (Pfurtscheller et al. 2010a). In designing a multisensory hybrid BCI, one challenge is ensuring that the desired brain patterns are enhanced by the multisensory stimuli. In the future, we may consider more combinations of multisensory stimuli involving visual, auditory, and tactile modalities. For hybrid BCIs based on multiple signals, one challenge is ensuring that the advantages of the different signals are fully exploited, thereby improving the system performance. Furthermore, one should also consider the real-time hybrid BCIs based on EEG and fMRI because of the following factors: high noise in EEG data (produced by fMRI scanner), slow BOLD responses, high dimension, and low time resolution of fMRI data. One potential application of this type of hybrid BCIs is in brain mechanism studies of BCIs. When designing hybrid BCIs for shared control, the paradigm of man–machine adaptation/learning for optimizing the coupling of the user and the machine and establishing a model that can effectively merge the user's intention and the machine's decision must be considered. Future studies should focus on these problems. Until now, most hybrid BCI systems, for example, BCI browsers and BCI wheelchairs, as discussed in this chapter, have been designed based on healthy subjects. These systems need to be extended for use by patients, carefully considering the major differences between healthy subjects and patients.

## ACKNOWLEDGMENTS

This work was supported by the National Key R&D Program of China under grant 2017YFB1002505; the National Natural Science Foundation of China under Grants 61633010, 91420302, and 61503143; the Guangdong Natural Science Foundation under Grants 2014A030312005 and 2014A030310244; and the Pearl River S&T Nova Program of Guangzhou under Grant 201710010038.

## REFERENCES

Allison, B., T. Luth, D. Valbuena, A. Teymourian, I. Volosyak, and A. Graser. 2010b. BCI demographics: How many (and what kinds of) people can use an SSVEP BCI? *IEEE Transactions on Neural Systems & Rehabilitation Engineering: A Publication of the IEEE Engineering in Medicine & Biology Society* no. 18 (2):107–116.

Allison, B. Z., C. Brunner, C. Altstätter, I. C. Wagner, S. Grissmann, and C. Neuper. 2012. A hybrid ERD/SSVEP BCI for continuous simultaneous two dimensional cursor control. *Journal of Neuroscience Methods* no. 209 (2):299.

Allison, B. Z. 2010. Toward ubiquitous BCIs. In *Brain–Computer Interfaces*, 357–387. Springer.

Allison, B. Z., C. Brunner, V. Kaiser, G. R. Müller-Putz, C. Neuper, and G. Pfurtscheller. 2010a. Toward a hybrid brain–computer interface based on imagined movement and visual attention. *Journal of Neural Engineering* no. 7 (2):026007.

Allison, B. Z., J. Jin, Y. Zhang, and X. Wang. 2014. A four-choice hybrid P300/SSVEP BCI for improved accuracy. *Brain–Computer Interfaces* no. 1 (1):17–26.

Allison, B. Z., E. W. Wolpaw, and J. R. Wolpaw. 2007. Brain–computer interface systems: Progress and prospects. *Expert Review of Medical Devices* no. 4 (4):463–474.

An, X., J. Höhne, D. Ming, and B Blankertz. 2014. Exploring combinations of auditory and visual stimuli for gaze-independent brain–computer interfaces. *Plos One* no. 9 (10):e111070.

Ang, K. K., C. Guan, K. S. Chua, B. T. Ang, C. W. Kuah, C. Wang, K. S. Phua, Z. Y. Chin, and H. Zhang. 2011. A large clinical study on the ability of stroke patients to use an EEG-based motor imagery brain–computer interface. *Clinical EEG and Neuroscience* no. 42 (4):253–258.

Ang, K. K., C. Guan, K. S. Phua, C. Wang, L. Zhou, K. Y. Tang, G. J. Ephraim Joseph, C. W. Kuah, and K. S. Chua. 2014. Brain–computer interface-based robotic end effector system for wrist and hand rehabilitation: Results of a three-armed randomized controlled trial for chronic stroke. *Frontiers in Neuroengineering* no. 7 (30):30.

Bai, L., T. Yu, and Y. Li. 2015. A brain computer interface-based explorer. *Journal of Neuroscience Methods* no. 244:2–7.

Belitski, A., J. Farquhar, and P. Desain. 2011. P300 audio-visual speller. *Journal of Neural Engineering* no. 8 (2):025022.

Brouwer, A. M., J. B. F. Van Erp, F. Aloise, and F. Cincotti. 2010. Tactile, visual, and bimodal P300s: Could bimodal P300s boost BCI performance? *Srx Neuroscience* no. 2010.

Capotosto, P., S. Spadone, A. Tosoni, C. Sestieri, G. L. Romani, S. Della Penna, and M. Corbetta. 2015. Dynamics of EEG rhythms support distinct visual selection mechanisms in parietal cortex: A simultaneous transcranial magnetic stimulation and EEG study. *Journal of Neuroscience* no. 35 (2):721.

Coyle, D. H., A. Carroll, J. Stow, A. Mccann, A. Ally, and J. Mcelligott. 2012. Enabling control in the minimally conscious state in a single session with a three channel BCI. *International Decoder Workshop*.

Cui, X., S. Bray, D. M. Bryant, G. H. Glover, and A. L. Reiss. 2011. A quantitative comparison of NIRS and fMRI across multiple cognitive tasks. *Neuroimage* no. 54 (4):2808.

Farwell, L. A., and E. Donchin. 1988. Talking off the top of your head: Toward a mental prosthesis utilizing event-related brain potentials. *Electroencephalography & Clinical Neurophysiology* no. 70 (6):510–523.

Fazli, S., J. Mehnert, J. Steinbrink, G. Curio, A. Villringer, K. R. Müller, and B. Blankertz. 2012. Enhanced performance by a hybrid NIRS–EEG brain computer interface. *Neuroimage* no. 59 (1):519–529.

Gürkök, H., and A. Nijholt. 2012. Brain–computer interfaces for multimodal interaction: A survey and principles. *International Journal of Human–Computer Interaction* no. 28 (5):292–307.

Guger, C., S. Daban, E. Sellers, C. Holzner, G. Krausz, R. Carabalona, F. Gramatica, and G. Edlinger. 2009. How many people are able to control a P300-based brain–computer interface (BCI)? *Neuroscience Letters* no. 462 (1):94.

Hoge, R. D., M. A. Franceschini, R. J. M. Covolan, T. Huppert, J. B. Mandeville, and D. A. Boas. 2005. Simultaneous recording of task-induced changes in blood oxygenation, volume, and flow using diffuse optical imaging and arterial spin-labeling MRI. *Neuroimage* no. 25 (3):701.

Horki, P., T. Solis-Escalante, C. Neuper, and G. Müller-Putz. 2011. Combined motor imagery and SSVEP based BCI control of a 2 DoF artificial upper limb. *Medical & Biological Engineering & Computing* no. 49 (5):567–577.

Iturrate, I., J. M. Antelis, A. Bler, and J. Minguez. 2009. A noninvasive brain-actuated wheelchair based on a P300 neurophysiological protocol and automated navigation. *IEEE Transactions on Robotics* no. 25 (3):614–627.

Jennett, B., and F. Plum. 1972. Persistent vegetative state after brain damage: A syndrome in search of a name. *The Lancet* no. 299 (7753):734–737.

Kauhanen, L., T. Nykopp, J. Lehtonen, P. Jylanki, J. Heikkonen, P. Rantanen, H. Alaranta, and M. Sams. 2006. EEG and MEG brain–computer interface for tetraplegic patients. *Neural Systems & Rehabilitation Engineering IEEE Transactions on* no. 14 (2):190–193.

Khan, M. J., M. J. Hong, and K. S. Hong. 2014. Decoding of four movement directions using hybrid NIRS–EEG brain–computer interface. *Frontiers in Human Neuroscience* no. 8 (1):244.

Koo, B., H. G. Lee, Y. Nam, H. Kang, C. S. Koh, H. C. Shin, and S. Choi. 2015. A hybrid NIRS–EEG system for self-paced brain computer interface with online motor imagery. *Journal of Neuroscience Methods* no. 244:26–32.

Krebs, H. I., and N. Hogan. 2006. Therapeutic robotics: A technology push. *Proceedings of the IEEE* no. 94 (9):1727–1738.

Leeb, R., H. Sagha, R. Chavarriaga, and J. R. Millán. 2011. A hybrid brain–computer interface based on the fusion of electroencephalographic and electromyographic activities. *Journal of Neural Engineering* no. 8 (2):025011.

Li, Y., K. A. Kai, and C. Guan. 2009. *Digital Signal Processing and Machine Learning*.

Li, Y., J. Long, T. Yu, Z. Yu, C. Wang, H. Zhang, and C. Guan. 2010. An EEG-based BCI system for 2-D cursor control by combining Mu/Beta rhythm and P300 potential. *IEEE Transactions on Biomedical Engineering* no. 57 (10):2495–2505.

Li, Y., J. Pan, J. Long, T. Yu, F. Wang, Z. Yu, and W. Wu. 2016. Multimodal BCIs: Target detection, multidimensional control, and awareness evaluation in patients with disorder of consciousness. *Proceedings of the IEEE* no. 104 (2):332–352.

Li, Y., J. Pan, F. Wang, and Z. Yu. 2013. A hybrid BCI system combining P300 and SSVEP and its application to wheelchair control. *IEEE Transactions on Biomedical Engineering* no. 60 (11):3156–3166.

Lin, K., A. Cinetto, Y. Wang, X. Chen, S. Gao, and X. Gao. 2016. An online hybrid BCI system based on SSVEP and EMG. *Journal of Neural Engineering* no. 13 (2):026020.

Long, J., Y. Li, H. Wang, T. Yu, J. Pan, and F. Li. 2012a. A hybrid brain computer interface to control the direction and speed of a simulated or real wheelchair. *IEEE Transactions on Neural Systems & Rehabilitation Engineering* no. 20 (5):720–729.

Long, J., Y. Li, T. Yu, and Z. Gu. 2012b. Target selection with hybrid feature for BCI-based 2-D cursor control. *IEEE Transactions on Biomedical Engineering* no. 59 (1):132–140.

Lulé, D., Q. Noirhomme, S. C. Kleih, C. Chatelle, S. Halder, A. Demertzi, M. A. Bruno, O. Gosseries, A. Vanhaudenhuyse, and C. Schnakers. 2012. Probing command following in patients with disorders of consciousness using a brain–computer interface. *Clinical Neurophysiology Official Journal of the International Federation of Clinical Neurophysiology* no. 124 (1):101–106.

Ma, J., Y. Zhang, A. Cichocki, and F. Matsuno. 2014. A novel EOG/EEG hybrid human–machine interface adopting eye movements and ERPs: Application to robot control. *IEEE Transactions on Biomedical Engineering* no. 62 (3):876.

Mehagnoul-Schipper, D. J., B. F. W. Van Der Kallen, W. N. J. M. Colier, M. C. Van Der Sluijs, L. J. Th. O. Van Erning, H. O. M. Thijssen, B. Oeseburg, W. H. L. Hoefnagels, and R. W. M. M. Jansen. 2002. Simultaneous measurements of cerebral oxygenation changes during brain activation by near-infrared spectroscopy and functional magnetic resonance imaging in healthy young and elderly subjects. *Human Brain Mapping* no. 16 (1):14–23.

Muller-Putz, G. R., R. Scherer, C. Neuper, and G. Pfurtscheller. 2006. Steady-state somatosensory evoked potentials: Suitable brain signals for brain–computer interfaces? *IEEE Transactions on Neural Systems & Rehabilitation Engineering* no. 14 (1):30–37.

Pan, J., Y. Li, R. Zhang, Z. Gu, and F. Li. 2013. Discrimination between control and idle states in asynchronous SSVEP-based brain switches: A pseudo-key-based approach. *IEEE Transactions on Neural Systems & Rehabilitation Engineering: A Publication of the IEEE Engineering in Medicine & Biology Society* no. 21 (3):435–443.

Panicker, R. C., S. Puthusserypady, and Y. Sun. 2011. An asynchronous P300 BCI with SSVEP-based control state detection. *IEEE Transactions on Biomedical Engineering* no. 58 (6):1781.

Pfurtscheller, G., B. Z. Allison, C. Brunner, G. Bauernfeind, T. Solis-Escalante, R. Scherer, T. O. Zander, G. Mueller-Putz, C. Neuper, and N. Birbaumer. 2010a. The hybrid BCI. *Frontiers in Neuroscience* no. 4 (30):30.

Pfurtscheller, G, and F. H. Lopes Da Silva. 1999. Event-related EEG/MEG synchronization and desynchronization: Basic principles. *Clinical Neurophysiology* no. 110 (11):1842–1857.

Pfurtscheller, G, T Solisescalante, R Ortner, P Linortner, and G. R. Müllerputz. 2010b. Self-paced operation of an SSVEP-based orthosis with and without an imagery-based "brain switch": A feasibility study towards a hybrid BCI. *IEEE Transactions on Neural Systems & Rehabilitation Engineering: A Publication of the IEEE Engineering in Medicine & Biology Society* no. 18 (4):409–414.

Punsawad, Y., Y. Wongsawat, and M. Parnichkun. 2010. Hybrid EEG–EOG brain–computer interface system for practical machine control. Paper read at the *International Conference of the IEEE Engineering in Medicine & Biology*.

Ramos-Murguialday, A., D. Broetz, M. Rea, L. Läer, O. Yilmaz, F. L. Brasil, G. Liberati, M. R. Curado, E. Garcia-Cossio, and A. Vyziotis. 2013. Brain–machine interface in chronic stroke rehabilitation: A controlled study. *Annals of Neurology* no. 74 (1):100–108.

Rebsamen, B., E. Burdet, Q. Zeng, H. Zhang, M. Ang, C. L. Teo, C. Guan, and C. Laugier. 2008. Hybrid P300 and mu-beta brain computer interface to operate a brain controlled wheelchair. Paper read at the *International Convention on Rehabilitation Engineering & Assistive Technology*.

Roy, A., B. Baxter, and B. He. 2014. High definition transcranial direct current stimulation induces both acute and persistent changes in broadband cortical synchronization: A simultaneous tDCS-EEG study. *IEEE Transactions on Biomedical Engineering* no. 61 (7):1967–1978.

Rutkowski, T. M., and H. Mori. 2015. Tactile and bone-conduction auditory brain computer interface for vision and hearing impaired users. *Journal of Neuroscience Methods* no. 244:45–51.

Soekadar, S. R., M. Witkowski, N. Vitiello, and N. Birbaumer. 2015. An EEG/EOG-based hybrid brain–neural computer interaction (BNCI) system to control an exoskeleton for the paralyzed hand. *Biomedical Engineering* no. 60 (3):199.

Sparing, R, and F. M. Mottaghy. 2008. Noninvasive brain stimulation with transcranial magnetic or direct current stimulation (TMS/tDCS)—From insights into human memory to therapy of its dysfunction. *Methods* no. 44 (4):329–337.

Stein, B. E., and T. R. Stanford. 2008. Multisensory integration: Current issues from the perspective of the single neuron. *Nature Reviews Neuroscience* no. 9 (4):255–266.

Strangman, G., J. P. Culver, J. H. Thompson, and D. A. Boas. 2002. A quantitative comparison of simultaneous BOLD fMRI and NIRS recordings during functional brain activation. *Neuroimage* no. 17 (2):719.

Thurlings, M. E., A. M. Brouwer, J. B. Van Erp, B. Blankertz, and P. J. Werkhoven. 2012. Does bimodal stimulus presentation increase ERP components usable in BCIs? *Journal of Neural Engineering* no. 9 (4):045005.

Wang, F., Y. He, J. Pan, Q. Xie, R. Yu, R. Zhang, and Y. Li. 2015. A novel audiovisual brain–computer interface and its application in awareness detection. *Scientific Reports* no. 5:9962.

Wang, H., Y. Li, J. Long, T. Yu, and Z. Gu. 2014. An asynchronous wheelchair control by hybrid EEG–EOG brain–computer interface. *Cognitive Neurodynamics* no. 8 (5):399–409.

Wolpaw, J. R., N. Birbaumer, D. J. Mcfarland, G. Pfurtscheller, and T. M. Vaughan. 2002. Brain–computer interfaces for communication and control. *Clinical Neurophysiology: Official Journal of the International Federation of Clinical Neurophysiology* no. 113 (6):767–791.

Xu, M., H. Qi, B. Wan, T. Yin, Z. Liu, and D. Ming. 2013. A hybrid BCI speller paradigm combining P300 potential and the SSVEP blocking feature. *Journal of Neural Engineering* no. 10 (2):026001.

Yin, E., T. Zeyl, R. Saab, D. Hu, Z. Zhou, and T. Chau. 2015. An auditory-tactile visual saccade-independent P300 brain–computer interface. *International Journal of Neural Systems* no. 26 (1):1650001.

Yin, E., Z. Zhou, J. Jiang, F. Chen, Y. Liu, and D. Hu. 2013. A novel hybrid BCI speller based on the incorporation of SSVEP into the P300 paradigm. *Journal of Neural Engineering* no. 10 (2):026012.

Yin, E., Z. Zhou, J. Jiang, F. Chen, Y. Liu, and D. Hu. 2014. A speedy hybrid BCI spelling approach combining P300 and SSVEP. *IEEE Transactions on Biomedical Engineering* no. 61 (2):473–483.

Yu, T., Y. Li, J. Long, and Z. Gu. 2012. Surfing the internet with a BCI mouse. *Journal of Neural Engineering* no. 9 (3):036012.

Yu, T., Y. Li, J. Long, and F. Li. 2013. A hybrid brain–computer interface-based mail client. *Computational and Mathematical Methods in Medicine* no. 2013.

Yu, T., J. Xiao, F. Wang, R. Zhang, Z. Gu, A. Cichocki, and Y. Li. 2015. Enhanced motor imagery training using a hybrid BCI with feedback. *IEEE Transactions on Biomedical Engineering* no. 62 (7):1706–1717.

Zhang, R., Y. Li, Y. Yan, H. Zhang, S. Wu, T. Yu, and Z. Gu. 2016. Control of a wheelchair in an indoor environment based on a brain–computer interface and automated navigation. *IEEE Transactions on Neural Systems & Rehabilitation Engineering: A Publication of the IEEE Engineering in Medicine & Biology Society* no. 24 (1):128–139.

# 28 Augmenting Attention with Brain–Computer Interfaces

*Mehdi Ordikhani-Seyedlar and Mikhail A. Lebedev*

## CONTENTS

28.1 Introduction .................................................................................................................549
28.2 Neuroscience of Attention ..........................................................................................550
28.3 Emergence of Attention-Based BCIs..........................................................................551
28.4 Neural Features for Attention-Based BCIs..................................................................552
    28.4.1 Importance of Feature Selection......................................................................552
    28.4.2 Neural Oscillations ..........................................................................................552
    28.4.3 Event-Related Potentials ..................................................................................553
    28.4.4 Steady-State Visual Evoked Potentials............................................................554
28.5 Future Directions.........................................................................................................554
28.6 Conclusions.................................................................................................................555
References.............................................................................................................................555

### Abstract

Brain–computer interfaces (BCIs) are rapidly gaining popularity. They can be employed in a clinic to treat neurological disorders and even to augment brain functions. Among clinical applications, BCIs can be used to treat disorders of attention. In this chapter, we review current attention-based BCIs, in particular the ones that operate in the domain of visual attention. Patients with attention deficits utilize such BCIs to improve their control of attention. We highlight the approaches for extraction of neural features relevant to attention-based BCIs. The efficiency of current clinical BCIs for augmenting attention is discussed. We conclude that although considerable advances have been made in attention-based BCIs, fundamental challenges for the optimization of such systems and their practical applications in the clinical world remain mostly unresolved.

## 28.1 INTRODUCTION

This chapter describes BCIs that operate in the domain of attention, a complex cognitive function. While attention has distinct neural manifestation, utilization of attention-related neural signals in BCIs is a difficult task because relevant signals may be obscured by irrelevant neural activities. A good understanding of neurophysiology of attention is needed to build better BCIs. Among them, extraction of relevant features is of high importance. This chapter delves into the basic neural mechanisms of attention, the ways they are manifested in the brain recordings, such as electroencephalography (EEG), features that can be extracted from these recordings, and their utilization in BCIs.

We focus mostly on visual attention because of the abundance of neurophysiological and BCI studies in this field. The visual system translates very complex input information from the external world into a stable neural representation. The emergence of such a representation can be described as a process of information reduction, where only behaviorally relevant visual inputs are processed (Sprague et al. 2015). For instance, for a driver moving toward a crossing point, it is essential to have the capacity to recognize traffic lights while disregarding insignificant light sources. Attention is the ability of the brain to suppress the superfluous sources of information and select only the relevant ones. This key brain function can suffer because of neurological conditions. Patients with disorders of attention have difficulty focusing on the relevant pieces of information and get easily distracted. Attention-deficit/hyperactivity disorder (ADHD) is a mental condition characterized by deteriorated attention, hyperactivity, and impulsivity (Biederman et al. 2000; Faraone et al. 2006). Treatment approaches to ADHD have been mostly pharmacological, such as the usage of psychostimulants. However, pharmacological treatment is often associated with unwanted side effects (Conners et al. 2001; Greenhill et al. 2001). There is also an associated substance abuse problem (Kollins 2008; Steiner et al. 2014a). Psychological therapy can be used as an alternative treatment for ADHD, but it is effective only in 30% of cases (Zarin et al. 1998).

BCIs offer a novel and potentially very effective strategy for treating attention deficits (Arns et al. 2009; Lim et al. 2010, 2012). BCIs link the brain and external devices in uni- or bidirectional ways (Donoghue et al. 2004; Lebedev 2014; Lebedev & Nicolelis 2006, 2017; Nicolelis & Lebedev 2009; Schwarz et al. 2014; Wolpaw et al. 2000). During BCI operation, neural signals are first recorded and then analyzed using mathematical methods. Following the analysis, certain features of the signals are selected and compared to template features based on control experiments in healthy subjects. Depending on how different the neural features are from the templates, the computer delivers an appropriate feedback to the person. In this context, the terms "neurofeedback," "neurofeedback therapy," "BCI," and "BCI therapy" are often used interchangeably. While many neural recording methods can be utilized by BCIs, EEG has been by far the most popular recording technology utilized in such applications (Bamdadian et al. 2014; De Vos et al. 2014; Kashihara 2014; Kus et al. 2013; Tonin et al. 2013; Yang et al. 2014). A distinct class of BCI/neurofeedback applications strives to improve attention in ADHD patients (Christiansen et al. 2014; Heinrich et al. 2014; Holtmann et al. 2014a,b; Micoulaud-Franchi et al. 2014; Steiner et al. 2014b). Optimizing attention-based BCI and making them practical is, however, quite challenging because the brain mechanisms of attention are highly sophisticated (Ming et al. 2009; Rossini et al. 2012) and it is not easy to dissociate attention-related neural activity from the other activities in the brain circuits (Sanei & Chambers 2008).

In this review, we first highlight the key findings of the neuroscience studies of attention. Next, we explain how BCIs could be used to treat attention deficits. We deliberate on several neural features that have been utilized in attention-based BCIs: neural oscillations, evoked potentials, and steady-state potentials. These considerations lead to the discussion of the problems in implementing attention BCIs and the ways these problems could be solved in the future.

## 28.2 NEUROSCIENCE OF ATTENTION

In our daily life, we constantly receive multiple sensory inputs from the external world; the amount of incoming sensory information is huge. The only way for the brain can process this information stream and generate proper behavioral responses is to filter out irrelevant incoming signals and leave only the important ones. As a result of such attentional filtering, only a tiny amount of the initial sensory information reaches higher-order areas of the brain (Posner 1994, 2012). The signals that are filtered out are still represented by neural modulations, especially at the early processing stages, but they are usually not perceived consciously. On the other hand, the relevant signals are selected by the brain attentional mechanism, and they enter the conscious processing stage. Such attentional selection is governed by a network of interconnected brain areas. One of these areas, the prefrontal cortex (PFC) has a particularly important role in the mechanisms of selective attention. PFC is activated during attentional tasks, and lesions to this area lead to attentional deficits (Ferrier 1876). Posner's laboratory has conducted a series of studies to identify the brain areas involved in attention (Fan et al. 2005; Petersen & Posner 2012; Posner & Rothbart 2007). These studies have demonstrated that multiple brain areas govern attention, and the same areas are also engaged in oculomotor control. In addition to PFC, the attentional brain network includes parietal cortical areas, the frontal eye field (FEF), subcortical nuclei, and, importantly, the superior colliculus.

Several types of attentional mechanisms have been defined in the literature. Overt and covert attention refer to attentional reactions performed with and without eye movements, respectively. According to Rizzolatti's premotor theory of attention (Rizzolatti et al. 1987), spatial attention (both overt and covert) is controlled by the same brain regions that move the eyes. The premotor theory of attention explains such overlap between the oculomotor and attentional areas in the following way: to produce overt shifts of attention, eye movements are first prepared and then executed; covert shifts of attention are also prepared by the same areas but not executed. Rizzolatti's theory gained some support from the functional magnetic resonance imaging studies that demonstrated an overlap between the cortical regions activated during both covert and overt shifts of attention (de Haan et al. 2008). Moreover, neurons in the superior colliculus, the area responsible for generation of saccades (rapid eye movement from one fixation point to another), have been shown to be involved in both overt and covert shifts of attention (Ignashchenkova et al. 2004).

Although the orientation of attention, the location of the target of movement, and gaze direction often coincide, the spatial location of attention focus can be disengaged from gaze direction (as in overt attention) and motor goals. Lebedev, Wise, and their colleagues investigated cortical representation of attention using experimental conditions that required monkeys to attend to one spatial location and also neutrally process the other as a potential target of movement. Two studies were conducted with this design. In the first study (Lebedev & Wise 2001), attention-related neuronal activity was recorded in dorsal premotor cortex (PMd). In this study, a robot served as an attention attractor, since its movements instructed monkeys when to initiate an arm-reaching movement. The arm movements were directed either to a feeder attached to the robot or a stationary feeder positioned differently from the robot. It was found that close to 20% of PMd neurons represented spatial attention instead of representing motor preparation or gaze direction. Such neurons could be involved in covert attentional shifts. In the second study (Lebedev et al. 2004), the researchers investigated how neurons in PFC represented attention and how this representation was different from the encoding of spatial locations in working memory. Monkeys were trained on an oculomotor task that required them to attend to one spatial location while remembering the other. A sizeable population of PFC neurons represented mostly attention, not the working memory. Taken together, these two series of findings indicate that a large number of frontal cortex neurons are tuned to the orientation of spatial attention.

In agreement with these findings in monkeys, human studies have shown that abnormalities of the frontal cortex have a key role in ADHDs (Dirlikov et al. 2015; Praamstra et al. 2005). In a brain imaging study by Dirlikov et al. (2015), the cortical structure was examined in 93 children with ADHD. Reductions in cortical surface were found in the PFC and premotor cortical areas (Dirlikov et al. 2015). The other neuroimaging studies demonstrated that, in ADHD, gray matter is affected in the FEF and the network of areas interconnected with it, particularly dorsal and ventral PFC, the inferior parietal cortex, and the dorsal anterior cingulate area (Szuromi et al. 2011; Valera et al. 2007). It has been suggested that the frontal lobe is involved in selective filtering of sensory information, since damage to this brain region causes ADHD (Jonkman et al. 2004). A study of resting-state EEG patterns in ADHD patients showed that frontal cortex abnormalities play a role in this disease (Keune et al. 2015).

## 28.3 EMERGENCE OF ATTENTION-BASED BCIS

After the emergence of the neurofeedback approach in the 1960s, many authors have proposed that neurofeedback could be utilized to treat attentional disorders (Elbert et al. 1980; Lutzenberger et al. 1980; Wolpaw et al. 1991). Modern attention-based BCIs employ advanced computer algorithms to decode neural signals associated with attention. In a typical BCI arrangement, subjects focus their attention on a video game. While they do so, the BCI extracts attention-related neural activities, processes them, and delivers the processed signals back to the subject, typically using visual feedback. Therapy sessions with such a BCI repeat several times, engage brain plasticity, and eventually normalize attention (Dobkin 2007; Rossini et al. 2012). Although attention-based BCIs have experienced a steady development, the outcomes of such treatment are not without controversy (Ordikhani-Seyedlar et al. 2016). Several reports described BCI training of attention as efficient (Gevensleben et al. 2009; Leins et al. 2007; Steiner et al. 2011; Wangler et al. 2011), but several other publications questioned this conclusion. Arns et al. (2009) called neurofeedback therapy for attention "efficient and specific" based on their literature analysis (Arns et al. 2009). Lofthouse et al. (2012) examined neurofeedback studies conducted from 1994 to 2010 and concluded that this approach was "probably efficacious" (Lofthouse et al. 2012). However, a different conclusion was reached by Vollebregt et at (2014a) based on a systematic review of BCIs for ADHD. They concluded that this approach had no effect on any neural functions affected by ADHD (Vollebregt et al. 2014a). Clearly, there is a need for further investigation into attention-based BCIs.

## 28.4 NEURAL FEATURES FOR ATTENTION-BASED BCIs

### 28.4.1 IMPORTANCE OF FEATURE SELECTION

Selection of neural features is an important part of BCI design (Shahid & Prasad 2011). During this signal processing stage, specific characteristics of neural activity are chosen, which are then sent to the decoding algorithm to produce neurofeedback. Depending on the BCI's principles of operation and recording method utilized, different features can be extracted from brain activity. Neuronal spikes recorded with implanted electrodes are usually converted into time-dependent discharge rates. EEG recordings are typically converted into spectral bands or event-related potentials (ERPs). The feature selection also depends on whether the BCI is endogenous (self-controlled) or exogenous (driven by an external stimulus). Subjects generate neural patterns at their will when operating endogenous BCIs, for example, using mental imagery (Nicolas-Alonso & Gomez-Gil 2012). In exogenous BCIs, external stimuli (e.g., objects shown on a screen) evoke neural responses, and subjects control these responses by directing attention and/or gaze to the stimulus of their choice.

### 28.4.2 NEURAL OSCILLATIONS

Analysis of oscillatory neural activity, for example, EEG rhythms sampled over different cortical areas, is a common method to extract neural features for endogenous BCIs. For example, EEG time-frequency analysis detects transient occurrences of neural oscillations, which in turn could be used to detect attentional shifts (Sanei & Chambers 2008). High-frequency oscillations (with a frequency greater than 30 Hz) indicate increased attention, as evident from EEG studies in humans (Kaiser & Lutzenberger 2005; Koelewijn et al. 2013; Musch et al. 2014) and intracranial recordings in monkeys (Fries et al. 2001).

Attention-related oscillations occur in the γ-band (30–80 Hz) and even higher-frequency bands (Crone et al. 2006). Ray et al. (2008) observed high-γ activity (80–150 Hz) in subjects presented with a sequence of auditory and tactile stimuli and instructed to attend to one of these modalities. Attentional shifts between the modalities resulted in high-γ activity in the cortical areas that correspond to the chosen modality, that is, auditory cortex for sounds and somatosensory cortex for tactile sensations. Furthermore, high-γ activity was elevated in PFC when subjects attended to any modality, which agrees with the suggestion that PFC is a part of the supramodal attentional system (Dirlikov et al. 2015; Keune et al. 2015). Oscillations at 350 Hz were reported in human frontal and centro-parietal regions, where they occurred in response to somatosensory stimulation (Ozaki et al. 2006). Several explanations have been proposed for the function of high-frequency oscillations during attentional shifts. According to one hypothesis, ultrahigh-frequency oscillations represent noise that has a modulatory function in neural processing (Benzi et al. 1982). Adding moderate amounts of noise to the activity of a brain circuit increases neural synchrony and decreases stimulus detection threshold (Ward et al. 2006), the effect known as stochastic resonance (Benzi et al. 1982). Similar modulations of brain circuits can be produced by adding noise to the brain activity using microstimulation (Medina et al. 2012).

Various EEG spectral bands have been utilized in the BCIs for controlling attention. For instance, human subjects can learn to modulate γ-oscillation in their superior parietal cortex by alternating between the rest state and attentive state (Grosse-Wentrup & Scholkopf 2014). In addition to using a single spectral band, attention-controlling BCIs have utilized the ratio of power in different bands as neural feature. Several BCI studies used the ratio $\beta/(\alpha + \theta)$ that increases with elevated attention (Nagendra et al. 2015). The ratio $\theta/\beta$ that decreases with elevated attention has been used as well (Clarke et al. 2013; Dupuy et al. 2013; Heinrich et al. 2014; Vollebregt et al. 2014b). In general, the slower waves such as $\theta$ and $\alpha$ rhythms are prominent in inattentive states and drowsiness, and $\beta$ rhythm increases in attentive states. In addition to EEG spectral bands, attention-based BCIs can utilize instantaneous phase of EEG oscillations as their feature (Busch et al. 2009). Busch et al. (2009) instructed subjects to detect a brief light flash that occurred either in an attended or unattended part of space. The performance on this task depended on the EEG phase at the time of stimulus occurrence. Additionally, detection errors increased in the presence of strong $\alpha$ activity, a finding that is consistent with several previous studies (Babiloni et al. 2006; Ergenoglu et al. 2004; Hanslmayr et al. 2007; Thut et al. 2006).

Several studies employed BCIs based on EEG rhythms as a treatment of ADHD. Lubar et al. (1995) treated children and adolescents with ADHD using a neurofeedback protocol that required increasing $\beta$ rhythms (16–20 Hz) and suppressing $\theta$ rhythms (4–8 Hz). Both parent ratings of their children and the performance on attention-demanding tasks improved following the training. More recently, Gevensleben et al. (2009) conducted a randomized controlled trial that assessed the efficacy of several neurofeedback protocols (based on $\theta$ and $\beta$ rhythms and slow cortical potentials) as a treatment for children with ADHD. The neurofeedback protocols were found to be more efficient compared to computerized attention skills training. In a meta-analysis study from five different studies, a total of 146 children with ADHD were considered, all trained using EEG-neurofeedback (Micoulaud-Franchi et al. 2014). This meta-analysis showed that ADHD symptoms were improved substantially after neurofeedback therapy.

### 28.4.3 Event-Related Potentials

ERPs consist of several deflections of an EEG trace after stimulus presentation; several of these deflections have been linked to attentional processing (Cohen 2013). Accordingly, ERPs have been used in numerous studies on neural mechanisms of attention (Gherri & Eimer 2011; Jones et al. 2013; Matheson et al. 2014; Wu et al. 2009; Zheng et al. 2014). ERPs recorded from cortical sensory areas increase in amplitude when the stimulus of the corresponding modality is attended to (Harter et al. 1984). For an ERP-based BCI to attain high performance, it is essential to select the optimal ERP components and scalp locations. Farwell and Donchin pioneered ERP-based BCIs in 1988 (Farwell & Donchin 1988). The participants of their experiments looked at a matrix of alphanumeric characters in a 6 × 6 arrangement. EEG activity was sampled with a single Pz electrode. The participants attended to one of the characters while the matrix columns and rows flashed. When the attended character flashed, an ERP, called P300, was evoked. Accordingly, the character could be recognized as the one that evoked the strongest P300. Approximately 30 repetitions of the character were needed to achieve good recognition accuracy.

ERP-based BCIs have a relatively slow performance, evaluated as information transfer rate (ITR). In Farwell and Donchin's experiments, the ITR of approximately 12 bits min$^{-1}$ was achieved (or 2.3 character per minute). Despite the advantage of requiring very little training time, surprisingly, P300-based BCIs have not yet been used for treatment of ADHD subjects. This is because the P300 characteristics substantially vary across trials conducted in the same subjects, as well as across different subjects. This variability is related to such factors as fatigue, mental state, motivation, and other nonstationary processes in the brain (McFarland & Wolpaw 2011). To cope with the variability, individualized calibration is needed for each subject and, additionally, calibration for different mental states of the same subject (Fazel-Rezai et al. 2012). Overall, fluctuations in P300 characteristics hinder their utilization for ADHD treatment (Furdea et al. 2009; Gonsalvez & Polich 2002; van der Waal et al. 2012).

### 28.4.4 STEADY-STATE VISUAL EVOKED POTENTIALS

Steady-state visual evoked potentials (SSVEPs) are another popular protocol used in exogenous BCIs (Lesenfants et al. 2014; Palomares et al. 2012; Reuter et al. 2015; Wu & Su 2014; Zhang et al. 2010). SSVEPs are evoked by flickering stimuli, for example, a flickering checkerboard (Punsawad & Wongsawat 2012). Such stimuli produce cortical responses that are entrained to the stimulus frequency. In BCIs, SSVEPs are typically recorded from the visual and parietal cortices. Such BCIs require a few seconds for the recognition of attended stimuli (Dmochowski et al. 2015). Several targets would flicker on a computer screen, each at a unique frequency, while a subject looks at one of the targets, and then the target with the strongest response would be identified using the analysis of the EEG spectral peaks (Bakhshayesh et al. 2011; Leins et al. 2007; Lim et al. 2010, 2012).

The performance of SSVEP-based BCIs is considerably better compared to the ERP-based BCIs (Muller-Putz & Pfurtscheller 2008). Bin et al. demonstrated an SSVEP-based BCI with an ITR of 58 ± 9.6 bits min$^{-1}$ and an accuracy of 95.3% (Bin et al. 2009). Flickering frequency of 6 Hz and higher is needed to achieve this level of performance. Recently, visual flicker of up to 100 Hz was implemented in a BCI demonstrated by Dreyer and Herrmann (2015). Subjects are comfortable with such high-frequency stimulation because they do not perceive flicker of 40 Hz and higher (Lin et al. 2012). Sakurada et al. (2015) reported that an SSVEP-based BCI with the frequency above 50–60 Hz eliminated visual fatigue while improving the performance (Sakurada et al. 2015). Training time also improves, notably in ADHD patients for whom the flicker is especially irritating (Kooij & Bijlenga 2014). In some cases, harmonics of the flicker frequency provide a better readout compared to the spectral band at the stimulation frequency (Allison et al. 2010; Muller-Putz & Pfurtscheller 2008; Ordikhani-Seyedlar et al. 2014). Additionally, SSVEP-based designs can be combined with ERP-based designs to improve the performance further. For example, Muller and Hillyard (2000) designed such an experiment where SSVEP and ERPs were captured at the same time. This study showed that there is a significant correlation between N1 and N2 components of ERP with SSVEP, whereas no such correlation was found between the P300 component.

An SSVEP-based BCI has been proposed as a potential method for training attention in ADHD patients (Ali & Puthusserypady 2015). The BCI settings incorporated a 3D classroom environment with 2D games played on the blackboard, and SSVEP features. Tests in healthy subjects showed that the attentional demands could be increased by changing the difficulty level of the game.

## 28.5 FUTURE DIRECTIONS

The development of the BCI field has been quite spectacular during the last decade. While the focus of many BCI studies has been on the enabling motor and sensory functions to disabled patients (Lebedev & Nicolelis 2006, 2017), the interest in BCIs that operate in the higher-order, cognitive domain has been steadily growing (Andersen et al. 2004; Mirabella & Lebedev Mcapital A 2017). Here, we reviewed the research on BCIs that work in the cognitive domain and strive to decode neural signals related to attentional control. Such attention-based BCIs have been already employed as an approach to treat ADHD, with positive results (Gevensleben et al. 2009; Leins et al. 2007;

Steiner et al. 2011; Wangler et al. 2011). In our opinion, the key future challenges for BCIs that treat attention disorders include the following:

1. Reducing noise and eliminating artifacts: Noise is common in EEG-based BCIs. It can be caused by electrical and mechanical artifacts, and it can be related to scalp muscle EMGs. Neural signals irrelevant to the targeted function can also be considered as noise because they hinder BCI operations. Dealing with noise is especially important for therapeutic BCIs because noise interference may result in unwanted functions being enhanced instead of the intended ones. As an example, the α-band is thought to be associated with the suppression of irrelevant inputs in attention tasks. However, drowsiness state also enhances the α-band, so the BCI based on this feature could increase drowsiness instead of improving attention. This issue can be handled by adding topographical information about the α-sources.

2. Improving the measurements of BCI training effects: The effectiveness of BCI-based therapy is typically evaluated using a comparison of neural features before and after the BCI training. However, such changes in neural features do not necessarily guarantee a functional improvement. For example, β-band power is often used as an indicator of a high attention level. However, different factors unrelated specifically to attention can cause an increase in β-band power, for example, suppression of voluntary movements (Zhang et al. 2008). Because of this possible confound, we suggest that the outcome of neurofeedback therapy should be evaluated using both EEG-derived measures and the measures of behavioral performance.

3. Taking individual variability into account: EEG data are variable across subjects. Variability can be manifested as intersubject differences in mental states, nonstationary EEG activity (Vidaurre et al. 2011), and variable responses to task events (Iturrate et al. 2013). Ideally, BCI algorithms should account for individual characteristics of subjects, including the way they respond to BCI training.

4. Ease of use: BCI-based training is currently conducted by an expert in EEG recordings and running BCI trials. In the future, more user-friendly ones need to be developed.

## 28.6 CONCLUSIONS

BCIs have significantly improved in recent years. They currently offer exciting opportunities not only as enablers of motor, sensory, and cognitive capabilities, but also as therapies for neural disorders. In particular, BCIs hold promise as a treatment for disorders of attention. While several BCI-based protocols for training attention have been already tested, there remain many challenges. We envision the development of BCIs for attention disorders as a multidisciplinary venture, where technical knowledge of BCIs is combined with Neuroscience and psychology expertise.

## REFERENCES

Ali, A., & Puthusserypady, S. (2015). *A 3D learning playground for potential attention training in ADHD: A brain computer interface approach.* Paper presented at the Engineering in Medicine and Biology Society (EMBC), 2015 37th Annual International Conference of the IEEE.

Allison, B. Z., Brunner, C., Kaiser, V., Muller-Putz, G. R., Neuper, C., & Pfurtscheller, G. (2010). Toward a hybrid brain–computer interface based on imagined movement and visual attention. *J Neural Eng, 7*(2), 1–9. doi:10.1088/1741-2560/7/2/026007

Andersen, R. A., Burdick, J. W., Musallam, S., Pesaran, B., & Cham, J. G. (2004). Cognitive neural prosthetics. *Trends Cogn Sci, 8*(11), 486–493. doi:10.1016/j.tics.2004.09.009

Arns, M., de Ridder, S., Strehl, U., Breteler, M., & Coenen, A. (2009). Efficacy of neurofeedback treatment in ADHD: The effects on inattention, impulsivity and hyperactivity: A meta-analysis. *Clin EEG Neurosci, 40*(3), 180–189.

Babiloni, C., Brancucci, A., Del Percio, C., Capotosto, P., Arendt-Nielsen, L., Chen, A. C., & Rossini, P. M. (2006). Anticipatory electroencephalography alpha rhythm predicts subjective perception of pain intensity. *J Pain, 7*(10), 709–717. doi:10.1016/j.jpain.2006.03.005

Bakhshayesh, A. R., Hansch, S., Wyschkon, A., Rezai, M. J., & Esser, G. (2011). Neurofeedback in ADHD: A single-blind randomized controlled trial. *Eur Child Adolesc Psychiatry, 20*(9), 481–491. doi:10.1007/s00787-011-0208-y

Bamdadian, A., Guan, C., Ang, K. K., & Xu, J. (2014). The predictive role of pre-cue EEG rhythms on MI-based BCI classification performance. *J Neurosci Methods, 235*, 138–144. doi:10.1016/j.jneumeth.2014.06.011

Benzi, R., Parisi, G., Sutera, A., & Vulpiani, A. (1982). Stochastic resonance in climatic change. *Tellus, 34*, 10–16.

Biederman, J., Mick, E., & Faraone, S. V. (2000). Age-dependent decline of symptoms of attention deficit hyperactivity disorder: Impact of remission definition and symptom type. *Am J Psychiatry, 157*(5), 816–818.

Bin, G., Gao, X., Wang, Y., Hong, B., & Gao, S. (2009). VEP-based brain–computer interfaces: Time, frequency, and code modulations. *IEEE Computational Intelligence Magazine, 4*(4), 22–26.

Busch, N. A., Dubois, J., & VanRullen, R. (2009). The phase of ongoing EEG oscillations predicts visual perception. *J Neurosci, 29*(24), 7869–7876. doi:10.1523/JNEUROSCI.0113-09.2009

Christiansen, H., Reh, V., Schmidt, M. H., & Rief, W. (2014). Slow cortical potential neurofeedback and self-management training in outpatient care for children with ADHD: Study protocol and first preliminary results of a randomized controlled trial. *Front Hum Neurosci, 8*, 943. doi:10.3389/fnhum.2014.00943

Clarke, A. R., Barry, R. J., Dupuy, F. E., McCarthy, R., Selikowitz, M., & Johnstone, S. J. (2013). Excess beta activity in the EEG of children with attention-deficit/hyperactivity disorder: A disorder of arousal? *Int J Psychophysiol, 89*(3), 314–319. doi:10.1016/j.ijpsycho.2013.04.009

Cohen, M. X. (2013). Overview of time-domain EEG analyses. *Analyzing Neural Time Series Data: Theory and Practice* (1st ed.): MIT Press.

Conners, C. K., Epstein, J. N., March, J. S., Angold, A., Wells, K. C., Klaric, J., ... Wigal, T. (2001). Multimodal treatment of ADHD in the MTA: An alternative outcome analysis. *J Am Acad Child Adolesc Psychiatry, 40*(2), 159–167. doi:10.1097/00004583-200102000-00010

Crone, N. E., Sinai, A., & Korzeniewska, A. (2006). High-frequency gamma oscillations and human brain mapping with electrocorticography. *Prog Brain Res, 159*, 275–295. doi:10.1016/S0079-6123(06)59019-3

de Haan, B., Morgan, P. S., & Rorden, C. (2008). Covert orienting of attention and overt eye movements activate identical brain regions. *Brain Res, 1204*, 102–111. doi:10.1016/j.brainres.2008.01.105

De Vos, M., Kroesen, M., Emkes, R., & Debener, S. (2014). P300 speller BCI with a mobile EEG system: Comparison to a traditional amplifier. *J Neural Eng, 11*(3), 036008. doi:10.1088/1741-2560/11/3/036008

Dirlikov, B., Shiels Rosch, K., Crocetti, D., Denckla, M. B., Mahone, E. M., & Mostofsky, S. H. (2015). Distinct frontal lobe morphology in girls and boys with ADHD. *Neuroimage Clin, 7*, 222–229. doi:10.1016/j.nicl.2014.12.010

Dmochowski, J. P., Greaves, A. S., & Norcia, A. M. (2015). Maximally reliable spatial filtering of steady state visual evoked potentials. *Neuroimage, 109*, 63–72. doi:10.1016/j.neuroimage.2014.12.078

Dobkin, B. H. (2007). Brain–computer interface technology as a tool to augment plasticity and outcomes for neurological rehabilitation. *J Physiol, 579*(Pt 3), 637–642. doi:10.1113/jphysiol.2006.123067

Donoghue, J. P., Nurmikko, A., Friehs, G., & Black, M. (2004). Development of neuromotor prostheses for humans. *Suppl Clin Neurophysiol, 57*, 592–606.

Dreyer, A. M., & Herrmann, C. S. (2015). Frequency-modulated steady-state visual evoked potentials: A new stimulation method for brain–computer interfaces. *J Neurosci Methods, 241*, 1–9. doi:10.1016/j.jneumeth.2014.12.004

Dupuy, F. E., Clarke, A. R., Barry, R. J., McCarthy, R., & Selikowitz, M. (2013). EEG differences between the combined and inattentive types of attention-deficit/hyperactivity disorder in girls: A further investigation. *Clin EEG Neurosci*. doi:10.1177/1550059413501162

Elbert, T., Rockstroh, B., Lutzenberger, W., & Birbaumer, N. (1980). Biofeedback of slow cortical potentials. I. *Electroencephalogr Clin Neurophysiol, 48*(3), 293–301.

Ergenoglu, T., Demiralp, T., Bayraktaroglu, Z., Ergen, M., Beydagi, H., & Uresin, Y. (2004). Alpha rhythm of the EEG modulates visual detection performance in humans. *Brain Res Cogn Brain Res, 20*(3), 376–383. doi:10.1016/j.cogbrainres.2004.03.009

Fan, J., McCandliss, B. D., Fossella, J., Flombaum, J. I., & Posner, M. I. (2005). The activation of attentional networks. *Neuroimage, 26*(2), 471–479. doi:10.1016/j.neuroimage.2005.02.004

Faraone, S. V., Biederman, J., & Mick, E. (2006). The age-dependent decline of attention deficit hyperactivity disorder: A meta-analysis of follow-up studies. *Psychol Med, 36*(2), 159–165. doi:10.1017/S003329170500471X

Farwell, L. A., & Donchin, E. (1988). Talking off the top of your head: Toward a mental prosthesis utilizing event-related brain potentials. *Electroencephalogr Clin Neurophysiol, 70*(6), 510–523.

Fazel-Rezai, R., Allison, B. Z., Guger, C., Sellers, E. W., Kleih, S. C., & Kubler, A. (2012). P300 brain computer interface: Current challenges and emerging trends. *Front Neuroeng, 5*, 14. doi:10.3389/fneng.2012.00014

Ferrier, D. (1876). *The Functions of the Brain*: London: Smith, Elder.

Fries, P., Reynolds, J. H., Rorie, A. E., & Desimone, R. (2001). Modulation of oscillatory neuronal synchronization by selective visual attention. *Science, 291*(5508), 1560–1563. doi:10.1126/science.291.5508.1560

Furdea, A., Halder, S., Krusienski, D. J., Bross, D., Nijboer, F., Birbaumer, N., & Kubler, A. (2009). An auditory oddball (P300) spelling system for brain–computer interfaces. *Psychophysiology, 46*(3), 617–625. doi:10.1111/j.1469-8986.2008.00783.x

Gevensleben, H., Holl, B., Albrecht, B., Vogel, C., Schlamp, D., Kratz, O., ... Heinrich, H. (2009). Is neurofeedback an efficacious treatment for ADHD? A randomised controlled clinical trial. *J Child Psychol Psychiatry, 50*(7), 780–789. doi:10.1111/j.1469-7610.2008.02033.x

Gherri, E., & Eimer, M. (2011). Active listening impairs visual perception and selectivity: An ERP study of auditory dual-task costs on visual attention. *J Cogn Neurosci, 23*(4), 832–844. doi:10.1162/jocn.2010.21468

Gonsalvez, C. J., & Polich, J. (2002). P300 amplitude is determined by target-to-target interval. *Psychophysiology, 39*(3), 388–396. doi:10.1017/S0048577201393137

Greenhill, L. L., Swanson, J. M., Vitiello, B., Davies, M., Clevenger, W., Wu, M., ... Wigal, T. (2001). Impairment and deportment responses to different methylphenidate doses in children with ADHD: The MTA titration trial. *J Am Acad Child Adolesc Psychiatry, 40*(2), 180–187. doi:10.1097/00004583-200102000-00012

Grosse-Wentrup, M., & Scholkopf, B. (2014). A brain–computer interface based on self-regulation of gamma-oscillations in the superior parietal cortex. *J Neural Eng, 11*(5), 056015. doi:10.1088/1741-2560/11/5/056015

Hanslmayr, S., Aslan, A., Staudigl, T., Klimesch, W., Herrmann, C. S., & Bauml, K. H. (2007). Prestimulus oscillations predict visual perception performance between and within subjects. *Neuroimage, 37*(4), 1465–1473. doi:10.1016/j.neuroimage.2007.07.011

Harter, M. R., Aine, C., & Schroeder, C. (1984). Hemispheric differences in event-related potential measures of selective attention. *Ann N Y Acad Sci, 425*, 210–211.

Heinrich, H., Busch, K., Studer, P., Erbe, K., Moll, G. H., & Kratz, O. (2014). EEG spectral analysis of attention in ADHD: Implications for neurofeedback training? *Front Hum Neurosci, 8*, 611. doi:10.3389/fnhum.2014.00611

Holtmann, M., Pniewski, B., Wachtlin, D., Worz, S., & Strehl, U. (2014a). Neurofeedback in children with attention-deficit/hyperactivity disorder (ADHD)—A controlled multicenter study of a non-pharmacological treatment approach. *BMC Pediatr, 14*, 202. doi:10.1186/1471-2431-14-202

Holtmann, M., Sonuga-Barke, E., Cortese, S., & Brandeis, D. (2014b). Neurofeedback for ADHD: A review of current evidence. *Child Adolesc Psychiatr Clin N Am, 23*(4), 789–806. doi:10.1016/j.chc.2014.05.006

Ignashchenkova, A., Dicke, P. W., Haarmeier, T., & Thier, P. (2004). Neuron-specific contribution of the superior colliculus to overt and covert shifts of attention. *Nat Neurosci, 7*(1), 56–64. doi:10.1038/nn1169

Iturrate, I., Montesano, L., & Minguez, J. (2013). Shared-control brain–computer interface for a two dimensional reaching task using EEG error-related potentials. *Conf Proc IEEE Eng Med Biol Soc, 2013*, 5258–5262. doi:10.1109/EMBC.2013.6610735

Jones, A., Hughes, G., & Waszak, F. (2013). The interaction between attention and motor prediction. An ERP study. *Neuroimage, 83*, 533–541. doi:10.1016/j.neuroimage.2013.07.004

Jonkman, L. M., Kenemans, J. L., Kemner, C., Verbaten, M. N., & van Engeland, H. (2004). Dipole source localization of event-related brain activity indicative of an early visual selective attention deficit in ADHD children. *Clin Neurophysiol, 115*(7), 1537–1549. doi:10.1016/j.clinph.2004.01.022

Kaiser, J., & Lutzenberger, W. (2005). Human gamma-band activity: A window to cognitive processing. *Neuroreport, 16*(3), 207–211.

Kashihara, K. (2014). A brain–computer interface for potential non-verbal facial communication based on EEG signals related to specific emotions. *Front Neurosci, 8*, 244. doi:10.3389/fnins.2014.00244

Keune, P. M., Wiedemann, E., Schneidt, A., & Schonenberg, M. (2015). Frontal brain asymmetry in adult attention-deficit/hyperactivity disorder (ADHD): Extending the motivational dysfunction hypothesis. *Clin Neurophysiol, 126*(4), 711–720. doi:10.1016/j.clinph.2014.07.008

Koelewijn, L., Rich, A. N., Muthukumaraswamy, S. D., & Singh, K. D. (2013). Spatial attention increases high-frequency gamma synchronisation in human medial visual cortex. *Neuroimage, 79*, 295–303. doi:10.1016/j.neuroimage.2013.04.108

Kollins, S. H. (2008). ADHD, substance use disorders, and psychostimulant treatment: Current literature and treatment guidelines. *J Atten Disord, 12*(2), 115–125. doi:10.1177/1087054707311654

Kooij, J. J., & Bijlenga, D. (2014). High prevalence of self-reported photophobia in adult ADHD. *Front Neurol, 5*, 256. doi:10.3389/fneur.2014.00256

Kus, R., Duszyk, A., Milanowski, P., Labecki, M., Bierzynska, M., Radzikowska, Z., ... Durka, P. J. (2013). On the quantification of SSVEP frequency responses in human EEG in realistic BCI conditions. *PLoS One, 8*(10), e77536. doi:10.1371/journal.pone.0077536

Lebedev, M. A. (2014). How to read neuron-dropping curves? *Front Syst Neurosci, 8*, 102. doi:10.3389/fnsys.2014.00102

Lebedev, M. A., Messinger, A., Kralik, J. D., & Wise, S. P. (2004). Representation of attended versus remembered locations in prefrontal cortex. *PLoS Biol, 2*(11), e365. doi:10.1371/journal.pbio.0020365

Lebedev, M. A., & Nicolelis, M. A. (2006). Brain–machine interfaces: Past, present and future. *Trends Neurosci, 29*(9), 536–546. doi:10.1016/j.tins.2006.07.004

Lebedev, M. A., & Nicolelis, M. A. (2017). Brain–machine interfaces: From basic science to neuroprostheses and neurorehabilitation. *Physiological Reviews, 97*(2), 767–837.

Lebedev, M. A., & Wise, S. P. (2001). Tuning for the orientation of spatial attention in dorsal premotor cortex. *Eur J Neurosci, 13*(5), 1002–1008.

Leins, U., Goth, G., Hinterberger, T., Klinger, C., Rumpf, N., & Strehl, U. (2007). Neurofeedback for children with ADHD: A comparison of SCP and theta/beta protocols. *Appl Psychophysiol Biofeedback, 32*(2), 73–88. doi:10.1007/s10484-007-9031-0

Lesenfants, D., Habbal, D., Lugo, Z., Lebeau, M., Horki, P., Amico, E., ... Noirhomme, Q. (2014). An independent SSVEP-based brain–computer interface in locked-in syndrome. *J Neural Eng, 11*(3), 035002. doi:10.1088/1741-2560/11/3/035002

Lim, C. G., Lee, T. S., Guan, C., Fung, D. S., Zhao, Y., Teng, S. S., ... Krishnan, K. R. (2012). A brain–computer interface based attention training program for treating attention deficit hyperactivity disorder. *PLoS One, 7*(10), e46692. doi:10.1371/journal.pone.0046692

Lim, C. G., Lee, T. S., Guan, C., Sheng Fung, D. S., Cheung, Y. B., Teng, S. S., ... Krishnan, K. R. (2010). Effectiveness of a brain–computer interface based programme for the treatment of ADHD: A pilot study. *Psychopharmacol Bull, 43*(1), 73–82.

Lin, F. C., Zao, J. K., Tu, K. C., Wang, Y., Huang, Y. P., Chuang, C. W., ... Jung, T. P. (2012). SNR analysis of high-frequency steady-state visual evoked potentials from the foveal and extrafoveal regions of human retina. *Conf Proc IEEE Eng Med Biol Soc, 2012*, 1810–1814. doi:10.1109/EMBC.2012.6346302

Lofthouse, N., Arnold, L. E., Hersch, S., Hurt, E., & DeBeus, R. (2012). A review of neurofeedback treatment for pediatric ADHD. *J Atten Disord, 16*(5), 351–372. doi:10.1177/1087054711427530

Lubar, J. F., Swartwood, M. O., Swartwood, J. N., & O'Donnell, P. H. (1995). Evaluation of the effectiveness of EEG neurofeedback training for ADHD in a clinical setting as measured by changes in T.O.V.A. scores, behavioral ratings, and WISC-R performance. *Biofeedback Self Regul, 20*(1), 83–99.

Lutzenberger, W., Elbert, T., Rockstroh, B., & Birbaumer, N. (1980). Biofeedback of slow cortical potentials. II. Analysis of single event-related slow potentials by time series analysis. *Electroencephalogr Clin Neurophysiol, 48*(3), 302–311.

Matheson, H., Newman, A. J., Satel, J., & McMullen, P. (2014). Handles of manipulable objects attract covert visual attention: ERP evidence. *Brain Cogn, 86*, 17–23. doi:10.1016/j.bandc.2014.01.013

McFarland, D. J., & Wolpaw, J. R. (2011). Brain–computer interfaces for communication and control. *Commun ACM, 54*(5), 60–66. doi:10.1145/1941487.1941506

Medina, L. E., Lebedev, M. A., O'Doherty, J. E., & Nicolelis, M. A. (2012). Stochastic facilitation of artificial tactile sensation in primates. *J Neurosci, 32*(41), 14271–14275. doi:10.1523/JNEUROSCI.3115-12.2012

Micoulaud-Franchi, J. A., Geoffroy, P. A., Fond, G., Lopez, R., Bioulac, S., & Philip, P. (2014). EEG neurofeedback treatments in children with ADHD: An updated meta-analysis of randomized controlled trials. *Front Hum Neurosci, 8*, 906. doi:10.3389/fnhum.2014.00906

Ming, D., Xi, Y., Zhang, M., Qi, H., Cheng, L., Wan, B., & Li, L. (2009). Electroencephalograph (EEG) signal processing method of motor imaginary potential for attention level classification. *Conf Proc IEEE Eng Med Biol Soc, 2009*, 4347–4351. doi:10.1109/IEMBS.2009.5332743

Mirabella, G., & Lebedev Mcapital A, C. (2017). Interfacing to the brain's motor decisions. *J Neurophysiol, 117*(3), 1305–1319. doi:10.1152/jn.00051.2016

Muller-Putz, G. R., & Pfurtscheller, G. (2008). Control of an electrical prosthesis with an SSVEP-based BCI. *IEEE Trans Biomed Eng, 55*(1), 361–364. doi:10.1109/TBME.2007.897815

Muller, M. M., & Hillyard, S. (2000). Concurrent recording of steady-state and transient event-related potentials as indices of visual-spatial selective attention. *Clin Neurophysiol, 111*(9), 1544–1552.

Musch, K., Hamame, C. M., Perrone-Bertolotti, M., Minotti, L., Kahane, P., Engel, A. K., ... Schneider, T. R. (2014). Selective attention modulates high-frequency activity in the face-processing network. *Cortex, 60*, 34–51. doi:10.1016/j.cortex.2014.06.006

Nagendra, H., Kumar, V., & Mukherjee, S. (2015). Cognitive behavior evaluation based on physiological parameters among young healthy subjects with yoga as intervention. *Comput Math Methods Med, 2015*, 821061. doi:10.1155/2015/821061

Nicolas-Alonso, L. F., & Gomez-Gil, J. (2012). Brain computer interfaces, a review. *Sensors (Basel), 12*(2), 1211–1279. doi:10.3390/s120201211

Nicolelis, M. A., & Lebedev, M. A. (2009). Principles of neural ensemble physiology underlying the operation of brain–machine interfaces. *Nat Rev Neurosci, 10*(7), 530–540. doi:10.1038/nrn2653

Ordikhani-Seyedlar, M., Lebedev, M. A., Sorensen, H. B. D., & Puthusserypady, S. (2016). Neurofeedback therapy for enhancing visual attention: State-of-the-art and challenges. *Front Neurosci, 10*(352). doi:10.3389/fnins.2016.00352

Ordikhani-Seyedlar, M., Sorensen, H. B., Kjaer, T. W., Siebner, H. R., & Puthusserypady, S. (2014). SSVEP-modulation by covert and overt attention: Novel features for BCI in attention neuro-rehabilitation. *Conf Proc IEEE Eng Med Biol Soc, 2014*, 5462–5465. doi:10.1109/EMBC.2014.6944862

Ozaki, I., Yaegashi, Y., Baba, M., & Hashimoto, I. (2006). High-frequency oscillatory activities during selective attention in humans. *Suppl Clin Neurophysiol, 59*, 57–60.

Palomares, M., Ales, J. M., Wade, A. R., Cottereau, B. R., & Norcia, A. M. (2012). Distinct effects of attention on the neural responses to form and motion processing: A SSVEP source-imaging study. *J Vis, 12*(10), 15. doi:10.1167/12.10.15

Petersen, S. E., & Posner, M. I. (2012). The attention system of the human brain: 20 years after. *Annu Rev Neurosci, 35*, 73–89. doi:10.1146/annurev-neuro-062111-150525

Posner, M. I. (1994). Attention: The mechanisms of consciousness. *Proc Natl Acad Sci USA, 91*, 7398–7403.

Posner, M. I. (2012). Attentional networks and consciousness. *Front Psychol, 3*, 64. doi:10.3389/fpsyg.2012.00064.

Posner, M. I., & Rothbart, M. K. (2007). Research on attention networks as a model for the integration of psychological science. *Annu Rev Psychol, 58*, 1–23. doi:10.1146/annurev.psych.58.110405.085516

Praamstra, P., Boutsen, L., & Humphreys, G. W. (2005). Frontoparietal control of spatial attention and motor intention in human EEG. *J Neurophysiol, 94*(1), 764–774. doi:10.1152/jn.01052.2004

Punsawad, Y., & Wongsawat, Y. (2012). Motion visual stimulus for SSVEP-based BCI system. *Conf Proc IEEE Eng Med Biol Soc, 2012*, 3837–3840. doi:10.1109/EMBC.2012.6346804

Ray, S., Niebur, E., Hsiao, S. S., Sinai, A., & Crone, N. E. (2008). High-frequency gamma activity (80–150 Hz) is increased in human cortex during selective attention. *Clin Neurophysiol, 119*(1), 116–133. doi:10.1016/j.clinph.2007.09.136

Reuter, E. M., Bednark, J., & Cunnington, R. (2015). Reliance on visual attention during visuomotor adaptation: An SSVEP study. *Exp Brain Res, 233*(7), 2041–2051. doi:10.1007/s00221-015-4275-z

Rizzolatti, G., Riggio, L., Dascola, I., & Umilta, C. (1987). Reorienting attention across the horizontal and vertical meridians: Evidence in favor of a premotor theory of attention. *Neuropsychologia, 25*(1A), 31–40.

Rossini, P. M., Noris Ferilli, M. A., & Ferreri, F. (2012). Cortical plasticity and brain computer interface. *Eur J Phys Rehabil Med, 48*(2), 307–312.

Sakurada, T., Kawase, T., Komatsu, T., & Kansaku, K. (2015). Use of high-frequency visual stimuli above the critical flicker frequency in a SSVEP-based BMI. *Clin Neurophysiol.* doi:doi:10.1016/j.clinph.2014.12.010

Sanei, S., & Chambers, J. (2008). Brain–computer interface. In S. Sanei & J. Chambers (Eds.), *EEG Signal Processing*: John Wiley & Sons.

Schwarz, D. A., Lebedev, M. A., Hanson, T. L., Dimitrov, D. F., Lehew, G., Meloy, J., ... Nicolelis, M. A. (2014). Chronic, wireless recordings of large-scale brain activity in freely moving rhesus monkeys. *Nat Methods, 11*(6), 670–676. doi:10.1038/nmeth.2936

Shahid, S., & Prasad, G. (2011). Bispectrum-based feature extraction technique for devising a practical brain-computer interface. *J Neural Eng, 8*(2), 025014. doi:10.1088/1741-2560/8/2/025014

Sprague, T. C., Saproo, S., & Serences, J. T. (2015). Visual attention mitigates information loss in small- and large-scale neural codes. *Trends Cogn Sci, 19*(4), 215–226. doi:10.1016/j.tics.2015.02.005

Steiner, H., Warren, B. L., Van Waes, V., & Bolanos-Guzman, C. A. (2014a). Life-long consequences of juvenile exposure to psychotropic drugs on brain and behavior. *Prog Brain Res, 211*, 13–30. doi:10.1016/B978-0-444-63425-2.00002-7

Steiner, N. J., Frenette, E. C., Rene, K. M., Brennan, R. T., & Perrin, E. C. (2014b). In-school neurofeedback training for ADHD: Sustained improvements from a randomized control trial. *Pediatrics, 133*(3), 483–492. doi:10.1542/peds.2013-2059

Steiner, N. J., Sheldrick, R. C., Gotthelf, D., & Perrin, E. C. (2011). Computer-based attention training in the schools for children with attention deficit/hyperactivity disorder: A preliminary trial. *Clin Pediatr (Phila), 50*(7), 615–622. doi:10.1177/0009922810397887

Szuromi, B., Czobor, P., Komlosi, S., & Bitter, I. (2011). P300 deficits in adults with attention deficit hyperactivity disorder: A meta-analysis. *Psychol Med, 41*(7), 1529–1538. doi:10.1017/S0033291710001996

Thut, G., Nietzel, A., Brandt, S. A., & Pascual-Leone, A. (2006). Alpha-band electroencephalographic activity over occipital cortex indexes visuospatial attention bias and predicts visual target detection. *J Neurosci, 26*(37), 9494–9502. doi:10.1523/JNEUROSCI.0875-06.2006

Tonin, L., Leeb, R., Sobolewski, A., & Millan Jdel, R. (2013). An online EEG BCI based on covert visuospatial attention in absence of exogenous stimulation. *J Neural Eng, 10*(5), 056007. doi:10.1088/1741-2560/10/5/056007

Valera, E. M., Faraone, S. V., Murray, K. E., & Seidman, L. J. (2007). Meta-analysis of structural imaging findings in attention-deficit/hyperactivity disorder. *Biol Psychiatry, 61*(12), 1361–1369. doi:10.1016/j.biopsych.2006.06.011

van der Waal, M., Severens, M., Geuze, J., & Desain, P. (2012). Introducing the tactile speller: An ERP-based brain–computer interface for communication. *J Neural Eng, 9*(4), 045002. doi:10.1088/1741-2560/9/4/045002

Vidaurre, C., Kawanabe, M., von Bunau, P., Blankertz, B., & Muller, K. R. (2011). Toward unsupervised adaptation of LDA for brain–computer interfaces. *IEEE Trans Biomed Eng, 58*(3), 587–597. doi:10.1109/TBME.2010.2093133

Vollebregt, M. A., van Dongen-Boomsma, M., Buitelaar, J. K., & Slaats-Willemse, D. (2014a). Does EEG-neurofeedback improve neurocognitive functioning in children with attention-deficit/hyperactivity disorder? A systematic review and a double-blind placebo-controlled study. *J Child Psychol Psychiatry, 55*(5), 460–472. doi:10.1111/jcpp.12143

Vollebregt, M. A., van Dongen-Boomsma, M., Slaats-Willemse, D., Buitelaar, J. K., & Oostenveld, R. (2014b). How the Individual alpha peak frequency helps unravel the neurophysiologic underpinnings of behavioral functioning in children with attention-deficit/hyperactivity disorder. *Clin EEG Neurosci.* doi:10.1177/1550059414537257

Wangler, S., Gevensleben, H., Albrecht, B., Studer, P., Rothenberger, A., Moll, G. H., & Heinrich, H. (2011). Neurofeedback in children with ADHD: Specific event-related potential findings of a randomized controlled trial. *Clin Neurophysiol, 122*(5), 942–950. doi:10.1016/j.clinph.2010.06.036

Ward, L. M., Doesburg, S. M., Kitajo, K., MacLean, S. E., & Roggeveen, A. B. (2006). Neural synchrony in stochastic resonance, attention, and consciousness. *Can J Exp Psychol, 60*(4), 319–326.

Wolpaw, J. R., Birbaumer, N., Heetderks, W. J., McFarland, D. J., Peckham, P. H., Schalk, G., ... Vaughan, T. M. (2000). Brain–computer interface technology: A review of the first international meeting. *IEEE Trans Rehabil Eng, 8*(2), 164–173.

Wolpaw, J. R., McFarland, D. J., Neat, G. W., & Forneris, C. A. (1991). An EEG-based brain–computer interface for cursor control. *Electroencephalogr Clin Neurophysiol, 78*(3), 252–259.

Wu, J., Li, Q., Bai, O., & Touge, T. (2009). Multisensory interactions elicited by audiovisual stimuli presented peripherally in a visual attention task: A behavioral and event-related potential study in humans. *J Clin Neurophysiol, 26*(6), 407–413. doi:10.1097/WNP.0b013e3181c298b1

Wu, Z., & Su, S. (2014). A dynamic selection method for reference electrode in SSVEP-based BCI. *PLoS One, 9*(8), e104248. doi:10.1371/journal.pone.0104248

Yang, L., Leung, H., Peterson, D. A., Sejnowski, T. J., & Poizner, H. (2014). Toward a semi-self-paced EEG brain computer interface: Decoding initiation state from non-initiation state in dedicated time slots. *PLoS One, 9*(2), e88915. doi:10.1371/journal.pone.0088915

Zarin, D. A., Suarez, A. P., Pincus, H. A., Kupersanin, E., & Zito, J. M. (1998). Clinical and treatment characteristics of children with attention-deficit/hyperactivity disorder in psychiatric practice. *J Am Acad Child Adolesc Psychiatry, 37*(12), 1262–1270. doi:10.1097/00004583-199812000-00009

Zhang, D., Maye, A., Gao, X., Hong, B., Engel, A. K., & Gao, S. (2010). An independent brain–computer interface using covert non-spatial visual selective attention. *J Neural Eng, 7*(1), 16010. doi:10.1088/1741-2560/7/1/016010

Zhang, Y., Chen, Y., Bressler, S. L., & Ding, M. (2008). Response preparation and inhibition: The role of the cortical sensorimotor beta rhythm. *Neuroscience, 156*(1), 238–246. doi:10.1016/j.neuroscience.2008.06.061

Zheng, H. Y., Peng, G., Chen, J. Y., Zhang, C., Minett, J. W., & Wang, W. S. (2014). The influence of tone inventory on ERP without focal attention: A cross-language study. *Comput Math Methods Med, 2014*, 961563. doi:10.1155/2014/961563

# Part V

## Human Factors, Design, and Evaluation in BCI

# 29 Toward Usability Evaluation for Brain–Computer Interfaces

*Ilsun Rhiu, Yushin Lee, Inchul Choi, Myung Hwan Yun, and Chang S. Nam*

## CONTENTS

29.1 Introduction ........................................................................................................564
29.2 Review Method......................................................................................................565
    29.2.1 Eligibility Criteria.....................................................................................565
    29.2.2 Study Selection .........................................................................................565
    29.2.3 Usability Framework .................................................................................566
29.3 Results....................................................................................................................569
    29.3.1 User Characteristics...................................................................................569
    29.3.2 Task Characteristics...................................................................................569
    29.3.3 Environment Characteristics .....................................................................571
    29.3.4 Technology Characteristics........................................................................573
    29.3.5 Method Characteristics..............................................................................575
    29.3.6 Measurement Characteristics ....................................................................575
29.4 Recommendations .................................................................................................579
29.5 Conclusion ............................................................................................................580
References.......................................................................................................................580

## Abstract

Along with the tremendous increase of studies related to usability in the field of human–computer interaction (HCI), researchers in brain–computer interfaces (BCI) agree that the usability is also an indispensable quality of BCI systems. From this perspective, several researchers are trying to conduct usability evaluation of BCI systems. However, many previous studies have been only focused on the performance measurement such as accuracy and information transfer rate. Moreover, among most of them, there is no well-structured usability framework that is widely used for BCI. Thus, a simple and useful framework for measuring BCI usability for researchers to conduct usability evaluation is necessary. This chapter reviews the state of the art of BCI related to usability evaluation. We conducted a systematic literature review in accord with PRISMA (Preferred Reporting Items for Systematic reviews and Meta-Analyses). A total of 279 articles from 2000 to January 2016 were obtained and reviewed. As a result, we proposed the usability framework for BCI in the perspective of User, Task, Environment, Technology, Method, and Measurement characteristics. Moreover, we provided recommendations for future usability studies of BCI that can motivate researchers and practitioners in the perspectives of human factors and ergonomics/HCI.

## 29.1   INTRODUCTION

Usability has been described by varying definitions (Nielsen 1994; Nielsen and Levy 1994; Shackel 1991) and discussed (Venkatesh et al. 2003) by both academic researchers and industrial practitioners for a long time. Those previous studies proposed that the key point of usability is that users can employ a particular technology artifact with relative ease according to a specified context of use. Moreover, usability has become an important factor in determining the acceptability and consequent success of products, computer software, user interfaces, and web pages (Nielsen 1994; Shneiderman 2010). In particular, the user interface could be a critical purchasing factor in highly competitive situations where many products have subtle difference regarding their functional capacity (Henderson et al. 1995). Users prefer to use well-designed interfaces that are easier and more comfortable to use since those interfaces allow more pleasant experiences. Thus, an attempt for evaluating the usability of user interfaces would be seen as an intrinsic element, especially for a new user interface.

Similarly, along with the tremendous increase of studies related to usability in the field of human–computer interaction (HCI), researchers in brain–computer interface (BCI) agree that the usability is also an indispensable quality of BCI systems (Bos et al. 2011a; Garcia et al. 2015; Holz et al. 2013; Kübler et al. 2014; Mora et al. 2015; Pasqualotto et al. 2015). From this perspective, several researchers are trying to conduct usability evaluation of BCI systems. Pasqualotto et al. (2012) proposed that BCI systems can be mainly evaluated in terms of efficiency, such as classification accuracy and communication speed. Moreover, several previous studies introduced the assessment of usability dimensions in their evaluation of BCI systems. With efficiency measures, Riccio et al. (2011) and Zander et al. (2010) have assessed workload and satisfaction. Also, Pasqualotto et al. (2011a,b) investigated error rate and learnability of a keyboard-controlled BCI prototype.

However, there are some limitations in those previous studies. First, many studies have been only focused on the performance measurement such as accuracy and information transfer rate (ITR). Because of the lack of previous qualitative studies related to heuristic evaluation for usability of BCI, it is difficult to figure out if proposed BCI systems can be easily used for the public. Second, there is no well-structured usability framework that is widely used for BCI. As Charlton and O'Brien (1996) mentioned, evaluations are not always planned systematically, but are often conducted based on the preference of the evaluator without careful considerations of various issues of usability evaluation. This is likely to result in irrelevant or useless results, and the evaluation efforts may turn out to be inefficient and unstructured. A practical support is particularly important for the measurement of usability. According to a widely accepted definition, usability should be measured in terms of effectiveness, efficiency, and satisfaction (ISO 1998). However, in some cases, it is not easy for the practitioners to figure out the exact measure stand for these three aspects. Thus, a simple and useful framework for measuring BCI usability for researchers to conduct usability evaluation is necessary.

This study aims to propose the usability framework for BCI and provide recommendations for future usability studies of BCI that can motivate researchers and practitioners. Therefore, the research question can be as follows: What are the key formation and evaluation dimensions of usability in BCI usability studies?

- To classify and summarize research relevant for BCI usability research
- To provide a usability framework for BCI based on the literature review
- To drive suggestions for conducting usability evaluation of BCI in the future

The remainder of the chapter is organized as follows: Section 29.2 presents a methodology to extract the articles and the proposed classification framework. Section 29.3 explains general characteristics of the collected literatures and describes each feature of the classification framework. Section 29.4 contains discussions and suggestions for future research. Finally, Section 29.5 concludes the paper with brief summaries and remarks.

## 29.2 REVIEW METHOD

In this study, we conducted a systematic literature review in accord with Preferred Reporting Items for Systematic reviews and Meta-Analyses (PRISMA) (Liberati et al. 2009). A total of 279 articles from 2000 to January 2016 were obtained and reviewed. The year 2000 was chosen as a start date since the first journal article related to BCI was published in 2000. Articles were found via computerized search. A detailed explanation of methodology for extracting articles follows.

### 29.2.1 ELIGIBILITY CRITERIA

These criteria were used to select and accept BCI usability articles. If the article did not meet the criteria, it was excluded. The three criteria are described as follows:

- Search keywords and databases: Keywords for the search engines were "Brain–computer interface" and "Usability." Various online journal databases were selected. A total of five online databases were searched (Engineering Village, IEEE Xplore, PubMed, Scopus, and Web of Science). Those covered not only engineering and medical perspectives but also broad-spectrum perspective (Powers et al. 2015).
- Publication year: This chapter surveys articles published from 2000 to January 2016. The reason for selecting this time period is that many journals have published research related to BCI since 2000.
- Publication type: The search covers only journal articles published in English. Other publication forms (e.g., proceeding papers, unpublished working papers, master's and doctoral dissertations, newspapers, and books, etc.) were not included. Since journal articles indicate a high level of research, journal articles can help both practitioners and academicians to obtain knowledge and spread their study findings.

### 29.2.2 STUDY SELECTION

The articles were selected according to the procedures shown in Figure 29.1. First, five online databases were searched for articles. The total number of articles found was 279. The number of articles

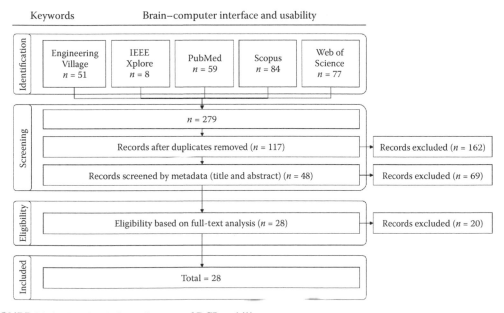

**FIGURE 29.1** PRISMA flow diagram of BCI usability.

by each online database is as follows: Engineering Village (51), IEEE Xplore (8), PubMed (59), Scopus (84), and Web of Science (77). On the other hand, 7636 articles were excluded because they did not have the words "Brain–computer interface" or "Usability" in the titles, abstracts, or research keywords. Next, the articles were carefully reviewed to select those that considered usability of BCI. As a result, a total of 28 articles for usability of BCI research met all the selection criteria.

### 29.2.3 USABILITY FRAMEWORK

Usability, according to a widely accepted definition, depends on a user, product, task, and environment (Jordan 1998; Shackel 1984). As such, a usability evaluation necessarily should include these elements as well. It is important that the conditions for usability evaluation are representative of important factors of the overall context of use (Bevan and Macelod 1994; Shami et al. 2005; Thomas and Macredie 2002). If the usability evaluation is not conducted in users' actual usage situation, it will be necessary to decide which attributes are to be represented in the actual context of use. However, it is less likely to come up with clearly specified users, goals, or context of use in BCI usability. Therefore, the selected attributes of context in BCI should be representative of the important aspects of the actual or intended context of use.

Several previous studies (Coursaris and Kim 2011; Han et al. 2001; Kim et al. 2008; Kwahk and Han 2002) proposed usability evaluation frameworks for various products (i.e., general consumer products, mobile device, ubiquitous computing device, etc.). While there may be other usability frameworks that identify contextual factors of usability evaluation, the frameworks cited here provide a representative set of work in the aspects of usability evaluation. From these frameworks, we adapted the framework proposed by Kwahk and Han (2002) and Coursaris and Kim (2011) because it offers reasonable and considerable detail for each dimension they identified.

On the basis of Kwahk and Han (2002) and Coursaris and Kim (2011), we propose a usability framework for a BCI environment. The framework is depicted in Figure 29.2 and contains four elements (i.e., User, User activity, Device, and Evaluation) for basic formation of usability and six attributes for context of use in BCI. Each element for basic formation of usability has contextual factors (i.e., User, Task, Environment, Technology, Method, and Measure). Although the basic structure is

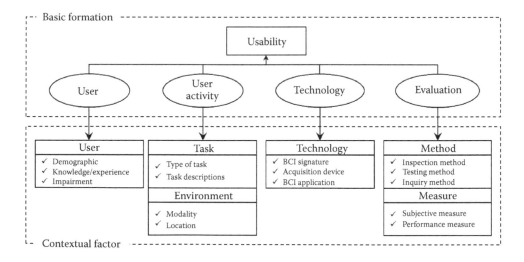

**FIGURE 29.2** A proposed BCI usability framework. (Modified from Kwahk, J., and S. H. Han. 2002. A methodology for evaluating the usability of audiovisual consumer electronic products. *Applied Ergonomics* 33 (5):419–431; Coursaris, C. K., and D. J. Kim. 2011. A meta-analytical review of empirical mobile usability studies. *Journal of Usability Studies* 6 (3):117–171.)

similar to that of Kwahk and Han (2002) and Coursaris and Kim (2011), some attributes and detail contextual information are modified for application to a BCI environment.

Compared to the framework proposed by Kwahk and Han (2002) and Coursaris and Kim (2011), there are several advantages of the suggested mobile usability framework. Although the previous framework proposed by Kwahk and Han (2002) is comprehensive, it is difficult to follow because of its complexity. Thus, in this paper, the proposed framework represents a simple yet direct way to identify and address the various contextual factors of BCI usability. In addition, we suggest three modifications in the basic formation of usability for BCI. First, "Device" replaces "Product," as the concept of BCI is closer to the system that a user may interact with various set of features (such as BCI signature, acquisition device, stimulus, etc.) than a product. Because user performance can change according to technologies of a BCI system (e.g., BCI signatures, acquisition devices, BCI applications, etc.), the technological factor of a BCI usability framework is an important and unique component that needs to be considered carefully. Second, "Environment" is moved to contextual factors of "User activity." Contexts of environment are highly related to users' activities and tasks since users' activities or tasks can change according to the location of the experiment, modality of stimuli, and feedback. Especially for a BCI environment, because of the current technology of BCI (e.g., difficulty of setup and performance of the system), there are many limitations in constructing the environment of usability evaluation. Thus, task and environment characteristics could be involved into contextual factors of "User activity." Finally, "Evaluation" is generated in the structure of basic formation of usability. The selection of rigorous methods and measures determines the quality of usability evaluation (Kwahk and Han 2002). Poor selection can result in irrelevant or useless results. Each attribute of basic formation for usability is related to others. Indeed, the usability evaluation requires careful consideration in defining usability dimensions and selecting appropriate evaluation methods. Therefore, method and measurement characteristics could be involved into contextual factors of "Evaluation."

We collected and summarized the main categories and subcategories of each contextual factor (i.e., user, task, environment, technology, method, measurement) from previous studies (Coursaris and Kim 2011; Ivory and Hearst 2001; Kwahk and Han 2002). As a result, a classification structure of contextual factors for BCI usability is presented in Table 29.1.

In User characteristics, demographic information, knowledge/experience, and perceptual/cognitive or physical limitation are selected as main categories (Coursaris and Kim 2011; Jordan 1998; Kwahk

**TABLE 29.1**

**A Suggested Classification Structure of BCI Usability**

| Context | Main Categories | Subcategories |
|---|---|---|
| User | Demographics | Age, number of participants, culture, etc. |
| | Knowledge/experience | Expert, end-user, general user, etc. |
| | Impairment | Physical, perceptual, cognitive limitation, etc. |
| Task | Type of task | Open task, closed task (self-managed, copy) |
| | Description of task | Spelling, rehabilitation, control task, mental task, etc. |
| Environment | Modality | Modality of stimulus, modality of feedback |
| | Location | Laboratory, hospital, etc. |
| Technology | BCI signature type | ERP, SMRs, SCP, cortical neuron, VEP, etc. |
| | Acquisition device | g.USBamp, BrainAmp, g.MOBIlab, Emotiv EPOC, etc. |
| | BCI application | Replacement, supplement, etc. |
| Method | Inspection method | Heuristics, cognitive walkthrough, guideline, etc. |
| | Testing method | Think aloud, log file analysis, performance, etc. |
| | Inquiry method | Questionnaires, self-reports, FGI, etc. |
| Measurement | Subjective measure | Efficiency, effectiveness, satisfaction, etc. |
| | Objective measure | Effectiveness, efficiency, etc. |

and Han 2002; Salvendy and Carayon 1997). Demographic information contains information about subjects such as age, gender, number of subjects, race/nationality, and occupation/career. Also, users can be categorized into expert, end-user, and general user according to knowledge and experience. Since the BCI system can provide alternate methods to interact with the outside world for patients, the information about subjects' physical, perceptual, and cognitive limitations could be important for constructing a usability evaluation.

In Task characteristics, collected articles were categorized according to the type and description of task. According to the goal of the task, we divided tasks into two types: open task and closed task. If user defines the outcome of the task, it can be involved in open task. Otherwise, in the case of closed task, the experimenter gives a predefined goal to users (Coursaris and Kim 2011). For example, freely using a program is considered as an open task but using the program according to predefined instruction is considered as a closed task. Again, we categorized closed tasks by the characteristics of the strategy. If a user can freely choose the strategy to achieve the predefined goal, it is a closed self-managing task. If users have no choice but to follow a predefined strategy, it is considered as a closed copying task. For example, typing words from users' own thoughts is considered as a closed self-managing task but typing provided words is considered as a closed copying task.

Moreover, the collected articles were categorized into seven tasks according to the description of a task. The Spelling task involves typing provided or free words via BCI systems. Movement control is the task to control the movement of a system. Gaming is the task to play a game. Selection control is the task to target and choose icons or buttons. Brain painting is a task to utilize a painting program. Mental task is engaging in a mental activity such as imagination, mental calculation, and so on. Finally, a Cognitive rehabilitation task is an activity to enhance intellectual capacity.

In Environment characteristics, modality and location are selected as main categories. Modality has two subcategories: Stimulus and Feedback. Modality of stimulus can be visual, auditory, or multimodal. Also, there can be no modality for BCI systems, like using motor or mental imagery. The location of a BCI system is usually a laboratory. However, in the case when a participant is a patient, studies can be conducted at a hospital or at the participant's home.

In Technology characteristics, BCI signature, acquisition device, and BCI application are main categories. There can be many types of signatures used for BCI systems such as event-related potential (ERP), sensorimotor rhythm (SMR), and steady-state evoked potential. According to the BCI signature and the purpose of the BCI system, various acquisition devices are utilized such as g.USBamp, BrainAmp, g.MOBIlab, and Emotiv EPOC. To categorize collected studies according to their application, the criteria of He et al. (2013) were adopted. The first application is replacing lost communication. BCIs for this application help people who have a problem interacting with an external environment (e.g., computer, electronic device, etc.) or communicating with other people. A second application is replacing lost motor function and promoting neuroplasticity to improve defective function. BCIs for this application help people who have a physical or psychological problem by providing direct assistance or rehabilitation. The last application is supplementing normal function. The BCIs for this application provide additional interaction rather than replacing a traditional one.

In Method characteristics, typical usability methods are selected: inspection method, testing method, and inquiry method. Usability inspection aims to find usability problems in a design (Mack and Montaniz 1994), though some methods also address issues like the severity of the usability problems and the overall usability of an entire design (Nielsen and Phillips 1993). In this method, identifying usability problems and improving the usability of an interface design are conducted by checking it against established standards (Holzinger 2005). This method includes heuristic evaluation, cognitive walkthroughs, and guideline checklist. Testing method is the most fundamental usability method. It provides information about how people use systems with a specific interface. There are several methods for testing usability, the most common being thinking aloud, field observation, and performance measurement. Similar to a testing method, an inquiry method enables gathering subjective input (e.g., preferences) from participants (Ivory and Hearst 2001). Typically, this method includes interviews, surveys, questionnaires, and focus group interview.

In Measurement characteristics, there are two main categories: subjective measures and objective measures. The subjective aspect is mostly concerned with user satisfaction and cognitive workload. Conversely, the objective aspect means "how efficient and effective a system/product is for a user to perform a task to achieve some intended goals." In the objective measures, the main purpose is to measure a user's task performance.

These six contextual variables (i.e., user, task, environment, technology, method, and measurement) were utilized for classification of previous studies related to the usability assessment of BCI systems. The benefit of using these variables for the literature review is as follows. The structure provides for the discussion to follow. Also, it helps highlight any areas that require further investigation.

## 29.3 RESULTS

### 29.3.1 User Characteristics

From Table 29.2, in the BCI usability studies, 12 studies tested only healthy subjects and 9 studies tested only patient subjects. Although this result showed that BCI usability studies were comparatively balanced by subject type, the number of subjects and their ages were not balanced.

When the studies were grouped into average age of their subjects, the studies enrolling subjects in their 20s were most prominent, and the number of studies enrolling subjects in their 30s, 40s, 50s, 60s, and 70s were 5, 7, 4, 4, and 1, respectively (Figure 29.3). Considering subject types, the average age of subjects was in their 20s or 30s in most studies with healthy subjects and 40s or 50s in most of studies with patient subjects. Also, classifying by number of subjects, most of the studies tested five to nine subjects (Figure 29.3). Considered by subject type, a small number of subjects were recruited in most of studies with patient subjects.

### 29.3.2 Task Characteristics

Most BCI usability studies were conducted using a closed type of task. However, only three studies used an open type of task. The most prominent type of task conducted in studies with a closed task was a copy task, and nine studies used a self-managed task. From Table 29.3, in the BCI usability studies, the spelling task was the most frequently used task. A control task (moving and selecting) is often used, too. In order of frequency of use, the game task, brain painting task, mental task, and cognitive rehabilitation task were used. In consideration of type of task, closed tasks were predominantly used and a closed copying task was used more than a self-managing task. The open type of

---

## TABLE 29.2
## Classification of Articles by the Type of Subject

| Subject Type | No. of Articles | References |
|---|---|---|
| Only healthy | 12 | Aloise et al. 2013; Baykara et al. 2016; Hohne and Tangermann 2014; Kos'Myna and Tarpin-Bernard 2013; Lee et al. 2013, 2015; Legény et al. 2011; Nam et al. 2010; Nijboer et al. 2015; Riccio et al. 2011; Simon et al. 2015; Weyand et al. 2015 |
| Only patient | 9 | Carabalona et al. 2012; Combaz et al. 2013; Holz et al. 2013, 2015; Morone et al. 2015; Pasqualotto et al. 2015; Schettini et al. 2015; Zickler et al. 2011, 2013 |
| Both healthy and patient | 6 | Daly et al. 2014; Deravi et al. 2015; Hortal et al. 2015; Kleih et al. 2015; Perdikis et al. 2014; Riccio et al. 2015 |
| No information | 1 | Joshi et al. 2012 |
| Total | 28 | |

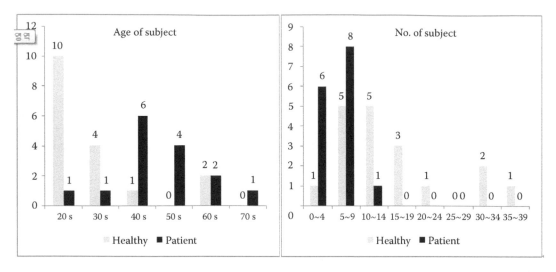

**FIGURE 29.3** Classification of articles by age and the number of subject.

**TABLE 29.3**

**Classification of Articles by Task Characteristics**

| Main Categories | Subcategories | No. of Articles | References |
|---|---|---|---|
| Type of task | Closed task (copy) | 21 | Aloise et al. 2013; Baykara et al. 2016; Carabalona et al. 2012; Daly et al. 2014; Deravi et al. 2015; Hohne and Tangermann 2014; Holz et al. 2013; Hortal et al. 2015; Joshi et al. 2012; Kleih et al. 2015; Legény et al. 2011; Nam et al. 2010; Nijboer et al. 2015; Pasqualotto et al. 2015; Perdikis et al. 2014; Riccio et al. 2015; Schettini et al. 2015; Simon et al. 2015; Weyand et al. 2015; Zickler et al. 2011, 2013 |
| | Closed task (self-managed) | 9 | Combaz et al. 2013; Holz et al. 2013; Lee et al. 2013, 2015; Riccio et al. 2011; Schettini et al. 2015; Simon et al. 2015; Weyand et al. 2015; Zickler et al. 2011 |
| | Open task | 3 | Holz et al. 2015; Kos'Myna and Tarpin-Bernard 2013; Morone et al. 2015 |
| Description of task | Spelling | 18 | Aloise et al. 2013; Baykara et al. 2016; Carabalona et al. 2012; Combaz et al. 2013; Daly et al. 2014; Deravi et al. 2015; Hohne and Tangermann 2014; Kleih et al. 2015; Nam et al. 2010; Nijboer et al. 2015; Pasqualotto et al. 2015; Perdikis et al. 2014; Riccio et al. 2011, 2015; Schettini et al. 2015; Simon et al. 2015; Zickler et al. 2011, 2013 |
| | Control (moving) | 7 | Daly et al. 2014; Hortal et al. 2015; Joshi et al. 2012; Legény et al. 2011; Morone et al. 2015; Riccio et al. 2011; Schettini et al. 2015 |
| | Game | 4 | Holz et al. 2013; Kos'Myna and Tarpin-Bernard 2013; Lee et al. 2013, 2015 |
| | Control (selecting) | 3 | Deravi et al. 2015; Riccio et al. 2011; Schettini et al. 2015 |
| | Brain painting | 2 | Holz et al. 2015; Zickler et al. 2013 |
| | Mental task | 2 | Aloise et al. 2013; Weyand et al. 2015 |
| | Cognitive rehabilitation task | 1 | Daly et al. 2014 |

task is found in only a few studies that used movement control, game, and brain painting as a task. In studies with a spelling and movement control task, a closed copying task was most frequently used. However, in the case of a game task, a closed self-managing task was more commonly used.

### 29.3.3 Environment Characteristics

Study results demonstrate that the stimulus modality most frequently used in previous studies was a visual stimulus (Table 29.4). Auditory stimuli and multimodal stimuli were used in four and three of the collected studies, respectively. The remaining studies did not use the stimuli for their BCI. The BCIs without stimuli used motor imagery, mental imagery, or attention level of subjects. Similarly, BCIs in most of the studies used visual feedback. Only two studies used auditory and multimodal feedback and one study did not use any feedback. Also, with respect to the location of

**TABLE 29.4**

**Classification of Articles by Environment Characteristics**

| Main Categories | Subcategories | No. of Articles | References |
|---|---|---|---|
| Modality of stimulus | Visual | 14 | Aloise et al. 2013; Carabalona et al. 2012; Combaz et al. 2013; Daly et al. 2014; Holz et al. 2015; Legény et al. 2011; Nam et al. 2010; Nijboer et al. 2015; Pasqualotto et al. 2015; Riccio et al. 2011; Schettini et al. 2015; Weyand et al. 2015; Zickler et al. 2011, 2013 |
| | Auditory | 4 | Baykara et al. 2016; Hohne and Tangermann 2014; Kleih et al. 2015; Simon et al. 2015 |
| | Multimodal | 3 | Kos'Myna and Tarpin-Bernard 2013; Perdikis et al. 2014; Riccio et al. 2015 |
| | No (motor imagery) | 5 | Deravi et al. 2015; Holz et al. 2013; Hortal et al. 2015; Joshi et al. 2012; Morone et al. 2015 |
| | No (mental imagery) | 2 | Hortal et al. 2015; Weyand et al. 2015 |
| | No (attention) | 2 | Lee et al. 2013, 2015 |
| Modality of feedback | Visual | 25 | Aloise et al. 2013; Baykara et al. 2016; Carabalona et al. 2012; Combaz et al. 2013; Daly et al. 2014; Deravi et al. 2015; Hohne and Tangermann 2014; Holz et al. 2013, 2015; Joshi et al. 2012; Kos'Myna and Tarpin-Bernard 2013; Lee et al. 2013, 2015; Legény et al. 2011; Morone et al. 2015; Nam et al. 2010; Nijboer et al. 2015; Pasqualotto et al. 2015; Perdikis et al. 2014; Riccio et al. 2011, 2015; Schettini et al. 2015; Weyand et al. 2015; Zickler et al. 2011, 2013 |
| | Auditory | 1 | Kleih et al. 2015 |
| | Multimodal | 1 | Hortal et al. 2015 |
| | No | 1 | Simon et al. 2015 |
| Location | Laboratory | 26 | Aloise et al. 2013; Baykara et al. 2016; Carabalona et al. 2012; Daly et al. 2014; Deravi et al. 2015; Hohne and Tangermann 2014; Holz et al. 2013; Hortal et al. 2015; Joshi et al. 2012; Kleih et al. 2015; Kos'Myna and Tarpin-Bernard 2013; Lee et al. 2013, 2015; Legény et al. 2011; Morone et al. 2015; Nam et al. 2010; Nijboer et al. 2015; Pasqualotto et al. 2015; Perdikis et al. 2014; Riccio et al. 2011, 2015; Schettini et al. 2015; Simon et al. 2015; Weyand et al. 2015; Zickler et al. 2011, 2013 |
| | Subject's home | 2 | Combaz et al. 2013; Holz et al. 2015 |

**TABLE 29.5**

**Classification of Articles by Technology Characteristics**

| Main Categories | Subcategories | No. of Articles | References |
|---|---|---|---|
| BCI signature type | ERP (P300) | 14 | Baykara et al. 2016; Carabalona et al. 2012; Combaz et al. 2013; Daly et al. 2014; Holz et al. 2015; Kleih et al. 2015; Nam et al. 2010; Nijboer et al. 2015; Pasqualotto et al. 2015; Riccio et al. 2011; Schettini et al. 2015; Simon et al. 2015; Zickler et al. 2011, 2013 |
| | ERP | 1 | Hohne and Tangermann 2014 |
| | ERP (gaze-independent BCI) | 1 | Aloise et al. 2013 |
| | EEG | 1 | Deravi et al. 2015 |
| | EEG (attention level) | 2 | Lee et al. 2013, 2015 |
| | VEP (SSVEP) | 2 | Combaz et al. 2013; Legény et al. 2011 |
| | Hemodynamic brain activity | 1 | Weyand et al. 2015 |
| | Hybrid BCI (EEG [oscillatory rhythms] + EMG) | 1 | Perdikis et al. 2014 |
| | Hybrid BCI (ERP [P300] + EMG) | 1 | Riccio et al. 2015 |
| | Hybrid BCI (VEP [SSVEP] + Eye tracker) | 1 | Kos'Myna and Tarpin-Bernard 2013 |
| | Hybrid BCI (ERD/S [Graz] + Eye tracker) | 1 | Kos'Myna and Tarpin-Bernard 2013 |
| | SMRs | 1 | Morone et al. 2015 |
| | SMRs (ERD/S [alpha, beta, delta]) | 1 | Holz et al. 2013 |
| | SMRs (ERD/S [mu rhythm]) | 1 | Joshi et al. 2012 |
| | SMRs (ERD/S [mu rhythm, beta]) | 1 | Hortal et al. 2015 |
| | SMRs (beta rebound) | 1 | Holz et al. 2013 |
| | SMRs (slower potential) | 1 | Holz et al. 2013 |
| Acquisition device | g.USBamp | 15 | Aloise et al. 2013; Baykara et al. 2016; Carabalona et al. 2012; Daly et al. 2014; Holz et al. 2015; Hortal et al. 2015; Kleih et al. 2015; Legény et al. 2011; Nam et al. 2010; Pasqualotto et al. 2015; Perdikis et al. 2014; Riccio et al. 2011, 2015; Zickler et al. 2011, 2013 |
| | Emotiv EPOC | 3 | Deravi et al. 2015; Kos'Myna and Tarpin-Bernard 2013; Nijboer et al. 2015 |
| | BrainAmp | 3 | Hohne and Tangermann 2014; Morone et al. 2015; Simon et al. 2015 |
| | g.MOBIlab | 1 | Schettini et al. 2015 |
| | Brain Vision amplifier | 1 | Holz et al. 2013 |
| | AD624 | 1 | Joshi et al. 2012 |
| | A prototype of an ultra low-power 8-channel miniature EEG amplifier | 1 | Combaz et al. 2013 |
| | A multichannel frequency domain NIRS system (Imagent Functional Brain Imaging System from ISS Inc., Champaign, Illinois) | 1 | Weyand et al. 2015 |
| | No information | 2 | Lee et al. 2013, 2015 |

*(Continued)*

**TABLE 29.5 (CONTINUED)**

**Classification of Articles by Technology Characteristics**

| Main Categories | Subcategories | No. of Articles | References |
|---|---|---|---|
| BCI application | Replacing lost communication | 17 | Aloise et al. 2013; Baykara et al. 2016; Combaz et al. 2013; Deravi et al. 2015; Hohne and Tangermann 2014; Kleih et al. 2015; Nam et al. 2010; Nijboer et al. 2015; Pasqualotto et al. 2015; Perdikis et al. 2014; Riccio et al. 2011, 2015; Schettini et al. 2015; Simon et al. 2015; Weyand et al. 2015; Zickler et al. 2011, 2013 |
| | Replacing lost motor function and promoting neuroplasticity to improve defective function | 4 | Hortal et al. 2015; Lee et al. 2013, 2015; Morone et al. 2015 |
| | Supplementing normal function | 6 | Carabalona et al. 2012; Holz et al. 2013, 2015; Joshi et al. 2012; Kos'Myna and Tarpin-Bernard 2013; Legény et al. 2011 |
| | All | 1 | Daly et al. 2014 |

the experiments, the most common collected studies were based on laboratory experiments. Only a few studies conducted field experiments in a subject's home.

### 29.3.4 TECHNOLOGY CHARACTERISTICS

From Table 29.5, many previous studies conducted usability evaluation on ERP-based BCI systems. Among them, P300 was the most prominent signal. In addition, few studies evaluated usability of VEP and hemodynamic brain activity–based BCI. There was also a special type of BCI that is known as hybrid BCI. Hybrid BCI involves a BCI system that uses a brain signal and an additional physiological signal. Four studies conducted usability evaluations on hybrid BCI systems. Each study used a different brain signal: EEG (oscillatory rhythms), ERP (P300), VEP (SSVEP), and ERD/S (Graz). To acquire the signal, eight kinds of devices were used. The most frequently used device was g.USBamp, Emotiv EPOC, and BrainAmp.

In BCI studies of communication, many previous studies used a speller system and gave a closed type of task to subjects to test usability of the system. Among the tasks of closed type, a copy-spelling task was used in all of these studies. Nijboer et al. (2015) developed a P300-based 6 × 6 speller and compared the usability of three headsets (Biosemi cap, Emotiv EPOC, and g.Sahara cap). For testing the usability, they provided subjects a short word such as "the" to type. Nam et al. (2010) also gave a similar task to subjects to identify the effect of background noise and interface color on performance and preference of a visual P300-based BCI system, specifically an 8 × 9 speller. Some studies used a speller with a closed type of task or only gave a self-managed spelling task to subjects. For instance, Simon et al. (2015) developed an auditory P300 speller based on bird sounds and tested the usability after conducting a copy-spelling task and free-spelling task. All studies applied various tasks for their own purpose to test the usability of a system, such as a control task, a mental task, and a brain painting task. However, the type of task was limited to closed type in these studies.

In the replacing motor function and rehabilitation application, four studies conducted a usability evaluation. One study aimed to develop and evaluate a BCI system for replacing lost motor function. Hortal et al. (2015) developed their own BCI to assist the subject's movement based on an exoskeleton system. They let subjects do a closed copy moving control task and then evaluated the usability.

**TABLE 29.6**

**Classification of Articles by Method Characteristics**

| Main Categories | Subcategories | No. of Articles | References |
|---|---|---|---|
| Inspection method | Heuristics evaluation | 2 | Schettini et al. 2015; Zickler et al. 2011 |
| | Pluralistic walkthrough | 1 | Morone et al. 2015 |
| | Not used | 25 | Aloise et al. 2013; Baykara et al. 2016; Carabalona et al. 2012; Combaz et al. 2013; Daly et al. 2014; Deravi et al. 2015; Hohne and Tangermann 2014; Holz et al. 2013, 2015; Hortal et al. 2015; Joshi et al. 2012; Kleih et al. 2015; Kos'Myna and Tarpin-Bernard 2013; Lee et al. 2013, 2015; Legény et al. 2011; Nam et al. 2010; Nijboer et al. 2015; Pasqualotto et al. 2015; Perdikis et al. 2014; Riccio et al. 2011, 2015; Simon et al. 2015; Weyand et al. 2015; Zickler et al. 2013 |
| Testing method | Performance measurement | 23 | Aloise et al. 2013; Baykara et al. 2016; Combaz et al. 2013; Daly et al. 2014; Deravi et al. 2015; Hohne and Tangermann 2014; Holz et al. 2013; Hortal et al. 2015; Joshi et al. 2012; Kleih et al. 2015; Kos'Myna and Tarpin-Bernard 2013; Legény et al. 2011; Nam et al. 2010; Nijboer et al. 2015; Pasqualotto et al. 2015; Perdikis et al. 2014; Riccio et al. 2011, 2015; Schettini et al. 2015; Simon et al. 2015; Weyand et al. 2015; Zickler et al. 2011, 2013 |
| | Log file analysis | 10 | Nam et al. 2010; Nijboer et al. 2015; Pasqualotto et al. 2015; Perdikis et al. 2014; Riccio et al. 2015; Schettini et al. 2015; Simon et al. 2015; Weyand et al. 2015; Zickler et al. 2011, 2013 |
| | Think-aloud | 1 | Morone et al. 2015 |
| | Not used | 4 | Carabalona et al. 2012; Holz et al. 2015; Lee et al. 2013, 2015 |
| Inquiry method | Questionnaires | 23 | Baykara et al. 2016; Carabalona et al. 2012; Combaz et al. 2013; Daly et al. 2014; Deravi et al. 2015; Hohne and Tangermann 2014; Holz et al. 2013, 2015; Kleih et al. 2015; Lee et al. 2013, 2015; Legény et al. 2011; Morone et al. 2015; Nam et al. 2010; Nijboer et al. 2015; Pasqualotto et al. 2015; Riccio et al. 2011, 2015; Schettini et al. 2015; Simon et al. 2015; Weyand et al. 2015; Zickler et al. 2011, 2013 |
| | Interview | 8 | Holz et al. 2013; Kleih et al. 2015; Kos'Myna and Tarpin-Bernard 2013; Lee et al. 2013, 2015; Riccio et al. 2011; Zickler et al. 2011, 2013 |
| | FGI | 4 | Holz et al. 2013; Kleih et al. 2015; Morone et al. 2015; Simon et al. 2015 |
| | Self-reports | 1 | Holz et al. 2015 |
| | Not used | 4 | Aloise et al. 2013; Hortal et al. 2015; Joshi et al. 2012; Perdikis et al. 2014 |

The rest were related to rehabilitation. Morone et al. (2015) developed a BCI for physical rehabilitation and designed an open moving control task experiment. Lee et al. (2013, 2015) developed a BCI for cognitive rehabilitation and gave a closed self-managed game task to subjects.

The studies that focused on supplementing normal function developed their own system such as a controller in a virtual environment, an input device for a computer, a speller, a game, and a painting program. For the usability evaluation, they gave specific tasks in accord with their predefined type of use. The type of these tasks was not only open but the tasks were of both open and closed type.

### 29.3.5 Method Characteristics

According to the usability evaluation method, the collected studies were classified into three categories: inspection method, testing method, and inquiry method (Table 29.6). The result showed that most studies used the testing method and inquiry method rather than the inspection method to evaluate the usability of BCI systems. Three studies used an inspection method with either heuristic evaluation (Schettini et al. 2015; Zickler et al. 2011) or pluralistic walkthrough (Morone et al. 2015). In the studies using the testing method, most employed a performance measurement method. In the studies using the inquiry method, the Questionnaires method was most commonly used. The interview, FGI, and self-reports were the next most common.

### 29.3.6 Measurement Characteristics

Since the objective of this study was to develop the usability dimensions measured in BCI usability studies, we collected and rearranged them in terms of usability dimensions. Table 29.7 presents a summary of these 40 measured subjective usability dimensions. A preliminary inspection of Table 29.7 shows that the constructs of satisfaction, cognitive workload, and ease of use are most commonly measured in BCI usability studies.

All measures were collected from 10 evaluation tools that were used in 28 BCI usability studies. The NASA Task Load Index (NASA-TLX), the Visual Analog Scale (VAS), the Assistive Technology Device Predisposition Assessment device form (ATD-PA device form), the System Usability Scale survey (SUS survey), Quebec User Evaluation of Satisfaction with assistive Technology 2.0 (QUEST 2.0), IBM's computer usability satisfaction questionnaire, the USE Questionnaire, and the Questionnaire for Current Motivation (QCM) were utilized. Last, some studies proposed and conducted their own evaluation tools.

NASA-TLX is a popular mental workload assessment technique that relies on a multidimensional construct. It derives overall workload based on six subscales: mental demand, physical demand, temporal demand, performance, effort, and frustration (Cao et al. 2009). VAS is one method for assessing a "feeling" (Ohnhaus and Adler 1975). It is usually conducted to assess the satisfaction of a system in BCI usability studies. The ATD-PA device form and QUEST 2.0 are specialized subjective assessment tools to evaluate assistive devices. ATD-PA is a set of questionnaires to assess the matching between person and assistive technology (Scherer and Craddock 2002). In BCI usability studies, only a set of 12 items, called ATD-PA device form, is usually utilized to ask users' views of 12 aspects of using a proposed BCI system as an assistive device. QUEST 2.0 is an instrument to evaluate users' satisfaction with assistive technology. It contains 12 items rated on a five-point satisfaction scale with respect to a device and services (Demers et al. 2002). The SUS survey and the USE Questionnaire are simple, yet effective tools for assessing the usability of various products. The SUS survey contains a 10-item scale giving a global view of usability (Bangor et al. 2009), and the USE Questionnaire contains a 14-item scale referring to four domains: satisfaction, ease of use, ease of learning, and usefulness (Lund 2001). IBM computer usability satisfaction questionnaires also measure user satisfaction with usability, but it is specialized to a computer system (Lewis 1995). QCM is a subjective assessment tool specialized to measuring users' motivations with respect to four motivational factors: mastery confidence, incompetence fear, challenge, and interest (Rheinberg et al. 2001).

Moreover, we recategorized performance measures (objective measures). Table 29.8 presents a summary of these 21 performance measures. From Table 29.8, task accuracy and ITR are the most commonly measured in BCI usability studies. Performance measures varied depending on study.

From Table 29.8, task accuracy and ITR were the most frequently used performance measures. The remaining measures related to brain activity (e.g., amplitude, latency), time-dependent variables (e.g., task speed, task time, and time for selection), and the difficulties of task completion (e.g., error rate, feasibility of finishing the task, and task completion rate). Also, there were some studies

**TABLE 29.7**

**Classification of Articles by Measurement Characteristics**

| Measures | References | Count |
|---|---|---|
| Satisfaction | Baykara et al. 2016; Carabalona et al. 2012; Combaz et al. 2013; Daly et al. 2014; Deravi et al. 2015; Hohne and Tangermann 2014; Holz et al. 2013; Hortal et al. 2015; Lee et al. 2013, 2015; Legény et al. 2011; Morone et al. 2015; Riccio et al. 2011, 2015; Schettini et al. 2015; Zickler et al. 2011, 2013 | 17 |
| Cognitive workload | Baykara et al. 2016; Combaz et al. 2013; Daly et al. 2014; Deravi et al. 2015; Holz et al. 2013, 2015; Morone et al. 2015; Pasqualotto et al. 2015; Riccio et al. 2011, 2015; Schettini et al. 2015; Simon et al. 2015; Zickler et al. 2011, 2013 | 14 |
| Ease of use | Carabalona et al. 2012; Deravi et al. 2015; Hohne and Tangermann 2014; Holz et al. 2013, 2015; Kleih et al. 2015; Lee et al. 2013, 2015; Pasqualotto et al. 2015; Simon et al. 2015; Weyand et al. 2015; Zickler et al. 2011, 2013 | 13 |
| Mental demand | Combaz et al. 2013; Holz et al. 2013, 2015; Kleih et al. 2015; Pasqualotto et al. 2015; Riccio et al. 2011, 2015; Simon et al. 2015; Zickler et al. 2011, 2013 | 10 |
| Comfort | Deravi et al. 2015; Holz et al. 2013, 2015; Lee et al. 2013, 2015; Legény et al. 2011; Nijboer et al. 2015; Zickler et al. 2011, 2013 | 9 |
| Effort | Combaz et al. 2013; Holz et al. 2013, 2015; Pasqualotto et al. 2015; Riccio et al. 2011, 2015; Simon et al. 2015; Zickler et al. 2011, 2013 | 9 |
| Frustration | Combaz et al. 2013; Holz et al. 2013, 2015; Pasqualotto et al. 2015; Riccio et al. 2011, 2015; Simon et al. 2015; Zickler et al. 2011, 2013 | 9 |
| Performance | Combaz et al. 2013; Holz et al. 2013, 2015; Pasqualotto et al. 2015; Riccio et al. 2011, 2015; Simon et al. 2015; Zickler et al. 2011, 2013 | 9 |
| Physical demand | Combaz et al. 2013; Holz et al. 2013, 2015; Pasqualotto et al. 2015; Riccio et al. 2011, 2015; Simon et al. 2015; Zickler et al. 2011, 2013 | 9 |
| Temporal demand | Combaz et al. 2013; Holz et al. 2013, 2015; Pasqualotto et al. 2015; Riccio et al. 2011, 2015; Simon et al. 2015; Zickler et al. 2011, 2013 | 9 |
| Efficiency | Holz et al. 2013, 2015; Riccio et al. 2011, 2015; Schettini et al. 2015; Simon et al. 2015; Zickler et al. 2011, 2013 | 8 |
| Learnability | Carabalona et al. 2012; Deravi et al. 2015; Holz et al. 2013, 2015; Pasqualotto et al. 2015; Simon et al. 2015; Zickler et al. 2011, 2013 | 8 |
| Usefulness | Carabalona et al. 2012; Deravi et al. 2015; Holz et al. 2013, 2015; Lee et al. 2013, 2015; Zickler et al. 2013 | 7 |
| Aesthetic | Deravi et al. 2015; Holz et al. 2013, 2015; Nijboer et al. 2015; Zickler et al. 2011, 2013 | 6 |
| Helpfulness | Deravi et al. 2015; Holz et al. 2013, 2015; Weyand et al. 2015; Zickler et al. 2011, 2013 | 6 |
| Predictability | Deravi et al. 2015; Holz et al. 2013, 2015; Pasqualotto et al. 2015; Simon et al. 2015; Zickler et al. 2013 | 6 |
| Effectiveness | Deravi et al. 2015; Holz et al. 2013, 2015; Zickler et al. 2011, 2013 | 5 |
| Responsiveness | Holz et al. 2013, 2015; Legény et al. 2011; Zickler et al. 2011, 2013 | 5 |
| Safety | Deravi et al. 2015; Holz et al. 2013, 2015; Zickler et al. 2011, 2013 | 5 |
| Adjustment | Holz et al. 2013, 2015; Zickler et al. 2011, 2013 | 4 |
| Enjoyment | Holz et al. 2013, 2015; Lee et al. 2013, 2015 | 4 |
| Operability | Deravi et al. 2015; Nijboer et al. 2015; Pasqualotto et al. 2015; Simon et al. 2015 | 4 |
| Physical accommodation | Holz et al. 2013, 2015; Zickler et al. 2011, 2013 | 4 |
| Reliability | Holz et al. 2013, 2015; Zickler et al. 2011, 2013 | 4 |
| Adaptability | Holz et al. 2013, 2015; Zickler et al. 2013 | 3 |
| Complexity | Legény et al. 2011; Pasqualotto et al. 2015; Simon et al. 2015 | 3 |
| Consistency | Deravi et al. 2015; Pasqualotto et al. 2015; Simon et al. 2015 | 3 |
| Exhaustion | Hohne and Tangermann 2014; Holz et al. 2013, 2015 | 3 |

*(Continued)*

**TABLE 29.7 (CONTINUED)**
## Classification of Articles by Measurement Characteristics

| Measures | References | Count |
|---|---|---|
| Expected technology benefit | Holz et al. 2013, 2015; Zickler et al. 2013 | 3 |
| Familiarity | Holz et al. 2013, 2015; Zickler et al. 2013 | 3 |
| Preference | Nam et al. 2010; Nijboer et al. 2015; Riccio et al. 2011 | 3 |
| Privacy | Holz et al. 2013, 2015; Zickler et al. 2013 | 3 |
| Security | Holz et al. 2013, 2015; Zickler et al. 2013 | 3 |
| Willing to use | Deravi et al. 2015; Pasqualotto et al. 2015; Simon et al. 2015 | 3 |
| Functionality | Deravi et al. 2015; Simon et al. 2015 | 2 |
| Recommendability | Lee et al. 2013, 2015 | 2 |
| Attractiveness | Deravi et al. 2015 | 1 |
| Clarity | Hohne and Tangermann 2014 | 1 |
| Controllability | Holz et al. 2015 | 1 |
| Mood | Morone et al. 2015 | 1 |

**TABLE 29.8**
## Classification of Articles by Performance Measures

| Measures | References | Count |
|---|---|---|
| Task accuracy | Aloise et al. 2013; Baykara et al. 2016; Combaz et al. 2013; Daly et al. 2014; Deravi et al. 2015; Hohne and Tangermann 2014; Holz et al. 2013; Hortal et al. 2015; Joshi et al. 2012; Kleih et al. 2015; Legény et al. 2011; Nam et al. 2010; Perdikis et al. 2014; Riccio et al. 2015; Schettini et al. 2015; Zickler et al. 2011, 2013 | 17 |
| Information transfer rate | Baykara et al. 2016; Combaz et al. 2013; Holz et al. 2013; Kleih et al. 2015; Nam et al. 2010; Pasqualotto et al. 2015; Riccio et al. 2015; Simon et al. 2015; Zickler et al. 2011, 2013 | 10 |
| Classification accuracy | Carabalona et al. 2012; Nijboer et al. 2015; Simon et al. 2015; Weyand et al. 2015 | 4 |
| Amplitude | Baykara et al. 2016; Kleih et al. 2015; Nam et al. 2010 | 3 |
| Error rate | Aloise et al. 2013; Hortal et al. 2015 | 2 |
| Latency | Baykara et al. 2016; Nam et al. 2010 | 2 |
| Proposed metric of efficiency | Aloise et al. 2013; Zickler et al. 2013 | 2 |
| Task speed | Joshi et al. 2012; Perdikis et al. 2014 | 2 |
| Task time | Kos'Myna and Tarpin-Bernard 2013; Legény et al. 2011 | 2 |
| Throughput time | Perdikis et al. 2014; Riccio et al. 2015 | 2 |
| Abstentions | Aloise et al. 2013 | 1 |
| Errors | Kos'Myna and Tarpin-Bernard 2013 | 1 |
| Hybrid system accuracy | Riccio et al. 2015 | 1 |
| Proposed metric of effectiveness | Riccio et al. 2011 | 1 |
| Real time to setup | Nijboer et al. 2015 | 1 |
| System accuracy | Hortal et al. 2015 | 1 |
| Task completion rate | Perdikis et al. 2014 | 1 |
| The feasibility of finishing the task | Legény et al. 2011 | 1 |
| Time for correct selection | Schettini et al. 2015 | 1 |
| Time for selection | Riccio et al. 2015 | 1 |
| W3 score | Weyand et al. 2015 | 1 |

that proposed new metrics for performance measures (e.g., effectiveness [Riccio et al. 2011], efficiency [Aloise et al. 2013; Zickler et al. 2013], and WS score [Weyand et al. 2015]).

Upon review of the measures' frequency in the collected articles, the three core constructs for the measurement of usability appear to be the following (Nielsen 1994):

- Efficiency: Degree to which the product enables the tasks to be performed in a quick, effective, and economical manner, or hinders performance
- Effectiveness: Accuracy and completeness with which specified users achieved specified goals in a particular environment
- Satisfaction: The degree to which a product gives contentment or makes the user satisfied

Most of the subjective measures are accounted for by Satisfaction and Efficiency. In particular, the metrics for evaluating cognitive workload by NASA-TLX were used for the assessment of the efficiency of BCI systems. Although various subjective measures were used and the definitions of each measure were different, the purpose of usage of the measures, except cognitive workload, is to assess user's satisfaction with a BCI system. Performance measures varied depending on the study. An accuracy measure was typically used to assess the effectiveness of BCI systems. According to the definition of effectiveness, error rate, errors, and task completion rate can also be involved in terms of effectiveness. Among the collected articles, ITR was typically used to assess the efficiency of BCI systems. Also, efficiency can involve how quickly and effectively a task is performed, task speed time, throughput time, the feasibility of finishing the task, or time for selection. The summary of usability dimensions is shown in Figure 29.4.

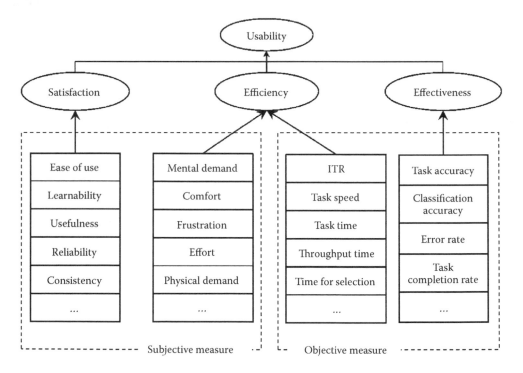

**FIGURE 29.4** Usability dimensions for BCI systems.

## 29.4 RECOMMENDATIONS

Previous studies of BCI usability have been mainly focused on cognitive workload or performance (objective measures). However, subjective measures can be helpful in identifying design problems involving human factors and ergonomics (HFE) and HCI. Since detecting diverse mental tasks in BCI systems for intuitive interaction is difficult, it is limited to enhancing ease of use in the design of BCI systems (Bos et al. 2011b). As the purpose of BCI systems is often to help persons with disabilities control interfaces, interaction between users and interfaces can be limited by users' physical/cognitive disabilities. Thus, diverse functions are difficult to accommodate in BCI systems. Moreover, if control methods for diverse functions do not take account of demands on users, users will feel physical and mental fatigue quickly (Blain-Moraes et al. 2012; Kübler et al. 2013a). Thus, by considering usability measures that are related to compatibility and scalability of BCI systems (e.g., predictability, adaptability, learnability, consistency, and familiarity), it is possible to identify problems and address these in the development of BCI systems.

Also, BCI systems are difficult to seamlessly incorporate into users' daily lives. Setup of BCI systems in daily life has limitations, such as poor calibration due to environment, connection of sensors, and time consuming in setting up hardware and software (Barros et al. 2015; Kübler et al. 2013a). Since BCI systems need space organization, the mobility of BCI systems is restricted (Botte-Lecocq et al. 2014; Kübler et al. 2013b). Moreover, because of the lack of scalability of BCI systems, it can be difficult to interact with other existing software and other devices (Barros et al. 2015; Blain-Moraes et al. 2012; Kübler et al. 2013a). To solve these issues, it is important to consider that usability measures, such as cognitive workload, learnability, adaptability, reliability, and ease of use, are necessary. Increasing the learnability, adaptability, and ease of use of BCI systems is also valuable.

The inspection method is one of the usability methods that have not been sufficiently adopted in assessing BCI usability. Through conducting the inspection method (e.g., heuristic evaluation, cognitive/pluralistic walkthrough, guideline checklist, etc.), it is possible to identify the usability problems of the user interface design in a detailed manner. It specifically involves evaluators (end-users or user interface experts) and is conducted in the context-of-use cases (typical user tasks) to provide feedback to the developers on the extent to which the interface is likely to be compatible with the intended users' needs and preferences. Therefore, future research on usability evaluation for BCI systems is necessary for identifying and solving usability problems.

Future research into the evaluation of user experiences (UX) with BCI systems is necessary. By evaluating and analyzing UX with BCI systems, it may be possible to increase usability and user acceptance of new technology. Some BCI researchers have started to apply User-Centered Design (UCD) to BCI systems (Lightbody et al. 2010; Zickler et al. 2009). UCD generally consists of user involvement in the design process, identification of user needs, and development of user/system requirements. Although, these previous studies involved users in the design process, they did not evaluate UX of BCI systems.

An interesting category of applications for BCI systems is enjoyment (e.g., games, creative expression). Most of the previous studies focused on proof of concepts (Jackson and Mappus 2010). Moreover, only task performance measures or mental task detection is usually used for those applications. Only few studies evaluated BCI systems for identification of the influence of different visuals and user tasks on the UX with a game experience questionnaire (Bos and Reuderink 2008; Van de Laar 2009).

## 29.5 CONCLUSION

We exhaustively reviewed recent literature on the usability of BCIs. To identify the key formation and evaluation dimensions of usability, we focused on contextual factors (user, activity, technology, and evaluation) of BCI usability. We classified and summarized BCI usability studies according to user, task, environment, technology, method, and measurement characteristics. Then, we proposed usability dimensions for BCI and offered suggestions for conducting usability evaluation of BCI in future research.

We found that previous studies of BCI usability have been mainly focused on evaluating the performance and cognitive workload of systems. From the review, we propose three core constructs for the measurement of usability: satisfaction, effectiveness, and efficiency. In satisfaction, all involved metrics are subjective measures. Those measures (e.g., ease of use, learnability, operability, helpfulness, etc.) are usually rated by a 5- or 7-point Likert scale. Also, all metrics in effectiveness are objective measures. The measures of effectiveness are mostly related to accuracy and completeness with which specified users achieved specified goals in a particular environment. In efficiency, there are both subjective and objective measures. Subjective measures in efficiency are related to users' cognitive workload, and NASA-TLX has been widely used to evaluate users' cognitive workload. Objective measures in efficiency are related to time and speed. Those measures aim to evaluate the degree to which the system enables the task to be performed in a quick, effective, and economical manner, or hinders performance. Moreover, most previous studies focused on a closed task of a speller with visual modality and ERP (P300) signature. Since a P300 signature has proven to be a reliable signal for controlling a BCI (Farwell and Donchin 1988), many studies have been conducted on speller tasks with P300.

The opportunities for further research were discussed in this study. Most previous studies have focused on cognitive workload and performance of systems. Thus, studies focused on subjective measures especially with the inspection method could be conducted in the future. Considering the proposed usability measures, it is possible to identify and solve design issues of BCI systems. Specifically, to enhance the compatibility and scalability of BCI systems, subjective measures (e.g., predictability, adaptability, learnability, consistency, and familiarity) should be considered for usability evaluation. Also, the proposed usability metrics, such as cognitive workload, learnability, adaptability, reliability, and ease of use, can be helpful to simplify the complexity of BCI systems. Therefore, suggestions for future research directions in this study can be helpful in establishing research directions and gaining insights to solve HFE/HCI design issues of BCI systems. BCI systems could be seamlessly integrated with traditional modalities while maintaining sufficiently reliable accuracy in the future. The next step will be to move beyond feasibility tests and prove that BCI is also applicable in real-world situations. The usability and UX study of BCI could lead us to make BCI systems well integrated under natural conditions (within realistic HCI settings and with naturally behaving users).

## REFERENCES

Aloise, F., P. Aricò, F. Schettini, S. Salinari, D. Mattia, and F. Cincotti. 2013. Asynchronous gaze-independent event-related potential-based brain–computer interface. *Artificial Intelligence in Medicine* 59 (2):61–69.

Bangor, A., P. Kortum, and J. Miller. 2009. Determining what individual SUS scores mean: Adding an adjective rating scale. *Journal of Usability Studies* 4 (3):114–123.

Barros, R. Q., G. Santos, C. Ribeiro, R. Torres, M. Q. Barros, and M. M. Soares. 2015. A usability study of a brain–computer interface apparatus: An ergonomic approach. *International Conference of Design, User Experience, and Usability*.

Baykara, E., C. Ruf, C. Fioravanti, I. Käthner, N. Simon, S. Kleih, A. Kübler, and S. Halder. 2016. Effects of training and motivation on auditory P300 brain–computer interface performance. *Clinical Neurophysiology* 127 (1):379–387.

Bevan, N., and M. Macleod. 1994. Usability measurement in context. *Behaviour and Information Technology* 13 (1–2):132–145.

Blain-Moraes, S., R. Schaff, K. L. Gruis, J. E. Huggins, and P. A. Wren. 2012. Barriers to and mediators of brain–computer interface user acceptance: Focus group findings. *Ergonomics* 55 (5):516–525.

Bos, D. P.-O., H. Gürkök, B. Van de Laar, F. Nijboer, and A. Nijholt. 2011a. User experience evaluation in BCI: Mind the gap!

Bos, D. P.-O., M. Poel, and A. Nijholt. 2011b. A study in user-centered design and evaluation of mental tasks for BCI. *International Conference on Multimedia Modeling.*

Bos, D. P.-O., and B. Reuderink. 2008. Brainbasher: A BCI game.

Botte-Lecocq, C., M.-H. Bekaert, J.-M. Vannobel, S. Leclercq, and F. Cabestaing. 2014. Considering human factors in BCI experiments: A global approach. *Journal Européen des Systèmes Automatisés (JESA)* 48 (4–6):283–301.

Cao, A., K. K. Chintamani, A. K. Pandya, and R. D. Ellis. 2009. NASA TLX: Software for assessing subjective mental workload. *Behavior Research Methods* 41 (1):113–117.

Carabalona, R., F. Grossi, A. Tessadri, P. Castiglioni, A. Caracciolo, and I. de Munari. 2012. Light on! Real world evaluation of a P300-based brain–computer interface (BCI) for environment control in a smart home. *Ergonomics* 55 (5):552–563.

Charlton, S. G., and T. G. O'Brien. 1996. The role of human factors testing and evaluation in systems development. *Handbook of Human Factors Testing and Evaluation*:13–26.

Combaz, A., C. Chatelle, A. Robben, G. Vanhoof, A. Goeleven, V. Thijs, M. M. Van Hulle, and S. Laureys. 2013. A comparison of two spelling brain–computer interfaces based on visual p3 and ssvep in locked-in syndrome. *PloS one* 8 (9):e73691.

Coursaris, C. K., and D. J. Kim. 2011. A meta-analytical review of empirical mobile usability studies. *Journal of Usability Studies* 6 (3):117–171.

Daly, J., E. Armstrong, E. Thomson, and S. Martin. 2014. Moving brain computer interfaces towards home based systems for people with acquired brain injury. *International Workshop on Ambient Assisted Living.*

Demers, L., R. Weiss-Lambrou, and B. Ska. 2002. The Quebec User Evaluation of Satisfaction with Assistive Technology (QUEST 2.0): An overview and recent progress. *Technology and Disability* 14 (3):101–105.

Deravi, F., C. S. Ang, M. H. B. Azhar, A. Al-Wabil, M. Philips, and M. Sakel. 2015. Usability and performance measure of a consumer-grade brain computer interface system for environmental control by neurological patients. *International Journal of Engineering and Technology Innovation (IJETI)* 5 (3):165–177.

Farwell, L. A., and E. Donchin. 1988. Talking off the top of your head: Toward a mental prosthesis utilizing event-related brain potentials. *Electroencephalography and Clinical Neurophysiology* 70 (6):510–523.

Garcia, L., V. Lespinet-Najib, S. Saioud, V. Meistermann, S. Renaud, J. Diaz-Pineda, J. M. André, and R. Ron-Angevin. 2015. Brain–computer interface: Usability evaluation of different P300 speller configurations: A preliminary study. *International Work-Conference on Artificial Neural Networks.*

Hohne, J., and M. Tangermann. 2014. Towards user-friendly spelling with an auditory brain–computer interface: The charstreamer paradigm. *PloS one* 9 (6):e98322.

Han, S. H., M. H. Yun, J. Kwahk, and S. W. Hong. 2001. Usability of consumer electronic products. *International Journal of Industrial Ergonomics* 28 (3):143–151.

He, B., S. Gao, H. Yuan, and J. R. Wolpaw. 2013. Brain–computer interfaces. In *Neural Engineering*, 87–151. Springer.

Henderson, R. D., M. C. Smith, J. Podd, and H. Varela-Alvarez. 1995. A comparison of the four prominent user-based methods for evaluating the usability of computer software. *Ergonomics* 38 (10):2030–2044.

Holz, E. M., L. Botrel, T. Kaufmann, and A. Kübler. 2015. Long-term independent brain–computer interface home use improves quality of life of a patient in the locked-in state: A case study. *Archives of Physical Medicine and Rehabilitation* 96 (3):S16–S26.

Holz, E. M., J. Höhne, P. Staiger-Sälzer, M. Tangermann, and A. Kübler. 2013. Brain–computer interface controlled gaming: Evaluation of usability by severely motor restricted end-users. *Artificial Intelligence in Medicine* 59 (2):111–120.

Holzinger, A. 2005. Usability engineering methods for software developers. *Communications of the ACM* 48 (1):71–74.

Hortal, E., D. Planelles, F. Resquin, J. M. Climent, J. M. Azorín, and J. L. Pons. 2015. Using a brain–machine interface to control a hybrid upper limb exoskeleton during rehabilitation of patients with neurological conditions. *Journal of Neuroengineering and Rehabilitation* 12 (1):1.

ISO. 1998. 9241-11. 1998. *Ergonomic Requirements for Office Work with Visual Display Terminals (VDTs)—Part II Guidance on Usability.*

Ivory, M. Y., and M. A. Hearst. 2001. The state of the art in automating usability evaluation of user interfaces. *ACM Computing Surveys (CSUR)* 33 (4):470–516.

Jackson, M. M., and R. Mappus. 2010. Neural control interfaces. In *Brain–Computer Interfaces*, 21–33. Springer.

Jordan, P. W. 1998. *An Introduction to Usability*: CRC Press.

Joshi, R., P. Saraswat, and R. Gajendran. 2012. A novel mu rhythm-based brain computer interface design that uses a programmable system on chip. *Journal of Medical Signals and Sensors* 2 (1):11.

Kübler, A., E. Holz, T. Kaufmann, and C. Zickler. 2013a. A user centred approach for bringing BCI controlled applications to end-users. *Brain–Computer Interface Systems—Recent Progress and Future Prospects* 1:19.

Kübler, A., E. M. Holz, A. Riccio, C. Zickler, T. Kaufmann, S. C. Kleih, P. Staiger-Sälzer, L. Desideri, E.-J. Hoogerwerf, and D. Mattia. 2014. The user-centered design as novel perspective for evaluating the usability of BCI-controlled applications. *PLoS One* 9 (12):e112392.

Kübler, A., C. Zickler, E. Holz, T. Kaufmann, A. Riccio, and D. Mattia. 2013b. Applying the user-centred design to evaluation of brain–computer interface controlled applications. *Biomedical Engineering/ Biomedizinische Technik*.

Kim, H. J., J. K. Choi, and Y. Ji. 2008. Usability evaluation framework for ubiquitous computing device. *Third International Conference on Convergence and Hybrid Information Technology, 2008. ICCIT'08*.

Kleih, S. C., A. Herweg, T. Kaufmann, P. Staiger-Sälzer, N. Gerstner, and A. Kübler. 2015. The WIN-speller: A new intuitive auditory brain–computer interface spelling application. *Frontiers in Neuroscience* 9.

Kos'Myna, N., and F. Tarpin-Bernard. 2013. Evaluation and comparison of a multimodal combination of BCI paradigms and Eye-tracking in a gaming context. *IEEE Transactions on Computational Intelligence and AI in Games (T-CIAIG)*:150–154.

Kwahk, J., and S. H. Han. 2002. A methodology for evaluating the usability of audiovisual consumer electronic products. *Applied Ergonomics* 33 (5):419–431.

Lee, T.-S., S. J. A. Goh, S. Y. Quek, R. Phillips, C. Guan, Y. B. Cheung, L. Feng, S. S. W. Teng, C. C. Wang, and Z. Y. Chin. 2013. A brain–computer interface based cognitive training system for healthy elderly: A randomized control pilot study for usability and preliminary efficacy. *PloS one* 8 (11):e79419.

Lee, T.-S., S. Y. Quek, S. J. A. Goh, R. Phillips, C. Guan, Y. B. Cheung, L. Feng, C. C. Wang, Z. Y. Chin, and H. Zhang. 2015. A pilot randomized controlled trial using EEG-based brain–computer interface training for a Chinese-speaking group of healthy elderly. *Clinical Interventions in Aging* 10:217.

Legény, J., R. V. Abad, and A. Lécuyer. 2011. Navigating in virtual worlds using a self-paced SSVEP-based brain–computer interface with integrated stimulation and real-time feedback. *Presence: Teleoperators and Virtual Environments* 20 (6):529–544.

Lewis, J. R. 1995. IBM computer usability satisfaction questionnaires: Psychometric evaluation and instructions for use. *International Journal of Human-Computer Interaction* 7 (1):57–78.

Liberati, A., D. G. Altman, J. Tetzlaff, C. Mulrow, P. C. Gøtzsche, J. P. Ioannidis, M. Clarke, P. J. Devereaux, J. Kleijnen, and D. Moher. 2009. The PRISMA statement for reporting systematic reviews and metaanalyses of studies that evaluate health care interventions: Explanation and elaboration. *Annals of Internal Medicine* 151 (4):W-65–W-94.

Lightbody, G., M. Ware, P. McCullagh, M. D. Mulvenna, E. Thomson, S. Martin, D. Todd, V. C. Medina, and S. C. Martinez. 2010. A user centred approach for developing brain–computer interfaces. *2010 4th International Conference on Pervasive Computing Technologies for Healthcare*.

Lund, A. M. 2001. Measuring Usability with the USE Questionnaire 12.

Mack, R., and F. Montaniz. 1994. Observing, predicting, and analyzing usability problems. In *Usability Inspection Methods*, 295–339. John Wiley & Sons.

Mora, N., I. De Munari, and P. Ciampolini. 2015. Improving BCI usability as HCI in ambient assisted living system control. *International Conference on Augmented Cognition*.

Morone, G., I. Pisotta, F. Pichiorri, S. Kleih, S. Paolucci, M. Molinari, F. Cincotti, A. Kübler, and D. Mattia. 2015. Proof of principle of a brain–computer interface approach to support poststroke arm rehabilitation in hospitalized patients: Design, acceptability, and usability. *Archives of Physical Medicine and Rehabilitation* 96 (3):S71–S78.

Nam, C. S., Y. Li, and S. Johnson. 2010. Evaluation of P300-based brain–computer interface in real-world contexts. *International Journal of Human–Computer Interaction* 26 (6):621–637.

Nielsen, J. 1994. *Usability Engineering*: Elsevier.

Nielsen, J., and J. Levy. 1994. Measuring usability: Preference vs. performance. *Communications of the ACM* 37 (4):66–75.

Nielsen, J., and V. L. Phillips. 1993. Estimating the relative usability of two interfaces: Heuristic, formal, and empirical methods compared. *Proceedings of the INTERACT'93 and CHI'93 Conference on Human Factors in Computing Systems*.

Nijboer, F., B. van de Laar, S. Gerritsen, A. Nijholt, and M. Poel. 2015. Usability of three electroencephalogram headsets for brain–computer interfaces: A within subject comparison. *Interacting with Computers*:iwv023.

Ohnhaus, E. E., and R. Adler. 1975. Methodological problems in the measurement of pain: A comparison between the verbal rating scale and the visual analogue scale. *Pain* 1 (4):379–384.

Pasqualotto, E., S. Federici, and M. O. Belardinelli. 2012. Toward functioning and usable brain–computer interfaces (BCIs): A literature review. *Disability and Rehabilitation: Assistive Technology* 7 (2): 89–103.

Pasqualotto, E., S. Federici, A. Simonetta, and M. Olivetti Belardinelli. 2011a. Usability of brain computer interfaces. *Assistive Technology Research Series*.

Pasqualotto, E., T. Matuz, S. Federici, C. A. Ruf, M. Bartl, M. O. Belardinelli, N. Birbaumer, and S. Halder. 2015. Usability and workload of access technology for people with severe motor impairment: A comparison of brain–computer interfacing and eye tracking. *Neurorehabilitation and Neural Repair*:1545968315575611.

Pasqualotto, E., A. Simonetta, V. Gnisci, S. Federici, and M. Olivetti Belardinelli. 2011b. Toward a usability evaluation of BCIs. *International Journal of Bioelectromagnetism* 13:121–122.

Perdikis, S., R. Leeb, J. Williamson, A. Ramsay, M. Tavella, L. Desideri, E.-J. Hoogerwerf, A. Al-Khodairy, and R. Murray-Smith. 2014. Clinical evaluation of BrainTree, a motor imagery hybrid BCI speller. *Journal of Neural Engineering* 11 (3):036003.

Powers, J. C., K. Bieliaieva, S. Wu, and C. S. Nam. 2015. The human factors and ergonomics of P300-based brain–computer interfaces. *Brain Sciences* 5 (3):318–356.

Rheinberg, F., R. Vollmeyer, and B. D. Burns. 2001. QCM: A questionnaire to assess current motivation in learning situations. *Diagnostica* 47 (2):57–66.

Riccio, A., E. M. Holz, P. Aricò, F. Leotta, F. Aloise, L. Desideri, M. Rimondini, A. Kübler, M. Mattia, and F. Cincotti. 2015. Hybrid P300-based brain–computer interface to improve usability for people with severe motor disability: Electromyographic signals for error correction during a spelling task. *Archives of Physical Medicine and Rehabilitation* 96 (3):S54–S61.

Riccio, A., F. Leotta, L. Bianchi, F. Aloise, C. Zickler, E. Hoogerwerf, A. Kübler, D. Mattia, and F. Cincotti. 2011. Workload measurement in a communication application operated through a P300-based brain–computer interface. *Journal of Neural Engineering* 8 (2):025028.

Salvendy, G., and P. Carayon. 1997. Data collection and evaluation of outcome measures. *Handbook of Human Factors and Ergonomics*:1451–1470.

Scherer, M. J., and G. Craddock. 2002. Matching person & technology (MPT) assessment process. *Technology and Disability* 14 (3):125–131.

Schettini, F., A. Riccio, L. Simione, G. Liberati, M. Caruso, V. Frasca, B. Calabrese, M. Mecella, A. Pizzimenti, and M. Inghilleri. 2015. Assistive device with conventional, alternative, and brain–computer interface inputs to enhance interaction with the environment for people with amyotrophic lateral sclerosis: A feasibility and usability study. *Archives of Physical Medicine and Rehabilitation* 96 (3):S46–S53.

Shackel, B. 1984. The concept of usability. In *Visual Display Terminals*, 45–88. Englewood Cliffs, NJ: Prentice-Hall, Inc.

Shackel, B. 1991. Usability-context, framework, definition, design and evaluation. *Human Factors for Informatics Usability*:21–37.

Shami, N. S., G. Leshed, and D. Klein. 2005. Context of use evaluation of peripheral displays (CUEPD). *IFIP Conference on Human–Computer Interaction*.

Shneiderman, B. 2010. *Designing the User Interface: Strategies for Effective Human–Computer Interaction*: Pearson Education India.

Simon, N., I. Käthner, C. A. Ruf, E. Pasqualotto, A. Kübler, and S. Halder. 2015. An auditory multiclass brain–computer interface with natural stimuli: Usability evaluation with healthy participants and a motor impaired end user. *Frontiers in Human Neuroscience* 8:1039.

Thomas, P., and R. D. Macredie. 2002. Introduction to the new usability. *ACM Transactions on Computer–Human Interaction (TOCHI)* 9 (2):69–73.

Van de Laar, B. L. 2009. Actual and imagined movement in BCI gaming.

Venkatesh, V., V. Ramesh, and A. P. Massey. 2003. Understanding usability in mobile commerce. *Communications of the ACM* 46 (12):53–56.

Weyand, S., L. Schudlo, K. Takehara-Nishiuchi, and T. Chau. 2015. Usability and performance-informed selection of personalized mental tasks for an online near-infrared spectroscopy brain–computer interface. *Neurophotonics* 2 (2):025001–025001.

Zander, T. O., M. Gaertner, C. Kothe, and R. Vilimek. 2010. Combining eye gaze input with a brain–computer interface for touchless human–computer interaction. *International Journal of Human–Computer Interaction* 27 (1):38–51.

Zickler, C., V. Di Donna, V. Kaiser, A. Al-Khodairy, S. Kleih, A. Kübler, M. Malavasi, D. Mattia, S. Mongardi, and C. Neuper. 2009. BCI applications for people with disabilities: Defining user needs and user requirements. *Assistive Technology from Adapted Equipment to Inclusive Environments, AAATE* 25:185–189.

Zickler, C., S. Halder, S. C. Kleih, C. Herbert, and A. Kübler. 2013. Brain painting: Usability testing according to the user-centered design in end users with severe motor paralysis. *Artificial Intelligence in Medicine* 59 (2):99–110.

Zickler, C., A. Riccio, F. Leotta, S. Hillian-Tress, S. Halder, E. Holz, P. Staiger-Sälzer, E.-J. Hoogerwerf, L. Desideri, and D. Mattia. 2011. A brain–computer interface as input channel for a standard assistive technology software. *Clinical EEG and Neuroscience* 42 (4):236–244.

# 30 Why User-Centered Design Is Relevant for Brain–Computer Interfacing and How It Can Be Implemented in Study Protocols

*Sonja C. Kleih and Andrea Kübler*

## CONTENTS

30.1 For Who Is This Chapter Most Relevant? .................................................................. 586
30.2 The Relevance of UCD ............................................................................................... 586
30.3 What Is UCD? ............................................................................................................. 586
30.4 UCD Realized in BCI Applications ............................................................................ 588
30.5 User-Oriented BCI Applications ................................................................................. 589
30.6 The Role of Evaluation ............................................................................................... 589
30.7 User Involvement ........................................................................................................ 589
30.8 Why the UCD Is Not Implemented in Applied BCI Research—Some Hypotheses .......... 590
30.9 Do-It-Yourself UCD and Evaluation—Getting Prepared ........................................... 591
30.10 Final Remarks ........................................................................................................... 591
References ............................................................................................................................. 592

**Abstract**

User-centered design (UCD) focuses on the needs and requirements of targeted users while developing assistive technology. Early inclusion of end-users may help to overcome the translational gap between BCI development and actual deployment by end-users. Despite its potential, the UCD is hardly followed in applied BCI research. In our book chapter, we describe how to implement the UCD in BCI studies, define usability, and how to incorporate evaluation as one component of the UCD. Different metrics to measure usability, that is, effectiveness, efficiency, and satisfaction, are readily available and should be regularly applied. To address specific BCI-controlled applications, new usability metrics can be easily integrated. We emphasize the importance to deliberately choose and define a BCI end-user group and to realize long-term field studies. Some exemplary studies with diverse clientele are presented as examples of successful UCD implementation in a BCI context.

## 30.1 FOR WHO IS THIS CHAPTER MOST RELEVANT?

Anyone who is aiming at bringing BCI to end-users of any kind, that is, the chapter is relevant for those who

- Are involved in applied BCI research
- Work with BCI end-users
- Are involved in the development or improvement of BCI-based applications
- Investigate the usability of BCI-based applications

In this chapter, we introduce user-centered design (UCD), which was standardized in ISO 9241–210 (ISO 2008) and present how to implement it in BCI research. We delineate why we consider UCD to play a major role in reaching the goal of BCI technology transfer to the end-user population for use in daily life. We focus on clinical end-users, mostly with motor impairments (for a definition of end-users, see EU project BNCI Horizon 2020 roadmap, http://bnci-horizon-2020.eu/roadmap).

## 30.2 THE RELEVANCE OF UCD

Even though an exponential increase in BCI research papers between 1988 (Farwell & Donchin 1988) and today is clearly observable (Kübler et al. 2015), BCI technology was only implemented in the daily lives of BCI end-users in very specific cases (Botrel et al. 2015; Holz et al. 2015b; Neumann & Kübler 2003; Sellers et al. 2010). Nevertheless, improvements in several aspects, such as accuracy and ease of use, have been achieved (e.g., Acqualagna et al. 2016; Allison et al. 2014; Faller et al. 2014; Kaufmann et al. 2013; Pfurtscheller et al. 2010; Townsend et al. 2010; Vidaurre et al. 2011). BCI applications are mostly developed and tested in healthy subjects, often students who volunteer for credits. The results of such research are relevant and valuable in the field of BCI, but they are barely transferrable to BCI end-users, who are mostly considered the target population for BCI (EU project BNCI Horizon: http://bnci-horizon-2020.eu/roadmap). BCI end-users may be diagnosed with (sometimes terminal) progressive muscular or neurological disease or traumatic brain injury (Grootenhuis et al. 2007; Mitchell & Borasio 2007), and some of them must be artificially ventilated, or fed, or both. Perceptual difficulties—for example in seeing—might occur (Palmowski et al. 1995) as well as cognitive impairment or fluctuation of consciousness (Bruno et al. 2011; Kübler & Kotchoubey 2007; Lulé et al. 2013). Therefore, BCI applications, which were developed in collaboration with healthy students, require changes, or improvement, or both to fulfill end-users' needs. The UCD approach directly addresses this problem: It describes the process of how end-users can be included in the design process of assistive technology from the beginning and thereby secure the creation of an application that is needed, accepted by, and adjusted to the end-user. UCD might therefore, after 30 years of BCI research, enable technology transfer that, and thereby, support overcoming the translational gap (Kübler et al. 2013; Nijboer 2015; Vaughan et al. 2012).

In non–BCI-based human–machine interaction, UCD is the standard procedure to be followed (ISO 2008). Therefore, it seems somehow surprising that in the BCI field, implementation of UCD has not yet been established and more intensively propagated, albeit the respective procedure is recommended and requested by others (e.g., Taherian et al. 2017). This is even more surprising as UCD has been adapted to BCI-controlled applications (Kübler et al. 2014). In the following sections, we will outline the UCD concept, address how to include UCD in BCI research, and hypothesize why it has not yet been broadly taken up by the community despite many declarations about BCIs being developed for end-users in need.

## 30.3 WHAT IS UCD?

The major goal of UCD is to focus on the needs and requirements of a specific target user while in the design process of an assistive technology or tool. Following the UCD, interfaces should be adaptable to individual needs and allow for high usability not only for skilled users but also for novices (Laux et al. 1996). UCD was defined by the International Organization for Standardization (ISO) as an

Approach to systems design and development that aims to make interactive systems more usable by focusing on the use of the system and applying human factors/ergonomics and usability knowledge and techniques. (https://www.iso.org/obp/ui/#iso:std:iso:9241:-210:ed-1:v1:en)

The ISO norm 9241-210:2010 released six principles concerning UCD for interactive systems: (1) understanding users, tasks, and environments; (2) users' involvement throughout the development process; (3) design being based on and adapted to the results of user-centered evaluation; (4) the adjustment process is iterative; (5) the user experience as a whole is taken into account; and (6) multidisciplinary skills and perspectives are included.

To follow the UCD, one needs to explicitly consider from the beginning the research goal or the purpose of an application and its implications for end-users. A research plan should be deduced in accordance with the UCD, such that the BCI application under investigation is presented to end-users early in the design process. Refinements are then based on end-users' feedback as assessed by evaluation metrics. Evaluation allows for comparison of the achieved solution with the requirements it is supposed to address. Actual use is possible and likely only if user requirements are met (for a recommendation on how to realize UCD for BCI-based application, please see Figure 30.1).

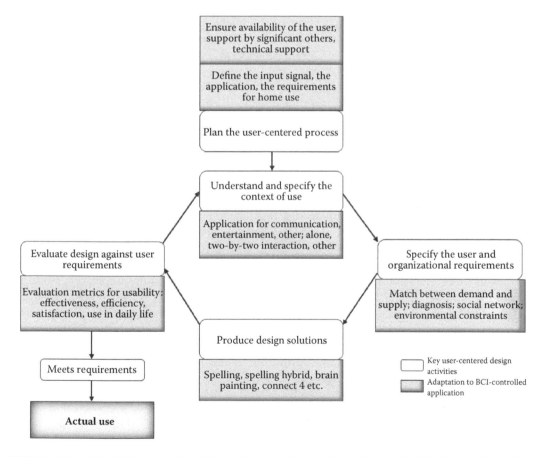

**FIGURE 30.1** The UCD adapted to BCI applications. (Adapted from Figure 4 in Kübler, A., E. M. Holz, A. Riccio, C. Zickler, T. Kaufmann, S. C. Kleih, P. Staiger-Sälzer, L. Desideri, E.-J. Hoogerwerf and D. Mattia. 2014. The user-centered design as novel perspective for evaluating the usability of BCI-controlled applications. *PLoS One* 9(12): e112392. doi:10.1371/journal.pone.0112392.)

Fortunately, examples in which BCI applications were developed based on the UCD process do exist and users' requirements were directly addressed (Holz et al. 2013; Rohm et al. 2013; Schreuder et al. 2013; Zickler et al. 2013). In other studies, user requirements were taken into account in the design of the BCI application or the choice of the protocol without explicitly emphasizing UCD (e.g., Morone et al. 2015; Riccio et al. 2015; Saeedi et al. 2016; Schettini et al. 2015; Vansteensel et al. 2016). In the Section 30.4, we present a nonconclusive review on examples for both approaches.

## 30.4   UCD REALIZED IN BCI APPLICATIONS

The importance of implementing UCD in BCI development and protocol elaboration was acknowledged not only in the clinical field but also in the BCI application areas of gaming and entertainment (e.g., Plass-Oude Bos et al. 2011). Plass-Oude Bos et al. (2011) interviewed BCI users about the strategies they would like to use (such as inner speech) to change brain states to control a character in the gaming environment. They implemented these requested changes in their BCI application. However, the authors do not report the success with which the BCI gamer controlled the application.

Scherer et al. (2015) investigated usability of a newly developed row–column scanning communication board for individuals with cerebral palsy. By iterating evaluation loops with persons with cerebral palsy, relatives, and caregivers, they adapted the regular spelling paradigm in several aspects according to the received information. The authors created a 3 × 3 matrix comprising symbols such as a soccer ball or a banana instead of the usually displayed letters to decrease paradigm complexity. Rows and columns were consecutively highlighted instead of randomly. This highlighting mode facilitated BCI use as the target population was already used to the scanning mode for operation of other assistive technologies. Motor imagery (MI) was chosen as an input signal because previous trials with evoked potentials were not as successful as MI BCI use, mostly due to strong muscle artifacts (Daly et al. 2013). Also in line with UCD, the authors report iterative BCI design development steps, which included testing a maximum-likelihood selection adaptable to the user. However, the adaptive BCI version that would provide an estimate of the symbol intended to be spelled was too confusing for end-users and therefore was abandoned during further trials. With the final BCI system, 6 of 11 participants performed above chance level.

In a report of two patients with ALS, the UCD approach was implemented to modify and adjust the artistic BCI application Brain Painting (BP) (Botrel et al. 2015; Holz et al. 2015a). The patients used the P300-based BP application at home with caregivers and relatives learning to provide the necessary assistance for home use that is independent from a local research support team. Data storage and BCI system control were adjusted to a remote connection such that the research team at the University of Würzburg could support the end-users from the laboratory. At the same time, relatives and caregivers were taught how to set up the BCI application as recommended in UCD. The paradigm itself was designed following UCD as the stimulation mode was changed from a regular flashing to the so-called face speller mode (Kaufmann et al. 2013). In this stimulation mode, letters are overlaid with faces instead of flashes, leading to ERPs related to face recognition in addition to increased P300 amplitudes (Chen et al. 2016). Less time was then needed by the end-users to paint, which increased usability and satisfaction. Visual analog scales were answered by the users after every use of the BCI application and questionnaires regularly after a defined amount of sessions, such that the system could be adapted continuously over time to the user's wishes. Evaluation revealed that the end-users would prefer more functions available in the application. Additional functions should allow for a higher level of artistic expression. Therefore, the software was changed according to the end-user wishes (Botrel et al. 2015). This new, more complex BP version was enthusiastically used by one end-user, while for the other, it was too complicated. Adjustments should therefore be realizable based on individual needs. Thus, a UCD-based BCI application ideally fulfills the criteria of generalizability and at the same time of adaptability (one prototype application that can be individually specified, e.g., Kleih et al. 2016).

## 30.5  USER-ORIENTED BCI APPLICATIONS

Some studies take into account end-user requirements but were not explicitly designed following the UCD. We will review two examples for such applications. In a BCI application that was developed for rehabilitation of motor function in the upper extremity, stroke patients imagined movements with their affected hand to trigger movement of a virtual hand representation that was projected on a white cloth placed on the affected hand (Morone et al. 2015; Picchiori et al. 2015). In this application, the BCI system detects MI and the virtual hand moves according to the imagined movement (opening or closing the hand as discrete feedback). The projection on the cloth was chosen as a feedback because patients had reported previously that the observation of a moving hand (instead of e.g., a cursor) would probably help them to imagine movements with their paralyzed hand. Moreover, different hand models (e.g., male and female) were developed. Participant feedback on the prototype hand model revealed that it was judged to represent a female hand. This perception would possibly hinder a male participant to accept the provided hand model as a representation of its own hand. Furthermore, patients reported being used to therapeutic support and to benefit from the interaction. Thus, a therapist was included in the BCI protocol to guide the BCI user through the training. The therapist supported the patients by giving continuous feedback on their performance in addition to the discrete feedback provided by the moving hand.

In a case study presented by Saeedi et al. (2016), the authors report BCI control by a tetraplegic, artificially ventilated end-user who used the BCI for 11 months. The participant's oculomotor muscles were completely paralyzed; thus, MI was chosen as an input signal. The participants' task was a two-class gaming task, which in later studies could be changed to a communication or navigation task. The authors tested an adaptive assistance approach and argued that such an approach could reliably take into account the cognitive state and brain signal—the so-called *internal context*. The adaptation consisted of a variable trial duration, and the adaptation level was determined by a performance estimator. Therefore, the BCI could directly use the information provided by the user (brain signal stability) and react to it.

## 30.6  THE ROLE OF EVALUATION

As often recommended (e.g., Laar et al. 2011; Schlögl et al. 2007; Vaughan et al. 2012), Kübler et al. (2014) suggested evaluation metrics for BCI applications based on the concept of usability. Usability is defined as the extent to which a product can be used by a specified target population to reach specific goals with effectiveness, efficiency, and satisfaction (ISO 2008). While effectiveness relates to the accuracy that can be achieved, efficiency refers to the cost and time invested in relation to effectiveness. Satisfaction assesses perceived accessibility, comfort of use, and product–user match (ISO 2008; Kübler et al. 2014; Laar et al. 2011). Transferring this concept to BCI use, Kübler and colleagues assessed effectiveness (accuracy = correct responses in relation to the number of total responses), efficiency (amount of information transferred per time unit and invested mental workload), and satisfaction in 19 end-users who operated BCI systems for spelling, painting, or gaming. They concluded that specific metrics yield informative results and that these metrics are applicable in end-users who are diagnosed with major motor impairment or even with the locked-in state. The framework proposed by Kübler et al. (2014) allows for integrating additional metrics depending on the application under investigation. As evaluation is the basis of the iterative UCD process, it should become a standard procedure in applied BCI research.

## 30.7  USER INVOLVEMENT

Even though involvement of end-users in the design process of assistive technologies was strongly recommended and supported by some authors (e.g., Elsma et al. 2004; Huggins et al. 2011; Kübler et al. 2014; Laar et al. 2011; Lightbody et al. 2010; Plass-Oude Bos et al. 2011; Vaughan et al. 2012), others argue that research should be independent of and not dictated by end-users' ideas (Newell & Gregor 2000). Newell and Gregor state that

> in User Centred Design although the needs and wants of users are the focus of the research, the user cannot be in control of the research, as is sometimes suggested by the proponents of PAR (Participatory Action Research). (Newell & Gregor, p. 40)

A potential conflict of interest is evident: On the one hand, the ultimate goal of the UCD is the development of a technological application for end-users reaching the best possible person–technology fit; on the other hand, potential dead ends that are not realizable or too complicated or not individually adjustable should be avoided. This implies that not every possible wish for technological changes or further investigation in the development process of an assistive device can be followed by the researchers; a modular hardware and software design may alleviate these issues. In this respect, applied clinical research must be distinguished from basic research, which, in our opinion, helps to resolve the conflict. Applied clinical research in the field of BCI aims at the development of solutions that can be used outside the laboratory, thereby overcoming the translational gap. This also comes with a potential loss of research possibilities as one route determines future paths to be investigated. Without a doubt, UCD should be followed in applied BCI research. Thus, we do not argue for applying the UCD in any BCI study, but for an unambiguous definition of the research goal—and if it is to provide BCI for end-users in the field, following the UCD is mandatory. This also includes a thorough definition of the end-user who can be manifold, such as doctors, paramedical staff, neurofeedback trainers, caregivers, or the patients themselves (for a thorough elaboration of end-users, see http://bnci-horizon-2020.eu/roadmap). Importantly, following the UCD in applied research does not exclude a realistic estimation and communication of possibilities to the end-user that can be realized at any point in time. However, if a BCI-controlled application was neither developed in cooperation with end-users nor took into account end-users' needs, it will not be used by the targeted population as is the case with almost all BCI-controlled applications, despite publications in high-impact journals (e.g., Hochberg et al. 2006). Therefore, applications as well as end-users should be carefully selected. To support such selection, Vaughan et al. (2012) provided some guidelines on end-user selection that were adopted and further developed by Kübler et al. (2015), who suggested an exemplary algorithm to select candidates for independent use of a BCI at home. Potential BCI candidates should be interested in BCI use, be in need of an assistive technology, be able to give informed consent, live in a supportive environment, and be cognitively able to operate a BCI system. If all these apply, the best-fitting stimulation modality (e.g., visual) and signal type (e.g., P300) can be identified. By following clearly defined selection criteria, generalizability of achieved results from the study sample to the entire population is more likely and lessons learnt might be transferrable to future translational studies in end-users' homes.

Basic research, on the other hand, generates research hypotheses and investigates fundamental principles. BCI prototypes that may not fulfill end-user criteria are tested and might provide meaningful input for later solutions applicable in end-users.

## 30.8  WHY THE UCD IS NOT IMPLEMENTED IN APPLIED BCI RESEARCH—SOME HYPOTHESES

While we consider UCD mandatory if applied BCI research seriously aims at bringing BCIs to end-users in the field, we are well aware of the problems that come along with it (Chavarriaga et al. 2017). Research with end-users, specifically those with disease, is effortful and requires appropriate financial and human resources, and studies need to adopt longitudinal designs—all requirements that are not easy to implement in a research environment that often appreciates most, a long publication list. The lack of funding for longitudinal studies adds to the problem.

Another possible reason why the UCD is only reluctantly taken up by the community is that researchers rather follow their own ideas of what may be valuable for an end-user. Garud and Ahlstrom (1994) suggested a Socio-Cognitive Model of Technology, pointing out the potential problem that researchers usually tend to create their research questions based on their own beliefs and experiences, leading to a technology that matches the researchers' rather than the end-users' needs. In comparison to the real needs of end-users, those of the researchers are often easier to achieve and evaluated accordingly because only convenient measures are used. Evaluation will, thus, most naturally, positively reinforce the created idea. Thereby, researchers might be limited by their own vision of end-users' needs instead of choosing potential new ways of improving and adjusting technology.

Furthermore, the end-user population is a vulnerable one, as BCI end-users who are really in need of assistive technologies are most likely also medically in a challenging state, some being artificially ventilated or fed, or both. Even with a perfectly planned data acquisition schedule, personal and health issues, family conflicts or interference with other therapies might occur and prevent fast and smooth data acquisition at the end-user's home. One is involved in the BCI end-user's personal history, is confronted with sometimes desperate relatives, and must try to create an atmosphere of mutual trust and collaboration in another person's home. This is challenging for researchers and end-users alike.

## 30.9    DO-IT-YOURSELF UCD AND EVALUATION—GETTING PREPARED

The first step always is and under all circumstances must be: Reading. Our experience is that results older than a few years or from different research groups or from fields not directly linked to the research question at hand are often neglected. This prevents integration of results and fosters reinventing the wheel albeit with a different tire.

Also, it is mandatory to get familiar with the end-user population you wish to work with. Ideally, one would spend some time with the (patient) end-users and attend focus groups or meetings of support groups. This will help to realize a BCI application that the targeted end-users' need indeed. Furthermore, in case your end-users have an idiosyncratic communication style (e.g., due to motor impairment), you must be ready to learn individual ways or codes of communication. We recommend following the advice given in the section "user involvement": cooperate with the family and staff and use their expertise as a resource for your research. Before starting BCI measurements, be very clear about the purpose of your work: Which goals would you like to achieve?

You also should plan extra time for data assessment with a clinical population. Because of sickness or hospital stays (Saeedi et al. 2016), measurements might be cancelled. You must, and even more in UCD-based studies, continuously check the assessed data to make sure that there are neither mistakes in the protocols nor major problems with the signal (e.g., artifacts caused by inflation of the anti-decubitus mattress). Finally, evaluate the BCI application you worked with and its usability, and use questionnaires to ensure systematic evaluation (Kübler et al. 2014).

## 30.10    FINAL REMARKS

We believe that overcoming the translational gap between BCI development and transfer to real-world use can be fostered by UCD implementation. This would support development of BCI devices that are (1) really needed, desired, and, thus, accepted by end-users; and (2) individually adjusted to the end-users' requirements. You as a scientist involved in applied BCI research can substantially contribute to bringing BCI technology to end-users. Become familiar with the UCD and the respective evaluation metrics. Ask for the needs and requirements of the target population and include from the beginning this information in your design of an application. Be ready to spend some time on readjustments and be convinced that the process is worth it, for the benefit of end-users in need.

## REFERENCES

Acqualagna, L., L. Botrel, C. Vidaurre, A. Kübler, and B. Blankertz. 2016. Large-scale assessment of a fully automatic co-adaptive motor imagery-based brain computer interface. *PloS One* 11(2): e0148886.

Allison, B.Z., J. Jin, Y. Zhang, and X. Wang. 2014. A four-choice hybrid P300/SSVEP BCI for improved accuracy. *Brain–Comput Interf* 1(1): 17–26.

Botrel, L., E.M. Holz, and A. Kübler. 2015. Brain Painting V2: Evaluation of P300-based brain–computer interface for creative expression by an end-user following the user-centered design. *Brain–Comput Interf* 2(2–3): 135–149. doi:10.1080/2326263X.2015.1100038.

Bruno, M.-A., A. Vanhaudenhuyse, A. Thibaut, G. Moonen, and S. Laureys. 2011. From unresponsive wakefulness to minimally conscious PLUS and functional locked-in syndromes: Recent advances in our understanding of disorders of consciousness. *J Neurol* 258(7): 1373–1384. doi:10.1007/s00415-011-6114-x.

Chavarriaga, R., M. Fried-Oken, S. Kleih, F. Lotte, and R. Scherer. 2017. Heading for new shores! Overcoming pitfalls in BCI design. *Brain–Comput Interf* 1–14. 10.1080/2326263X.2016.1263916.

Chen, L., J. Jin, I. Daly, Y. Zhang, X. Wang, and A. Cichocki. 2016. Exploring combinations of different color and facial expression stimuli for gaze-independent BCIs. *Front Comput Neurosci* 10(5): 10.3389/fncom.2016.00005.

Daly, I., M. Billinger, J. Laparra-Hernandez, F. Aloise, M.L. Garcia, J. Faller, R. Scherer, and G. Müller-Putz. 2013. On the control of brain–computer interfaces by users with cerebral palsy. *Clin Neurophysiol* 124(9): 1787–1797. doi:10.1016/j.clinph.2013.02.118.

Eisma, R., A. Dickinson, J. Goodman, A. Syme, L. Tiwari, and A.F. Newell. 2004. Early user involvement in the development of information technology-related products for older people. *Univ Access Inform Soc* 3(2): 131–140.

EU project BNCI Horizon homepage: http://bnci-horizon-2020.eu/roadmap.

Faller, J., R. Scherer, E.V. Friedrich, U. Costa, E. Opisso, J. Medina, and G.R. Müller-Putz. 2014. Non-motor tasks improve adaptive brain–computer interface performance in users with severe motor impairment. *Front Neurosci* 8: 10.3389/fnins.2014.00320.

Farwell, L.A., and Donchin, E. 1988. Talking off the top of your head: Toward a mental prosthesis utilizing event-related brain potentials. *Electroencephalogr Clin Neurophysiol* 70: 512–523.

Garud, R., and D. Ahlstrom. 1994. A socio-cognitive model of technology evolution: The case of cochlear implants. *Org Sci* 5(3): 344–362. doi:10.1287/orsc.5.3.344.

Grootenhuis, M.A., J. de Boone, and A.J. van der Kooi. 2007. Living with muscular dystrophy: Health related quality of life consequences for children and adults. *Health Qual Life Outcomes* 5(1): 31. doi:10.1186/1477-7525-5-31.

Hochberg, L.R., M.D. Serruya, G.M. Friehs, J.A. Mukand, M. Saleh, A.H. Caplan, A. Branner, D. Chen, R.D. Penn, and J.P. Donoghue. 2006. Neuronal ensemble control of prosthetic devices by a human with tetraplegia. *Nature* 442(7099): 164–171.

Holz, E.M., L. Botrel, T. Kaufmann, and A. Kübler. 2015a. Long-term independent brain–computer interface home use improves quality of life of a patient in the locked-in state: A case study. *Arch Phys Med Rehabil* 96(3 Suppl): S16–26. doi:10.1016/j.apmr.2014.03.035.

Holz, E.M., L. Botrel, and A. Kübler. 2015b. Independent home use of Brain Painting improves quality of life of two artists in the locked-in state diagnosed with amyotrophic lateral sclerosis. *Brain–Comput Interf* 2(2–3): 117–134. doi:10.1080/2326263X.2015.1100048.

Holz, E.M., J. Höhne, P. Staiger-Sälzer, M. Tangermann, and A. Kübler, A. 2013. Brain–computer interface controlled gaming: Evaluation of usability by severely motor restricted end-users. *Artif Intel Med* 59(2): 111–120. doi:http://dx.doi.org/10.1016/j.artmed.2013.08.001.

Huggins, J.E., P.A. Wren, and K.L. Gruis. 2011. What would brain–computer interface users want? Opinions and priorities of potential users with amyotrophic lateral sclerosis. *Amyotroph Lateral Scler* 12(5): 318–324.

ISO (2008). ISO 9241–210 (2008) Ergonomics of human system interaction—Part 210: Human-centred design for interactive systems (formerly known as 13407). International Organization for Standardization (ISO) Switzerland.

Kaufmann, T., S.M. Schulz, A. Köblitz, G. Renner, C. Wessig, and A. Kübler. 2013. Face stimuli effectively prevent brain–computer interface inefficiency in patients with neurodegenerative disease. *Clin Neurophysiol* 124(5): 893–900. doi:http://dx.doi.org/10.1016/j.clinph.2012.11.006.

Kleih, S.C., L. Gottschalt, E. Teichlein, and F.X. Weilbach. 2016. Toward a P300 based brain-computer interface for aphasia rehabilitation after stroke: Presentation of theoretical considerations and a pilot feasibility study. *Front Hum Neurosci* 10: 10.3389/fnins.2014.00320.

Kübler, A., E.M. Holz, A. Riccio, C. Zickler, T. Kaufmann, S.C. Kleih, P. Staiger-Sälzer, L. Desideri, E.-J. Hoogerwerf, and D. Mattia. 2014. The user-centered design as novel perspective for evaluating the usability of BCI-controlled applications. *PLoS One* 9(12): e112392. doi:10.1371/journal.pone.0112392.

Kübler, A., and B. Kotchoubey. 2007. Brain–computer interfaces in the continuum of consciousness. *Curr Opin Neurol* 20(6): 643–649. doi:10.1097/WCO.0b013e3282f14782.

Kübler, A., D. Mattia, R. Rupp, and M. Tangermann. 2013. Facing the challenge: Bringing brain–computer interfaces to end-users. *Artif Intell Med* 59(2): 55–60. doi:10.1016/j.artmed.2013.08.002.

Kübler, A., G. Müller-Putz, and D. Mattia. 2015. User-centred design in brain–computer interface research and development. *Ann Phys Rehabil Med* 58(5): 312–314. doi:10.1016/j.rehab.2015.06.003.

Laar, B., F. Nijboer, H. Gürkök, D. Plass-Oude Bos, and A. Nijholt. 2011. User experience evaluation in BCI: Bridge the gap. *Int Bioelectromagn* 13(3): 157–158.

Laux, L.F., P.R. McNally, M.G. Paciello, and G.C. Vanderheiden. 1996. Designing the World Wide Web for people with disabilities: A user centered design approach. In *Proceedings of the Second Annual ACM Conference on Assistive Technologies*, pp. 94–101. ACM, 1996.

Lightbody, G., M. Ware, P. McCullagh, M.D. Mulvenna, E. Thomson, S. Martin, D. Todd, V.C. Medina, and S.C. Martinez. 2010. A user centred approach for developing Brain–Computer Interfaces. In *2010 4th International Conference on Pervasive Computing Technologies for Healthcare*: 1–8.

Lulé, D., Q. Noirhomme, S.C. Kleih, C. Chatelle, S. Halder, A. Demertzi, M.-A. Bruno, O. Gosseries, A. Vanhaudenhuyse, C. Schnakers, M. Thonnard, A. Soddu, A. Kübler, and S. Laureys. 2013. Probing command following in patients with disorders of consciousness using a brain–computer interface. *Clin Neurophysiol* 124(1): 101–106. doi:http://dx.doi.org/10.1016/j.clinph.2012.04.030.

Mitchell, J.D., and G.D. Borasio. 2007. Amyotrophic lateral sclerosis. *Lancet,* 369(9578): 2031–2041. doi:10.1016/s0140-6736(07)60944-1.

Morone, G., I. Pisotta, F. Pichiorri, S. Kleih, S. Paolucci, M. Molinari, F. Cincotti, A. Kübler and D. Mattia. 2015. Proof of principle of a brain–computer interface approach to support poststroke arm rehabilitation in hospitalized patients: Design, acceptability, and usability. *Arch Phys Med Rehabil* 96(3, Supplement): S71–S78. doi:http://dx.doi.org/10.1016/j.apmr.2014.05.026.

Neumann, N., and A. Kübler. 2003. Training locked-in patients: A challenge for the use of brain–computer interfaces. *IEEE Trans Neural Syst Rehabil Eng* 11(2): 169–172. doi:10.1109/TNSRE.2003.814431.

Newell, A.F., and P. Gregor. "User sensitive inclusive design"—In search of a new paradigm. In *Proceedings on the 2000 Conference on Universal Usability*: 39–44. ACM, 2000.

Nijboer, F. 2015. Technology transfer of brain–computer interfaces as assistive technology: Barriers and opportunities. *Ann Phys Rehabil Med* 58(1): 35–38.

Palmowski, A., W.H. Jost, J. Prudlo, J. Osterhage, B. Käsmann, K. Schimrigk, and K.W. Ruprecht. 1995. Eye movement in amyotrophic lateral sclerosis: A longitudinal study. *Ger Ophthalmol* 4(6): 355–362.

Pfurtscheller, G., T. Solis-Escalante, R. Ortner, P. Linortner, and G.R. Müller-Putz. 2010. Self-paced operation of an SSVEP-based orthosis with and without an imagery-based "brain switch:" A feasibility study towards a hybrid BCI. *IEEE Trans Neural Syst Rehabil Eng* 18(4): 409–414.

Pichiorri, F., Morone, G., Petti, M., Toppi, J., Pisotta, I., Molinari, M., Paolucci, S., Inghilleri, M., Astolfi, L., Cincotti, F., and Mattia, D. 2015. Brain–computer interface boosts motor imagery practice during stroke recovery. *Ann Neurol* 77(5): 851–865.

Plass-Oude Bos, D., H. Gürkök, B.L.A. Van de Laar, F. Nijboer, and A. Nijholt. 2011. User experience evaluation in BCI: Mind the gap! *Int Bioelectromagn* 13(1): 48–49.

Riccio, A., E.M. Holz, P. Aricò, F. Leotta, F. Aloise, L. Desideri, L., ... and F. Cincotti. 2015. Hybrid P300-based brain–computer interface to improve usability for people with severe motor disability: Electromyographic signals for error correction during a spelling task. *Arch Phys Med Rehabil* 96(3, Supplement): S54–S61. doi:http://dx.doi.org/10.1016/j.apmr.2014.05.029.

Rohm, M., M. Schneiders, C. Müller, A. Kreilinger, V. Kaiser, G.R. Müller-Putz, and R. Rupp. 2013. Hybrid brain–computer interfaces and hybrid neuroprostheses for restoration of upper limb functions in individuals with high-level spinal cord injury. *Artif Intel Med* 59(2): 133–142. doi:http://dx.doi.org/10.1016/j.artmed.2013.07.004.

Saeedi, S., R. Chavarriaga, and J.D.R. Millan. 2016. Long-term stable control of motor-imagery BCI by a locked-in user through adaptive assistance. *IEEE Trans Neural Syst Rehabil Eng.*

Scherer, R., M. Billinger, J. Wagner, A. Schwarz, D.T. Hettich, E. Bolinger, E., ... and G. Müller-Putz. 2015. Thought-based row–column scanning communication board for individuals with cerebral palsy. *Ann Phys Rehabil Med,* 58(1): 14–22. doi:http://dx.doi.org/10.1016/j.rehab.2014.11.005.

Schettini, F., A. Riccio, L. Simione, G. Liberati, M. Caruso, V. Frasca, V., ... and F. Cincotti. 2015. Assistive device with conventional, alternative, and brain–computer interface inputs to enhance interaction with the environment for people with amyotrophic lateral sclerosis: A feasibility and usability study. *Arch Phys Med Rehabil* 96(3 Supplement): S46–S53. doi:http://dx.doi.org/10.1016/j.apmr.2014.05.027.

Schlögl, A., J. Kronegg, J.E. Huggins, and S.G. Mason. 2007. Evaluation criteria for BCI research. In G. Dornhege, J. del R. Millan, T. Hinterberger, D. McFarland, and K.R. Müller (Eds.). *Toward Brain Computer Interfacing*. MIT Press. pp. 327–342.

Schreuder, M., A. Riccio, M. Risetti, S. Dähne, N. Ramsay, J. Williamson, M. Tangermann. 2013. User-centered design in brain–computer interfaces—A case study. *Artif Intel Med* 59(2): 71–80. doi:http://dx.doi.org/10.1016/j.artmed.2013.07.005.

Sellers, E.W., T.M. Vaughan, and J.R. Wolpaw. 2010. A brain–computer interface for long-term independent home use. *Amyotroph Lateral Scler* 11(5): 449–455. doi:10.3109/17482961003777470.

Taherian, S., Selitskiy, D., Pau, J. et al. (2017). Are we there yet? Evaluating commercial grade brain–computer interface for control of computer applications by individuals with cerebral palsy. *Disabil Rehabil Assist Technol* (12): 165–174.

Townsend, G., B.K. LaPallo, C.B. Boulay, D.J. Krusienski, G.E. Frye, C.K. Hauser, N.E. Schwartz, T.M. Vaughan, J.R. Wolpaw, and E.W. Sellers. A novel P300-based brain–computer interface stimulus presentation paradigm: Moving beyond rows and columns. *Clin Neurophysiol* 121, no. 7 (2010): 1109–1120.

Vansteensel, M.J., E.G. Pels, M.G. Bleichner, M.P. Branco, T. Denison, Z.V. Freudenburg, P. Gosselaar, S. Leinders, T.H. Ottens, M.A. Van Den Boom, and P.C. Van Rijen. 2016. Fully implanted brain–computer interface in a locked-in patient with ALS. *N Engl Med* 375(21): 2060–2066.

Vaughan, T., E. Sellers, and J. Wolpaw. 2012. Clinical evaluation of BCIs. In J. Wolpaw and E. Winter Wolpaw (Eds.). *Brain–Computer Interfaces Principles and Practice*. Oxford University Press: New York. pp. 325–336.

Vidaurre, C., C. Sannelli, K.R. Müller, and B. Blankertz. 2011. Co-adaptive calibration to improve BCI efficiency. *J Neural Eng* 8(2): 025009.

Zickler, C., S. Halder, S.C. Kleih, C. Herbert, and A. Kübler. 2013. Brain Painting: Usability testing according to the user-centered design in end users with severe motor paralysis. *Artif Intell Med* 59(2): 99–110. doi:10.1016/j.artmed.2013.08.003.

# 31 A Generic Framework for Adaptive EEG-Based BCI Training and Operation

*Jelena Mladenović, Jérémie Mattout\*, and Fabien Lotte\**

## CONTENTS

31.1 Introduction .................................................................................................................596
31.2 Adaptive BCI Systems—Motivations and Principles................................................597
    31.2.1 Reasons for Adaptation...................................................................................597
        31.2.1.1 Causes of Signal Variability .........................................................597
    31.2.2 Main Principles of Adaptation........................................................................598
        31.2.2.1 Machine Learning...........................................................................598
        31.2.2.2 Human Learning .............................................................................598
31.3 Framework .................................................................................................................599
    31.3.1 The System Pipeline .......................................................................................600
        31.3.1.1 Literature Review on Adaptive Signal Processing/Machine Learning .....601
    31.3.2 The User and the Task Model........................................................................603
        31.3.2.1 User Model......................................................................................604
        31.3.2.2 Task Model......................................................................................605
    31.3.3 Machine Output ..............................................................................................606
        31.3.3.1 Feedback .........................................................................................606
        31.3.3.2 Instructions and Stimuli.................................................................606
    31.3.4 Conducting Adaptation with the Conductor .................................................606
31.4 Perspectives and Challenges......................................................................................607
31.5 Conclusion .................................................................................................................607
Acknowledgment ..................................................................................................................608
References..............................................................................................................................608

**Abstract**

Adaptive BCIs have shown promising results by reaching higher performances and robustness. However, existing methods lack guidelines in their manner of addressing the problem. Most of the current adaptive techniques simply handle challenges at hand by dynamically adjusting the machine to signal variability, often not entirely taking into account the human factors. To our knowledge, there has not been any work done in creating a taxonomy for adaptive BCIs, one that acknowledges and arranges known BCI components in a comprehensive and structured way. We propose a conceptual framework that encompasses adaptation approaches for both the user and the machine, that is, using instructional design observations as well as the usual machine learning techniques. This framework not only provides a coherent review of such extensive literature but also allows the readers to clearly visualize which component is being adapted and for what reason. Moreover, it enables the readers to perceive gaps in current BCIs

---

\* Both authors contributed equally to this manuscript.

and grasp the adaptive system in its entirety. Our proposal hopefully contributes as a guideline for a computational implementation of a fully adaptive BCI and an overall improvement.

## 31.1 INTRODUCTION

Thanks to the technological advancements, the interest in brain–computer interfaces (BCIs) has grown immensely during the last decades. BCIs are mainly used to facilitate the interaction between people with different disabilities and their environment (Millán et al. 2010; Perrin 2012). However, there has been outreach in nonclinical domains such as gaming and art (Lotte 2013a; Tan and Nijholt 2010).

There are two main paradigms in BCI, depending on the type of extracted physiological markers. (1) Spontaneous BCIs (synchronous or self-paced) paradigms typically measure oscillatory EEG activity, and the event-related desynchronization/synchronization (ERD/ERS) in sensorimotor rhythms (SMRs) (Pfurtscheller 2006). They are mainly related to motor imagery (MI) BCI, for instance, imagining left or right hand movements (Pfurtscheller 2006), and to mental imagery, such as mental object rotation or calculations (Faradji 2009). Spontaneous BCI paradigms may also rely on slow cortical potentials (Birbaumer and Kübler 2000). (2) Evoked responses or ERP (event-related potential)-based BCI paradigms are based on the attentional selection of an external stimulus among many. Be it in the visual (V), the auditory (A), or the somatosensory (S) modality, this approach can give rise to various types of well-known responses such as the P300 component (Donchin et al. 2000) or steady-state sensory evoked potentials (SS(V/A/S)EP) (Middendorf et al. 2000). Those BCIs follow the same rationale; they typically consist of (i) a calibration phase, in which the classifier "learns" to discriminate and translate signal features into commands, (ii) a training phase, in which the user learns to manipulate the system and to regulate his or her EEG patterns, and (iii) the application, in which the user has hopefully control over the system. A general opinion is that there is very little need for user training with ERP-based BCIs (Fazel-Rezai et al. 2012), even though the user can improve his or her P300 marker with training (Baykara 2016). However, the system calibration is often mandatory (Fazel-Rezai et al. 2012) and lasts about 10 min. Furthermore, for MI BCIs, user training is a necessary and often cumbersome process, during which novel functional circuits for action are created, referred to as the "neuroprosthetic skill" (Orsborn 2014; Shenoy and Carmena 2014). Also, SMR with higher signal-to-noise ratio have been observed as a consequence of learning during such training (Gaume et al. 2016; Kober et al. 2013).

There are two main approaches engaged in improving BCI systems: (i) improving the machine learning techniques (Makeig et al. 2012; Müller et al. 2008) and the newly introduced (ii) improving human learning, by using the knowledge from instructional design and positive psychology (Lotte 2013b; Lotte and Jeunet 2015). Both agree that the system needs to be adapted to the user but rely on different sources of adaptation: the machine for the former and the brain for the latter. In particular, machine learning algorithms should adapt to nonstationary brain signals, while human learning approaches assist in the production of stable EEG patterns of the user or in the adaptability of the brain to the machine. This implies that these approaches should guide the machine adaptation according to the various users' skills and profiles. Including both aspects of adaptation, a symbiotic coadaptation (Sanchez et al. 2009) could give rise to a system ready to be used in real-life conditions.

However, a major obstacle lies in the large spectrum of sources of variability during BCI use, ranging from (i) imperfect recording conditions: environmental noise, humidity, static electricity, and so on (Maby 2016) to (ii) the fluctuations in the user's psychophysiological states, as a result of fatigue, motivation, attention, and so on (Jeunet et al. 2016). For these reasons, a BCI has not yet proven to be reliable enough to be used outside the laboratory (Wolpaw and Wolpaw 2012). In particular, it is still almost impossible to create one BCI design effective for every user, owing to large intersubject variability (Allison and Neuper 2010). Therefore, the main concerns are to create a more robust system with the same high level of success for everyone, at all times, and to improve the current usability of the system (Lotte 2013b; Wolpaw and Wolpaw 2012). This calls for adaptive BCI training and operation.

To our knowledge, there is no work devoted to classifying the literature on adaptive BCI in a comprehensive and structured way. Hence, we propose a conceptual framework that encompasses most important approaches to fit them in such a way that a reader can clearly visualize which elements can be adapted and for what reason. In the interest of having a clear review of the existing adaptive BCIs, this framework considers adaptation approaches for both the user and the machine, that is, referring to instructional design observations as well as the usual machine learning techniques. It not only provides a coherent review of the extensive literature but also enables the reader to perceive gaps and flaws in current BCI systems, which would, hopefully, bring novel solutions for an overall improvement. BCIs, which use noninvasive electroencephalography (EEG) as a measuring tool, will be in the center of our attention throughout this chapter. Nevertheless, the proposed solutions for adaptation can be applied to other techniques such as invasive recordings, functional near-infrared spectroscopy (fNIRS), or magnetoencephalography (MEG).

This chapter is organized as follows. Section 31.2 discusses the reasoning behind creating adaptive BCIs; it will guide the reader through the aspects of human and machine learning that call for adaptive methods. Section 31.3 presents our contribution to the field, a comprehensive framework to design and study adaptive BCI systems. We show that the framework encompasses most techniques of adaptive BCIs, which we briefly review. In Section 31.4, we describe the challenges and future work. Finally, Section 31.5 is the concluding section of this chapter.

## 31.2 ADAPTIVE BCI SYSTEMS—MOTIVATIONS AND PRINCIPLES

For the sake of understanding the reasons for adaptation, we develop prominent variabilities that cause low BCI performance and present the main principles used for adaptation.

### 31.2.1 REASONS FOR ADAPTATION

Currently, adaptation is mainly done by using different signal processing techniques without including the human factors (Allison and Neuper 2010; Makeig et al. 2012). However, the user's success in mastering the BCI skill appears to be a key element for BCI robustness. If the user is not able to produce stable and distinct EEG patterns, then no signal processing algorithm would be able to recognize them (Lotte 2013b).

Up to a certain extent, machine learning techniques can adapt to the signal variability. However, most of those techniques are blind to the causes of signal variability. Identifying those causes, accounting for them and possibly acting directly on them may help design more advanced and more robust approaches. Such causes may act at different time scales, for instance, a person's drop of attention may have a sudden and dramatic impact, while learning rather operates on the long run.

The term *variability* is somewhat used to describe the user, environment, and equipment "variability" and, more frequently, the signal variability. These two variabilities are often confounded, as one being the cause and the other being the effect, respectively. Throughout this chapter, we mostly address the user variability as the main cause and denote its various expressions as *components*.

### 31.2.1.1 Causes of Signal Variability

Variability can be distinguished as (1) short term (Schlögl et al. 2010), that is, signal variabilities within trials or runs caused by, for example, fluctuations in attention, mood, and muscle tension (Jeunet et al. 2016; Schumacher 2015), or (2) long term (Schlögl et al. 2010), such as regulations of SMRs over sessions because of learning (Kober et al. 2013). EEG variability can be provoked by many causes, as follows:

The equipment and experimental context:

1. Equipment sensitivity or magnetic field present in the environment (Maby 2016; Niedermeyer and da Silva 2005)
2. Quality of the instructions given to the user to follow through the task (Neuper et al. 2005)

Short-term user *components*:

1. Attention, mood (Jeunet et al. 2016; Nijboer et al. 2008), and muscle tension (Schumacher 2015), naturally evolving during, and somewhat driven by, the interaction with a BCI system.
2. In the case of no specific instruction, user's mental command itself can be a cause of signal variability. For instance, during a MI task, the user may be using kinesthetic or visual MI as strategy for mental commands (Neuper et al. 2005).

Long-term user *components*:

1. The user's learning capacity to control the machine depending on memory span, intrinsic motivation, curiosity, user profiles, and skills (Jeunet et al. 2016).

A negative or positive loop in learning progression could occur (see instructional design—Keller 2010; Oudeyer et al. 2016). For instance, a positive loop concerns a motivated user in whom being motivated has a higher attention level, which would, in turn, ideally enhance learning and control and finally induce higher motivation, and so complete the (virtuous) cycle (Mattout et al. 2014).

### 31.2.2 Main Principles of Adaptation

When considering adaptation, we mean adaptation of the machine to reduce the negative effect of some user's fluctuations onto the measured signals. In practice, (i) reducing the impact of **signal variability** would require the use of advanced machine learning techniques, such as adaptive spatial filters (Woehrle et al. 2015); (ii) influencing the **user variability** would require adapting the machine output (feedback and instructions) in order to keep the user in an optimal psychological state. The latter could follow instructional design theories by simplifying the layout or diminishing the task difficulty if the user is in a state of fatigue (Hattie and Timperley 2007; Sweller et al. 1998). Ideally, the BCI system should be (i) set *a priori* for each subject, for instance, based on their stable characteristics (skills or profile), and also (ii) dynamically readjusted during the usage, according to their evolving cognitive and affective states.

#### 31.2.2.1 Machine Learning

The BCI community has long been aware of the need for adaptive signal processing and classification (Krusienski et al. 2011; Schlögl et al. 2010). Experimental results have confirmed that using adaptive features and classifiers significantly improves BCI performances, both offline and online (Mattout et al. 2014; McFarland et al. 2011). Signal processing adaptation appears to be particularly useful for spontaneous BCI such as MI (McFarland et al. 2011). However, they can also be useful to reduce calibration time in ERP-based BCI by starting with generic, subject-independent classifiers, and then adapting them to each user during BCI use (Kindermans et al. 2014).

#### 31.2.2.2 Human Learning

It is shown that one's capacity to create distinct EEG patterns depends, among others, on one's psychological *components* as motivation, mood, skills, personality traits, and so on (Hammer et al. 2012; Jeunet et al. 2016). In that way, those patterns are more or less detectable and as such influence the BCI performance accuracy (Wolpaw 2002). To assist the users to produce clear EEG patterns is to assist in their learning. To do that, we consider adapting the BCI output (feedback and instructions) by considering a specter of users' psychological *components* in order to keep them motivated and for them to perform well and to be efficient and effective. As in any discipline, a well-designed and well-adapted feedback on one's progress from a tutor is what enables further development, intrinsic motivation, and learning (derived from cognitive developmental theories with Vygotsky 1978, and refined through instructional design theories [Keller 2010]). It is important to design a feedback that would encourage motivation and learning (Lumsden et al. 2016) and thus good BCI performance. Moreover, if inappropriate feedback is provided, subjects can learn incorrectly or have negative emotional reactions, which could impair performance and discourage further skill development (Barbero and Grosse-Wentrup 2010).

In order to minimize fatigue and induce motivation in BCI, we should investigate the instructional design theories (Lotte 2013b). These theories could be useful for finding and guiding the adaptation of tasks to users' skills, profiles, and cognitive abilities. Indeed, it has been shown that, for instance, visual–motor coordination and the ability to concentrate (Hammer et al. 2012); age, gender, practicing sports, gaming, or playing a musical instrument (Randolph 2012); moods and motivation (Nijboer et al. 2008); or spatial abilities (abilities to create, manipulate, and transform mental images) (Jeunet et al. 2016) were all positively correlated to MI BCI performances (classification accuracy). It is likely that some other factors may affect BCI performances, e.g., mental workload, which is known to affect learning in general (Sweller et al. 1998). Accounting for the variety of users' psychological *components* would lead to a better BCI feedback design and task adaptation, further assisting them in learning to control a BCI. This way, the EEG patterns would be regulated, which implies that to assist in the user's learning also means to assist in the machine learning techniques.

## 31.3 FRAMEWORK

We introduce a conceptual framework that can be used as a tool for a clear visualization of the elements being adapted, as well as of the missing methods that could possibly lead to optimal adaptive BCI design. It emphasizes existing solutions encompassing all the information possibly used for creating a fully adaptive BCI system. The framework (see Figure 31.1) has a hierarchical structure,

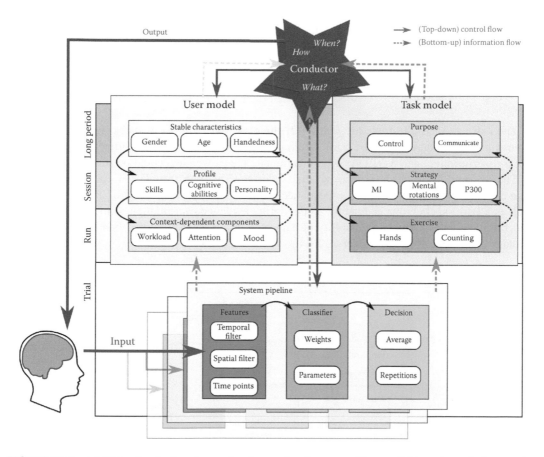

**FIGURE 31.1** Multiple signals (input) may be observed and processed in parallel in order to infer complementary states or intents, at the trailwise time scale. All the information extracted from these parallel pipelines may trigger the updating of the user or task model, which, in turn, might yield a decision from the conductor to take action, such as adapting one of the systems or the output, or modifying the task or the user model.

from the lowest-level elements that endure rapid changes to the highest-level elements that change at a much slower rate.

It is composed of four major elements, presented bottom-up: (1) the **system pipeline** presents the path that the raw EEG signal goes through when manipulated by the computer; (2a) the **user model** is an abstraction of the user's states, skills, and stable characteristics; (2b) the **task model** is a detailed representation of the BCI task; (3) the **conductor** masters the adaptation process by deciding the moment, the manner, and the elements of the whole system (pipeline, task, user, output) to adapt. The input of the system pipeline comes from (neuro)physiological activity patterns measured on the user, while the output of the system (feedback and instructions) is handled by the conductor and employed by the user. As they undergo rapid changes, input and output take place in the bottom level, as summarized in Figure 31.1.

To our knowledge, for the first time, we conceptualize a possibility of having an intelligent agent that could eventually replace the experimenter. For the sake of readability, we introduce step by step each element of the framework, starting bottom-up.

### 31.3.1 THE SYSTEM PIPELINE

The system pipeline, as in Figure 31.2 includes: (1) **EEG features** extracted from the raw signal (the input), possibly passing through

- A temporal filter: to filter noise or to choose an optimal frequency band for instance
- A spatial filter: combining those electrodes that lead to more discriminating signals, such as common spatial pattern (CSP) filter and its variants
- Signal epoching: selecting a time window to target an event of interest (a motor command or a stimulation)

The extracted EEG features are sent to (2) **the classifier**, which translates signal features into the estimated mental commands, using different machine learning classification methods, such as linear discriminant analysis (LDA), whose parameters (e.g., weights) could be adapted.

The accumulation of classification labels over several time samples or epochs give rise to (3) **a decision**, which often defines a speed–accuracy trade-off. Typically, with ERP-based systems such as a P300-speller, this is done by accumulating evidence over multiple stimulus repetition, to select a given letter when its probability of being the target letter is higher than a given threshold (Kindermans et al. 2014; Mattout et al. 2014).

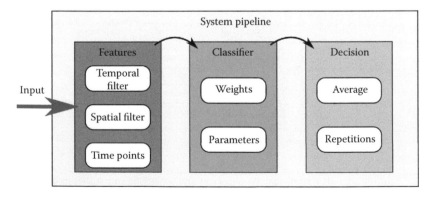

**FIGURE 31.2** The system pipeline, acquiring and processing one of the input signals measured with, for example, EEG.

In order to maintain or improve BCI performances, one requires accommodating the signal variability, by adapting either one or several elements of the pipeline:

- Feature extraction, in order to adapt to fast (e.g., a sudden faulty sensor) or slow (e.g., change in the frequency of the signal of interest) changes
- Classification, in order to change the number of classes, or to change the mapping between each class label and signal features
- Decision, in order to optimize performance, by adjusting the speed–accuracy trade-off for instance

### 31.3.1.1    Literature Review on Adaptive Signal Processing/Machine Learning

#### 31.3.1.1.1    Adaptive Feature Extraction

In order to extract features that adapt to the signal variability, a number of adaptive filters have been proposed for BCI. To the best of our knowledge, they are all supervised; that is, they require the actual EEG class label. Most of the proposed adaptive filters were spatial filters and, in particular, adaptive CSP for MI-based BCI applications. For instance, Sun and Zhang (2006) and Shenoy et al. (2006) proposed to reoptimize the CSP filters as a new batch of labeled data becomes available. Later, Zhao et al. (2008) and Song et al. (2013) proposed new algorithms to incrementally update the CSP spatial filters without the need to reoptimize everything. Tomioka et al. (2006) proposed a method to adapt spatial filters to changing EEG data class distribution. Finally, an incrementally adaptive version of the xDAWN spatial filter was proposed (Woehrle et al. 2015), dedicated to ERP-based BCI.

Adaptive temporal filters were proposed in Thomas et al. (2011). In this work, the optimal frequency bands for discriminating MI tasks were regularly re-estimated, and the temporal filters were adapted accordingly. It is worth noting that all these adaptive filter algorithms were evaluated only in offline experiments. Thus, it is unknown how changing the filters influences the users.

Features extracted from EEG signals can also be computed adaptively (Vidaurre and Schlogl 2008). In particular, there are a couple of methods used to estimate features adaptively, with each new EEG sample measured, rather than estimating them as the average feature from a full window of samples in a fixed way. For instance, Adaptive AutoRegressive (AAR) features estimate AR parameters and use them as features for each new EEG sample (Schlögl et al. 2010), which was proven superior to (fixed) AR parameters estimated on a full time window of samples, including for online experiments. Another example of adaptive features is Adaptive Gaussian Representation, which uses as features time-frequency weights that are adaptively estimated for each time window (Costa and Cabral 2000).

Finally, compensating for the features change is possible through the estimation of this change before it is used as the classifier input. As such, the corrected features will follow, more or less, the same distribution over time, and thus a classifier trained on features at $t - 1$ will still be relevant to classify features at time $t + 1$. For instance, Satti et al. (2010) proposed a "Covariate Shift minimization," which firsts estimates a polynomial function, modeling the moving of the features' distribution center within time. Then, they subtracted this function value at time $t$ from the features at the same $t$, to correct for the deviation due to time, which led to improvement of the classification accuracy.

#### 31.3.1.1.2    Adaptive Classifiers

The majority of the work on adaptive signal processing for BCI was so far on the design of adaptive classifiers, that is, classifiers whose parameters were incrementally re-estimated over time. Both supervised and unsupervised (not having the class labels) adaptive classifiers were proposed.

In the supervised category, multiple classifiers were explored offline including Gaussian classifiers (Buttfield 2006), LDA, or quadratic discriminant analysis (QDA) (Schlögl et al. 2010; Shenoy et al.

2006) for mental imagery–based BCI. For ERP-based BCI, Woehrle et al. (2015) explored adaptive support vector machine (SVM), adaptive LDA, a stochastic gradient-based adaptive linear classifier, and online passive-aggressive algorithms. Online, still in a supervised way, only the LDA/QDA (Vidaurre et al. 2007) and an adaptive variational Bayesian classifier (Sykacek et al. 2004) were explored.

Unsupervised adaptation of the classifiers is obviously much more difficult since the class labels, hence the class specific variability, is unknown. Thus, unsupervised methods were proposed that try to estimate the class labels of the new incoming samples first, before adapting the classifier based on this estimation. This was explored offline in Blumberg et al. (2007) and Gan (2006) for an LDA classifier with MI data. Another simple unsupervised adaptation of the LDA classifier for MI data was proposed and evaluated both offline and online in Vidaurre et al. (2011a). The idea is not to incrementally adapt all the LDA parameters, but only its bias, which can be estimated without knowing the class labels if we know that the data are balanced, that is, with the same number of samples per class.

For ERP-based BCI, semi-supervised learning also proved useful for adaptation. Semi-supervised learning consists in using a supervised classifier to estimate the labels of unlabeled data, that is, adapting this classifier based on these initially unlabeled data. This was explored with SVM and enabled to calibrate P300 spellers with less data than with a fixed, nonadaptive classifier (Li et al. 2008; Lu et al. 2009).

Finally, both offline and online, Kindermans et al. (2014) proposed a probabilistic method to adaptively estimate the parameters of a linear classifier in P300-based spellers, which led to a drastic reduction in calibration time, essentially removing the need for the initial calibration altogether. This method exploited the specific structure of the P300 speller, and notably the frequency of samples from each class at each time, to probabilistically estimate the most likely class label. In a related work, Grizou et al. (2014) proposed a generic method to adaptively estimate the parameters of the classifier without knowing the true class labels by exploiting any structure that the application may have.

### 31.3.1.1.3  Fully Adaptive Signal Processing

It is possible to use fully adaptive BCI signal processing pipelines. Several groups have explored BCI designs with both adaptive features and classifiers.

Offline adaptive xDAWN and several adaptive classifiers for ERP-based BCIs are studied in Woehrle et al. (2015), showing that each improved performances as compared to a nonadaptive version. Even so, combining them both improved the classification accuracy even further.

Online for MI-based BCI, Vidaurre et al. (2007) explored using both AAR features with an adaptive LDA. Later, she also explored co-adaptive training, where both the machine and the user are continuously learning, by using adaptive features and an adaptive LDA classifier (Vidaurre et al. 2011b). This enabled some users, who were initially unable to control the BCI, to reach classification performances better than by chance. This work was later refined in Faller et al. (2012) by using a simpler but fully adaptive setup with auto-calibration, which proved to be efficient including for users with disabilities (Faller et al. 2014). Co-adaptive training, using adaptive CSP patches, proved to be even more efficient (Sannelli et al. 2016).

Altogether, these studies clearly stress the benefits of adaptive signal processing for EEG-based BCI at the feature extraction, classifier, and decision levels. However, these works often omit the human factors.

### 31.3.1.1.4  Adaptive Decision Methods

The decision can be adaptive as well, by adapting the speed–accuracy trade-off for wheelchair control (Saedi 2015), or adapting the number of repetitions in a P300 speller (Mattout et al. 2014). While monitoring the user's state, it is also possible to inhibit BCI interaction until specific requirements, such as the user attention level, are met (George et al. 2011).

Monitoring the user during the BCI task could be useful for revealing a way to adapt features over time, such as an increase in workload that can affect MI features (Gerjets et al. 2015). Hence, we introduce the user, and the task they have to do, as a guide for adapting the system.

### 31.3.2 THE USER AND THE TASK MODEL

In order to adapt all the elements of the system pipeline with respect to the user skills and states, it is useful to consider a user model (Figure 31.3). We assume that the user *components* have a degree of changeability within certain time intervals and also react to the machine output. Hence, we categorized the user model according to time, within a timeline based on three time scales: runs, sessions, and a loosely long time period. Creating a complete automatic adaptation would mean refining the machine to manage more precisely the user's responses. For that purpose, we created a task model (Figure 31.4), containing the necessary BCI task information, whose components follow the same time intervals as the user model.

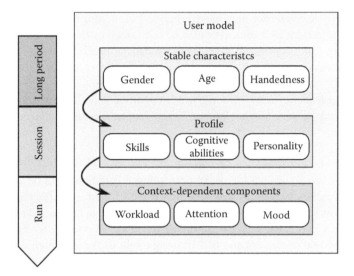

**FIGURE 31.3** User model, containing three levels, arranged from the least stable (context dependent) to the most stable components (stable characteristics).

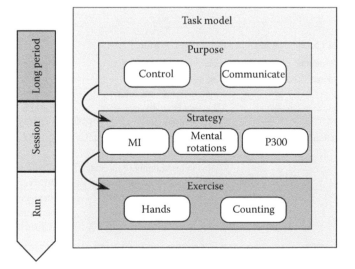

**FIGURE 31.4** Task model, arranged within three time scales.

The timeline prescribes how often the system should be adapted/updated and according to which element. Notably, the time intervals are chosen as they are commonly used in the BCI community, but it is not necessary to have them fixed as such.

#### 31.3.2.1 User Model

We customized Scherrer's classification of affective states (Martín et al. 2013) for BCI purposes and arranged them in the user model. Namely, the user model is an abstraction of the user, where their skills, states, and stable characteristics are arranged according to the time needed for them to change. The more we climb up, the more stable the components are.

- *Stable user characteristics*: gender, age, culture, background, genetic predispositions (handedness), and so on. These elements can assist in accounting for intersubject variability.
- *User profile*: (i) A given user may have developed particular (non-BCI or BCI) skills that may help in the current BCI context or may be reinforced by the ongoing practice. Same for (ii) personality traits (openness, conscientiousness, extraversion, agreeableness, neuroticism, flow proneness, etc.) and (iii) cognitive abilities (memory span, imagination, attention span, etc.).
- *Context-dependent characteristics*: the user's cognitive and affective state (attention level, fear, stress, etc.) are very much related to the current task set and environmental situation.

*31.3.2.1.1 A Brief Literature Review of "Adaptive Methods" Related to the User Model*

There are many attempts to predict the users' performance (predictors) in order to fully customize the system to users' needs. Hence, by knowing that some of their already acquired skills relate to the BCI skills, such as spatial abilities (Teillet et al. 2016), they can be trained and improved beforehand, without using a BCI. This way, by improving those skills, one improves a BCI skill as well. Table 31.1 gathers several predictors and BCI training methods for each element of our user model. For a detailed report on predictors, see Jeunet et al. (2016).

---

**TABLE 31.1**

**Examples of Predictors and User Training Methods Regarding Each User Model Component**

| | Stable Characteristics | Profile | Context-Dependent Components |
|---|---|---|---|
| Predictors | Age-determining performance (Zich et al. 2016) | Acquired skill (gaming, sport; Randolph 2012) | Mood and motivation, confidence (Nijboer et al. 2008) |
| | Paraplegic (Vuckovic et al. 2014) | Visual–motor coordination (Hammer et al. 2012) | Attention (Hammer et al. 2012) |
| | Gender (Randolph 2012) | Spatial abilities (Jeunet et al. 2016) | Fear of BCIs (Witte et al. 2013) |
| | | High θ and low α powers reveal illiteracy (Ahn et al. 2013) | γ oscillations (Grosse-Wentrup and Scholkopf 2012) |
| Training adaptation | | Spatial ability training (Teillet et al. 2016) | Mindfulness training (Tan et al. 2014) |
| | | | Attenuating γ power for good BCI performance (attention) (Grosse-Wentrup 2011) |

### 31.3.2.2 Task Model

The goal of the task model is to assist the BCI user in accomplishing his or her goal (communication/control, rehabilitation, amusement, or artistic expression). Similarly to the user model, the task model can be organized hierarchically according to the following three time scales: runs, sessions, and long period.

Components of the task model are typically determined beforehand, by the experimenter, and are not changed during the BCI session. Nevertheless, we envision the possibility to adapt each of these elements within the timeline. The task model is composed of the following:

- *Purpose of a BCI*: (1) a tool to control: prostheses, wheelchairs, and other devices; (2) a communication device: writing words on a screen, and so on; (3) a tool for rehabilitation: after stroke (Birbaumer and Cohen 2007), for paraplegic patients (Vuckovic et al. 2014), for autistic and ADHD children (Friedrich et al. 2014), and others; (4) a tool for artistic expression (creating music or paintings) or entertainment (Lécuyer et al. 2008), and so on.
- *Strategy*: the most used strategies include mental imagery, P300, or SSEP. The strategy will influence the choice of the initial signal processing and classification techniques, for instance, using the MI BCI strategy, the band power initially considered could be 8–12 Hz (mu rhythm) and 13–30 Hz (beta rhythm), measured on the electrodes placed over the sensorimotor cortex, while P300 would mean considering band-pass–filtered time series (between 1 and 20 Hz) on fronto-central, parietal, and occipital regions.
- *Exercise*: it indicates the mental command to be used given a strategy; as for MI strategies, an exercise is chosen between various motor imageries such as feet, hands, or tongue movements.

The strategy and exercise, initialized by the BCI purpose, can be adapted automatically based on the evolution of the user's need or state, as informed by bottom-up message passing. For instance, the user's performance being lower than a certain threshold could indicate the need to change strategy or exercise.

#### 31.3.2.2.1 A Brief Literature Review of Adaptive Methods Related to the Task Model

*Purpose*: Depending on the purpose of the BCI, the adaptation methods will differ. Rehabilitation will favor methods engaged in learning and self-regulation, communication will favor methods that improve accuracy and speed, while application for entertainment will favor design and innovation, and so on. We have not found literature fostering this idea; thus, it should be left as a perspective for future adaptive BCIs.

*Strategies*: A strategy can be switched to another, favoring the one in which the user produces the clearest EEG patterns and has the highest performance. In Müller-Putz et al. (2015) and Pfurtscheller et al. (2010), the use of hybrid BCIs is suggested, that is, switching between or using multiple BCI strategies (e.g., P300, MI, SSEP), combining different measuring techniques (e.g., M/EEG or fNIRS), or using tools apart from those in BCI, such as eye trackers, electrocardiograms, and so on. Accounting for these possible hybrid BCIs is why there are multiple instances of the system pipeline in Figure 31.1.

*Exercises*: An exercise depends on the chosen strategy. Exercises can be adapted within runs, such as variating between hand and foot imagination, choosing the one that had better performance (Friedrich et al. 2013; Fruitet et al. 2013). Adaptation is possible in larger time intervals such as within sessions, for example, switching from 1D, 2D, to 3D MI BCI tasks (McFarland et al. 2010), changing everything related to it (the instructions and feedback).

### 31.3.3 Machine Output

Along with feedback, instructions are what the user can receive from the machine. They can be adapted by the conductor based on the information flowing bottom-up, from the various signal processing pipelines or systems, through the user and task models.

#### 31.3.3.1 Feedback

The feedback is usually a representation of the classifier's output, managed by the decision. It can be seen as the machine's response to the user's performance or states. It is useful or even necessary for the user's self-regulation process or learning, to be informed on his or her progress when accomplishing the task. There are many different types of feedback, supporting emotional or cognitive states of the user, possibly given in (i) **different modalities**, typically visual (Neuper et al. 2005), but also vibrotactile (Jeunet et al. 2015), a tangible interface (Frey et al. 2014), or an immersive virtual environment (Vourvopoulos et al. 2016); and (ii) **degrees of assistance** (biased feedback—Barbero and Grosse-Wentrup 2010). A feedback could be designed to target some *stable user characteristics*, such as applications for autistic children (Friedrich et al. 2014), or *context-dependent* user components, such as inducing motivation in a social context (Bonnet 2013) or catching the user's attention with video games (Ron-Angevin 2008).

Adapting feedback could potentially bring benefits that favor ergonomy, minimize fatigue, and optimize learning. This mostly remains to be explored.

#### 31.3.3.2 Instructions and Stimuli

These are, for instance, the stimuli (flashing letters) in P300 spellers or arrows indicating the user to perform left or right hand MI in MI BCI. The instructions could be presented/adapted, independently from the classifier's output in (i) **different modality**: visual, auditive, or tactile; or (ii) **difficulty**:

- Speed—the speed of instruction's appearance might decrease over time, if we assume the user's fatigue (decreasing the task difficulty).
- Order of appearance—it would be interesting to investigate whether presenting a block of instructions for one-class MI (arrow left-hand) and then a block of the other class (right hand) is easier for some users than presenting them in an alternate manner (left–right).

### 31.3.4 Conducting Adaptation with the Conductor

As each of the framework elements can be adapted/updated separately, or in combination, using various algorithms or criteria, we explicitly refer to a controlling agent in our framework, which would preferably be created for a global adaptive BCI. It gathers all the information available from the user, the task, and the signal processing pipelines, in order to decide the how, when, and what to adapt. The conductor would need an objective function, upon which it would make its decisions. We draw an analogy with Intelligent Tutoring Systems (ITS), which are methods creating objective metrics and computational models for learning with digital environment. With our adaptive framework, our user is the ITS student, the conductor is the ITS tutor, and the task is the ITS expert (NKambou et al. 2010).

ITS adapt content and activities for the purpose of challenging and guiding students in an optimal way, that is, preventing them from being too overwhelmed with difficult material or too bored with easy or repetitive material (Murray and Arroyo 2002). There are many methods dealing with adapting the content of the task to keep students' attention and motivation up, and most of them are inspired by the following two approaches: (i) maintaining the zone of proximal development (ZPD) (Vygotsky 1978) and (ii) being in flow (Nakamura and Csikszentmihalyi 2014). The first, based on cognitive developmental theory for instructional design (Luckin 2001), may guide an indirect estimation of the person's cognitive resources (Allal and Ducrey 2000). Flow, originating from positive psychology, is an autotelic (self-rewarding) state, where one is immersed in a task so that one loses the sense of time, of self, and of the environment. They both concord with theories of intrinsic motivation, which suggest that motivation and learning improve if the proposed exercises are at a level that is slightly higher than the current user's skill level.

Choosing automatically the optimal task, in real time, while considering the user and task models, could bring promising results for BCI training and operation. For instance, the conductor, as for some ITS, could use Multi-Armed Bandit algorithms to select an optimal sequence of tasks and outputs (Clement et al. 2015).

## 31.4   PERSPECTIVES AND CHALLENGES

The perspectives we consider here correspond to some gaps we noticed while confronting the literature we are aware of, to the proposed new framework. First of all, the gaps in the user model: training methods (outside the BCI context), and feedback and instructions (during the BCI task) should adapt considering the following: (i) the user's *stable characteristics*—considering patients with different disorders (paraplegic, after stroke, autistic, etc.), also considering different preferences (between children and adults, women and men, etc.); (ii) the user's *profile*—for individuals who differ in their skills or personality traits; (iii) the user's *context-dependent characteristics*, favoring those methods that increase attention level, motivation, and so on.

Another important matter, instead of adapting the nature of the exercise based on the user's performance only (typically the classifier's output), we could also account for context-dependent components, such as the user's attention or workload level, as monitored with some passive BCI pipeline or with other physiological sensors (e.g., skin conductance).

The challenges we encounter when considering the full adaptation with the conductor are as follows: (1) identifying metrics and criteria to optimize depending on the task, to ensure relevant adaptation, that is, favoring those adaptation methods that most concur to user's needs; (2) designing computational models of the user and task models; (3) testing the adaptive BCI online and validating it with real experiments; (4) designing unsupervised adaptive features and classifiers, and validating them online (most of them are supervised and only evaluated offline so far); (5) propose adaptive feedback and exercises.

As for the conductor, beside the algorithm that should decide when and how to perform the adaptations, the criteria for adapting the whole system is hidden in the "purpose" of the BCI, or what one wishes to achieve. Hence, will the conductor aim for flow or ZPD as an objective function (by adapting the task difficulty or by presenting a biased feedback for example) or for system's performance and speed (by favoring higher classification accuracy). Finally, we need to ensure that adapting the system will not impede the inevitable user adaptation (human learning) and thus lead to a virtuous coadaptation.

## 31.5   CONCLUSION

Throughout this chapter, we emphasized the crucial need for adaptive methods in order to optimize the design and online performance of BCI. We stressed out the fact that, in order to create an overall adaptive system, it is not sufficient to consider adapting the signal processing and classification techniques, but also the output and the task parameters, in order to fully accommodate the user's variability in terms of needs and psychophysiological states. Following that requirement, we created a framework, composed of (i) one or several BCI systems/pipelines; (ii) a user model, whose elements are arranged according to different time scales; (iii) a task model, enabling the system adaptation with respect to the user model; and (iv) the conductor, an intelligent agent that implements the adaptive control of the whole system. For the first time, we conceptualize a fully adaptive BCI system, with respect to the user needs and states. The existing adaptation methods are described through an extensive literature review of each element of both types of models (user and task) and of possible low-level pipelines for raw signal processing.

The potential benefits of using this framework are numerous; for one, it enables clear and methodological visualization of all the BCI system components, their possible interaction, and the way and the context in which they could be adapted. Although invasive brain activity recording approaches (e.g., ECoG or intracortical electrodes array) consider different signal processing algorithms from those presented in our pipeline, the same principles for co-adaptivity (Sanchez et al. 2009) and the rest of the framework structure and methods apply for any BCI system, be it invasive or not. Moreover, this framework is also convenient for mapping the literature onto each of its components in order to understand current issues in BCI in general, and to visualize the gaps to be filled by future studies in order to further improve BCI usability. We believe that this framework will contribute to delve possible future research paths and give rise to novel challenges and ventures.

## ACKNOWLEDGMENT

This work was supported by the French National Research Agency with the REBEL project and grant ANR-15-CE23-0013-0.

## REFERENCES

Ahn, M., Cho, H., Ahn, S., and Jun, S.C. 2013. High theta and low alpha powers may be indicative of BCI-illiteracy in motor imagery. *PLoS ONE* 8(11): e80886. doi:10.1371/journal.pone.0080886

Allal, L., and Ducrey, G.P. 2000. Assessment of—or in—the zone of proximal development. *Learn Instr* 10: 137–152.

Allison, B., and Neuper, C. 2010. *Could Anyone Use a BCI?* Springer, London.

Barbero, Á., and Grosse-Wentrup, M. 2010. Biased feedback in brain–computer interfaces. *Journal Neuroeng Rehabil* 7: 34.

Baykara, E., Ruf, C.A., Fioravanti, C., Käthner, I., Simon, N., Kleih, S.C., Kübler, A., Halder, S. 2016. Effects of training and motivation on auditory P300 brain–computer interface performance. *Clin Neurophys* 127(1): 379–387. doi: 10.1016/j.clinph.2015.04.054.

Birbaumer, N., Cohen, L.G. 2007. Brain–computer interfaces: Communication and restoration of movement in paralysis. *J Phys* 579: 621–636.

Birbaumer, N., and Kübler, A. 2000. The thought translation device (TTD) for completely paralyzed patients. *IEEE Trans Rehab Eng*, 8: 190–193.

Blumberg, J., Rickert, J., Waldert, S., Schulze-Bonhage, A., Aertsen, A., and Mehring, C. 2007. Adaptive classification for brain computer interfaces. *Proc EMBC*, 2536–2539.

Bonnet, L., Lotte, F., and Lécuyer, A. 2013. Two brains, one game: Design and evaluation of a multiuser BCI video game based on motor imagery. *IEEE Transactions on Computational Intelligence and AI in Games* 5(2): 185–198.

Buttfield, A., Ferrez, P., and Millan, J. 2006. Towards a robust BCI: Error potentials and online learning. *IEEE Trans Neur Sys Rehab Eng* 14: 164–168.

Clement, B. et al. 2015. Multi-armed bandits for intelligent tutoring systems. *Journal of Educational Data Mining* 7.2: 20–48.

Costa, E., and Jr, E. Cabral. 2000. EEG-based discrimination between imagination of left and right hand movements using adaptive Gaussian representation. *Med Eng & Physics* 22: 345–348.

Donchin, E, Spencer, K.V., and Wijesinghe, R. 2000. The mental prosthesis: Assessing the speed of a P300-based brain–computer interface. *IEEE Trans Rehab Eng* 8(2): 174–179.

Faller, J., Scherer, R., Costa, U., Opisso, E., Medina, J., and Müller-Putz, G.R. 2014. A co-adaptive brain–computer interface for end users with severe motor impairment. *PLoS ONE* 9: e101168.

Faller, J., Vidaurre, C., Solis-Escalante, T., Neuper, C., and Scherer, R. 2012. Autocalibration and recurrent adaptation: Towards a plug and play online ERD-BCI. *IEEE Trans Neural Sys Rehab Eng* 20: 313–319.

Faradji, F., Ward, R.K., and Birch, G.E. 2009. Plausibility assessment of a 2-state self-paced mental task-based BCI using the no-control performance analysis. *J Neurosci Methods*, 180: 330–339.

Fazel-Rezai, R., Allison, B., Guger, C., Sellers, E., Kleih, S., and Kübler, A. 2012. P300 brain computer interface: Current challenges and emerging trends. *Front Neuroeng* 5.

Frey, J., Gervais, R., Fleck, S., Lotte, F., and Hachet, M. 2014. Teegi: Tangible EEG interface. In *Proc 27th ACM Symposium UIST* (pp. 301–308).

Friedrich, E.V., Neuper, C., and Scherer, R. 2013. Whatever works: A systematic user-centered training protocol to optimize brain–computer interfacing individually. *PLoS ONE*, 8(9): e76214.

Friedrich, E.V., Suttie, N., Sivanathan, A., Lim, T., Louchart, S., and Pineda, J.A. 2014. Brain–computer interface game applications for combined neurofeedback and biofeedback treatment for children on the autism spectrum. *Front Neuroeng* 7: 21. doi: 10.3389/fneng.2014.00021. eCollection 2014.

Fruitet, J., Carpentier, A., Munos, R., and Clerc, M. 2013. Automatic motor task selection via a bandit algorithm for a brain-controlled button. *J Neuroeng* 10(1): 016012.

Gan, J. 2006. Self-adapting BCI based on unsupervised learning. In *Proc. Int. BCI Workshop.*

Gaume, A., Vialatte, A., Mora-Sánchez, A., Ramdani, C., and Vialatte, F.B. 2016. A psychoengineering paradigm for the neurocognitive mechanisms of biofeedback and neurofeedback. *Neuroscience & Biobehavioral Reviews* 68: 891–910.

George, L., Bonnet, L., and Lécuyer, A. 2011. Freeze the BCI until the user is ready: A pilot study of a BCI inhibitor. In *5th International BCI Workshop.*

Gerjets, P., Walter, C., Rosenstiel, W., Bogdan, M., and Zander, T.O. 2015. Cognitive state monitoring and the design of adaptive instruction in digital environments: Lessons learned from cognitive workload assessment using a passive brain–computer interface approach. *Front Neurosci* 8: 35.

Grosse-Wentrup, M. 2011. Neurofeedback of fronto-parietal gamma-oscillations. In *5th International BCI Conf* (pp. 172–175).

Grosse-Wentrup, M., and Scholkopf, B. 2012. High gamma-power predicts performance in SMR BCIs. *J NeuroEng.*

Grizou, J., Iturrate, I., Montesano, L., Oudeyer, P.-Y., and Lopes, M. 2014. Calibration-free BCI based control. *Proc AAAI*, 1–8.

Hammer, E.M., Halder, S., Blankertz, B., Sannelli, C., Dickhaus, T., Kleih, S., ..., and Kübler, A. 2012. Psychological predictors of SMR-BCI performance. *Biological Psychology* 89(1): 80–86.

Hattie, J., and Timperley, H. 2007. The power of feedback. *Review of Educational Research* 77: 81–112.

Jeunet, C., N'Kaoua, B., and Lotte, F. 2016. Advances in user-training for mental-imagery-based BCI control: Psychological and cognitive factors and their neural correlates. *Progress in Brain Research* 228: 3–35.

Jeunet, C., Vi, C., Spelmezan, D., N'Kaoua, B., Lotte, F., and Subramanian, S. 2015. *Continuous Tactile Feedback for Motor-Imagery Based Brain–Computer Interaction in a Multitasking Context.* HCI (pp. 488–505). Springer International Publishing.

Keller, J. 2010. *Motivational Design for Learning and Performance: The ARCS Model Approach* Springer.

Kindermans, P.J., Tangermann, M., Müller, K.-R., and Schrauwen, B. 2014. Integrating dynamic stopping, transfer learning and language models in an adaptive zero-training ERP speller. *Journal of Neural Engineering* 11: 035005.

Kober, S.E., Witte, M., Ninaus, M., Neuper, C., and Wood, G. 2013. Learning to modulate one's own brain activity: The effect of spontaneous mental strategies. *Front Hum Neurosci* 7: 695.

Krusienski, D., Grosse-Wentrup, M., Galán, F., Coyle, D., Miller, K., Forney, E., and Anderson, C. 2011. Critical issues in state-of-the-art brain–computer interface signal processing. *J NeuoEng* 8: 025002.

Lécuyer, A., Lotte, F., Reilly, R.B., Leeb, R., Hirose, M., and Slater, M. 2008. Brain–computer interfaces, virtual reality, and videogames. *IEEE Computer* 41(10): 66–72.

Li Y., Guan, C., Li, H., and Chin, Z. 2008. A self-training semi-supervised SVM algorithm and its application in an EEG-based brain computer interface speller system. *Pattern Recognition Letters* 29: 1285–1294.

Lotte, F., Faller, J., Guger, C., Renard, Y., Pfurtscheller, G., Lécuyer, A., and Leeb, R. 2013a. Combining BCI with virtual reality: Towards new applications and improved BCI. In *Towards Practical Brain–Computer Interfaces.* pp. 197–220. Springer Berlin Heidelberg.

Lotte, F., and Jeunet, C. 2015. Towards improved BCI based on human learning principles. In *3rd International Winter Conference on Brain–Computer Interface* (pp. 1–4). IEEE.

Lotte, F., Larrue, F., and Mühl, C. 2013b. Flaws in current human training protocols for spontaneous brain–computer interfaces: Lessons learned from instructional design. *Front Hum Neurosci* 7: 568.

Lu, S., Guan, C., and Zhang, H. 2009. Unsupervised brain computer interface based on inter-subject information and online adaptation. *IEEE Transactions on Neural Systems and Rehabilitation Engineering* 17: 135–145.

Luckin, R. 2001. Designing children's software to ensure productive interactivity through collaboration in the zone of proximal development (zpd). *Info Tech in Childhood Education Annual* 1: 57–85.

Lumsden, J., Edwards, E., Lawrence, N., Coyle, D., and Munafò, M. 2016. Gamification of cognitive assessment and cognitive training: A systematic review of applications and efficacy. *JMIR Serious Games* 4(2): e11.

Maby, E. 2016. Chapter 7. Sensors: Theory and innovation, Chapter 8. Technical requirements for high quality EEG recordings. In *Brain–Computer Interfaces 2: Technology and Applications*, Eds. Clerc, M., Bougrain, L., and Lotte, F. ISTE-Wiley.

Makeig, S., Kothe, C., Mullen, T., Bigdely-Shamlo, N., Zhang, Z., and Kreutz-Delgado, K. 2012. Evolving signal processing for brain–computer interfaces. *Proceedings of the IEEE* 100: 1567–1584.

Martín, E., Haya, P.A., and Carro, R.M. 2013. *Modeling and Adaptation for Daily Routines: Providing Assistance to People with Special Needs*. Springer Sci & Bus Media.

Mattout, J., Perrin, M., Bertrand, O., Maby, E. 2014. Improving BCI performance through co-adaptation: Applications to the P300-speller. *Ann Phys Rehabil Med* 58(1): 23–28. doi: 10.1016/j.rehab.2014.10.006.

McFarland, D., Sarnacki, W., and Wolpaw, J. 2010. Electroencephalographic (EEG) control of three-dimensional movement. *J NeurEng* 7(3); 036007.

McFarland, D., Sarnacki, W., and Wolpaw, J. 2011. Should the parameters of a BCI translation algorithm be continually adapted? *Journal of Neuroscience Methods* 199: 103–107.

Middendorf, M., McMillan, G., Calhoun, G., and Jones, S.K. 2000. Brain–computer interfaces based on the steady-state visual-evoked response. *IEEE Trans Rehab Eng* 8(2): 211–214.

Millán, J.d.R., Rupp, R., MüllerPutz, G., Murray, R., Smith, R., Giugliemma, C., Tangermann, M., Vidaurre, C., Cincotti, F., Kübler, A., Leeb, R., Neuper, C., Müller, K.R., and Mattia, D. 2010. Combining brain–computer interfaces and assistive technologies: Stateoftheart and challenges. *Front Neurosci*, 4.

Müller-Putz, G., Leeb, R., Tangermann, M., Höhne, J., Kübler, A., Cincotti, F., ..., and Millán, J. D.R. 2015. Towards noninvasive hybrid brain–computer interfaces: Framework, practice, clinical application, and beyond. *Proc IEEE*, 103(6): 926–943.

Murray, T., and Arroyo, I. 2002. Toward measuring and maintaining the zone of proximal development in adaptive instructional systems. In *Inter Conf on ITS*.

Müller, K. R., Tangermann, M., Dornhege, G., Krauledat, M., Curio, G., and Blankertz, B. 2008. Machine learning for real-time single-trial EEG-analysis: From brain–computer interfacing to mental state monitoring. *J Neurosci Methods* 167(1): 82–90.

Nakamura, J., and Csikszentmihalyi, M. 2014. The concept of flow. In *Flow and the Foundations of Positive Psychology* (pp. 239–263). Springer, Netherlands.

Neuper, C., Scherer, R., Reiner, M., and Pfurtscheller, G. 2005. Imagery of motor actions: Differential effects of kinesthetic and visual-motor mode of imagery in single-trial EEG. *Brain Res Cogn Brain Res* 25(3): 668–677.

Niedermeyer, E., and da Silva, F.L. 2005. *Electroencephalography: Basic Principles, Clinical Applications, and Related Fields*. Lippincott Williams & Wilkins.

Nijboer, F., Furdea, A., Gunst, I., Mellinger, J., McFarland, D. J., Birbaumer, N., and Kübler, A. 2008. An auditory brain–computer interface (BCI). *Journal of Neuroscience Methods* 167(1): 43–50.

NKambou, R., Mizoguchi, R., and Boudreau, J. 2010. *Advances in Intelligent Tutoring Systems*. Vol. 308. Springer.

Orsborn, A.L., Moorman, H.G., Overduin, S.A., Shanechi, M.M., Dimitrov, D.F., and Carmena, J.M. 2014. Closed-loop decoder adaptation shapes neural plasticity for skillful neuroprosthetic control. *Neuron* 82(6): 1380–1393.

Oudeyer, P.-Y., Gottlieb, J., and Lopes, M. 2016. Intrinsic motivation, curiosity, and learning: Theory and applications in educational technologies. *Prog Brain Res* 229: 257–284.

Perrin, M., Maby, E., Daligault, S., Bertrand, O., and Mattout, J. 2012. Objective and subjective evaluation of online error correction during P300-based spelling. *Adv HCI* 2012, 578295:1–578295:13.

Pfurtscheller, G., Allison, B.Z., Bauernfeind, G., Brunner, C., Solis Escalante, T., Scherer, R., ..., and Birbaumer, N. 2010. The hybrid BCI. *Front Neurosci* 4: 3.

Pfurtscheller, G., Brunner, C., Schlögl, A., and Lopes da Silva, F.H. 2006. Mu rhythm (de)synchronization and EEG single-trial classification of different motor imagery tasks. *NeuroImage* 31: 153–159.

Randolph, A.B. 2012. Not all created equal: Individual technology fit of brain–computer interfaces. In: *45th Hawaii International Conference on System Science HICSS*, pp. 572–578.

Ron-Angevin, R., and Díaz-Estrella, A. 2009. Brain–computer interface: Changes in performance using virtual reality techniques. *Neuroscience Letters*, 449(2): 123–127.

Saeedi, S., Chavarriaga, R., Leeb, R., and Millán, J.D.R. 2016. Adaptive assistance for brain-computer interfaces by online prediction of command reliability. IEEE Computational Intelligence Magazine, 11(1): 32–39.

Sanchez, J.C., Mahmoudi, B., DiGiovanna, J., and Principe, J.C. 2009. Exploiting co-adaptation for the design of symbiotic neuroprosthetic assistants. *Neural Networks* 22: 305–315.

Sannelli, C., Vidaurre, C., Müller, K.R., and Blankertz, B. 2016. Ensembles of adaptive spatial filters increase BCI performance: An online evaluation. *J Neuroeng* 13: 046003.

Satti, A., Guan, C., Coyle, D., and Prasad, G. 2010. A covariate shift minimisation method to alleviate nonstationarity effects for an adaptive brain–computer interface. *Proc ICPR*.

Schlögl, A., Vidaurre, C., and Müller, K.-R. 2010. Adaptive methods in BCI research—An introductory tutorial. In *Brain–Computer Interfaces*. pp. 331–335. Springer.

Schumacher, J., Jeunet, C., and Lotte, F. 2015. *Towards Explanatory Feedback for User Training in Brain-Computer Interfaces*, (IEEE SMC).

Shenoy, K.V., and Carmena, J.M., 2014. Combining decoder design and neural adaptation in brain–machine interfaces. *Neuron* 84(4): 665–680.

Shenoy, P., Krauledat, M., Blankertz, B., Rao, R., and Müller, K.R. 2006. Towards adaptive classification for BCI. *J NeuroEng*, 3: R13.

Song, X., Yoon, S.-C., and Perera, V. 2013 Adaptive Common Spatial Pattern for single-trial EEG classification in multi subject BCI. *Proc. IEEE EMBS NER*, 411–414.

Sun, S., and Zhang, C. 2006. Adaptive feature extraction for EEG signal classification. *Med Biol Eng Comput* 44: 931–935.

Sweller, J., van Merrienboer, J., and Pass, F. 1998. Cognitive architecture and instructional design. *Educational Psychology Review* 10: 251–296.

Sykacek, P., Roberts, S. J., and Stokes, M. 2004. Adaptive BCI based on variational Bayesian Kalman filtering: An empirical evaluation. *IEEE Transactions on Biomed Eng* 51: 719–729.

Tan D., and Nijholt A. 2010. *Brain–Computer Interaction: Applying our Minds to HCI*. London: Springer-Verlag.

Tan, L.F., Dienes, Z., Jansari, A., and Goh, S.Y. 2014. Effect of mindfulness meditation on brain–computer interface performance. *Consciousness and Cognition* 23: 12–21.

Teillet, S., Lotte, F., N'Kaoua, B., and Jeunet, C. 2016. Towards a spatial ability training to improve motor imagery based brain–computer interfaces (MI-BCIs) performance: A pilot study. *Proc IEEE SMC*.

Thomas, K., Guan, C., Lau, C., Prasad, V., and Ang, K. 2011. Adaptive tracking of discriminative frequency components in EEG for a robust brain–computer interface. *J NeuroEng* 8: 1–15.

Tomioka, R., Hill, J., Blankertz, B., and Aihara, K. 2006. Adapting spatial filtering methods for nonstationary BCIs. *Proc IBIS*, 65–70.

Vidaurre, C., Kawanabe, M., Von Bunau, P., Blankertz, B., and Muller, K. 2011a. Toward unsupervised adaptation of LDA for brain–computer interfaces. *IEEE Transactions on Biomedical Engineering* 58: 587–597.

Vidaurre, C., Sannelli, C., Müller, K.-R., and Blankertz, B. 2011b. Co-adaptive calibration to improve BCI efficiency. *J Neuroeng* 8, 025009.

Vidaurre, C., and Schlogl, A. 2008. Comparison of adaptive features with linear discriminant classifier for brain computer interfaces. *Proc EMBC*, 173–176.

Vidaurre, C., Schlogl, A., Cabeza, R., Scherer, R., and Pfurtscheller, G. 2007. Study of on-line adaptive discriminant analysis for EEG-based brain computer interfaces. *IEEE Transactions on Biomedical Engineering* 54: 550–556.

Vourvopoulos, A., Ferreira, A., and Bermudez S. 2016. NeuRow: An immersive VR environment for motor-imagery training with the use of brain–computer interfaces and vibrotactile feedback. In *Proc PhyCS*.

Vuckovic, A., Pineda, J., La Marca, K., Gupta, D., and Guger, C. 2014. Interaction of BCI with the underlying neurological conditions in patients: Pros and cons. *Front Neuroeng*.

Vygotsky, L.S. 1978. *Mind in Society: The Development of Higher Psychological Processes*. Harvard University Press.

Witte, M., Kober, S.E., Ninaus, M., Neuper, C., and Wood, G. 2013. Control beliefs can predict the ability to up-regulate sensorimotor rhythm during neurofeedback training. *Front Hum Neurosci* 7: 478.

Woehrle, H., Krell, M.M., Straube, S., Kim, S.K., Kirchner, E.A., and Kirchner, F. 2015. An adaptive spatial filter for user-independent single trial detection of event-related potentials. *IEEE Transactions on Biomedical Engineering* 62: 1696–1705.

Wolpaw, J.R., and Wolpaw, E.W. 2012. *BCI: Principles and Practice*. Oxford University Press.

Wolpaw, J.R., McFarland, D.J., Pfurtscheller, G. and Vaughan, T.M. 2002. Brain–computer interfaces for communication and control. *Clinical Neurophysiology* 113(6):767–791.

Zhao, Q., Zhang, L., Cichocki, A., and Li, J. 2008. Incremental common spatial pattern algorithm for BCI. *Proc IJCNN* 2656–2659.

Zich, C., Debener, S., Chen, L.C., and Kranczioch, C. 2016. FV 10. Motor imagery supported by neurofeedback: Age-related changes in EEG and fNIRS lateralization patterns. *Clinical Neurophysiology* 127(9), e215.

# 32 Mind the Traps! Design Guidelines for Rigorous BCI Experiments

*Camille Jeunet, Stefan Debener, Fabien Lotte,*
*Jérémie Mattout, Reinhold Scherer, and Catharina Zich*

## CONTENTS

32.1 Introduction .................................................................................................................. 614
32.2 Acquisition of the Signals ............................................................................................ 615
    32.2.1 How to Choose the Appropriate Sensor Type, Location, and Number
        Depending on What We Want to Measure ......................................................... 615
    32.2.2 What Can We Infer from the Activation of One Electrode? Concept
        of Spatial Resolution ........................................................................................ 616
    32.2.3 How Muscular Activity Can Interfere with EEG Activity and Why It Should
        Be Controlled for to Avoid Confounds ............................................................ 617
    32.2.4 What Kinds of Mental States Can Be Used? .................................................... 618
32.3 Data Processing ............................................................................................................ 619
    32.3.1 Which Classifier Can We Use Depending on the Distribution of the Data? ........... 619
    32.3.2 Why Is It Important to Separate the Training Data Set from the Testing Data Set? ... 620
    32.3.3 How to Determine the Chance Level for the Classified Data ........................... 620
    32.3.4 To Which Extent Can Commercial Algorithms Be Trusted? ............................ 622
    32.3.5 How to Determine the Relevance of Neurophysiological Markers ................... 622
    32.3.6 Why Is It Important to Correct for Multiple Comparisons? ............................. 623
32.4 Experimental Design and the User Component ............................................................ 624
    32.4.1 What to Have in Mind When Designing a New BCI Experiment ..................... 624
    32.4.2 Why and How to Have a Good Control Group? ............................................... 625
    32.4.3 How to Avoid Biases: Concepts of Counterbalancing, Sham Control, Double
        Blindness, and Randomization ......................................................................... 626
    32.4.4 How to Select the Appropriate Statistical Tests .............................................. 627
32.5 Summary and Conclusion ............................................................................................. 629
Acknowledgments ................................................................................................................. 630
References .............................................................................................................................. 630

## Abstract

Designing brain–computer interface (BCI) experiments requires knowledge in many different disciplines: from neurosciences to signal processing and machine learning, through psychology. However, very few people have skills in all these disciplines. Yet, a lack of knowledge in a single aspect of BCIs is likely to result in flaws in the experimental design, statistical analyses, or the interpretation of the results. Moreover, because the BCI field is relatively young, no widely accepted guidelines are available yet, while at the same time an exponentially increasing number of research teams contribute to this field and would benefit from such guidelines. Thus, the objective of this chapter is to propose, in a pedagogical way, step-by-step guidance to design a rigorous BCI experiment. We name potential pitfalls and explain how to avoid them using concrete examples. This chapter could be seen as a checklist of points that should be addressed when the aim is to design rigorous and scientifically valid BCI studies and experiments. It is structured into three categories: (1) the acquisition of brain signals, (2) data processing issues, and (3) the experimental design and consideration of the BCI user.

## 32.1  INTRODUCTION

Brain–computer interfaces (BCIs) enable users to control an application using their brain activity alone. Such control can be achieved following different paradigms. Mainly, BCIs can be active, reactive, or passive. Active BCIs rely on modifications of the amplitude of brain rhythms in different frequency bands while users perform an explicit task, such as mental imagery. The most common active BCI paradigm is based on motor imagery: users are asked to perform a motor imagery task (i.e., to imagine movements of their limbs), which lowers the amplitude of sensorimotor rhythms (SMRs) in the mu (8–12 Hz) and beta (12–30 Hz) frequency bands in the sensorimotor cortex. By detecting this spatio-spectral signal change, the system may be able to infer the mental task performed by the user and in return associate to it a command for the application. For instance, by performing left- and right-hand motor imagery tasks, one can make a wheelchair turn left or right, respectively (Millán et al. 2010). On the other hand, reactive BCIs rely on the detection of brain potentials generated in response to a stimulus. The most popular BCI application is probably the P300 speller (Farwell and Donchin 1988). The P300 speller was first designed to enable communication for the paralyzed. A matrix of letters is displayed on a screen. The rows and columns of this matrix flash sequentially in a random order. The user has to focus on the letter he or she wants to spell. When this letter flashes, a positive cortical potential is generated around 300 ms later. This way, after several repetitions, by intersecting the rows and columns, the flashing of which triggered a P300, the system will be able to infer the target letter. Finally, passive BCIs are systems that enable the user's mental state to be measured in order to adapt an application/interface accordingly (Zander and Kothe 2011). Here, users do not follow specific instructions or voluntary interact with the BCI; in other words, they do not send conscious commands. Instead, their cognitive (e.g., workload), emotional (e.g., frustration), or motivational states are inferred from their ongoing electroencephalography (EEG) signals, which can also be related to other physiological and behavioral data to identify a particular mental state. A passive BCI application automatically adapts to fluctuations in user states.

BCIs are very promising for a wide range of applications, from assistive technologies to communication devices. Beyond their obvious potential for patients with motor impairments, BCIs also offer new possibilities in different fields, ranging from sports to video games (Lécuyer et al. 2008) through education (Frey et al. 2014) and rehabilitation (Kübler et al. 2013) to name only a few examples. Thus, not only engineers and psychologists are interested in using such technologies, but also medical doctors, neuroscientists, teachers, or specialists in sports science, business, physiotherapy or linguistics, between many others. Yet, designing BCI experiments requires knowledge in many different disciplines: neurosciences to understand the properties of the brain signals used to control the BCI, signal processing to extract the relevant information from these brain signals, machine learning to make the system able to learn which brain patterns correspond to which mental command, psychology to understand the factors influencing users' ability to control a BCI, and human–computer interaction to design usable and efficient BCI protocols. However, very few people have skills in all these disciplines. Yet, a lack of knowledge in a single aspect of BCIs is likely to result in flaws in the experimental design, statistical analyses, or the interpretation of the results. Moreover, because the BCI field is relatively young, no widely accepted guidelines are available yet, while at the same time an exponentially increasing number of research teams contribute to this field and thus would benefit from such guidelines.

The objective of this chapter is to propose, in a pedagogical way, step-by-step guidance to design a rigorous BCI experiment. We do not propose a perfect experimental design, but rather name potential pitfalls, and explain how to avoid them. This chapter could be seen as a checklist of points that should be addressed when the aim is to design rigorous and scientifically valid BCI studies and experiments. Therefore, this chapter targets more specifically the numerous researchers, professionals, passionate people, or patients and their families who start using BCIs and want to avoid the current traps surrounding BCIs. This chapter does not claim to be exhaustive but rather aims (1) at naming the important elements to be considered while designing a BCI experiment and (2) at guiding the reader toward relevant pieces of literature if they want to investigate further some specific elements.

The next part of this chapter is structured into three sections. The first section focuses on the acquisition of brain signals. Here, we will focus on EEG-based BCIs, simply because this is the most popular input modality for BCIs. The second section deals with data processing issues, while the third one will introduce important points concerning the experimental design and the target individuals, the BCI users.

To illustrate these different points, we propose to design a BCI experiment all along the chapter, following the recommendations point by point. Let us say that our research question is the following:

We want to evaluate the relevance and reliability of new tasks to control a Mental Imagery–based BCI (MI-BCI), namely, "remembering a positive vs. negative emotional souvenir."

The object of providing this example is not to undertake a real research study or to answer a specific research question. Thus, no data or statistical analyses will be described. Rather, the aim is to provide the reader with a clear application so that they know in which context the recommendations could be applied. For specific applications of BCIs for therapeutic purposes, please refer to Guger et al. (2018) and McFarland (2018).

At the end of each subsection, we will discuss which tools/methods are the most relevant in the context of this research question.

## 32.2 ACQUISITION OF THE SIGNALS

### 32.2.1 How to Choose the Appropriate Sensor Type, Location, and Number Depending on What We Want to Measure

Typical EEG signals refer to voltage fluctuations in the direct current to approximately 40 Hz frequency range, with amplitudes ranging from a few tens of microvolts to below 1 µV. To capture these miniature signals, sensors are placed on the scalp and a conducting gel is applied to lower the skin-electrode impedance to approximately <20 kΩ. However, wet sensors have the disadvantage that individuals have to wash their hair after the EEG recording, to remove the conductive gel. Therefore, new sensor types have been developed, such as active wet electrodes, active dry electrodes, or miniature sensors requiring no or very small amounts of gel only (Debener et al. 2015). Typical EEG recordings require the use of several electrodes (the minimum number is 3, common are 32, 64, 128, or even 256 channel recordings), which are placed with a cap or net on the scalp. Different sensor types have their advantages and disadvantages. The signal quality and wearing comfort of dry electrodes, for instance, are typically inferior to conventional wet electrodes, but the benefits are the faster setup time and that hair washing is not required after the end of the recording. While alternative materials and electrodes may suffice for some EEG signals, we recommend the use of sintered Ag/AgCl electrodes, which, when used as wet electrodes and applied correctly, provide good signal characteristics. They do not generate voltage fluctuations on their own and do not cause frequency distortion, which are two problems that should be avoided when measuring biosignals with microvolt amplitude. The international 10–20 system is the standard for electrode placement. Depending on the type of brain signals that should be recorded, appropriate electrode locations should be used.

Which sensor positions are important? The answer depends on the class of BCI that one wants to implement. However, as outlined in Section 32.2.2, a good spatial sampling is generally helpful even if only a few channels are used. For BCIs that detect sensory evoked responses, electrodes should be placed such that known topographical representations of sensory evoked potential are captured. This includes placing electrodes over posterior and occipital sites for capturing visual evoked responses and placing electrodes over fronto-central sites for capturing auditory evoked responses. However, the most discriminative information does not necessarily overlap spatially with locations giving the best signal-to-noise ratio. Moreover, to optimally classify signals, it is also helpful to place electrodes away from the signal of interest, in order to cancel out irrelevant activity, as explained by Blankertz et al. (2011). Accordingly, for BCIs that detect the neural correlates of motor imagery, electrodes should be located over sensorimotor areas, and, in order to disentangle sensorimotor mu from occipital alpha,* some sensors should be placed over posterior scalp sites as well. In summary, multichannel EEG (32+ channels) acquisition from sensors covering wider parts of the head is beneficial, although for practical applications and for economic reasons, a limited setup is often used, under ideal circumstance, without much loss of performance.

*And for our experiment?* In our case, since we do not have a precise idea of the relevant brain areas for the tasks (remembering positive/negative emotional souvenirs), we will use at least 32 or 64 electrodes, placed all over the scalp. Also, because we want to maximize signal quality, we will use wet Ag/AgCl electrodes (i.e., with conductive gel).

### 32.2.2 WHAT CAN WE INFER FROM THE ACTIVATION OF ONE ELECTRODE? CONCEPT OF SPATIAL RESOLUTION

It is important to understand the concept of differential amplification when voltage is measured. EEG signals reflect voltage fluctuations over time, and voltage fluctuations can be best captured as the difference between two locations, say one electrode placed on the top of the head (vertex) and another one behind the ear (mastoid). Even though one electrode is often defined as the reference electrode (mastoid), the recorded signal cannot be regarded as reflecting electrical activity from the patch of brain underneath the other electrode (vertex). Likewise, since the whole body conducts current fairly well (with different tissues having different conductivity properties), it is not required to place electrodes close to the heart to measure the electrocardiogram. The reason for that is that EEG measures the synchronized electrical activity of adjacent pyramidal cells aligned in parallel, which rise to electrical fields that are strong enough to be captured with electrode placed on the skin. Accordingly, all brain signals captured by EEG result from relatively large and highly synchronized patches of cortex. Each patch of cortex contributing to the EEG may be best regarded as an equivalent current dipole. If the aim is to capture the electrical activity of such a dipole, it is important to understand that dipole orientation is at least as important as dipole location. In fact, two electrodes placed very close to a dipolar generator may not record any activity if placed in the wrong orientation. On the other hand, two electrodes placed further away from the generator may capture its signature nicely.

Given that an unknown number of brain (and non-brain, e.g., electrocardiogram) generators contribute to the scalp EEG, one can safely assume that the number of generators contributing to the mixed recorded signal is much higher than the number of channels used to record the signals, even if high-density EEG acquisition is performed. The inverse problem means that one cannot determine the brain source of any particular EEG signal for sure. Inferring the number and locations of active brain regions that caused the recorded EEG signals on scalp is sometimes compared to

---

* The 8–12 Hz frequency range in the literature is referred to as mu rhythm when related to sensorimotor activity; otherwise, it is referred to as alpha rhythm.

the problem of guessing what 3D shape created an observed shadow on a wall. It is a so-called ill-posed problem that has no unique solution. However, good guesses are possible, and EEG source localization and spatial filtering procedures—which combine the signals from multiple electrodes; see Blankertz (2008) and Chapter 18 ("Gentle Introduction to Signal Processing and Classification for Single-Trial EEG Analysis")—can be used to confirm ideas about brain sources contributing to the EEG, with reasonable spatial resolution and precision. To this end, making use of multiple EEG channels can help. The rich spatial detail of multichannel recordings has two key advantages. First, it is much easier to disentangle brain from non-brain contributions to the measured EEG signal, and second, it is much easier to identify, and disentangle, different brain signals from each other.

*And for our experiment?* To be able to disentangle the brain area(s) involved in each of the tasks, we will apply, offline, source localization procedures (i.e., source reconstruction algorithms).

### 32.2.3 How Muscular Activity Can Interfere with EEG Activity and Why It Should Be Controlled for to Avoid Confounds

As stated in Section 32.2.2, EEG sensors measure all electrical currents at the sensor location, not only those coming from the brain. In particular, muscle tensions and eye movements generate electrical currents, known respectively as electromyography (EMG) and electrooculography (EOG), that are of much larger magnitude than currents of cortical origin, that is, signals originating from the brain (Fatourechi et al. 2007) (see Figure 32.1). EOG signals may dominate the EEG at frontal scalp sites (near the eyes), while EMG signals are common for electrodes placed near muscles (Goncharova et al. 2003), contributing broad band and in particular high-frequency activity (Whitham et al. 2007).

EOG/EMG artifacts can corrupt EEG signals and result in poor BCI performance. However, EMG and EOG can also contribute to BCI control and lead to high classification accuracy if their presence or amplitude happens to be correlated with that of the mental states decoded by the BCI. In other words, EOG and EMG are typical confounding factors in BCI experiments. Thus, one may conclude that a given mental state can be decoded from EEG when it is actually decoded from EMG/EOG.

Such a risk of EMG/EOG confound can, for instance, be found when decoding emotions from EEG signals (Mühl et al. 2014b). Indeed, a given emotion often appears with a given facial expression, for example, by frowning when experiencing anger. This would lead to specific facial muscle contractions and thus to specific EMG signatures that would be picked up by EEG sensors. Thus, a BCI classifier based on these EEG signals may actually recognize facial expressions from EMG

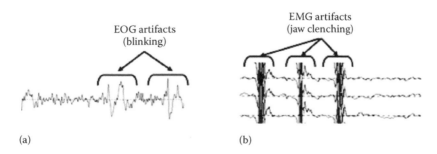

EOG artifacts
(blinking)

EMG artifacts
(jaw clenching)

(a)                                    (b)

**FIGURE 32.1** Examples of EOG (a) and EMG (b) measured by EEG sensors. (From Lotte, F. 2015. Signal processing approaches to minimize or suppress calibration time in oscillatory activity-based brain–computer interfaces. *Proceedings of the IEEE*, 103(6), 871–890.)

signals rather than actual emotions from cortical brain signals. As Mühl and colleagues pointed out, if one wants to ensure that the classification is truly based on cortical signals, it is necessary to control for EMG or EOG activity when classifying emotions from EEG recordings (Mühl et al. 2014b).

This is only one example, and ideally all BCIs, relying solely on brain activity, should be controlled for EOG/EMG confounds. While there is no perfect solution, minimizing such confounds can be done by

- Designing protocols limiting eye and motor/facial movements
- Using manual or automatic EOG/EMG cleaning techniques (Islam et al. 2016) (note that existing techniques are still improvable)
- Studying and reporting the spatial and spectral EEG topographies for each condition, to ensure they differ from that of EMG/EOG (Goncharova et al. 2003)
- Classifying directly EOG/EMG to see if they contain class-related information (if so, there is a risk of confound)
- Performing classification on high-frequency EEG signals, likely to contain EMG, to estimate EMG impact (see, e.g., Mühl et al. 2014a)
- Reanalyzing BCI data, offline, after removal of artifactual signals

*And for our experiment?* Here, we will definitely measure EOG and EMG of the face during the experiment as we use emotional tasks that are most likely related to facial expressions. Then, we will apply EOG/EMG cleaning techniques online. Afterward, we will classify EOG/EMG (offline) to ensure that they do not contain class-related information and also classify artifact-corrected EEG data (offline) to verify that BCI performance is above chance (and as high as possible).

### 32.2.4  What Kinds of Mental States Can Be Used?

The question of what kinds of mental states can be used to operate a BCI goes back to the question of what kinds of mental states can be detected with the neuroimaging technique at hand, which, in turn, is simply a matter of the signal-to-noise-ratio. In other words, if the neural signature of a mental state is larger than the background noise, the mental state can be detected and used to operate a BCI. Although some mental states can be detected on a single-trial level, generally the signal-to-noise ratio, and thus the reliability of the BCI output, can be increased with more repetitions. And although more repetitions typically increase the single-trial classification accuracy, repetitions may come at the expense of a lower information transfer rate. Consequently, while theoretically every mental state that can be detected with the neuroimaging technique used can be employed to operate a BCI, the actual range is narrowed down by practical considerations such as the reliability of the neural signature, the speed and accuracy of the BCI system, as well as the BCI application.

The variety of types of mental states that can be used within BCIs has led to classify BCIs from active over reactive up to passive (Mühl et al. 2009; Zander and Kothe 2011). As raised in Section 32.1, active BCIs require direct and conscious modulation of brain activity, whereby external stimulations serve at most as cues. Motor imagery, the mental imagination of movements, is a prominent active BCI paradigm (Pfurtscheller et al. 1997). Contrariwise, reactive BCIs rely on the indirect modulation of brain activity as a reaction to an external stimulation. Well-known examples for reactive BCIs are the P300 speller (De Vos et al. 2014; Farwell and Donchin 1988) and BCIs that are based on steady-state visual/somatosensory evoked potentials (Lalor et al. 2005; Müller-Putz et al. 2005, 2006). Finally, passive BCIs use brain activity arising without the users' conscious modulation or without external stimulation, such as in the detection of error potentials (Zander and Kothe 2011). Additionally, different kinds of BCIs can be combined together, to make what is called a hybrid BCI (see Pfurtscheller et al. 2010 and Chapter 27 ["Hybrid Brain–Computer Interfaces and Their Applications"]). Given a BCI application, it is advisable to use the mental state that optimally balances accuracy and speed for the target application.

*And for our experiment?* Our experiment aims at investigating whether or not remembering positive/negative emotional souvenirs is reliable enough to control a BCI: thus, we are focusing on active BCIs. In other words, we want to investigate the feasibility of discriminating both these tasks on a single-trial basis. Importantly, the length of the trial will be limited: the system has to be able to discriminate the tasks in a few seconds. In other words, the information transfer rate must be at least as good as with standard motor imagery tasks for these new tasks to be useful for BCI control.

## 32.3  DATA PROCESSING

### 32.3.1  WHICH CLASSIFIER CAN WE USE DEPENDING ON THE DISTRIBUTION OF THE DATA?

The choice of a machine learning algorithm significantly affects the BCI decoding accuracy. To obtain optimal performance, the algorithm capabilities and the data properties have to match. Statistical classifiers are mainly used in BCI (Lotte et al. 2007). In order to discriminate EEG signals into different classes (commands), such classifiers rely on the EEG feature data distribution, that is, on their probability density function. There are different ways to estimate such density and to infer classifiers from them. Most importantly, the classifier type should be selected based on this data distribution. In general, linear methods such as linear discriminant analysis (LDA) or support vector machines (SVMs) are used for classification of EEG signals. Such methods use linear hyperplanes to subdivide the feature space into regions belonging to the different classes/commands. The position and orientation of the hyperplanes are typically computed using the mean and covariance of the EEG features. During subsequent online BCI use, new and unseen data, that is, independent data, are then assigned to the label of their area, as defined by the hyperplanes. Linear methods are successful when the feature density follows a normal distribution. If it does not, the features can be transformed to be so. For example, applying a logarithm transformation converts band power estimates extracted from EEG (the power is the square of the amplitude and hence not a linear measure) into a normal-like distribution. A linear hyperplane between two normal distributions can therefore potentially lead to reasonable performance. An advantage of linear methods is that they do not need a lot of training data compared to nonlinear methods and thus a shorter calibration time when used online. Since the lack of sufficient training data is a common issue in BCI (Lotte 2015), linear methods are leading. As far as LDA is concerned, when little data are available, regularized LDA (notably shrinkage LDA) should be used preferably to LDA, as they were shown to lead to higher accuracy (Blankertz et al. 2011; Lotte 2015). Nonlinear methods can separate data using curves instead of "just" (hyper)planes and thus can better capture the shape of the feature density, which may lead to good generalization. Generalization is the ability of a classifier to achieve good results also with independent data. Generalizing is different from memorizing the data (a.k.a. overfitting): more details on this point are provided in Section 32.3.2. Recent nonlinear methods that are somewhat robust against overfitting are Random Forest (Steyrl et al. 2016) and neural networks such as Restricted Boltzmann Machines (Kobler and Scherer 2016). These methods do not make any assumption about the data distribution and, as such, are likely to be increasingly used for BCI in the future and to give potentially better performances. Proving superior performances nonetheless require a proper evaluation of the algorithms and notably the use of separate training and testing data sets.

As for classifiers, the other algorithms used in the data processing pipeline, for example, preprocessing or feature extraction, should also match the data properties. For instance, the common spatial pattern (CSP) spatial filter (Blankertz 2008) can be used to classify oscillatory activity data (EEG rhythm band power) but is suboptimal to classify event-related potentials such as the P300 (Lotte 2014). For the latter, dedicated spatial filters such as xDAWN should be used (Rivet et al. 2009). For a complete review of the signal processing and machine learning methods used in BCI, please refer to Blankertz (2018) and Chevallier (2018).

*And for our experiment?* We do not want the calibration of the classifier to be too long. Thus, we will choose a linear classifier, as it requires fewer training data. Moreover, to obtain features respecting the properties of a standard LDA or SVM classifier, we will operate the following transformation of the features in order to obtain a normal-like distribution: (1) compute the power of the signal and (2) take the log of this power.

### 32.3.2  WHY IS IT IMPORTANT TO SEPARATE THE TRAINING DATA SET FROM THE TESTING DATA SET?

When evaluating BCIs offline, the classification system should be calibrated using only the data from a training data set, and the resulting calibrated system should then be evaluated on completely different and independent data, which represent the testing data set (Lemm et al. 2011). Such evaluation ensures that the classifier can indeed generalize to unseen data and has not just memorized the training data set class labels. Failure to use distinct and independent training and testing data sets may lead to much higher classification performance than the "real" performance that would be obtained on unseen data (Olivetti et al. 2010) or even to better than chance performance on random data with no class information (Dominguez 2009).

Therefore, not a single parameter of the machine learning algorithm should have been calibrated with the knowledge of the testing data set. This means the choice of channels, features, hyperparameters, and normalization should be done using only the training data. In particular, when using cross-validation (CV),* all these should **not** be selected on all the data before applying CV to assess the classifier. Rather, they should be selected separately for each fold of the CV. Misuse of this procedure could result in erroneously concluding that some mental states can be discriminated from brain signals, when they cannot. Such a bias was revealed by Luu and Chau (2008), who claimed that it was possible to predict from functional near-infrared spectroscopy (fNIRS) which object among two a user was going to choose before they could see them. The authors claimed that they could discriminate the preferred object from the nonpreferred one, based on fNIRS signals preceding their presentation, with 80% of average CV classification accuracy (Luu and Chau 2008). Unfortunately, feature selection was performed not for each fold of the CV, as it should have, but only once on all the data. Dominguez (2009) revealed that by applying the exact same incorrect CV evaluation procedure on completely randomly generated noise—with no class information—he could obtain the same classification accuracy. Subsequently, when correcting their approach, and performing feature selection only on each training CV fold, the authors of the original paper obtained a classification accuracy as low as 56% (vs. 80% before), that is, essentially chance level, thus disproving their initial claim (Chau and Damouras 2009). This stresses once more the need for an independent testing data set, that is, a data set that no part of the machine learning algorithm has ever used.

*And for our experiment?* In order to assess whether remembering a positive emotional souvenir can be distinguished in EEG signals from remembering a negative one, we will use machine learning algorithms such as feature selection, spatial filter optimization, and LDA/SVM. To assess the achievable classification accuracy, we will use $K$-fold CV (a typical value of $K$ would be 10). Therefore, we will run the training algorithm, the feature selection algorithm, the spatial filter optimization algorithm, and the LDA/SVM on $K - 1$ folds and evaluate the obtained parameters on the remaining fold (i.e., the testing data set). This training/testing procedure should thus be done $K$ times, for the classifier training, feature selection, and filter optimization.

### 32.3.3  HOW TO DETERMINE THE CHANCE LEVEL FOR THE CLASSIFIED DATA

In the example introduced just above, we state that 56% of classification accuracy was basically chance level. But how do we know from which accuracy onward we can consider a result to be above

---

\* CV is a procedure that divides a data set randomly into K folds of equal size, and then spatial filter optimization, feature selection, and classifier training are performed on all but one part, and the obtained predictions are compared to the real labels of the remaining part.

chance? It is indeed an important question to determine whether a classification result, the decoding accuracy, deviates from chance level or not. Chance level refers to the rate achieved by random classification. For a two-class problem, the theoretical chance level is 50%; for a four-class problem, it is 25%, and so on. However, achieving a classification result of 70% in a two-class scenario may or may not indicate a valid above chance classification accuracy. It is important to recognize that the theoretical chance level is valid only for a large number of samples (or trials). Imagine flipping a coin once; the result could be either head or tails. Now assume you flip the coin four times in a row. By chance alone, it may be that the outcome is four times head. At least, and even though the coin would not be biased, it is not at all certain that the result will be two times head and two times tail. Because of the small number of trials, a strong deviation of the observed rate from the theoretical chance level can occur. Only with a sufficient number of trials does the outcome of heads become more and more unlikely—and for a sufficient number of observations, the frequency of heads and tails will approach the theoretical chance level of 50%. Thus, if the theoretical chance level can be exceeded by chance alone, how could it be determined whether a particular classification result is significantly above chance? Analytical (binomial statistic) and empirical approaches (permutation tests) are available to answer this question, as summarized in Combrisson and Jerbi (2015) and Müller-Putz et al. (2008). By assuming that classification errors follow a cumulative binomial distribution, one can apply the inverse binomial cumulative distribution to figure out whether a particular classification result is above a particular significance threshold. The critical number of correctly classified trials that could arise by chance alone is determined by

$$\text{Crit\_trials} = \text{binoinv}(1 - p, n, 1/c) * 100/n.$$

Here, $p$ refers to the significance threshold (e.g., $p = 0.05$), $n$ indicates the number of trials, and $c$ denotes the number of classes (assuming equal class occurrence). The binoinv function is available for instance in MATLAB® (Mathworks Inc., Natick, Massachusetts). According to this equation, for a two-class problem, $p = 0.05$ and $n = 20$ trials, the critical number of correctly classified trials is 70%. Hence, only a classification accuracy exceeding 70% can be interpreted as a result significant above chance level. A corresponding look-up table is provided by Müller-Putz et al. (2008) and Combrisson and Jerbi (2015) for different $p$ values; two-, four-, and eight-class scenarios; and different trial counts. As discussed by Combrisson and Jerbi (2015), the analytical approach has some theoretical limitations, whereas the empirical approach comes at the expense of high computational costs. However, for random noise data, both suggest similar thresholds.

The procedure just described refers to random data, typically resulting in balanced class labels for a sufficient number of trials. However, in unbalanced two-class situations where one class occurs in the majority of all trials (e.g., 90% nontarget class trials, 10% target class trials in paradigms of reactive BCIs such as the P300 speller, when measuring single-trial P300 detection performances), the calculation of accuracies across all trials can be highly misleading. If one always goes with the majority vote, the resulting accuracy may falsely indicate very high recognition rate: Imagine a classifier always voting 1, then the accuracy would be incorrectly calculated as 90%! In those cases, the confusion or error matrix should be reported, which makes it easy to evaluate which classes are confused. One simple solution is the calculation of a corrected accuracy given as the mean across all recognition rates for all classes. In the above example, for class 1, the recognition rate would be 100%; for class 2, the recognition rate would be 0%, and the average of both is then 50%—the corrected classification accuracy. Another frequently used performance metric in that case is the area under the receiver operating characteristic curve (Bradley 1997). The interested reader can refer to the tutorial in Thompson et al. (2014) for more information on classification performance metrics. Alternatively or additionally, the end application performances can also be reported, for example, the percentage of correctly selected characters in the P300 speller, which is a balanced problem.

*And for our experiment?* Once our CV process performed, we will have to answer the following question: Can remembering a positive emotional souvenir be distinguished from remembering a negative one, in EEG? The answer depends on whether the obtained classification accuracy is above or below chance level. If it is above, it means that these two tasks can actually be distinguished; otherwise, it means that the classifier did not manage to separate them. To know the chance level, it is enough to have a look at the tables introduced here-above and look at the chance level for two classes (because here we have positive vs. negative emotional souvenirs). The chance level will also depend on the number of trials per class. This should thus encourage collecting as many trials as possible (the higher the number of trials, the lower the chance level).

### 32.3.4  To What Extent Can Commercial Algorithms Be Trusted?

Consumer-grade EEG and BCI systems, such as the popular Neurosky (www.neurosky.com), Emotiv (www.emotiv.com), or many other devices, are increasingly used. Many commercial BCI systems come with ready-to-use algorithms to detect mental states such as attention, emotions, or meditation. Such algorithms are often used as they are, as a ground truth value, notably in human–computer interaction research. This could sometimes be an issue when designing rigorous BCI experiments for a number of reasons.

First, many (but fortunately not all) of these algorithms claim to be able to measure such mental states but have never been scientifically validated. It does not mean that they do not work, but rather that one does not know if they work. As such, if they were not independently and rigorously validated in a scientific journal publication (whose rigor standards are usually higher than that of conferences), such algorithms cannot be used as reliable measures. For instance, an independent evaluation of the Emotiv emotion recognition algorithms revealed that "the data is unreliable and incoherent" (Jorgensen et al. 2017).

Second, such algorithms are most often black boxes, meaning one does not know how they work and which features they use. This makes a study using them potentially unreproducible with other EEG devices. Moreover, it also prevents us from assessing whether these algorithms are really BCI, based only on signals from cortical origin, or whether they are based on confounding factors such as EOG/EMG (see also Section 32.2.3). For instance, Neurosky and Emotiv algorithms are believed to or even admit they use EMG/EOG and thus are not real BCI (Singer 2008).

Even for algorithms that are scientifically validated and purely based on signals from cortical origin, it should be noted that EEG signals are changing heavily because of their context of use (Brandl et al. 2016; Mühl 2014a). As such, they should be validated again in their target context, if this context is different from the one in which the validation was performed. Finally, even for such algorithms, like any other BCI system, they are not perfect and make frequent mistakes when estimating users' mental states. Therefore, they should be treated as such, and not as perfect mental state decoders.

Overall, using commercial algorithms is thus not a problem per se and can even be very useful and convenient, but it should be done with care. In particular, they should be used in rigorous scientific BCI experiments only if they were scientifically validated, including in the target context of use, and if the algorithm is known (i.e., not a black box).

*And for our experiment?* Since some commercial algorithms claim to be able to recognize various emotion-related mental states, or even any user-defined mental states in EEG, we might be tempted to compare the performances they obtain for positive versus negative emotional souvenir, to the one we obtain with our own data and algorithms. However, we should refrain from doing so, at least with algorithms being black box, because we do not know whether they rely on pure EEG signals, or whether they use EMG/EOG as well. In the latter case, any comparison would be unfair and meaningless since we use only EEG.

### 32.3.5  How to Determine the Relevance of Neurophysiological Markers

One crucial issue when designing BCIs is the choice of features used to encode messages. Features that do not contain relevant information add noise to the system. If the machine learning algorithm is not robust, then adding noise or redundant information may decrease the BCI decoding accuracy. One way to prevent this from happening is feature reduction or selection. This means that only features that lead to high decoding performance are given to the machine learning algorithm. Note that to ensure that such features do not lead to overfitting, that is, that they can generalize to new unseen data, it is necessary to assess them on a different data set than the one on which they were selected, as indicated in Section 32.3.2. The most crucial point, however, is that the selected features are neurophysiologically meaningful. Machine learning methods generally cannot judge whether the used features are neurophysiologically meaningful. For instance, artifacts not originating from the brain (e.g., EMG) may be strongly correlated with the BCI task and would be easier to detect given their higher amplitudes. An algorithm exploiting them would, however, not be considered as a pure BCI, as discussed in Section 32.2.3. A relevant concept in machine learning is "Garbage in, Garbage out," which means that if the used features are meaningless, even the best machine learning algorithm will not be able to find patterns that can be discriminated.

One way to check whether there are significant differences between conditions in the spontaneous EEG is to compute time/frequency event-related desynchronization (ERD—relative amplitude decrease in a specific frequency band over defined brain areas) and event-related synchronization (ERS—relative amplitude increase) maps (Pfurtscheller and Da Silva 1999). These maps show statistically significant changes as a function of time. In other words, they show which oscillatory components undergo significant amplitude changes. If identified components are in agreement with patterns reported in the literature, then the process was successful. For instance, for a motor imagery experiment, in agreement with the literature would mean ERD in the alpha and beta range over sensorimotor areas (Pfurtscheller et al. 1997), while for a steady-state visual evoked potential experiment, it would mean ERS at the stimulation frequencies over occipital areas (Vialatte et al. 2010). As mentioned before, if the experiment consists in exploring a new mental task for BCI, then such analyses are even more necessary to ensure that the machine learning algorithm is not in fact using artifacts (see also Section 32.2.3).

Finally, it should be stressed that the weights obtained by training the machine learning algorithms cannot necessarily be used directly to identify the involved brain areas. Indeed, most classifier weights are actually "filters" and can thus give high weights to sources of noise in order to cancel them (Haufe et al. 2014). Rather, the weights should be transformed into "patterns" before interpretation (see notably Haufe et al. 2014 for the linear case).

*And for our experiment?* In addition to the offline classification of EOG/EMG introduced in Section 32.3.1, we will perform a time/frequency ERD/ERS analysis in order to determine the neurophysiological features involved. We hope that some neurophysiological features related to emotions (positive vs. negative valence) based on the literature, such as the frontal asymmetry (Dolcos et al. 2004; Schmidt and Trainor 2001), will be involved whereas frontal and occipital high frequencies (gamma) will not be involved, as they are most likely related to EMG (Goncharova et al. 2003).

### 32.3.6 WHY IS IT IMPORTANT TO CORRECT FOR MULTIPLE COMPARISONS?

The aim of most experiments is to test and compare alternative hypotheses. In BCI, typical hypotheses may arise from questions such as the following: When is the sensorimotor desynchronization significantly different from baseline? Where on scalp can the beta rebound be best captured after motor imagery? In which frequency band can we observe a significant difference between two mental states? Or what signal features best discriminate between the desired alternative commands?

Although quite different, those questions share a common goal (feature identification) and a common procedure (statistical hypothesis testing). Importantly, when the data space is large, such as with EEG data that unfold in space, time, and frequency, feature identification involves multiple hypothesis testing. As the size of the space of possible features increases, the number of tests or comparisons to be performed increases. And as the number of tests increases, so does the risk of concluding to a significant effect in at least one of those comparisons, by mistake. The latter means that an effect could be suggested to be significant whereas this effect does not truly exist.

Controlling for that risk (called the risk alpha or type I error) is very important since wrongly identifying an effect would typically yield a choice of BCI features that would not work in practice. The risk alpha at the level of multiple tests relates to the risk alpha at the level of a single comparison. In classical statistics, there is a wide agreement to keep that risk below 5%. This number has been chosen somewhat arbitrarily and could be chosen otherwise. What is important is to define that limit before testing, so as not to bias this choice and the ensuing conclusion; 5% means that the probability $p$ of mistakenly rejecting the null hypothesis is equal to or less than 0.05.

A classic example of multiple comparisons is the two-sided $t$ test, when comparing the means of two populations, say $\mu_1$ and $\mu_2$. The null hypothesis states that $\mu_1 = \mu_2$. The test to reject this null is two-sided when one tests for both alternatives: $\mu_1 > \mu_2$ and $\mu_1 < \mu_2$. In that case, the risk alpha for each comparison is typically set to 2.5% so that the risk alpha of mistakenly rejecting the null is 5%. Hence, the family risk is equal to the number of comparisons ($n = 2$) times the risk alpha at the single test level (2.5%).

The same rationale applies to $n$ multiple comparisons with $n > 2$ so that the risk for a single test is set to $0.05/n$ and guarantees that the family risk remains 5%. This is known as the Bonferroni correction. However, this correction is often too conservative, since it relies on the a priori assumption that the multiple comparisons are mutually independent, which is rarely true in practice, at least when dealing with neurophysiological or neuroimaging data. For instance, scalp EEG data are known to be spatially blurred so that nearby sensors will likely display highly similar activities. These spatial correlations should be accounted for in order to increase the sensitivity of the statistical analysis. Similarly, EEG signals exhibit strong temporal correlations and most reliable significant effects typically expand over several tens of milliseconds. Methods have been developed so as to optimize the corrections for multiple comparisons in the particular context of brain functional data. The most popular ones are available in main academic software packages (see, for instance, Litvak et al. 2011 and Oostenveld et al. 2011 and other articles in that same special issue). These are the corrections based on random field theory (see Worsley 2006) to control for the familywise error rate or on approaches to control for the false discovery rate (see Nichols 2006). Note that the former is typically made for statistical inference on parametric images. However, nonparametric or permutation approaches are also very much used for the analysis of electrophysiological data (Maris and Oostenveld 2007).

To sum up, as the number of comparisons increases, the risk of mistakenly rejecting the null hypothesis in one of these comparisons increases. A correction is needed to reliably identify a useful feature for BCI. Be it at the individual or group level, feature identification will often require multiple testing. This reminds us very importantly that whenever prior knowledge is available to reduce the search space to the most likely relevant features, the correction for multiple comparisons will be less drastic and the ensuing identification will be more sensitive.

*And for our experiment?* Here, to complete the time/frequency analysis, we would like to know if, in accordance to the literature, the frontal asymmetry varies depending on the valence of the emotional memory and if this asymmetry enables us to classify reliably enough our data. Thus, we will divide the frequency range and subbands, for instance, delta (1–4 Hz), theta (4–8 Hz), low alpha (8–10 Hz), high alpha (10–12 Hz), low beta (12–24 Hz), and high beta (24–30 Hz). Then, we will compare the frontal asymmetry for each of these frequency bands. Because we perform several comparisons, we will apply a correction, for instance, the false discovery rate, in order to adjust the significance threshold.

## 32.4 EXPERIMENTAL DESIGN AND THE USER COMPONENT

### 32.4.1 What to Have in Mind When Designing a New BCI Experiment

Along the long road to develop and validate a new application, BCI experiments may have different purposes. At an early stage, offline experiments may be required to explore the neural correlates of some targeted mental processes and their potential usefulness. For instance, significant ERDs or ERSs in specific frequency bands will be investigated in a population of subjects, between two conditions that we wish to distinguish (e.g., low vs. high mental workload).

Then, online experiments are typically designed to evaluate or compare the performance of a BCI or of one of its component (a neurophysiological marker, an algorithm, a feedback, etc.). In that case, typically, the same subjects will be tested under two or more conditions in order to answer questions such as the following: Is it useful to include the early N170 visual component in the classification to improve P300-based spelling? Which classifier provides the best performance? Does it make a different if we move from a 2D to a 3D visual feedback? Note that some of these questions can be partially answered with offline experiments in which many tests can be performed a posteriori, based on the same data. However, a full evaluation will require an online study where the different conditions to be compared will have to be evaluated in separate trials.

BCI experiments may also aim at assessing a learning curve over several sessions or at comparing groups of users. Although not mutually exclusive, these questions are very different from each other and point toward different design parameters. In particular, the former will require defining the number of sessions for each subject, while the latter will require defining the number of subjects in each group.

Finally, at a later stage of development, validation of a BCI may take the form of a randomized controlled trial (e.g., for neurofeedback training applications), which will have to be carefully designed to efficiently demonstrate and help quantify the desired effect. An important question, in particular, will be to control for putative confounders and ensure that the observed effect is indeed produced by the intended manipulation (e.g., in BCI, that the control is based on brain and not muscular activity, or in neurofeedback, that the effect is specific to the modulation of the targeted neural activity).

Hence BCI experiments cover pretty much the whole spectrum of possible designs that one may encounter in empirical science. The crucial question of how to optimally design a BCI experiment can thus rely on principles derived from applied statistical works in the fields of experimental psychology, cognitive neurosciences, and neuroimaging (e.g., Daunizeau et al. 2011; Henson 2006).

Put simply, designing an experiment first requires one to clearly state the alternative hypothesis to be tested. If properly done, this greatly constrains the experimental conditions one should consider and naturally points toward confounds that should be carefully controlled. In other words, this early and seemingly simple first step is essential to enable finding natural and proper answers to most important design questions that come next about the control group (Section 32.4.2), the control condition (Section 32.4.3) and the appropriate statistical tests (Section 32.4.4).

An often overlooked aspect in BCI though, like in many other fields, relates to the sampling issue. How many subjects should I test? And how many trials per subject should I record? Answering those questions is crucial for guaranteeing the reproducibility of BCI results.

Interestingly, the theoretical field of design optimization is still very active and BCI already motivated methodological innovations in that field, be it for maximizing design efficiency with respect to hypothesis testing or parameter estimation, by optimizing the stimuli or the number of samples (trials and subjects) (see, for instance, Sanchez et al. 2016 and Melinscak and Montesano 2016).

*And for our experiment?* Here, our objective is to "explore the neural correlates of some targeted mental processes and their potential usefulness," the mental process being remembering positive/negative emotional souvenirs. Given the high between-subject and intrasubject variability in terms of BCI performance, in order to obtain a statistically significant response to our hypothesis, we need an important number of participants (at least 20 would be good) and many trials (a typical BCI session would be 4 runs of 20 trials per class, i.e., 80 trials per class in total).

## 32.4.2 Why and How to Have a Good Control Group?

Broadly speaking, one can distinguish between feasibility studies and controlled studies. As the name indicates, feasibility studies, also referred to as proof-of-concept studies, analyze the viability of an idea. Often, feasibility studies are designed to pave the way for future controlled studies. To take but one example, Gharabaghi et al. (2014) demonstrated that closing the loop between mental states, cortical stimulation, and haptic feedback is feasible. Building on this, larger (clinical) controlled studies are necessary to evaluate the utility of this approach for the rehabilitation of lost motor function after stroke. It is not unusual that, at the beginning of a scientific achievement, a higher rate of feasibility studies is performed, which, at success, are followed by controlled studies. Contrary to most feasibility studies, controlled studies comprise an experimental group and a control group, whereby the nature of the control group largely depends on the research question. For instance, if one wants to assess the effect of age on the accuracy of a motor imagery–based BCI, the experimental group could comprise older individuals and the control group could comprise younger individuals. If one is, however, interested in the consequences of stroke on the ability to steer a motor imagery–based BCI, the experimental group could consist of stroke patients and the control group could consist of healthy individuals. If, to name another example, one wants to examine the rehabilitative effects of motor imagery–based BCI training after stroke, both experimental and control group should consist of stroke patients, whereby the experimental group receives real feedback and the control group receives sham feedback during the BCI training (for details on the aspects of sham feedback, see Section 32.4.3). In all cases, the experimental group and the control group differ ideally only with regard to the independent variable. This can be achieved by matching individuals on variables of putative importance but of noninterest, such as gender, age, or education, or, ideally, if possible, by employing a within-subject design. Taken together, well-controlled studies have the potential to isolate the effect of the independent variable of interest on dependent variable(s).

*And for our experiment?* We are proposing a feasibility study: the goal being to investigate whether or not it is possible to control a BCI using the remembrance of positive/negative emotional souvenirs. This step being preliminary, a control group is not mandatory. Nonetheless, we also aim to assess the relevance of these tasks in comparison to more standard motor imagery tasks such as imagining left- and right-hand movements. This is why we will propose a within-subject design with two conditions: in some runs, participants will perform the new tasks (remembering positive vs. negative emotional souvenirs), while in other intermixed runs, they will perform standard left- and right-hand motor imagery tasks. To keep a high number of trials per class (as required), participants will take part in two sessions of four runs.

### 32.4.3  How to Avoid Biases: Concepts of Counterbalancing, Sham Control, Double Blindness, and Randomization

In order to avoid biases, a couple of concepts can be useful. One of these is to compare the effects of real feedback with the effects of sham feedback. The so-called sham-controlled designs enable one to better evaluate the effectiveness and specificity of the feedback. In other words, the inclusion of a sham-control group is crucial to control for nonspecific factors such as motivation, expectancy, and practice effects. Based on these principles, there seems to be a general agreement that the inclusion of a sham-control group is of advantage. However, at present, there are no common criteria for the optimal sham-control condition. The existing sham-control conditions can be mainly assigned into five groups: (1) no feedback (Kadosh et al. 2016; Zich et al. 2015); (2) feedback based on activity stemming from a different brain region (Harmelech et al. 2015; Lee et al. 2012; Paret et al. 2016; Yao et al. 2016; Zotev et al. 2016); (3) feedback based on the activity from a different point in time, for example, different trial or session (Braun et al. 2016; Okazaki et al. 2015); (4) feedback based on activity from a different user (Chiew et al. 2012; Engelbregt et al. 2016; Escolano et al. 2014; Kober et al. 2014; Ros et al. 2013; Witte et al. 2013); and (5) feedback based on artificially created irrelevant randomized signals (Arnold et al. 2012; Mihara et al. 2012, 2013). Furthermore, Gevensleben et al. (2014) designed for their learning study a particular exceptional sham-control condition. In brief, feedback was based on data from a previous study, providing a variety of different feedback curves, which were additionally weighted by coefficients to control the development over time (Gevensleben et al. 2014). To the best of our knowledge, there is no ideal sham-control condition* at the present time, which is why it is even more important to indicate in detail what kind of sham-control condition was used. Furthermore, the ethical concerns of sham-control conditions should be considered; this particularly applies for clinical research where standard treatment exists (La Vaque and Rossiter 2001; Vernon et al. 2004).

For sham-control designs, but also other group comparisons (e.g., two different mental strategies), the question arises whether to employ a within-subject design or a between-subject design. Each has its advantages and disadvantages; for instance, while a between-subject design avoids order and carryover effects, interindividual variation introduces nonspecific differences between the experimental groups. In each case, it is advisable to (pseudo-)randomize and counterbalance the conditions, ideally in a double-blind manner. While no randomization and counterbalancing can introduce order effects, no blinding can compromise the objectivity of the evaluation.

*And for our experiment?* Here, we are performing offline analyses. In other words, we do not classify online the data and therefore do not propose a closed-loop BCI. Thus, participants will not be provided with a feedback. Furthermore, as we propose a within-subject design with the comparison of two pairs of mental imagery tasks, we have to choose to either randomize or counterbalance the conditions in order to avoid order effects. Given the low number of participants, it will be more relevant to counterbalance the conditions. The experiment will be conducted in a single-blind manner: the experimenter is blind to the order of the two mental imagery tasks.

### 32.4.4 How to Select the Appropriate Statistical Tests

The type of statistical test to use depends on the research question, that is, more precisely on the hypothesis. Typically, a dependency analysis is performed: we want to find either differences (univariate analyses) or correlations (bivariate analyses). There are two cases if one looks for differences. The samples are either independent or related (paired). For instance, if we have a variable with two modalities, A and B, (1) in a between-subject design, group 1 will use modality A and group 2 will use modality B: the samples will be independent; (2) in a within-subject design, all the participants will use both modalities: the samples will be related/paired. Then, it is also important to pick the method based on the distribution of the data: if the data have a normal distribution, it will be possible to use parametric tests; otherwise, nonparametric tests should be used (although it is worth noting that parametric tests are fairly robust to deviations from the normal distribution). Concerning bivariate analyses, if the data's distribution is normal, a Pearson correlation analysis should be performed; otherwise, a Spearman rank correlation should be used. Concerning univariate analyses, for a better readability, we propose a table (Table 32.1) to find the appropriate statistical test depending on (1) the number of variables, (2) the fact that the samples are independent or not, and (3) the distribution of the data.

Then, when we have three or more groups, if the analysis shows significant effects (for instance, $p < 0.05$), post-tests can be performed for which correction for multiple comparisons should be applied (see Section 32.3.6).

*And for our experiment?* In our experiment, we want to investigate the difference of BCI performance between the tasks "remembering positive/negative emotional souvenirs" and "imagining left/right-hand movements." Thus, we will do a univariate analysis. Also, we have one variable "MI tasks" with two modalities: "remembering emotional souvenirs" and "performing motor imagery"; we use a within-subject design and counterbalance the conditions to avoid order effects. Thus, we will average the performance obtained at the four runs of each condition in order to obtain one measure of performance for each pair of tasks, for each participant. We will analyze the distribution of the data, but given the small sample (20 participants), we will most likely have to use a

---

* Indeed, the abovementioned control conditions do not control exactly for the same aspects/effects; therefore, it would be hard if not impossible to imagine a sham condition that would control for all of them.

**TABLE 32.1**

**Type of Statistical Test to Be Performed as a Function of the Study Design (Type and Number of Samples) and of the Distribution of the Data**

| | Independent/Unpaired Samples | Paired Samples |
|---|---|---|
| **Parametric Tests** | | |
| 2 Samples | *Variances assumed equal*: Student $t$ test<br>*Otherwise:* Welch $t$ test | Paired $t$ test |
| 3+ Samples | *Variances assumed equal*: $n$-way ANOVA<br>*Otherwise:* Kruskal–Wallis test | ANOVA for repeated measures |
| **Nonparametric Tests** | | |
| 2 Samples | Mann–Whitney $U$ test | Wilcoxon signed-rank test |
| 3+ Samples | Kruskal–Wallis test | Friedman test |

nonparametric test. Thus, we will do a univariate nonparametric test for two paired samples: a Wilcoxon signed-rank test.

## 32.5 SUMMARY AND CONCLUSION

To conclude, we propose, in Table 32.2, a summary of the key points to be considered to design a rigorous BCI experiment. Once again, we do not claim to be exhaustive, but hope that we tackled the key points that will enable the reader to understand how to avoid common pitfalls when designing a BCI experiment. Nonetheless, it has to be noted that designing a rigorous experiment is often not enough to guarantee the significance and relevance of the latest. It is also of the utmost importance to question the scientific relevance of the study, to carefully acknowledge the impact of the user training and feedback (Kleih and Kübler 2018; Mladenovic et al. 2018), as well as to consider the impact of social and relational aspects, that is, of the way the study is performed and the relationship between the experimenter and the participant/patient.

**TABLE 32.2**

**Key Points to Design Rigorous BCI Experiments**

| | Acquisition of the Signals |
|---|---|
| How to choose the appropriate sensor type, location, and number depending on what we want to measure | Currently, a trade-off has to be done between the comfort/ease of use and the quality of the signal. Ag/AgCl wet electrodes offer the highest quality of signal. Using the 10–20 system with at least 32 electrodes enables a large coverage of the scalp. Nonetheless, for economical/practical reasons, lighter setups can be used. |
| What can we infer from the activation of one electrode? Concept of spatial resolution | Given that an unknown number of brain (and non-brain) generators contribute to the scalp EEG, one cannot determine the brain source of any particular EEG signal for sure only based on the activity measure at one electrode location. EEG source localization procedures can be used to confirm ideas about brain sources contributing to the EEG. |
| How muscular activity can interfere with EEG activity and why it should be controlled for to avoid confounds | Ocular (EOG) and muscular (EMG) activity are also measured by EEG sensors. They are typical confounding factors in BCI experiments, when correlated with the EEG patterns used by the BCI. They should thus be controlled for in any study. |

*(Continued)*

**TABLE 32.2 (CONTINUED)**
**Key Points to Design Rigorous BCI Experiments**

| | |
|---|---|
| What kinds of mental states can be used? | Theoretically, any mental state can be used while its neural signature is larger than the background noise. Then, the mental state should be selected depending on the information transfer rate and on the classification accuracy required for the target application. |

**Data Processing**

| | |
|---|---|
| Which classifier can we use depending on the distribution of the data? | When a few data are available for the calibration, linear classifiers such as LDA or SVM should be used (to avoid overfitting). It should be reminded that to be allowed to use these classifiers, a transformation of the features must be performed to obtain a normal-like distribution. |
| Why is it important to separate the training data set from the testing data set? | During offline analyses, cross-validation procedures should use testing data sets that are independent from the training data set to ensure that the algorithm can indeed generalize to unseen data and has not just memorized the training data set class labels. |
| How to determine the chance level for the classified data | The chance level depends on the number of classes and of the number of trials per class. To know the chance level, it is enough to have a look at the tables presented in the papers cited in this section. |
| To which extent can commercial algorithms be trusted? | Using commercial algorithms can be very useful and convenient, but it should be done with care. In particular, these algorithms should be used in rigorous scientific BCI experiments only if they were scientifically validated, including in the target context of use. |
| How to determine the relevance of neurophysiological markers | One way to determine the relevance of neurophysiological markers is to do time/frequency analyses of ERD and ERS and to compare the highlighted features to the literature. |
| Why is it important to correct for multiple comparisons? | As the number of tests increases, so does the risk of concluding to a significant effect in at least one comparison by mistake. Controlling for that risk (called the risk alpha or type I error) is very important since wrongly identifying an effect would typically yield a choice of BCI features that would not work in practice. |

**Experimental Design and the User Component**

| | |
|---|---|
| What to have in mind when designing a new BCI experiment | Designing an experiment first requires to clearly state the alternative hypotheses to be tested. If properly done, this greatly constrains the experimental conditions one should consider and naturally points toward confounds that should be carefully controlled. |
| Why and how to have a good control group? | Control groups are required to prove the efficiency of a new paradigm/approach. The nature of this control group should be defined depending on the hypotheses and on the goal of the experiment. |
| How to avoid biases: Concepts of counterbalancing, sham control, double blindness, and randomization | The so-called sham-controlled designs enable one to better evaluate the effectiveness and specificity of the feedback. Also, it is advisable to randomize or counterbalance the conditions, ideally in a double-blind manner. While no randomization and counterbalancing can introduce order effects, no blinding can compromise the objectivity of the evaluation. |
| How to select the appropriate statistical tests | The type of statistical test to use depends on the research question and more precisely on the hypothesis. Typically, a dependency analysis is performed: either we want to find differences or correlations. Then, to determine which test to perform, 3 questions should be answered: (1) Is the distribution of the data normal-like? (2) Are the samples paired? (3) How many groups are involved? |

## ACKNOWLEDGMENTS

CJ and FL were supported by the French National Research Agency with the REBEL project (grant ANR-15-CE23-0013-01). JM is supported by the LabEx Cortex ("Construction, Function and Cognitive Function and Rehabilitation of the Cortex," grant ANR-11-LABX-0042) of Université de Lyon.

## REFERENCES

Arnold, L.E., Lofthouse, N., Hersch, S., Pan, X., Hurt, E., Bates, B., Kassouf, K., Moone, S., & Grantier, C. 2012. EEG neurofeedback for ADHD: Double-blind sham-controlled randomized pilot feasibility trial. *Journal of Attention Disorders*, 17(5), 410–419.

Blankertz, B. 2018. Gentle introduction to signal processing and classification for single-trial EEG analysis. In: *Brain–Computer Interfaces Handbook—Technological and Theoretical Advances*.

Blankertz, B., Lemm, S., Treder, M., Haufe, S., & Müller, K.R. 2011. Single-trial analysis and classification of ERP components—A tutorial. *NeuroImage*, 56(2).

Bradley, A.P. 1997. The use of the area under the ROC curve in the evaluation of machine learning algorithms. *Pattern Recognition*, 30(7), 1145–1159.

Brandl, S., Frølich, L., Höhne, J., Müller, K.R., & Samek, W. 2016. Brain–computer interfacing under distraction: An evaluation study. *Journal of Neural Engineering*, 13(5), 056012.

Braun, N., Emkes, R., Thorne J.D., & Debener, S. 2016. Embodied neurofeedback with an anthropomorphic robotic hand, *Sci Rep*, 6, 37696.

Chau, T., & Damouras, S. 2009. Reply to: On the risk of extracting relevant information from random data. *Journal of Neural Engineering*, 6(5).

Chevallier, S. 2018. Riemannian classification for SSVEP based BCI: Offline versus online implementations. In: *Brain–Computer Interfaces Handbook—Technological and Theoretical Advances*.

Chiew, M., LaConte, S.M., & Graham, S.J. 2012. Investigation of fMRI neurofeedback of differential primary motor cortex activity using kinesthetic motor imagery, *NeuroImage*, 61(1), 21–31.

Combrisson, E., & Jerbi, K. 2015. Exceeding chance level by chance: The caveat of theoretical chance levels in brain signal classification and statistical assessment of decoding accuracy. *Journal of Neuroscience Methods*, 250, 126–136.

Daunizeau, J., Preuschoff, K., Friston, K., & Stephan, K. 2011. Optimizing experimental design for comparing models of brain function. *PLoS Comput. Biol*, 7(11), e1002280.

Debener, S., Emkes, R., De Vos, M., & Bleichner, M. (2015). Unobtrusive ambulatory EEG using a smartphone and flexible printed electrodes around the ear. *Scientific Reports*, 5, 16743.

De Vos, M., Kroesen, M., Emkes, R., & Debener, S. 2014. P300 speller BCI with a mobile EEG system: Comparison to a traditional amplifier. *Journal of Neural Engineering*, 11(3), 036008.

Dolcos, F., LaBar, K.S., & Cabeza, R. 2004. Dissociable effects of arousal and valence on prefrontal activity indexing emotional evaluation and subsequent memory: An event-related fMRI study. *NeuroImage*, 23(1), 64–74.

Dominguez, L.G. 2009. On the risk of extracting relevant information from random data. *Journal of Neural Engineering*, 6(5), 058001.

Engelbregt, H.J., Keeser, D., van Eijk, L., Suiker, E.M., Eichhorn, D., Karch, S., Deijen J.B., Pogarell, O. 2016. Short and long-term effects of sham-controlled prefrontal EEG-neurofeedback training in healthy subjects, *Clinical Neurophysiology*, 127(4), 1931–1937.

Escolano, C., Navarro-Gil, M., Garcia-Campayo, J., & Minguez, J. 2014. The effects of a single session of upper alpha neurofeedback for cognitive enhancement: A sham-controlled study. *Applied Psychophysiology and Biofeedback*, 39(3), 227–236.

Farwell, L., & Donchin, E. 1988. Talking off the top of your head: Towards a mental prosthesis utilizing event-related brain potentials. *Electroencephalography and Clinical Neurophysiology*, 70, 510–523.

Fatourechi, M., Bashashati, A., Ward, R., & Birch, G. 2007. EMG and EOG artifacts in brain computer interface systems: A survey, 118, 480–494.

Frey, J., Gervais, R., Fleck, S., Lotte F., & Hachet, M., 2014. Teegi: Tangible EEG interface. In: *Proceedings of the 27th Annual ACM Symposium on User Interface Software and Technology*. ACM, pp. 301–308.

Gevensleben, H., Albrecht, B., Lütcke, H., Auer, T., Dewiputri, W.I., Schweizer, R., Moll, G., Heinrich, H., & Rothenberger, A. 2014. Neurofeedback of slow cortical potentials: Neural mechanisms and feasibility of a placebo-controlled design in healthy adults. *Front Hum Neurosci*, 8, 990.

Gharabaghi, A., Kraus, D., Leao, M.T., Spüler, M., Walter, A., Bogdan, M., Rosenstiel, W., Naros, G., & Ziemann, U. 2014. Coupling brain–machine interfaces with cortical stimulation for brain-state dependent stimulation: Enhancing motor cortex excitability. *Frontiers in Human Neuroscience*, 8(122).

Goncharova, I., McFarland, D., Vaughan, T., & Wolpaw, J. 2003. EMG contamination of EEG: Spectral and topographical characteristics. *Clinical Neurophysiology*, 114, 1580–1593.

Guger, C., Spataro, R., Annen, J., Ortner, R., Irimia, D., Allison, B., La Bella, V., Cho, W., Edlinger, G., & Laureys, S. 2018. Brain–computer interfaces for motor rehabilitation, DOC assessment and communication. In: *Brain–Computer Interfaces Handbook—Technological and Theoretical Advances*.

Harmelech, T., Friedman, D., & Malach, R. 2015. Differential magnetic resonance neurofeedback modulations across extrinsic (visual) and intrinsic (default-mode) nodes of the human cortex. *The Journal of Neuroscience*, 35(6), 2588–2595.

Haufe, S., Meinecke, F., Görgen, K., Dähne, S., Haynes, J.D., Blankertz, B., & Bießmann, F. 2014. On the interpretation of weight vectors of linear models in multivariate neuroimaging. *Neuroimage*, 87, 96–110.

Henson, R. 2006. Efficient experimental design for fMRI. In: Karl Friston, John Ashburner, Stefan Kiebel, Thomas Nichols, and William Penny, editors, *Statistical Parametric Mapping: The Analysis of Functional Brain Images*, pp. 193–210. Elsevier.

Islam, M.K., Rastegarnia, A., & Yang, Z. 2016. Methods for artifact detection and removal from scalp EEG: A review. *Neurophysiologie Clinique/Clinical Neurophysiology*, 46(4), 287–305.

Jorgensen, M., Bakland, T., & Thorsen, E. 2017. *Satisfaction Measured Emotiv*, University of Oslo Technical Report, INF2260, 2012.

Kadosh, K.C., Luo, Q., de Burca, C., Sokunbi, M.O, Feng, J., Linden, D.E., & Lau, J.Y. 2016. Using real-time fMRI to influence effective connectivity in the developing emotion regulation network. *NeuroImage*, 15(125), 616–626.

Kleih, S.C., & Kübler, A. 2018. Why user-centered design is relevant for brain–computer interfacing and how it can be implemented in study protocols. In: *Brain–Computer Interfaces Handbook—Technological and Theoretical Advances*.

Kober, S.E., Wood, G., Kurzmann, J., Friedrich, E.V.C., Stangl, M., Wippel, T., Väljamäe, A., & Neuper, C. 2014. Near-infrared spectroscopy based neurofeedback training increases specific motor imagery related cortical activation compared to sham. *Biological Psychology*, 95, 21–30.

Kobler, R., & Scherer, R. 2016. Restricted Boltzmann machines in sensory motor rhythm brain–computer interfacing: A study on inter-subject transfer and co-adaptation. In: *IEEE International Conference on Systems, Man and Cybernetics SMC 2016*.

Kübler, A., Mattia, D., Rupp, R., & Tangermann, M. 2013. Facing the challenge: Bringing brain–computer interfaces to end-users. In: *Artificial Intelligence in Medicine*.

La Vaque, T.J., & Rossiter, T. 2001. The ethical use of placebo controls in clinical research: The Declaration of Helsinki. *Applied Psychophysiology and Biofeedback*, 26(1), 23–37.

Lalor, E.C., Kelly, S.P., Finucane, C., Burke, R., Smith, R., Reilly, R.B., & Mcdarby, G. 2005. Steady-state VEP-based brain–computer interface control in an immersive 3D gaming environment. *EURASIP Journal on Applied Signal Processing*, 2005, 3156–3164.

Lécuyer, A., Lotte, F., Reilly, R., Leeb, R., Hirose, M. and Slater, M. 2008. Brain–computer interfaces, virtual reality and videogames. *IEEE Computer*, 41.10, 66–72.

Lee, J.H., Kim, J., & Yoo, S.S. 2012. Real-time fMRI-based neurofeedback reinforces causality of attention networks. *Neuroscience Research*, 72(4), 347–354.

Lemm, S., Blankertz, B., Dickhaus, T., & Müller, K.R. 2011. Introduction to machine learning for brain imaging. *NeuroImage*, 56(2), 387–399.

Litvak, V., Mattout, J., Kiebel, S., Phillips, C., Henson, R., Kilner, J., Barnes, G., Oostenveld, R., Daunizeau, J., Flandin, G., Penny, W., & Friston, K. 2011. EEG and MEG data analysis in SPM8. *Comput Intell Neurosci*, Article ID 852961.

Lotte, F. 2014. A tutorial on EEG signal-processing techniques for mental-state recognition in brain–computer interfaces. In: Eduardo Reck Miranda and Julien Castet, editors *Guide to Brain-Computer Music Interfacing*, pp. 133–161. Springer, London.

Lotte, F. 2015. Signal processing approaches to minimize or suppress calibration time in oscillatory activity-based brain–computer interfaces. *Proceedings of the IEEE*, 103(6), 871–890.

Lotte, F., Congedo, M., Lécuyer, A., Lamarche, F., & Arnaldi, B. 2007. A review of classification algorithms for EEG-based brain–computer interfaces. *Journal of Neural Engineering*, 4(2), R1.

Luu S., & Chau, T. 2008. Decoding subjective preference from single trial near-infrared spectroscopy signals. *Journal of Neural Engineering*, 6(1).

Maris, E., & Oostenveld, R. 2007. Nonparametric statistical testing of EEG- and MEG-data. *Journal of Neuroscience Methods*, 164(1), 177–190.

McFarland, D.J. 2018. Therapeutic applications of BCI technologies. In: *Brain–Computer Interfaces Handbook—Technological and Theoretical Advances*.

Melinscak, F., & Montesano, L. 2016. Beyond *p*-values in the evaluation of brain–computer interfaces: A Bayesian estimation approach. *J Neurosci Methods*, 270, 30–45.

Mihara, M., Hattori, N., Hatakenaka, M., Yagura, H., Kawano, T., Hino, T., & Miyai, I. 2013. Near-infrared spectroscopy-mediated neurofeedback enhances efficacy of motor imagery-based training in poststroke victims. *Stroke*, 44, 1091–1098.

Mihara, M., Miyai, I., Harrori, N., Hatakenaka, M., Yagura, H., Kawano, T., Okibayashi, M., Danjo, N., Ishikawa, A., Inoue, Y., & Kubota, K. 2012. Neurofeedback using real-time near-infrared spectroscopy enhances motor imagery related cortical activation. *PLoS One*, 7(3), e32234.

Millán, J.D.R., Rupp, R., Mueller-Putz, G., Murray-Smith, R., Giugliemma, C., Tangermann, M., ... & Neuper, C. 2010. Combining brain–computer interfaces and assistive technologies: State-of-the-art and challenges. *Frontiers in Neuroscience*, 4, 161.

Mladenovic, J., Mattout, J., & Lotte, F. 2018. A generic framework for adaptive EEG-based BCI training and operation. In: *Brain–Computer Interfaces Handbook—Technological and Theoretical Advances*.

Mühl, C., Allison, B., Nijholt, A., & Chanel, G. 2014a. A survey of affective brain computer interfaces: Principles, state-of-the-art, and challenges. *Brain–Computer Interfaces*, 1–19.

Mühl, C., Bos, P.D., Thurlings, M.E., Scherffig, L., Duvinage, M., Elbakyan, A.A., ... Heylen, D. 2009. Bacteria hunt: A multimodal, multiparadigm BCI game. In: *Workshop Report for the Interface Workshop* (pp. 1–22). Genova, Italy.

Mühl, C., Jeunet, C., & Lotte, F. 2014b. EEG-based workload estimation across affective contexts. *Frontiers in Neuroscience, Section Neuroprosthetics*, 8, 114.

Müller-Putz, G.R., Scherer, R., Brauneis, C., & Pfurtscheller, G. 2005. Steady-state visual evoked potential (SSVEP)-based communication: Impact of harmonic frequency components. *Journal of Neural Engineering*, 2(4), 123–130.

Müller-Putz, G.R., Scherer, R., Brunner, C., Leeb, R., & Pfurtscheller, G. 2008. Better than random: A closer look on BCI results. *International Journal of Bioelectromagnetism*, 10, 52–55.

Müller-Putz, G.R., Scherer, R., Neuper, C., Pfurtscheller, G. 2006. Steady-state somatosensory evoked potentials: Suitable brain signals for brain–computer interfaces? *Neural Systems and Rehabilitation Engineering IEEE Transactions*, 14, 30–37.

Nichols, T. 2006. False discovery rate procedures. In: Karl Friston, John Ashburner, Stefan Kiebel, Thomas Nichols, and William Penny, editors, *Statistical Parametric Mapping: The Analysis of Functional Brain Images*, pp. 246–252. Elsevier.

Okazaki, Y.O., Horschig, J.M., Luther, L., Oostenveld, R., Murakami, I., & Jensen, O. 2015. Real-time MEG neurofeedback training of posterior alpha activity modulates subsequent visual detection performance. *NeuroImage*, 107, 323–332.

Olivetti, E., Mognon, A., Greiner, S., & Avesani, P. 2010. Brain decoding: Biases in error estimation. In: *IEEE First Workshop on Brain Decoding: Pattern Recognition Challenges in Neuroimaging (WBD)*, 40–43.

Oostenveld, R., Fries, P., Maris, E., & Schoffelen, J.-M. 2011. FieldTrip: Open source software for advanced analysis of MEG, EEG, and invasive electrophysiological data. *Comput Intell Neurosci*, Articles ID 156869.

Paret, C., Ruf, M., Gerchen, M.F., Kluetsch, R., Demirakca, T., Jungkunz, M., Bertsch, K., Schmahl, C., & Ende, G. 2016. fMRI neurofeedback of amygdala response to aversive stimuli enhances prefrontal–limbic brain connectivity. *NeuroImage*, 15(125), 182–188.

Pfurtscheller, G., Allison, B.Z., Brunner, C., Bauernfeind, G., Solis-Escalante, T., Scherer, R., ... Birbaumer, N. 2010. The hybrid BCI. *Frontiers in Neuroscience*, 4, 42. http://doi.org/10.3389/fnpro.2010.00003

Pfurtscheller, G., & Da Silva, F.L. 1999. Event-related EEG/MEG synchronization and desynchronization: Basic principles. *Clinical Neurophysiology*, 110(11), 1842–1857.

Pfurtscheller, G., Neuper, C., Flotzinger, D., & Pregenzer, M. 1997. EEG-based discrimination between imagination of right and left hand movement. *Electroencephalography and Clinical Neurophysiology*, 103(6), 642–651.

Rivet, B., Souloumiac, A., Attina, V., & Gibert, G. 2009. xDAWN algorithm to enhance evoked potentials: Application to brain–computer interface. *IEEE Transactions on Biomedical Engineering*, 56, 2035–2043.

Ros, T., Theberge, J., Frewen, P.A., Kluetsch, R., Densmore, M., Calhoun, V.D., Lanius, R.A. 2013. Mind over chatter: Plastic up-regulation of the fMRI salience network directly after EEG neurofeedback. *NeuroImage*, 65, 324–335.

Sanchez, G., Lecaignard, F., Otman, A., Maby, E., & Mattout, J. 2016. Active SAmpling Protocol (ASAP) to optimize individual neurocognitive hypothesis testing: A BCI-inspired dynamic experimental design. *Front Hum Neurosci*, 10.

Schmidt, L.A., & Trainor, L.J. 2001. Frontal brain electrical activity (EEG) distinguishes valence and intensity of musical emotions. *Cognition & Emotion*, 15(4), 487–500.

Singer, E. 2008. Brain games. *Technology Review*, 111(4), 82–84.

Steyrl, D., Scherer, R., Faller, J., & Müller-Putz, G.R. 2016. Random forests in non-invasive sensorimotor rhythm brain–computer interfaces: A practical and convenient non-linear classifier. *Biomedizinische Technik. Biomedical Engineering*, 61(1), 77–86.

Thompson, D.E., Quitadamo, L.R., Mainardi, L., Gao, S., Kindermans, P.J., Simeral, J.D., ... & Chestek, C.A. 2014. Performance measurement for brain–computer or brain–machine interfaces: A tutorial. *Journal of Neural Engineering*, 11(3), 035001.

Vernon, D., Frick, A., & Gruzelier, J. 2004. Neurofeedback as a treatment for ADHD: A methodological review with implications for future research. *Journal of Neurotherapy*, 8(2), 53–82.

Vialatte, F.B., Maurice, M., Dauwels, J., & Cichocki, A. 2010. Steady-state visually evoked potentials: Focus on essential paradigms and future perspectives. *Progress in Neurobiology*, 90(4), 418–438.

Whitham, E.M., Pope, K.J., Fitzgibbon, S.P., Lewis, T., Clark, C.R., Loveless, S., Broberg, M., Wallace, A., DeLosAngeles, D., Lillie, P. et al. 2007. Scalp electrical recording during paralysis: Quantitative evidence that EEG frequencies above 20 Hz are contaminated by EMG. *Clinical Neurophysiology*, 118, 1877–1888.

Witte, M., Kober, S.E., Ninaus, M., Neuper, C., & Wood, G. 2013. Control beliefs can predict the ability to up-regulate sensorimotor rhythm during neurofeedback training, *Frontiers in Human Neuroscience*, 7, 478.

Worsley, K. 2006. Random field theory. In: Karl Friston, John Ashburner, Stefan Kiebel, Thomas Nichols, and William Penny, editors, *Statistical Parametric Mapping: The Analysis of Functional Brain Images*, pp. 232–236. Elsevier.

Yao, S., Becker, B., Geng, Y., Zhao, Z., Xu, X., Zhao, W., Ren, P., & Kendrick, K.M. 2016. Voluntary control of anterior insula and its functional connections is feedback-independent and increases pain empathy. *NeuroImage*, 130, 230–240.

Zander, T.O., & Kothe, C. 2011. Towards passive brain–computer interfaces: Applying brain–computer interface technology to human–machine systems in general. *Journal of Neural Engineering*, 8(2), 25005.

Zich, C., Debener, S., De Vos., M., Frerichs, S., Maurer, S., & Kranczioch, C. 2015. Lateralization patterns of covert but not overt movements change with age: An EEG neurofeedback study. *NeuroImage*, 1(116), 80–91.

Zotev, V., Yuan, H., Misaki, M., Phillips, R., Young, K.D., Feldner, M.T., & Bodurka, J. 2016. Correlation between amygdala BOLD activity and frontal EEG asymmetry during real-time fMRI neurofeedback training in patients with depression. *NeuroImage*, 11, 224–238.

# 33 Evaluation and Performance Assessment of the Brain–Computer Interface System

*Md Rakibul Mowla, Jane E. Huggins, and David E. Thompson*

## CONTENTS

33.1 Introduction .................................................................................................................636
33.2 General Framework .......................................................................................................636
33.3 Discrete BCI .................................................................................................................637
    33.3.1 Binary Classification Accuracy versus Task Accuracy ...................................637
        33.3.1.1 Confusion Matrix.................................................................................638
        33.3.1.2 Binomial Models for Accuracy............................................................638
    33.3.2 Information Gain ...............................................................................................639
        33.3.2.1 Information Transfer Rate.....................................................................639
        33.3.2.2 Rate of Information Gain......................................................................640
    33.3.3 BCI Utility........................................................................................................640
        33.3.3.1 Utility for P300 Speller .......................................................................641
    33.3.4 Data Scarcity and Predicted Accuracy .............................................................642
        33.3.4.1 Projected Accuracy Metric ..................................................................643
        33.3.4.2 Classifier-Based Latency Estimation ..................................................644
33.4 Continuous BCI .............................................................................................................644
    33.4.1 Fitts's Law and Information Theory ..................................................................645
        33.4.1.1 Shannon's Theory ................................................................................645
        33.4.1.2 Fitts's Law ...........................................................................................645
    33.4.2 Shannon–Welford Model .................................................................................646
33.5 Discussion......................................................................................................................647
References.................................................................................................................................647

**Abstract**

Performance assessment has a pivotal role in the development of brain–computer interface (BCI) systems and algorithms. A large number of performance-measuring metrics exist in the literature, and the choice of best metric may be difficult for researchers. The main objective of this chapter is to demonstrate different performance assessment criteria as well as to report the most widely accepted system performance metrics. This chapter will also help readers to choose suitable performance-measuring metrics for a specific type of BCI. Performance measurement and evaluation criteria are different for discrete and continuous BCIs; these systems will be discussed separately. The chapter should help researchers and BCI system developers to compare systems side by side with existing technologies.

## 33.1 INTRODUCTION

Measuring system performance is a vital step in brain–computer interface (BCI) system development. Measuring performance includes assessing the success of the design process as well as evaluating algorithm performance. Another goal of performance measurement is to compare system performance with existing systems. All of these goals are achieved through the use of "metrics" or measurement tools for performance.

However, performance measurement is not easy. One problem with performance measurement is the diversity of modalities, experimental methods, data analysis approaches, and personal/team preferences for performance-measuring metrics. This diversity has led to the creation of many different performance metrics, many of which are not commensurate. This creates ambiguity when attempting to understand and compare the performance of one group with others, as their reported metrics are not similar.

Additionally, BCIs tend to be very slow compared to other forms of communication or control. As a result, the amount of data that can reasonably be gathered in a given experiment is small. Inconvenience of using EEG (or other modalities) to monitor brain activity is also a strong factor for data scarcity. This data scarcity can complicate the calculation of performance metrics, in some cases leading to such large confidence bounds that comparisons between systems are statistically meaningless. Data scarcity is a significant problem in most BCI studies and particularly in spelling systems.

Performance measurement does not end with choice of metric; readers are invited to look at Thompson et al. (2014) for a recent consensus regarding some significant measurement-related issues. That paper, in addition to including a discussion of some of the metrics presented here, includes concepts such as task descriptions and timing details that can be important when calculating metrics. Here, we will focus more on binomial modeling, confidence intervals, data scarcity, and performance metrics—including newer metrics such as projected accuracy and Shannon–Welford's model as an alternative to Fitts's law.

The overall goal of this chapter is to discuss potential solutions of the abovementioned problems, as well as to report the most widely accepted system performance metrics. This chapter should thus be a useful introduction for researchers seeking to measure performance of a BCI system. The first step in measuring BCI performance is understanding the output of the BCI system, specifically, if the output is discrete or continuous. Discrete outputs make a selection from a measurable number of choices—as an example, the letters on a keyboard. Continuous BCIs, by contrast, have many possible outputs—often, the output is a 1- or 2-D cursor movement. High degree-of-freedom prosthetic control would be another application for continuous BCI. Performance measurement for discrete system will be discussed in Section 33.3.

Performance measurement for continuous-output BCIs is still evolving in the field. Many groups use a task that converts the continuous output into a discrete-output system (e.g., using a cursor movement to select letters; Neuper et al. 2003), which allows the calculation of discrete-output metrics. Other groups use targeting tasks adapted from human–computer interface device research and adapt the metric from that field known as Fitts's law (Section 33.4.1) for performance measurement. Performance measurement for continuous BCI will be discussed in Section 33.4.

This chapter has five sections including this introduction. Section 33.2 discusses the general framework of a BCI system to guide big-picture understanding. Sections 33.3 and 33.4 discuss different performance measurement metrics for discrete and continuous BCI system, respectively. Section 33.5 presents concluding thoughts and discussion.

## 33.2 GENERAL FRAMEWORK

Figure 33.1 shows a general framework of a BCI system. The first stage, called the transducer (TR) level, includes signal acquisition, preprocessing, and classification. The next level, which converts

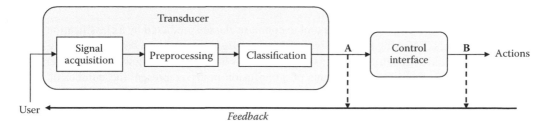

**FIGURE 33.1**  A general framework of BCI systems. **A** and **B** are points where performance of a BCI system can be measured.

TR output into a control output, is referred to as the control interface (CI) (Dal Seno et al. 2010; Thompson et al. 2014); for example, in a BCI for spelling, the task of CI is to combine the classification outputs from the TR level in order to find the target character. CI may also incorporate other assistive tools such as a word prediction software in P300 speller BCI (Ryan et al. 2010). A third level, consisting of the human experience of using the BCI, has been suggested (Thompson et al. 2014), but is not the focus of this chapter.

In Figure 33.1, **A** and **B** represent the outputs of the TR and CI, respectively. Performance can be measured at **A** or **B**, and the two measurements are related but far from identical. For example, in P300-based BCIs for spelling, the accuracy metric at **A** is the binary accuracy of the classifier, whereas at **B**, the accuracy is the percentage of correctly spelled characters. Not only are the two accuracies different, an increase in binary classification performance may not lead to increased task performance at the CI level. CI-level performance is typically more intuitive and useful (being expressed in units such as characters per minute or selections per minute), but may be difficult to compare between tasks. Hence, BCI performance measurements at different levels are incomparable. Further, while TR-level performance may sometimes be comparable as long as the same performance metric is used, different CIs can make the same performance metrics measured at the CI level incomparable.

## 33.3  DISCRETE BCI

This section discusses different concepts and utility metrics for discrete BCI systems. The P300 speller system is used several times in this section as an example of a discrete system, to demonstrate the calculation of performance measurement metrics.

Similarly, derivations and final expressions for BCI utility in Section 33.3.3 and projected accuracy in Section 33.3.4.1 use the P300 speller as an example. Please note that those metrics are not limited to speller systems. With proper assumptions, both BCI utility and projected accuracy metrics can be used with other discrete BCI systems.

### 33.3.1  Binary Classification Accuracy versus Task Accuracy

As we mentioned earlier, accuracy of a BCI system can be calculated for both TR outputs and CI outputs. In most cases, we can label the acquired data in two groups. The task of the classifier is to classify target and nontarget data, a task commonly known as binary or binomial classification. TR outputs can be binary outputs, or the classifier "scores"—the distance between the observation and the boundary the classifier draws between classes. Evaluation of accuracy on TR outputs is binary classification accuracy. In contrast, evaluation of accuracy on CI outputs is task accuracy. Accuracy is the most popular evaluation criteria (Schlogl et al. 2007), but task accuracy is more meaningful for BCI systems than binary accuracy. To interpret and compare performance based on accuracy, Cohen's κ coefficient and confusion matrices might be helpful.

### 33.3.1.1  Confusion Matrix

A confusion matrix (Stehman 1997) is a tool to compare classes predicted by a classification system to the actual labels. Referring back to Figure 33.1, a confusion matrix can be built by using CI outputs as columns and actual (true) labels as rows. The cells hold a count of how often the intersecting events occur. Thus, the diagonal elements of a confusion matrix represent the number of correct outputs. Meanwhile, Cohen's κ coefficient (κ statistic) (Cohen 1960) is a measure of agreement between the BCI control module output and the expected/correct output and can be computed from a confusion matrix.

However, neither the confusion matrix nor the κ statistic accounts for time per selection. Hence, both are unable to provide any measure of throughput. Both metrics can be useful to measure classifier reliability and error patterns, and may see application in self-paced BCI, but are of limited use when comparing performance between systems. In these self-paced systems, receiver operating characteristic curves are also often used for comparing different systems. Self-paced BCI system's performance measurement is not discussed in this chapter, but interested readers are referred to the review article by Eoin Thomas (Thomas et al. 2013).

Further, for BCI systems with a large number of targets (e.g., a simple P300 speller with 36 or possible selections), the confusion matrix will be very large (with 36 rows and 36 columns, it will have 1296 cells). Each row of the matrix will require its own data with large trial numbers; we will discuss the required number of trials in Section 33.3.4. Thus, for spellers or other BCIs with large numbers of possible outputs, these metrics are not recommended because of data scarcity. In BCIs with a very limited number of outputs—perhaps five or fewer—a confusion matrix might be a useful tool for measuring and reporting performance. Hence, both confusion matrix and Cohen's κ coefficient are widely used in self-paced BCI systems, which tend to drive two-class outputs such as controlling a physical switch.

The extended confusion matrix (ECM) was presented in Bianchi et al. (2007); this metric extends confusion matrices by adding support for classifier "abstentions," where the classifier is allowed to abstain from making a selection if it is uncertain what class the data belong to. Additionally, that paper proposed an accompanying metric, $Eff_{sys}$, which includes time information. These metrics should be used in place of regular confusion matrices in BCI systems with limited possible outputs. However, ECM is derived from confusion matrix and shares the same data requirements; neither are suitable for large numbers of classes with current-generation BCIs.

### 33.3.1.2  Binomial Models for Accuracy

Accuracy is the simplest and most intuitive metric for discrete BCI performance. However, measuring accuracy is a parameter estimation problem and requires careful treatment. This section will present a frequentist perspective, although Bayesian interpretations are also possible.

If we consider a discrete BCI output as either correct (success) or incorrect (failure), then each discrete output is a Bernoulli trial, and the BCI can be considered a Bernoulli random process. Assuming that the user's accuracy is fixed during some duration, the number of correct and incorrect outputs during that duration is then a binomial random variable. Given one or more observations of this random variable, the task is then to estimate the user's accuracy. Note that this modeling scheme also assumes that the probability of correct selection does not depend on the selection itself; in other words, there are no outputs that are easier to select than others.

Consider a binomial distribution with $x$ number of success out of $n$ Bernoulli trials:

$$x \sim B(n, p) \, (n \geq 1, 0 < p < 1). \tag{33.1}$$

The maximum likelihood (ML) estimate for the probability of success is $x/n$. Thus, the ML estimate for classification accuracy is $p = x/n$. Now, consider random chance accuracy, $p_0 = 1/N$, where $N$ is the number of possible outputs, assuming uniform distribution of selections

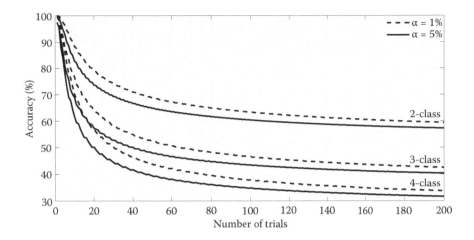

**FIGURE 33.2**  Upper confidence limits (Clopper–Pearson method) of chance results for two-, three-, and four-class classification accuracy for $\alpha = 1\%$ and $5\%$.

in the absence of control. Demonstrating BCI control requires showing performance significantly better than chance. In this case, the upper limit of the confidence interval of the binomial distribution for different numbers of trial sets the minimum detectable accuracy (Müller-Putz et al. 2008). Figure 33.2 shows that minimum accuracy requires to be obtained at different numbers of trials for two-class, three-class, and four-class classification task at $\alpha = 1\%$ and $\alpha = 5\%$.

As an example, for a two-class classification with 60 trials and chance accuracy of 50%, BCI accuracy must be above 63.5% and 67.25% to say that the classifier performed better than random chance with 95% and 99% confidence, respectively. From the figure, it is clear that the minimum detectable accuracy depends heavily on the number of trials, and hence it has been advised to report number of trials while reporting accuracy (Yuan et al. 2013).

### 33.3.2  Information Gain

#### 33.3.2.1  Information Transfer Rate

The information transfer rate (ITR), or simply bit rate, is another widely used performance measurement metric derived from Shannon's channel theory (Shannon's theory will be discussed in Section 33.4.1.1) by Wolpaw (Wolpaw et al. 1998). The ITR is intended to be more meaningful than accuracy, since it accounts for both the number of choices and time per selection. The ITR can be calculated from Equation 33.2:

$$\text{ITR} = \frac{1}{c}\left\{\log_2 n + p\log_2 p + (1-p)\log_2\left(\frac{1-p}{n-p}\right)\right\}, \tag{33.2}$$

where the ITR is in bits per second, $c$ is the time per selection, $n$ is the number of choices per trial, and $p$ is the classifier accuracy. The ITR equation was derived based on a few assumptions:

- User will have $n$ finite number of discrete choices to target.
- User will choose, and successfully select, each choice with equal probability.
- System accuracy, $p$, will remain constant over time.
- Errors will be uniformly distributed over all nontarget outputs.

While the ITR is the most common way to calculate transfer rate, it has some limitations. The primary limitation is that the assumptions in the ITR often do not hold in practical BCI systems (Yuan et al. 2013), because users do not use BCI systems with an equal rate over time and also do not choose all choices with equal probability. Further, Shannon's channel theorem gives the maximum achievable transfer rate over a noisy channel. While in digital communication it is possible to achieve bit rates close to Shannon's limit, BCI involves human subjects at one end of the system and hence the actual transfer rate is often far below the theoretical limit. Thus, ITR comparisons may not reflect practical differences between two systems since the ITR reflects theoretical, rather than achieved, channel capacity.

### 33.3.2.2 Rate of Information Gain

In a recent study, N.J. Hill proposed another metric named rate of information gain ($RIG_B$) to generalize the equation for computing the ITR (Hill et al. 2014):

$$RIG_B = \text{sign}\,(p - p_0)\left[ p\log_2 \frac{p}{p_0} + (1-p)\log_2 \left(\frac{1-p}{1-p}\right)\right]\Big/\bar{t}\,, \tag{33.3}$$

where $p$ is the observed accuracy (classification accuracy), $p_0$ is the chance performance, and $\bar{t}$ is the mean duration of a trial. The term inside the square bracket is also a generalized term of Wolpaw's ITR equation. Estimation of $p_0$ is a crucial factor to calculate $RIG_B$. For discrete BCI with $n$ choices, the naive estimation of $p_0$ is $1/n$. If we substitute $p_0 = 1/n$ in the square term of Equation 33.3,

$$
\begin{aligned}
&p\log_2 \frac{p}{p_0} + (1-p)\log_2 \left(\frac{1-p}{1-p}\right) \\
&= p\log_2 (np) + (1-p)\log_2 \left(\frac{1-p}{n-1}n\right) \\
&= p\log_2 n + p\log_2 p + (1-p)\log_2 \left(\frac{1-p}{n-1}\right) + (1-p)\log_2 n \\
&= \log_2 n + p\log_2 p + (1-p)\log_2 \left(\frac{1-p}{n-1}\right),
\end{aligned}
\tag{33.4}
$$

which is identical to the ITR equation. As stated in Section 33.3.2.1, ITR assumed that errors were uniformly distributed $p_0 = 1/n$. But this may not happen in all BCI systems. Hence, $RIG_B$ provides the flexibility to model and estimate $p_0$.

Hill recommends estimating $p_0$ with a Monte Carlo simulation of random control. First, a *scope* for $p_0$ should be defined—typically, this is the set of trials over which one wishes to estimate $p_0$, such as all trials for a particular user under one experimental condition. Then, each trial is simulated many times with an artificial input to the BCI: a random walk. For each trial simulation, the BCI begins with the same initial parameter/adjustment as it was during the online experiment, which is particularly important for BCI systems that perform online learning. Finally, $p_0$ may be estimated by taking the average across trials of the simulated chance accuracies.

### 33.3.3 BCI Utility

The goal of the BCI utility metric is to find the quantifiable benefits for a user of a BCI system. The metric was originally proposed by Dal Seno et al. (2010). The utility metric provides a quantitative measure of BCI system throughput by considering user benefit. To find the utility metric, we need to measure the expected average benefit over time:

$$U = \mathbb{E}\left[\lim_{T \to \infty} \frac{\int_0^T b(t)\,dt}{T}\right]. \tag{33.5}$$

Here, $b(t)$ is the benefit function, which takes a positive or negative value based on whether the BCI outputs match or mismatch the user's intentions. Now, for discrete BCI, utility can be derived from Equation 33.5 as (Dal Seno et al. 2010)

$$U = \mathbb{E}\left[\frac{\mathbb{E}[b_i]}{\mathbb{E}[\Delta t_i]}\right] = \frac{\mathbb{E}[b_i]}{\mathbb{E}[\Delta t_i]}, \tag{33.6}$$

where $\Delta t_i = t_i - t_{i-1}$ for $i > 1$, $\Delta t_1 = t_1$, and $b_i$ represents the benefit for the $i$th target. The system that gives the same benefit with the shortest possible time is the better system according to this metric. The benefit function, the numerator in Equation 33.6, can be computed in two different ways:

a. Assigning a positive or negative 1 for each correct or wrong output, respectively. In this case, the unit of $U$ will be *correct selections/time*.
b. Benefit can also be considered as the amount of information transferred at each time that the system gives a correct (user intended) output (often $\log_2 N$). In this case, the units of $U$ will be *bits/time*.

### 33.3.3.1 Utility for P300 Speller

Consider a P300 speller paradigm with $n$ characters including a backspace. A user will focus on backspace only if the system types a wrong character. Hence, the information conveyed by the system is $b_c = \log_2(n - 1)$ assuming equal probability of each character. Now let $c$ be the time for a single trial, $T_c$ be the time to select a character correctly, and $p$ be the probability of selecting a character correctly. If the system outputs an incorrect character, then the user will need to select backspace first and then select the target character. Thus, the general expression for the time to select a character correctly:

$$\begin{aligned} T_c &= pc + (1-p)(c + T_b + T_c) \\ &= c + (1-p)(T_b + T_c). \end{aligned} \tag{33.7}$$

Here, $T_b$ is the time to type backspace. If the backspace is mistyped, then an additional backspace will be required. Hence, the time for backspace can be written as

$$\begin{aligned} T_b &= pc + (1-p)(c + T_b + T_b) \\ &= c + (1-p)2T_b. \end{aligned} \tag{33.8}$$

By subtracting Equation 33.8 from Equation 33.7, we will get $p(T_b - T_c) = 0$. But $p \neq 0$, as the probability of selecting a correct character cannot be zero, so $T_b = T_c$. Now from Equation 33.7,

$$\begin{aligned} T_c &= c + (1-p)2T_c \\ 2pT_c - T_c &= c \\ T_c &= \frac{c}{2p-1}. \end{aligned} \tag{33.9}$$

Here, for $p < 0.5$, we will get a negative $T_c$, and for $p = 0.5$, we will get infinite time, which means practically it is not possible to type a target character correctly if $p \leq 0.5$. The expression for $T_c$ in Equation 33.9 is only valid for $p > 0.5$. Thus, the utility becomes

$$U = \frac{b_c}{T_c} = \frac{2p-1}{c} \log_2 (n-1), \tag{33.10}$$

where $p$ is the classification accuracy, $c$ is the time per trial, and $n$ is the number of choices. For example, for a $6 \times 6$ P300 speller, $n = 36$.

## 33.3.4 Data Scarcity and Predicted Accuracy

Lets assume, we have an existing *method 1* and another newly developed *method 2*. The observed accuracy at CI for any particular subject with *method 1* is $p_1$ and that with *method 2* is $p_2$. Now, for instance, we want to claim *method 2* is better than the existing method for this particular subject because $p_2 = 0.90$ and $p_1 = 0.80$ for $n$ number of trials. Here, we will check how accurate the claim is using a hypothesis test. Our null hypothesis is both observed accuracies are equal, with an alternate hypothesis that they are different.

$$H_0 : p_1 = p_2 \quad \text{and} \quad H_1 : p_1 \neq p_2.$$

Now, we have to find our test statistic for binomials $B(n,p_2)$ and $B(n,p_2)$. But if $n \cdot \min(p, 1-p)$ is greater than 10, then the approximation of $B(n,p)$ can be expressed by $N(np, np(1-p))$ (Brown et al. 2001); hence, the test statistic is

$$z = \frac{p_2 - p_1}{\sqrt{\hat{p}(1-\hat{p})\left(\dfrac{1}{n_1} + \dfrac{1}{n_2}\right)}}, \quad \text{where} \quad \hat{p} = \frac{n_1 p_1 + n_2 p_2}{n_1 + n_2}.$$

Here, in our example, we assumed *method 1* and *method 2* are tested on the same number of trials, which implies $n = n_1 = n_2$. If $n_1$ and $n_2$ are different, then we have to calculate the test statistic using their individual values. Thus, in this example, $\hat{p} = (p_1 + p_2)/2 = 0.85$.

$$z = \frac{0.90 - 0.80}{\sqrt{0.85 \times 0.15 \times \dfrac{2}{n}}} = \frac{0.10\sqrt{n}}{\sqrt{0.255}}.$$

Our goal is to reject the null hypothesis with a given confidence level. For example, we want 95% confidence level to reject the null hypothesis. At this level, the critical region value is $z_{\alpha/2} = 1.96$, and to reject the null hypothesis, we need $z > z_{\alpha/2}$, which implies

$$z > 1.96$$

$$\Rightarrow \frac{0.10\sqrt{n}}{\sqrt{0.255}} > 1.96$$

$$\Rightarrow n > 97.96.$$

Thus, we need at least 98 trials (per method) to claim *method 2* is better than *method 1*, even with *method 2* having 10% higher observed accuracy. If the observed accuracy difference is only 5%, for example, if $p_2 = 0.85$, then the required number of trials is approximately 444.

In many experiments, even 98 trials per method is impractical because of the low throughput of BCI systems. Currently, most researchers combine data across participants to compare methods, although the differences found are often much smaller than those between any two participants. Some recent studies have proposed methods to estimate and predict BCI accuracy using substantially fewer trials, including the projected accuracy metric and classifier-based latency estimation.

### 33.3.4.1  Projected Accuracy Metric

Colwell proposed a method to estimate P300 speller accuracy at CI based on the observed probability of selecting rows ($p_r$) and columns ($p_c$) correctly (Colwell et al. 2014). Then, the *projected accuracy* can be expressed as $p = p_r \times p_c$. If $x_i$ is the classifier score and $y_i \in \{0, 1\}$ is the class label for the $i$th flash response, then the mean of classifier scores for target and nontarget rows can be written as

$$\bar{T}_r = \frac{1}{s}\sum_{i=1}^{s}[x_i \mid y_i = 1] \quad \text{and} \quad \bar{U}_r^{(k)} = \frac{1}{s}\sum_{j=1}^{s}\left[x_j^{(k)} \mid y_j = 0\right],$$

where, $k = \{1,\ldots, R - 1\}$. Here $S$ and $R$ represent the number of sequences per character and the number of rows, respectively and $C$ will represent the number of columns. Sequences are complete sets of stimuli; in the P300 speller, sequences per character is the number of times each row and column is flashed, per spelled character. Now, $p_r$ can be written as

$$p_r = P\left(\bigcap_{k=1}^{R-1}\left\{\bar{T}_r > \bar{U}_r^{(k)}\right\}\right) \tag{33.11}$$

$$p_r = \int_{-\infty}^{\infty}\left[\prod_{k=1}^{R-1}P\left(\bar{T}_r > \bar{U}_r^{(k)} \mid \bar{T}_r \mid \bar{T}_r\right)\right]p(\bar{T}_r)\,d\bar{T}_r \tag{33.12}$$

$$= \int_{-\infty}^{\infty}\left[\prod_{k=1}^{R-1}\int_{-\infty}^{\bar{T}_r} p\left(\bar{U}_r^{(k)}\right)d\bar{U}_r^{(k)}\right]p(\bar{T}_r)d\bar{T}_r \tag{33.13}$$

$$= \int_{-\infty}^{\infty}\left(F_{\bar{U}_r(t)}\right)^{R-1} f_{\bar{T}_r}(t)\,dt. \tag{33.14}$$

Here, $F_{\bar{U}_r}$ is the cumulative distribution function of $\bar{U}_r$ and $f_{\bar{T}_r}$ is the probability density function of $\bar{T}_r$. Expressions for $p_c$ are similar to $p_r$. If the rows and columns are presented an equal number of times for each character spelled ($S_r = S_c$), then we can assume the distributions for row and column will be the same, which implies $\bar{T}_r \sim \bar{T}_c$ and $\bar{U}_r \sim \bar{U}_c$, and can be written as $\bar{T}$ and $\bar{U}$, respectively. Hence, the projected accuracy ($p$) can be written as

$$p = \int_{-\infty}^{\infty}(F_{\bar{U}(t)})^{R-1} f_{\bar{T}}(t)\,dt \times \int_{-\infty}^{\infty}(F_{\bar{U}(t)})^{C-1} f_{\bar{T}}(t)\,dt. \tag{33.15}$$

Now, to find the projected accuracy, we only need the distributions of $\bar{T}$ and $\bar{U}(k)$, and it has been shown that those distributions usually follow Gaussian distributions (Speier et al. 2011). Hence, the distributions can be written as

$$\bar{T} \sim \mathcal{N}(x_i \mid \mu_1, \sigma_1) \quad \text{and} \quad \bar{U}^{(k)} \sim \mathcal{N}(x_i \mid \mu_0, \sigma_0)$$

$$\Rightarrow \bar{T} \sim \mathcal{N}(x_i \mid \mu_1, \sigma_1) \quad \text{and} \quad \bar{U}^{(k)} \sim \mathcal{N}(x_i \mid \mu_0, \sigma_0).$$

To compute the value of $p$, we then need only the parameters $R$, $C$, $S$, and the means and variances for target and nontarget score distributions.

### 33.3.4.2 Classifier-Based Latency Estimation

Classifier-based latency estimation (CBLE) is a technique developed by Thompson et al. (2012), originally intended to estimate the latency of a P300 event-related potential. However, a strong predictive relationship was found between observed latency variation on small (five-character) data sets and same-day accuracy from much larger (23+ character) data sets.

CBLE works by presenting many time-varying versions of the event-related potential to a classifier. These versions are offset in time relative to the stimulus by a predefined set of values. Alternatively, CBLE may be conceptualized by picturing a classifier being applied on a sliding time window. The time offset producing the largest classifier score is considered to be the difference between the latency of the observed event-related potential and the latency that the classifier was trained on. The variance of target character time offsets measured by this method is termed vCBLE. In Thompson et al. (2012), accuracy (Acc) was shown to depend strongly on vCBLE. Here, we have performed two linear regressions to derive equations for predicted accuracy based on that data set. The result of a simple linear regression is the formula

$$\text{Acc} = 122 - 0.0149 * \text{vCBLE}, \tag{33.16}$$

where Acc is in percentage and vCBLE in milliseconds squared. Note that since the relationship in Equation 33.16 was derived from a simple linear model, it could predict accuracy greater than 100%. If this happens, then the predicted accuracy will be 100% for Acc > 100%. Another alternative formula can be given using a piecewise-linear model

$$\text{Acc} = \begin{cases} 95\%, & \text{vCBLE} < 2440 \\ 95 - 0.0215(\text{vCBLE} - 2440), & \text{otherwise.} \end{cases} \tag{33.17}$$

One advantage of CBLE is that it should work with any classifier; however, the particular relationship between vCBLE and accuracy was found for a least-squares classifier with particular settings. If a different classifier is used, groups are encouraged to investigate the relationship between vCBLE and accuracy using offline analysis of existing databases.

## 33.4 CONTINUOUS BCI

This section will focus on Fitts's law, as the previous section's metrics can be used for any discrete-output BCI—even if an intermediate stage included continuous control.

### 33.4.1 FITTS'S LAW AND INFORMATION THEORY

In 1954, Fitts proposed a performance measurement equation for pointing devices (Douglas et al. 1999; Fitts 1954). Fitts's law gained attention in the field of human–computer interaction (MacKenzie 1992; Newell and Card 1985) and recently in the BCI field to measure the performance of continuous BCIs (Felton et al. 2009; Simeral et al. 2011). The basis of Fitts's law was Shannon's Theorem 17 (Shannon and Weaver 1949), and from the beginning, Fitts attributed information theory and Shannon's theorem as the inspiration of his law. But later on, researchers found demonstrable difference with Shannon's original theory (Soukoreff et al. 2011) and Welford suggested that Fitts's law did not fit properly with empirical data (Welford 1960). To address these problems, researchers suggested several modifications to Fitts's law. The latest model of modified Fitts's law is the Shannon–Welford model (Shoemaker et al. 2012), which has been used recently to measure the performance of continuous BCI (Matlack et al. 2016). In this part, we will discuss and derive the Shannon–Welford model, beginning from Shannon and Fitts results.

#### 33.4.1.1 Shannon's Theory

Shannon's channel capacity theorem (Shannon and Weaver 1949) gives an expression to find the maximum ITR, $C$, through a noisy channel of bandwidth $B$. The formulation is

$$C = B \log_2 \frac{S+N}{N},$$ (33.18)

where $S$ and $N$ are the signal power and noise power, respectively. Now, in the case of BCI, it is not as straightforward as in telecommunications. To measure human performance, Fitts proposed a new term called *index of performance* (IP), which is analogous to channel capacity ($C$) in Shannon's theorem.

#### 33.4.1.2 Fitts's Law

Fitts's law was originally inspired by Shannon's channel capacity theorem but the novelty was to introduce the concept that psychological task difficulty can be measured in terms of ITR. In this case, information transfers through a human channel. Fitts introduced an *index of difficulty* (ID), which is a slightly rearranged version of Shannon's channel capacity equation, and defined the *index of performance* (IP) as the ratio of ID to *movement time* (MT) (Fitts 1954). Fitts used movement distance ($d$) and width of the region within which movement terminates ($w$) to replace the signal power ($S$) and noise power ($N$) in Equation 33.18:

$$\text{IP} = \frac{\text{index of difficulty (ID)}}{\text{movement time (MT)}}$$ (33.19)

$$\text{ID} = \log_2 \left( \frac{2d}{w} \right)$$ (33.20)

$$\text{MT} = \frac{\text{ID}}{\text{IP}}.$$ (33.21)

Now, IP can be computed by regressing MT on ID. This can be written as

$$MT = \theta_0 + \theta_1(ID)$$
$$= \theta_0 + \theta_1 \log_2\left(\frac{2d}{w}\right), \tag{33.22}$$

where $\theta_0$ and $\theta_1$ are the regression coefficients. Fitts's law is a standard technique to measure the performance of pointing tasks, either physical or virtual (Standard 1998). Since the most common application of continuous BCI is cursor movement, Fitts's law has been used considerably in BCI (Flint et al. 2013; Gilja et al. 2012; Kim et al. 2015; LaFleur et al. 2013; Pino et al. 2003).

### 33.4.2 Shannon–Welford Model

While Fitts's law is now the preferred method for measuring pointing task performance, it does not match well with empirical data for low ID. Observing this mismatch, Welford suggested a slight modification of Fitts's law (Welford 1960). Welford's modified Fitts's law is

$$MT = \theta_0 + \theta_1 \log_2\left(\frac{d + 0.5w}{w}\right). \tag{33.23}$$

This equation is more similar to Shannon's original equation (Equation 33.18). However, as signal-to-noise ratio through a human channel is low, Mackenzie suggested keeping Shannon's original formulation (MacKenzie 1989, 1992), which is

$$MT = \theta_0 + \theta_1 \log_2\left(\frac{d + w}{w}\right). \tag{33.24}$$

All of the above mentioned formulations have two degrees of freedom and an additive and a multiplicative constant for both $d$ and $w$. Recently, researchers have suggested another modified version of Fitts's law, which combines Shannon's original formulation and Welford's model (Shoemaker et al. 2012). The purpose of the new formulation is to consider the effect of $d$ and $w$ separately in MT. This new model, called the Shannon–Welford model, has three degrees of freedom:

$$MT = \theta_0 + \theta_{11} \log_2(d + w) - \theta_{12} \log_2(w) \tag{33.25}$$

$$= \theta_0 + \theta_1 \log_2\left(\frac{d + w}{w^k}\right). \tag{33.26}$$

Here, $k = \theta_{11}/\theta_{12}$, and when $k = 1$, this model becomes identical to Shannon's formulation of Fitts's law. However, $k$ can take any value in the range 0.2–1.8 (Shoemaker et al. 2012). Matlack, in a very recent study (Matlack et al. 2016), as well as in his doctoral dissertation (Matlack 2014), reported that the Shannon–Welford model fits well with continuous BCI data and was a significantly better performance measurement model than Fitts's original model. However, the Shannon–Welford model is prone to overfitting if the experimental design does not include a range of $d$ and $w$ values—if fixed target sizes are used, the estimation of $k$ may produce large errors. If a range of values are available, then the Shannon–Welford model is preferable to the original Fitts's formulation.

## 33.5  DISCUSSION

For both discrete and continuous BCIs, it is recommended to use one or more of the abovementioned metrics. In the case of discrete BCI, ITR has been most frequently chosen by researchers. However, the underlying assumptions of ITR are rarely met (Yuan et al. 2013), and it is no longer suggested as a primary reporting metric (Thompson et al. 2014). Whenever ITR is used, alternative candidates should be reported as well; the BCI utility metric is the suggested throughput measure for spellers in particular. In the case of a continuous BCI, Fitts's law has seen the most use, but in some studies (MacKenzie 1989, 1992; Shoemaker et al. 2012), it has been shown that the modified Fitts's law better matches experimental data. This modified Fitts's law, also termed the Shannon–Welford model (Shoemaker et al. 2012), has recently been used in continuous BCI to measure performance of a BCI system (Matlack 2014). Hence, the Shannon–Welford model may become a suitable alternative for Fitts's law to measure performance of continuous BCI. However, using the Shannon–Welford model requires task data from several different target widths, which may present difficulties during offline analysis of previous experiments.

Certainly, performance measure metrics are not limited to only the abovementioned methods. Reporting of these metrics is suggested so that the work is comparable to other studies. Researchers might need to use or introduce other types of performance-measuring metrics for particular tasks. For example, Karl LaFleur et al. tested a BCI system to operate a quadcopter in three-dimensional space under a controlled environment using a series of ring-shaped targets (LaFleur et al. 2013). As a standard of performance-measuring metric, they have reported ITR using MacKenzie's formulation of Fitts's law (Equation 33.24). But additionally, they also have introduced several other performance-measuring metrics for their unconventional system. Task-specific metrics may be often necessary in order to capture and describe the improvement from some BCI design changes, and they can be reported in parallel with more standard metrics that allow for some comparison with other studies. Researchers should consider these aspects carefully, particularly when using a BCI for a nontraditional task.

Finally, the main purpose of performance metrics is to help people understand systems and compare those systems side by side. This chapter provided information about performance measurement metrics for discrete BCIs (ITR, BCI utility, projected accuracy) and continuous BCIs (Fitts's law, Shannon–Welford model) separately. ITR, BCI utility, Fitts's law, and the Shannon–Welford model all provide us performance in terms of *bits/time*. But often, some additional units will help people from other fields to better understand the performance of the system. For example, in spelling BCIs, *characters per minute* or *words per minute* might be more familiar to many people and reporting performance in those units along with ITR and BCI utility will make the performance of the system more understandable.

## REFERENCES

Bianchi, Luigi, Lucia Rita Quitadamo, Girolamo Garreffa, Gian Carlo Cardarilli, and Maria Grazia Marciani. 2007. Performances evaluation and optimization of brain computer interface systems in a copy spelling task. *IEEE Transactions on Neural Systems and Rehabilitation Engineering* 15 (2): 207–216.

Brown, Lawrence D., T. Tony Cai, and Anirban DasGupta. 2001. Interval estimation for a binomial proportion. *Statistical Science* 101–117.

Cohen, Jacob. 1960. A coefficient of agreement for nominal scale. *Educational and Psychological Measurement* 20: 37–46.

Colwell, Kenneth, Chandra Throckmorton, Leslie Collins, and Kenneth Morton. 2014. Projected accuracy metric for the P300 speller. *IEEE Transactions on Neural Systems and Rehabilitation Engineering* 22 (5): 921–925.

Dal Seno, Bernardo, Matteo Matteucci, and Luca T. Mainardi. 2010. The utility metric: A novel method to assess the overall performance of discrete brain–computer interfaces. *IEEE Transactions on Neural Systems and Rehabilitation Engineering* 18 (1): 20–28.

Douglas, Sarah A., Arthur E. Kirkpatrick, and I. Scott MacKenzie. 1999. Testing pointing device performance and user assessment with the ISO 9241, Part 9 Standard. ACM.

Felton, E. A., R. G. Radwin, J. A. Wilson, and J. C. Williams. 2009. Evaluation of a modified Fitts law brain–computer interface target acquisition task in able and motor disabled individuals. *Journal of Neural Engineering* 6 (5): 056002.

Fitts, Paul M. 1954. The information capacity of the human motor system in controlling the amplitude of movement. *Journal of Experimental Psychology* 47 (6): 381.

Flint, Robert D., Zachary A. Wright, Michael R. Scheid, and Marc W. Slutzky. 2013. Long term, stable brain machine interface performance using local field potentials and multiunit spikes. *Journal of Neural Engineering* 10 (5): 056005.

Gilja, Vikash, Paul Nuyujukian, Cindy A. Chestek, John P. Cunningham, M. Yu Byron, Joline M. Fan, Mark M. Churchland, Matthew T. Kaufman, Jonathan C. Kao, and Stephen I. Ryu. 2012. A high-performance neural prosthesis enabled by control algorithm design. *Nature Neuroscience* 15 (12): 1752–1757.

Hill, N. Jeremy, Ann-Katrin Häuser, and Gerwin Schalk. 2014. A general method for assessing brain–computer interface performance and its limitations. *Journal of Neural Engineering* 11 (2): 026018.

Kim, Minho, Byung Hyung Kim, and Sungho Jo. 2015. Quantitative evaluation of a low-cost noninvasive hybrid interface based on EEG and eye movement. *IEEE Transactions on Neural Systems and Rehabilitation Engineering* 23 (2): 159–168.

LaFleur, Karl, Kaitlin Cassady, Alexander Doud, Kaleb Shades, Eitan Rogin, and Bin He. 2013. Quadcopter control in three-dimensional space using a noninvasive motor imagery-based brain–computer interface. *Journal of Neural Engineering* 10 (4): 046003.

MacKenzie, I. Scott. 1992. Fitts' law as a research and design tool in human–computer interaction. *Human–Computer Interaction* 7 (1): 91–139.

MacKenzie, I. Scott. 1989. A note on the information-theoretic basis for Fitts' law. *Journal of Motor Behavior* 21 (3): 323–330.

Matlack, Charles Bruce. 2014. Adaptation for brain–computer interfaces. University of Washington.

Matlack, Charles, Howard Chizeck, and Chet T. Moritz. 2016. Empirical movement models for brain computer interfaces. *IEEE Transactions on Neural Systems and Rehabilitation Engineering.*

Müller-Putz, Gernot, Reinhold Scherer, Clemens Brunner, Robert Leeb, and Gert Pfurtscheller. 2008. Better than random: A closer look on BCI results. *International Journal of Bioelectromagnetism* 10 (EPFL-ARTICLE-164768): 52–55.

Neuper, C., G. R. Müller, A. Kübler, N. Birbaumer, and G. Pfurtscheller. 2003. Clinical application of an EEG-based brain–computer interface: A case study in a patient with severe motor impairment. *Clinical Neurophysiology* 114 (3): 399–409.

Newell, Allen and Stuart K. Card. 1985. The prospects for psychological science in human-computer interaction. *Human–Computer Interaction* 1 (3): 209–242.

Pino, Alexandros, Eleftherios Kalogeros, Elias Salemis, and Georgios Kouroupetroglou. 2003. Brain computer interface cursor measures for motion-impaired and able-bodied users. HCI International 2003: The 10th International Conference on Human–Computer Interaction, Heraklion, Crete, Greece, Vol. 4, pp. 1462–1466.

Ryan, David B., G. E. Frye, G. Townsend, D. R. Berry, S. Mesa-G, Nathan A. Gates, and Eric W. Sellers. 2010. Predictive spelling with a P300-based brain–computer interface: Increasing the rate of communication. *Intl Journal of Human–Computer Interaction* 27 (1): 69–84.

Schlogl, Alois, Julien Kronegg, J. Huggins, and S. Mason. 2007. 19 Evaluation criteria for BCI research. *Toward Brain–Computer Interfacing.*

Shannon, Claude E. and Warren Weaver. 1949. *The Mathematical Theory of Information. Urbana: University of Illinois Press*, pp. 104–107.

Shoemaker, Garth, Takayuki Tsukitani, Yoshifumi Kitamura, and Kellogg S. Booth. 2012. Two-part models capture the impact of gain on pointing performance. *ACM Transactions on Computer–Human Interaction (TOCHI)* 19 (4): 28.

Simeral, J. D., Sung-Phil Kim, M. J. Black, J. P. Donoghue, and L. R. Hochberg. 2011. Neural control of cursor trajectory and click by a human with tetraplegia 1000 days after implant of an intracortical microelectrode array. *Journal of Neural Engineering* 8 (2): 025027.

Soukoreff, R. William, Jian Zhao, and Xiangshi Ren. 2011. *The Entropy of a Rapid Aimed Movement: Fitts' Index of Difficulty Versus Shannon's Entropy.* Springer.

Speier, William, Corey Arnold, Jessica Lu, Ricky K. Taira, and Nader Pouratian. 2011. Natural language processing with dynamic classification improves P300 speller accuracy and bit rate. *Journal of Neural Engineering* 9 (1): 016004.

Standard, I. 1998. Ergonomic requirements for office work with visual display terminals (Vdts)—Part 11: Guidance on Usability. ISO Standard 9241-11: 1998. International Organization for Standardization.

Stehman, Stephen V. 1997. Selecting and interpreting measures of thematic classification accuracy. *Remote Sensing of Environment* 62 (1): 77–89.

Thomas, Eoin, Matthew Dyson, and Maureen Clerc. 2013. An analysis of performance evaluation for motor-imagery based BCI. *Journal of Neural Engineering* 10 (3): 031001.

Thompson, David E., Lucia R. Quitadamo, Luca Mainardi, Shangkai Gao, Pieter-Jan Kindermans, John D. Simeral, Reza Fazel-Rezai, Matteo Matteucci, Tiago H. Falk, and Luigi Bianchi. 2014. Performance measurement for brain–computer or brain–machine interfaces: A tutorial. *Journal of Neural Engineering* 11 (3): 035001.

Thompson, David E., Seth Warschausky, and Jane E. Huggins. 2012. Classifier-based latency estimation: A novel way to estimate and predict BCI accuracy. *Journal of Neural Engineering* 10 (1): 016006.

Welford, Alan Traviss. 1960. The measurement of sensory-motor performance: Survey and reappraisal of twelve years' progress. *Ergonomics* 3 (3): 189–230.

Wolpaw, Jonathan R., Herbert Ramoser, Dennis J. McFarland, and Gert Pfurtscheller. 1998. EEG-based communication: Improved accuracy by response verification. *IEEE Transactions on Rehabilitation Engineering* 6 (3): 326–333.

Yuan, Peng, Xiaorong Gao, Brendan Allison, Yijun Wang, Guangyu Bin, and Shangkai Gao. 2013. A study of the existing problems of estimating the information transfer rate in online brain–computer interfaces. *Journal of Neural Engineering* 10 (2): 026014.

# Part VI

## Emerging Issues and Future BCIs

# 34 Privacy and Ethics in Brain–Computer Interface Research

*Eran Klein and Alan Rubel*

## CONTENTS

34.1 Introduction: Privacy and BCI.................................................................................653
34.2 BCI and Definitions of Privacy...............................................................................654
34.3 Mental Privacy.........................................................................................................656
34.4 BCI and Privacy Opportunity..................................................................................660
34.5 Privacy and BCI Big Data .......................................................................................662
34.6 Conclusion ...............................................................................................................664
References.............................................................................................................................665

**Abstract**

Neural engineers and clinicians are starting to translate advances in electrodes, neural computation, and signal processing into clinically useful devices to allow control of wheelchairs, spellers, prostheses, and other devices. In the process, large amounts of brain data are being generated from research participants, including intracortical, subdural, and extracranial sources. Brain data are a vital resource for brain–computer interface (BCI) research but concerns have been raised about whether the collection and use of these data generate risk to privacy. Further, the nature of BCI research involves understanding and making inferences about device users' mental states, thoughts, and intentions. This, too, raises privacy concerns by providing otherwise unavailable direct or privileged access to individuals' mental lives. And BCI-controlled prostheses may change the way in which clinical care is provided and the type of physical access caregivers have to patients. This, too, has important privacy implications for patients and caregivers. Our goal in this chapter is to examine several of these privacy concerns in light of prominent views of the nature and value of privacy. We argue that increased scrutiny needs to be paid to privacy concerns arising from Big Data and decoding of mental states, but that BCI research may also provide opportunity for individuals to enhance their privacy.

## 34.1 INTRODUCTION: PRIVACY AND BCI

Brain–computer interface (BCI) technology has advanced considerably in the last several decades, presenting substantial opportunities for treatments (Shih et al. 2012; Soekadar et al. 2014). Research in BCI is leading to unprecedented accumulation of brain data, the need to better understand the neural structures and mental states of research participants and patients, and potential changes in how BCI users, caregivers, and researchers interact. Each of these carries important privacy considerations.

BCI can be defined as "a computer-based system that acquires brain signals, analyzes them, and translates them into commands that are relayed to an output device to carry out a desired action" (Shih et al. 2012). And this volume is a testament to the fact that research and implementation of BCI are both promising and growing. But despite the fact that BCI research is advancing steadily, there is still relatively little scholarship dedicated to privacy considerations. Among those who have discussed privacy and BCI (see, e.g., Finn et al. 2013; Jebari 2013), no consensus approach has emerged. More importantly, though, commentary on BCI and privacy tends not to address *why* privacy in the context of BCI is (or is not) morally important. In a chapter devoted to privacy issues in new and emerging technologies, Finn et al. describe a number of facets of privacy that BCI may affect. They "carry the potential to impact upon privacy of the person, privacy of behavior and action, privacy of communication, privacy of data and image and privacy of thoughts and feelings." For example, privacy of behavior and action may be diminished if BCI information is used to predict behaviors or as a means of gaining marketing influence. Finn et al. also suggest that communications privacy may be affected if data are vulnerable to interception. As plausible as such concerns are, there is a further question as to *why* they matter. Part of our task here is to consider not just how privacy may be affected by BCI and BCI research, but what kinds of privacy effects are morally considerable, and why.

There are several potential reasons why privacy in BCI has not been addressed more extensively, each based on some questionable assumptions. First, there may be an implicit assumption on the part of researchers, clinicians, and policy-makers that loss of privacy or heightened risk to privacy is a worthwhile or inevitable trade-off of developing devices with enormous potential health benefits. The promise of a BCI device that would allow someone locked-in to speak or someone who is tetraplegic to reanimate a limb or control a robotic limb is compelling and might seem to make privacy concerns trivial in comparison. Second, more BCI data are collected than is currently interpretable (Finn et al. 2013). Until more is known about what's in BCI data, concerns with privacy can seem premature (Hallinan et al. 2014). Third, implantable and non-implantable BCI research with human research participants takes place within academic institutions that have strict data protection policies and informed consent regulation that requires seeking prior consent or authorization of participants; this may lead some to believe that privacy risks are already in some sense adequately addressed.

Each of these reasons for dismissing or minimizing the importance of privacy considerations rests on questionable assumptions. (1) Recent work exploring the perspectives of end users and potential end users of BCI has shown that much is still unknown about what constitutes acceptable trade-offs in BCI (Blabe et al. 2015; Blain-Moraes et al. 2012; Collinger et al. 2013; Huggins et al. 2011; Lahr et al. 2015). (2) Waiting until better data analysis methods are available before taking privacy concerns seriously may hinder the goal of developing anticipatory guidance for privacy norms and regulations. (3) While policies and practices of informed consent are already in place in BCI research, the extent to which research informed consent achieves meaningful consent has been challenged, and BCI research may need to include atypical risks (like identity, agency, and stigma) that are not a standard part of the informed consent process (Klein 2015).

From here, the paper is organized as follows. We begin, in Section 34.2, by outlining several key conceptions of privacy relevant to BCI. We then turn to key moral considerations with respect to privacy. In Section 34.3, we address issues of mental privacy. In Section 34.4, we consider opportunities that BCI presents for carving out important domains of privacy for users. And in Section 34.5, we consider implications of large amounts of data collected in BCI research. Finally, we conclude by offering some preliminary recommendations for next steps in addressing the kinds of privacy concerns identified.

## 34.2 BCI AND DEFINITIONS OF PRIVACY

There is a substantial literature on privacy across a wide range of scholarly disciplines, and just how to define privacy remains controversial. Nonetheless, a key step in addressing privacy concerns is to clarify the concept of privacy itself. Here, we describe several important facets of privacy that reflect important threads in privacy scholarship. To begin, it is useful to think of privacy as involving three parts: (1) some person who has, or lacks, privacy; (2) some form or domain of privacy;

and (3) some other person or persons who limit the first person's privacy (Blaauw 2013; Matheson 2007; Rubel and Biava 2014). Among the forms of privacy scholars have identified are informational (what others can learn about a person), physical (the degree to which others can physically access one's person), associational (whether others can control the people with whom one associates), and decisional (whether others can limit the range of important decisions one can make for oneself) (Allen 1988; DeCew 1997; Nissenbaum 2010). It is useful for our purposes to focus on three of these forms (see Table 34.1). Note that these forms of privacy do not entail anything about the conditions under which privacy is morally important (or indeed whether it is morally valuable at all). We will address those questions below.

Much privacy discussion centers on informational privacy, or the extent to which others may learn about, access information about, or make inferences regarding a person. Informational privacy is protected in research and clinical care by physician–patient confidentiality, health information privacy laws [such as HIPAA (1996) and GINA (2008) in the United States], general privacy laws [e.g., EU Directive 95/46/EC (1995)], human subject protections in research, and data security laws. Here, it is worth noting that because BCI research often involves international collaboration, it is likely to implicate (inter alia) U.S. sectoral privacy laws and EU general data protection laws.

The extent to which BCI-derived data can be used to generate health or other personal information about a user is only beginning to be understood. For example: Can BCI reveal incidental findings of clinical significance (such as a proclivity to seizures or early tumor) or correlate with disease, such as Alzheimer's disease (Soekadar et al. 2014)? Can neural activity patterns be used to detect attention or motivation, which are critical to the success of BCI training (Curran and Stokes 2003) and also may say something about the underlying personality of the person using the BCI? Already, BCI data are collected alongside and could, in principle, be correlated with actions or circumstances with implications for privacy, such as a desire to use the bathroom, discussions with loved ones, or outbursts of emotion. The extent to which associated BCI data could be used to infer mental states or personality characteristics is uncertain, but raises legitimate concern.

Informational privacy is distinct from (though related to) physical privacy. Physical privacy is the condition of having one's body or personal spaces protected from intrusion by others. Thus, for example, one may desire a degree of physical solitude or to remain free of video surveillance, regardless of whether one is concerned about information gathering. Being subjected to physical examination is an imposition on one's physical privacy, independently of the degree to which new information is gained by the person conducting the examination.

Participation in BCI research involves the loss of some physical privacy. Placement of electro-encephalography (EEG) electrodes onto the skull involves a loss of physical privacy in this regard,

## TABLE 34.1
## Types of Privacy in BCI

| Types of Privacy | Definition | BCI Examples |
|---|---|---|
| Physical | The condition in which others' access to one's person (by sight, sound, touch, and presence) is limited | Ability to attend some activities of daily living with less intensive intervention by others<br>Physical access to skull<br>Being pulled aside in security screening |
| Informational | The condition in which others' ability to learn about one, or to make inferences about one, is limited | Potential for neural recording to expose thoughts, dispositions, and intentions<br>Unknown inferences from troves of data currently stored |
| Decisional | The ability of a person to make important, intimate decisions without excessive influence or control by others | Storage of intimate BCI conversations<br>Being prohibited from entering studies based on exclusion criteria regarding, for example, reproductive decisions |

but the loss of physical privacy is more obviously the case with implantable BCI research where neurosurgeons must temporarily traverse or remove part of the skull in order to place electrodes into, atop, or in proximity to the brain. This is an intrusion, albeit voluntary, of the body and hence involves a loss of physical privacy. Even after surgery, physical privacy remains an issue insofar as an implanted device facilitates easier physical access to a person's body. Participants in the BrainGate trial, for instance, have a pedestal attached to their skull that serves as an access port for attaching a data recording cable during BCI experiments (Hochberg et al. 2012). Facilitated physical access is not just a feature of the laboratory, though, but of the presence of a device and the bodily residuals of having been implanted with it. For instance, individuals with deep brain stimulators are subject to special screening at airports. Being pulled aside from standard metal detectors or other detection devices and showing one's cranial scar or subcutaneous bulge of a battery placed under the chest wall as evidence of a pmed (personal medical electronic device) are forms of physical accessibility to which others are not subject.* Individuals with implantable BCI devices are likely to face similar kinds of physical privacy loss.

Decisional privacy concerns whether others can limit the range of important decisions one can make for oneself. In the United States, decisional privacy is often discussed in the context of access to birth control [*Griswald v. Connecticut*, 381 U.S. 479 (1965)], abortion [*Roe v. Wade*, 410 U.S. 113 (1973)], legal restrictions on same-sex partners [*Lawrence v. Texas*, 539 U.S. 558 (2003)], and "conscience clauses" (whether health care professionals must provide services to which they have moral objections). Some commentators object that decisional privacy is better understood as individual autonomy, but others note that legal limits on birth control, abortion, sexual partners, and actions of conscience require surveillance and information-gathering practices, and are hence deeply entwined with informational and physical privacy (DeCew 2016).

Participation in BCI research can require that volunteers engage in or forego certain activities or make certain decisions. Most obviously, this involves adhering to current medical therapy, such as taking one's medications as prescribed, in order that no additional risks of research participation are incurred. But the kinds of decisions required for research participation can also straddle the medical versus lifestyle divide. For instance, in her autobiography *On My Feet Again*, Jennifer French describes the difficult decision to forego having biological children in order to participate in a trial of an implanted neural device (functional electrical stimulation [FES]) (French 2012).† Establishing similar inclusion criteria in BCI research may be reasonable given lack of pregnancy safety data, but does represent a significant restriction on an important life choice. Of course, what constitutes an important life choice varies by individual. In a recent study of deep brain stimulation (DBS) for depression or obsessive–compulsive disorder (OCD) conducted by one us (Klein), one research participant lamented that he had been told to avoid roller coasters so long as he had an implanted device. It is as yet unclear which life choices individuals with BCI devices will be subject to and whether BCI devices will include technology for monitoring BCI performance that will provide concomitant surveillance data on adherence to restrictions (e.g., accelerometer embedded within a BCI device that identifies a roller coaster versus an automobile ride). Hence, it seems clear that BCI research will implicate questions of informational and decisional privacy.

## 34.3  MENTAL PRIVACY

The prospect of a device capable of reading the contents of minds has long generated popular appeal and philosophical interest (Levy 2007). While far from that imagined in science fiction movies and philosophical thought experiments, BCI shows that it is possible to use thought to control devices. As early as the 1960s, research participants were able to learn to send Morse code by modulating

---

* In the United States, the Transportation Security Administration (TSA) issues notification cards that can be shown to screeners, but this does not exempt individuals from additional screening.
† The FES device was not a BCI, but similar rationale for study exclusion could be applied to BCI research.

alpha oscillations measured by EEG (Dewan 1967). More recent work in BCI demonstrates the possibility of using information gathered from scalp or surgically implanted electrodes to control prostheses, wheelchairs, and computer spellers, among other devices. The ability to decode intentions is currently limited but improving in accuracy, and the range of potential applications is expanding.

Advances in neuroimaging in recent decades helped pave the way for BCI work on decoding brain states. While computed tomography and magnetic resonance imaging have provided increasingly detailed diagnostic information about structural features of the brain, the development of functional magnetic resonance imaging (fMRI) is a critical advance in understanding mental activity. fMRI allows for measurement of brain activity (indirectly through measures of blood flow) during certain mental processes or in conjunction with the experience of certain mental states. This has allowed researchers to determine, for instance, which visual image someone is viewing (even being able to reconstruct the image (Schoenmakers et al. 2013) or what implicit attitudes correlate with moral decision-making (Greene et al. 2001). It has also allowed for measurement of specific intentions (Haynes et al. 2007).

Intentions are of particular interest in BCI insofar as they can be used to control an output device. Measurement electrodes placed on the scalp (EEG), on the cortex (electrocorticography [ECoG]), in the cortex (penetrating cortical electrode arrays), or in deep regions of the brain (deep brain electrodes) can be used to gather data with high temporal resolution on neural processes associated with preparing for, reflecting on, or acting on intentions. How complex intentions or goals are represented in neural networks is an active area of research. The central idea is that pattern-recognition algorithms can be used to decipher what neural activity underlies a particular intention. In other words, BCI can be used to determine what a person is thinking (or planning) at a given moment.

BCI offers the prospect of accessing other minds, in some sense, *directly*. We typically ascribe mental states—perceptions, beliefs, memories, attitudes, emotions—based on what can be observed, such as what people tell us they are thinking and what we observe in their body language or behavior. And we make further ascriptions of personality traits or characteristics such as sociability, honesty, procrastination, suspicion of authority, and so on. But the prospect of decoding mental states opens a new window on mental life. The animating, even if unduly simplistic, metaphor is that the development of radiographs let us look past the skin to the bones and tissues beneath, and now advances in BCI will allow us to peer not just into the brain, but into the mental life buzzing within it (or less colloquially, "supervening upon it").

The prospect of decoding intentions raises concerns about informational privacy. Some of these informational privacy concerns resonate with broader concerns about "mental privacy" arising from work in neuroimaging (Farah and Wolpe 2004; Ryberg 2016).* There are related terms for this, including "neural privacy," "brain privacy," "cognitive privacy," "thought privacy," and "cognitive liberty" (Illes and Racine 2005; Räikkä 2010; Schneider et al. 2012; Trimper et al. 2014). Richmond distinguishes between two uses of "mental privacy" in the literature—an older, philosophical sense in which "mental states are (descriptively) private, accessed by the subject in a distinctive first-personal way" and one more involved with civil rights debates concerned with "invasions of the (normatively) private area of the mind" (Richmond 2012, p. 186, n. 2). It is this latter use, often underwritten by a folk psychological notion that the mind contains inner monologues, judgments, eidetic memories capable of being exposed for all to see, that has been taken up in debates about wholesale mind reading or brainotyping of personality (Illes and Racine 2005). Two examples of debates related to the "invasion" sense of mental privacy are lie detection (which is a matter of informational privacy) and neuromarketing (which involves use of information to influence individuals' decision-making, and hence affects decisional privacy).

---

* It should be noted that, at present, the ability to discern mental states using fMRI is significantly more advanced than that of BCI. It is too early to say whether this difference in capabilities is a contingent or inherent feature of these two technologies. Regardless, the use of fMRI to infer mental states provides an instructive example for thinking through considerations of privacy in BCI research.

Advances in neuroscience will have effects on the law.* One area that has attracted significant attention is the use of neuroimaging and neural recording to assist or replace testimony (Wolpe et al. 2005). Memory and eye witness testimony are fallible forms of forensic evidence subject to numerous kinds of psychological biases and errors (for substantial review, see Lacy and Stark 2013). Direct neural recording through EEG (or implantable electrodes if available) may provide an alternative source of forensic information. For instance, if neural patterns are discovered that correlate with deception or feeling of guilt or recognition of people, places, or events, these patterns could be introduced as evidence. There has been significant legal and ethical resistance to using neuroscience in this way (Greely and Illes 2007). Even if not admissible in court, correlations between neural data and mental states could be used in military or anti-terrorism contexts (Finn et al. 2013; Tennison and Moreno 2012), employee surveillance (Jebari 2013), or social interactions (e.g., verifying veracity of personal information posted on a dating site).

The application of neuroscience to improve products and advertising has been termed neuromarketing (Ariely and Berns 2010). Neural recording could be used in various ways to gather data of value to companies (Jebari 2013). Data gathered on reward-processing regions of the brain (such as the nucleus accumbens) are used to fine-tune advertising to particular individuals or groups of individuals (Haynes 2012). Neural data also could be gathered early in the design process to make products that better fit user needs. Further, the commercialization of devices capable of measuring neural data (e.g., portable EEGs), such as for gaming or wellness, may create a wide conduit for collection of neural data by companies. At present, neuromarketing represents a relatively unregulated commercial area. As techniques for measuring and finding patterns in neural activity continue to improve, legitimate concerns will be raised about whether neuromarketing technologies are akin to acceptable forms of persuasion or whether they constitute a kind of manipulation or hijacking of the subconscious.

These kinds of privacy concerns do not seem particularly relevant to the current state of BCI decoding of intentions. This is for two reasons. The first is that decoding of intentions is largely a *willed* process in which participants engage in arduous training to learn to isolate and execute an intention for a given task (e.g., to move a cursor, activate a prosthetic). This process can take weeks (or longer) to have a desired effect on the world (e.g., to control a prosthetic, computer screen, stimulation levels of implanted electrodes, etc.). Second, this process is *voluntary* and done with the consent of the participant. As Owen (2012) notes with regard to fMRI, "[L]ike raising an arm in response to the instruction to do so, activating the brain by, say, imagining playing tennis, is a voluntary response, which can be suppressed at will....[and thus] poses no more of an ethical issue than observing that same participant outside the scanner and asking them to raise their left arm when told to do so" (Owen 2012, pp. 84–85). A BCI motor intention task might be viewed similarly. If we confine ourselves to voluntary and deliberate decoding of intentions in a research setting—and not to talk of brain translating machines (Edwards 2012)—are there still privacy concerns?

Privacy concerns can still arise in the context of voluntary participation in BCI research if *additional* information about brain function can be gathered alongside the conduct of the primary experiment. For instance, BCI can be used to covertly monitor other cognitive processes while a research participant is engaged in BCI research task (Zander and Jatzev 2009). Participants may be wholly unaware of this additional monitoring and may even deny that they are engaging in the cognitive activity being monitored at all (e.g., subconsciously attending to some background feature of the environment). Further, passive BCI monitoring can be combined with interventions to modulate or manipulate cognitive states. For instance, a BCI has been used to measure affective states (e.g., happiness, tranquility) and select music via algorithm that modulates these affective states (Daly et al. 2016).

Even if we confine ourselves to the decoding of motor intentions, different kinds of privacy concerns are relevant. The first might be what we call a *voyeuristic* concern. This is the concern that someone might peer into a private realm (one's private intentions) without invitation (an intrusion upon

---

* See, for example, http://www.lawneuro.org/, accessed October 30, 2016.

informational privacy) and the individual might feel violated. There are protections against this in the context of research. The second we might call a *maliciousness* concern. Here, the concern is that knowing someone's intention could allow external actors to pry the lid off one's mental life, so to speak, and muck around with vicious intent, implicating a person's decisional privacy. Again, research protections are in place to prevent this. But there is another kind of concern here, what might be called a *collateral information* concern. The idea with the collateral concern is that additional information collected alongside targeted neural data has relevance to privacy (Haynes and Rees 2006). This is our focus here.

An obvious kind of collateral information from BCI studies of intention is incidental diagnostic findings. Electrode recording may turn up patterns of activity that indicate pathology. Consider two examples. First, changes in delta, theta, and beta band frequencies have been associated with Alzheimer's dementia (Soekadar et al. 2014). Further, EEG in BCI studies could identify people with lower thresholds for future seizures. Second, neuroimaging needed to localize brain regions for electrode placement can identify brain pathology (e.g., tumor). Some of the ethical challenges of neuroimaging incidental findings in research are well recognized (Edwards 2012). As the BCI field develops, there will be more opportunity to correlate electrophysiologic data with signs and symptoms of clinical significance. As of now, this is rare but perhaps suggests that there should be mechanisms put in place in the future to collect this information.

An important and underappreciated privacy risk of collateral information is the effect on identity and sense of self. Take the example of someone in the BrainGate trial conjuring up a motor intention ("I will try to move my right hand NOW"). Imagine what other information might be gathered in the process of learning to decode the relevant intention. Perhaps information about one's concentration or level of interest in a task might become evident (Curran and Stokes 2003). Perhaps a neural pattern portending an inability to master a BCI task (sometimes inaccurately called "BCI illiteracy") could become apparent (Blankertz et al. 2010). Could this lead to stigmatization or demoralization? Or maybe there is a neural signature when someone (e.g., a particular research assistant) walks in the room and this is found to correlate with BCI performance. Could this "extra fact" be used to motivate (or manipulate) research participants or allow research teams to infer something about an individual's attitude toward race, attractiveness, or authority?

One can get a sense of the challenge here by thinking about the close connection between intention and action. Imagine a BCI device capable of decoding intentions for operating an electronic wheelchair ("go left," "speed up," "avoid hitting the pedestrian," "stop"). It is important not just that intentions be accurately decoded and implemented, but that there be "checks" on putting intentions into action. For instance, if my nemesis walks into a room, I would not want my pre-reflective intention "I really want to run over his foot" to immediately be an operative command for the wheelchair. Even if able to override the intention with another, the fact that the wheelchair moves in his direction *says something about me* ("I'm hotheaded," "not as collegial as I purport to be," or worse).

This challenge is made even more evident by decoding intentions related to communication. Though one might want a BCI for communication to be fast to facilitate fluid conversation, there is a risk of all intentions getting through, for instance, "I never intend to see you again!" The risk of not filtering or a failure to adequately filter actionable intentions is profound. Telling a stranger this may be very different compared to telling one's life partner, who might reasonably think: "I never thought you would be the kind of person who would say such a thing." Neurotechnologies, like BCI, make us "answerable" for a wider range of our mental life (Richmond 2012). We are responsible not only for what we verbalize or our body language but also for what can be decoded. Part of this may be addressed by developing BCI error detection mechanisms, but the challenge is not merely technical. What counts as an actionable intention, in part, depends on who I take myself to be and how I project myself into the future. This will be particularly hard to incorporate into a decision algorithm.*

---

* Note that this is a case that blurs the distinction between informational and decisional privacy. There is information conveyed about persons' decision procedures, but at root the issue is about what kinds of intentions suffice to render something a decision to act.

It is also important to recognize that device output controlled by intentions can magnify the identity concern. DBS has been investigated as a potential treatment of medication-refractory depression and OCD. BCI control is being investigated as a way to modulate DBS to meet clinical need. For instance, an individual could increase stimulation when feeling depressed by forming a particular intention. There are potential benefits to such control, including battery conservation and enhanced patient sense of agency. Higher levels of DBS stimulation in particular brain regions have known side effects, however, including hypomania, which can lead to gambling, hypersexuality, and overspending. An individual who has control of DBS stimulation levels is likely be to viewed as responsible in part for these effects. What might before have been viewed as unfortunate side effects of DBS may come instead to be viewed as the outcome of choice: "You must be the kind of person who wants to engage in such behavior." This implicates decisional privacy in that others may view one as accountable for DBS stimulation levels and hence responsible for underlying side effects, which puts constraints (viz., disapproval) on their ability to undergo DBS in the first place.

## 34.4 BCI AND PRIVACY OPPORTUNITY

A different way of understanding the privacy implications of BCI is as a kind of *opportunity for* privacy. Much of the literature addressing privacy in the context of clinical research, clinical care, commercial transactions, employment, law enforcement, security, and so forth addresses ways in which individuals' privacy may be diminished and the conditions under which such privacy loss is morally, legally, or socially problematic. Under this "loss model," individuals have privacy (to some degree) and others may infringe that privacy to the individuals' detriment. There are a couple of ways, however, in which the loss model is inadequate, and this has implications for BCI.

First, the loss model implies that privacy always has a positive moral value, and hence that any loss of privacy demands a justification. Compare this with other moral goods, such as freedom of expression or freedom of conscience. Any instance in which a person's ability to express herself freely or in which her ability to exercise matters of conscience is limited is prima facie bad and demands some kind of reason. That is not to say that such limitations are unjustified—far from it. Rather, it just means that the limitations require *some* kind of justification. For example, limitations of free expression may be justifiable to prevent harm or fraud. Privacy, though, is not like that. Given the definition we offer above, once we determine that some person's privacy is diminished, there is a further question as to whether that diminution is negative at all. Thus, when a person walks down a grocery store aisle, his privacy regarding his food choices are diminished with respect to others in the store. But there is no sense in which this simple fact presents a moral problem or demands a justification.

To understand why this is important in the context of BCI, it is useful to consider Ruth Gavison's seminal article examining the concept and value of privacy. Similar to our approach in this paper, Gavison's view is that "privacy is a limitation of others' access to an individual" (Gavison 1980, p. 428). Perfect privacy, then, is a condition in which one "is completely inaccessible to others… no one has any information about X, no one pays any attention to X, and no one has physical access to X" (Gavison 1980, p. 428). On this view, Gavison notes, having *too much* privacy is undesirable, and indeed people "may resent privacy that is imposed on them against their will" (Gavison 1980, p. 428, n. 24).

Now consider locked-in syndrome (LIS), a rare neurological disorder, often caused by a vascular or traumatic brain stem injury or by late-stage amyotrophic lateral sclerosis (ALS or "Lou Gehrig's disease") (Walter 2010). Patients with LIS have voluntary motor paralysis and are hence unable to communicate by speaking or movement, though unless they have complete LIS they are usually able to move their eyes and eyelids (Walter 2010, p. 62).* Despite physical paralysis, people with LIS typically retain consciousness, self- and environmental awareness, and cognitive function.

---

* LIS may be classified by severity, ranging from total immobility (including eye and eyelid movement), classic LIS (quadriplegia, anarthria, eye movement), and incomplete LIS (some degree of voluntary movement beyond eyes and eyelids) (Walter 2010).

The experience of LIS is recounted in Jean Dominique Bauby's book *The Diving Bell and Butterfly*, the content of which Bauby conveyed to a transcriber by blinking a code for letters of the alphabet (Bauby 1998). The book conveys Bauby's frustrations with being unable to share both his most basic needs and desires (e.g., physical comfort) and his more complex and nuanced thoughts. Until he can actually communicate (via blinking, a code, and a skilled transcriber), his mental states are "completely inaccessible to others… no one has any information about [his thoughts], [and] no one pays any attention to" his thoughts. He has, in other words, almost perfect informational and physical privacy regarding his conscious life, with respect to *all* others. And this is profoundly alienating. Denise Dudzinski explains that Bauby realizes that he "can be apprehended by others as an object in their world to be ignored or to be noticed," and that this affects Bauby's understanding of himself and his identity (Dudzinski 2001, p. 37).

Recent work in BCI has demonstrated that a patient with LIS following a brainstem stroke could communicate successfully using an EEG BCI (Sellers et al. 2010), and this has generated optimism for further work on the basis of "the tremendous potential of non-invasive BCIs to cope with the unbearable condition of complete isolation from the social environment" (Chaudhary and Birbaumer 2015). Further, studies with communication devices controlled by implantable electrodes are underway.* The benefits of such advances are undeniable; our point here is that the benefit is constituted in substantial part by *decreasing* privacy.

A second way in which BCI presents a privacy opportunity focuses on relational aspects of privacy. In Section 34.2, we explain that it is useful to think of privacy as a three-part relation between some person, some domain, and some other person or persons with respect to whom the first person has privacy. Specifying particular privacy relationships is key to understanding one of privacy's main values—its effects on personal relationships. In an early article outlining moral foundations for privacy claims, James Rachels argues that privacy is vital in fostering many and varied social relationships. Thus, one might wish to have substantial privacy regarding one's family life with respect to one's work colleagues so as to maintain a professional distance, and one defining feature of intimate relationships is that they involve sharing important things (which privacy facilitates) (Rachels 1975). Indeed, what one shares (information, access to one's person) is a defining feature of different kinds of relationships.

Now consider patients with severe spinal cord injuries (SCIs). Dreer et al. (2007) explain that because life expectancy of people with SCIs has been significantly extended due in part to improvements in medical technology, "family members often become the primary sources of assistance for various activities of daily living, such as feeding, dressing, transfers, and bowel and bladder care" (Dreer et al. 2007, p. 2). In Collinger et al.'s study of attitudes toward BCI in persons with SCI, nearly 20% of participants with tetraplegia and over 30% of those with paraplegia received unpaid assistance with self-care activities or mobility by family members or others (Collinger et al. 2013). More generally, there is substantial evidence that many family members taking on caregiving roles encounter a range of difficulties: emotional, psychological, physical, and financial. Providing care, of course, may have positive effects as well, such as fostering deeper, more meaningful relationships with loved ones, and evidence shows that in many cases patients and caregivers value the way care provision functions in their relationship (Donelan et al. 2002). This range of experience within caregiving has led some to propose increased support and training for family caregivers to allow caregiving to be both less difficult and more rewarding (Donelan et al. 2002).

BCI-controlled devices, like neuroprosthetics in SCI, will have significant effects on caregiving. Though the scope of such effects may vary by condition and device, current effects of BCI research on family and caregivers are instructive. For example, wearable EEG-based BCI devices can require extensive involvement of caregivers in daily setup, calibration, and removal (Mak and Wolpaw 2009). In one study of patients with ALS and their caregivers, the time and effort of caregivers in BCI setup was a significant concern (Blain-Moraes et al. 2012). Implantable BCI devices

---

* See, for example, http://neuroprosthesis.edu; Hochberg NIH#5R01DC009899-05.

would substantially reduce BCI setup demands and thereby offer greater independence. This may explain interest in implantable devices found in studies of persons with SCI and ALS (Collinger et al. 2013; Huggins et al. 2011). Blain-Mores et al. (2012) quote one person with ALS as saying "If it made it easier on the caretaker, I'd go with the implant" (Blain-Moraes et al. 2012, p. 520). Caregivers also recognize that BCI-controlled devices, by affording their loved ones a greater ability to manage their own activities of daily living, could reduce caregiving demands. "It can alleviate concerns that you have, it could give you, the caregiver, more time to maybe take care of things that you need done" (Blain-Moraes et al. 2012, p. 521). BCI-controlled devices need not yield functional independence or completely obviate the need for care provision in order to have benefits for both users and caregivers. BCI-controlled devices may allow patients and their families to structure caregiving in a way that decreases the intensity of the need, allowing for a patient to have greater physical privacy in some areas of their life (e.g., eating or toileting), and thus diminish the stress upon family caregivers. Moreover, that greater opportunity for physical privacy may allow patients and family caregivers to better appreciate the aspects of caregiving that they already value, and hence to better foster the relationship overall. In other words, to the extent that BCI-controlled devices increase a patient's physical privacy regarding some aspects of daily living, they may help support other values—caregiver well-being and flourishing relationships.

## 34.5  PRIVACY AND BCI BIG DATA

Neural data sets from BCI research, particularly EEG or intracortical single- or multi-neuron recordings, constitute a kind of "big data." Big data can refer to both the complexity of analyzing large quantities of data and to large data sets themselves (Mittelstadt and Floridi 2016). BCI data sets can be "big" in both procedural and quantitative terms, with single research participant studies generating uncompressed data in gigabyte or terabyte quantities, and the capacity to dramatically increase quantity and complexity by adding electrodes or recording channels. Similar to other kinds of "big data" in neuroscience, such as neuroimaging, neurogenetics, and behavioral data, BCI data hold promise for improving diagnosis, treatment, and prevention of disease, but present challenges of collection, storage, analysis, and transmission. Informational privacy is a central challenge to the rapid accretion of BCI data.

The next big advances in neuroscience will come from integration (across measuring technologies, laboratories, neuroscientific subdisciplines, target problems, data analysis techniques), and this integration "will require a cultural shift in the way that data are shared across labs" (Sejnowski et al. 2014). While there are countervailing pressures to data sharing in neuroscience—such as a lack of uniform attitudes toward data sharing across subdisciplines (Van Horn and Ball 2008) or unsettled publishing and data ownership norms (Poldrack and Poline 2015)—neuroscientific data sharing in general maximizes the contribution of research participants, generates new scientific questions, enhances reproducibility, improves research practices, provides a test bed for new analysis methods, reduces the cost of doing science, and protects valuable scientific resources (Poldrack and Gorgolewski 2014).

Several forces push in the direction of data sharing in BCI research. For instance, data from implantable BCI can be expensive to generate because of costs associated with building an implantable device as well as costs associated with developing surgical implantation and other kinds of related expertise. Implantable human BCI research has tended to be confined to a small number of academic centers. In addition, the cohorts within dedicated implantable BCI studies can be small, involving only several research participants at a time or can piggyback on coincident clinical procedures (e.g., temporary placement of implanted electrodes for presurgical epilepsy localization; Blakely et al. 2014).

BCI data can be shared in different ways, which raise different kinds of privacy concerns. First, BCI data can be shared informally between laboratories or through formal laboratory data-sharing agreements. Sharing of raw neural data between BCI laboratories can spur development and facilitate reproducibility of new analytic methods, lead to further collaborations, and reduce financial and ethical costs of redundancy within a small field. Sharing of deidentified neural data sets can raise security concerns if not encrypted or procedures are not in place to prevent reassociation with identity-compromising data (e.g., MRI images used for lead placement if not scrubbed by de-facing software). Second, BCI data can be shared through large data repositories. Repositories aggregate data sets explicitly for research purposes to allow for complex forms of data linking and mining. Neuroimaging repositories provide an example of this (Ozyurt et al. 2010) as does the Human Connectome Project. Of particular relevance to BCI, efforts have been made to collect EEGs and make these available to researchers (https://www.nedcdata.org/drupal/). Privacy concerns raised about data repositories more generally (Poldrack and Gorgolewski 2014; Sorani et al. 2015) will arise with BCI as well. Third, BCI data can be shared through new forms of scientific practice, such as crowd sourcing or coding contests using donated BCI data (for instance, the "Decoding Brain Signals" contest sponsored by Microsoft).* Particularly challenging questions about ownership of data (and corresponding analytic methods) can be raised by novel forms of scientific activity. Who owns the data and the analytic methods in this context—the researcher ("contestant"), laboratory, institution, research participant, sponsor?

BCI big data raise privacy concerns related to deidentification. Research regulations require the stripping of identifiers from BCI data. There are questions about the technical adequacy of deidentification, particularly when one form of data (e.g., BCI neural data) can be combined with other data—genetic or microbiomic sequencing data, biological specimens, electronic medical records, administrative hospital data, or other forms of neural data (e.g., MRI for localizing lead placement). A more specific concern in BCI research is risk of reidentification of research participants because of the small size of BCI research studies and media publicity that such studies attract (Neergaard 2016; Pelley 2012). Publications that list research participant gender, age, or type of medical condition (e.g., SCI versus ALS) add to this risk of reidentification.

The concern about identification or reidentification of research participants has less to do with what can currently be inferred from BCI data and more to do with the potential that these data may hold. At present, what can be inferred from a neural data set of voltage spikes of a single implanted electrode, for instance, is very narrow (e.g., intending a specific body movement at time $T$). A log of blood pressure and heart rate readings allows for more inference at present (Undergoing a stress response? Have a pacemaker? Taking a beta blocker antihypertensive? Autonomic dysfunction from a disease like diabetes or Parkinson's disease?), but even here, a log of deidentified readings contains little in the way of private information about personality or behavior. For instance, one cannot infer from such a log absent other information whether your blood pressure goes up when you see your spouse or a member of a different race. BCI data stripped of identifiers and context might seem to be as innocuous as a deidentified blood pressure log.

But there are important differences. The first is that we don't know how much one *could* possibly infer from a log of neural data given advances in decoding algorithms. We have a pretty good sense of the range of possible inferences from deidentified and decontextualized cardiac data; the same cannot be said of brain data. There may be a lot more *in there* to be decoded. At present, we just don't know. And, what could be in there are patterns that are revelatory of important—and private—aspects of the self. Hence, maybe BCI data could be decoded not only to indicate a stress response (as a cardiac log might) but also to associate it with some emotion or personality characteristic (e.g., shame, animus, jealousy, and sexual desire). These kinds of personality and behavioral inferences would have significant implications for privacy. BCI may also contain more fine-grained information. For instance, given a data set from a BCI speller, it might be possible to decode what an individual was saying by reverse engineering the linguistic content from the data. Decoding that a research participant thought "left" or "thirsty" or "bored" might be uninteresting, but thoughts of the sort "I (no longer) love my husband" or "This is boring... and my life is empty" might reveal

---

* See https://gallery.cortanaintelligence.com/Competition/e9d67f7668e048328b8bb3a4a81fa5e7. Accessed November 1, 2016.

thoughts that are certainly of a private character. Thus, the *potential* of BCI data matters for privacy. BCI data are stored not only because they are valuable *now*, but because they are of uncertain, yet potentially large, value in the future. But it is this potential value that also carries with it potential privacy risks.

Now, these privacy concerns reflect some of the issues that we have outlined in previous sections. One of the key issues in the large-scale collection of BCI data is that the repercussions (if any) would be years in the future, yet decisions about collection will be made in the present. And those future privacy issues cannot effectively be addressed by current research informed consent regimes. In a literature review of ethical concerns in biomedical big data, Mittelstadt and Floridi (2016) outline several key concerns about informed consent to collection, analysis, and use of big data that are applicable to BCI. One is that the notion of consent as an ability to control personal information is based on an assumption that people can reasonably infer what data will reveal. But of course, even researchers don't know this, and hence any research participant's conjectures are at least as limited. Likewise, the idea behind collecting and storing large volumes of BCI data is the potential to develop algorithms to find unforeseen connections; this, too, makes meaningful, explicit consent implausible (Choudhury et al. 2014).

One might argue that *broad* consent—to collect and use data for any purpose—is possible (Mittelstadt and Floridi 2016, citing Clayton 2005; Ioannidis 2013). That, however, may conflict with the paradigm that informed consent be based on individual, autonomous decisions. Refinements to broad consent, such as tiered consent—letting research participants select among options for how data will be used—or opt-out consent—presuming broad consent unless subjects explicitly designate unacceptable uses for data—may be of limited value. For instance, the boundaries between different areas of and uses for BCI may be too porous to support tiers or specific opt-outs in practice, for example, to help people with SCI reanimate a limb but not to contribute to BCI control of exoskeletons for potential military uses. More generally, current consent paradigms consider potential ramifications for the individual while ignoring how such research may affect groups to which individuals are a part. Thus, if BCI currently targets certain populations (e.g., SCI, ALS)—which it does—then this research may have effects on the group (e.g., discrimination, stigmatization) that are not considered as part of the consent process. It needs to be noted that many of the challenges for informed consent described here are not unique to BCI. The important point to recognize is that while informed consent processes in BCI are important and valuable, they do not provide ready solutions to problems of privacy in BCI research. More work will need to be done.

## 34.6  CONCLUSION

Summing up, we can see a number of ways in which privacy is important in BCI. BCI implicates physical, informational, and decisional privacy. More importantly, BCI raises a number of morally significant privacy issues, including mental or cognitive privacy, potential for privacy opportunity, and unknown, downriver effects of large-scale collection, analysis, and use of BCI research data, the effects of which neither researchers nor research participants can discern now.

Our focus here has been on exploring and delineating privacy issues raised by BCI research and their ethical implications. Getting clear on what privacy means in BCI research and ways in which it is (or is not) valuable is an important step in the development of strategies for addressing privacy concerns. There are models for this further step of developing privacy policies and practices from which the BCI community can benefit. For instance, the NIH Genomic Data Sharing Policy provides an example of how to address data privacy concerns through the granting process (National Institutes of Health 2014). In addition, the INCF Task Force on Neuroimaging Datasharing provides an example of how an emerging neuroscientific field (i.e., neuroimaging) can develop and articulate privacy and data sharing standards (Poline et al. 2012). And the Genetic Information Nondiscrimination Act (GINA 2008) in the United States is an example of a legal and regulatory framework for protecting privacy related to genetic information. Even with such models, more work will need to be done to develop privacy policies tailored to the particular features of BCI research data and practice.

But we have had to put aside several important debates. One is that different modes of brain data collection (ECoG, EEG, and intracortical electrodes) currently yield brain data of different quality, quantity, cost, and reproducibility. While these differences may have privacy implications, it is difficult to anticipate how developments in technology will affect these and, as such, for simplicity we have considered these together as a source of BCI data. Another is the philosophical question of whether decoding neural activity to infer mental states is conceptually coherent or misguided. There is a rich debate in the philosophy of mind about the relation between neural activity and mental states, such as that about the theory of extended mind, which also has implications for BCI (Heersmink 2013). While the extension of one's mind out into a neuroprosthetic, for instance, may have implications for privacy (is confiscating a prosthetic an invasion of physical privacy?), we think that such questions can be tabled for now. Last, BCI raises concern not only about privacy but also about *security* (or "neurosecurity") and hacking of data and devices (Bonaci et al. 2014; Denning et al. 2009; Ienca and Haselager 2016). That is clearly an important and far-reaching issue; we have focused on privacy here because security is important either for reasons that are independent of privacy (e.g., harms to patients or compromise of devices) or *because of* the importance of privacy. We take security to be significant in part because of the importance of privacy, and we assume that to the extent that privacy is valuable, security is all the more important.

## REFERENCES

Allen, Anita L. 1988. *Uneasy Access: Privacy for Women in a Free Society.* Totowa, N.J.: Rowman & Littlefield.

Ariely, Dan, and Gregory S. Berns. 2010. Neuromarketing: The hope and hype of neuroimaging in business. *Nat Rev Neurosci* 11 (4): 284–292.

Bauby, Jean-Dominique. 1998. *The Diving Bell and the Butterfly: A Memoir of Life in Death.* Vintage Books.

Blaauw, Martijn. 2013. The epistemic account of privacy. *Episteme* 10 (Special Issue 02): 167–177. doi:10.1017/epi.2013.12.

Blabe, Christine H., Vikash Gilja, Cindy A. Chestek, Krishna V. Shenoy, Kim D. Anderson, and Jaimie M. Henderson. 2015. Assessment of brain–machine interfaces from the perspective of people with paralysis. *J Neural Eng* 12 (4): 043002. doi:10.1088/1741-2560/12/4/043002.

Blain-Moraes, Stefanie, Riley Schaff, Kirsten L. Gruis, Jane E. Huggins, and Patricia A. Wren. 2012. Barriers to and mediators of brain–computer interface user acceptance: Focus group findings. *Ergonomics* 55 (5): 516–525.

Blakely, Tim M., Jared D. Olson, Kai J. Miller, Rajesh P.N. Rao, and Jeffrey G. Ojemann. 2014. Neural correlates of learning in an electrocorticographic motor-imagery brain–computer interface. *Brain–Comput Interf* 1 (3–4): 147–157.

Blankertz, Benjamin, Claudia Sannelli, Sebastian Halder, Eva M. Hammer, Andrea Kübler, Klaus-Robert Müller, Gabriel Curio, and Thorsten Dickhaus. 2010. Neurophysiological predictor of SMR-based BCI performance. *NeuroImage* 51 (4): 1303–1309. doi:10.1016/j.neuroimage.2010.03.022.

Bonaci, Tamara, Ryan Calo, and Howard J. Chizeck. 2014. App stores for the brain: Privacy & security in brain–computer interfaces. In *Ethics in Science, Technology and Engineering, 2014 IEEE International Symposium on*, 1–7. IEEE. http://ieeexplore.ieee.org/xpls/abs_all.jsp?arnumber=6893415.

Chaudhary, Ujwal, and Niels Birbaumer. 2015. Communication in locked-in state after brainstem stroke: A brain–computer-interface approach. *Ann Translat Med* 3 (Suppl 1). http://www.ncbi.nlm.nih.gov/pmc/articles/PMC4437925/.

Choudhury, Suparna, Jennifer R. Fishman, Michelle L. McGowan, and Eric T. Juengst. 2014. Big data, open science and the brain: Lessons learned from genomics. *Front Hum Neurosci* 8. doi:10.3389/fnhum.2014.00239.

Clayton, Ellen Wright. 2005. Informed consent and biobanks. *Law Med Ethics* 33 (1): 15–21. doi:10.1111/j.1748-720X.2005.tb00206.x.

Collinger, Jennifer L., Michael L. Boninger, Tim M. Bruns, Kenneth Curley, Wei Wang, and Douglas J. Weber. 2013. Functional priorities, assistive technology, and brain–computer interfaces after spinal cord injury. *J Rehabil Res Dev* 50 (2): 145.

Curran, Eleanor A., and Maria J. Stokes. 2003. Learning to control brain activity: A review of the production and control of EEG components for driving brain–computer interface (BCI) systems. *Brain Cogn* 51 (3): 326–336.

Daly, Ian, Duncan Williams, Alexis Kirke, James Weaver, Asad Malik, Faustina Hwang, Eduardo Miranda, and Slawomir J. Nasuto. 2016. Affective brain–computer music interfacing. *J Neural Eng* 13 (4): 046022. doi:10.1088/1741-2560/13/4/046022.

DeCew, Judith. 1997. *In Pursuit of Privacy: Law, Ethics, and the Rise of Technology*. Ithaca, N.Y.: Cornell University Press.

DeCew, Judith. 2016. Connecting tort, fourth amendment, and constitutional privacy. In *Privacy, Security, and Accountability*, edited by Moore, Adam D, 73–88. New Jersey: Rowman & Littlefield.

Denning, Tamara, Yoky Matsuoka, and Tadayoshi Kohno. 2009. Neurosecurity: Security and privacy for neural devices. *Neurosurg Focus* 27 (1): E7.

Dewan, Edmond M. 1967. Occipital alpha rhythm eye position and lens accommodation. *Nature* 214: 975–977.

Donelan, Karen, Craig A. Hill, Catherine Hoffman, Kimberly Scoles, Penny Hollander Feldman, Carol Levine, and David Gould. 2002. Challenged to care: Informal caregivers in a changing health system. *Health Affairs* 21 (4): 222–231. doi:10.1377/hlthaff.21.4.222.

Dreer, Laura E., Timothy R. Elliott, Richard Shewchuk, Jack W. Berry, and Patricia Rivera. 2007. Family caregivers of persons with spinal cord injury: Predicting caregivers at risk for probable depression. *Rehabil Psychol* 52 (3): 351. doi:10.1037/0090-5550.52.3.351.

Dudzinski, Denise. 2001. The diving bell meets the butterfly: Identity lost and remembered. *Theoret Med Bioethics* 22 (1): 33–46. doi:10.1023/A:1009981213630.

Edwards, Sarah J.L. 2012. Protecting privacy interests in brain images: The limits of consent. In *I Know What You're Thinking: Brain Imaging and Mental Privacy*, edited by Sarah Richmond, Sarah J.L. Rees, and Sarah J.L. Edwards, 245–260. Oxford: Oxford University Press.

European Union. 1995. Council Directive 95/46, on the Protection of Individuals with Regard to the Processing Personal Data and on the Free Movement of Such Data, 1995 O.J. (L281) 31 (EU).

Farah, Martha J., and Paul R. Wolpe. 2004. Monitoring and manipulating brain function: New neuroscience technologies and their ethical implications. *Hastings Cent Rep* 34: 34–45.

Finn, Rachel L., David Wright, and Michael Friedewald. 2013. Seven types of privacy. In *European Data Protection: Coming of Age*, 3–32. Springer. http://link.springer.com/chapter/10.1007/978-94-007-5170-5_1.

French, Jennifer. 2012. *On My Feet Again: My Journey out of the Wheelchair Using Neurotechnology*. San Francisco: Neurotech Press.

Gavison, Ruth. 1980. Privacy and the limits of law. *Yale Law J* 89 (3): 421–471. doi:10.2307/795891.

*Genetic Information Nondiscrimination Act of 2008*. (GINA) 2008. *U.S.C.* Vol. 42.

Greely, Henry T., and Judy Illes. 2007. Neuroscience-based lie detection: The urgent need for regulation. *Am JL Med* 33: 377.

Greene, Joshua D., R. Brian Sommerville, Leigh E. Nystrom, John M. Darley, and Jonathan D. Cohen. 2001. An fMRI investigation of emotional engagement in moral judgment. *Science* 293 (5537): 2105–2108.

Hallinan, Dara, Michael Friedewald, Philip Schütz, and Paul de Hert. 2014. Neurodata and neuroprivacy: Data protection outdated? *Surveill Soc* 12 (1): 55.

Haynes, John-Dylan. 2012. Brain reading. In *I Know What You're Thinking: Brain Imaging and Mental Privacy*, edited by Sarah Richmond, Geraint Rees, and Sarah J.L. Edwards, 29–40. Oxford: Oxford University Press.

Haynes, John-Dylan, and Geraint Rees. 2006. Decoding mental states from brain activity in humans. *Nat Rev Neurosci* 7 (7): 523–534.

Haynes, John-Dylan, Katsuyuki Sakai, Geraint Rees, Sam Gilbert, Chris Frith, and Richard E. Passingham. 2007. Reading hidden intentions in the human brain. *Curr Biol* 17 (4): 323–328.

*Health Insurance Portability and Accountability Act* (HIPAA). 1996. *U.S.C.* Vol. 29.

Heersmink, Richard. 2013. Embodied tools, cognitive tools and brain-computer interfaces. *Neuroethics* 6 (1): 207–219.

Hochberg, Leigh R., Daniel Bacher, Beata Jarosiewicz, Nicolas Y. Masse, John D. Simeral, Joern Vogel, Sami Haddadin et al. 2012. Reach and grasp by people with tetraplegia using a neurally controlled robotic arm. *Nature* 485 (7398): 372–375.

Huggins, Jane E., Patricia A. Wren, and Kirsten L. Gruis. 2011. What would brain–computer interface users want? Opinions and priorities of potential users with amyotrophic lateral sclerosis. *Amyotroph Lateral Scler* 12 (5): 318–324.

Ienca, Marcello, and Pim Haselager. 2016. Hacking the brain: Brain–computer interfacing technology and the ethics of neurosecurity. *Ethics Inform Technol* 1–13.

Illes, Judy, and Eric Racine. 2005. Imaging or imagining? A neuroethics challenge informed by genetics. *Am J Bioeth* 5 (2): 5–18.

Ioannidis, John P. A. 2013. Informed consent, big data, and the oxymoron of research that is not research. *Am Bioeth*, March. http://www.tandfonline.com/doi/abs/10.1080/15265161.2013.768864.

Jebari, Karim. 2013. Brain machine interface and human enhancement—An ethical review. *Neuroethics* 6 (3): 617–625.

Klein, Eran. 2015. Informed consent in implantable BCI research: Identifying risks and exploring meaning. *Sci Eng Ethics* 1–19.

Lacy, Joyce W., and Craig E. L. Stark. 2013. The neuroscience of memory: Implications for the courtroom. *Nat Rev Neurosci* 14 (9): 649–658. doi:10.1038/nrn3563.

Lahr, Jacob, Christina Schwartz, Bernhard Heimbach, Ad Aertsen, Jörn Rickert, and Tonio Ball. 2015. Invasive brain–machine interfaces: A survey of paralyzed patients' attitudes, knowledge and methods of information retrieval. *J Neural Eng* 12 (4): 043001.

Levy, Neil. 2007. *Neuroethics*. Cambridge, UK; New York: Cambridge University Press.

Mak, Joseph N., and Jonathan R. Wolpaw. 2009. Clinical applications of brain–computer interfaces: Current state and future prospects. *IEEE Rev Biomed Eng* 2: 187–199.

Matheson, David. 2007. Unknowableness and informational privacy. *J Philos Res* 32: 251–267.

Mittelstadt, Brent Daniel, and Luciano Floridi. 2016. The ethics of big data: Current and foreseeable issues in biomedical contexts. *Sci Eng Ethics* 22 (2): 303–341. doi:10.1007/s11948-015-9652-2.

National Institutes of Health. 2014. Supplemental Information to the National Institutes of Health Genomic Data Sharing Policy. https://gds.nih.gov/pdf/supplemental_info_GDS_Policy.pdf.

Neergaard, Lauran. 2016. Obama shakes mind-controlled robot hand wired to sense touch. *US News & World Report*, October 13. http://www.usnews.com/news/news/articles/2016-10-13/paralyzed-man-feels-touch-through-mind-controlled-robot-hand.

Nissenbaum, Helen Fay. 2010. *Privacy in Context: Technology, Policy, and the Integrity of Social Life*. Stanford, California: Stanford Law Books.

Owen, Adrian. 2012. When thoughts become actions: Neuroimaging in non-responsive patients. In *I Know What You're Thinking: Brain Imaging and Mental Privacy*, edited by Sarah Richmond, Sarah J.L. Rees, and Sarah J.L. Edwards, 73–88. Oxford: Oxford University Press.

Ozyurt, I. Burak, David B. Keator, Dingying Wei, Christine Fennema-Notestine, Karen R. Pease, Jeremy Bockholt, and Jeffrey S. Grethe. 2010. Federated web-accessible clinical data management within an extensible neuroimaging database. *Neuroinformatics* 8 (4): 231–249.

Pelley, Scott. 2012. Paralyzed woman uses mind-control technology to operate robotic arm. *60 Minutes*. http://www.cbsnews.com/news/paralyzed-woman-uses-mind-control-technology-to-operate-robotic-arm/.

Poldrack, Russell A., and Krzysztof J. Gorgolewski. 2014. Making big data open: Data sharing in neuroimaging. *Nat Neurosci* 17 (11): 1510–1517.

Poldrack, Russell A., and Jean-Baptiste Poline. 2015. The publication and reproducibility challenges of shared data. *Trends Cogn Sci* 19 (2): 59–61.

Poline, Jean-Baptiste, Janis L. Breeze, Satrajit Ghosh, Krzysztof Gorgolewski, Yaroslav O. Halchenko, Michael Hanke, Christian Haselgrove et al. 2012. Data sharing in neuroimaging research. *Front Neuroinform* 6: 9. doi:10.3389/fninf.2012.00009.

Rachels, James. 1975. Why privacy is important. *Philos Publ Affairs* 4 (4): 323–333. doi:10.2307/2265077.

Räikkä, Juha. 2010. Brain imaging and privacy. *Neuroethics* 3 (1): 5–12.

Richmond, Sarah. 2012. Brain imaging and the transparency scenario. In *I Know What You're Thinking: Brain Imaging and Mental Privacy*, edited by Sarah Richmond, Sarah J.L. Rees, and Sarah J.L. Edwards, 185–204. Oxford: Oxford University Press.

Rubel, Alan, and Ryan Biava. 2014. A framework for analyzing and comparing privacy states. *J Assoc Inform Sci Technol* 65 (12): 2422–2431. doi:10.1002/asi.23138.

Ryberg, Jesper. 2016. Neuroscience, mind reading and mental privacy. *Res Publ* doi:10.1007/s11158-016-9343-0.

Schneider, Mary-Jane, Joseph J. Fins, and Jonathan R. Wolpaw. 2012. Ethical issues in BCI research. *Brain–Comput Interf Principles Pract*, 373–383.

Schoenmakers, Sanne, Markus Barth, Tom Heskes, and Marcel van Gerven. 2013. Linear reconstruction of perceived images from human brain activity. *NeuroImage* 83: 951–961.

Sejnowski, Terrence J., Patricia S. Churchland, and J. Anthony Movshon. 2014. Putting big data to good use in neuroscience. *Nat Neurosci* 17 (11): 1440–1441.

Sellers, Eric W., Theresa M. Vaughan, and Jonathan R. Wolpaw. 2010. A brain computer interface for long-term independent home use. *Amyotroph Lateral Scler* 11 (5): 449–455.

Shih, Jerry J., Dean J. Krusienski, and Jonathan R. Wolpaw. 2012. Brain–computer interfaces in medicine. In *Mayo Clinic Proceedings*, 87: 268–279. Elsevier. http://www.sciencedirect.com/science/article/pii /S0025619612001231.

Soekadar, Surjo R., Leonardo G. Cohen, and Niels Birbaumer. 2014. Clinical brain–machine interfaces. In *Cognitive Plasticity in Neurologic Disorders*, edited by Tracy, Joseph I., Hamstead, Bejamin M., and Sathian, K., 347–362. Oxford: Oxford University Press.

Sorani, Marco D., John K. Yue, Sourabh Sharma, Geoffrey T. Manley, Adam R. Ferguson, Shelly R. Cooper, Kristen Dams-O'Connor et al. 2015. Genetic data sharing and privacy. *Neuroinformatics* 13 (1): 1–6.

Tennison, Michael N., and Jonathan D. Moreno. 2012. Neuroscience, ethics, and national security: The state of the art. *PLoS Biol* 10 (3): e1001289.

Trimper, John B., Paul Root Wolpe, and Karen S. Rommelfanger. 2014. When 'I' becomes 'We': Ethical implications of emerging brain-to-brain interfacing technologies. *Front Neuroeng* 7. http://www.ncbi .nlm.nih.gov/pmc/articles/PMC3921579/.

Van Horn, John Darrell, and Catherine A. Ball. 2008. Domain-specific data sharing in neuroscience: What do we have to learn from each other? *Neuroinformatics* 6 (2): 117–121.

Walter, Sven. 2010. Locked-in syndrome, BCI, and a confusion about embodied, embedded, extended, and enacted cognition. *Neuroethics* 3 (1): 61–72. doi:10.1007/s12152-009-9050-z.

Wolpe, Paul R., Kenneth R. Foster, and Daniel D. Langleben. 2005. Emerging neurotechnologies for lie-detection: Promises and perils. *Am Bioeth* 5 (2): 39–49.

Zander, Thorsten O., and Sabine Jatzev. 2009. Detecting affective covert user states with passive brain–computer interfaces. In *2009 3rd International Conference on Affective Computing and Intelligent Interaction and Workshops*, 1–9. doi:10.1109/ACII.2009.5349456.

# 35 Associative Plasticity Induced by a Brain–Computer Interface Based on Movement-Related Cortical Potentials

*Natalie Mrachacz-Kersting, Ning Jiang, Kim Dremstrup, and Dario Farina*

## CONTENTS

35.1 Introduction ..................................................................................................... 669
35.2 The Movement-Related Cortical Potential ....................................................... 671
    35.2.1 MRCPs during Sensorimotor Behavior ................................................. 673
        35.2.1.1 Type of Movement ................................................................ 673
        35.2.1.2 Speed/Velocity of Movement ............................................... 673
        35.2.1.3 Force ...................................................................................... 674
    35.2.2 MRCP during Motor Imagery ............................................................... 674
    35.2.3 Detection of the MRCP during Motor Tasks and Imagery ................... 675
    35.2.4 Detection of the MRCP during Gait ...................................................... 676
35.3 MRCP-Based Associative BCIs ....................................................................... 677
    35.3.1 Effects of Type of Neurofeedback as Part of the Associative BCI ........ 678
    35.3.2 Potential and Challenges of MRCP-Based Associative BCI ................. 679
References ................................................................................................................. 680

### Abstract

This chapter presents the basic concepts of a brain–computer-interface (BCI) designed for neuromodulation that is based on known theories of memory storage and learning. Initially, an overview is provided of the control signal, the movement-related cortical potential (MRCP), its advantages over other signal modalities, and its neural generators. This is followed by a detailed account of factors that affect the MRCP morphology such as task parameters, shifts in user attention and plasticity, and insights into algorithm design for both detection and classification in an online self-paced BCI. Finally, the applications of this type of associative BCI to more complex tasks such as human gait and in the clinical environment with patients are presented.

## 35.1 INTRODUCTION

A brain–computer interface (BCI) system designed for neuromodulation aims at inducing plasticity in neural structures. Since the initial reports by Daly et al. (2009), many research groups have documented the feasibility of this concept (Ang et al. 2010; Broetz et al. 2010; Cincotti et al. 2012; Daly et al. 2009; Kasashima-Shindo et al. 2015; Li et al. 2014; Mrachacz-Kersting et al. 2016a [p. 248],b; Mukaino et al. 2014; Pichiorri et al. 2015; Ramos Murguialday et al. 2013; Young et al. 2014).

Relearning motor tasks because of motor impairments requires correlated activations of neural cells (Hebb 1949). According to this, synapses that experience correlated activation of two converging inputs are strengthened, whereas those weakened by uncorrelated activity are lost. Hebb's theorem was subsequently substantiated by in vitro experiments in the dentate area of the anaesthetized rabbit (Bliss and Lomo 1973). This phenomenon, called long-term potentiation (LTP), remains one of the candidate cellular mechanisms for learning and memory storage and has been extensively investigated in the hippocampus of rats. In the year 2000, Stefan and colleagues provided the first proof that LTP-like plasticity can be induced noninvasively in the intact human nervous system (Stefan et al. 2000). They applied a single stimulation of the peripheral nerve that innervates the target muscle (in their case the abductor pollicis brevis [APB]) followed 25 ms later by a single magnetic stimulation of that area on the motor cortex that controls the APB. The continuous pairing of these two stimuli at the appropriate interstimulus interval of 25 ms led to a significant increase of the excitability of the cortical projections to the APB that outlasted the stimulation period, was long lasting, specific to the target muscles, and dependent on both NMDA receptors and Ca2+ channel activation. Within BCIs, this concept requires that artificially provided sensory feedback is associated to the decoded motor commands. Thus, the afferent feedback generated by the artificial stimulus (whether via electrical stimulation or the activation of a robotic device that produces the movement intended by the motor command) has to be timed such that it will arrive at the motor cortex at the time of its maximum activation. Only then will strengthening of the synapse and thus learning be achieved. For this purpose, the movement intent needs to be detected before movement execution, reliably trial by trial. One signal modality that has been used for this aim is the movement-related cortical potential (MRCP), which is naturally and physiologically associated with the movement (Kuhtz-Buschbeck et al. 2003; Leifert-Fiebach et al. 2013; Salinet et al. 2012), does not require user training, is repeatable between trials, and, most importantly, is generated 1–1.5 s before movement execution.

In the last decade, we have implemented, tested, and clinically applied in subacute and chronic stroke patients an associative BCI based on the MRCP (Mrachacz-Kersting et al. 2012a, 2016a [p. 248],b). Its components are shown in Figure 35.1. According to this approach, the user imagines or attempts to perform a task, such as ankle dorsiflexion, while electroencephalography (EEG) is measured from the motor, sensory, frontal, and parietal cortex. The initiation of the movement generates the MRCP, which is detected before movement execution and used to trigger either an

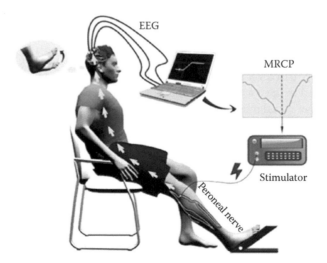

**FIGURE 35.1** Schematic of the associative brain–computer interface. (Modified from Mrachacz-Kersting, N., N. Jiang, S. Aliakbaryhosseinabadi, R. Xu, L. Petrini, R. Lontis, K. Dremstrup, and D. Farina. 2015. The changing brain: Bidirectional learning between algorithm and user. In Brain–Computer Interface Research: A State-of-the-Art Summary-4, edited by C. Guger, B. Z. Allison and G. Edlinger: Springer.)

electrical stimulator or an exoskeleton that induces afferent feedback timed to arrive at the peak negative (PN) phase of the MRCP. The PN represents the time of the maximum activation of the motor cortex. After a limited number of trials, significant plasticity and physiological and behavioral changes are induced. This associative BCI is based on an initial characterization of the MRCP morphology (do Nascimento et al. 2005a,b, 2006; Gu et al. 2009c, 2013), followed by the proposal of a novel associative intervention (Mrachacz-Kersting et al. 2012a, 2016a [p. 248],b) and by the developments of signal processing techniques for highly accurate and timely detection of the MRCP (Lin et al. 2016; Niazi et al. 2011; Xu et al. 2014a, 2016). Moreover, efforts were devoted to minimize or eliminate the need for user training (Niazi et al. 2013).

In this chapter, we will first introduce the MRCP and its neural generators, as well as the task parameters that influence its characteristics. Then, we will present the development of the associative BCI both for cued and self-paced motor tasks in healthy and impaired populations.

## 35.2 THE MOVEMENT-RELATED CORTICAL POTENTIAL

The first demonstration of a slow MRCP was reported by Walter in 1964. Participants were required to press a button in response to a series of flashes (the imperative cue) that occurred 1 s after a warning stimulus (a single clicking sound). This resulted in a slow negative potential that was termed the contingent negative variation (CNV) (Walter et al. 1964). Generally, motor acts can be considered as either responses to external stimuli and thus reactions to our environment or volitional and thus spontaneous actions on the environment. The latter may also be guided by a stimulus (e.g., thirst will prompt us to drink a glass of water) though this is internally motivated. Thus, while reactions will induce a CNV, spontaneous actions are accompanied by a different type of slow cortical potential, the Bereitschaftspotential (BP) (Kornhuber and Deecke 1965). Both the CNV and the BP may be referred to as an MRCP, which is the term we will use in the remaining of the chapter. The initial slow shift in the MRCP is attributed to the planning and preparation of the impeding movement while the more rapid change is thought to reflect the execution of the movement itself.

Since the CNV is preceded by a warning stimulus and an imperative cue, both an early and a late CNV have been described (Walter et al. 1964). The early CNV commences immediately after the warning stimulus (Hamano et al. 1997) while the late CNV appears 1 to 0.5 s before the imperative cue (Hamano et al. 1997). The BP on the other hand commences approximately 800 ms before unilateral movement onset and is distributed bilaterally over the precentral and parietal cortex (Deecke et al. 1969, 1976; Kornhuber and Deecke 1965). Approximately 400 ms later, the BP distribution is predominantly unilateral over the contralateral precentral cortex, which attains significance 150 ms before movement onset. Interestingly, during bimanual movements, the BP predominance is seen in the nondominant precentral cortex (Kristeva et al. 1979), which has been explained by a greater effort to perform the task by the nondominant limb with respect to the dominant limb. In general, bilateral movements are associated to greater BP amplitudes, as it could be expected by the greater number of neurons to be activated to achieve the task. The BP may be further subdivided into several components; the readiness potential (RP), the pre-movement potential (PMP), and the motor potential (MP) occur 800 ms, 150 ms, and 50–60 ms before movement onset, respectively. A reafferent potential may be observed just after task execution (Deecke et al. 1976).

In the associative BCI we have developed, significant plasticity was induced irrespective of whether the BP or the CNV was used as the control signal. However, the BP and CNV may differ in form, shape, and topographical distribution according to the experimental paradigm implemented. The CNV has a frontal distribution, which is absent in the BP, owing to the focus on an external stimulus and its relation to the internal cue to commence the movement (Deecke et al. 1976). Sensory information from both the visual and auditory association area converges, with afferents from the limbic system in the frontal cortex (Groenewegen and Uylings 2000). In addition, the CNV is typically distributed bilaterally and thus may be recorded from both hemispheres even for unilateral motor tasks (Deecke et al. 1984). The cue provided to the participant likely changes the neural contributors to the CNV since the initial warning stimulus prompts the participant to move while he or she is on hold. This holding of a movement is not a passive process but rather requires an active inhibition of neurons (Deecke et al. 1976, 1984). The BP also commences bilaterally, but from approximately 400 ms before movement onset, it becomes lateralized.

When the time between the warning and the imperative cue is greater than 5 s, the shape of the late CNV is identical to that of the BP (Deecke et al. 1976). Moreover, if the warning and imperative cue are auditory, the CNV is not present in parietal regions while it is recorded from these sites when the cue is visual (Deecke et al. 1976, 1984). The dependence of the topographical distribution according to the experimental paradigm implemented has important consequences for the use of the CNV within a BCI.

Since the CNV occurs as a response to a cue, it can be used in cue-based BCIs designed for neuro-rehabilitation (Mrachacz-Kersting et al. 2016a [p. 248],b). Patients who have suffered a cerebral incident can perform motor tasks significantly more accurately when a cue is provided (Heremans et al. 2009), making the CNV an ideal candidate for such applications.

As has been outlined above, within the current literature, there remains controversy if the BP and CNV may be considered similar direct current shifts in relation to movement execution. As has been outlined above, there are several distinct differences between the generators of these two potentials. However, in our associative BCI, we time the peripheral afferent volley at the PN component of the MRCP, and in this time interval, the consensus is that activation of the motor cortex (M1) and the direct corticospinal tract (Deecke et al. 1976) are the main generators for both the CNV and the BP. Nonetheless, for triggering the afferent activity, the movement intent has to be detected in the preparation and planning phase, which differ between the two signals.

MRCPs have been recorded for movements of hands (Brunia and Van den Bosch 1984b; Deecke and Kornhuber 1978; Gu et al. 2009a,b, 2013; Lang et al. 1988; Slobounov et al. 1999, 2000), feet (do Nascimento and Farina 2008; do Nascimento et al. 2005b; Mrachacz-Kersting et al. 2012a; Terada et al. 1999; Xu et al. 2014b), mouth (Deecke et al. 1986; Uhl et al. 1988), and eyes (Becker et al. 1972). Although the optimal electrode recoding sites differ for the different tasks (e.g., Cz for foot movements, C3 or C4 for finger movements), it is striking that the MRCPs have consistently the same morphology and onset across tasks (Figure 35.2). In all cases, the MRCP develops bilaterally until approximately 500 ms before movement onset and has a widespread distribution. Despite general similarity in morphology, small but consistent differences in MRCPs are observed in relation to the purpose or context of the task (i.e., whether they are reactions or actions), to the body part(s) to

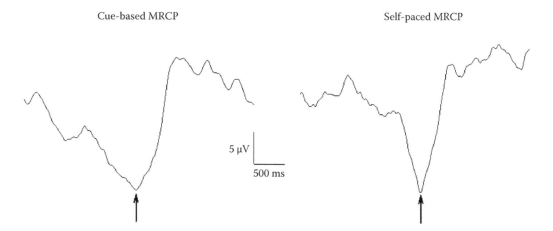

**FIGURE 35.2** The MRCP following either cue-based or self-paced ankle dorsiflexion. Data are the average of 20 repetitions for one participant tested with both paradigms on the same day. The vertical arrows indicate movement onset.

be moved (i.e., whether they are unilateral or bilateral, or rhythmic or complex, performed with the dominant or nondominant side), and to the characteristics of the movement (i.e., flexion/extension, fast/slow, level of force required). These factors of influence have been extensively examined in the literature, also in the context of BCI design.

## 35.2.1 MRCPs DURING SENSORIMOTOR BEHAVIOR

### 35.2.1.1 Type of Movement

Animal studies have revealed that different sets of neurons and activity are responsible for flexion versus extension tasks (e.g., extensor neurons fire at approximately twice the rate of flexor neurons) (Fetz and Cheney 1979; Georgopoulos et al. 1986). In addition, as force demand increases, so do the number of neurons that fire (Ashe 1997; Georgopoulos et al. 1992). Several groups have thus attempted to differentiate flexion and extension movements as well as different levels of force and speed of a movement from the MRCP.

Index finger flexion and extension correspond to similar early components of the MRCP (RP and PMP), but extension presents with significantly larger MPs (the only unilateral potential of the three) (Deecke et al. 1980). In conditions when the participant receives feedback on the correct response that is either predictable or not, the RP and the MP attain higher amplitudes for the unpredictable condition (Hink et al. 1982). Interestingly, when both task uncertainty and force levels were varied, the RP and MP were significantly larger for all force levels in the uncertain condition. The amplitudes in the uncertain conditions were similar to those at the greatest force level in the predictable condition, indicating that participants prepare for heavy resistance when confronted with force uncertainty (Hink et al. 1983). Surprisingly, no significant differences occur for toe flexion and extension (Boschert et al. 1983). A similar discrepancy occurs for differentiating between contraction and active relaxation. When participants actively relax their wrist extensor after a wrist flexion, the BP commences earlier and is significantly larger in amplitude over contralateral parieto-temporal electrode locations (Terada et al. 1995). This has been attributed to relaxation requiring a longer preparation time. For foot muscles, this difference is not evident and the amplitude of the BP is smaller during relaxation as compared to contraction (Terada et al. 1999). The origin of this discrepancy between upper and lower limb muscles is unclear. However, the representation of foot muscles is located deep in the interhemispheric fissures and further the anatomical organization is not as consistent as in the upper limb. For example, Penfield and Jasper (1954) showed that ankle movements may be elicited either by stimulation within the fissure or on the lateral aspect of the motor cortex. Thus, while the RP is bilaterally symmetrical for both finger and toe movements, the MP of finger movements is lateralized toward the contralateral precentral cortex while toe movements are lateralized toward the ipsilateral precentral cortex (Brunia and van den Bosch 1984a). This has significant implications for the location of the recording electrodes during the design of a BCI.

### 35.2.1.2 Speed/Velocity of Movement

Fast, ballistic movements are regulated differently compared to slow movements because, contrary to slow movements, afferent feedback cannot adjust the ongoing ballistic movement performance. The effects of movement velocity on the MRCP morphology have been little investigated in the past and reveals conflicting findings. In slow hand movements, the MRCP commences earlier (500 ms) and has greater amplitude compared to fast ballistic hand movements (Becker et al. 1976). However, during discrete and repetitive finger tapping, only the late component of the MRCP (the MMP) is higher in amplitude for fast speeds irrespective of the force required (Slobounov and Ray 1998). In an effort to better discriminate between rates of force development, Ray et al. (2000) quantified the lateralized RP, which is considered a measure of motor preparation, by subtracting the ipsilateral from the contralateral potential. They reported that higher rates of force development are significantly related to an increased amplitude of the lateralized RP during an index finger pressing task

(Ray et al. 2000). In a BCI, detection of motor intent should ideally occur before movement execution to allow an association to be formed between the intent to move and the artificial generation of the movement through the external device (Figure 35.1). Thus, discrimination between tasks during the preparation phase is desirable. The finding of a larger size of the MRCP during high versus low rates of torque development has also been reported for isometric ankle plantarflexion (do Nascimento et al. 2005b). In fact, movement speed has been discriminated from all components of the MRCP, following averaging over a large number of trials. Gu et al. (2009a) were the first to demonstrate that speed can be decoded from single-trial MRCPs as well. Participants were asked to imagine either extension or rotation of the dominant wrist at one of two speeds, as controlled by an online visual cue. The reafferent phase of the MRCP was significantly larger for fast compared to slow speeds and this difference was also observed in patients suffering from ALS (Gu et al. 2009b).

### 35.2.1.3 Force

A movement requiring higher force would presumably activate a larger number of cortical cells, at least in the execution phase. It is well known that force is encoded in the motor cortex (Ashe 1997) and it is thus not surprising that various studies have documented force to also be encoded in the MRCP. Extending the forearm against a large force induces a larger reafferent phase of the MRCP compared to an extension against low force (Wilke and Lansing 1973). Squeezing a ball with the dominant or nondominant hand at 25%, 50%, or 7% of the maximal force showed significant differences in the MRCP amplitude 500 ms before movement onset (Kutas and Donchin 1974). Similarly, Slobounov et al. (1999) demonstrated significant changes in the MRCP that commenced 100 ms before finger flexion at variable forces, particularly the activation at electrode sites located across frontal and precentral areas. For tasks involving the lower limb, the early components of the MRCP (the RP) are significantly related to force (do Nascimento et al. 2005b). Contrary to the all above studies that focused on averaged MRCPs, the force could be decoded from single-trial MRCPs by do Nascimento et al. (2008).

In summary, both force and speed of movement influence the morphology of the MRCP. The possibility of extracting such movement characteristics from single trials, as recently shown, may be used for the design of a BCI. On the one hand, it is well known that learning under variable conditions by altering force and speed is more effective than repeating the same movement across trials. On the other hand, for BCI control, decoding movement characteristics may enlarge the number of commands.

### 35.2.2 MRCP DURING MOTOR IMAGERY

One of the goals of a BCI for neuromodulation is to aid locked-in patients to perform an intended movement generated artificially by functional electrical stimulation (FES) or a robotic exoskeleton. The advantage of using the MRCP as the control signal is that it occurs both during actual and imaginary movement (Beisteiner et al. 1995; do Nascimento et al. 2006). Evidence suggests that imagery of a motor task activates the same physiological processes as the actual movement (Decety 1996a,b; Decety and Jeannerod 1995; Jeannerod and Decety 1995).

During imagery of the kinaesthetics of a movement, the preparation and execution phases of the MRCP are similar to when performing an actual movement (Beisteiner et al. 1995; Cunnington et al. 1996; do Nascimento et al. 2006). However, without the movement execution, there is no afferent inflow and thus the reafferent phase of the MRCP is not present (do Nascimento et al. 2006). Moreover, in healthy subjects, the MRCP amplitude during both hand and foot motor imagery is smaller with respect to motor execution (Beisteiner et al. 1995; do Nascimento et al. 2006). This difference is, however, not observed in patients with a complete spinal cord injury (Lacourse et al. 1999). The attenuation of the MRCP in healthy participants during motor imagery may be related to the activation of two conflicting neural assemblies, one to move and one to hold or stop moving (Deecke et al. 1976; Lacourse et al. 1999). Since the final signal recorded at each electrode is the summation of the overall activity of the underlying neuronal structures, a cancelling effect will lead to an attenuated overall MRCP. This explanation is in agreement with the data on spinal cord–injured patients where the injury has weakened the inhibitory processes (Lacourse et al. 1999).

Despite these significant differences in the amplitude of the MRCP elicited during motor execution and imagery, it is possible to classify the rate of force development and level of force in both cases from single-trial MRCPs in healthy and impaired populations (do Nascimento and Farina 2008; Gu et al. 2009a,b,c; Jochumsen et al. 2013).

### 35.2.3 Detection of the MRCP during Motor Tasks and Imagery

The characteristics of MRCPs can be well identified by averaging over several trials. In this way, the relatively poor signal-to-noise ratio of single trials increases with the square root of the number of averages. Usually, tens to hundreds of trials have been used for the averaging. As discussed above, by averaging, it has been demonstrated that MRCPs generated during both executed movements and motor imagery are influenced by the speed and force of the motor task (do Nascimento and Farina 2008; do Nascimento et al. 2005a,b). The differences attributed to motor task characteristics were small and mainly associated to the negative slope during movement preparation and the rebound rate. do Nascimento et al. also reported averaged MRCPs during gait initiation and showed that they differed depending on the direction (forward or backward) of gait (do Nascimento et al. 2005a).

The signal-to-noise ratio of MRCPs from single trials is much poorer than after averaging. Moreover, the frequency content of MRCPs corresponds to that of artifacts, such as those due to eye blinking. Therefore, extracting information from these signals on a single-trial basis is challenging. Nonetheless, Farina et al. (2007) showed that it is possible to classify MRCPs associated to different characteristics (force and speed) of a plantarflexion motor task on a single-trial basis. For this purpose, they projected the single-trial EEG traces into a discrete wavelet basis function and classified the wavelet coefficients with a support vector machine. They proved that, by optimizing the parameters of the transformation on the training set, it was possible to classify signals in the test set associated to different speeds and forces of the task with accuracy for two classes of approximately 70%. These results were later extended to motor imagery of ankle joint movements instead of motor execution (do Nascimento and Farina 2008) and to wrist tasks (extension and rotation in healthy participants and ALS patients) (Gu et al. 2009a,b, 2013). Consistently, single-trial MRCPs could be classified with accuracy above the chance level in both executed and imagined movements. These studies proved the feasibility of using MRCPs as a signal modality for BCI. The advantage of this signal modality was in the feasibility of classifying movement parameters, such as speed, which could add more degrees of freedom for BCI control.

Detection of MRCPs from the background noise is a similar challenge to classification. It is indeed the classification between a signal class and a noise class. Methods for single-trial MRCP detection have been proposed with the aim of developing a fast brain switch that can accurately detect the user motor intention with very short latency (i.e., less than a few hundreds of milliseconds). The rationale for this approach came from the studies on averaged MRCPs that showed that the negative deflection associated to movement preparation commenced as early as 1–1.5 s before the actual movement execution. In principle, this property can be used to detect movement intention with very short latency and therefore to obtain a fast brain switch that can trigger external devices. The simplest approach for detecting MRCPs in single trials consists in designing a matched filter and thresholding the filtered EEG signals. This approach was proposed by Niazi et al. (2011) who designed a matched filter based on the averaged first portion of the MRCPs from a training set of signals and then applied this filter to test data. Occurrences were detected when the filtered signal passed a threshold. This approach is equivalent to projecting the signal on a waveform basis function that maximally resembles the event to be detected and imposing a simple threshold classifier on the extracted projection, sample by sample. Interestingly, this approach provided results that were similar to the classification of MRCPs according to speed or force; that is, the MRCPs could be differentiated from noise with a rate of true positives of approximately 70%. However, for detection, the signal is continuously classified (and not only classified in intervals corresponding to a cue, as in MRCP classification of movement parameters), and this was associated to a relatively high number of false positives. Of course, true positives and false positives could be tuned by adjusting the threshold (Niazi et al. 2011), which has an opposite effect on these two metrics. The approach of the matched filter for MRCP detection has the interesting property that the filter can be universal; that is, it can be the same across different subjects, since the shape of the MRCPs is very similar across subjects. For example, Niazi et al. (2013) showed that the performance in detection did not degrade substantially when the matched filter was the same for all subjects investigated with respect to the case of subject-specific filters.

Several further studies attempted to improve the performance of single-trial MRCP detection (Ibanez et al. 2014; Lin et al. 2016; Xu et al. 2016). The common characteristic of these studies was the proposal of projection methods for the EEG signals and the identification of the presence of MRCPs from a noisy background with classification of the projected signals, for example, with linear discriminant analysis (LDA). For example, Xu et al. (2014a) used the locality preserving projection (LPP) for extracting signal features. LPP is a manifold learning method for dimensionality reduction, which preserves the local intrinsic structure of the data in the original high dimension. The method identifies a linear weights matrix "$W$" that applies to the signal "$X$" in the original high-dimensional space (time samples) and projects it into a lower-dimensional space where the projection $y$ maintains the geometrical relations of the original space. With this transformation, followed by LDA, the sensitivity and specificity in detection were improved with respect to the matched filter, with an average rate of true positives reaching approximately 80%. With a similar approach that used a locality sensitive discriminant analysis as the transformation for signal projection, Lin et al. (2016) further improved the performance with respect to the use of LPP, specifically in terms of reduction of false positives.

With respect to the above methods that are all based on features extracted from MRCPs, that is, in the very low frequency band of EEG (<1 Hz), detection methods of motor intention have also been proposed by using features from the full EEG signal bandwidth. For example, Ibanez et al. (2014) used features extracted from the MRCP waveforms as well as from sensorimotor rhythms (event-related synchronization and desynchronization [ERS and ERD, respectively]) for detecting movement intention with low latency and improved the performance with respect to the use of MRCP features only. The results were partly confirmed in a study that systematically analyzed the frequency bands and features that led to best detection results (Xu et al. 2016).

In all the above approaches, one important constraint has been the maintenance of detection latency within a small delay, so that detection usually occurred tens to hundreds of milliseconds before the peak negativity. This ensured the possibility of triggering external devices with physiological delay (Mrachacz-Kersting et al. 2016a [p. 248],b; Niazi et al. 2012; Xu et al. 2014b).

## 35.2.4 DETECTION OF THE MRCP DURING GAIT

An interesting application of MRCP detection is in gait initiation. do Nascimento et al. (2005a) showed that averaged MRCPs associated to gait initiation have similar characteristics to those generated during ankle dorsiflexion. However, the peak amplitude of the MRCP occurs significantly later during gait initiation as compared to standing, sitting, or foot dorsiflexion (Yazawa et al. 1997). On the basis of these observations, Jiang et al. (2014) applied a matched filter approach, as the one described above, for detecting the instant of gait initiation in healthy individuals. They showed similar results in terms of accuracy and latency as in the more standardized conditions of detection of ankle dorsiflexion. The average detection accuracy was >75% with ICA preprocessing, thus providing the possibility to develop a brain switch to control robotic systems for walking rehabilitation in stroke patients.

The challenge of detecting gait initiation from MRCPs has been addressed with other approaches that aimed at increasing the intersession and intersubject transfer. For example, Sburlea et al. (2017)

extracted both the phase and amplitude of the MRCPs as features for detection in both healthy subjects and stroke, showing superior performance with respect to the use of amplitude only. They also reported that self-initiated walking movement intention can be detected from EEG without session-to-session recalibration (Sburlea et al. 2015). In that experiment, the participants were asked to stand on a wooden stage with their right foot on a foot switch and to relax in that posture for 10 s. After this, a fixation cross appeared on a screen in front of them, cueing them to commence walking with the initiation of the right leg. The pre-movement state was detected from a combination of MRCPs and ERDs, resulting in a detection accuracy of approximately 70% within a session. However, only one type of gait initiation was detected from EEG signals and participants were restricted as to which leg initiated the task.

## 35.3   MRCP-BASED ASSOCIATIVE BCIs

The first introduction of the associative BCI developed by our group was presented in 2011 (Mrachacz-Kersting et al. 2011) and later fully published in 2012 (Mrachacz-Kersting et al. 2012a). In this paradigm, healthy participants were asked to imagine a simple dorsiflexion task timed to a visual cue (Figure 35.3) in two sets of 25 trials each. EEG signals were recorded continuously over C1, Cz, C2, and CPz, according to the international 10–20 system, and divided into epochs from −2 to +2.5 s in relation to the cue during offline analysis. The time of the PN phase of the MRCP was extracted and used for the subsequent BCI intervention. The BCI intervention was composed of an artificial stimulation to the deep branch of the common peroneal nerve timed such that the generated afferent signal would reach the motor cortex at the time of PN of the MRCP as the participants were imagining the movement. In this way, a causal relation was established between the intent of the participant (measured as the MRCP) and the artificial reproduction of the intended movement (the peripheral stimulus) that led to cortical plasticity. Through a number of control experiments, we were able to show conclusively that the effects of this BCI intervention were strongly dependent on the correct timing of the afferent signal in relation to the PN, that the effects evolved rapidly, outlasting the intervention period by at least 30 min, and were specific to the target muscle. This associative BCI thus satisfied many of the properties of LTP, thought to underlie memory formation and learning (Bliss and Collingridge 1993; Bliss and Cooke 2011; Bliss and Lomo 1973; Cooke and Bliss 2006).

After this initial proof-of-concept study in healthy participants, we sought to test this associative BCI in a group of chronic stroke patients (Mrachacz-Kersting et al. 2012b, 2016b). Patients were allocated to either a $BCI_{associative}$ or a $BCI_{non-associative}$ group. Both groups attended three separate testing sessions separated by >48 h. During each session, they were instructed to attempt 50 ballistic dorsiflexion movements while EEG signals were continuously monitored from FP1, F3, F4, Fz, Pz, P3, P4, C3, C4, and Cz. During offline analysis, EEG data were divided into epochs from 2 s before to 1 s after the visual cue for each attempted movement and subsequently a Laplacian

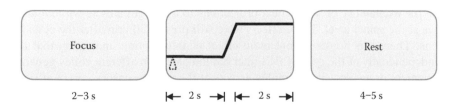

**FIGURE 35.3**   The visual cue provided to the user. FOCUS appeared on the screen initially followed by the schematic of a step function. Subjects were required to start the attempted movement once the moving cursor (triangle) reached the upward slope. The word REST appeared last on the screen.

channel (McFarland et al. 1997) was used to enhance the MRCP in each epoch. Significant cortical plasticity, as assessed through noninvasive transcranial magnetic stimulation, was induced only in the BCI$_{associative}$ group. Similarly, behavioral (10 m walking speed and foot tapping frequency) and clinical (Fugl–Meyer score) measures improved significantly only for the BCI$_{associative}$ group, further highlighting the importance of the precise coupling between the brain command and the afferent signal in the associative BCI.

This coupling was later also demonstrated for a fully self-paced BCI (Mrachacz-Kersting et al. 2011; Niazi et al. 2012) where movement detection occurred before the imagined movement onset. Upon online single-trial detection, a peripheral electric stimulation was delivered to the common peroneal nerve, timed at the PN of the MRCP. Even though the detection accuracy attained values of only approximately 65% (true positive rate), with a relatively high false-positive rate of >20%, significant plasticity was induced within the motor cortical representation of the target muscle (Niazi et al. 2012).

In these initial studies, the peripherally generated afferent signal was relatively weak and just above motor threshold. At such intensities, the primary afferents recruited were the muscle spindle Ia afferents that are the fastest-conducting neurons in the human nervous system. In addition, the electrical stimulation of a peripheral nerve leads to a very synchronous afferent volley. However, during natural movements, the Ia afferent activity is relatively small with respect to spindle group II afferents, sensitive to changes in the amplitude of stretch of a muscle, or group Ib afferents, arising from Golgi tendon organs and sensitive to force (Nielsen and Sinkjaer 2002; Sinkjaer et al. 2000, 2001). In the relearning of tasks such as required in stroke rehabilitation, it may thus be desirable to generate more natural afferent feedback. In an effort to test this idea, we used an active motorized ankle foot orthosis that was triggered as part of a self-paced associative BCI. This intervention also induced significant plasticity in the motor cortex (Xu et al. 2014b), similar to our original study (Mrachacz-Kersting et al. 2012a).

### 35.3.1 Effects of Type of Neurofeedback as Part of the Associative BCI

As outlined above, significant plasticity using our associative BCI may be induced irrespective of whether the peripheral stimulus that is artificially elicited comprises a single electrical stimulus delivered at an intensity just above motor threshold (Mrachacz-Kersting et al. 2012a) or a passive dorsiflexion movement induced by an exoskeleton (Xu et al. 2014b). For this BCI to be used within the daily clinical routine, it would be desirable to provide the feedback that is typically used in the existing therapies. These include both FES and passive ankle angle movements provided by a robotic device (for a review, see Laffont et al. 2014).

In a preliminary study, we sought to compare the plasticity induced at the motor cortex following the use of the cue-based associative BCI where afferent feedback was generated by a direct nerve stimulation to generate movement or an ankle angle movement (Mrachacz-Kersting 2016). Cortical plasticity was assessed using noninvasive transcranial magnetic stimulation. An example of the changes induced at the motor cortex before and immediately after either type of feedback is shown in Figure 35.4. Both nerve FES and passive changes in ankle angle led to significant increases in the excitability of the cortical projections to the target muscle without any concomitant changes at the spinal level. These effects were still present 30 min after the cessation of both interventions. There was no significant main effect of intervention, indicating that the changes occurred independently of the type of BCI intervention used. An afferent volley generated from a passive movement or an electrical stimulus arrives at the somatosensory cortex at similar times. It is thus likely that the similar effects observed here are strictly attributed to the tight coupling in time between the afferent inflow and the PN of the MRCP. This provides further support to the associative nature of the BCI system.

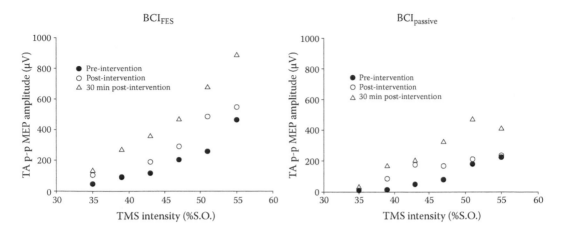

**FIGURE 35.4** Changes in motor output after the $BCI_{associative}$ intervention for a single representative participant receiving either single nerve stimulation ($BCI_{FES}$) or passive movements ($BCI_{passive}$). The motor evoked potential (MEP) size of the tibialis anterior (TA) is expressed as the peak-to-peak amplitude (p-p MEP) and the TMS intensity as a percentage of the stimulator output (S.O.). Each data point represents the average of 12 stimuli. All data are for $n = 1$.

### 35.3.2 POTENTIAL AND CHALLENGES OF MRCP-BASED ASSOCIATIVE BCI

Although closed-loop BCI systems for neuromodulation have recently been proposed according to several paradigms (Cincotti et al. 2012; Ono et al. 2013; Ramos-Murguialday et al. 2013; Varkuti et al. 2012), the BCI system described in this chapter is unique. Its main characteristic is the precise temporal association between motor commands and afferent volley. This association is possible because of the small latency in detection of MRCPs with respect to movement onset. So far, no other EEG signal modalities allow the detection of movement intention before movement onset without user training. This unique feature of MRCP-based brain switches results in the translation of the concept of associative plasticity to the system level. Our results on the timing needed for cortical plasticity (Mrachacz-Kersting et al. 2012a) indicate how crucial this characteristic is. In this view, it is perhaps not surprising that the proposed system has shown significant effects in patients, both functional and cortical excitability, with substantially shorter interventions (Mrachacz-Kersting et al. 2016a [p. 248],b) with respect to other methods (Cincotti et al. 2012; Ono et al. 2013; Ramos-Murguialday et al. 2013; Varkuti et al. 2012). Indeed, despite the fact that the basic concept of other interventions is similar to ours, that is, an afferent volley is triggered by brain activity decoded by a BCI, the system we developed is the only one for which the delay between motor commands and afferent volley is exactly quantified and maintained within a very precise interval.

However, while the exact timing of afferent volley is crucial for the system we propose, it also makes the system design extremely challenging. The need for a short latency has a direct impact on the accuracy in detection. Reaching high sensitivity and specificity with short latency is not always possible, and this affects the intervention. Moreover, the MRCP has a very small frequency band, which overlaps with artifacts and drifts. The reduction of these unwanted signal components in a fully automatic way and in real time is necessary for clinical applications outside the laboratory, but it is still an open issue. In addition, as for other BCI signal modalities, the plasticity induction (Mrachacz-Kersting et al. 2015a) and attention state (Aliakbaryhosseinabadi et al. 2017) of the user significantly affect the signal. Finally, as also with other BCI systems, the portability of EEG sensors and of the actuators for inducing afferent feedback is fundamental for clinical translation.

These challenges make it unlikely that a BCI therapeutic system as the one we propose will be used at home independently by patients. However, it is conceivable that clinical operators can be trained to apply this system on patients in a hospital environment. Indeed, our recent studies (Mrachacz-Kersting et al. 2016a [p. 248],b) have been fully conducted in hospitals and with physiotherapists. The substantial functional improvements that the proposed system determines and the relatively short intervention sessions needed for such an effect may well justify an investment in training clinical therapists to its use.

## REFERENCES

Aliakbaryhosseinabadi, S., V. Kostic, A. Pavlovic, S. Radovanovic, E. Nlandu Kamavuako, N. Jiang, L. Petrini, K. Dremstrup, D. Farina, and N. Mrachacz-Kersting. 2017. Influence of attention alternation on movement-related cortical potentials in healthy individuals and stroke patients. *Clinical Neurophysiology: Official Journal of the International Federation of Clinical Neurophysiology* 128 (1): 165–175.

Ang, K. K., C. Guan, K. S. Chua, B. T. Ang, C. Kuah, C. Wang, K. S. Phua, Z. Y. Chin, and H. Zhang. 2010. Clinical study of neurorehabilitation in stroke using EEG-based motor imagery brain–computer interface with robotic feedback. *Conference Proceedings: Annual International Conference of the IEEE Engineering in Medicine and Biology Society. IEEE Engineering in Medicine and Biology Society. Annual Conference* 2010: 5549–5552.

Ashe, J. 1997. Force and the motor cortex. *Behavioural Brain Research* 86: 1–15.

Becker, W., O. Hoehne, K. Iwase, and H. H. Kornhuber. 1972. Readiness potential, pre-motor positivity and other changes of cortical potential in saccadic eye movements. *Vision Research* 12 (3): 421–436.

Becker, W., K. Iwase, R. Juergens, and H. H. Konrhuber. 1976. Brain potentials preceding slow and rapid hand movements. In *The Responsive Brain*, edited by W. C. McCallum and J. R. Knott. 1st ed., 99–102. Bristol: J. Wright and Son.

Beisteiner, R., P. Hollinger, G. Lindinger, W. Lang, and A. Berthoz. 1995. Mental representations of movements. Brain potentials associated with imagination of hand movements. *Electroencephalography and Clinical Neurophysiology* 96 (2): 183–193.

Bliss, T. V. P. and G. L. Collingridge. 1993. A synaptic model of memory: Long-term potentiation in the hippocampus. *Nature* 361 (6407): 31–39.

Bliss, T. V. P. and S. F. Cooke. 2011. Long-term potentiation and long-term depression: A clinical perspective. *Clinics (Sao Paulo)* 66 Suppl 1 (1980-5322; 1807-5932): 3–17.

Bliss, T. V. P. and T. Lomo. 1973. Long-lasting potentiation of synaptic transmission in the dentate area of the anaesthetized rabbit following stimulation of the perforant path. *The Journal of Physiology* 232 (2): 331–356.

Boschert, J., P. Brickett, H. Weinberg, and L. Deecke. 1983. Movement-related potentials preceding toe plantarflexion and dorsiflexion. *Human Neurobiology* 2 (2): 87–90.

Broetz, D., C. Braun, C. Weber, S. R. Soekadar, A. Caria, and N. Birbaumer. 2010. Combination of brain–computer interface training and goal-directed physical therapy in chronic stroke: A case report. *Neurorehabilitation and Neural Repair* 24 (7): 674–679.

Brunia, C. H. and W. E. Van den Bosch. 1984a. Movement-related slow potentials. I. A contrast between finger and foot movements in right-handed subjects. *Electroencephalography and Clinical Neurophysiology* 57 (6): 515–527.

Brunia, C. H. and W. E. van den Bosch. 1984b. The influence of response side on the readiness potential prior to finger and foot movements. A preliminary report. *Annals of the New York Academy of Sciences* 425: 434–437.

Cincotti, F., F. Pichiorri, P. Arico, F. Aloise, F. Leotta, F. de Vico Fallani, R. Millan Jdel, M. Molinari, and D. Mattia. 2012. EEG-based brain–computer interface to support post-stroke motor rehabilitation of the upper limb. *Conference Proceedings: Annual International Conference of the IEEE Engineering in Medicine and Biology Society. IEEE Engineering in Medicine and Biology Society. Annual Conference* 2012: 4112–4115.

Cooke, S. F. and T. V. P. Bliss. 2006. Plasticity in the human central nervous system. *Brain* 129: 1659–1673.

Cunnington, R., R. Iansek, J. L. Bradshaw, and J. G. Phillips. 1996. Movement-related potentials associated with movement preparation and motor imagery. *Experimental Brain Research* 111 (3): 429–436.

Daly, J. J., R. Cheng, J. Rogers, K. Litinas, K. Hrovat, and M. Dohring. 2009. Feasibility of a new application of noninvasive brain computer interface (BCI): A case study of training for recovery of volitional motor control after stroke. *Journal of Neurologic Physical Therapy* 33 (1557-0584; 1557-0576; 4): 203–211.

Decety, J. 1996a. Do imagined and executed actions share the same neural substrate? *Brain Research. Cognitive Brain Research* 3 (2): 87–93.

Decety, J. 1996b. The neurophysiological basis of motor imagery. *Behavioural Brain Research* 77 (1–2): 45–52.

Decety, J. and M. Jeannerod. 1995. Imagery and its neurological substrate. *Revue Neurologique* 151 (8–9): 474–479.

Deecke, L., T. Bashore, C. H. Brunia, E. Grunewald-Zuberbier, G. Grunewald, and R. Kristeva. 1984. Movement-associated potentials and motor control. Report of the EPIC VI Motor Panel. *Annals of the New York Academy of Sciences* 425: 398–428.

Deecke, L., H. Eisinger, and H. H. Kornhuber. 1980. Comparison of bereitschaftspotential, pre-motion positivity and motor potential preceding voluntary flexion and extension movements in man. *Progress in Brain Research* 54: 171–176.

Deecke, L., M. Engel, W. Lang, and H. H. Kornhuber. 1986. Bereitschaftspotential preceding speech after holding breath. *Experimental Brain Research* 65 (1): 219–223.

Deecke, L., B. Grozinger, and H. H. Kornhuber. 1976. Voluntary finger movement in man: Cerebral potentials and theory. *Biological Cybernetics* 23 (2): 99–119.

Deecke, L. and H. H. Kornhuber. 1978. An electrical sign of participation of the mesial 'supplementary' motor cortex in human voluntary finger movement. *Brain Research* 159 (2): 473–476.

Deecke, L., P. Scheid, and H. H. Kornhuber. 1969. Distribution of readiness potential, pre-motion positivity, and motor potential of the human cerebral cortex preceding voluntary finger movements. *Experimental Brain Research* 7 (2): 158–168.

do Nascimento, O. F. and D. Farina. 2008. Movement-related cortical potentials allow discrimination of rate of torque development in imaginary isometric plantar flexion. *IEEE Transactions on Bio-Medical Engineering* 55 (1558-2531; 0018-9294; 11): 2675–2678.

do Nascimento, O. F., K. D. Nielsen, and M. Voigt. 2005a. Influence of directional orientations during gait initiation and stepping on movement-related cortical potentials. *Behavioural Brain Research* 161 (0166-4328; 0166-4328; 1): 141–154.

do Nascimento, O. F., K. D. Nielsen, and M. Voigt. 2005b. Relationship between plantar-flexor torque generation and the magnitude of the movement-related potentials. *Experimental Brain Research* 160 (0014-4819; 0014-4819; 2): 154–165.

do Nascimento, O. F., K. D. Nielsen, and M. Voigt. 2006. Movement-related parameters modulate cortical activity during imaginary isometric plantar-flexions. *Experimental Brain Research* 171 (1): 78–90.

Farina, D., O. F. do Nascimento, M. F. Lucas, and C. Doncarli. 2007. Optimization of wavelets for classification of movement-related cortical potentials generated by variation of force-related parameters. *Journal of Neuroscience Methods* 162 (1–2): 357–363.

Fetz, E. E. and P. D. Cheney. 1979. Muscle fields and response properties of primate corticomotoneuronal cells. *Progress in Brain Research* 50: 137–146.

Georgopoulos, A. P., J. Ashe, N. Smyrnis, and M. Taira. 1992. The motor cortex and the coding of force. *Science* 256: 1692–1695.

Georgopoulos, A. P., A. B. Schwartz, and R. E. Kettner. 1986. Neuronal population coding of movement direction. *Science (New York, N.Y.)* 233 (4771): 1416–1419.

Groenewegen, H. J. and H. B. Uylings. 2000. The prefrontal cortex and the integration of sensory, limbic and autonomic information. *Progress in Brain Research* 126: 3–28.

Gu, Y., K. Dremstrup, and D. Farina. 2009a. Single-trial discrimination of type and speed of wrist movements from EEG recordings. *Clinical Neurophysiology* 120 (1872-8952; 1388-2457; 8): 1596–1600.

Gu, Y., D. Farina, A. R. Murguialday, K. Dremstrup, and N. Birbaumer. 2013. Comparison of movement related cortical potential in healthy people and amyotrophic lateral sclerosis patients. *Frontiers in Neuroscience* 7: 65.

Gu, Y., D. Farina, A. R. Murguialday, K. Dremstrup, P. Montoya, and N. Birbaumer. 2009b. Offline identification of imagined speed of wrist movements in paralyzed ALS patients from single-trial EEG. *Frontiers in Neuroscience* 3 (1662-453; 1662-453): 62.

Gu, Y., O. do Nascimento, M. F. Lucas, and D. Farina. 2009c. Identification of task parameters from movement-related cortical potentials. *Medical and Biological Engineering and Computing* 47 (12): 1257–1264.

Hamano, T., H. O. Luders, A. Ikeda, T. F. Collura, Y. G. Comair, and H. Shibasaki. 1997. The corti-cal generators of the contingent negative variation in humans: A study with subdural electrodes. *Electroencephalography and Clinical Neurophysiology/Evoked Potentials Section* 104 (3): 257–268.

Hebb, D. O. 1949. *The Organization of Behavior: A Neuropsychological Theory*, edited by M. E. Hebb. Vol. 1. Mahwah, NJ: Lawrence Erlbaum Associates Inc.

Heremans, E., W. F. Helsen, H. J. De Poel, K. Alaerts, P. Meyns, and P. Feys. 2009. Facilitation of motor imagery through movement-related cueing. *Brain Research* 1278: 50–58.

Hink, R. F., L. Deecke, and H. H. Kornhuber. 1983. Force uncertainty of voluntary movement and human movement-related potentials. *Biological Psychology* 16 (3–4): 197–210.

Hink, R. F., H. Kohler, L. Deecke, and H. H. Kornhuber. 1982. Risk-taking and the human bereitschaftspoten-tial. *Electroencephalography and Clinical Neurophysiology* 53 (4): 361–373.

Ibanez, J., J. I. Serrano, M. D. del Castillo, E. Monge-Pereira, F. Molina-Rueda, I. Alguacil-Diego, and J. L. Pons. 2014. Detection of the onset of upper-limb movements based on the combined analysis of changes in the sensorimotor rhythms and slow cortical potentials. *Journal of Neural Engineering* 11 (5): 056009-2560/11/5/056009. Epub 2014 Aug 1.

Jeannerod, M. and J. Decety. 1995. Mental motor imagery: A window into the representational stages of action. *Current Opinion in Neurobiology* 5 (6): 727–732.

Jiang, N., L. Gizzi, N. Mrachacz-Kersting, K. Dremstrup, and D. Farina. 2014. A brain computer inter-face for single-trial detection of gait initiation from movement related cortical potentials. *Clinical Neurophysiology*.

Jochumsen, M., I. K. Niazi, N. Mrachacz-Kersting, D. Farina, and K. Dremstrup. 2013. Detection and classi-fication of movement-related cortical potentials associated with task force and speed. *Journal of Neural Engineering* 10 (1741-2552; 1741-2552; 5): 056015.

Kasashima-Shindo, Y., T. Fujiwara, J. Ushiba, Y. Matsushika, D. Kamatani, M. Oto, T. Ono et al. 2015. Brain–computer interface training combined with transcranial direct current stimulation in patients with chronic severe hemiparesis: Proof of concept study. *Journal of Rehabilitation Medicine* 47 (4): 318–324.

Kornhuber, H. H. and L. Deecke. 1965. Changes in the brain potential in voluntary movements and pas-sive movements in man: Readiness potential and reafferent potential. *Pflugers Arch Gesamte Physiol Menschen Tiere* 284 (0365-267; 0365-267): 1–17.

Kristeva, R., E. Keller, L. Deecke, and H. H. Kornhuber. 1979. Cerebral potentials preceding unilateral and simultaneous bilateral finger movements. *Electroencephalography and Clinical Neurophysiology* 47 (2): 229–238.

Kuhtz-Buschbeck, J. P., C. Mahnkopf, C. Holzknecht, H. Siebner, S. Ulmer, and O. Jansen. 2003. Effector-independent representations of simple and complex imagined finger movements: A combined fMRI and TMS study. *European Journal of Neuroscience* 18 (12): 3375–3387.

Kutas, M. and E. Donchin. 1974. Studies of squeezing: Handedness, responding hand, response force, and asymmetry of readiness potential. *Science (New York, N.Y.)* 186 (4163): 545–548.

Lacourse, M. G., M. J. Cohen, K. E. Lawrence, and D. H. Romero. 1999. Cortical potentials during imagined movements in individuals with chronic spinal cord injuries. *Behavioural Brain Research* 104 (1–2): 73–88.

Laffont, I., K. Bakhti, F. Coroian, L. van Dokkum, D. Mottet, N. Schweighofer, and J. Froger. 2014. Innovative technologies applied to sensorimotor rehabilitation after stroke. *Annals of Physical and Rehabilitation Medicine* 57 (8): 543–551.

Lang, W., M. Lang, F. Uhl, C. Koska, A. Kornhuber, and L. Deecke. 1988. Negative cortical DC shifts preced-ing and accompanying simultaneous and sequential finger movements. *Experimental Brain Research* 71 (3): 579–587.

Leifert-Fiebach, G., A. Welfringer, R. Babinsky, and T. Brandt. 2013. Motor imagery training in patients with chronic neglect: A pilot study. *NeuroRehabilitation* 32 (1): 43–58.

Li, M., Y. Liu, Y. Wu, S. Liu, J. Jia, and L. Zhang. 2014. Neurophysiological substrates of stroke patients with motor imagery-based brain–computer interface training. *The International Journal of Neuroscience* 124 (6): 403–415.

Lin, C., B. Wang, N. Jiang, R. Xu, N. Mrachacz-Kersting, and D. Farina. 2016. Discriminative manifold learn-ing based detection of movement-related cortical potentials. *IEEE Transactions on Neural Systems and Rehabilitation Engineering: A Publication of the IEEE Engineering in Medicine and Biology Society*.

McFarland, D. J., L. M. McCane, S. V. David, and J. R. Wolpaw. 1997. Spatial filter selection for EEG-based communication. *Electroencephalography and Clinical Neurophysiology* 103 (3): 386–394.

Mrachacz-Kersting, N. 2016. Effect of feedback type on the effectiveness of a novel associative BCI protocol targeting the tibialis anterior muscle. *Converging Clinical and Engineering Research on Neurorehabilitation II: Proceedings of the 3rd International Conference on NeuroRehabilitation, ICNR 2016*, 18–21 October 2016, Segovia, Spain, 13–17.

Mrachacz-Kersting, N., N. Jiang, S. Aliakbaryhosseinabadi, R. Xu, L. Petrini, R. Lontis, K. Dremstrup, and D. Farina. 2015a. The changing brain: Bidirectional learning between algorithm and user. In *Brain–Computer Interface Research: A State-of-the-Art Summary 4*, edited by C. Guger, B. Z. Allison and G. Edlinger: Springer.

Mrachacz-Kersting, N., N. Jiang, A. J. Stevenson, I. K. Niazi, V. Kostic, A. Pavlovic, S. Radovanovic et al. 2016b. Efficient neuroplasticity induction in chronic stroke patients by an associative brain–computer interface. *Journal of Neurophysiology* 115 (3): 1410–1421.

Mrachacz-Kersting, N., S. R. Kristensen, I. K. Niazi, and D. Farina. 2012a. Precise temporal association between cortical potentials evoked by motor imagination and afference induces cortical plasticity. *The Journal of Physiology* 590 (Pt 7): 1669–1682.

Mrachacz-Kersting, N., I. K. Niazi, and D. Farina. 2011. Movement related cortical potentials: Asynchronous versus synchronous brain computer interfaces. *Clinical Neurophysiology* 122: S16, No. W5.3.

Mrachacz-Kersting, N., I. K. Niazi, N. Jiang, A. M. Pavlovic, S. Radovanovic, V. S. Kostiç, D. B. Popovic, K. Dremstrup, and D. Farina. 2012b. A novel brain–computer interface for chronic stroke patients. *Converging Clinical and Engineering Research on Neurorehabilitation*, pp. 837–841.

Mrachacz-Kersting, N., A. J. T. Stevenson, S. Aliakbaryhosseinabadi, A. C. Lundgaard, H. R. Jørgensen, K. Severinsen, and D. Farina. 2016a. An associative brain–computer-interface for acute stroke patients. *Converging Clinical and Engineering Research on Neurorehabilitation II*, pp. 841–845.

Mukaino, M., T. Ono, K. Shindo, T. Fujiwara, T. Ota, A. Kimura, M. Liu, and J. Ushiba. 2014. Efficacy of brain–computer interface-driven neuromuscular electrical stimulation for chronic paresis after stroke. *Journal of Rehabilitation Medicine* 46 (4): 378–382.

Niazi, I. K., N. Jiang, M. Jochumsen, J. F. Nielsen, K. Dremstrup, and D. Farina. 2013. Detection of movement-related cortical potentials based on subject-independent training. *Medical & Biological Engineering & Computing* 51 (5): 507–512.

Niazi, I. K., N. Jiang, O. Tiberghien, J. Feldbæk-Nielsen, K. Dremstrup, and D. Farina. 2011. Detection of movement intention from single-trial movement-related cortical potentials. *Journal of Neural Engineering* 8 (6): 066009.

Niazi, I. K., N. Mrachacz-Kersting, N. Jiang, K. Dremstrup, and D. Farina. 2012. Peripheral electrical stimulation triggered by self-paced detection of motor intention enhances motor evoked potentials. *IEEE Transactions on Neural Systems and Rehabilitation Engineering* 20 (1558-0210; 1534-4320; 4): 595–604.

Nielsen, J. B. and T. Sinkjaer. 2002. Afferent feedback in the control of human gait. *Journal of Electromyography Kinesiology* 12 (1050-6411; 3): 213–217.

Ono, T., M. Mukaino, and J. Ushiba. 2013. Functional recovery in upper limb function in stroke survivors by using brain–computer interface: A single case A-B-A-B design. *Conference Proceedings:...Annual International Conference of the IEEE Engineering in Medicine and Biology Society. IEEE Engineering in Medicine and Biology Society Annual Conference* 2013: 265–268.

Penfield, W. and H. Jasper. 1954. *Epilepsy and the Functional Anatomy of the Human Brain*. Boston, MA: Little, Brown.

Pichiorri, F., G. Morone, M. Petti, J. Toppi, I. Pisotta, M. Molinari, S. Paolucci et al. 2015. Brain–computer interface boosts motor imagery practice during stroke recovery. *Annals of Neurology* 77 (5): 851–865.

Ramos-Murguialday, A., D. Broetz, M. Rea, L. Laer, O. Yilmaz, F. L. Brasil, G. Liberati et al. 2013. Brain–machine interface in chronic stroke rehabilitation: A controlled study. *Annals of Neurology* 74 (1531-8249; 0364-5134; 1): 100–108.

Ray, W. J., S. Slobounov, J. T. Mordkoff, J. Johnston, and R. F. Simon. 2000. Rate of force development and the lateralized readiness potential. *Psychophysiology* 37 (6): 757–765.

Salinet, A. S. M., Thompson G. Robinson, and R. B. Panerai. 2012. Reproducibility of cerebral and peripheral haemodynamic responses to active, passive and motor imagery paradigms in older healthy volunteers: A fTCD study. *Journal of Neuroscience Methods* 206 (2): 143–150.

Sburlea, A. I., L. Montesano, and J. Minguez. 2015. Continuous detection of the self-initiated walking pre-movement state from EEG correlates without session-to-session recalibration. *Journal of Neural Engineering* 12 (3): 036007-2560/12/3/036007. Epub 2015 Apr 27.

Sburlea, A. I., L. Montesano, and J. Minguez. 2017. Advantages of EEG phase patterns for the detection of gait intention in healthy and stroke subjects. *Journal of Neural Engineering* 14 (3): 036004-2552/aa5f2f.

Sinkjaer, T., J. B. Andersen, M. Ladouceur, L. O. Christensen, and J. B. Nielsen. 2000. Major role for sensory feedback in soleus EMG activity in the stance phase of walking in man. *The Journal of Physiology* 523 Pt 3 (0022-3751): 817–827.

Sinkjaer, T., J. B. Nielsen, M. Voigt, M. Ladouceur, M. J. Grey, and J. B. Andersen. 2001. Muscle afferent feedback during human walking. Chap. 9, In *Motor Neurobiology of the Spinal Cord*, edited by T. C. Cape, 215–229. London: CRC Press.

Slobounov, S., M. Rearick, and H. Chiang. 2000. EEG correlates of finger movements as a function of range of motion and pre-loading conditions. *Clinical Neurophysiology: Official Journal of the International Federation of Clinical Neurophysiology* 111 (11): 1997–2007.

Slobounov, S., R. Tutwiler, M. Rearick, and J. H. Challis. 1999. EEG correlates of finger movements with different inertial load conditions as revealed by averaging techniques. *Clinical Neurophysiology: Official Journal of the International Federation of Clinical Neurophysiology* 110 (10): 1764–1773.

Slobounov, S. M. and W. J. Ray. 1998. Movement-related potentials with reference to isometric force output in discrete and repetitive tasks. *Experimental Brain Research* 123 (0014-4819; 0014-4819; 4): 461–473.

Stefan, K., E. Kunesch, L. G. Cohen, R. Benecke, and J. Classen. 2000. Induction of plasticity in the human motor cortex by paired associative stimulation. *Brain* 123 (3): 572–584.

Terada, K., A. Ikeda, T. Nagamine, and H. Shibasaki. 1995. Movement-related cortical potentials associated with voluntary muscle relaxation. *Electroencephalography and Clinical Neurophysiology* 95: 335–345.

Terada, K., A. Ikeda, S. Yazawa, T. Nagamine, and H. Shibasaki. 1999. Movement-related cortical potentials associated with voluntary relaxation of foot muscles. *Clinical Neurophysiology: Official Journal of the International Federation of Clinical Neurophysiology* 110 (3): 397–403.

Uhl, F., W. Lang, M. Lang, A. Kornhuber, and L. Deecke. 1988. Cortical slow potentials in verbal and spatial tasks—The effect of material, visual hemifield and performing hand. *Neuropsychologia* 26 (5): 769–775.

Varkuti, B., C. Guan, Y. Pan, K. S. Phua, K. K. Ang, C. W. K. Kuah, K. Chua, B. T. Ang, N. Birbaumer, and R. Sitaram. 2012. Resting state changes in functional connectivity correlate with movement recovery for BCI and robot-assisted upper-extremity training after stroke. *Neurorehabilitation and Neural Repair*.

Walter, W. G., R. Cooper, V. J. Aldridge, W. C. McCallum, and A. L. Winter. 1964. Contingent negative variation: An electric sign of sensorimotor association and expectancy in the human brain. *Nature* 203 (0028-0836; 0028-0836): 380–384.

Wilke, J. T. and R. W. Lansing. 1973. Variations in the motor potential with force exerted during voluntary arm movements in man. *Electroencephalography and Clinical Neurophysiology* 35 (3): 259–265.

Xu, R., N. Jiang, C. Lin, N. Mrachacz-Kersting, K. Dremstrup, and D. Farina. 2014a. Enhanced low-latency detection of motor intention from EEG for closed-loop brain-computer interface applications. *IEEE Transactions on Bio-Medical Engineering* 61 (1558-2531; 0018-9294; 2): 288–296.

Xu, R., N. Jiang, N. Mrachacz-Kersting, K. Dremstrup, and D. Farina. 2016. Factors of influence on the performance of a short-latency non-invasive brain switch: Evidence in healthy individuals and implication for motor function rehabilitation. *Frontiers in Neuroscience* 9: 527.

Xu, R., N. Jiang, N. Mrachacz-Kersting, C. Lin, G. Asin Prieto, J. C. Moreno, J. L. Pons, K. Dremstrup, and D. Farina. 2014b. A closed-loop brain-computer interface triggering an active ankle-foot orthosis for inducing cortical neural plasticity. *IEEE Transactions on Bio-Medical Engineering* 61 (7): 2092–2101.

Yazawa, S., H. Shibasaki, A. Ikeda, K. Terada, T. Nagamine, and M. Honda. 1997. Cortical mechanism underlying externally cued gait initiation studied by contingent negative variation. *Electroencephalography and Clinical Neurophysiology* 105 (0013-4694; 0013-4694; 5): 390–399.

Young, B. M., Z. Nigogosyan, L. M. Walton, J. Song, V. A. Nair, S. W. Grogan, M. E. Tyler et al. 2014. Changes in functional brain organization and behavioral correlations after rehabilitative therapy using a brain–computer interface. *Frontiers in Neuroengineering* 7: 26.

# 36 Past and Future of Multi-Mind Brain–Computer Interfaces

*Davide Valeriani and Ana Matran-Fernandez*

## CONTENTS

36.1 Introduction..........................................................................................................686
36.2 Theoretical Aspects of Multi-Mind BCIs............................................................687
    36.2.1 History of Multi-Mind BCIs....................................................................687
    36.2.2 Implementing a Collective Brain..............................................................688
    36.2.3 How Many Minds Are Needed?................................................................689
    36.2.4 Influence of Participant Similarity When Forming Groups......................689
    36.2.5 Challenges.................................................................................................690
36.3 Applications.........................................................................................................690
    36.3.1 Communication ........................................................................................691
    36.3.2 Control of External Devices......................................................................691
    36.3.3 Video Games ............................................................................................692
    36.3.4 Target Detection and Decision Making.....................................................693
    36.3.5 Music........................................................................................................694
36.4 Tutorial.................................................................................................................695
    36.4.1 Application................................................................................................695
    36.4.2 Number of Users ......................................................................................695
    36.4.3 Real-Time Requirement............................................................................696
    36.4.4 Operation Mode........................................................................................696
    36.4.5 Fusion of Brain Signals............................................................................696
36.5 Future Directions.................................................................................................697
References.......................................................................................................................698

### Abstract

The great improvements in brain–computer interface (BCI) performance that are brought upon by merging brain activity from multiple users have made this a popular strategy that allows even for human augmentation. These *multi-mind BCIs* have contributed in changing the role of BCIs from assistive technologies for people with disabilities into tools for human enhancement. This chapter reviews the history of multi-mind BCIs that have their root in the hyperscanning technique; the *collaborative* and *competitive* approaches; and the different ways that exist to integrate the brain signals from multiple people and optimally form groups to maximize performance. The main applications of multi-mind BCIs, including control of external devices, entertainment, and decision making, are also surveyed and discussed, in order to help the reader understand what are the most promising avenues and find the gaps that are worthy of future exploration. The chapter also provides a step-by-step tutorial to the design and implementation of a multi-mind BCI, with theoretical guidelines and a sample application.

## 36.1 INTRODUCTION

Brain–computer interfaces (BCIs) have traditionally been employed to help people with disabilities communicate or control prostheses (Wolpaw et al. 2002; see Chapter 4 ["Brain–Computer Interfaces for Motor Rehabilitation, Assessment of Consciousness, and Communication"] by Guger et al. and Chapter 5 ["Therapeutic Applications of BCI Technologies"] by McFarland in this handbook). Many advances have been done in research in the last few decades that have allowed for the development of more reliable BCIs (see Chapter 6 ["Advances in Neuroprosthetics: Past, Present, and Future"] by Dambrot). For example, new hardware has improved the signal-to-noise ratio of brain signals recorded and used to control BCIs, while innovative algorithms and machine learning techniques have boosted classification performance. As a result, innovative applications of BCIs have been proposed, targeting a broader range of users (van Erp et al. 2012).

One of the main focuses of this new line of investigation is the development of new BCIs based on the brain activity recorded from *multiple users* simultaneously. These devices have been introduced as *hyperscanning* systems when used for passive applications, such as monitoring the brain activity (Babiloni and Astolfi 2014), and as *multi-mind* (also called *multi-brain* or *multi-user*) *BCIs* for active control, for example, to improve human performance in target detection (Wang and Jung 2011). Despite the fact that this area of research has just recently appeared, a high number of papers have been published in this field. Multi-mind BCIs have shown the potential of improving the performance of single-user BCIs for people with disabilities (Li and Nam 2016), as well as augmenting human performance (Wang and Jung 2011). While this research field is relatively new, much effort has been put in investigating different modalities of implementing a collective brain (Cecotti and Rivet 2014a; Wang and Jung 2011), so that current and future researchers could focus on innovative applications of these technologies.

The aim of this chapter is to provide the reader with an overview of multi-mind BCIs based on electroencephalography (EEG). We assume that the reader is familiar with BCIs (for a detailed introduction to these systems, please refer to Chapter 1 ["Brain–Computer Interface: An Emerging Interaction Technology"] by Nam et al.). We will consider as multi-mind BCIs all those devices that use *the brain activity of at least two participants* to perform an active task (i.e., the BCI is actively being used to achieve a goal, and not only for monitoring, e.g., to move a prosthetic arm or make a selection on the screen). These include both collaborative and competitive BCIs, as long as the state of the interface depends on the brain signals of multiple people. If the users are trying to reach a common goal, the multi-mind BCI will be categorized as a *collaborative BCI*, regardless of the way in which the information from their brains is fused. If, on the contrary, users are competing against each other or are given individual goals that do not allow collaboration between them, we will consider this to be a *competitive BCI*. Both collaborative and competitive BCIs are *active BCIs*, since the brain activity of the participants has a direct impact on the state of the interface. Passive multi-mind BCIs (or hyperscanning systems, see Chapter 3 ["Passive Brain–Computer Interfaces: A Perspective on Increased Interactivity"] by Krol et al.), traditionally used to monitor the brain activity of multiple users while performing a certain task, will not be covered in this chapter.

Occasionally, the name "collaborative BCIs" has been associated with systems where the output depends on a combination of artificial intelligence and single-user BCIs (Göhring et al. 2013; Katyal et al. 2014) and not on the brain signals of multiple users. Such systems are more commonly described as hybrid BCIs (see Chapter 27 ["Hybrid Brain–Computer Interfaces and Their Applications"] by Pan and Li), a term that can refer either to shared control with an artificial agent— for example, when controlling a wheelchair, sensors will stop it if they detect an obstacle (Philips et al. 2007)—or to situations in which multiple (different) signals from the user are used to control the BCI—for example, physiological signals (e.g., amount of sweat and heart rate), behavioral measures (e.g., key presses), or different types of EEG-evoked responses (Müller-Putz et al. 2011). Nevertheless, this definition does not exclude the possibility of creating multi-mind hybrid BCIs.

The organization of this chapter is as follows. Section 36.2 reviews the origin and development of multi-mind BCIs and describes the techniques that have been used in this field, introducing the main technological challenges and open issues. Section 36.3 presents an overview of the main applications of multi-mind BCIs found in the literature. Section 36.4 provides a tutorial on how to build a multi-brain BCI. Finally, in Section 36.5, we outline some suggestions for future developments of BCIs based on brain signals of multiple users.

## 36.2 THEORETICAL ASPECTS OF MULTI-MIND BCIs

This section reviews different aspects of multi-mind BCIs from a theoretical point of view. We will start by providing a short summary of the origin and evolution of these systems over the last few decades and then consider different features that reflect the state of the art in multi-mind BCIs.

### 36.2.1 HISTORY OF MULTI-MIND BCIs

The origin of multi-mind BCIs can be found in *hyperscanning*, a technique to measure and analyze the brain activity of two or more people while they participate in a common activity, for example, playing cards (Astolfi et al. 2010). The first EEG hyperscanning results date from 1965 (Babiloni and Astolfi 2014; Duane and Behrendt 1965). Hyperscanning allowed researchers to discover that collaborative and competitive tasks have different effects on the connections in the brains of participants performing behavioral experiments. For a review on hyperscanning, we refer the reader to Babiloni and Astolfi (2014).

The hyperscanning technique was primarily conceived as a way of measuring, at a neurological level, the effects of social interaction. The idea of monitoring multiple people was later used in what can be considered as *passive multi-mind BCIs*. Examples of this can be found in the work of Hasson et al. (2004) and Hasson et al. (2008), in which the authors assessed the effects of feature films on brain activity during free movie watching. The main result of their work was to show that aspects such as movie content, editing, and directing style have a direct impact on the level of control over the viewer's brain activity. Later studies used passive multi-mind BCIs to show the high level of intersubject correlation during natural vision (Bridwell et al. 2015). This discovery made it possible to study the brain's naive responses to stimuli by averaging signals across multiple users, hence increasing the low signal-to-noise ratio that is typical in EEG-based BCIs. Moreover, the high time resolution provided by EEG systems allows researchers to use this technique also for *active multi-mind BCIs*, for example, in those based on event-related potentials (ERPs), which traditionally rely on multiple repetitions of a stimulus in single-user interfaces (Farwell and Donchin 1988; Jiang et al. 2015; Kapeller et al. 2014; Korczowski et al. 2015; Matran-Fernandez and Poli 2015; Vidal 1973).

Multi-mind BCIs started being developed in the 2000s using mainly a competitive form. Ilstedt Hjelm and Browall (2000) conceived a multi-mind BCI as a neurofeedback tool to help people learn how to relax through gamification. Babiloni et al. (2007) also employed the competitive approach in a game with the aim of shortening user training times in modulating alpha and mu rhythms. They were also the first ones to include disabled participants in their study, showing that multi-mind BCIs can also be useful to the disabled community (e.g., for user training). During the following years, the focus was placed mostly on collaborative BCIs, especially for augmenting human capabilities. As we will show below, research in the 2010s was devoted to studying different ways of merging evidence from multiple people (Cecotti and Rivet 2014a,b; De Vico Fallani et al. 2010), identifying an optimal group size (Cecotti and Rivet 2014a; Eckstein et al. 2012; Poli et al. 2014), and, as in the case of single-user BCIs, reducing the number of electrodes while maintaining good levels

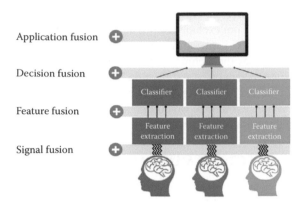

**FIGURE 36.1**   Different strategies to merge the brain activity in multi-mind BCIs.

of performance (Cecotti and Rivet 2014a). Hence, most of the recent research followed an *offline*\*
approach, in which no interaction from the users was considered.

### 36.2.2   Implementing a Collective Brain

A traditional single-user BCI is usually composed by a *signal acquisition* module, a *feature extraction* module, and a *decision* module. The brain activity of multiple users can thus be combined at four different levels: *signal*, *feature*, *decision*, and *application* levels (see Figure 36.1).

The simplest mode of combining evidence from multiple users is at the *signal level*. At this level, EEG signals of different users are averaged and either fed into a unique classifier directly, without extracting any feature (Cecotti and Rivet 2014a,b; Jiang et al. 2015; Kapeller et al. 2014; Korczowski et al. 2015; Matran-Fernandez and Poli 2014; Matran-Fernandez et al. 2013; Poli et al. 2013a), or used to perform multi-user analyses, taking advantage of the increased signal-to-noise ratio that can be achieved by averaging trials from multiple users (De Vico Fallani et al. 2010; Matran-Fernandez and Poli 2015).

In a second scenario, features extracted from each user's EEG signals could be merged. The fusion can be done by simple concatenation to form a unique feature vector or any other combination (Eckstein et al. 2012; Wang and Jung 2011), so that only one classifier is used.

Third, the outputs of individually tailored classifiers can be merged. At this level, we should mention the work from Cecotti and Rivet (2014a,b), who studied different modes of combining the BCI decisions on a P300-based collaborative BCI and a steady-state visual evoked potential (SSVEP) multi-mind BCI. Their strategies for merging the classifiers' outputs included majority voting, average of classifiers' outputs, and maximum and minimum values. They found that averaging the classifiers' outputs provided the best performance.

Bonnet et al. (2013) also proposed an additional level of integration of brain signals called the application level. In this case, the implementation of the multi-mind BCI is not done by the BCI itself but by the application operated by the BCI. This is very common in competitive scenarios, where the outputs of different single-user BCIs may be (a) used to control different avatars in a game (e.g., Li et al. 2013), (b) compared to control a unique aspect of the interface according to the intentions of the "winner" (e.g., Ling and Vučković 2016), or (c) taken into account independently for shared control of a unique interface (Bonnet et al. 2013; Le Groux et al. 2010; Li and Nam 2016;

---

\* When talking about offline/online BCIs, we follow the traditional definition: online (multi-brain) BCIs are those in which the brain signals of the users are being processed at the time of collection to control the BCI. On the contrary, an offline BCI is that in which the brain activity of the users is recorded for posterior analysis, and the state of the interface is either static or manipulated by the experimenters.

Schultze-Kraft et al. 2013). Other possible ways of making a final decision in a multi-mind system at the application level include choosing the fastest available output (e.g., if speed is a requirement of the system and it can be safely assumed that faster responders are also more accurate, perhaps in the form of a collaborative hybrid BCI), the most consistent brain activity, or the strongest one (Nijholt and Poel 2016).

A considerable amount of work has been conducted to establish which level of fusion is optimal, obtaining quite consistent results across laboratories and applications. In particular, the two approaches that are often compared are the single-trial averages across participants (i.e., signal level) and fusion at the decision level (usually averaging classifiers' outputs to send a command). Since most of this work has been done based on different ERPs, given the intersubject differences in latencies and amplitudes, it is not surprising that the best performance is obtained when information is merged at the decision level (Cecotti and Rivet 2014a,b; Matran-Fernandez and Poli 2014; Wang and Jung 2011). Such differences in performance are statistically significant (Matran-Fernandez and Poli 2014, 2017), even at the lowest level of fusion.

### 36.2.3   How Many Minds Are Needed?

Years of research in decision making have shown that bigger groups tend to lead to better decisions (Kerr and Tindale 2004). The aggregation of information from different sources can help reduce bias and increase certainty in the system's final output. In general, this is also true in the field of collaborative BCIs, where increasing group sizes has steadily led to better classification performance (Cecotti and Rivet 2014a,b; Matran-Fernandez and Poli 2017; Wang and Jung 2011) and group decisions (Eckstein et al. 2012; Poli et al. 2014; Valeriani et al. 2016). However, this increase in performance does not follow a linear relationship with the number of people included in the BCI. Indeed, there is a tipping point at group sizes between 5 and 10 users (Eckstein et al. 2012), above which the addition of a new member to a group might not be cost-effective (i.e., the small increase in performance brought upon by this member does not justify the expenses required for the additional hardware). This tipping point will vary depending on the complete system and should be studied depending on the specific application at hand. For example, Eckstein et al. (2012) found that seven brains were required to match the mean behavioral accuracy of a single observer (not using a BCI) when making perceptual decisions.

As we will show in Section 36.2.4, it might be possible to reduce the number of users of a collaborative BCI by finding users who perform similarly. Hence, in some applications, it may be worth developing a study of potential candidates and select them to perform the task at hand to obtain a small group of users that are able to outperform a bigger one at a fraction of the total cost.

### 36.2.4   Influence of Participant Similarity When Forming Groups

Depending on the level of information fusion, taking into account how similar the brain's responses from multiple users are may boost performance when creating collaborative BCIs, regardless of the metric used to assess it. This was first mentioned by Matran-Fernandez et al. (2013) in a target detection task following a rapid serial visual protocol. The authors noticed that the increase in performance obtained by pairs of observers was higher when the classification accuracy of their individual BCIs was similar, irrespective of the actual individual accuracy values. Korczowski et al. (2015) also noticed a high correlation between user similarity and BCI performance but did not explore further.

Perhaps the most comprehensive study of this effect to date is that of Matran-Fernandez and Poli (2017), who showed numerically that the biggest gains for groups of sizes between 2 and 11 can be obtained when participants are very similar, both at the signal and the classifier fusion levels, and that these gains are statistically significant even when compared against the best individual of the group. The higher gains achieved when merging the brain signals at the decision level (with respect to the signal level) could be due to the fact that the groups were created based on classification performance, which might give an inherent advantage to this fusion strategy. When fusion is done at the signal level, the differences in peak latencies and amplitudes between different users could be employed to form the groups based on similarity of their ERPs, which might yield better BCI performance (Matran-Fernandez and Poli 2016).

It should be noted that the results described above are referred to collaborative BCIs. To the best of our knowledge, there is no study of participant similarity/dissimilarity and its effects in competitive BCIs. Competitive BCIs could highly benefit from grouping participants according to their level of control, especially when used to reduce training times—for example, when learning to control the mu and alpha rhythms (Babiloni et al. 2007)—which may increase the motivation of the users.

### 36.2.5 CHALLENGES

There are some challenges that apply to BCIs, regardless of the number of users needed to control it. For example, in cue-based BCIs, there is the need of synchronizing the whole system, from the display to the acquisition modules and, possibly, also to the processing and feedback parts of the BCI. This problem is accentuated in multi-mind BCIs, both self-paced and cue-based, as the synchronization needs to be done to multiple displays (if applicable), acquisition devices, and processing nodes (Cecotti and Rivet 2014b). This issue is particularly important in online systems, where a small jitter might have a large impact in performance of both collaborative (e.g., if merging information at the signal level) and competitive (e.g., where the difference in timing may result in an advantage for one of the users) systems.

Moreover, online systems are less flexible than offline ones for posterior data analysis, especially those that involve some sort of interaction between the users. If the communication between the participants modifies in some way their behavior, regrouping users (a technique widely used in offline collaborative BCIs) might be a hard task. However, offline studies do not allow investigating the impact of such interaction, which might play a crucial role in the final online BCI. Unfortunately, this aspect remains unexplored in multi-mind BCIs of the collaborative type.

Online multi-mind BCIs also require multiple acquisition devices, which increases the overall cost of the system, as opposed to the single piece of EEG equipment that is necessary for running offline experiments. Despite the recent appearance of low-cost EEG systems, which aim at reducing preparation times, using a multi-mind BCI remains quite costly, in terms of both time and money.

There are also difficulties associated with the different levels of merging information in the multi-mind system. Leaving aside those of precisely synchronizing all the devices that are part of the multi-mind BCI, the signals from multiple users will vary in amplitude and latency due to electrode positioning and functional anatomy. Thus, it is necessary to normalize the EEG signals from each participant, especially when fusion occurs at the signal level. The same applies to other levels of fusion, where either features or classifier's outputs should be on the same scale to guarantee that the differences between them do not affect performance.

Another challenge that arises in multi-mind BCIs is that of finding a metric that can be used to compare such systems with single-user BCIs. Measures such as accuracy or the area under the receiving operating characteristic are still valid. However, if time should be considered (as it is done, e.g., by including the number of repetitions needed to control a speller in the information transfer rate [ITR], a standard of BCI performance), the formula for the ITR needs to be modified accordingly to allow for the number of users (Cecotti and Rivet 2014a).

### 36.3 APPLICATIONS

The first BCI using data recorded from multiple brains to augment performance dates back to 2011, when Wang and Jung (2011) proposed a collaborative framework for BCIs in which data from multiple participants performing a movement planning task were fused together. Since then, multi-mind BCIs have been applied to a variety of contexts, which are reviewed in this section.

### 36.3.1 COMMUNICATION

The first single-user BCIs—the matrix spellers—were developed to help people with severe disabilities communicate (Farwell and Donchin 1988). Despite recent advances (Townsend and Platsko 2016), the single-trial performance of such systems (typically based on the P300 ERP) is still far from perfect (see Chapter 18 ["Gentle Introduction to Signal Processing and Classification for Single-Trial EEG Analysis"] by Blankertz). Although averaging brain signals across a number of repetitions of the same stimulus leads to higher accuracy, this approach also reduces speed as it requires to record the ERPs associated to the same stimulus multiple times. However, BCI spellers might represent the only opportunity for locked-in patients to communicate, so every little step to improve reliability and practicality of these systems could represent a great benefit to their users.

P300-based BCIs are an attractive test bed for multi-mind BCIs, since they rely on the presence or absence of a relatively large EEG component. Since the original speller from Farwell and Donchin (1988) relied on this ERP, several researchers have tested the performance of multi-mind BCIs on spellers, admitting that it is not a realistic application of such devices, due to the need for the multiple users to agree on what to spell beforehand (Cecotti and Rivet 2014a; Kapeller et al. 2014).

Cecotti and Rivet (2014a) showed in an offline analysis how a cooperative BCI could be used to improve the accuracy of the P300 speller using different methods (summarized in Section 36.2.4). Their results suggested that averaging the BCI outputs seemed to be the best method for implementing a cooperative BCI. Increasing the group size led to better performance, as would have been the case if the number of repetitions of each row/column of the speller had been increased in a single-user BCI, although they showed that single-trial multi-mind BCIs perform better than multi-trial single-mind BCIs. However, that study did not investigate a combined approach where collaborative BCIs are based on the aggregation of trials over time and over participants.

The performance of a collaborative P300-based BCI speller was validated online by Kapeller et al. (2014), who showed that the aggregation of EEG signals of eight participants could allow a single-trial BCI to reach perfect performance. However, it was not stated what the performance would have been with fewer participants, and it raises the question of whether perfect accuracy is really needed or if it is possible to sacrifice some of the performance for a lower number of users.

Although the two studies presented in this section recognized that communication is not a practical application for collaborative BCI, their results helped show the potential of multi-mind BCIs, opening the way to more practical applications.

### 36.3.2 CONTROL OF EXTERNAL DEVICES

Another traditional application of BCIs is to control external devices (Wolpaw et al. 2002). Current single-user BCI systems can achieve reasonable performance for *simple control* tasks, such as controlling a cursor (Citi et al. 2008; Wolpaw et al. 1991) or using a robotic arm to reach and grasp an object (Hochberg et al. 2012), but they might not be accurate enough to control *complex devices*, such as manipulators with many degrees of freedom. In order to enhance accuracy of such complex devices, researchers have developed hybrid BCIs that take into account domain knowledge from the area to automatize certain tasks (Müller-Putz et al. 2011; Philips et al. 2007).

Multi-mind BCIs have also been introduced in this area to guarantee reliable control of external devices based only on neural signals. Three main approaches have been explored in this area: (a) single BCI users take turns to operate a shared external device, (b) a collaborative BCI is used to control the whole device, or (c) multiple single-user BCIs control different parts of a shared device (e.g., roll, pitch and yaw in a plane). The strategy of taking turns does not seem to be very promising as groups of users either perform on par (Li and Nam 2016) or worse (Nam et al. 2013) than single BCI users. Therefore, this section will mainly focus on strategies (b) and (c).

Collaborative BCIs were first applied to simple control tasks, such as a movement-planning task (Wang and Jung 2011) where participants were told the type of movement to perform (saccade to target, reach without eye movements, or reach with eye movements) and the direction (left, right, or center). Merging information from 20 participants at the signal, feature, and classifier levels yielded accuracies of up to 95% (accuracy in the single-user case was 66%) when predicting the direction of the movement (left vs. right) up to 250 ms before the actual motor response.

Poli et al. (2013a) developed a collaborative online ERP-based BCI where the neural signals from two users were used jointly to control a spacecraft simulator through an analog BCI. They used the normalized path length and the absolute angle deviation to compare the performance of their multi-mind BCI with that of single-user BCIs, showing that the former was significantly better than the latter. This suggests that collaborative BCIs could provide a better control of the simulator than single-user BCIs. Moreover, they showed that the success rate of single-user BCIs was much higher (67.5%) than that of a random controller (6.2%).

Other researchers developed SSVEP-based collaborative BCIs that allowed pairs of participants to operate a robot by sending target sequences of commands (Li and Nam 2016). The EEG signals of the two participants were processed by two independent BCIs and then aggregated following a majority rule. The robot knew the sequence of tasks and reacted only to correct commands, so no error correction was needed in case of BCI misclassification. An interesting aspect of those studies was the fact that they included a cohort of patients with amyotrophic lateral sclerosis, who were also able to operate the system with better accuracy and in less time than single BCI users.

The studies presented in this section showed that multi-mind BCIs can be used to control a broad range of external devices. We envision that other innovative applications will be proposed in the following years. For example, multi-mind BCIs could be used to jointly control an exoskeleton by a physiotherapist and a patient, to enhance the training of the latter. Still within the scope of rehabilitation, competitive multi-mind BCIs can also be used to improve the level of engagement of the patient while reducing training times (Ling and Vučković 2016). Finally, multi-mind BCIs could also be used as a switch to decide which agent should have the control (e.g., in an aircraft operated by an automated system and two pilots, the BCI could be used to temporarily override the artificial intelligence in case of perceived hazards).

### 36.3.3 VIDEO GAMES

Games provide a nice framework for testing the performance of a BCI while keeping users motivated and entertained. Gaming was one of the first nonmedical applications of BCIs (see Chapter 11 ["BCI and Games: Playful, Experience-Oriented Learning by Vivid Feedback?"] by Kober et al.), showing a growing interest by both researchers and the entertainment industry (Bos et al. 2010; Marshall et al. 2013; Nijholt et al. 2009; van Erp et al. 2012). Of course, there are many varieties of games, each with different interaction modalities. Some games only allow a low number of commands (e.g., arcade games), making BCI control feasible (Marshall et al. 2013). More complex games (e.g., simulation or role-playing games) might require users to quickly react to different events, or provide them with a myriad of possible actions. In the latter case, BCIs could be used as an additional alternative input, for example, to change the shape of the avatar in World of Warcraft (van de Laar et al. 2013).

The high number of actions supported by the majority of video games suggest that a promising way of using multi-mind BCIs in this area could be by sharing the control (see Section 36.2.2). This was one of the approaches tested by Schultze-Kraft et al. (2013), where pairs of participants navigated through a 2-D maze by controlling one dimension each.

Multi-mind BCIs have also been used in sports video games. Bonnet et al.'s (2013) BrainArena involved pairs of users that scored goals on the left or right side of the screen using two motor imagery BCIs. The outputs of the individual classifiers were aggregated to produce the command to be sent to the game. They tested a cooperative and a competitive manner. The performance achieved by the paired users in the cooperative mode was compared with that obtained by (a) paired users in the competitive mode and (b) single BCI users. Although no significant differences in performance between the three methods were found, comparisons in the three forms using only the best participant of each pair showed that his or her performance was significantly better in collaborative mode with respect to single-user mode.

The application fusion mode used in the competitive approach investigated by Bonnet et al. (2013) compared the outputs of the individual classifiers to decide which user's command to use to control the ball (a unique avatar). An alternative approach in competitive multi-mind BCIs would be to have users controlling different avatars in the game through independent BCIs, for example, to control multiple cars in a racing game (Li et al. 2013) or play BrainPong (Babiloni et al. 2007) and BrainBall (Ilstedt Hjelm and Browall 2000). This is also the approach that was used in the BCI race of Cybathlon 2016 (see www.cybathlon.com), where paralyzed participants used a self-paced BCI to overcome different virtual obstacles.

Multi-mind BCIs have also been employed to develop innovative video games where users score points based on their ability to modulate their brain activity. In this direction, Ling and Vučković (2016) developed a cooperative and a competitive video game. In the former, users had to modulate their alpha band powers to be as similar as possible to score a point, while in the latter, the user with the highest power would win.

Another category of video games where multi-mind BCIs have been applied is arcade games. Korczowski et al. (2015) developed a two-user BCI video game based on *Space Invaders* in which users scored extra points if they were able to reduce the number of repetitions needed for successful selection of a target. They fused information at the classifier level, using a novel method based on the assumption that the EEG signals recorded from users performing the same trials are *not* independent. While this is a reasonable assumption when users share a common goal and are presented the same stimuli, it would not be valid for competitive scenarios. However, this application shows how multi-mind BCIs could make classic games even more exciting.

Multi-mind BCIs increase the range of possible applications of BCIs in the game industry. Various types of multi-mind BCIs have been proposed in the last few years, adopting different approaches to competitive and collaborative gaming. For a review, the reader could refer to Nijholt and Poel (2016) and Nijholt (2015). Even though playing a video game using only a BCI is still difficult due to the high effort needed to control the BCI, which, could also affect the social interaction between users (Obbink et al. 2012), multi-mind BCIs could be used with very simple games to increase engagement of users while learning to modulate their brainwaves. However, shared-control multi-mind BCIs could already be used as a complementary input for complex video games. We envisage that future applications of multi-mind BCIs in games will be in these two contexts.

### 36.3.4 TARGET DETECTION AND DECISION MAKING

Decision making is one of the most promising applications of multi-mind BCIs. Every day, we have to make decisions in various situations, some of which are critical and making the wrong choice could result in dramatic consequences. Research in decision making has established that groups generally make better decisions than individuals due to group's abilities to integrate multiple percepts and information (Kerr and Tindale 2004). On the basis of these findings, BCI researchers have started investigating the possibility of using collaborative BCIs to keep the advantages of groups in decision accuracy and the intrinsic ability of the BCI to bypass the motor channels and accelerate decision making.

Considering the broad range of applications of decision making and the influence of psychology experiments on BCI research, researchers have mostly applied multi-mind BCI to target detection tasks, where groups of users have to decide whether a target object/person is present or not in a scene. A first attempt in this direction was made by Wang et al. (2011), who integrated EEG signals from multiple participants performing a detection task. Users were asked to release a button when they saw a target stimulus. The detection accuracy achieved by the collaborative BCI was significantly superior to that obtained with single-user BCIs. Furthermore, as in the case of Wang and Jung (2011), the multi-mind BCI was able to accelerate the decision with respect to the motor action. A following study (Yuan et al. 2013) validated these results with an online BCI with groups of six participants, showing that the multi-mind BCI was more accurate than the actual key releases.

These studies demonstrated the potential of collaborative BCIs to improve and accelerate target detection. However, the results were obtained with very simple tasks. In recent years, multi-mind BCIs have been applied to progressively more complex and challenging decision-making tasks, including face recognition (Jiang et al. 2015), detection of visual targets in slow (Yuan et al. 2012) and rapid presentation of images (Matran-Fernandez et al. 2013; Stoica et al. 2013), and target localization within images (Matran-Fernandez and Poli 2014, 2017). Studies from Matran-Fernandez and collaborators also found that pairing participants on the basis of their similarity in performance could further enhance the accuracy of the multi-mind BCI.

The studies mentioned so far used multi-mind BCIs to improve the performance of single-user BCIs. However, in order to present BCIs as an alternative way to make decisions, their performance should be compared with that obtained using behavioral decisions. In a study on decoding the neural patterns of collective wisdom (discriminating between pictures of cars and faces), Eckstein et al. (2012) compared the performance obtained by a multi-mind BCI with that achieved by non-BCI observers. While the multi-mind BCI was faster than the behavioral decision, it required at least seven users to achieve the same accuracy of individual observers. With such results, the authors stated that it was hard to envision scenarios for which the neural voting would replace standard behavioral voting practices.

In order to overcome the limitations of the multi-mind BCI shown by Eckstein et al. (2012), Poli et al. (2013b) proposed a *hybrid* collaborative BCI that recorded the behavioral responses from multiple participants and used the neural signals to estimate the probability of each individual decision to be correct and provide a measure of "confidence" for each user. The confidence was then used to weigh individual responses and obtain group decisions. This approach was tested with a visual pattern matching task (Poli et al. 2014). The authors showed that, for most group sizes (up to 10 users), the decisions made using the hybrid collaborative BCI were superior to those made by the best individual and those made by equally sized non-BCI groups using the standard majority. Similar results were obtained in visual search tasks using geometrical shapes (Valeriani et al. 2016) and realistic stimuli (Valeriani et al. 2015, 2017b) and for face recognition (Valeriani et al. 2017a).

Applications of multi-mind BCIs to decision making are among the most promising avenues for this technology. Hybrid collaborative BCIs could be used to assist groups, especially in critical scenarios where erroneous decisions could cause loss of lives or money. Focus should be placed on validating these approaches with online experiments, using more realistic decision-making tasks to accelerate the deployment of these technologies.

### 36.3.5  MUSIC

Repairing or augmenting human cognitive or sensorimotor functions is one of the major applications of BCIs. However, biomedical engineers and neuroscientists have occasionally joined forces with artists to use BCIs as an alternative way to produce and perform music (Miranda and Castet 2014; see Chapter 10 ["BCI for Music Making: Then, Now, and Next"] by Williams and Miranda) and other arts (Zioga et al. 2014; see Chapter 9 ["Toward Practical BCI Solutions for Entertainment and Art Performance"] by Pradhapan et al.).

In music, single-user BCIs have been used to produce melodies from the EEG. However, music could also be made by several people, for example, in an orchestra where every member plays a different instrument, hence adjusting to our definition of multi-mind BCIs. This idea was proposed by Le Groux et al. (2010). Their "multimodal brain orchestra" was composed of four members, two of them controlling an SSVEP-based BCI that modulated the articulation and accentuation of pre-composed sounds, and the other two equipped with a P300-based BCI that allowed the addition of discrete sound events, plus a director with a Wii Remote whose accelerometer controlled the tempo and decided which sound should be played. This framework showed how paradigms developed for common BCI applications (e.g., the P300 speller) could also be used in other contexts.

Music can also be used to evoke emotions. This is what Eaton et al. (2015) envisioned: valence and arousal can be derived from EEG data, so they proposed a music generator that would generate a piece based on the current states of two users in order to drive them to a common state. However, to the best of our knowledge, this idea was not brought to life.

In other arts, multi-mind BCIs have been used to support and guide the creation of polygons through interactive genetic algorithms (Kattan et al. 2015), an application that could easily lead to the production of abstract paintings.

## 36.4 TUTORIAL

The previous sections provided an introduction to the theory behind multi-mind BCIs and the main applications that have been explored for this technology. On the basis of this information, here we summarize the main design choices that a researcher should make when implementing a multi-mind BCI. Some of these are related, as they result from decisions made at an earlier stage. Hence, a bad design choice made at an initial stage could lead to major drawbacks later on. However, it is always possible to revert to a previous design choice and attempt a different path.

To help the reader follow this tuning process, we will use an example scenario in this section: the design of a multi-mind BCI to assist investors in deciding whether or not to buy a stock. At the end of each step of the tutorial, we will describe the design decision we would make in this context.

### 36.4.1 APPLICATION

The first step of designing a system is deciding the problem that it should solve. This decision involves the area of application and will influence most of the following decisions regarding the technical implementation of the system. Most of the applications you may have in mind could be fitted in one of the main categories described in Section 36.3, which might help in deciding which approach to follow. This decision will also determine the type of output the BCI should provide: a continuous output is usually appropriate for control applications, while a discrete one is adopted by most decision-making applications, where the number of possible outcomes is limited.

Example: the application would clearly fall under the decision-making category (see Section 36.3), as the BCI has to support investors to make a decision. Also, the type of output of the BCI would be binary, as the possible decisions available are either to buy or not that stock (to simplify, we assume the investors could only buy one stock, as the problem of deciding which or how many stocks to buy would be different).

### 36.4.2 NUMBER OF USERS

Deciding the number of users that will operate the multi-mind BCI is another important step of the design, directly related to the requirements of the system. On the one hand, as we showed in Section 36.2.3, a higher number of users results in better performance. On the other hand, more users also require more resources for data acquisition (e.g., electrodes and amplifiers), processing, and classification, which will in turn increase the *cost* of the multi-mind BCI.

This design choice is also highly dependent on the application of the multi-mind BCI. For most purposes, a few users are usually sufficient for adequate control and communication applications while keeping the system practical. When it comes to decision making, however, a higher number of users might be needed, especially when considering critical decision making (e.g., in finance, health, or defense). If there is a non-BCI application that the multi-mind is supposed to replace, a good starting point is to choose this number based on the non-BCI number of people needed and adjust the number afterward.

Example: the decision to be made is critical, especially if the amount to invest is large. At the same time, bigger groups will lower individual profits. Hence, our choice is to use a group of between two and four investors to operate the multi-mind BCI.

### 36.4.3 REAL-TIME REQUIREMENT

A BCI would usually work *offline* or *online*. Offline BCIs are generally used for testing and analysis purposes, allowing the brain signals to be acquired at one time and process them at a different time. On the contrary, online BCIs must satisfy real-time requirements, which may change depending on the application: a few seconds can be acceptable in some areas, while for control of external devices, the BCI response should arrive within milliseconds.

There is a trade-off between the time needed to issue a command and the accuracy of that command. In the case of single-trial decisions, it might be preferable to increase the number of users operating the multi-mind BCI to enhance the accuracy. In this way, the BCI would still benefit from quick outputs without sacrificing speed. As in the case of single-user BCIs, it is a good idea to first test a system offline to determine and adjust the requirements and then transition to online operation. However, this transition may not be straightforward, as it may be necessary to change some processing methods that are too computationally heavy for the resources available.

Example: the fast-changing nature of stock markets implies that our multi-mind BCI needs to be able to produce quick outputs (possibly with a few seconds of margin). Given that most of the approaches found in the literature rely on algorithms that are capable of dealing with single-trial decisions in real time, the system could first be validated through an offline analysis (to help decide the number of users required) but quickly migrate to an online system for it to be relevant.

### 36.4.4 OPERATION MODE

This is the core step of the design process, as it requires choosing what type of signals the multi-mind is going to work with, together with the algorithms needed for processing the neural signals and, if necessary, provide relevant feedback to the users. If using evoked potentials, as is the case of target detection systems, a way of displaying the information is needed. Most of the decisions required for the implementation of the BCI, however, are the same required to implement a single-user BCI, so we will not analyze them here, referring the reader to the relevant literature (e.g., Chapter 23 of this handbook). It should also be noted that, in the case of online operation, training data are needed to tune the machine learning component of the BCI.

Example: investors will be shown graphs representing the past story of the stock that they are trying to decide on. They could be given the opportunity to select how far into the past they want the information and also the evolution of prices for other related stocks. In order to train the BCI, investors could be asked to decide whether to buy or not at different points of the timeline (with no information of the future evolution from that point).

### 36.4.5 FUSION OF BRAIN SIGNALS

As explained in Section 36.2.4, the brain signals from multiple people could be fused at different levels. Even if the literature shows that voting methods outperform signal and feature fusion, different multi-mind BCIs might benefit from different strategies, and it is up to the developer to study which one is the most suitable for his or her purposes. For example, if the aim of the BCI is to exploit the cognition processes of the group, it may be better to average EEG data directly instead.

If the signals are combined at the decision level, a myriad of approaches is still possible (e.g., simple majority, weighted majority, second-layer classifiers, etc.). This choice will have an impact on the complexity of the whole system. An important aspect to consider is how to deal with the special case where a tie is generated, which might be frequent if using simple majority or impossible if using a classifier.

Example: considering the low number of operators chosen and the possibility of having only two of them, in order to avoid ties, we decided to adopt a weighted majority approach to fuse the decisions of the investors. In this case, the weights could be given by their levels of expertise or assigned through machine learning.

## 36.5 FUTURE DIRECTIONS

Less than a decade ago, the idea of fusing brain signals from multiple people to control a device looked like it was taken from a science fiction movie. Recent advances in neuroscience and BCI research have now made it possible through multi-mind BCIs, which, in turn, have given rise to many interesting applications. However, multi-mind BCIs have still many challenges to face, suggesting that further advances are needed in this field. One of the issues to be investigated is related to the sociological aspects of multi-mind BCIs (Bonnet et al. 2013; Cecotti and Rivet 2014a,b; Nijholt and Poel 2016). Although several groups have compared individual performance when alternating between collaborative and competitive scenarios with a multi-mind BCI (e.g., Bonnet et al. 2013), to date, very little research has been conducted on how team design, collaboration, and motivation can influence task performance in collaborative BCIs (e.g., Schultze-Kraft et al. 2013). Multi-mind BCIs give us the opportunity to study motivation and reward using ERP characteristics, for example, in competitive or collaborative modes (Cecotti and Rivet 2014a). Moreover, the fact that the performance of the system would depend on the group and not on a single individual might have an impact on how success or failure is reflected in the neural signals (Cecotti and Rivet 2014b).

Some of the applications presented in Section 36.3 will likely be explored and studied in the following years, while others may progressively be left out because they are naturally single-user (e.g., communication). We believe that using multi-mind BCIs for decision making is the most promising application, since it is directly applicable to a range of daily problems. The transition from target detection tasks used in current research to more advanced decision-making tasks (e.g., including several possible answers) will not be easy. We believe that the advances in the understanding of the human brain will help researchers identify and better characterize the processes associated with the formation of a decision and develop multi-mind BCIs that are more capable of decoding the intentions of the users. Developing low-cost EEG headsets will also affect the adoption of these systems, especially in video games and other entertainment applications that are naturally multi-user and are interesting for the general public. Furthermore, multi-mind BCIs also have the potential to be used to control devices that are too complex to operate for a single person. This could be in the form of assisting manual operations (e.g., passive systems that monitor attention or active ones for enhancing human performance) or fully operating a device via brain signals.

Multi-mind BCIs could also be used as tools to replicate social situations and give us a better understanding of social psychology (Cecotti and Rivet 2014a), to access collective mental states (Eckstein et al. 2012; cf. Chapter 8 ["Affective Brain–Computer Interfacing and Methods for Affective State Detection"] by Daly), or as a tool for neuro-marketing. In a futuristic world, they could be used in classrooms or theaters to give feedback to teachers or performers about the cognitive state of the listeners (Cecotti and Rivet 2014a). If movies produce high intersubject correlations (Bridwell et al. 2015), is the same true for real-life experiences such as a live performance?

New and established researchers in multi-mind BCIs should not limit their imagination to traditional applications and continue to conceive innovative uses of this technology, hence shaping the future of human enhancement and new interfaces.

# REFERENCES

Astolfi, L., J. Toppi, F. De Vico Fallani et al. 2010. Neuroelectrical hyperscanning measures simultaneous brain activity in humans. *Brain Topography* 23 (3): 243–256.

Babiloni, F., and L. Astolfi. 2014. Social neuroscience and hyperscanning techniques: Past, present and future. *Neuroscience & Biobehavioral Reviews* 44 (2014): 76–93.

Babiloni, F., F. Cincotti, M. G. Marciani et al. 2007. The estimation of cortical activity for brain–computer interface: Applications in a domotic context. *Computational Intelligence and Neuroscience* 2007 (91651): 1–7.

Bonnet, L., F. Lotte, and A. Lécuyer. 2013. Two brains, one game: Design and evaluation of a multi-user BCI video game based on motor imagery. *IEEE Transactions on Computational Intelligence and AI in Games* 5 (2): 185–198.

Bos, D. P.-O., B. Reuderink, B. van de Laar et al. 2010. Brain–computer interfacing and games. In *Brain–Computer Interfaces*, edited by D. S. Tan and A. Nijholt, 149–178. London: Springer.

Bridwell, D. A., C. Roth, C. N. Gupta, and V. D. Calhoun. 2015. Cortical response similarities predict which audiovisual clips individuals viewed, but are unrelated to clip preference. *PLoS ONE* 10 (6): e0128833.

Cecotti, H., and B. Rivet. 2014a. Subject combination and electrode selection in cooperative brain–computer interface based on event related potentials. *Brain Sciences* 4 (2): 335–355.

Cecotti, H., and B. Rivet. 2014b. Performance estimation of a cooperative brain–computer interface based on the detection of steady-state visual evoked potentials. In *2014 IEEE International Conference on Acoustics, Speech and Signal Processing*, 2059–2063.

Citi, L., R. Poli, C. Cinel, and F. Sepulveda. 2008. P300-based BCI mouse with genetically-optimized analogue control. *IEEE Transactions on Neural Systems and Rehabilitation Engineering* 16 (1): 51–61.

De Vico Fallani, F., V. Nicosia, R. Sinatra et al. 2010. Defecting or not defecting: How to "Read" human behavior during cooperative games by EEG measurements. *PLoS ONE* 5 (12): e14187.

Duane, T. D., and T. Behrendt. 1965. Extrasensory electroencephalographic induction between identical twins. *Science*, 150 (3694): 367.

Eaton, J., D. Williams, and E. Miranda. 2015. The space between us. Evaluating a multi-user affective brain–computer music interface. *Brain–Computer Interfaces* 2 (2–3): 103–116.

Eckstein, M. P., K. Das, B. T. Pham, M. F. Peterson, and C. K. Abbey. 2012. Neural decoding of collective wisdom with multi-brain computing. *NeuroImage* 59 (1): 94–108.

Farwell, L. A., and E. Donchin. 1988. Talking off the top of your head: Toward a mental prosthesis utilizing event-related brain potentials. *Electroencephalography and Clinical Neurophysiology* 70 (6): 510–523.

Göhring, D., D. Latotzky, M. Wang, and R. Rojas. 2013. Semi-autonomous car control using brain computer interfaces. In *Proceedings of the 12th International Conference on Intelligent Autonomous Systems (IAS)*, 393–408.

Hasson, U., O. Landesman, B. Knappmeyer, I. Vallines, N. Rubin, and D. J. Heeger. 2008. Neurocinematics: The neuroscience of film. *Projections* 2 (1): 1–26.

Hasson, U., Y. Nir, I. Levy, G. Fuhrmann, and R. Malach. 2004. Intersubject synchronization of cortical activity during natural vision. *Science* 303 (5664): 1634–1640.

Hochberg, L. R., D. Bacher, B. Jarosiewicz et al. 2012. Reach and grasp by people with tetraplegia using a neurally controlled robotic arm. *Nature* 485 (7398): 372–375.

Ilstedt Hjelm, S., and C. Browall. 2000. Brainball—Using brain activity for cool competition. In *Proceedings of NordiCHI 2000*, 177–188.

Jiang, L., Y. Wang, B. Cai, Y. Wang, W. Chen, and X. Zheng. 2015. Rapid face recognition based on single-trial event-related potential detection over multiple brains. In *7th Annual International IEEE EMBS Conference on Neural Engineering*, 106–109.

Kapeller, C., R. Ortner, G. Krausz et al. 2014. Toward multi-brain communication: Collaborative spelling with a P300 BCI. In *International Conference on Augmented Cognition*, 47–54.

Kattan, A., F. Doctor, and M. Arif. 2015. Two brains guided interactive evolution. In *2015 IEEE International Conference on Systems, Man, and Cybernetics (SMC)*, 3203–3208.

Katyal, K. D., M. S. Johannes, S. Kellis et al. 2014. A collaborative BCI approach to autonomous control of a prosthetic limb system. In *IEEE International Conference on Systems, Man and Cybernetics*, 1479–1482.

Kerr, N., and R. Tindale. 2004. Group performance and decision making. *Annual Review of Psychology* 55 (1): 623–655.

Korczowski, L., M. Congedo, and C. Jutten. 2015. Single-trial classification of multi-user P300-based brain–computer interface using Riemannian geometry. In *37th Annual International Conference of IEEE Engineering in Medicine and Biology Society*, 1769–1772.

Le Groux, S., J. Manzolli, and P. F. M. J. Verschure. 2010. Disembodied and collaborative musical interaction in the multimodal brain orchestra. In *Proceedings of the International Conference on New Interfaces for Musical Expression*, 309–314.

Li, J., Y. Liu, Z. Lu, and L. Zhang. 2013. A competitive brain computer interface: Multi-person car racing system. In *Proceedings of the Annual International Conference of the IEEE Engineering in Medicine and Biology Society (EMBS)*, 2200–2203.

Li, Y., and C. S. Nam. 2016. Collaborative brain–computer interface for people with motor disabilities. *IEEE Computational Intelligence Magazine* 11 (3): 56–66.

Ling, P., and A. Vučković. 2016. Competitive and collaborative multiuser BCI. In *Proceedings of the 6th International Brain–Computer Interface Meeting*, 228.

Marshall, D., D. Coyle, S. Wilson, and M. Callaghan. 2013. Games, gameplay, and BCI: The state of the art. *IEEE Transactions on Computational Intelligence and AI in Games* 5 (2): 82–99.

Matran-Fernandez, A., and R. Poli. 2014. Collaborative brain–computer interfaces for target localisation in rapid serial visual presentation. In *6th Computer Science and Electronic Engineering Conference (CEEC 2014)*, 127–132.

Matran-Fernandez, A., and R. Poli. 2015. Event-related potentials induced by cuts in feature movies and their exploitation for understanding cut efficacy. In *7th International IEEE EMBS Conference on Neural Engineering*, 74–77.

Matran-Fernandez, A., and R. Poli. 2016. Brain–computer interfaces for detection and localisation of targets in aerial images. *IEEE Transactions on Biomedical Engineering* 64 (6): 959–969.

Matran-Fernandez, A., and R. Poli. 2017. Towards the automated localisation of targets in rapid image-sifting by collaborative brain–computer interfaces. *PLoS ONE* 12 (5): e0178498.

Matran-Fernandez, A., R. Poli, and C. Cinel. 2013. Collaborative brain–computer interfaces for the automatic classification of images. In *6th International IEEE EMBS Conference on Neural Engineering (NER)*, 1096–1099.

Miranda, E. R., and J. Castet. 2014. *Guide to Brain–Computer Music Interfacing*. London: Springer.

Müller-Putz, G. R., C. Breitwieser, F. Cincotti et al. 2011. Tools for brain–computer interaction: A general concept for a hybrid BCI. *Frontiers in Neuroinformatics* 5: 30.

Nam, C. S., J. Lee, and S. Bahn. 2013. Brain–computer interface supported collaborative work: Implications for rehabilitation. In *35th Annual International Conference of the IEEE Engineering in Medicine and Biology Society (EMBC)*, 269–272.

Nijholt, A. 2015. Competing and collaborating brains: Multi-brain computer interfacing. In *Brain–Computer Interfaces*, ed. A. E. Hassanien, and A. T. Azar, 313–335. Springer International Publishing.

Nijholt, A., and M. Poel. 2016. Multi-brain BCI: Characteristics and social interactions. In *Proceedings of the 10th International Conference on Foundations of Augmented Cognition: Neuroergonomics and Operational Neuroscience*, 79–90.

Nijholt, A., B. Reuderink, and D. O. Bos. 2009. Turning shortcomings into challenges: Brain–computer interfaces for games. *Entertainment Computing* 1 (2): 85–94.

Obbink, M., H. Gürkök, D. P.-O. Bos, G. Hakvoort, M. Poel, and A. Nijholt. 2012. Social interaction in a cooperative brain–computer interface game. In *2012 International Conference on Intelligent Technologies for Interactive Entertainment*, 183–192. Springer Berlin Heidelberg.

Philips, J., J. del R. Millán, G. Vanacker et al. 2007. Adaptive shared control of a brain-actuated simulated wheelchair. In *2007 IEEE 10th International Conference on Rehabilitation Robotics (ICORR)*, 408–414. IEEE.

Poli, R., C. Cinel, A. Matran-Fernandez, F. Sepulveda, and A. Stoica. 2013a. Towards cooperative brain–computer interfaces for space navigation. In *Proceedings of the 2013 International Conference on Intelligent User Interfaces*, 149–160. ACM.

Poli, R., C. Cinel, F. Sepulveda, and A. Stoica. 2013b. Improving decision-making based on visual perception via a collaborative brain–computer interface. In *2013 IEEE International Multi-Disciplinary Conference on Cognitive Methods in Situation Awareness and Decision Support (CogSIMA)*, 1–8. IEEE.

Poli, R., D. Valeriani, and C. Cinel. 2014. Collaborative brain–computer interface for aiding decision-making. *PLoS ONE* 9 (7): e102693.

Schultze-Kraft, R., K. Görgen, M. Wenzel, J.-D. Haynes, and B. Blankertz. 2013. Cooperating brains: Joint control of a dual-BCI. In *Proceedings of the Fifth International Brain–Computer Interface Meeting 2013.*

Stoica, A., A. Matran-Fernandez, D. Andreou et al. 2013. Multi-brain fusion and applications to intelligence analysis. In *Proceedings of SPIE 8756, Multisensor, Multisource Information Fusion: Architectures, Algorithms, and Applications.* doi:10.1117/12.2016456.

Townsend, G., and V. Platsko. 2016. Pushing the P300-based brain–computer interface beyond 100 bpm: Extending performance guided constraints into the temporal domain. *Journal of Neural Engineering* 13 (2): 026024.

Valeriani, D., C. Cinel, R. Poli. 2017a. Augmenting group performance in target-face recognition via collaborative brain–computer interfaces for surveillance applications. In *8th International IEEE EMBS Neural Engineering Conference*, 415–418. IEEE.

Valeriani, D., C. Cinel, R. Poli. 2017b. Group augmentation in realistic visual-search decisions via a hybrid brain–computer interface. *Scientific Reports* 7 (7772): 1–12.

Valeriani, D., R. Poli, and C. Cinel. 2015. A collaborative brain–computer interface for improving group detection of visual targets in complex natural environments. In *7th International IEEE EMBS Neural Engineering Conference*, 25–28. IEEE.

Valeriani, D., R. Poli, and C. Cinel. 2016. Enhancement of group perception via a collaborative brain–computer interface. *IEEE Transactions on Biomedical Engineering* 64 (6): 1238–1248.

van de Laar, B., H. Gürkök, D. Plass-Oude Bos, M. Poel, and A. Nijholt. 2013. Experiencing BCI control in a popular computer game. *IEEE Transactions on Computational Intelligence and AI in Games* 5 (2): 176–184.

van Erp, J., F. Lotte, and M. Tangermann. 2012. Brain–computer interfaces: Beyond medical applications. *Computer* 45 (4): 26–34.

Vidal, J. J. 1973. Toward direct brain–computer communication. *Annual Review of Biophysics and Bioengineering* 2(1), 157–180.

Wang, Y., and T.-P. Jung. 2011. A collaborative brain–computer interface for improving human performance. *PLoS ONE* 6 (5): e20422.

Wang, Y., Y.-T. Wang, T.-P. Jung, X. Gao, and S. Gao. 2011. A collaborative brain–computer interface. In *2011 4th International Conference on Biomedical Engineering and Informatics (BMEI)*, 583–86. IEEE.

Wolpaw, J. R., N. Birbaumer, D. J. McFarland, G. Pfurtscheller, and T. M. Vaughan. 2002. Brain–computer interfaces for communication and control. *Clinical Neurophysiology* 113 (6): 767–791.

Wolpaw, J. R., D. J. McFarland, G. W. Neat, and C. A. Forneris. 1991. An EEG-based brain–computer interface for cursor control. *Electroencephalography and Clinical Neurophysiology* 78 (3): 252–259.

Yuan, P., Y. Wang, X. Gao, T.-P. Jung, and S. Gao. 2013. A collaborative brain–computer interface for accelerating human decision making. In *International Conference on Universal Access in Human-Computer Interaction*, 672–681. Springer Berlin Heidelberg.

Yuan, P., Y. Wang, W. Wu, and H. Xu. 2012. Study on an online collaborative BCI to accelerate response to visual targets. In *Proceedings of the 34th Annual International IEEE EMBS Conference*, 1736–1739. IEEE.

Zioga, P., M. Ma, P. Chapman, and F. Pollick. 2014. A wireless future: Performance art, interaction and the brain–computer interfaces. In *Proceedings of the ICLI 2014—Interface: International Conference on Live Interfaces*, 220–230.

# 37 Bidirectional Neural Interfaces

*Mikhail A. Lebedev and Alexei Ossadtchi*

## CONTENTS

37.1 Introduction ........................................................................................................ 701
37.2 Types of Neural Interfaces ................................................................................ 702
37.3 Neural Recordings ............................................................................................. 704
37.4 Decoding Neural Signals ................................................................................... 705
37.5 Motor Neural Interfaces .................................................................................... 708
37.6 Artificial Sensation ........................................................................................... 709
37.7 Bidirectional Neural Interfaces ......................................................................... 710
37.8 Futuristic Ideas ................................................................................................. 711
37.9 Concluding Remarks ......................................................................................... 712
References ..................................................................................................................... 712

### Abstract

Bidirectional neural interfaces link the nervous system to external devices, itself, or even the nervous systems of different individuals to treat a neural disorder, augment brain functions, or provide a means for entertainment. Such interfaces combine an efferent loop that handles information derived from neural activity and an afferent loop that delivers signals to the brain. For example, a sensorized neuroprosthetic limb can be controlled by the brain motor activity while sending signals from the prosthetic sensors back to the brain. In this chapter, we review the basic components needed for bidirectional interfaces and consider several implementations of such systems. Among the large number of relevant methodologies, we highlight electrocorticographic grids as an approach particularly suitable for developing practical interfaces for patients suffering from sensory and motor disabilities.

## 37.1 INTRODUCTION

Of all organs in the human body, the brain is clearly the most unique. Composed of billions of neurons, the brain circuits constantly process multiple streams of information, perform motor and sensory functions, produce thoughts, and generate a vivid subjective experience of being conscious. We usually take for granted that we can effortlessly perform such complex tasks as commanding our body to move, walking, maintaining balance, generating speech, perceiving the visual world, and recognizing familiar faces. Unfortunately, this flawless neural processing can go wrong when neurological trauma or disease disrupt brain processing, making a person unable to speak, move, feel, attend, or remember. Currently, there is no cure for many devastating neurological conditions, such as spinal cord injury, stroke and amyotrophic lateral sclerosis.

Neural interfaces (NIs), interchangeably called brain–machine interfaces, brain–computer interfaces, or neural prostheses, are an ambitious attempt to revolutionize treatment of neural disorders by linking the brain circuits to artificial components, such as limb prostheses, communication devices, computers, and electrical stimulators of the nervous tissue (Lebedev & Nicolelis 2006). For example, spinal cord injury can be bypassed by an NI that directly connects the motor cortex to a prosthetic limb (Bouton et al. 2016; Collinger et al. 2013; Hochberg et al.

2006, 2012). The list of neuroprosthetic components for connecting to neural circuitry is constantly growing. These are sensors for recording brain signals, devices for stimulating the brain, wireless transmitters and receivers, and electronic chips that process brain signals. The range of external devices to which NIs could connect is growing, as well. These include computer cursors (Carmena et al. 2003; Lebedev et al. 2005), spelling devices (Akram et al. 2014; Pan et al. 2013), robotic arms (Carmena et al. 2003; Collinger et al. 2013; Velliste et al. 2008), powered exoskeletons (Contreras-Vidal & Grossman 2013; Gancet et al. 2011; Kwak et al. 2015), virtual-reality systems (Bermudez i Badia et al. 2013), motorized wheelchairs (Chai et al. 2014; Galán et al. 2008), drones (LaFleur et al. 2013), and even brain-controlled automobiles (Göhring et al. 2013). Moreover, NIs can nowadays enable communication between individual brains (Pais-Vieira et al. 2013; Rao et al. 2014).

In this review, we consider NIs that simultaneously handle two streams of information: (1) the flow of information from the brain to an external device, and (2) an afferent information stream from the external devices to the brain. Such NIs are called bidirectional. We review the main component needed to build such bidirectional NIs and consider several implementations of such systems in animals and human subjects. We also discuss the feasible ways for developing clinically relevant bidirectional NIs.

## 37.2 TYPES OF NEURAL INTERFACES

Several NI classifications have been proposed in the literature (Lebedev 2014). Most relevant to this review, NIs can be classed into (1) *efferent NIs* that extract information from the brain, (2) *afferent or sensory NIs* that deliver information to the brain, and (3) *bidirectional NIs* that combine information extraction and delivery. The information handled by efferent, afferent, and bidirectional NIs can be of different kinds: motor, somatosensory, visual, auditory, cognitive, and so on.

The majority of efferent NIs that have been developed so far work in the motor domain. Such motor NIs enact movements of the upper (Carmena et al. 2003; Collinger et al. 2013; Velliste et al. 2008; Wessberg et al. 2000) and lower limbs (Fitzsimmons et al. 2009). Additionally, several types of non-motor efferent NIs have started to develop, for example, *cognitive neural prosthesis*, an umbrella term for NIs that extract higher-order representations from neural activity (Andersen et al. 2004, 2010; Mirabella & Lebedev 2017).

Afferent NIs include a variety of systems that interfere with different sensory modalities. Neural prostheses for restoration of hearing are currently the most advanced NI of this type, with hundreds of thousands of deaf people receiving these implants and restoring their hearing (House 1976). Afferent NIs have been also developed for vision (Dobelle 1994; Normann et al. 2009), somatosensory sensations (Bensmaia & Miller 2014), and vestibular function (Merfeld & Lewis 2012).

It should be clarified that by bidirectional NIs, we do not designate any NI system that communicates bidirectionally with the external world. Generally speaking, bidirectional communications take place practically in any NI implementation as a combination of both artificial and natural communication channels. For example, a motor NI could be linked to an external device through an artificial control loop while receiving feedback information through natural senses, such as vision. Instead of considering bidirectional NIs in this very broad sense, we use a narrow definition: Bidirectional NI is a system where both efferent and afferent loops are artificial and directly interfaced to the nervous system.

Figure 37.1 illustrates a bidirectional NI implemented using electrocorticographic (ECoG) recordings. The ECoG grid is placed over both the motor and somatosensory cortical areas. The grid portion overlying the motor area is used to extract motor commands that are sent to a prosthetic hand. The prosthetic hand is equipped with touch and position sensors whose signals are sent to the somatosensory portion of the grid. Electrical stimulation of the somatosensory cortex through the ECoG electrodes generates the sensory feedback needed to improve the control of the prosthetic hand.

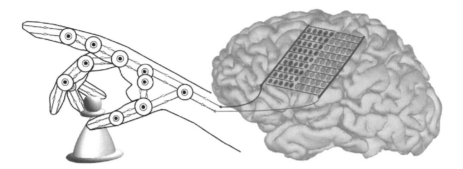

**FIGURE 37.1** Bidirectional neural interface implemented using an ECoG grid. Here, a sensorized neuro-prosthetic hand is controlled by the motor commands extracted from the grid portion overlying the motor cortex (red). The signals from the prosthetic sensors are sent back to the grid portion overlying the somatosensory cortex (blue). Electrical stimulation of the ECoG electrodes evokes somatosensory sensations needed to improve the control of the neuroprosthetic hand.

In addition to the classification by the direction of information flow, NIs are often classified as *invasive* and *noninvasive*. Noninvasive NIs are obviously much safer compared to invasive ones, but invasive systems offer potentially much better accuracy and speed of decoding.

In this review, we give a special emphasis to an invasive approach, called electrocorticography (ECoG). ECoG requires an invasive surgical procedure to open the skull but it is safer compared to brain implants because ECoG recording sensors do not penetrate into the brain tissue. An ECoG grid is placed over the brain surface epidurally or subdurally (Reid 1989; Schalk 2010; Walker et al. 1949). ECoG-based NIs may become an optimal clinical solution because they combine the advantages of a minimally invasive implantation procedure with better temporal and spatial resolution compared to the mainstream noninvasive NIs based on EEG recordings. ECoG grids can be implanted chronically (Weinand et al. 1994; Wyler et al. 1991).

The other useful classification of NIs is the division into *endogenous* and *exogenous* systems. In endogenous NIs, users initiate actions at will, at the time when they want to issue a command, for example, by engaging mental imagery (Obermaier et al. 2001; Pfurtscheller & Neuper 2006). Although endogenous NIs' tasks are often guided by external stimuli, they can be, in principle, performed without any external triggers. By contrast, external stimulation is necessary for the operation of exogenous NIs (Fazel-Rezai et al. 2012; Sellers et al. 2006) because they are based on the detection of modified evoked neural responses, such as EEG P300 responses evoked by attended stimuli (Brunner et al. 2011; Donchin et al. 2000; Piccione et al. 2006).

Recently, a new NI design has been proposed, called *passive NI* (Zander et al. 2010) (see Chapter 3 ["Passive Brain–Computer Interfaces: A Perspective on Increased Interactivity"]). Passive NIs do not require any active effort from the subject, to control an external device with brain activity. Instead, they collect brain signals while subjects interact with a technical system and strive to improve this interaction by adjusting the system parameters based on the recorded brain activity.

Finally, NIs can be classified by the parts of the nervous system to which they connect: cortex, subcortical areas, peripheral nerves, or spinal motoneurons. The activity of spinal motoneurons is conventionally measured using electromyographic (EMG) recordings.

## 37.3  NEURAL RECORDINGS

Many recording approaches have been utilized for interfacing to the brain, and the list of recording techniques is constantly growing. Historically, invasive recordings with microelectrodes have been a mainstream technique for studying neurophysiological mechanisms in awake, behaving animals. Currently, this method is used in NIs for both animals and humans. Edward Evarts used this method in the mid-1960s to conduct single-unit recordings in awake, behaving monkeys performing motor tasks (Evarts et al. 1962). Evarts' key demonstration was that the discharge rates of motor cortical neurons correlate with the parameters of movements, such as movement onset and force applied to a manipulandum.

In Evarts' classical settings, usually just one neuron would be recorded at a time. This is fine for certain neurophysiological inquiries but insufficient to achieve an accurate performance of an NI in real time. In the mid-1990s, Miguel Nicolelis and John Chapin pioneered recordings from many neurons simultaneously using multielectrode implants (Chapin et al. 1999; Nicolelis et al. 1995); they were also the first to incorporate this method in an NI (Chapin et al. 1999). Currently, multielectrode recordings are the mainstream approach to NIs in nonhuman primates (Krüger et al. 2010; Schwarz et al. 2014). Multielectrode NIs have also been tested in humans (Bouton et al. 2016; Collinger et al. 2013; Hochberg et al. 2006, 2012) using the implant, called Utah array (Campbell et al. 1991). Chronically implanted microelectrode arrays can both record and electrically stimulate brain tissue (Bensmaia & Miller 2014; O'Doherty et al. 2011; Tabot et al. 2013).

There is an ongoing research into making implanted microelectrodes thinner, more flexible, and less traumatic to the brain. For this purpose, polymer-based microelectrodes have been developed (Agorelius et al. 2015; Kozai & Kipke 2009). Additionally, increasing the neuronal yield of an electrode can be achieved by incorporating many recording points in the electrode shaft (Najafi et al. 1985; Vetter et al. 2004). Research is also ongoing into carbon nanotubes as the way to improve recording quality and biocompatibility (Berthing et al. 2011; Kotov et al. 2009).

ECoG grids placed over the cortical surface appear to be a particularly promising approach for implementing NIs in humans (Figure 37.1). This method is much more safe and reliable compared to invasive recordings with microelectrodes. ECoG methods allow multichannel recordings of field potentials from several cortical areas simultaneously (Crone et al. 2006; Hill et al. 2012; Leuthardt et al. 2006). The quality of these recordings is much better compared to EEG. In particular, the ECoG method allows recording high-frequency cortical rhythms that are particularly informative for NI decoding. Currently, ECoG methods are widely used in epileptic patients for diagnostics. Various NI designs can be tested in these patients.

Despite the direct contact with the cortical tissue, the ECoG electrodes cannot capture specific sources of neural activity in cortical gyri and instead record a superposition of activity of many sources located beneath the grid. Mathematically, measurements on each electrode can be described as a sum of sources weighted by different scaling factors (Figure 37.2). The scaling factors depend on the local conductivity profiles and can be estimated by solving the Maxwell equations in the quasi-static approximation (Nunez & Srinivasan 2006). Next, using the methods for solving the inverse problem, the measured signals can be decomposed to improve the spatial resolution by estimating the activity of sources located in the nodes of a virtual grid. The virtual grid's step can be smaller than the step of the real ECoG grid. This method allows one to estimate the activity of neural sources located at a distance from the ECoG electrodes, including those located in the gyri. This approach has been explored (Pascarella et al. 2016; Zhang et al. 2006), including solving the inverse problem using the method of minimum norm (Hämäläinen & Ilmoniemi 1994), and a significant improvement in spatial resolution has been achieved.

Recently, several solutions have been proposed for increasing the density of the electrodes in the grid and using embedded electronics for recordings (Bleichner et al. 2016; Mendoza et al. 2016; Viventi et al. 2011; Zippo et al. 2015). Furthermore, flexible recording mesh has recently been developed that was injected in the rodent brain with a syringe and proved to be efficient for long-term recordings (Fu et al. 2016).

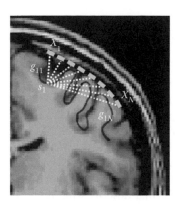

**FIGURE 37.2** Neural sources of ECoG activity. ECoG recordings represent a superposition of activity of many cortical sources beneath the ECoG grid. Mathematically, the $j$th electrode scales the $i$th source with a weight $g_{ij}$ that depends on the local conductivity profile. The weights can be estimated by solving the Maxwell equations in the quasi-static approximation and then used to obtain a generating equation for signals, $x$, generated by sources, $s$. Next, using the methods for solving the inverse problem, the measured signals can be decomposed into the contribution from the individual sources.

Notwithstanding the potential advantages of ECoG, EEG recordings remain the most popular recording method in human NIs. EEG-based NIs of both endogenous and exogenous types have been developed. In endogenous EEG-based NIs, subjects voluntarily modulate their EEG rhythms (Ang et al. 2011; Blakely et al. 2014; Muller-Putz et al. 2014; Pfurtscheller & Neuper 2001) (see Chapter 23 ["A Step-by-Step Tutorial for a Motor Imagery–Based BCI"]). In exogenous systems, external stimuli, most often visual stimuli, trigger EEG responses, which the user can modify by attending to some parts of the stimuli (Brunner et al. 2011; Donchin 1979; Donchin et al. 2000; Eason 1981; Farwell & Donchin 1988) (see Chapter 26 ["Issues and Challenges in Designing P300 and SSVEP Paradigms"]).

In addition to sampling electrical potentials generated by brain neurons, NIs can employ a variety of other recording methods, including functional magnetic resonance imaging (fMRI) (Cohen et al. 2014; Yoo et al. 2004), magnetoencephalography (MEG) (Buch et al. 2008; Lal et al. 2005), and functional near-infrared spectroscopy (fNIRS) (Naseer & Hong 2015; Sitaram et al. 2009; Tai & Chau 2009). Neural activity can be recorded from peripheral nerves as well (Navarro et al. 2005; Yoo & Durand 2005). Finally, EMG recordings are a very practical way for connecting to spinal motoneurons (Farry et al. 1996; Jiang et al. 2012; Linderman et al. 2009; Okorokova et al. 2015).

## 37.4 DECODING NEURAL SIGNALS

The main idea of efferent NIs is that relevant information can be extracted directly from neural recordings, analyzed, and then converted into messages or control commands, which are then sent to an external device.

Neural decoding is performed by mathematical algorithms, called decoders. Ideally, the decoder design should be based on good understanding on the functional role of the recorded neural signals. In practice, this is possible only to a certain degree because we still know very little about the neural representation and processing of information. Current NIs rely on the existing theories of brain processing, some of them traditional and the others more innovative. In the motor domain, the most traditional view is that motor regions of the brain form a hierarchy and, depending on the hierarchical rankings of the regions involved in controlling a particular behavior, the behavior would be more or less automated (Bernstein 1967). The most automated motor behaviors, such as spinal reflexes (Sherrington 1906) and locomotion generation (Guertin 2009), are controlled by the spinal circuits, somewhat more complex behaviors engage the brainstem, and the most complex voluntary movements are controlled by cortical areas. Many current NIs utilize cortical recordings, so that they can be thought of as NIs mimicking voluntary motor control.

Going beyond reflexes and voluntary movements, some developers of robots (Hoffmann et al. 2010), prostheses (Pazzaglia & Molinari 2016), and NIs (Alimardani et al. 2016; Lebedev & Nicolelis 2006) build their ideas around the concept of body schema. This concept was proposed by Head and Holmes (1911) as an explanation of how the brain integrates multiple streams of information from peripheral sensors to form a coherent model of the body (Maravita & Iriki 2004; Maravita et al. 2003). The internal model theory (Kawato 1999; Wolpert et al. 1995) is a modern version of the body schema theoretical framework. The internal model theory delineates two components: the controlled object (e.g., a body part) and the neural controller. To optimize the performance, the controller builds an internal model that describes the properties of the object. When planning a movement, the controller utilizes the internal model to form an expectation of how the body part would move. Next, during motor execution, afferent information from the body part is compared with the expectation, and a correcting command is issued if the incoming sensory information is different from the expected state. It has been proposed that NI should utilize an internal model to perform better (Cui 2016; Golub et al. 2012). Similar optimization ideas can be found in the theory of optimal feedback control (Todorov 2004; Todorov & Jordan 2002) that was recently applied to NI design (Benyamini & Zacksenhouse 2015; Shanechi et al. 2016).

All decoding algorithms assume that neural activity represents behavioral parameters of interest, such as limb position and velocity, joint torque, and so on. In practice, one cannot be certain that the recorded neural signals represent the parameters being decoded directly instead of being related to them in an indirect way. This problem, however, does not stop NI developers from utilizing any correlation between the neural activity and behavioral variables for neural decoding and real-time NI control. One way to partly avoid the use of the indirect information is to rely only on the causal processing by using only the neuronal activity from the immediate past to predict the current dynamics of the behavioral variables.

The phrase "neural tuning" is often used to refer to the correlation between neuronal modulations and a behavioral parameter. For example, if the firing rate of a neuron is different for different directions of arm movements, such a neuron is described as directionally tuned. Apostolos Georgopoulos and his coworkers contributed considerably to our current understanding of neuronal tuning to motor parameters. They described tuning of motor cortical neurons as a cosine of arm-movement direction (Georgopoulos 1987; Schwartz et al. 1988). Georgopoulos also proposed a model of how a population of cosine-tuned neurons could encode movement direction. In this model, called population vector, the contribution of each neuron is represented by a vector pointing in the preferred direction for that neuron and with the length proportional to the neuron's firing rate. The population vector is the sum of individual neuronal contributions. Modern NI decoders utilize somewhat similar principles of decoding, and they also incorporate improvements to minimize decoding errors. In other words, these decoders are optimized according to some criteria.

Optimal linear decoders, often referred to as Wiener filters, were first introduced to NI research by Humphrey and his colleagues for offline decoding of neuronal data (Humphrey et al. 1970) and were later employed by others for real-time NI control (Carmena et al. 2003; Wessberg et al. 2000). The Kalman filter (Kalman 1960), another linear algorithm, offers several additional advantages (Kim et al. 2006; Okorokova et al. 2015; Serruya et al. 2003) by separating the filter variables into the state variables that describe the object (e.g., prosthetic limb) and the observed variables represented by neuronal rates. Neuronal tuning is described by the Kalman filter tuning model. The characteristics of state transitions, such as arm inertia, are described by the state model. A nonlinear modification of the Kalman filter, called the unscented Kalman filter (UKF) (Li et al. 2009) offers additional advantages by capturing nonlinear relationship between neuronal rates and the state variables. Additionally, point-process algorithms (Eden et al. 2004; Li 2014) and artificial neural networks (Chapin et al. 1999; Kim et al. 2005; Sanchez et al. 2003; Wessberg et al. 2000) have been applied to NI decoding.

A typical NI session consists of a training part, when data are collected to train an NI decoder, and a real-time control part, when the decoder output is connected to an external device, for example, a robotic arm. The training part may consist of a manual performance of a behavioral task (Carmena et al. 2003; Ifft et al. 2013; Wessberg et al. 2000) or passive observation of the task replay (Ifft et al. 2013; Tkach et al. 2008; Wahnoun et al. 2006). In some settings, the training part can be eliminated and replaced by arbitrary decoder settings (Ganguly & Carmena 2009), followed by neural and/or algorithmic adaptation to real-time NI control. A variety of adaptive algorithms have been introduced for this purpose, including co-adaptive algorithm for a population-vector decoder (Taylor et al. 2002), Bayesian regression (Li et al. 2011), and several others (Dangi et al. 2013; Shanechi et al. 2014; Suminski et al. 2013). Reinforcement learning has also been employed for decoder adaptation (DiGiovanna et al. 2009).

Figure 37.3 illustrates an analysis, where we causally decoded finger movements in humans from a strip of epidural ECoG electrodes. The strip was placed over the cortical area representing the

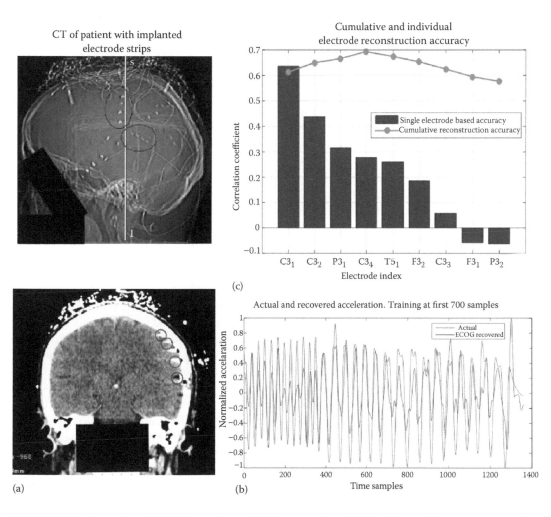

**FIGURE 37.3** Decoding of ECoG recordings. (a) Placement of an ECoG strip over the motor cortex of an epileptic patient. (b) Reconstruction of finger acceleration from ECoG recordings. The blue trace represents the actual finger acceleration and the red trace represents acceleration reconstruction based on the four most relevant ECoG channels. (c) Cumulative and individual-electrode reconstruction accuracy. Using a single electrode, the correlation coefficient for reconstruction accuracy can be as high as 0.65.

wrist. The correlation coefficient of 0.7 was achieved between the estimated and the actual finger acceleration. These decoding results were obtained using a convolutional neural network trained using the absolute values of the Morlet wavelet coefficients. A small amount of training data (1 min) was used for this decoding.

In addition to continuous decoding methods, various types of discrete classifiers, such as linear discriminant analysis (LDA) (Fisher 1936) and more advanced algorithms, have been popular in noninvasive NIs, such as EEG-based systems. Discrete decoding is appropriate because these NIs typically require selection from two or more choices instead of continuous control of an external device (Halder et al. 2010; Placidi et al. 2015) (see Chapter 18 ["Gentle Introduction to Signal Processing and Classification for Single-Trial EEG Analysis"]).

## 37.5 MOTOR NEURAL INTERFACES

A now classical example of a motor NI is the NI that allows subject to control movements performed by a robotic arm or some other robotic manipulator. The first such NI was demonstrated in rats (Chapin et al. 1999), followed by demonstrations in owl monkeys (Wessberg et al. 2000) and rhesus monkeys (Carmena et al. 2003; Lebedev et al. 2005; Taylor et al. 2002; Velliste et al. 2008). More recently, multielectrode recordings with invasive Utah arrays were employed to demonstrate similar controls in humans (Hochberg & Donoghue 2006; Hochberg et al. 2012), including very sophisticated control of a multiple degree of freedom robotic arm (Collinger et al. 2013). While the majority of motor NIs enable arm movements, some progress has been attained in the development of NIs for lower limbs (Cheng et al. 2007; Fitzsimmons et al. 2009; Foster et al. 2012, 2014; Schwarz et al. 2014; Zhang et al. 2010).

Motor NIs can reanimate the subject's own body by connecting to the motor nerves and evoking movements using functional electrical stimulation (FES). Such FES-based NIs have been demonstrated in monkeys, where FES was triggered by cortical activity recorded with intracortical electrodes (Ethier et al. 2012; Moritz et al. 2008; Pohlmeyer et al. 2009), and humans using EEG-based (Pfurtscheller et al. 2003, 2005) and intracranial array-based (Ajiboye et al. 2017; Bouton et al. 2016) NIs.

Notwithstanding the progress in multielectrode-based NIs that restore mobility to paralyzed patients, ECoG-based NIs could be a more practical solution for humans, at least in the nearest future (Schalk 2010; Schalk & Leuthardt 2011; Slutzky & Flint 2017; Wilson et al. 2006). Indeed, ECoG is much safer compared to intracortical implants, and it is also more reliable. Additionally, developing fully implantable ECoG systems is easier from the engineering point of view compared to the systems that record spiking activity from large populations of neurons (Foerster et al. 2012; Hirata et al. 2011; Pistor et al. 2013). Motor NIs based on ECoG recordings have already been demonstrated, for example, systems for screen cursor control (Felton et al. 2007; Leuthardt et al. 2004, 2006; Wang et al. 2013). ECoG-based spellers have been developed as well (Brunner et al. 2011; Korostenskaja et al. 2014; Song et al. 2012).

A very significant step in the development of clinical ECoG-based NIs was recently made by Mariska Vansteensel and her colleagues (Vansteensel et al. 2016) who implemented a fully implantable NI of this type in a patient with locked-in syndrome, unable to move but with normal cognitive functions. Their fully implantable NI incorporated a subdural ECoG grid placed over the motor cortex and a transmitter implanted in the thorax. The patient regained the ability to communicate with the external world by imagining moving the hand on the side contralateral to the cortical implant. Since the NI was fully implantable, it was suitable for everyday use at home.

Myoelectric interface is a good practical solution in many cases (Farry et al. 1996; Jiang et al. 2012). For example, we applied this method for decoding handwritten characters (Linderman et al. 2009). EMG activity was recorded from the hand and forearm muscles while subjects wrote characters on a digitizing tablet. Linear algorithms were applied to reconstruct pen trace from multi-channel EMG recordings. Additionally, LDA was used to extract font characters from the EMGs.

Utilization of a Kalman filter additionally improved continuous decoding of pen traces from EMG activity (Okorokova et al. 2015).

## 37.6 ARTIFICIAL SENSATION

A variety of artificial sensations have been developed using afferent NIs, and many more systems will likely be developed in the future. Cochlear implant is undoubtedly the most successful story of an afferent NI, with hundreds of thousands of people restoring hearing using this type of neural prosthesis (Shannon 2012; Wilson & Dorman 2008). This implant evokes auditory sensations by applying electrical pulses to the cochlear nerve. Implanted patients can recognize speech, different voices, and even music.

Visual prostheses hold promise of restoring vision to the blind (Fernandes et al. 2012). Several types of visual prostheses have been developed, which are applicable to different cases of blindness. Retinal prostheses (epiretinal, subretinal, transchoroidal, and optic nerve) are applicable to eye pathologies that spare parts of the optic nerve. Non-retinal prostheses employ electrical stimulation of cortical and subcortical visual areas. They are applicable to cases where the eye and/or optic nerve is severely damaged. Electrical stimulation of visual cortex to restore vision has been pioneered by William Dobelle (Dobelle et al. 1974).

Here, we focus on efferent NIs for producing artificial somatosensory sensations because this type of afferent channel has already been implemented in several bidirectional NIs. Historically, Harvey Cushing was the first to report clinical cases, where he evoked somatosensory sensations by stimulating the surface of human postcentral cortex (Cushing 1909). Significantly, the stimulation did not evoke movements. Wilder Penfield and his colleagues conducted a series of studies where they stimulated different sites in the human cortex (Penfield & Boldrey 1937). When stimulated in the postcentral cortex, patients usually described their perceptions as sensations of tingling or numbness or tingling. Ranulfo Romo employed intracortical stimulation (ICMS) of postcentral cortex in monkeys to produce somatosensory sensations (Romo et al. 1998). He argued that monkeys experienced sensations that were similar to sensations of vibration. Indeed, his monkeys learned a sensory discrimination task where they compared the frequency of hand vibration to the frequency of ICMS applied to their somatosensory cortex. For stimulation, Romo used a single electrode, which he inserted anew on each recording day.

Nathan Fitzsimmons and his colleagues conducted a study in owl monkeys, where they used multi-electrode cortical arrays implanted to apply ICMS (Fitzsimmons et al. 2007). With this approach, they investigated monkeys' learning to utilize ICMS as an artificial sensation over the course of many training days. ICMS instructed a binary choice of a target for arm reaching movements. It took owl monkeys several weeks to learn to respond to the presence of ICMS. Next, they were required to discriminate different temporal patterns of ICMS. Surprisingly, it took the animals just a few days to learn this difficult task. Even more surprisingly, the monkeys learned almost immediately a spatiotemporal discrimination task, where spatiotemporal ICMS patterns were delivered through multiple implanted electrodes. Thus, the more the animals practiced with ICMS, the more readily could they discriminate the fine patterns of this artificial somatosensory sensation.

Similar experiments were performed by O'Doherty et al. (2009) and Tabot et al. (2013) in rhesus monkeys chronically implanted with multielectrode arrays in the primary somatosensory cortex. O'Doherty's monkeys responded to ICMS patterns with different directions of arm movements. Tabot applied ICMS to different sites of the hand representing areas of the somatosensory cortex, and monkeys responded with eye movements in different directions depending where on the hand they felt the stimulation. It was also shown that rhesus monkeys could learn an initially unfamiliar pattern of multichannel ICMS that signaled the location of an unseen target (Dadarlat et al. 2015).

Flesher and her colleagues implanted a multielectrode array in a tetraplegic patient and applied ICMS to evoke somatotopically organized sensations that corresponded to different hand locations

(Flesher et al. 2016). The patient described his sensations as a close to natural feeling of pressure from the skin surface and below the skin.

Importantly, ECoG implants, a much less invasive approach, has been successfully utilized to evoke somatosensory sensations (Borchers et al. 2012; Cronin et al. 2016; Hiremath et al. 2017; Johnson et al. 2013; Nii et al. 1996; Pistohl et al. 2008). Particularly encouraging results were recently obtained by stimulation through a high-density ECoG grid (60 electrodes in a 4 × 4 cm area) (Hiremath et al. 2017). The subject of this study localized different spatial patterns of stimulation, felt as buzz or tingling, to different hand locations. Sensation intensity increased monotonically with the amplitude and frequency of electrical pulses. The authors concluded that temporal and spatial resolution of this method of stimulation was good enough to be utilized for generation of somatosensory feedback in neuroprosthetic applications.

Peripheral nerve stimulation is another method to produce somatosensory sensations. Different types of stimulation have been developed, including nerve cuff electrodes (Tan et al. 2014) and Utah arrays inserted in nerves (Davis et al. 2016; Raspopovic et al. 2014).

In addition to electrical stimulation as the method to produce somatosensory sensations, several studies employed optogenetic methods for this purpose (May et al. 2014; Yazdan-Shahmorad et al. 2016).

## 37.7 BIDIRECTIONAL NEURAL INTERFACES

Bidirectional NIs that simultaneously control the movements of an artificial device, for example, a robotic arm, and enable somatosensory sensations from the device are highly desirable by people suffering from paralysis because only such sensorized NIs can achieve good quality of motor control and provide patients with the appropriate perceptions. In such bidirectional interfaces, motor commands are extracted from a component of the motor system of the brain, and sensory feedback is enabled as stimulation of somatosensory areas of the brain or peripheral nerves.

O'Doherty and his colleagues has demonstrated a bidirectional NI implemented using cortical multielectrode implants in monkeys (O'Doherty et al. 2009, 2011). In these experiments, monkeys controlled reaching movements, performed by a virtual hand on a computer screen, by their motor cortical activity decoded using a UKF. Monkeys used the virtual hand to scan through several screen objects that appeared identical visually but had different virtual textures mimicked by ICMS. Each time the virtual hand touched an object, a temporal pattern of ICMS was applied to the somatosensory cortex. A unique ICMS pattern corresponded to each artificial pattern. Monkeys successfully learned to use this type of active tactile exploration, enabled by a bidirectional NI, to find the artificial texture for which they were rewarded with fruit juice. In this study, each ICMS pulse evoked an electrical artifact that occluded the recordings. To prevent interference between the recordings and ICMS delivery, time was split into 50-ms bins; one bin was used for recordings, the next one for ICMS, and so on. Although this solution removed half of the neural data, monkeys still performed well.

While the bidirectional interface of O'Doherty et al. required cable connections to the implant, fully implantable interfaces for both recording and stimulation have been developed and tested in monkeys (Greenwald et al. 2016; Jackson et al. 2006; Su et al. 2016).

Several recent studies have demonstrated bidirectional NIs in humans. Raspopovic et al. (2014) developed a myoelectric interface that controlled grasping movements performed by a robotic hand. This interface was tested in amputees. Somatosensory feedback of grasp force was delivered by electrically stimulating median and ulnar nerves. Subjects learned to maintain a required force level without visual feedback from the robotic hand.

Davis et al. (2016) demonstrated such an NI by connecting to peripheral nerves. They implanted Utah slanted arrays in two amputees. One subject received an implant in the median nerve and the other received an implant in the ulnar nerve. The implants recorded neural activity when the subjects intended with their phantom fingers. The intended movements were decoded by a Kalman filter. The output of this NI was connected to a virtual hand. The authors demonstrated decoding of 13 different movements offline and two movements during real-time performance. In addition to such decoding of motor commands, electrical stimulation was applied through the nerve implants to more than 80 different sensations.

As to using ECoG implants in bidirectional NIs, we have seen several conference presentations but no published papers yet. As a step in this direction, an ECoG-based sensory NI was recently demonstrated, where subjects adjusted their movements based on an artificial sensory feedback (Cronin et al. 2016). Electrical stimulation was applied through ECoG electrodes placed over the somatosensory cortex. Human subjects wore a data glove that tracked their hand aperture. The aperture was fed back to the subjects using electrical stimulation. The subjects successfully utilized the "abstract sensation of the hand" provided by this feedback to adjust their hand aperture to a required target value.

The examples presented above represent cases, where bidirectional interfaces consisted of a motor loop for controlling external devices by brain activity and an artificial sensory loop for transmitting sensory information from an external device to the brain sensory areas or sensory nerves. In a more general sense, bidirectional interface is a system that simultaneously records neural signals and stimulates neural circuits (Fetz 2015). Such bidirectional interfaces could work, for example, as artificial parts inserted in brain circuits. While all possible varieties of such interfaces are beyond the scope of this manuscript, several recent developments are worth mentioning.

In recent years, noninvasive stimulation methods have gained popularity, such as transcranial magnetic stimulation and transcranial electrical stimulation utilized to augment various brain functions (Bennabi et al. 2014; Davis & van Koningsbruggen 2013; Horvath et al. 2014; Krause & Kadosh 2014). Bidirectional implementations of these methods have also started to develop, where neural activity triggers noninvasive stimulation (Karabanov et al. 2016; Sun & Morrell 2014). The idea here is that stimulation parameters can be adjusted based on the effect the stimulation has on neural activity.

In the invasive NI domain, a "brain–spine interface" has been demonstrated for restoration of quadrupedal locomotion in monkeys with unilateral spinal cord lesions (Capogrosso et al. 2016). In this study, unilateral lesions were made to the spinal cord of rhesus monkeys, leading to a paralysis of one of the lower limbs. Consequently, the monkeys had great difficulty walking quadrupedally. Multielectrode implants were placed in the lower-limb representing areas of the monkey's motor cortex, contralateral to the lesion site. Additionally, epidural stimulating electrodes were placed over the spinal cord. Next, motor cortical activity was set to trigger electrical stimulation of the spinal cord, which resulted in movements of the paralyzed lower limb. After adjusting the stimulation parameters, the researchers managed to restore near-normal locomotion patterns with this bidirectional NI.

At the level of cortical microcircuits, Prsa and his colleagues operantly conditioned single neurons in mouse motor cortex using a bidirectional NI (Prsa et al. 2017). Neuronal activity was recorded using two-photon imaging, whereas stimulation was applied optogenetically. The mice were trained to activate the neuron chosen by the experimenters. A continuous feedback of the neuronal firing was provided by the stimulation of the somatosensory cortex. Aided by this artificial somatosensory feedback, the mice learned to control the firing of the motor cortical neuron. Curiously, the conditioning effect was specific to that single neuron as the other neurons in the motor cortical population did not change their activity levels.

## 37.8   FUTURISTIC IDEAS

Among the currently discussed futuristic ideas, one is the possibility of a bidirectional interface for cognitive functions and emotions (Andersen et al. 2010; Mirabella & Lebedev 2017). For example, Widge and Moritz proposed a closed-loop stimulation system, where activity recorded in the prefrontal cortex regulates emotional states by controlling the stimulation in the medial forebrain bundle (Widge & Moritz 2014).

Bidirectional communications between the brains of several subjects is another futuristic idea. Such direct brain-to-brain communications have been demonstrated in rats (Pais-Vieira et al. 2013), where the neural representation of decision-making of one rat was transmitted to another rat using ICMS. Human demonstrations have been conducted as well (Grau et al. 2014; Rao et al. 2014). In these experiments, one subject operated an EEG-based NI, and the output of that NI was sent to the brain of the other subject using transcranial magnetic stimulation as a delivery method.

Although brain-to-brain interfaces are at their early stage of development and all current demonstrations are relatively simple and unpractical, we foresee that such systems will become more practical in the near future. They could be used, for example, for patient–therapist interactions. For the longer term, we would not exclude any futuristic scenario, even the possibility that these technologies will evolve into a "global brain" (Kyriazis 2015).

## 37.9 CONCLUDING REMARKS

We have shown that a bidirectional interface is a system composed of two components: an efferent component that decodes neural activity and an afferent component that delivers information to the brain circuits. However, once these two components are combined, the resulting NI is much more than a sum of parts. It offers many more functional capacities compared to merely efferent and afferent NIs. Indeed, practically any area of the nervous system communicates with the other area bidirectionally and uses predictive processing in such communication: the processing of incoming information is a comparison with the expectation of the input. If future bidirectional NIs are capable of reproducing such modes of processing, they could be seamlessly integrated with the neural circuits to augment, repair, and rehabilitate brain functions.

## REFERENCES

Agorelius, J., Tsanakalis, F., Friberg, A., Thorbergsson, P. T., Pettersson, L. M. E., & Schouenborg, J. (2015). An array of highly flexible electrodes with a tailored configuration locked by gelatin during implantation—Initial evaluation in cortex cerebri of awake rats. *Frontiers in Neuroscience, 9*. doi:10.3389 /fnins.2015.00331

Ajiboye, A. B., Willett, F. R., Young, D. R., Memberg, W. D., Murphy, B. A., Miller, J. P., ... Keith, M. W. (2017). Restoration of reaching and grasping movements through brain-controlled muscle stimulation in a person with tetraplegia: A proof-of-concept demonstration. *The Lancet, 389*(10081), 1821–1830.

Akram, F., Han, H. S., & Kim, T. S. (2014). A P300-based brain computer interface system for words typing. *Comput Biol Med, 45*, 118–125. doi:10.1016/j.compbiomed.2013.12.001

Alimardani, M., Nishio, S., & Ishiguro, H. (2016). Removal of proprioception by BCI raises a stronger body ownership illusion in control of a humanlike robot. *Scientific Reports, 6*.

Andersen, R. A., Burdick, J. W., Musallam, S., Pesaran, B., & Cham, J. G. (2004). Cognitive neural prosthetics. *Trends Cogn Sci, 8*(11), 486–493. doi:10.1016/j.tics.2004.09.009

Andersen, R. A., Hwang, E. J., & Mulliken, G. H. (2010). Cognitive neural prosthetics. *Annu Rev Psychol, 61*, 169–190, C161–163. doi:10.1146/annurev.psych.093008.100503

Ang, K. K., Guan, C., Wang, C., Phua, K. S., Tan, A. H., & Chin, Z. Y. (2011). Calibrating EEG-based motor imagery brain–computer interface from passive movement. *Conf Proc IEEE Eng Med Biol Soc, 2011*, 4199–4202. doi:10.1109/IEMBS.2011.6091042

Bennabi, D., Pedron, S., Haffen, E., Monnin, J., Peterschmitt, Y., & Van Waes, V. (2014). Transcranial direct current stimulation for memory enhancement: From clinical research to animal models. *Frontiers in Systems Neuroscience, 8*.

Bensmaia, S. J., & Miller, L. E. (2014). Restoring sensorimotor function through intracortical interfaces: Progress and looming challenges. *Nature Reviews Neuroscience, 15*(5), 313–325.

Benyamini, M., & Zacksenhouse, M. (2015). Optimal feedback control successfully explains changes in neural modulations during experiments with brain–machine interfaces. *Front Syst Neurosci, 9*, 71. doi:10.3389 /fnsys.2015.00071

Bermudez i Badia, S., Garcia Morgade, A., Samaha, H., & Verschure, P. F. (2013). Using a hybrid brain computer interface and virtual reality system to monitor and promote cortical reorganization through motor activity and motor imagery training. *IEEE Trans Neural Syst Rehabil Eng, 21*(2), 174–181. doi:10.1109 /TNSRE.2012.2229295

Bernstein, N. A. (1967). The co-ordination and regulation of movements.

Berthing, T., Bonde, S., Sørensen, C. B., Utko, P., Nygård, J., & Martinez, K. L. (2011). Intact mammalian cell function on semiconductor nanowire arrays: New perspectives for cell-based biosensing. *Small, 7*(5), 640–647.

Blakely, T. M., Olson, J. D., Miller, K. J., Rao, R. P., & Ojemann, J. G. (2014). Neural correlates of learning in an electrocorticographic motor-imagery brain–computer interface. *Brain Comput Interfaces (Abingdon), 1*(3–4), 147–157. doi:10.1080/2326263X.2014.954183

Bleichner, M., Freudenburg, Z., Jansma, J., Aarnoutse, E., Vansteensel, M., & Ramsey, N. (2016). Give me a sign: Decoding four complex hand gestures based on high-density ECoG. *Brain Structure and Function, 221*(1), 203–216.

Borchers, S., Himmelbach, M., Logothetis, N., & Karnath, H.-O. (2012). Direct electrical stimulation of human cortex—The gold standard for mapping brain functions? *Nature Reviews Neuroscience, 13*(1), 63–70.

Bouton, C. E., Shaikhouni, A., Annetta, N. V., Bockbrader, M. A., Friedenberg, D. A., Nielson, D. M., ... Rezai, A. R. (2016). Restoring cortical control of functional movement in a human with quadriplegia. *Nature.* doi:10.1038/nature17435

Brunner, P., Ritaccio, A. L., Emrich, J. F., Bischof, H., & Schalk, G. (2011). Rapid communication with a "P300" matrix speller using electrocorticographic signals (ECoG). *Front Neurosci, 5*, 5. doi:10.3389 /fnins.2011.00005

Buch, E., Weber, C., Cohen, L. G., Braun, C., Dimyan, M. A., Ard, T., ... Fourkas, A. (2008). Think to move: A neuromagnetic brain–computer interface (BCI) system for chronic stroke. *Stroke, 39*(3), 910–917.

Campbell, P. K., Jones, K. E., Huber, R. J., Horch, K. W., & Normann, R. A. (1991). A silicon-based, three-dimensional neural interface: Manufacturing processes for an intracortical electrode array. *Biomedical Engineering, IEEE Transactions on, 38*(8), 758–768.

Capogrosso, M., Milekovic, T., Borton, D., Wagner, F., Moraud, E. M., Mignardot, J.-B., ... Xing, D. (2016). A brain–spine interface alleviating gait deficits after spinal cord injury in primates. *Nature, 539*(7628), 284–288.

Carmena, J. M., Lebedev, M. A., Crist, R. E., O'Doherty, J. E., Santucci, D. M., Dimitrov, D. F., ... Nicolelis, M. A. (2003). Learning to control a brain–machine interface for reaching and grasping by primates. *PLoS Biol, 1*(2), E42. doi:10.1371/journal.pbio.0000042

Chai, R., Ling, S. H., Hunter, G. P., Tran, Y., & Nguyen, H. T. (2014). Brain–computer interface classifier for wheelchair commands using neural network with fuzzy particle swarm optimization. *IEEE J Biomed Health Inform, 18*(5), 1614–1624. doi:10.1109/JBHI.2013.2295006

Chapin, J. K., Moxon, K. A., Markowitz, R. S., & Nicolelis, M. A. (1999). Real-time control of a robot arm using simultaneously recorded neurons in the motor cortex. *Nat Neurosci, 2*(7), 664–670. doi:10.1038/10223

Cheng, G., Fitzsimmons, N., Morimoto, J., Lebedev, M., Kawato, M., & Nicolelis, M. (2007). *Bipedal locomotion with a humanoid robot controlled by cortical ensemble activity.* Paper presented at the Abstr. Soc. Neurosci.

Cohen, O., Koppel, M., Malach, R., & Friedman, D. (2014). Controlling an avatar by thought using real-time fMRI. *J Neural Eng, 11*(3), 035006. doi:10.1088/1741-2560/11/3/035006

Collinger, J. L., Wodlinger, B., Downey, J. E., Wang, W., Tyler-Kabara, E. C., Weber, D. J., ... Schwartz, A. B. (2013). High-performance neuroprosthetic control by an individual with tetraplegia. *Lancet, 381*(9866), 557–564. doi:10.1016/S0140-6736(12)61816-9

Contreras-Vidal, J. L., & Grossman, R. G. (2013). NeuroRex: A clinical neural interface roadmap for EEG-based brain machine interfaces to a lower body robotic exoskeleton. *Conf Proc IEEE Eng Med Biol Soc, 2013*, 1579–1582. doi:10.1109/EMBC.2013.6609816

Crone, N. E., Sinai, A., & Korzeniewska, A. (2006). High-frequency gamma oscillations and human brain mapping with electrocorticography. *Progress in Brain Research, 159*, 275–295.

Cronin, J. A., Wu, J., Collins, K. L., Sarma, D., Rao, R. P., Ojemann, J. G., & Olson, J. D. (2016). Task-specific somatosensory feedback via cortical stimulation in humans. *IEEE Transactions on Haptics, 9*(4), 515–522.

Cui, H. (2016). Forward prediction in the posterior parietal cortex and dynamic brain–machine interface. *Frontiers in Integrative Neuroscience, 10.*

Cushing, H. (1909). A note upon the faradic stimulation of the postcentral gyrus in conscious patients 1. *Brain, 32*(1), 44–53.

Dadarlat, M. C., O'Doherty, J. E., & Sabes, P. N. (2015). A learning-based approach to artificial sensory feedback leads to optimal integration. *Nature Neuroscience, 18*(1), 138–144.

Dangi, S., Orsborn, A. L., Moorman, H. G., & Carmena, J. M. (2013). Design and analysis of closed-loop decoder adaptation algorithms for brain–machine interfaces. *Neural Comput, 25*(7), 1693–1731. doi:10.1162/NECO_a_00460

Davis, N. J., & van Koningsbruggen, M. G. (2013). "Non-invasive" brain stimulation is not non-invasive. *Frontiers in Systems Neuroscience, 7.*

Davis, T. S., Wark, H. A., Hutchinson, D. T., Warren, D. J., O'Neill, K., Scheinblum, T., ... Greger, B. (2016). Restoring motor control and sensory feedback in people with upper extremity amputations using arrays of 96 microelectrodes implanted in the median and ulnar nerves. *J Neural Eng, 13*(3), 036001. doi:10.1088/1741-2560/13/3/036001

DiGiovanna, J., Mahmoudi, B., Fortes, J., Principe, J. C., & Sanchez, J. C. (2009). Coadaptive brain–machine interface via reinforcement learning. *IEEE Transactions on Biomedical Engineering, 56*(1), 54–64.

Dobelle, W. H. (1974). Introduction to sensory prostheses for the blind and deaf. *Trans Am Soc Artif Intern Organs, 20*(B), 761–764.

Dobelle, W. H. (1994). Artificial vision for the blind. The summit may be closer than you think. *ASAIO J, 40*(4), 919–922.

Donchin, E. (1979). Event-related brain potentials: A tool in the study of human information processing *Evoked Brain Potentials and Behavior* (pp. 13–88): Springer.

Donchin, E., Spencer, K. M., & Wijesinghe, R. (2000). The mental prosthesis: Assessing the speed of a P300-based brain–computer interface. *IEEE Trans Rehabil Eng, 8*(2), 174–179.

Eason, R. G. (1981). Visual evoked potential correlates of early neural filtering during selective attention. *Bulletin of the Psychonomic Society, 18*(4), 203–206.

Eden, U. T., Frank, L. M., Barbieri, R., Solo, V., & Brown, E. N. (2004). Dynamic analysis of neural encoding by point process adaptive filtering. *Neural Computation, 16*(5), 971–998.

Ethier, C., Oby, E. R., Bauman, M., & Miller, L. E. (2012). Restoration of grasp following paralysis through brain-controlled stimulation of muscles. *Nature, 485*(7398), 368–371.

Evarts, E. V., Bental, E., Bihari, B., & Huttenlocher, P. R. (1962). Spontaneous discharge of single neurons during sleep and waking. *Science, 135*(3505), 726–728.

Farry, K. A., Walker, I. D., & Baraniuk, R. G. (1996). Myoelectric teleoperation of a complex robotic hand. *IEEE Transactions on Robotics and Automation, 12*(5), 775–788.

Farwell, L. A., & Donchin, E. (1988). Talking off the top of your head: Toward a mental prosthesis utilizing event-related brain potentials. *Electroencephalography and Clinical Neurophysiology, 70*(6), 510–523.

Fazel-Rezai, R., Allison, B. Z., Guger, C., Sellers, E. W., Kleih, S. C., & Kubler, A. (2012). P300 brain computer interface: Current challenges and emerging trends. *Front Neuroeng, 5*, 14. doi:10.3389/fneng.2012.00014

Felton, E. A., Wilson, J. A., Williams, J. C., & Garell, P. C. (2007). Electrocorticographically controlled brain–computer interfaces using motor and sensory imagery in patients with temporary subdural electrode implants: Report of four cases. *Journal of Neurosurgery, 106*(3), 495–500.

Fernandes, R. A., Diniz, B., Ribeiro, R., & Humayun, M. (2012). Artificial vision through neuronal stimulation. *Neurosci Lett, 519*(2), 122–128. doi: 10.1016/j.neulet.2012.01.063

Fetz, E. E. (2015). Restoring motor function with bidirectional neural interfaces. *Prog Brain Res, 218*, 241–252. doi:10.1016/bs.pbr.2015.01.001

Fisher, R. A. (1936). The use of multiple measurements in taxonomic problems. *Annals of Eugenics, 7*(2), 179–188.

Fitzsimmons, N. A., Drake, W., Hanson, T. L., Lebedev, M. A., & Nicolelis, M. A. (2007). Primate reaching cued by multichannel spatiotemporal cortical microstimulation. *J Neurosci, 27*(21), 5593–5602. doi:10.1523/JNEUROSCI.5297-06.2007

Fitzsimmons, N. A., Lebedev, M. A., Peikon, I. D., & Nicolelis, M. A. (2009). Extracting kinematic parameters for monkey bipedal walking from cortical neuronal ensemble activity. *Front Integr Neurosci, 3*, 3. doi:10.3389/neuro.07.003.2009

Flesher, S. N., Collinger, J. L., Foldes, S. T., Weiss, J. M., Downey, J. E., Tyler-Kabara, E. C., ... Gaunt, R. A. (2016). Intracortical microstimulation of human somatosensory cortex. *Science Translational Medicine, 8*(361), 361ra141–361ra141.

Foerster, M., Porcherot, J., Bonnet, S., Van Langhenhove, A., Robinet, S., & Charvet, G. (2012). *Integration of a state of the art ECoG recording ASIC into a fully implantable electronic environment.* Paper presented at the Biomedical Circuits and Systems Conference (BioCAS), 2012 IEEE.

Foster, J. D., Nuyujukian, P., Freifeld, O., Gao, H., Walker, R., Ryu, S. I., ... Shenoy, K. V. (2014). A freely-moving monkey treadmill model. *Journal of Neural Engineering, 11*(4), 046020.

Foster, J. D., Nuyujukian, P., Freifeld, O., Ryu, S. I., Black, M. J., & Shenoy, K. V. (2012). A framework for relating neural activity to freely moving behavior. *Conf Proc IEEE Eng Med Biol Soc, 2012*, 2736–2739. doi:10.1109/EMBC.2012.6346530

Fu, T.-M., Hong, G., Zhou, T., Schuhmann, T. G., Viveros, R. D., & Lieber, C. M. (2016). Stable long-term chronic brain mapping at the single-neuron level. *Nature Methods*.

Galán, F., Nuttin, M., Lew, E., Ferrez, P. W., Vanacker, G., Philips, J., & Millán, J. d. R. (2008). A brain-actuated wheelchair: Asynchronous and non-invasive brain–computer interfaces for continuous control of robots. *Clinical Neurophysiology, 119*(9), 2159–2169.

Gancet, J., Ilzkovitz, M., Cheron, G., Ivanenko, Y., van der Kooij, H., van der Helm, F., ... Thorsteinsson, F. (2011). *MINDWALKER: A brain controlled lower limbs exoskeleton for rehabilitation. Potential applications to space.* Paper presented at the 11th Symposium on advanced space technologies in robotics and automation.

Ganguly, K., & Carmena, J. M. (2009). Emergence of a stable cortical map for neuroprosthetic control. *PLoS Biol, 7*(7), e1000153. doi:10.1371/journal.pbio.1000153

Georgopoulos, A. P. (1987). Cortical mechanisms subserving reaching. *Ciba Found Symp, 132*, 125–141.

Göhring, D., Latotzky, D., Wang, M., & Rojas, R. (2013). Semi-autonomous car control using brain computer interfaces. *Intelligent Autonomous Systems 12*, 393–408.

Golub, M. D., Byron, M. Y., & Chase, S. M. (2012). *Internal models engaged by brain-computer interface control.* Paper presented at the 2012 Annual International Conference of the IEEE Engineering in Medicine and Biology Society.

Grau, C., Ginhoux, R., Riera, A., Nguyen, T. L., Chauvat, H., Berg, M., ... Ruffini, G. (2014). Conscious brain-to-brain communication in humans using non-invasive technologies. *PLoS One, 9*(8), e105225.

Greenwald, E., Masters, M. R., & Thakor, N. V. (2016). Implantable neurotechnologies: Bidirectional neural interfaces—Applications and VLSI circuit implementations. *Medical & Biological Engineering & Computing, 54*(1), 1–17.

Guertin, P. A. (2009). The mammalian central pattern generator for locomotion. *Brain Research Reviews, 62*(1), 45–56.

Halder, S., Rea, M., Andreoni, R., Nijboer, F., Hammer, E. M., Kleih, S. C., ... Kubler, A. (2010). An auditory oddball brain–computer interface for binary choices. *Clin Neurophysiol, 121*(4), 516–523. doi:10.1016/j.clinph.2009.11.087

Hämäläinen, M. S., & Ilmoniemi, R. J. (1994). Interpreting magnetic fields of the brain: Minimum norm estimates. *Medical and Biological Engineering and Computing, 32*(1), 35–42.

Head, H., & Holmes, G. (1911). Sensory disturbances from cerebral lesions. *Brain, 34*(2–3), 102–254.

Hill, N. J., Gupta, D., Brunner, P., Gunduz, A., Adamo, M. A., Ritaccio, A., & Schalk, G. (2012). Recording human electrocorticographic (ECoG) signals for neuroscientific research and real-time functional cortical mapping. *J Vis Exp*(64). doi:10.3791/3993

Hirata, M., Matsushita, K., Suzuki, T., Yoshida, T., Fumihiro, S., Morris, S., ... Yoshimine, T. (2011). A fully-implantable wireless system for human brain–machine interfaces using brain surface electrodes: W-HERBS. *IEICE Transactions on Communications, 94*(9), 2448–2453.

Hiremath, S. V., Tyler-Kabara, E. C., Wheeler, J. J., Moran, D. W., Gaunt, R. A., Collinger, J. L., ... Boninger, M. L. (2017). Human perception of electrical stimulation on the surface of somatosensory cortex. *PLoS One, 12*(5), e0176020.

Hochberg, L. R., Bacher, D., Jarosiewicz, B., Masse, N. Y., Simeral, J. D., Vogel, J., ... Donoghue, J. P. (2012). Reach and grasp by people with tetraplegia using a neurally controlled robotic arm. *Nature, 485*(7398), 372–375. doi:10.1038/nature11076

Hochberg, L. R., & Donoghue, J. P. (2006). Sensors for brain–computer interfaces. *IEEE Eng Med Biol Mag, 25*(5), 32–38.

Hochberg, L. R., Serruya, M. D., Friehs, G. M., Mukand, J. A., Saleh, M., Caplan, A. H., ... Donoghue, J. P. (2006). Neuronal ensemble control of prosthetic devices by a human with tetraplegia. *Nature, 442*(7099), 164–171. doi:10.1038/nature04970

Hoffmann, M., Marques, H., Arieta, A., Sumioka, H., Lungarella, M., & Pfeifer, R. (2010). Body schema in robotics: A review. *IEEE Transactions on Autonomous Mental Development, 2*(4), 304–324.

Horvath, J. C., Carter, O., & Forte, J. D. (2014). Transcranial direct current stimulation: Five important issues we aren't discussing (but probably should be). *Frontiers in Systems Neuroscience, 8*.

House, W. F. (1976). Cochlear implants. *Annals of Otology, Rhinology & Laryngology, 85*(3_suppl), 3–3.

Humphrey, D. R., Schmidt, E. M., & Thompson, W. D. (1970). Predicting measures of motor performance from multiple cortical spike trains. *Science, 170*(3959), 758–762.

Ifft, P. J., Shokur, S., Li, Z., Lebedev, M. A., & Nicolelis, M. A. (2013). A brain–machine interface enables bimanual arm movements in monkeys. *Sci Transl Med, 5*(210), 210ra154. doi:10.1126/scitranslmed.3006159

Jackson, A., Mavoori, J., & Fetz, E. E. (2006). Long-term motor cortex plasticity induced by an electronic neural implant. *Nature, 444*(7115), 56–60. doi:10.1038/nature05226

Jiang, N., Dosen, S., Muller, K.-R., & Farina, D. (2012). Myoelectric control of artificial limbs—Is there a need to change focus?[In the spotlight]. *IEEE Signal Processing Magazine, 29*(5), 152–150.

Johnson, L., Wander, J., Sarma, D., Su, D., Fetz, E., & Ojemann, J. G. (2013). Direct electrical stimulation of the somatosensory cortex in humans using electrocorticography electrodes: A qualitative and quantitative report. *Journal of Neural Engineering, 10*(3), 036021.

Kalman, R. E. (1960). A new approach to linear filtering and prediction problems. *Journal of Basic Engineering, 82*(1), 35–45.

Karabanov, A., Thielscher, A., & Siebner, H. R. (2016). Transcranial brain stimulation: Closing the loop between brain and stimulation. *Current Opinion in Neurology, 29*(4), 397.

Kawato, M. (1999). Internal models for motor control and trajectory planning. *Current Opinion in Neurobiology, 9*(6), 718–727.

Kim, S.-P., Rao, Y. N., Erdogmus, D., Sanchez, J. C., Nicolelis, M. A., & Principe, J. C. (2005). Determining patterns in neural activity for reaching movements using nonnegative matrix factorization. *EURASIP Journal on Applied Signal Processing, 2005*, 3113–3121.

Kim, S. P., Sanchez, J. C., Rao, Y. N., Erdogmus, D., Carmena, J. M., Lebedev, M. A., ... Principe, J. C. (2006). A comparison of optimal MIMO linear and nonlinear models for brain–machine interfaces. *J Neural Eng, 3*(2), 145–161. doi:10.1088/1741-2560/3/2/009

Korostenskaja, M., Kapeller, C., Prueckl, R., Ortner, R., Chen, P.-C., Guger, C., & Lee, K. H. (2014). Improving ECoG-based P300 speller accuracy. Proceedings of the 6th International Brain–Computer Interface Conference 2014.

Kotov, N. A., Winter, J. O., Clements, I. P., Jan, E., Timko, B. P., Campidelli, S., ... Prato, M. (2009). Nanomaterials for neural interfaces. *Advanced Materials, 21*(40), 3970–4004.

Kozai, T. D. Y., & Kipke, D. R. (2009). Insertion shuttle with carboxyl terminated self-assembled monolayer coatings for implanting flexible polymer neural probes in the brain. *Journal of Neuroscience Methods, 184*(2), 199–205.

Krause, B., & Kadosh, R. C. (2014). Not all brains are created equal: The relevance of individual differences in responsiveness to transcranial electrical stimulation. *Frontiers in Systems Neuroscience, 8*.

Krüger, J., Caruana, F., & Rizzolatti, G. (2010). Seven years of recording from monkey cortex with a chronically implanted multiple microelectrode. *Frontiers in Neuroengineering, 3*, 6.

Kwak, N. S., Muller, K. R., & Lee, S. W. (2015). A lower limb exoskeleton control system based on steady state visual evoked potentials. *J Neural Eng, 12*(5), 056009. doi:10.1088/1741-2560/12/5/056009

Kyriazis, M. (2015). Systems neuroscience in focus: From the human brain to the global brain? *Frontiers in Systems Neuroscience, 9*.

LaFleur, K., Cassady, K., Doud, A., Shades, K., Rogin, E., & He, B. (2013). Quadcopter control in three-dimensional space using a noninvasive motor imagery-based brain–computer interface. *Journal of Neural Engineering, 10*(4), 046003.

Lal, T. N., Schröder, M., Hill, N. J., Preissl, H., Hinterberger, T., Mellinger, J., ... Birbaumer, N. (2005). *A brain computer interface with online feedback based on magnetoencephalography*. Paper presented at the Proceedings of the 22nd international conference on Machine learning.

Lebedev, M. (2014). Brain–machine interfaces: An overview. *Translational Neuroscience, 5*(1), 99–110.

Lebedev, M. A., Carmena, J. M., O'Doherty, J. E., Zacksenhouse, M., Henriquez, C. S., Principe, J. C., & Nicolelis, M. A. (2005). Cortical ensemble adaptation to represent velocity of an artificial actuator controlled by a brain–machine interface. *J Neurosci, 25*(19), 4681–4693. doi:10.1523/JNEUROSCI.4088-04.2005

Lebedev, M. A., & Nicolelis, M. A. (2006). Brain–machine interfaces: Past, present and future. *Trends Neurosci, 29*(9), 536–546. doi:10.1016/j.tins.2006.07.004

Leuthardt, E. C., Miller, K. J., Schalk, G., Rao, R. P., & Ojemann, J. G. (2006). Electrocorticography-based brain computer interface—The Seattle experience. *IEEE Trans Neural Syst Rehabil Eng, 14*(2), 194–198. doi:10.1109/TNSRE.2006.875536

Leuthardt, E. C., Schalk, G., Wolpaw, J. R., Ojemann, J. G., & Moran, D. W. (2004). A brain–computer interface using electrocorticographic signals in humans. *Journal of Neural Engineering, 1*(2), 63.

Li, Z. (2014). Decoding methods for neural prostheses: Where have we reached? *Front Syst Neurosci, 8*, 129. doi:10.3389/fnsys.2014.00129

Li, Z., O'Doherty, J. E., Hanson, T. L., Lebedev, M. A., Henriquez, C. S., & Nicolelis, M. A. (2009). Unscented Kalman filter for brain–machine interfaces. *PLoS One, 4*(7), e6243. doi:10.1371/journal.pone.0006243

Li, Z., O'Doherty, J. E., Lebedev, M. A., & Nicolelis, M. A. (2011). Adaptive decoding for brain–machine interfaces through Bayesian parameter updates. *Neural Comput, 23*(12), 3162–3204. doi:10.1162/NECO_a_00207

Linderman, M., Lebedev, M. A., & Erlichman, J. S. (2009). Recognition of handwriting from electromyography. *PLoS One, 4*(8), e6791.

Maravita, A., & Iriki, A. (2004). Tools for the body (schema). *Trends in Cognitive Sciences, 8*(2), 79–86.

Maravita, A., Spence, C., & Driver, J. (2003). Multisensory integration and the body schema: Close to hand and within reach. *Current Biology, 13*(13), R531–R539.

May, T., Ozden, I., Brush, B., Borton, D., Wagner, F., Agha, N., ... Nurmikko, A. V. (2014). Detection of optogenetic stimulation in somatosensory cortex by non-human primates—Towards artificial tactile sensation. *PLoS One, 9*(12), e114529.

Mendoza, G., Peyrache, A., Gámez, J., Prado, L., Buzsaki, G., & Merchant, H. (2016). Recording extracellular neural activity in the behaving monkey using a semi-chronic and high-density electrode system. *Journal of Neurophysiology*, jn. 00116.02016.

Merfeld, D. M., & Lewis, R. F. (2012). Replacing semicircular canal function with a vestibular implant. *Current Opinion in Otolaryngology & Head and Neck Surgery, 20*(5), 386–392.

Mirabella, G., & Lebedev, M. A. (2017). Interfacing to the brain's motor decisions. *Journal of Neurophysiology, 117*(3), 1305–1319.

Moritz, C. T., Perlmutter, S. I., & Fetz, E. E. (2008). Direct control of paralysed muscles by cortical neurons. *Nature, 456*(7222), 639–642. doi:10.1038/nature07418

Muller-Putz, G. R., Daly, I., & Kaiser, V. (2014). Motor imagery-induced EEG patterns in individuals with spinal cord injury and their impact on brain-computer interface accuracy. *J Neural Eng, 11*(3), 035011. doi:10.1088/1741-2560/11/3/035011

Najafi, K., Wise, K. D., & Mochizuki, T. (1985). A high-yield IC-compatible multichannel recording array. *Electron Devices, IEEE Transactions on, 32*(7), 1206–1211.

Naseer, N., & Hong, K.-S. (2015). fNIRS-based brain–computer interfaces: A review. *Frontiers in Human Neuroscience, 9*. doi:10.3389/fnhum.2015.00003

Navarro, X., Krueger, T. B., Lago, N., Micera, S., Stieglitz, T., & Dario, P. (2005). A critical review of interfaces with the peripheral nervous system for the control of neuroprostheses and hybrid bionic systems. *Journal of the Peripheral Nervous System, 10*(3), 229–258.

Nicolelis, M. A., Baccala, L. A., Lin, R. C., & Chapin, J. K. (1995). Sensorimotor encoding by synchronous neural ensemble activity at multiple levels of the somatosensory system. *Science, 268*(5215), 1353–1358.

Nii, Y., Uematsu, S., Lesser, R. P., & Gordon, B. (1996). Does the central sulcus divide motor and sensory functions? Cortical mapping of human hand areas as revealed by electrical stimulation through subdural grid electrodes. *Neurology, 46*(2), 360–367.

Normann, R. A., Greger, B., House, P., Romero, S. F., Pelayo, F., & Fernandez, E. (2009). Toward the development of a cortically based visual neuroprosthesis. *J Neural Eng, 6*(3), 035001. doi:10.1088/1741-2560/6/3/035001

Nunez, P. L., & Srinivasan, R. (2006). *Electric Fields of the Brain: The Neurophysics of EEG*: Oxford University Press, USA.

O'Doherty, J. E., Lebedev, M. A., Hanson, T. L., Fitzsimmons, N. A., & Nicolelis, M. A. (2009). A brain–machine interface instructed by direct intracortical microstimulation. *Front Integr Neurosci, 3*, 20. doi:10.3389/neuro.07.020.2009

O'Doherty, J. E., Lebedev, M. A., Ifft, P. J., Zhuang, K. Z., Shokur, S., Bleuler, H., & Nicolelis, M. A. (2011). Active tactile exploration using a brain–machine–brain interface. *Nature, 479*(7372), 228–231. doi:10.1038/nature10489

Obermaier, B., Neuper, C., Guger, C., & Pfurtscheller, G. (2001). Information transfer rate in a five-classes brain–computer interface. *IEEE Trans Neural Syst Rehabil Eng, 9*(3), 283–288. doi:10.1109/7333.948456

Okorokova, E., Lebedev, M., Linderman, M., & Ossadtchi, A. (2015). A dynamical model improves reconstruction of handwriting from multichannel electromyographic recordings. *Frontiers in Neuroscience, 9*.

Pais-Vieira, M., Lebedev, M., Kunicki, C., Wang, J., & Nicolelis, M. A. (2013). A brain-to-brain interface for real-time sharing of sensorimotor information. *Sci Rep, 3*, 1319. doi:10.1038/srep01319

Pan, J., Li, Y., Gu, Z., & Yu, Z. (2013). A comparison study of two P300 speller paradigms for brain–computer interface. *Cogn Neurodyn, 7*(6), 523–529. doi:10.1007/s11571-013-9253-1

Pascarella, A., Todaro, C., Clerc, M., Serre, T., & Piana, M. (2016). Source modeling of ElectroCortico Graphy (ECoG) data: Stability analysis and spatial filtering. *Journal of Neuroscience Methods, 263*, 134–144.

Pazzaglia, M., & Molinari, M. (2016). The embodiment of assistive devices—From wheelchair to exoskeleton. *Physics of Life Reviews, 16*, 163–175.

Penfield, W., & Boldrey, E. (1937). Somatic motor and sensory representation in the cerebral cortex of man as studied by electrical stimulation *Brain: A Journal of Neurology*.

Pfurtscheller, G., Müller, G. R., Pfurtscheller, J., Gerner, H. J., & Rupp, R. (2003). 'Thought'—Control of functional electrical stimulation to restore hand grasp in a patient with tetraplegia. *Neuroscience Letters, 351*(1), 33–36.

Pfurtscheller, G., & Neuper, C. (2001). Motor imagery and direct brain–computer communication. *Proceedings of the IEEE, 89*(7), 1123–1134.

Pfurtscheller, G., & Neuper, C. (2006). Future prospects of ERD/ERS in the context of brain–computer interface (BCI) developments. *Prog Brain Res, 159*, 433–437. doi:10.1016/S0079-6123(06)59028-4

Pfurtscheller, J., Rupp, R., Muller, G. R., Fabsits, E., Korisek, G., Gerner, H. J., & Pfurtscheller, G. (2005). [Functional electrical stimulation instead of surgery? Improvement of grasping function with FES in a patient with C5 tetraplegia]. *Unfallchirurg, 108*(7), 587–590. doi:10.1007/s00113-004-0876-x

Piccione, F., Giorgi, F., Tonin, P., Priftis, K., Giove, S., Silvoni, S., ... Beverina, F. (2006). P300-based brain computer interface: Reliability and performance in healthy and paralysed participants. *Clin Neurophysiol, 117*(3), 531–537. doi:10.1016/j.clinph.2005.07.024

Pistohl, T., Ball, T., Schulze-Bonhage, A., Aertsen, A., & Mehring, C. (2008). Prediction of arm movement trajectories from ECoG-recordings in humans. *J Neurosci Methods, 167*(1), 105–114. doi:10.1016/j.jneumeth.2007.10.001

Pistor, J., Hoeffmann, J., Rotermund, D., Tolstosheeva, E., Schellenberg, T., Boll, D., ... Kreiter, A. (2013). *Development of a fully implantable recording system for ECoG signals.* Paper presented at the Proceedings of the Conference on Design, Automation and Test in Europe.

Placidi, G., Petracca, A., Spezialetti, M., & Iacoviello, D. (2015). Classification strategies for a single-trial binary brain computer interface based on remembering unpleasant odors. *Conf Proc IEEE Eng Med Biol Soc, 2015*, 7019–7022. doi:10.1109/EMBC.2015.7320008

Pohlmeyer, E. A., Oby, E. R., Perreault, E. J., Solla, S. A., Kilgore, K. L., Kirsch, R. F., & Miller, L. E. (2009). Toward the restoration of hand use to a paralyzed monkey: Brain-controlled functional electrical stimulation of forearm muscles. *PLoS One, 4*(6), e5924.

Prsa, M., Galiñanes, G. L., & Huber, D. (2017). Rapid integration of artificial sensory feedback during operant conditioning of motor cortex neurons. *Neuron, 93*(4), 929–939. e926.

Rao, R. P., Stocco, A., Bryan, M., Sarma, D., Youngquist, T. M., Wu, J., & Prat, C. S. (2014). A direct brain-to-brain interface in humans. *PLoS One, 9*(11), e111332. doi:10.1371/journal.pone.0111332

Raspopovic, S., Capogrosso, M., Petrini, F. M., Bonizzato, M., Rigosa, J., Di Pino, G., ... Fernandez, E. (2014). Restoring natural sensory feedback in real-time bidirectional hand prostheses. *Science Translational Medicine, 6*(222), 222ra219-222ra219.

Reid, S. A. (1989). Toward the ideal electrocorticography array. *Neurosurgery, 25*(1), 135–137.

Romo, R., Hernández, A., Zainos, A., & Salinas, E. (1998). Somatosensory discrimination based on cortical microstimulation. *Nature, 392*(6674), 387–390.

Sanchez, J. C., Erdogmus, D., Rao, Y., Principe, J. C., Nicolelis, M., & Wessberg, J. (2003). *Learning the contributions of the motor, premotor, and posterior parietal cortices for hand trajectory reconstruction in a brain machine interface.* Paper presented at the Neural Engineering, 2003. Conference Proceedings. First International IEEE EMBS Conference on.

Schalk, G. (2010). Can electrocorticography (ECoG) support robust and powerful brain–computer interfaces? *Front Neuroeng, 3*, 9. doi:10.3389/fneng.2010.00009

Schalk, G., & Leuthardt, E. C. (2011). Brain–computer interfaces using electrocorticographic signals. *IEEE Reviews in Biomedical Engineering, 4*, 140–154.

Schwartz, A. B., Kettner, R. E., & Georgopoulos, A. P. (1988). Primate motor cortex and free arm movements to visual targets in three-dimensional space. I. Relations between single cell discharge and direction of movement. *J Neurosci, 8*(8), 2913–2927.

Schwarz, D. A., Lebedev, M. A., Hanson, T. L., Dimitrov, D. F., Lehew, G., Meloy, J., ... Nicolelis, M. A. (2014). Chronic, wireless recordings of large-scale brain activity in freely moving rhesus monkeys. *Nat Methods, 11*(6), 670–676. doi:10.1038/nmeth.2936

Sellers, E. W., Krusienski, D. J., McFarland, D. J., Vaughan, T. M., & Wolpaw, J. R. (2006). A P300 event-related potential brain–computer interface (BCI): The effects of matrix size and inter stimulus interval on performance. *Biol Psychol, 73*(3), 242–252. doi:10.1016/j.biopsycho.2006.04.007

Serruya, M., Shaikhouni, A., & Donoghue, J. (2003). *Neural decoding of cursor motion using a Kalman filter.* Paper presented at the Advances in Neural Information Processing Systems 15: Proceedings of the 2002 Conference.

Shanechi, M. M., Orsborn, A., Moorman, H., Gowda, S., & Carmena, J. M. (2014). High-performance brain–machine interface enabled by an adaptive optimal feedback-controlled point process decoder. *Conf Proc IEEE Eng Med Biol Soc, 2014*, 6493–6496. doi:10.1109/EMBC.2014.6945115

Shanechi, M. M., Orsborn, A. L., & Carmena, J. M. (2016). Robust brain–machine interface design using optimal feedback control modeling and adaptive point process filtering. *PLoS Comput Biol, 12*(4), e1004730. doi:10.1371/journal.pcbi.1004730

Shannon, R. V. (2012). Advances in auditory prostheses. *Curr Opin Neurol, 25*(1), 61–6. doi: 10.1097/WCO .0b013e32834ef878

Sherrington, C. S. (1906). *The Integrative Action of the Nervous System.* New York: C. Scribner's Sons.

Sitaram, R., Caria, A., & Birbaumer, N. (2009). Hemodynamic brain–computer interfaces for communication and rehabilitation. *Neural Networks, 22*(9), 1320–1328.

Slutzky, M. W., & Flint, R. D. (2017). Physiological properties of brain machine interface input signals. *Journal of Neurophysiology*, jn. 00070.02017.

Song, H., Zhang, D., Ling, Z., Zuo, H., & Hong, B. (2012). *High gamma oscillations enhance the subdural visual speller.* Paper presented at the Engineering in Medicine and Biology Society (EMBC), 2012 Annual International Conference of the IEEE.

Su, Y., Routhu, S., Moon, K. S., Lee, S. Q., Youm, W., & Ozturk, Y. (2016). A wireless 32-channel implantable bidirectional brain machine interface. *Sensors, 16*(10), 1582.

Suminski, A. J., Fagg, A. H., Willett, F. R., Bodenhamer, M., & Hatsopoulos, N. G. (2013). *Online adaptive decoding of intended movements with a hybrid kinetic and kinematic brain machine interface.* Paper presented at the 2013 35th Annual International Conference of the IEEE Engineering in Medicine and Biology Society (EMBC).

Sun, F. T., & Morrell, M. J. (2014). Closed-loop neurostimulation: The clinical experience. *Neurotherapeutics, 11*(3), 553–563.

Tabot, G. A., Dammann, J. F., Berg, J. A., Tenore, F. V., Boback, J. L., Vogelstein, R. J., & Bensmaia, S. J. (2013). Restoring the sense of touch with a prosthetic hand through a brain interface. *Proceedings of the National Academy of Sciences, 110*(45), 18279–18284.

Tai, K., & Chau, T. (2009). Single-trial classification of NIRS signals during emotional induction tasks: Towards a corporeal machine interface. *Journal of Neuroengineering and Rehabilitation, 6*(1), 1.

Tan, D. W., Schiefer, M. A., Keith, M. W., Anderson, J. R., Tyler, J., & Tyler, D. J. (2014). A neural interface provides long-term stable natural touch perception. *Science Translational Medicine, 6*(257), 257ra138–257ra138.

Taylor, D. M., Tillery, S. I., & Schwartz, A. B. (2002). Direct cortical control of 3D neuroprosthetic devices. *Science, 296*(5574), 1829–1832. doi:10.1126/science.1070291

Tkach, D., Reimer, J., & Hatsopoulos, N. G. (2008). Observation-based learning for brain–machine interfaces. *Curr Opin Neurobiol, 18*(6), 589–594. doi:10.1016/j.conb.2008.09.016

Todorov, E. (2004). Optimality principles in sensorimotor control. *Nature Neuroscience, 7*(9), 907–915.

Todorov, E., & Jordan, M. I. (2002). Optimal feedback control as a theory of motor coordination. *Nature Neuroscience, 5*(11), 1226–1235.

Vansteensel, M. J., Pels, E. G., Bleichner, M. G., Branco, M. P., Denison, T., Freudenburg, Z. V., ... Van Den Boom, M. A. (2016). Fully implanted brain–computer interface in a locked-in patient with ALS. *N Engl J Med, 2016*(375), 2060–2066.

Velliste, M., Perel, S., Spalding, M. C., Whitford, A. S., & Schwartz, A. B. (2008). Cortical control of a prosthetic arm for self-feeding. *Nature, 453*(7198), 1098–1101. doi:10.1038/nature06996

Vetter, R. J., Williams, J. C., Hetke, J. F., Nunamaker, E. A., & Kipke, D. R. (2004). Chronic neural recording using silicon-substrate microelectrode arrays implanted in cerebral cortex. *Biomedical Engineering, IEEE Transactions on, 51*(6), 896–904.

Viventi, J., Kim, D.-H., Vigeland, L., Frechette, E. S., Blanco, J. A., Kim, Y.-S., ... Vanleer, A. C. (2011). Flexible, foldable, actively multiplexed, high-density electrode array for mapping brain activity *in vivo. Nature neuroscience, 14*(12), 1599–1605.

Wahnoun, R., He, J., & Tillery, S. I. H. (2006). Selection and parameterization of cortical neurons for neuro-prosthetic control. *Journal of Neural Engineering, 3*(2), 162.

Walker, A. E., Johnson, H. C., & Marshall, C. (1949). Electrocorticography. *Bull Johns Hopkins Hosp, 84*(6), 583.

Wang, W., Collinger, J. L., Degenhart, A. D., Tyler-Kabara, E. C., Schwartz, A. B., Moran, D. W., ... Ashmore, R. C. (2013). An electrocorticographic brain interface in an individual with tetraplegia. *PLoS One, 8*(2), e55344.

Weinand, M. E., Hermann, B., Wyler, A. R., Carter, L. P., Oommen, K. J., Labiner, D., ... Herring, A. (1994). Long-term subdural strip electrocorticographic monitoring of ictal deja vu. *Epilepsia, 35*(5), 1054–1059.

Wessberg, J., Stambaugh, C. R., Kralik, J. D., Beck, P. D., Laubach, M., Chapin, J. K., ... Nicolelis, M. A. (2000). Real-time prediction of hand trajectory by ensembles of cortical neurons in primates. *Nature, 408*(6810), 361–365. doi:10.1038/35042582

Widge, A. S., & Moritz, C. T. (2014). Pre-frontal control of closed-loop limbic neurostimulation by rodents using a brain–computer interface. *Journal of Neural Engineering, 11*(2), 024001.

Wilson, B. S., & Dorman, M. F. (2008). Cochlear implants: A remarkable past and a brilliant future. *Hear Res, 242*(1–2), 3–21. doi: 10.1016/j.heares.2008.06.005

Wilson, J. A., Felton, E. A., Garell, P. C., Schalk, G., & Williams, J. C. (2006). ECoG factors underlying multimodal control of a brain–computer interface. *IEEE Transactions on Neural Systems and Rehabilitation Engineering, 14*(2), 246–250.

Wolpert, D. M., Ghahramani, Z., & Jordan, M. I. (1995). An internal model for sensorimotor integration. *Science, 269*(5232), 1880.

Wyler, A. R., Walker, G., & Somes, G. (1991). The morbidity of long-term seizure monitoring using subdural strip electrodes. *J Neurosurg, 74*(5), 734–737. doi:10.3171/jns.1991.74.5.0734

Yazdan-Shahmorad, A., Diaz-Botia, C., Hanson, T. L., Kharazia, V., Ledochowitsch, P., Maharbiz, M. M., & Sabes, P. N. (2016). A large-scale interface for optogenetic stimulation and recording in nonhuman primates. *Neuron, 89*(5), 927–939.

Yoo, P. B., & Durand, D. M. (2005). Selective recording of the canine hypoglossal nerve using a multicontact flat interface nerve electrode. *IEEE Transactions on Biomedical Engineering, 52*(8), 1461–1469.

Yoo, S. S., Fairneny, T., Chen, N. K., Choo, S. E., Panych, L. P., Park, H., ... Jolesz, F. A. (2004). Brain–computer interface using fMRI: Spatial navigation by thoughts. *Neuroreport, 15*(10), 1591–1595.

Zander, T. O., Kothe, C., Jatzev, S., & Gaertner, M. (2010). Enhancing human–computer interaction with input from active and passive brain-computer interfaces. *Brain–Computer Interfaces* (pp. 181–199): Springer.

Zhang, H., Ma, C., & He, J. (2010). *Predicting lower limb muscular activity during standing and squatting using spikes of primary motor cortical neurons in monkeys.* Paper presented at the 2010 Annual International Conference of the IEEE Engineering in Medicine and Biology.

Zhang, Y., Ding, L., van Drongelen, W., Hecox, K., Frim, D. M., & He, B. (2006). A cortical potential imaging study from simultaneous extra-and intracranial electrical recordings by means of the finite element method. *Neuroimage, 31*(4), 1513–1524.

Zippo, A. G., Romanelli, P., Torres Martinez, N. R., Caramenti, G. C., Benabid, A. L., & Biella, G. E. M. (2015). A novel wireless recording and stimulating multichannel epicortical grid for supplementing or enhancing the sensory-motor functions in monkey (*Macaca fascicularis*). *Frontiers in Systems Neuroscience, 9*(73). doi:10.3389/fnsys.2015.00073

# 38 Perspectives on Brain–Computer Interfaces

*Gerwin Schalk*

## CONTENTS

38.1 Future Development.................................................................................................722
38.2 Summary ............................................................................................................723

**Abstract**

The field of brain–computer interfaces (BCIs) began in the 1960s and has produced substantial excitement and engagement by scientists, funding agencies, and the public for more than 20 years. Despite these efforts, clinically and commercially successful examples of BCI technology are rare. This issue has been recognized for several years and has usually been attributed to specific technical difficulties (such as low information transfer rates) that need to be addressed. This perspective chapter draws attention to other issues of translational research that impede the widespread adoption of BCI technology.

The exciting and emerging field of brain–computer interface (BCI) research that is the subject of this book is developing devices that interact with electrical signals from the nervous system and thereby realize entirely new diagnostic or treatment options for nervous system disorders. Such devices are completely novel, because they use electrical interactions rather than chemicals to make beneficial changes to the nervous system. Possible examples for the application of BCI devices include the restoration of communication function in people with amyotrophic lateral sclerosis, treatment of movement disorders, detection and suppression of epileptic seizures, rehabilitation of chronic stroke survivors, or treatment of people with severe chronic pain. The substantial excitement for BCI research is documented by the large and growing academic research in this area, several dedicated conference series, as well as large funding initiatives in the United States, Europe, and elsewhere.

The important opportunities of BCI research are opened up and supported by a confluence of three drivers. The first driver is the recognition that the nervous system can change in response to appropriate training protocols. The second driver is the growing abundance of cheap computing power and the miniaturization of sensor and stimulation devices. The third driver is the recent and increasing recognition of the commercial opportunities of BCI devices. Together, these drivers produced the motivation for BCI research, which began with an initial demonstration of brain-controlled devices in the 1960s and 1970s, and has now evolved into a diverse research and development enterprise.

In accord with many other studies over the past decades, the research described and summarized in this book has provided ample evidence that signals recorded invasively or noninvasively from the brain can be used to give information about the motor, sensory, cognitive, or affective state of a user, that such information can be decoded from the brain in real time, and that the results of this decoding can produce stimulation of the nervous system to replace, restore, enhance, supplement, or improve human functions.

## 38.1 FUTURE DEVELOPMENT

Previous research has produced exciting technical demonstrations of BCI technologies. At the same time, despite more than 20 years of intense research funded by substantial and sustained support from funding agencies, and the undeniable fascination for the topic by scientists, the media, and the public, only very few BCI technologies have been translated into new clinically and commercially successful diagnostic or treatment options.

This problem has been recognized for many years. Contemporary discussions of this topic usually focus on the necessity for additional scientific understanding or further technical improvements. These discussions imply that the current lack of those improvements in understanding or technology is the reason for the lack in commercial adoption of BCI technologies. This logic suggests that the critical issue at hand is to further improve BCI technologies and our understanding of the brain but does not provide any suggestions about which aspects of technology or understanding should be improved.

In this context, it is helpful to remember the differing goals of basic versus translational research. The goal of basic neuroscientific research is to produce additional knowledge about brain function, irrespective of the immediate utility of that increase in understanding. In contrast, the goal of translational research is to use existing neuroscientific understanding to design, implement, and apply new neurotechnologies that address an important clinical or other problem. Most of the contemporary work in BCI research could be considered translational. Thus, in determining those aspects of technology or understanding that is in most dire need of improvement, it appears to be helpful to consider that the perhaps most important requirement for any successful new technology is that its benefit exceeds its cost.

In this way, an assessment of benefit should not primarily be concerned with optimizing a particular technical specification, but rather carefully consider the realistic benefit of the BCI technology relative to all existing (BCI or other) diagnostic or treatment options as well as the number of individuals that are interested in using it. For example, a BCI-based communication device may support brain-based spelling at a rate of a few characters per minute. This capacity to spell using the brain may be inspiring and statistically well above chance, but it may not provide a clinically relevant improvement over existing augmentative communication devices or may provide such improvement to only very few people. Likewise, an assessment of the cost of BCI technologies should consider not only the hardware cost of a BCI device but also the risks and costs of regulatory approvals, intellectual property strategies and other legal activities, development of new sales/marketing channels, product development, support, and the complexities associated with the change to the BCI technologies from the traditional technologies that they replace. If the aggregated benefit does not exceed the aggregated cost, commercialization is unlikely.

Finally, it is important to recognize that successful commercialization in the medical sector requires not only knowledgeable individuals but also legal, commercial, and procedural frameworks that guide their fruitful interaction. For example, a clinician needs to be aware of different BCI options and needs to understand how it can be prescribed, reimbursed, acquired, supported, and serviced. The corresponding knowledge and people required for successful commercialization, as well as the medical, corporate, and legal arrangements necessary to support this process, have existed for decades for traditional medical devices and pharmaceuticals. This critical infrastructure is in a very early stage for BCI systems, but will require substantial cost, effort, and thus time to conceive, implement, and optimize.

BCIs to replace, restore, or enhance functions, such as those that restore movements, support communication functions, or automatically brake a car, face a principal challenge in that they need to derive an assessment of the user's brain state very rapidly and accurately. Unfortunately, all currently available brain signal sensors can only either produce unreliable measurements quickly or reliable measurements very slowly. Given this principal limitation, the number of users that can benefit from these types of BCI technologies using current sensor technologies is small, and/or those users often already have access to non-BCI alternatives. For this reason, it is quite possible that successful commercialization of these types of BCIs may require the development of currently unknown sensor technologies that can simultaneously produce rapid and reliable brain signal measurements.

At the same time, BCIs to improve functions, such as those that rehabilitate chronic stroke survivors or people with incomplete spinal cord injury, have attracted increasing interest over the past several years. They use appropriate BCI protocols to induce beneficial plasticity in specific central nervous system circuits and usually have more relaxed requirements with respect to rapidity and reliability. The number of users that can benefit from those BCI technologies can be large, and there are often no satisfactory alternatives to BCI approaches. Thus, it appears that, with additional development and validation, and with development of proper regulatory, reimbursement, and commercialization strategies, these types of BCIs may have a more direct trajectory toward successful translation and commercialization.

## 38.2 SUMMARY

Real-time interaction with the brain using BCI technologies is opening up fundamentally new, important, and potentially highly impactful possibilities for improving the lives of people with and eventually without nervous system disorders. Appropriate focus on the needs of end users and on legal, regulatory, and commercial realities should help hasten the realization of development of BCI systems that not only can succeed in the realm of academia but also can create a whole range of completely new and clinically and commercially successful diagnosis and treatment options.

# Conclusion: Moving Forward in Brain–Computer Interfaces

*Chang S. Nam, Fabien Lotte, and Anton Nijholt*

Thirty-eight chapters ago, we started this handbook with an introduction that began with brain–computer interface (BCI) technology trends and historical events that have broken ground for BCI research and development. We thought that the world is ready for a new handbook that comprehensively addresses the recent and rapid changes in the field of BCIs. However, this handbook was not intended to provide a single blueprint for BCIs. Rather, it highlighted a synopsis of key findings and technological and theoretical advances directly applicable to brain–computer interfacing technologies, readily understood and applied by individuals with no formal training in BCI research and development.

It is timely given the important role that BCI researchers play in the improvement of people's lives by replacing, restoring, supplementing, enhancing, and improving motor and cognitive actions, and by understanding the neural bases of such functions as seeing, hearing, attending, remembering, deciding, and planning in relation to technologies and their functioning in the real world. By including up-to-date techniques (Parts II and III), BCI paradigms (Part IV), and diverse applications (Part I), and taking into account the views of stakeholders throughout the process (Part V) and emerging issues (Part VI), BCI systems can be designed and developed with the overall goal of supporting a wide range of users for a wide range of applications. This notably includes impaired users for assistive technology and rehabilitation, as well as various other existing or new potential healthy user groups such as gamers, artists, or IT professionals for applications in the domestic domain, human–computer interaction, robotics, and team performance, among many others. Passive BCIs are also expected to be very promising tools to bring many of such applications to the real world and to the market.

Overall, we hope that this handbook gave our readers the tools and the inspiration to bring BCI usability and reliability to the next level, as well as to identify and design new applications that can be used outside the laboratory. To do so, we also hope that this handbook encouraged collaborative work among researchers from various disciplines, which is key to innovative and relevant results in the field.

# Author Index

**A**

Aakula, R., 457
Aarnoutse, E., 300, 301, 303, 304, 305, 309, 310, 313, 334
Aarts, R. M., 15, 24, 136, 373, 465
Abad, R. V., 241
Abarbanel, A., 27
Abdulkader, S. N., 463
Abenstein, M., 21
Abhari, Kamyar, 504
Abootalebi, V., 74
Abosch, A., 34
Absil, P.-A., 378
Abu-Alqumsan M., 329
à Campo, S., 176, 177, 181
Acharya, S., 257, 300, 303
Achyuta, A. K. H, 122
Acimovic, R., 116
Acosta, S., 150
Acqualagna, L., 464, 506, 586
Adali, T., 420
Adami, H., 37t
Adams, D. L., 313
Adamski, T., 309
Adler, R., 575
Adolphs, R., 149
Aertsen, A., 21, 300, 303
Afergan, D., 78
Afsari, B., 362
Afshar, P., 305, 309
Aftanas, L., 152, 153
Aggarwal, V., 257
Aggensteiner, P., 105
Agnew, W. F., 303
Agorelius, J., 704
Agostini, M., 102, 106
Agrafioti, F., 149
Aguilar, J. M., 33
Ahlstrom, D., 591
Ahmad, S. K., 125
Ahmad, Waqas, 503
Ahmar, N., 35t
Ahmedian, P., 171
Ahn, M., 60, 257, 260, 447f, 448f, 449, 449f, 450t, 451, 453, 457, 462, 517
Ahn, S., 257, 259, 260, 447f, 448f, 449, 449f, 450t, 451, 453, 457
Ai, Q., 134, 373, 375
Aigen, K., 195
Aihara, K., 377, 453
Air, E. L., 302, 306, 307, 308
Ajiboye, A. B., 708
Akram, F., 702
Alamdari, Nasim, 508
Alamgir, M., 431, 432
Albrecht, B., 15
Aldridge, D., 195
Alhaddad, M. J., 27

Ali, A., 554
Aliakbaryhosseinabadi, S., 679
Alicea, B., 236, 238
Alimardani, M., 706
Allal, L., 607
Allefeld, C., 362
Allen, Anita L., 655
Allen, E. A., 302
Alley, R.L., 228
Allison, B., 461, 462, 463, 464, 465, 527, 528, 535, 554, 586, 596, 597
Allison, B. Z., 4, 13, 15, 17, 25, 89–90, 94, 95, 97, 147, 151, 154, 155, 156, 171, 210, 211, 220, 238, 241, 242, 243, 305, 329, 332, 334, 408
Aloise, F., 38t, 39, 257, 258, 259, 260, 334, 479, 578
*Alpha WoW*, 240
Altenmüller, E., 150
Altun, Y., 431, 432
AlZoubi, O., 152, 153, 154, 195
Amari, S. I., 409, 412
Ambadar, Z., 150
American Speech-Language-Hearing Association, 115
Amir, N., 150
Amiri, S., 465, 467, 479, 507, 514
Amma, C., 468
Amore, M., 107
An, X., 535
An, X.-W., 19
Anantram, M. P., 125
Andersen, R. A., 468, 470, 554, 702, 711
Andersen, S., 373
Anderson, A. K., 149
Anderson, C. A., 27
Anderson, C. W., 3, 28, 31, 32, 362, 408
Anderson, K. D., 126
Anderson, K. L., 300
Anderson, N., 4, 299, 300, 301, 303, 304, 313, 334
Ando, T., 382
Andor, Minodora, 198
Andreasen, D., 280, 283, 289, 292
Andreessen, L. M., 82
Andreev, A., 362, 377, 378, 386, 517
Andreoni, G., 4, 244, 331, 332, 479
Andujar, M., 4
Ang, B. T., 408
Ang, K. K., 4, 105, 152, 153, 366, 408, 409, 410, 418, 451, 453, 542, 543, 669, 705
Anghelescu, A., 38t
Anikeeva, P., 120
Ansari-Asl, Karim, 200
Antelis, J., 35t
Antley, A., 218, 224, 227
Anumanchipalli, G. K., 305, 313
Aoki, F., 299
Appelhans, B. M., 149
Appriou, A., 331
Aranibar, A., 54
Aranyi, G. G., 152

Arbabian, A., 123
Arbib, M. A., 21
Arbizu, J., 373, 465
Archer, J., 309, 312
Arciniegas, D. B., 27
Ard, T., 105, 334
Ardolino, G., 306
Argunsah, A. Ö., 33, 34t
Aricò, P., 38t, 39, 334, 479
Arieli, A., 299
Ariely, Dan, 658
Arlotti, M., 306
Armilio, M. L., 105
Arnaldi, B., 30, 33, 60, 70, 240, 362, 408, 456
Arnegard, R. J., 73
Arnemann, K., 211
Arnett, C., 309
Arnold, L. E., 626
Arnold, M. M., 224, 300
Arns, M., 181, 211, 550, 552
Arra, S., 123
Arroyo, I., 606
Arroyo A., 3
Arsenin, V., 58
Arsigny, V., 383, 384
Artieda, J., 373, 465
Arvaneh, M., 410
Arzabal, P., 381
Asadpour, V., 479
Asaka, Y., 103, 107
Asama, H., 222
Asare, Philip, 201
Ascari, L., 171
Aschenbrenner-Scheibe, R., 300
Asghari-Esfeden, S., 152, 154
Ash, B., 123
Ashe, J., 673
Ashkan, K., 306
Ashmore, R. C., 270, 303, 313, 330
Asin, G., 95
Astolfi, L., 90, 95, 102, 105, 334, 446, 451, 686, 687
Aström, T., 152, 153
Atencio, C. A., 118
Atia, A., 463
Atkins, M. D., 270
Attias, H. T., 420
Auais, M. A., 133
Auer, T., 15
Augath, M., 299
Auguste, K., 299, 300
Avestruz, A., 305, 309
Ayache, N., 383, 384
Ayaz, H., 221
Ayton, L. N., 119f
Azinfar, L., 465
Aziz, T. Z., 306

**B**

Babacan, S. D., 410
Babiloni, F., 3, 33, 257, 334, 553, 686, 687, 690, 693
Babyak, M. A., 74
Baccino, T., 467
Bacher, D., 280, 293, 479

Bachhuber, D. R. W., 29
Baciu, M., 299
*Bacteria Hunt*, 240
Badakva, A. M., 256
Bae, Jae Hwan, 517
Bahn, S., 13, 34
Bahramisharif, A., 347
Bai, O., 171, 408, 462, 528, 534
Baier, G., 196, 198
Bailes, F., 194
Baillet, S., 57, 58, 59, 61, 63
Bainbridge, W. S., 114
Bakardjian, H., 33, 152, 420
Bakay, R. A. E., 280, 283
Baker, M. A., 292, 293
Bakhshayesh, A. R., 554
Balakrishnan, D., 33
Balderas, D., 211, 220, 237, 240
Baldwin, C.L., 457
Ball, K. R., 394
Ball, T., 21, 300, 303
Ballard, D. H., 35t, 216, 240, 241
Ball, Catherine A., 662
Bamdad, M., 133
Bamdadian, A., 550
Bamidis, P. D., 152
Banbury, S., 73
Bangor, A., 575
Baniasad, M. H., 152, 153
Barachant, A., 362, 377, 378, 385, 386, 428, 429
Barbara, R., 330
Barbaro, N., 299, 302, 307, 313
Barbeau, H., 117
Barber, D., 29
Barberini, C., 306
Barbero, Á., 598, 606
Barbieri, R., 152, 153, 154
Barbosa, M. A., 167
Barbour, D. L., 305, 334
Barefoot, L., 280, 293
Bareket, L., 118, 119
Barfield, W., 237
Barkley, G. L., 309, 311, 373, 465
Baron, J.-C., 102, 105
Barreto, A. B., 33
Barrett, L. F., 148, 149, 150
Barros, R. Q., 579
Barry, E., 181
Bartels, J., 280, 283, 289, 292
Bartenstein, P., 21
Barthélemy, Q., 382, 386
Bartl, M., 466
Bartneck, C., 219
Bartolomei, F., 102
Bartsch, A., 211
Bascil, M. S., 33
Bashashati, A., 30
Bastos-Filho, T. F., 15
Basyul, I., 35t, 36
Bathia, R., 377
Batista, A. P., 63
Battles, B., 167
Bauby, Jean-Dominique, 661
Bauer, R., 243

Bauernfeind, G., 4, 15, 94, 151, 154, 155, 238, 242, 461
Baumgartner, J., 334
Baykara, E., 239, 596
Bayliss, J. D., 35t, 216, 227, 240, 241
Bayoudh, S., 347, 355, 401, 409
bcisociety.org, 4
Bearden, T. S., 102
Beck, P. D., 70
Becker, W., 672, 673
Beckmann, C.F., 211
Beek, P. J., 179
Begault, D. R., 237
Behrendt, T., 687
Beisteiner, R., 674
Belardinelli, M. O., 151
Belardinelli, P., 114
Belda-Lois, J. M., 95
Belitski, A., 535
Bell, C. J., 35t, 36, 334
Bell, M. L., 314
Bellamkonda, R., 22
Bellgrove, M. A., 181
Belliveau, J. W., 54
Benabid, A.-L., 22, 309, 311
Bench, C. J., 211
Benedetti, F., 215, 227
Benedik, M., 116
Bengio, S., 33, 34t
Benitez, R., 198
Benítez-Burraco, A., 114
Bennabi, D., 711
Bennett, K. P., 31, 32
Bensch, M., 35t, 134, 334, 408
Bensmaia, S. J., 120, 702, 704
Benyamini, M., 706
Benz, H. L., 300, 303
Benzi, R., 553
Berar, M., 377, 378
Berg, A., 82
Berg, P., 105
Berger, H., 2, 16
Berger, M. S., 299, 313
Berger, T. W., 121
Berhanu, E., 280, 293
Berka, C., 152, 153, 154
Berkovic, S. F., 309, 312
Berman, B. D., 211
Bermejo-Bosch, I., 95
Bermúdez i Badia, S., 226, 243, 702
Berns, Gregory S., 658
Bernstein, N. A., 705
Berry, S. D., 103, 107
Berthing, T., 704
Berthoumieu, Y., 394
Bertrand, A., 168
Bertrand, O., 4, 299, 331, 449, 457
Besio, G., 449
Besserve, M., 61
Betler, T., 330
Bevan, N., 566
Beveridge, R., 13
Beyerer, J., 467
Bhatia, R., 362, 377, 384
Bhatt, M. B., 106

Bhattacharyya, S., 16, 21
Bi, L., 38
Bi, N., 409, 412
Bianchi, L., 4, 90, 244, 332, 334, 449, 479, 638
Bianchini, F., 125
Biava, Ryan, 655
Bidet-Caulet, A., 299, 307
Biederman, J., 550
Bieger, J., 15, 24, 136, 373, 465
Bieliaieva, E., 305
Bieliaieva, K., 14
Bießmann, F., 74, 347, 365
Bigand, Emmanuel, 194
Bigdely-Shamlo, N., 4, 82, 152, 153, 154, 155, 167, 177
Bijlenga, D., 554
Billinger, M., 28, 38t, 220, 225
Billinghurst, M., 237
Bin, G., 347, 366, 403, 458, 554
Bink, H., 309
Bink, M., 181
Biocca, F. A., 236, 238
Birbaumer, N., 3, 4, 12, 13, 15, 20, 23, 24, 35t, 36, 39, 70,
      72, 75, 80, 82, 89, 90, 94, 101, 102, 104, 105,
      106, 108, 133, 134, 151, 154, 155, 210, 236, 242,
      244, 259, 299, 303, 304, 305, 313, 314, 330, 331,
      332, 334, 347, 349, 362, 373, 408, 426, 446,
      449, 455, 456, 457, 461, 462, 463, 464, 466,
      596, 605, 661
Birch, G. E., 30, 332, 362, 449, 468
Birkle, S. M., 25
Birman, D., 362
Bischof, H., 32, 211, 218, 226, 239, 298, 300, 301, 303,
      305, 313, 334, 466
Bishop, C. M., 355, 410, 413
Blaauw, M., 655
Blabe, C. H., 126
Blabe, Christine H., 654
Black, A. H., 104
Black, M. J., 280, 293
Blain-Moraes, S., 579, 654, 661, 662
Blake, A., 410
Blakely, Tim M., 303, 304, 313, 334, 662, 705
Blakeslee, S., 80
Blanca-Mena, M. J., 240
Blank, F., 125
Blanke, O., 238
Blankertz, B., 3, 4, 15, 29, 35t, 61, 70, 72, 74, 78, 90, 174,
      210, 211, 221, 244, 258, 259, 260, 305, 332,
      344, 347, 349, 350, 352, 353, 355, 360, 361, 362,
      364, 365, 366, 381, 408, 409, 418, 434, 451, 453,
      456, 457, 461, 462, 463, 464, 466, 467, 468,
      479, 503, 506, 586, 616, 617, 619, 659
Blatt, R., 38t
Bledowski, C., 22
Bleichner, M. G., 64, 303, 304, 305, 309, 310, 313, 334,
      704
Bleuel, M., 82
Bleuler, H., 246
Bliquez, L. J., 114
Bliss, T. V. P., 677
Blumberg, J., 602
Boas, D. A., 20
Boatman, D., 299
Boatman-Reich, D., 299, 300

Bock, S. W., 20
Bocker, K. B. E., 104
Boe, S., 102
Boecker, H., 21
Boeckx, C., 114
Boehm, S. G., 210
Bogacz, R., 211
Bogdan, M., 73, 78, 134, 210, 303, 314, 334
Bogdancd, M., 35t
Bogojeski, M., 344
Bohannon, A. W., 238, 394, 464, 468
Bohil, C. J., 236, 238
Boland, Daniel, 517
Boldrey, E., 709
Bolinger, E., 38t, 220, 225
Boly, M., 90
Bompas, A., 4
Bond, K., 37t
Bongers, I., 181
Boninger, M. L., 13, 126, 270, 299, 330
Bonnet, L., 38t, 39, 226, 606, 688, 692, 697
Bonnet, M., 377, 386
Bonnet, S., 362, 377, 378, 385
Boon, P., 168
Boonstra, T. W., 107
Borasio, G. D., 586
Borchers, S., 710
Bordoloi, S., 38t
Bortfeld, H., 20
Borton, D., 117
Bos, D. P.-O., 4, 76, 242, 464, 564, 579, 692
Bos, N., 127
Bos, P.-O. D., 242
Boschert, J., 673
Bostanov, V., 31
Botrel, L., 35t, 36, 334, 586, 588
Botte-Lecocq, C., 579
Böttiger, C., 20
Botvinick, M., 244
Bouchard, K. E., 305, 313
Bougrain, L., 458
Boulay, C. B., 35t, 102, 106, 334
Bourget, D., 309
Bouton, C. E., 701, 704, 708
Bovermann, T., 176
Bowden, T., 115
Bowen, S., 106
Bower, G. H., 150
Bowers, C. W., 299
Bowman, D. A., 237
Bowsher, K., 330
Boye, A. T., 28
Bradley, A. P., 621
Bradley, M. M., 150, 152, 155
Bradley, W. E., 116
Bragdon, H. R., 54
Bragin, A., 21
Brainwave Music, 193
Brammar, R., 115
Branco, M. P., 305, 309, 310, 334
Brandeis, D., 104, 105
Brandl, S., 622
Branner, A., 4
Braren, M., 54

Brasil, F. L., 102, 106
Bratsas, C., 152
Brauchle, D., 243
Braun, C., 105, 300, 334
Braun, M., 78
Braun, N., 626
Brauneis, C., 36, 37t, 462
Breimhorst, M., 211
Breitwieser, B., 244
Breitwieser, C., 4, 151, 259, 260, 261, 331, 332, 479
Brennan, C., 469
Brennan, R. T., 105
Breshears, J., 305, 334
Bressler, S. L., 299
Breteler, M., 211
Bridwell, D. A., 37t, 687, 697
Briggs, K. E., 152, 155
Briskin, S., 466
Broccard, F. D., 117
Brockmeier, A. J., 171
Brodbeck, C., 327
Broderick, A. J., 74
Broetz, D., 102, 106, 669
Bronkhorst, A. W., 73
Brönstrup, J., 70, 80
Bronte-Stewart, H., 306
Brookes, M. J., 59
Brookhuis, K. A., 73
Brooks, D. J., 211
Brooks, J. O., 228
Brose, S. W., 299
Bross, D., 35t, 36, 70, 334
Brosschot, J. F., 149
Brotz, D., 108
Brouwer, A. M., 13, 15, 22, 35t, 70, 73, 76, 152, 153, 156,
        196, 256, 258, 259, 260, 261, 527, 535, 538
Brovelli, A., 171
Browall, C., 76, 687, 693
Brown, E., 420
Brown, E. H. P., 330
Brown, E. N., 152, 153, 154
Brown, K. A., 102, 106
Brown, Lawrence D., 642
Brown, P., 107, 306
Brown, R., 305, 313
Brown, S., 243
Bruckner, M., 329
Brühl, A. B., 211
Brühlmann, F., 211
Brumberg, J. S., 283, 289, 292
Brunia, C. H., 672, 673
Brunner, C., 4, 15, 90, 94, 95, 151, 154, 155, 241, 243, 244,
        332, 408, 461, 463, 464, 479
Brunner, P., 298, 299, 300, 301, 303, 305, 313, 334, 466,
        703, 705, 708
Bruno, M.-A., 90
Bruno, P., 27
Bruns, T. M., 126
Bryant, D., 13
Bryson, S. E., 181
Buch, E., 105, 334, 705
Buell T. J., 118
Bufalari, F. S., 334
Bufalari, S., 334

Buitelaar, J. K., 181
Bullara, L. A., 303
Bunce, S., 221
Bundy, D., 313, 314, 334
Bunts, R. C., 116
Burges, C. J., 31
Burgess, A. P., 352
Burke, B. C., 21
Burke, J. F., 103
Burke, R., 37t, 217, 465
Burnett, W. H., 116
Busch, N. A., 553
Buss, M., 60, 366
Buttaro, T. M., 116
Buttfield, A., 464, 601
Buzsáki, G., 300
Byblow, W. D., 451
Byrne, E. A., 78

## C

Cabestaing, F., 347, 355, 401, 409
Cabral, 601
Cacciola, L., 167
Cacioppo, J. T., 152, 155
Cage, John, 193, 195
Cagnoni, S., 171
Cai, Z., 462
Caldera, K., 105
Calhoun, G., 3, 197, 216, 241
Calhoun, V. D., 37t, 211, 224, 302
Callaghan, M., 133
Calvo, R. A., 152, 153, 154, 195
Cameirão, M., 226
Campbell, C., 31, 32
Campbell, J. M., 237
Campbell, N., 150
Canady, B., 211
Canli, T., 152
Canolty, R. T., 299, 302, 307
Cantor, D. S., 16
Cao, A., 575
Cao, J., 33
Cao, T., 15, 37t, 138
Cao, Y., 168
Caplan, A., 4
Caplan, J. B., 300
Capogrosso, M., 117, 711
Caporusso, N., 210
Capotosto, P., 543
Carabalona, R., 22, 462
Carayon, P., 568
Card, Stuart K., 645
Carey, H. L., 237
Caria, A., 95, 102, 105, 106, 108, 211, 236, 334
Caridakis, G., 150
Carlson, D., 305, 309
Carlson, T., 408, 516
Carmeli, C., 28
Carmena, J. M., 596, 702, 707, 708
Carmien, S. P., 147
Carney, P. R., 299
Carp, J., 75
Carrette, E., 168

Carter, M., 211
Caruso, D., 150
Casanova, M. F., 121
Cascino, G. D., 314
Cash, S., 64, 280, 293
Caspary, E., 196
Cassady, K., 38t, 240, 334
Cassel, T., 150
Cassisi, J. E., 102
Castaño-Candamil, S., 19, 59
Castellanos-Dominguez, G., 19
Castermans, T., 21, 22
Castet, 694
Castet, Julien, 73, 193, 197
Castillo, J., 33
Catenacci Volpi, N., 215, 227
Cauwenberghs, G., 36, 82, 168, 327
Cavazza, M. M., 152
Cavinato, M., 101, 259
Cavrini, F., 479
Ceballos-Baumann, A. O., 21
Cecotti, H., 37t, 135, 137, 139, 334, 462, 469, 476, 686,
        687, 688, 689, 690, 691, 697
Cerutti, S., 152, 153, 154
Cervenka, M. C., 117, 299, 300
Cetin, A. E., 34
Çetin, M., 33, 34t
Cetnarski, R., 105
Chai, R., 702
Chaisanguanthum, K. S., 305, 313
Chakrabarti, S., 305
Chalodhorn, R., 35t, 36, 334
Chamberlain, L., 74
Chambers, J., 550, 552
Chanel, G., 4, 13, 17, 147, 151, 152, 155, 156, 200
Chang, E. F., 299, 300, 305, 306, 313
Chang, M., 462
Chang, R., 78
Chang, T. C., 123
Chan Jun, S., 257, 260
Chao, Z. C., 303
Chapin, J. K., 3, 70, 704, 707
Chapman, M. G., 270
Chapman, P., 167
Chapman, R. M., 54
Charles, F. F., 152
Charlton, S. G., 564
Charthad, U., 123
Charvet, G., 22, 309, 311
Chase, S. M., 63
Chatelle, C., 90
Chatrian, G., 300
Chatterjee, A., 257
Chaturvedi, A., 306
Chau, T., 222, 259, 620, 705
Chaudhary, U., 408, 661
Chauncey, K., 4
Chavarriaga, R., 76, 80, 171, 464, 590
Chen, C.-H., 329
Chen, D., 4
Chen, F., 15, 334, 463
Chen, Jyh-Horng, 200
Chen, K., 134, 373, 375
Chen, M., 313

Chen, N.-K., 223
Chen, P.-C., 334
Chen, X., 17, 366, 376, 377, 393, 404, 405, 408, 464, 508, 588
Chen, Y. H., 168
Chen, Z., 408, 420
Cheney, 673
Cheng, M., 136, 465, 516, 708
Cheng, R., 334
Cheng, S., 194, 200
Cherng, R.-J., 237
Cheron, G., 21, 22
Cherubini, A., 244, 334
Cheshin, A., 127
Chestek, C. A., 126
Cheung, B., 254
Cheung, C., 313
Cheung, S. W., 118
Chevallier, S., 376, 382, 386, 619
Chew, Yee Chieh (Denise), 196
Chhatbar, P., 117
Chi, M., 167, 177
Chi, Y. M., 36, 82, 117, 168, 327
Chiappa, S., 29, 33, 34t
Chiew, M., 626
Childers, D., 3
Chimeno, M. F., 168
Chimica, D., 20
Chin, J. M., 211, 224
Chin, Z. Y., 366, 408, 418, 453
Chiu, Y.-J., 137
Chizeck, H. J., 117
Cho, B.-H., 211, 213, 224, 225, 227
Cho, H., 257, 260, 447f, 448f, 449, 449f, 450t, 451, 453, 457
Cho, J.-H., 37t
Cho, W., 90, 97, 102, 106
Cho, Y., 257
Choi, B., 244
Choi, B. C., 125
Choi, H., 36, 37t, 136
Choi, I., 13, 15, 37t, 39
Choi, K., 38t
Choi, S., 19, 32, 260, 409, 420, 431, 465, 468
Choi, W. I., 125
Cholewiak, R. W., 254
Choo, S.-E., 223
Chou, H.-C., 38
Chou, S. N., 116
Choudhury, S., 664
Chouinard, P. A., 108
Christakis, N. A., 127
Christiansen, H., 550
Christoff, K., 227
Christoforou, C., 171
Chu, S. L., 175
Chua, K. S. G., 105, 408
Chumerin, N., 37t, 409, 472
Chung, C. E., 175
Chung, H.-Y., 329
Cichocki, A., 38t, 134, 152, 155, 213, 239, 260, 373, 408,
        409, 410, 413, 414, 416, 418, 420, 462, 465
Cincotti, F., 3, 4, 33, 38t, 39, 60, 90, 95, 102, 105, 151, 210,
        256, 257, 258, 259, 260, 334, 446, 449, 451,
        464, 479, 669, 679

Cinel, C., 511
Cinetto, A., 464
Cipolla, R., 410
Cipresso, P., 152, 153, 154
Cisotto, G., 101
Citi, L., 17, 19, 20, 489, 691
Ciurea, A. V., 38t
Clair, Alicia Ann, 195
Clanton, S. T., 330
Clark, C. R., 300
Clarke, A. R., 553
Clarke, Arthur C., 114
Clatterbuck, R., 303
Clayton, E. W., 664
Clerc, M., 32, 394, 458
Clerx, M., 169, 182
Coenen, T., 211
Coffey, E. B. J., 256
Coffey, R. J., 116
Coghlan, Niall, 197
Cogiamanian, F., 306
Cohen, A. A., 152
Cohen, J., 244
Cohen, L. G., 102, 105, 106, 108, 299, 334, 553, 605, 638,
        705
Cohn, J. F., 150
Co-investigator, N., 13
Colbert, A.P., 102, 106
Cole, A. J., 299, 300, 309, 311
Cole, S. W., 211
Collet, C., 451
Collinger, J. L., 4, 13, 126, 270, 299, 303, 313, 330, 654,
        661, 662, 701, 702, 704, 708
Collingridge, G. L., 677
Collins, J. J., 125
Collins, L. M., 402
Colon, E., 37t
Colwell, K. A., 402, 495, 643
Combaz, A., 37t, 409, 472
Combrisson, E., 621
Comstock, J. R. J., 73
Conant, D. F., 305, 313
Conforto, A. B., 108
Cong, P., 305, 309
Congedo, M., 30, 33, 35t, 70, 134, 242, 331, 362, 377, 378,
        385, 386, 394, 408, 429, 449, 456, 457, 517
Conio, B., 107
Conners, C. K., 550
Conrad, B., 21
Contreras-Vidal, J. L., 117, 243, 279, 702
Cook, J. C., 334
Cook, M. J., 309, 312
Cooke, S. F., 677
Cools, R., 106
Cooper, R., 300
Coovert, M. D., 254
Cornelius, R., 150
Cornelsen, S., 108
Cornwell, T. B., 148
Corralejo, R., 35t, 36
Correia, J., 82, 167
Cortese, F., 306
Cortese, M., 70
Cortese, S., 105

Cossio, E. G., 102
Costa, U., 210, 237, 240, 601
Cott, A., 104
Courchesne, E., 299
Coursaris, C. K., 566, 567, 568
Courtine, G., 117
Cover, 489
Cowan, N., 78
Cowie, R., 150, 156, 157
Cox, C., 300
Coyle, D., 13, 38t, 102, 103, 105, 133, 211, 408
Coyle, D. H., 537
Coyle, S. M., 15, 20, 222
Craddock, G., 575
Craggs, M., 116
Craighero, L., 226
Crainiceanu, C. M., 299
Crawford, C. S., 4
Creasey, G., 116
Crespi, V., 33
Crisler, M. C., 228
Crone, N. E., 299, 300, 303, 305, 552, 704
Cronin, J. A., 710, 711
Crosbie, J., 102, 103, 105
Crowell, A. L., 302
Cruz-Neira, C., 237
Csikszentmihályi, M., 77, 224, 606
Cuénod, M., 28
Cui, H., 706
Cui, X., 540
Cumlí C, M. U., 464
Cunningham, D. A., 108
Cunningham, J. A., 242
Cunningham, V. J., 211
Cunnington, R., 674
Curado, M. R., 102, 106
Curio, G., 3, 15, 29, 70, 72, 78, 107, 174, 210, 211, 305, 347, 349, 362, 363, 366, 409, 451, 453, 456, 462, 464
Curley, K., 126
Curran, E. A., 33
Cushing, H., 709
Cuthbert, B. N., 152, 155
Cutillo, B. A., 299
Cutrell, E., 70, 155
Cybenko, G., 33

D

Daban, S., 22, 462
da Cruz, L., 118, 138
Dadarlat, M. C., 709
Daffertshofer, A., 107
Dagher, A., 21, 211
Dahlwi, F., 27
Dahmen, B., 223
Dähne, S., 74, 136, 347, 362, 365, 464
Dai, W., 457
Daia, C., 38t
Daibhis, A., 181
Dalal, S., 299, 302, 307
D'albis, T., 38t
Dale, A. M., 20, 56, 59
Daley, D., 105
Dal Seno, 637, 640, 641

Daly, I., 149, 152, 153, 154, 155, 156, 196, 199, 200, 201, 202, 221, 331, 588, 658, 669
Daly, J. J., 22, 101, 107, 334
Damaraju, E., 37t
Damasevicius, R., 331
Dambrot, S. M., 108, 114, 125
Damouras, S., 620
Dan, I., 18
Danas, E., 237
Dancer, C., 15
Dangi, 707
Dani, S., 305, 309
Daniel, M., 73
D'Anna, S., 303
Danóczya, M., 62, 451
Dario, P., 17, 19, 20
Darling, R. D., 103, 107
da Rocha, J. D., 151
Darvas, F., 63, 270, 271, 299, 313
Darzi, A. W., 75
Das, U. N., 116
Dashuber, R., 70
da Silva, F. H. Lopes, 446, 452, 453, 526, 597, 623
da Silva, F. L., 16, 22, 236
Daskalakis, J. Z., 116
Daudet, C., 102
Daunizeau, J., 4, 625
Dauwels, J., 373
David, S. V., 27, 363
Davidson, R. J., 29
Davis, 710, 711
de, Strehl, U., 211
Dean, Roger T., 194
Deardeuff, K., 13
Debener, S., 64, 615
De Boulogne, Duchenne, 115
De Bruin, H., 378
De Campo, A., 176
Decety, 674
DeCew, 655, 656
deCharms, R. C., 223, 227
Deecke, L., 171, 362, 671, 672, 673, 674
DeFanti, T. A., 237
DeFelipe, Javier, 198
De Filippis, M., 70
Degenhart, A. D., 270, 303, 313, 330
Deger, M., 121
de Haan, B., 551
de Hemptinne, C., 302, 306, 307, 308
Dehghani, M., 122
Deisenroth, M., 456
de Juan, E. J., 303
Delannoy, V., 134, 242, 331, 449, 457
del Millán, J. R., 171
Delorme, A., 327, 451, 456
De Massari, D., 259, 347
Demers, L., 575
Demertzi, A., 90
Demetriou, S., 211
de Munch, J., 61
Deng, Y., 125
Denison, T., 117, 305, 309, 310, 334
Denissen, A., 181
den Nijs, M., 299, 304, 307, 313, 334

Dennis, T. A., 152, 153
Densmore, M., 211, 224
Denys, D., 106
Deouell, L. Y., 299
de Pasquale, F., 59
de Pesters, A., 305, 334
Desai, S., 303
Desain, P., 23, 35t, 36, 37t, 258, 259
Desideri, L., 4, 38, 408
Desimone, R., 300
Desmond, J. E., 152, 299
de Vico Fallani, F., 38t, 39, 334, 687, 688
Devlaminck, D., 60, 430
Devor, A., 20
De Vos, M., 64, 550, 618
Dewan, 657
Dewhurst, R., 468, 470
Dewiputri, W. I., 15
Dezhong, Y., 177
Díaz-Estrella, A., 213, 220, 227, 240
Dichter, B., 305, 313
Dickerson, J., 149
Dickerson, Robert F., 201
Dickhaus, T., 210, 349, 362, 363, 451
Dienes, Z., 224
Di Fonzo, A., 306
Di Gennaro, G., 167
DiGiovanna, 707
Di Lazzaro, V., 306
Dimitrievic, A., 106
Dimyan, M. A., 105, 334
Ding, L., 60
Ding, M., 300
Dirlikov, B., 551, 552
Dirnagl, U., 20
Diserens, K., 409, 413
Ditton, T., 236
Djouani, K., 376, 382, 386
Djourno, André, 117
D'Mello, S., 156
Dmochowski, J. P., 554
Do, K. Q., 28
Dobelle, 702, 709
Dobkin, B. H., 101, 102, 106, 552
Dobson, K., 176
Dohring, M., 334
Dolcos, 623
Dominguez, 620
do Nascimento, O. F., 28
Donchin, E., 2, 3, 15, 34, 35t, 36, 54, 70, 71, 74, 257, 347,
    349, 398, 408, 409, 462, 504, 505, 513, 515,
    553, 596, 614, 618, 674, 687, 691, 703, 705
Donelan, 661
Dong, X., 476, 479
Dong, Y.-Z., 17
Donner, E. J., 300
Donnerer, M., 241
Donoghue, J. P., 4, 22, 280, 293, 550, 708
Dorman, 709
Dorn, J. D., 118
Dornhege, G., 70, 72, 78, 174, 347, 362, 366, 409, 451, 453
Dostrovsky, J. O., 306
Doud, A. J., 38t, 60, 211, 214, 240, 334
Douglas-Cowie, E., 150, 156, 157, 645

Do Valle, B., 64
Dove, G. O., 344
Dow, M., 116
Dowling, J., 299, 334
Downar, Z., 116
Downey, J. E., 4, 330
Downs, J., 211
Doyle, John, 117
Doyon, J., 451
Drechsler, R., 104, 105
Dreer, 661
Dremstrup, K., 95, 334
Dreyer, A. M., 554
Drmic, I. E., 181
d R Millán, J., 38
Dronkers, N., 299
D'Souza, W., 309, 312
Duane, 687
Duann, Jeng-Ren, 200
Duchenne, G.-B., 115
Duckrow, R., 299, 300
Ducrey, G. P., 607
Duda, R. O., 31, 355
Dudzinski, 661
Duh, H. B.-L., 237
Duin, R. P., 31
Dum, R. P., 108
Duncan, Alexander, 196
Duncan, N. W., 107
Dunn, A. K., 20
Dunn, S., 89–90, 332, 334, 462, 463, 464
Dupont-Hadwen, J., 106
Dupuy, F. E., 553
Durand, 705
Durka, P., 462, 472
Dürschmid, S., 300
Dutoit, T., 21, 22
Duun-Henriksen, J., 270
Duvinage, M., 21, 22, 242
Duysens, J., 23, 37t, 259
Dzaack, J., 70, 71, 75

**E**

Eason, 705
Eaton, Joel, 194, 196, 197, 200, 516, 695
Eaton, Manford L., 195
Ebisch, B., 299
Ebner, T. J., 300
Ebrahimi, T., 31, 409, 413
Eckhardt, H., 123
Eckstein, 687, 688, 689, 694
Eden, 707
Edlinger, G., 22, 35t, 241, 327, 455, 462, 515
Edwards, D. F., 105
Edwards, E., 211, 299, 302, 307
Edwards, Sarah J. L., 658
Eerola, T., 150, 200
Ehirim, P., 280, 283, 289, 292
Ehrsson, H. H., 244
Eimer, M., 553
Eisen, M. D., 117
Eisma, R., 589
Ekman, P., 149

Elbakyan, A. A., 242
Elbert, T., 152, 154, 349, 551
Elger, C., 17, 303, 305, 313, 345
Elias, D., 33
Elias, W. J., 118
Elliott, A., 37t
Elliott, L. R., 254
Ellison, C., 280, 293
Ellsworth, P., 150
Elmer, S., 152, 153
Elsas, S., 182
Emkes, R., 64
Emmert, K., 211
Emrich, J. F., 298, 300, 301, 303, 305, 313, 334
Endsley, M. R., 78
Eng, K., 242, 243
Engel, A. K., 15, 260
Engel, J., 21
Engelbregt, 626
Engell, A. D., 299
Engemann, D. A., 327
Enghoff, S., 299
Enriquez-Geppert, S., 102
Erb, M., 236
Erba, G., 373, 465
Erfanian, A., 15, 516
Ergenoglu, T., 553
Erkkila, J., 150
Ermer, J. J., 57, 61, 63
Ernest, T., 240
Escelsior, A., 107
Escolano, 626
Eskandar, E., 280, 293
Eskandari, Parvaneh, 516
Espina-Hernandez, J. H., 37t
Essig, K., 468
Ethier, 708
Etzel, J. A., 149
Eugster, M. J. A., 467
Evans, J. R., 16, 27
Evarts, Edward, 704
Eyriès, Charles, 117

F

Fabinyi, G., 309, 312
Fadiga, L., 21
Fagen, Trudy Shulman, 195
Fahle, M., 79
Fairclough, S. H., 81
Fairneny, T., 223
Faisal, A., 456
Falco, C., 167
Fallani, d. V. F., 334
Faller, J., 37t, 210, 211, 220, 237, 238, 240, 241, 242, 243, 246, 464, 468, 479, 586, 602
Fallgatter, A., 108
Fan, J., 550
Fan, X., 38
Fantini, S., 4
Faradji, F., 596
Farah, 657
Faraone, S. V., 550
Farina, 672, 675

Farina, D., 28, 95, 117
Farokhzad, O. C., 125
Farquhar, J., 23, 37t, 258, 259, 451
Farry, 705, 708
Farwell, L. A., 2, 34, 35t, 54, 70, 71, 74, 257, 347, 349, 398, 409, 462, 504, 505, 515, 553, 614, 618, 687, 691, 705
Fatourechi, M., 30, 468, 617
Fazel-Rezai, R., 305, 465, 479, 489, 503, 504, 505, 506, 508, 509, 511, 517, 554, 560, 596, 703
Fazli, S., 62, 211, 451, 464, 515, 538, 540
Federici, S., 466
Fedorova, A. A., 76
Fei, D.-Y., 408
Feijs, L. M. G., 219
Feldman, J. M., 280, 293
Felix, L. B., 33, 34t
Fellenz, W., 150
Fellner, D. W., 239, 242
Felton, E. A., 303, 313, 334, 645, 708
Felzer, T., 33
Fernandes, 709
Fernaud, Isabel, 198
Ferree, T. C., 169
Ferreira, V. M., 167
Ferrez, P. W., 29, 70
Ferrier, D., 550
Ferrin, M., 105
Fetz, 673, 711
Fetz, E. E., 106, 107, 292, 293, 299, 304, 307, 313, 334
Ficke, R., 12
Fidopiastis, Cali M., 516
Fiebig, Karl-Heinz, 435, 438
Fifer, M. S., 300, 303
Figueiredo, M. A., 420
Filho, S. A. S., 33, 34t
Fillard, P., 383, 384
Filley, C. M., 27
Finch, J., 114
Finke, A., 35t, 468, 517
Finn, 654, 658
Fins, J. J., 90
Finucane, C., 37t, 217, 241, 465
Fioravanti, C., 239
Fischer, G., 79
Fischl, B., 57, 59
Fisher, R. A., 401
Fisher, R. S., 373, 465, 508
Fitter, M. J., 491
Fitts, 645
FitzGerald, J., 306
Fitzgerald, M., 181
Fitzgibbon, S. P., 300
Fitzsimmons, 702, 708, 709
Fleck, M., 82
Flesher, S. N., 120, 710
Fletcher, P.T., 384
Flinker, A., 299
Flint, 646, 708
Flint, R. D., 305, 334
Flor, H., 3, 13
Floridi, 662, 664
Florio, M., 114
Flotzinger, D., 3, 101

Flyvbjerg, H., 174
Focacci, F., 17, 19, 20
Foerster, M., 22, 309, 311, 708
Fogelson, N., 299
Foldes, S. T., 330
Foltynie, T., 306
Fonlupt, P., 299
Fonseca, C., 167
Fontaine, J. R., 150
Foote, K., 302, 306, 307
Forgas, J., 150
Forlani, G., 179
Formisano, R., 90
Forneris, C. A., 2, 54, 101, 349, 446
Forney, E., 408
Forrester, L., 279
Forslund, P., 32
Forster, K., 21
Forster, P., 381
Fortunato de Barros Filho, M., 108
Foster, J., 226, 708
Fourkas, A., 334
Fourkias, A., 105
Fox, N. A., 152
Fox, P. T., 20
Foy, N., 394
Francis, G., 37t
Franco, F., 200
Frank, S., 211
Franks, E., 115
Frantzidis, C. A., 152
Franz, J. R., 25
Franzco, B. S., 115
Franzé, M., 3
Frear, M., 150
Freeman, W. J., 21, 299
Freisleben, B., 33
French, L. A., 116
Frenette, E. C., 105
Freudenberg, Z., 305, 309, 310, 313, 334
Frewen, P. A., 211, 224
Frey, J., 4, 73, 331, 606, 614
Freytag, S.-C., 82
Friberg, A., 704
Fried, I., 21, 299
Friedman, D., 15, 216, 218, 224, 227, 237, 239
Friedman, J. H., 355, 361
Friedrich, 605, 606
Friedrich, E. V., 102, 106, 210, 211, 212, 219, 220, 226
Friehs, G., 4, 280, 293, 300
Fries, P., 300, 327, 456, 552
Friesen, C., 102
Friman, O., 465
Friston, K. J., 59, 106
Froke, R., 22
Fruitet, 605
Fruitet, J., 32
Frye, G. E., 35t, 334
Fu, 704
Fu, F., 127
Fu, Y., 152, 154
Fuchs, M., 61
Fuchs, T., 104
Füchtemeier, M., 20

Fuentes Cabrera, A., 334
Fujii, G., 303
Fujii, N., 303
Fujikado T., 119f
Fujisawa, J., 4
Fujisawa, S., 300
Fujiwara, T., 38t
Fukuda, T., 238
Fukunaga, K., 363, 374, 381, 453
Furdea, A., 15, 35t, 36, 70, 171, 210, 334, 347, 554
Furlani, S., 171, 462
Furness, T. A. III, 246
Furukawa, K., 167
Fusini, L., 179

## G

Gabrieli, J. D., 152, 223, 227
Gabrielsson, A., 149
Gadeyne, S., 168
Gaertner, M., 13, 155, 467, 469
Galán, F., 29, 408, 702
Galante, D., 179
Galifianakis, N. B., 302, 306, 307, 308
Gallagher, A. G., 238
Gallagher, L., 181
Gallivan, E. M., 280, 293
Galuske, R., 299
Galway, L., 469
Gambrell, C., 293
Gan, J., 602
Gan, T. T., 175
Gancet, J., 702
Ganguly, K., 707
Ganin, I., 35t, 36
Gantner, I. S., 35t, 90
Gao, J.-H., 20, 29
Gao, S., 4, 15, 24, 27, 29, 136, 260, 334, 347, 349, 366, 376,
    377, 393, 403, 404, 405, 408, 420, 458, 464,
    465, 476
Gao, X., 4, 15, 24, 27, 29, 136, 260, 347, 349, 366, 375,
    376, 377, 392, 393, 403, 404, 405, 408, 420,
    458, 464, 465, 476, 507
Gaona, C., 299, 305, 334
Garabaghi, A., 303, 314
Garau, M., 218, 224, 227, 239
Garcia, J., 38t
Garcia, M. L., 220, 221, 225, 226
Garcia, P. A., 302, 307, 308
Garcia-Cossio, E., 102, 106, 259
Garcia-Molina, G., 13, 15, 24, 31, 465, 466, 564
Gardner, E. P., 260
Garell, P. C., 313, 334
Garnero, L., 61
Garrett, D., 31, 32
Gärtner, M., 76
Garud, R., 591
Gasche, Y., 270
Gates, J. R., 300
Gaume, A., 596
Gaunt, R., 13
Gaunt, R. A., 330
Gavett, Scott, 489, 503
Gavison, Ruth, 660

Gayraud, N., 394
Gean, A. D., 299, 307
Gehring, W. J., 75
Gelbard, H., 299
Gelernter, J., 302
Gembler, F., 133, 134, 135, 136, 137, 138, 139, 140, 141, 373, 465, 466, 472
Gemetti, A., 20
Genna, C., 259
George, L., 602
Georgopoulos, A. P., 673, 706
Gergondet, P., 244
Gerhardt, L. A., 299, 300, 301, 303, 334
Gerjets, P., 73, 78, 602
Gerking, J. M., 174
Gerloff, C., 108
Gerner, H. J., 211
Gershenfeld, N., 176
Gerson, A. D., 70, 75, 453, 468
Gerstner, W., 121
Gethmann, J., 20
Geuze, J., 35t, 36, 258, 259, 489, 491, 498
Gevensleben, H., 15, 25, 552, 553, 554, 626, 627
Gevins, A., 73
Gevins, A. S., 299
Ghacibeh, G. A., 300
Ghanayim, N., 3, 13, 70
Gharabaghi, A., 102, 103, 105, 243, 255, 256, 626
Gherri, E., 553
Ghosh, J., 33, 34
Ghosh, P., 16, 21
Ghovanloo, M., 123
Giabbiconi, C. M., 15
Giacino, J. T., 90
Giacobbe, P., 116
Giardini, M. E., 20
Gibbs, M., 211
Gibert, G., 134, 242, 244, 331, 449, 457
Gibson, D. G., 125
Gibson, D. J., 299
Gielen, C., 23, 37t
Giftakis, J., 305, 309
Gilbert, J. E., 4
Gilja, V., 126, 646
Gill, M., 181
Gilroy, S. W. S., 152
Girard, C., 123
Girouard, A., 4, 242
Giugliemma, C., 4, 210, 464
Gizzi, L., 108
Gladden, M. E., 126
Glover, G. H., 152, 223, 227
Goebel, R., 22, 210, 223
Goertz, M., 118
Goh, S.Y., 224
Göhring, 686, 702
Gold, L., 20
Goldberg, J. O., 181
Goldrick, M., 305
Goldstein, R., 107
Golenia, J.-E., 467
Goli, A., 37t
Gollakota, S., 123
Gollee, H., 466

Golub, M. D., 63, 706
Gómez, C., 70
Gomez-Gil, J., 17, 20, 24, 25, 29, 30, 508, 552
Gomez-Rodriguez, M., 102, 103, 105, 255, 256
Goncharova, 617, 618, 623
Goncharova, I. I., 105
Gonsalvez, C. J., 554
Gonzalez-Mendoza, A., 37t
Goodenough, R. R., 228
Goodsell, R., 226
Gordon, B., 299, 300
Gordon, S., 82
Görgen, K., 74, 347, 362, 365
Gorgolewski, 662
Gosselaar, P., 305, 309, 310, 334
Gosseries, O., 90, 223
Goth, G., 104
Gottman, J. M., 150
Goudeseune, Camille, 195
Goverdovsky, V., 82
Gowen, A. H., 211
Goyat, M., 35t
Grabham, Tim, 199
Graesser, A., 156
Grafton, S. T., 21
Graimann, B., 25, 31, 151, 299
Gramann, K., 60, 75, 80, 82, 366
Gramatica, F., 462
Gramfort, A., 58, 59, 327
Grandjean, D., 149, 150, 200
Grasby, P. M., 211
Gräser, A., 135, 136, 137, 138, 139, 334, 465, 466, 469, 476
Grau, C., 712
Gray, C. M., 300
Graybiel, A. M., 299
Grayer, A., 115
Greely, Henry T., 658
Green, A. L., 306
Greene, Joshua D., 657
Greenhill, L. L., 550
Greenwald, E., 710
Greger, B., 305, 313
Gregor, P., 590
Greischar, L. L., 29
Grewe, O., 150
Gribetz, M., 244
Grierson, M., 35t, 197
Grieshofer, P., 102, 104, 106, 210
Griffin, A. L., 103, 107
Griffioen, R., 169, 182
Grill, W. M., 116, 117
Grimm, F., 243
Grizou, J., 602
Grob, A., 148, 149
Grodd, W., 20
Grönegress, C., 35t, 241
Grootenhuis, M. A., 586
Großekathöfer, U., 171, 174, 176, 177, 181
Gross, J. J., 148, 149
Gross, R. E., 116
Grosse-Wentrup, M., 60, 61, 102, 103, 105, 118, 167, 255, 256, 366, 408, 431, 432, 434, 553, 598, 606
Grossman, 702

Grosswindhager, B., 329
Groten, J., 176
Grozea, C., 38t, 451
Gruber, T., 15, 152, 154
Grundlehner, B., 166, 167, 168, 169, 171, 179
Grünzinger, C., 334
Gruss, L. F., 24
Gruzelier, J. H., 104, 106, 210, 214, 224, 226, 227, 352
Grzeska, K., 221
Gu, Y., 671, 672, 674, 675
Gu, Z., 38, 408, 409, 412, 420
Guan, C., 4, 61, 105, 236, 366, 408, 410, 418, 420, 430, 431, 451, 453, 456, 457
Guenther, F. H., 259, 283, 289, 292
Guertin, P. A., 705
Guger, C., 4, 22, 33, 34t, 35t, 61, 90, 95, 97, 116, 211, 216, 218, 224, 227, 239, 241, 258, 259, 305, 327, 329, 332, 334, 347, 366, 449, 455, 461, 462, 463, 464, 515, 535, 615
GugerTec, 272
Guigue, V., 32, 409
Guillot, A., 451
Guiraud, D., 117
Gumnit, R. J., 300
Gunasekera, B., 22
Gunduz, A., 299, 300, 302, 303, 305, 306, 307, 334
Gunn, R. N., 211
Gunst, I., 15
Guo, F., 347
Gupta, C. N., 37t
Gupta, D., 334
Gupta, R., 305, 309
Gürkök, H., 76, 211, 242, 527
Gururajan, A., 60
Gwak, K., 33, 254, 257
Gwinn, R. P., 309, 311
Gyulai, F. E., 330

H

Habes, I., 210
Hachet, M., 4, 73, 331
Hadi, A., 27
Hadjileontiadis, L., 152, 153, 154
Haegens, S., 300
Hagemann, K., 78
Haider, Ali, 505
Hairston, W. D., 82
Hakkani-Tur, D., 150
Halder, S., 35t, 36, 70, 90, 171, 210, 211, 212, 239, 241, 334, 347, 408, 451, 466, 708
Hall, D., 31
Haller, S., 210, 211
Hallett, M., 171, 462
Hallinan, 654
Hallowell, J., 149, 152, 153, 154, 196, 199
Hämäläinen, M., 19, 56, 57, 58, 59, 327
Hämäläinen & Ilmoniemi, 704
Hamam, Y., 376, 382, 386
Hamano, T., 167, 671
Hammer, B. U., 102, 106
Hammer, E. M., 35t, 210, 334
Hammer, E. M., 451, 598, 599
Hammond, D. C., 102, 211

Hampson, R. E., 121
Han, C., 37t
Han, J. H., 15
Han, S. H., 566, 567
Hancock, P. A., 73
Hancu, M., 198
Handy, T. C., 155
Hanger, James, 115
Hansen, J. C., 373
Hansen, L. K., 105
Hansen, S. T., 105
Hanser, Suzanne B., 195
Hanslmayr, S., 553
Hao, L., 299
Haralick, R., 171
Harandi, M., 377
Harchick, E. A., 330
Harding, G., 373, 465
Hardoon, D. R., 376, 465
Hari, R., 19
Hariz, M., 306
Harkam, W., 455
Harmelech, 626
Harrington, D., 330
Harrison, L., 78
Harrop, M., 211
Hart, D., 226
Hart, J. C., 237, 299
Hart, P. E., 31, 355
Hartley, R., 377
Hartmann, M., 465
Hartson, K.A., 211, 224
Haselager, P., 464
Haselsteiner, E., 33
Haslinger, B., 21
Haslwanter, Thomas, 255
Hassanein, K., 228
Hasson, U., 299, 687
Hastie, T., 355
Hata, N., 244
Hattie, J., 598
Hatzinakos, D., 149
Hauberg, S., 105
Haufe, S., 19, 74, 211, 347, 350, 355, 360, 361, 362, 365, 381, 409, 464, 623
Häuser, A.-K., 15, 23
Hauser, C. K., 35t, 334
Hautzinger, M., 25
Haviland, D. B., 115
Hawkins, J., 80
Hayashi, Y., 171
Hayashibe M., 117
Haylock, C., 115
Haynes, J.-D., 74, 347, 362, 365, 657, 658, 659
Hazarika, S. M., 38t
Hazrati, M. K., 15, 240
He, B., 15, 60, 211, 214, 240, 334, 451
He, T., 38
He, Y., 243
Head, M., 228, 706
Healy, D., 210
Hearst, M. A., 567, 568
Hebb, 670
Heck, C. N., 309, 311

Heetderks, W. J., 3, 72
Heger, D., 305, 334
Heikkila, J., 123
Heikkonen, J., 3
Heilinger, A., 90, 97
Heinrich, H., 25, 550, 553
Heinze, H.-J., 300, 305
Helder, J. B., 330
Hemmes, T., 330
Henderson, J. M., 126
Hendler, T. T., 152
Henkel, G., 115, 117, 118
Henle, C., 21
Hennrich, J., 428
Henshaw, J., 463
Henson, 625
Herbert, C., 334
Heremans, 672
Herff, C., 305, 334
Herman, J., 17
Herman, P., 102, 103, 105
Hermann, T., 198
Hermes, D., 303, 304, 307, 313
Hernando, D., 33
Herrmann, C. S., 102, 373, 554
Herron, J., 117
Herweg, A., 35t, 258, 259, 334
Hesse, C., 59
Hestenes, J., 239
Hettich, D. T., 38t, 220, 225
Hettinger, L. J., 242
Hewstone, M., 127
Heylen, D., 13, 152, 153, 242
Hild, J., 467
Hiley, Jonathon B., 513
Hill, B. C., 306, 640, 704
Hill, J., 102, 103, 105, 255, 256, 303, 305, 313, 491, 493
Hill, N. J., 15, 23, 36, 37t, 300, 334
Hillyard, S. A., 373, 554
Himes, D., 309, 312
Hines, E. L., 33
Hinic, V., 35t
Hink, 673
Hinrichs, H., 300
Hinterberger, T., 3, 13, 39, 70, 104, 134, 196, 198, 210, 242, 244, 303, 305, 313, 330, 331, 332, 362, 446, 449, 455, 456, 457, 462
Hintermüller, C., 259, 329, 517
Hirata, 708
Hirata, A., 108
Hiremath, 710
Hirose, M., 4, 237
Hirshfield, L. M., 4
Hjelm, 687
Ho, A. C., 118
Hochberg, L. R., 4, 22, 280, 293, 590, 656, 691, 701, 704, 708
Hoechstetter, K., 22
Hoekstra, Rolf, 115
Hoffmann, 706
Hoffmann, D., 299
Hofmann, U. G., 147, 240, 409, 503
Hogan, N., 540, 542, 543
Hoge, R. D., 540

Hogervorst, M., 156
Höhne, J., 4, 19, 35t
Holdgraf, C., 305
Holland, Simon, 198
Hollands, J. G., 73
Holmes, M. D., 21, 299, 706
Holmquest, H. J., 116
Holmqvist, K., 468, 470
Holper, L., 242, 243
Holtmann, M., 105, 550
Holz, E. M., 4, 35t, 36, 261, 334, 564, 569t, 570t–577t, 586, 588
Holzinger, A., 568
Holzner, C., 22, 35t, 241, 462
Homan, R. W., 17
Homer, M. L., 22, 280, 293
Honey, C., 304, 307
Hong, 705
Hong, B., 4, 15, 24, 260, 347, 349, 366, 403, 458, 465, 476
Hong, Dezhi, 201
Hong, J. H., 60
Hong, K.-S., 13
Hong, L. E., 37t
Hoogerwerf, E.-J., 4
Hori, G., 33
Horki, P., 528, 531, 543
Hornik, K., 33
Horovitz, S. G., 211
Hortal, E., 573
Horton, J. C., 313
Horvath, 711
Hoshi, Y., 4
Hosking, S., 309, 312
Hösle, A., 35t, 36, 171
Hotelling, H., 375
House, P., 305, 313
House, William, 117
Howard, M. W., 300
Howard-Jones, P., 211
Howells, P. J., 238
Hoya, T., 33
Hrovat, K., 334
Hsiao, C. T., 175
Hsiao, S. S., 299
Hsu, S.-H., 327
Hsu, W.-Y., 134
Hu, D., 15, 38, 259, 334, 463
Huang, B., 468
Huang, C.-N., 329
Huang, D., 408
Huang, Z., 107
Hucek, C., 270
Huettel, S. A., 22, 299
Huggins, J. E., 4, 299, 589, 654, 662
Humayun, M. S., 119f, 303
Hummel, F., 108
Humphrey, 706
Hunt, Andy, 195
Hunt, K. J., 466
Hunt, W. A., 149
Hunter, Patrick G., 200
Huron, D., 200
Huster, R. J., 102
Hutchison, W. D., 306

Hwang, F., 149, 152, 153, 154, 155, 156, 196, 199, 201, 202
Hwang, H. J., 19, 36, 37t, 136, 217, 465, 468
Hyttinen, J., 276
Hyvärinen, A., 29

**I**

Ibanez, 676
Ifft, P. J., 246, 707
Ignashchenkova, A., 551
Ihme, K., 76, 82, 167, 260
Ikeda, S., 238
Ilioi, E. C., 102, 106
Ille, N., 105
Illes, Judy, 657, 658
Ilmoniemi, R. J., 19, 58
Ilstedt Hjelm, S., 76, 693
Im, C. H., 19, 36, 37t, 136, 217, 462, 465, 468
Ince, N. F., 34
Inchingolo, P., 27
Inghilleri, M., 95, 102, 105, 446, 451
Ingle, D., 3
Inglese, A., 107
Inlow, M., 182
Inoue, A., 214, 224, 226, 227
Insola, A., 306
*In Tune*, 197
Inverso, S. A., 241
Ioannidis, 664
Ioannou, S., 150
Ionescu, G., 35t
Iosa, M., 95
Irazoqui, P. P., 280, 293
Iriki, 706
Irimia, D. C., 95
Irizarry, R., 299
Ishikawa, A., 4
Ishwaran, H., 420
Islam, 618
Israni, Shweta, 200
Ito, M., 105
Ito, R., 4
Ito, T., 152, 155
Iturrate, I., 35t, 76, 80, 305, 334, 516, 542, 554
Iversen, I., 3, 70
Iversen, J., 13, 167, 177
Ives, J. R., 270
Ivory, M. Y., 567, 568

**J**

Jackont, G. G., 152
Jackson, F., 4
Jackson, M. M., 15, 465, 579, 710
Jacob, R. J. K., 4, 78, 242
Jacobs, J., 103, 299
Jacobs, R., 115
Jacques, S., 303
Jahanpour, E., 211, 331
Jaimovich, Javier, 197
Jain, A. K., 31
Jain, K. K., 125
Jäncke, L., 152, 153
Jang, H., 451

Jangraw, D. C., 238, 244, 246, 464, 468
Jansari, A., 224
Jarodzka, H., 468, 470
Jarosiewicz, B., 280, 293, 479
Jaskowski, P., 347
Jasper, H. H., 17, 63, 345, 673
Jatzev, S., 13, 70, 73, 76, 80, 82, 147, 155, 167, 658
Jayaram, Vinay, 426, 431, 432, 438
Jayasumana, S., 377
Jeannerod, 674
Jebari, 654, 658
Jeglic, A., 116
Jeng, Shyh-Kang, 200
Jenner, A., 151
Jennett, B., 532, 606
Jensen, O., 13, 59, 106, 299, 300
Jensen, R. M., 305, 309
Jeon, Y., 34, 39
Jerbi, 621
Jessell, T. M., 254
Jetha, M. K., 181
Jeunet, 596
Jeunet, C., 4, 73, 211, 257, 331, 597, 598, 599, 604
Jeyalakshmi, C., 118
Jezernik, S., 116
Jha, R., 330
Ji, Q., 33, 34, 300
Ji, S., 15
Jia, C., 15, 24, 366, 458, 465
Jia, W., 408
Jiang, J., 15, 38, 334, 463, 687, 688, 694, 705, 708
Jiang, N., 95
Jiang, Xiaofan, 201
Jiao, Y., 211, 215, 224
Jin, J., 134, 408, 409, 410, 413, 414, 416, 418, 420, 462,
        463, 465, 489, 491, 498
Jo, S., 244
Jobst, B. C., 309, 311
Jochumsen, 675
Johannes, M. S., 330
Johnsen, E. L., 149
Johnson, 710
Johnson, B., 237
Johnson, K., 305, 313
Johnson, K. A., 181
Johnson, L., 270, 271
Johnson, R. R., 152, 153, 154
Johnson, S. L., 13, 14, 34
Johnston, J., 334
Johnston, S., 210, 211
Johri, A., 244
Jolesz, F. A., 223
Jones, A., 553
Jones, C. M., 149
Jones, K. A., 241
Jones, Keith S., 197, 216
Jones, T., 211
Jonkman, L., 551
Jordà, Sergio, 198
Jordan, 706
Jordan, L. R., 313
Jordan, M. A., 210, 334
Jordan, M. I., 116
Jordan, P. W., 566, 567

Jorgensen, 622
Joseph, G. J. E., 105
Joshi, S., 384, 466
Joutsen, A., 276
Juan, Octavio, 198
Juhl, C. B., 270
Jun, S. C., 60, 259, 260, 447f, 448f, 449, 449f, 450t, 451, 453, 457, 462
Jung, K.-Y., 37t
Jung, T.-P., 36, 82, 136, 168, 175, 182, 200, 299, 327, 366, 404, 405, 410, 420, 456, 686, 688, 689, 692, 694
Jung, Y.-J. J., 36, 37t, 136
Jurcak, V., 18
Jurewicz, K., 105
Juslin, Patrik N., 200
Jutten, C., 35t, 362, 377, 378, 385, 386, 394
Jylänki, P., 210

**K**

Kaas, A. L., 61
Kadosh, 626, 711
Kahana, M. J., 103, 117, 299, 300
Kahane, P., 299
Kaido, T., 116
Kaila, K., 168
Kaiser, D. A., 211
Kaiser, J., 13, 89, 104, 299, 552
Kaiser, V., 242
Kajinami, T., 237
Kakuda, N., 260
Kalcher, J., 3, 101, 351
Kalman, 706
Kaloko, F., 200
Kalunga, E. K., 376, 382, 386
Kam, J., 299
Kamel, M., 27
Kamiya, J., 2, 15
Kamousi, B., 60
Kandel, E. R., 254
Kaneko, Y., 116
Kang, H., 409, 431
Kang, S., 242
Kanoh, S., 4, 244, 331, 332, 479
Kansaku, K., 244
Kapeller, 687, 688, 691
Kapeller, C., 258, 329, 334
Kapetanovic, A., 125
Kaplan, A., 35t, 36
Kapoor, A., 516
Karabanov, 711
Karcher, H., 382
Karim, Ahmed A., 513
Karkar, A., 133
Karpouzis, K., 150
Karumbaiah, L., 22
Kasashima-Shindo, 669
Kashihara, K., 550
Kastner, S., 105
Käthner, I., 239, 241, 334
Kato, K., 107
Katsaggelos, A. K., 410
Kattan, 695
Katyal, 686

Katyal, K. D., 330
Kaufman, D., 467, 489, 586, 588
Kaufmann, T., 4, 35t, 258, 259, 261, 334, 408
Kauhanen, L., 257, 538
Kawanabe, M., 29, 349, 352, 353, 364, 366, 408, 418, 430, 453, 456
Kawasaki, T., 107
Kawashima, K., 105
Kawato, 706
Kayser, J., 27, 28
Keavey, M., 181
Keil, A., 24, 152, 154
Keinrath, C., 211, 218, 224, 226, 227, 239
Keller, J., 598
Keller, J. M., 211, 228
Keller, S., 211, 226
Kellis, S., 305, 313
Kelly, J. W., 270, 330, 461
Kelly, S. P., 37t, 181, 217, 241, 465
Kenemans, J. L., 104
Kennedy, P. R., 280, 283, 289, 292, 293
Kennedy, Philip R., 12, 120
Kenyon, R. V., 237
Kern, M., 21
Kerr, 689, 693
Kerth, T., 82, 168, 327
Kesavarajan, Indu, 200
Kesser, B. W., 118
Kessous, L., 150
Keune, P. M., 551, 552
Key, A. P., 344
Keynan, N. J. N. J., 152
Khalil, A., 13, 167, 177
Khalilzadeh, M. A., 74
Khambhati, A., 305, 309
Khan, M. J., 13, 538
Khasnobish, A., 16, 21
Kheddar, A., 244
Khosla, A., 330
Khosrowabadi, R., 152, 153
Khullar, S., 37t
Kiani, M., 123
Kidmose, P., 82
Kiefer, Chris, 197
Kiehl, K. A., 302
Kienzle, S., 15, 23
Kierkels, J. J., 152
Kilavik, B. E., 171
Kilborn, Kerry, 196
Kilgore, K. L., 327
Kim, 646, 706
Kim, C.-H., 244
Kim, D.-G., 244
Kim, D. J., 566, 567, 568
Kim, D.-S., 33, 254, 257
Kim, D.-W., 37t, 462
Kim, I. Y., 211, 213, 224, 225, 227, 462
Kim, J. G., 451
Kim, Ji Yun, 517
Kim, K., 259
Kim, K.-T., 37t
Kim, Min-Ki, 434
Kim, N. Y., 13
Kim, S., 19, 151, 211, 213, 224, 225, 227, 465, 468

Kim, S. I., 211, 213, 224, 225, 227
Kim, S. K., 79
Kim, S. P., 280, 293
Kim, W., 299
Kim, Y-J., 34, 39
Kimura, A., 38t, 105
Kimura, K., 107
Kincses, W., 78
Kindermans, P. J., 61, 389, 435, 598, 600, 602
King, B., 280, 293
King-Stephens, D., 309, 311
Kiper, D., 242, 243
Kipke, 704
Kirchner, E. A., 79
Kirchner, F., 79
Kirchner, W. L., 73
Kiris, E. O., 78
Kirk, Ross, 195
Kirke, A., 149, 152, 153, 154, 155, 156, 195, 196, 199, 200, 201, 202
Kirsch, H., 299, 302, 307
Kjaer, T. W., 270
Klaver, E. R. G., 219
Kleih, S., 4, 35t, 36, 38t, 90, 134, 171, 210, 211, 212, 239, 334
Kleih, S. C., 588
Klein, 654
Klein, E., 12, 126, 408
Klein, N. D., 228
Klem, G. H., 17, 345
Klinger, C., 104
Klippel, M. D., 76
Klostermann, F., 107
Klovatch, I. I., 152
Kluetsch, R., 211, 224
Kluge, T., 465
Knapp, R. Benjamin, 195, 197, 201
Knight, R. T., 299, 300, 302, 305, 307, 313, 334
Knutson, B., 74, 211
Knuutila, J., 19
Knyazeva, M. G., 28
Kober, 596, 626, 692
Kober, S. E., 102, 104, 106, 210, 211, 215, 224, 226, 227, 228, 597
Kobler, 619
Kobler, R., 126
Köblitz, A., 334
Koblitz, Neal, 505
Koch, C., 118
Koelewijn, L., 553
Koelstra, S., 152, 153, 154
Koene, R. A., 147
Koepp, M. J., 211
Kogalur, U., 420
Koh, C. S., 409
Kohl-Bareis, M., 20
Kohlmorgen, J., 78
Kok, A., 73
Koka, K., 457
Koles, Z. J., 363, 453
Kollias, K., 150
Kollias, S., 150
Kollins, S. H., 550
Kollreider, A., 329

Kondo, T., 171
Konger, C., 3
Konicar, L., 259
Konigsmark, B. W., 303
Kono, S., 35t, 259
Konstantinidis, E., 152
Koo, B., 260, 409, 538
Kooij, J. J., 554
Koon, B. L., 228
Koop, M. M., 306
Kooper, R., 227
Koopmans, P. J., 106
Kopel, R., 211
Kopell, N. J., 299
Kopiez, R., 150
Koppenhaver, A. M., 29
Koppes, R. A., 120
Koprinska, Irena, 195
Korczowski, L., 517, 687, 688, 689, 693
Korisek, G., 211, 219
Kornhuber, 671, 672
Kornhuber, H. H., 171, 362
Korostenskaja, M., 334, 708
Korteling, J. E., 73
Korzeniewska, A., 299, 300
Koschutnig, K., 210, 211
Kosmyna, Nataliya, 517
Kostov, A., 33, 101
Kotchoubey, B., 3, 25, 35t, 70, 89, 334
Kothe, 614, 618
Kothe, C. A., 4, 13, 39, 70, 71, 72, 76, 82, 152, 153, 154, 155, 167, 175, 237, 238, 244, 245, 255, 256, 260, 327, 332, 449, 463, 464, 467, 469, 479
Kotov, 704
Kotwas, I., 102
Kozai, 704
Kozyrskiy, B. L., 76
Kragel, P. A., 107
Kralik, J. D., 70
Kramer, M. A., 299
Krämer, N., 361
Krämer, U. M., 300
Kranczioch, C., 4, 64
Kratz, O., 25
Krauledat, M., 61, 72, 221, 347, 366, 409, 451, 453, 457
Krause, C. M., 152, 153, 711
Krausz, G., 22, 211, 219, 329, 462
Krebs, H. I., 540, 542, 543
Kreilinger, A., 76
Krell, M. M., 79
Krepki, R., 15
Kreutz-Delgado, K., 4
Krieg, T., 313
Krishnamurthi, V., 118
Kristeva, 671
Kristiansen, U. Q., 28
Krol, L. R., 70, 75, 76, 80, 82, 686
Kronegg, Julien, 200
Kronmal, R., 355
Krüger, 704
Krumhansl, C., 150
Krusienski, D. J., 25, 28, 32, 35t, 36, 37t, 70, 210, 242, 305, 334, 347, 355, 362, 401, 408, 409, 462, 495, 598

Kryger, M. A., 330
Kryger, Michael., 517
Ksendzovsky, A., 118
Kuah, C. W. K., 105, 408
Kubánek, J., 299, 300, 301, 303, 334
Kübler, A., 3, 4, 13, 15, 35t, 36, 70, 89, 90, 134, 171, 210,
   211, 212, 239, 241, 258, 259, 261, 305, 334, 408,
   451, 461, 463, 464, 516, 564, 579, 586, 589, 590,
   591, 596, 614
Kübleraf, A., 35t
Kublik, E., 105
Kubota, Y., 299
Kühl, M., 20
Kuhn, A. A., 107
Kühnle, C., 467
Kuhtz-Buschbeck, 670
Kullback, S., 493
Kunzmann, V., 347, 451
Kuo, C.-H., 38
Kuperman, R., 299, 300
Kupsch, A., 107
Kus, R., 462, 472, 550
Kushki, A., 222
Kutas, 674
Kwahk, J., 566, 567, 702
Kwon, K., 217
Kwon, M., 447f, 448f, 449, 449f, 450t
Kyriazis, 712

**L**

Laakso, I., 108
Laar, B., 589
LaBar, K. S., 107
La Bella, V., 90, 97
Lachaux, J. P., 155, 299
Lacourse, 674
Lacroix, J. M., 211
Lacy, 658
Laer, L., 102, 106
Laffont, I., 242, 678
LaFleur, K., 38t, 240, 334, 646, 647, 702
Lago, M. C. P., 20
Lahn, B. T., 114
Lahr, 654
Lal, T., 303, 305, 313, 705
Lalor, E. C., 217, 241, 465, 618
Lalor, E. E. C., 37t
Lamarche, F., 4, 30, 33, 70, 240, 362, 408, 456
Lampl, I., 299
Lan, H., 211, 215, 224
Lance, B. J., 238, 394, 464, 468
Lancelle, M., 242
Landis, C., 149
Landvogt, N., 21
Lang, P. J., 149, 152, 155, 672
Lanius, R. A., 211, 224
Lansbergen, M., 181
Lansbergen, M. M., 104
Lansing, 674
LaPallo, B. K., 35t, 334
Large, Edward W., 198
Larrue, F., 4, 211
Larson, E., 59, 61, 62, 63, 327

Larson, P. S., 306
Lartillot, O., 150
Laschi, C., 17, 19, 20
Laubach, M., 70
Lauer, R. T., 327
Laukka, Petri, 200
Laureys, S., 35t, 90, 223, 259
Lauritzen, T. Z., 118
LaVaque, T. J., 104, 106, 627
Law, R., 283, 289, 292
Lawhern, V. J., 238, 394, 464, 468
Lawrence, A. D., 211
Lawrence, N. S., 211
Laxer, K. D., 299
Lazarewicz, M., 305, 309
Leach, J. B., 122
Leahy, R. M., 57, 58, 59, 61, 63
Lebedev, M. A., 4, 116, 117, 246, 550, 551, 554, 702
Lechner, A., 35t, 90
Lécuyer, A., 4, 30, 33, 38t, 39, 60, 70, 217, 226, 227, 228,
   239, 240, 241, 244, 331, 332, 362, 408, 449,
   456, 457, 479, 605, 614
Ledoit, O., 361, 381
Lee, A., 59, 61, 62, 63
Lee, F., 32, 211, 218, 226, 239
Lee, H., 32, 420
Lee, H.-G., 409
Lee, H.-N., 457
Lee, H.-Y., 237
Lee, I., 39
Lee, J.-C., 462
Lee, J. H., 211, 213, 224, 225, 227
Lee, J.-Y., 13, 25
Lee, J. H., 626
Lee, K. H., 334
Lee, N., 74
Lee, P.-L., 137
Lee, P.-S., 244
Lee, S., 244, 457, 516
Lee, S. M., 211, 213, 224, 225, 227
Lee, S. W., 33, 34t, 36, 37t, 136, 420
Lee, S.-Y., 223
Lee, T.-S., 574
Lee, Y., 13
Leeb, R., 4, 15, 33, 38, 89–90, 151, 210, 211, 216, 218, 224,
   226, 227, 237, 239, 241, 242, 243, 254, 257, 332,
   334, 350, 408, 461, 462, 463, 464, 538, 539,
   540, 543
Leff, D. R., 75
Legény, J., 241
Legrain, V., 37t
Le Groux, Sylvain, 200, 688, 695
Lehne, M., 76, 82, 167, 260
Lei, X., 409
Leibler, R. A., 493
Leifert-Fiebach, 670
Leijten, F., 303, 304, 313
Leinders, S., 305, 309, 310, 334
Leins, U., 104, 552, 554
Leithner, C., 20
Lemay, M., 117
Lemm, S., 29, 347, 350, 352, 353, 355, 360, 361, 362, 364,
   366, 381, 408, 409, 418, 453, 456, 620
Lempka, S. F., 306

Lenhardt, A., 35t
Lenz, F. A., 299
Leon, E., 147
Leonards, U., 211
Leotta, F., 38t, 39, 151, 334
Lepski, G., 102
Leroy, Charles, 115
Lesenfants, D., 554
Leskinen, J., 123
Leslie, G., 13, 152, 153, 154, 155, 167, 177, 200
Lesser, R. P., 299, 300
Lettich, E., 299
Leuthardt, E. C., 4, 21, 270, 299, 300, 301, 302, 303, 304, 305, 313, 314, 334, 704, 708
Levenson, R. W., 150
Levin, O., 451
Levine, S. P., 299
Levy, J., 564, 656
Levy, R., 306
Lew, E., 29, 171
Lewis, 702
Lewis, J. R., 575
Leyde, K., 309, 312
Li, 686
Li, C., 15, 37t, 177
Li, C.-K., 382
Li, H., 377
Li, J., 516, 528, 529, 543, 688, 693
Li, Kun, 526
Li, M., 331, 669
Li, Q., 489, 503
Li, Qiang, 201
Li, W., 331
Li, X., 224
Li, Y., 13, 14, 15, 34, 37t, 38, 39, 378, 408, 409, 412, 420, 458, 516, 527, 528, 532, 543, 686, 688, 692, 707
Li, Z., 707
Lia, X., 33
Liang, J.-M., 137
Liberati, A., 565
Liberati, G., 102, 106, 151
Liberson, W. T., 116
Liefhold, C., 60, 366
Liew, S.-L., 108
Lifshitz, M., 105, 210
Lightbody, G., 37t, 462, 469, 470, 579, 589
Lightfoot, P., 309, 312
Lim, C. G., 550, 554
Lim, D. A., 302
Lim, J.-H., 36, 37t, 136
Lim, S., 13
Lim, T., 102, 106, 211, 212, 219, 226
Lim, Y., 382
Limbrick, D., 299, 300, 301, 303, 334
Limousin, P., 306
Lin, A.-L., 20
Lin, C., 95, 671, 676
Lin, C.-H., 237
Lin, C.-T., 82
Lin, Chih-Yi, 194, 200
Lin, F. C., 554
Lin, F.-H., 59
Lin, J., 299
Lin, K., 464, 538, 539

Lin, P., 171, 462
Lin, Y.-P., 36, 82, 200
Lin, Y.-T., 38
Lin, Z., 347, 375, 376, 392, 393, 465
Linakis, V., 227
Lindauer, U., 20
Linde, D., 305, 309
Linden, D. E., 14, 22, 210, 211
Linden, M., 104, 106
Linderman, 705, 708
Lindquist K. A., 26
Ling, 688, 692
Ling, G. S. F., 330
Lin L., 121
Linortner, P., 38t
Lipsman, N., 116
Lisman, J., 300
Litewka, L., 309, 312
Litinas, K., 334
Litt, B., 299, 300
Little, S., 306
Litvak, 624
Liu, B., 420
Liu, J., 224, 280, 293, 302
Liu, J.-Q., 17
Liu, M., 105, 211, 215, 224
Liu, Q., 134, 373, 375
Liu, T., 347
Liu, V., 123
Liu, W., 463
Liu, Y., 15, 75, 334, 463
Liu, Z., 60, 211, 215, 224, 334
Lively, M. W., 115
Li Y, 602
Lloria Garcia, M., 220, 225
Lo, A. H. P., 468
Loeb, G. E., 115, 303
Loewenstein, G., 74
Lofthouse, N., 552
Logan, W. C., 228
Logemann, H. N. A., 104
Logothetis, N. K., 299
Lombard, M., 236
Lomo, T., 677
London, B. M., 256
Long, J., 38, 408, 528, 532, 534, 541
Long, Z., 211
Looney, D., 82, 270
Lopes, S. F. H., 408
Lopes da Silva, F. H., 17, 56, 57, 106, 182, 271, 351, 363, 373
Lorenz, R., 70, 75, 80, 102
Losch, F., 347, 451, 453
Lotte, F., 4, 30, 33, 38t, 39, 60, 61, 70, 72, 73, 134, 211, 217, 226, 227, 228, 239, 240, 242, 244, 255, 257, 331, 362, 366, 377, 378, 408, 409, 430, 431, 449, 451, 456, 457, 458, 464, 596, 597, 599, 619
Lotto, B., 224
Louchart, S., 102, 106, 211, 212, 219, 226
Lounasmaa, O. V., 19
Loup-Escande, E., 217, 226, 227, 228
Lozano, A. M., 116, 306
Lu, C., 384

Lu, H., 20, 224
Lu, J., 489
Lu, Na, 428
Lu, S., 602
Lubar, J. F., 102, 104, 106, 553
Lucas, J. P., 38t, 214, 240, 334
Lucas, T. H., 106, 107
Lucier, Alvin, 192–193, 194, 195
Luck, G., 150
Luck, S. J., 73
Luckin, 606
Luders, H., 17
Lüders, H. O., 345
Ludlow, D., 223
Ludolph, A. C., 151
Luecken, L. J., 149
Luessi, M., 327
Lugato, N., 108
Lugo, Z. R., 35t, 90, 259
Lulé, D., 90, 151, 537
Lumsden, J., 211, 598
Luna, R., 300
Luo, J.-X., 242
Lusted, Hugh S., 195
Lütcke, H., 15
Lüth, T., 135, 138, 465
Lutz, A., 155
Lutzenberger, W., 104, 349, 551, 552
Luu, 620
Luu, P. L., 169
Luu, T. P., 243
Lv, Y., 211, 215, 224
Ly, V. Q., 237
Lynch, T. M., 300, 301, 334
Lynn, S., 104, 106
Lyon, Eric, 197

**M**

Ma, 543
Ma, J., 538, 539, 540
Ma, M., 167
Maby, E., 4, 134, 242, 331, 449, 457, 597
Machado, A. G., 108
Machado, Sergio, 512
Mack, R., 568
MacKay, D. J., 413, 414, 489, 491
MacKay, W. A., 171
MacKenzie, 645, 646, 647
Mackenzie, L., 300
Mackey, S. C., 223
Macleod, M., 566
Macredie, R. D., 566
Madsen, J. R., 300
Madsen, R. E., 270
Maeda, F., 223
Maeder, C., 211, 464
Magagnin, V., 152, 153, 154
Magee, Wendy L., 194
Maggi, L., 331
Magioncaldo, P., 107
Maguire, M. J., 344
Mahalanobis, P. C., 359
Mahmud, M., 125

Mahony, R., 378
Maia, C. A., 33, 34t
Maia, M., 303
Maier, C., 36
Mailis, T., 150
Mainardi, L., 152, 153, 154
Mainsah, B. O., 491, 493, 498
Majek, Joseph A., 200
Majerus, S., 90
Mak, 489, 661
Mak, P. I., 15, 37t
Mak, P. U., 15, 37t
Makeig, S., 4, 39, 82, 152, 153, 154, 155, 182, 244, 245,
        299, 327, 332, 410, 420, 449, 451, 456, 479, 596,
        597
Makela, A., 150
Makhnev, V., 152, 153
Makino, S., 35t, 259, 462
Malach, R., 299
Malechka, T., 135, 136, 139, 465, 469
Malibary, H., 27
Malik, A., 149, 152, 153, 154, 155, 156, 196, 199, 201, 202
Malik, W. Q., 280, 293
Malinowski, P., 373
Malmivuo, J., 276
Malouin, F., 451
Mandic, D. P., 82, 152, 155, 270
Manley, G. T., 299, 307
Manning, C. D., 31
Manning, J., 299
Mantione, D. D. M., 116
Manuel, Peter, 200
Manunta, Y., 467
Manyakov, N. V., 37t, 409, 472
Manzolli, Jonatas, 200
Mao, H., 280, 283, 289, 292
Mao, J., 31
Mao, X., 331
Mapelli, A., 179
Mappus, R., 579
Marathe, A. R., 237
Maravita, 706
Marceglia, S., 306
Marchal, M., 217, 226, 227, 228
Marchetti, M., 90
Marchioro, G., 468
Marciani, A. G., 33
Marciani, M. G., 257, 334
Margalit, E., 303
Marimon, Xavier, 198
Marinelli, M., 17, 19, 20
Maris, 624
Maris, E., 299, 327, 456
Markham, C. M., 15, 20, 21, 222, 329
Markowitz, R. S., 3
Marozzi, V., 107
Marque, C., 176
Marques de Sa, J. P., 167
Marsh, W. R., 314
Marshall, 692
Marshall, D., 13, 133
Martens, 489
Martens, S. M. M., 489, 491, 492, 493, 498
Martin, F. H., 152, 155

Martin, J.-C., 156
Martin, S., 305, 334, 462, 470, 604
Martin da Silva, A., 167
Martinerie, J., 61, 155
Martinez-Vargas, J.-D., 19
Martino, M., 107
Martins, R. E., 167
Martisius, I., 331
Martz, G. U., 270
Marzelli, M. J., 151
Marzinzik, F., 107
Masdeu, J. C., 373, 465
Mason, S. G., 332
Masse, N., 479
Masse, N. Y., 280, 293
Massey, A. D., 309, 311
Matheson, 655
Matheson, H., 553
Mathewson, K. J., 181
Mathiak, K., 20
Mathias, R., 382
Matlack, 645, 646, 647
Matran-Fernandez, 687, 688, 689, 690, 694
Matsumoto, A., 167, 168, 169
Matsumoto, Y., 462
Matsuura, K., 59
Matsuyama, H., 222
Matteucci, M., 38t
Matthews, F., 21, 329
Mattia, C. F., 334
Mattia, D., 4, 33, 38t, 39, 90, 95, 102, 105, 118, 210, 226,
        239, 256, 257, 334, 446, 451, 461, 463, 464,
        479
Mattout, J., 4, 63, 598, 600, 602
Matuz, T., 210, 334, 347, 466
Maudoux, A., 223
Maunsell, J., 299
Mauri, M., 152, 153, 154
Maurice, M., 373
Maurus, M., 79
Maxwell, J. S., 29
Maxwell, R., 300
May, 710
Mayberg, H. S., 116
Maye, A., 15, 260
Mayer, J., 150
Mazaheri, A., 106, 299, 300
Mazumder, A., 16, 21
Mazzone, P., 306
McAllister, G., 462
McCane, L. M., 27, 363
McCarthy, G., 22, 299
McClelland, J. L., 32
McCormick, D. A., 17, 73
McCoy, A., 167, 177
McCrea, D., 117
McCullagh, P., 462, 469, 470
McCullagh, P. J., 37t
McDaid, A. J., 37t, 38
McDarby, G., 37t, 217, 465
McDonough, S., 102, 103, 105
McDowell, K., 82
McFarland, D. J., 446, 449, 455, 456, 457, 462, 465, 476,
        502, 554, 598, 605, 615, 678

McFarland, Dennis J., 2, 3, 4, 12, 15, 23, 24, 25, 27, 28, 32, 35t,
        39, 54, 70, 72, 89, 101, 102, 104, 105, 106, 107, 108,
        116, 133, 134, 211, 242, 244, 304, 330, 331, 332,
        334, 347, 349, 355, 362, 363, 373, 401, 408, 409, 426
McGee, J. R., 117
McGinnity, T. M., 38t
McGonigal, A., 102
McIlwain, Doris, 200
McInnes, K., 102
McIntyre, C. C., 306
McKeown, G., 150
McLachlan, A. J., 466
McMahon, E., 150, 156, 157
McMahon, R., 37t
McMenamin, B. W., 29
McMillan, G., 3, 197, 216, 241
McMorland, A. J. C., 330
Mcneal, D., 116
McRoberts, A., 462
McRorie, M., 150
Meador, K. J., 300
Mealla, Sebastian, 198
Medina, J., 70
Medina, L. E., 553
Meena, Y. K., 469
Meghanathan, R. N., 468
Mehagnoul-Schipper, D. J., 540
Mehrabian, A., 150
Mehring, C., 300, 303
Meinecke, F., 74, 347, 365
Meinecke, F. C., 60
Meinecke, F. C., 451
Mekler, E. D., 211
Melinscak, 625
Meller, D. M., 119
Mellinger, J., 15, 17, 21, 27, 105, 210, 244, 332, 334, 449,
        462, 479
Memmott, Jenny, 195
Mena-del Horno, S., 95
Mendoza, 704
Meng, J., 257
Menon, V., 299
Mercier-Ganady, J., 217, 226, 227, 228
Merfeld, 702
Merkow, M. B., 103
Mesgarani, N., 313
Mesquita, B., 148, 149
Messinger, D. S., 150
Mestais, C. S., 22, 309, 311
Meyer, F. B., 314
Micouland-Franchi, J. A., 102
Micoulaud-Franchi, J. A., 550, 553
Middendorf, M., 3, 197, 216, 241, 596
Middleton, S., 37t
Miglioretti, D. L., 299, 300
Mihajlovic, V., 166, 167, 168, 169, 171, 174, 176, 177, 179,
        181, 182, 465, 466
Mihalas, Georges I., 198
Mihara, 626
Milekovic, T., 117
Mill, R., 462
Millán, J., 334
Millán, J. D. R., 3, 4, 29, 33, 70, 76, 80, 89–90, 210, 254,
        257, 305, 362, 408, 461, 463, 464, 516, 596, 610

Millán, JR., 332, 334
Miller, J., 299, 303, 334
Miller, K., 4, 270, 299, 300, 301, 303, 304, 305, 307, 313, 334
Miller, K. J., 302, 303, 304, 307, 308, 313, 334, 408
Miller, L. E., 256, 313, 702, 704
Miller, N. V., 256
Mills, M., 115
Miltner, W. H., 300
Min, B.-K., 151
Minces, V., 167, 177
Ming, D., 550
Minguez, J., 35t, 76, 80
Mininel, S., 27
Minotti, L., 299
Mirabella, G., 554, 702, 711
Miralles, F., 4, 90, 461, 463, 464
Miranda, Eduardo R., 36, 149, 152, 153, 154, 155, 156, 175, 177, 193, 194, 195, 196, 197, 198, 199, 200, 201, 202, 516, 694
Mirbozorgi, S. A., 123
Mirghasemi, Hamed, 508
Mirica, Nicoleta, 198
Mirra, S., 280, 283
Mirsattari, S. M., 270
Mishara, A. L., 302
Mitchell, J. D., 586
Mitra, P. P., 300
Mitra, S., 167, 168, 169
Mitsukura, Y., 376, 377, 392
Mittelstadt, 662, 664
Mitzdorf, U., 299
Miyamoto, K., 331
Miyawaki, Y., 33
Mlnn, Á. L. V. Q. Á., 33
Moakher, M., 362, 383, 384
Mochty, U., 210, 334
Mogul, D. J., 313
Mohamed, A., 133
Moinuddin, A., 15, 23
Moitzi, G., 221
Mokom, Z. N., 102
Molina, G. G., 136, 373
Molina, R., 410
Molinari, 706
Molinari, M., 38t, 95, 102, 105, 226, 334, 446, 451
Moll, G. H., 25
Molnar, G. F., 305, 309
Monacelli, E., 376, 382, 386
Monastra, V. J., 104, 106
Montaniz, F., 568
Montesano, 625
Montesano, L., 76, 80
Moonen, G., 90
Moonen, M., 168
Moore, M., 12, 15, 37t, 39
Mora, N., 564
Moradi, M. H., 74
Morales, Juan, 198
Moran, D. W., 4, 21, 270, 299, 300, 301, 303, 304, 305, 309, 313, 314, 330, 334
Moran, R. J., 106
Morash, V., 171, 462
Moreno, 658

Moreno, J. C., 95
Morgade, A. G., 243
Morgan, S. T., 373
Morganti, F., 228
Mori, H., 35t, 259, 462, 535, 538
Mori, K., 462
Morin, F. O., 147
Moritz, 708, 711, 712
Morokoff, A., 309, 312
Morone, G., 38t, 95, 102, 105, 226, 243, 446, 451, 574, 575, 588, 589
Morrell, 711
Morris, J., 150
Morris, R., 150
Mosher, J. C., 57, 58, 59, 61, 63
Mostafa, M. S. M., 463
Mottaghy, F. M., 544
Mouraux, A., 37t
Mowla, Rakibul, Md, 122
Moxon, K. A., 3
Mozaffar, S., 29
Mrachacz-Kersting, N., 95, 669, 670, 671, 672, 676, 677, 678, 679, 680
Mrazek, M. D., 211, 224
Mudry, A., 115
Muehlemann, T., 242, 243
Mueller, K. R., 464
Mugler, E. M., 35t, 305, 334, 408
Mugler, Emily M., 517
Mühl, C., 4, 13, 17, 73, 147, 151, 152, 153, 154, 155, 156, 211, 242, 331, 517, 617, 618, 622
Mukaino, 669
Mukaino, M., 38t
Mukamel, R., 299
Mukand, J., 4
Mukesh, 465
Mulder, T., 226
Mullen, T., 4, 13, 82, 117, 152, 153, 154, 155, 167, 175, 177, 200, 327
Müller, G. R., 31, 211
Müller, K. R., 3, 4, 15, 28, 29, 60, 61, 62, 70, 72, 136, 174, 210, 211, 221, 347, 349, 350, 352, 353, 355, 360, 361, 362, 363, 364, 366, 377, 381, 408, 409, 410, 418, 430, 451, 453, 456, 457, 464, 596
Müller, M. M., 152, 154, 373, 554
Muller, S. M. T. S., 15
Müller, U. J., 116
Müller-Dahlhaus, F., 114
Müller-Gerking, J., 3, 27, 62, 70, 349, 363, 446, 447, 453
Müller-Putz, G. R., 4, 15, 35t, 36, 37t, 38t, 70, 76, 90, 94, 126, 134, 151, 152, 154, 155, 210, 211, 219, 220, 221, 225, 226, 237, 239, 241, 244, 259, 260, 261, 331, 332, 461, 462, 463, 464, 479, 514, 526, 554, 605, 618, 621, 639, 687, 691, 705
Mulvenna, M. D., 37t, 462, 470
Munafò, M. R., 211
Münßinger, J. I., 35t, 36, 171, 517
Muntean, Danina, 198
Murguialday, A. R., 257
Murphy, M., 309, 312
Murray, 606
Murray-Smith, R., 4, 210, 464

Murthy, S. K., 122
Musch, K., 553
*Music for Solo Performer*, 192, 194, 195
Musiek, F. E., 22
Mutschler, I., 21

**N**

Nácher, V., 300
Nagarajan, S. S., 299, 302, 307, 420
Nagasaka, Y., 303
Nagel, F., 150
Nagendra, H., 553
Naim, A., 299
Nair, D. R., 309, 311
Nair, V. A., 105
Najafi, 704
Nakada, T., 171
Nakagame, S., 243
Nakamura, 606
Nakanishi, M., 366, 376, 377, 392, 404, 405
Nakayashiki, K., 171
Nallapati, R., 31
Nam, C. S., 12, 13, 14, 15, 25, 26, 34, 37t, 39, 166, 305,
        408, 686, 692
Nam, Y., 260, 409
Nan, N., 127
Nansen, B., 211
Naros, G., 243, 303, 314
Narumi, T., 237
Nascimento, 671, 672, 674, 676
Naseer, 705
Nashman, V., 3
Nasiri, A., 60
Nasuto, Slawomir J., 149, 152, 153, 154, 155, 156, 195, 196,
        199, 200, 201, 202
National Research Council, 114, 125
Navarro, J., 220, 225, 705
Neal, S., 306
Neat, G. W., 2, 54, 101, 349, 446
Neergaard, 663
Nelson, W. T., 242
Neumann, N., 210, 462, 586
Neuper, C., 4, 15, 31, 33, 34t, 35t, 36, 37t, 71, 76, 94, 95,
        102, 104, 106, 151, 154, 155, 171, 210, 211, 215,
        218, 219, 224, 226, 227, 228, 239, 241, 243, 259,
        260, 331, 362, 451, 461, 462, 463, 464, 507,
        596, 597, 598, 606, 636, 703
Newell, 645
Newell, A. F., 590
Newell, K. M., 237
Nguyen, M. K., 214
Nguyen, T., 449
Nguyen, V. A., 451
Niazi, I. K., 671, 675, 676, 678
Nichols, 624
Nicolás-Alonso, L., 17, 20, 24, 25, 29, 30, 35t, 36, 508, 552
Nicolelis, M. A. L., 3, 4, 70, 246, 550, 554, 704
Niebur, E., 299
Niedermayer, I., 455, 597
Niedermeyer, E., 16, 22, 182, 271, 373
Nielsen, J., 470, 509, 564, 578, 678
Niessing, J., 299
Niessing, M., 299

Nieto-Castanon, A., 283, 289, 292
Nigogosyan, Z., 105
Nii, 710
Nijboer, F., 15, 35t, 36, 70, 82, 147, 152, 153, 167, 210, 211,
        212, 334, 464, 573, 586, 598, 599
Nijholt, A., 2, 4, 12, 13, 17, 76, 89–90, 147, 151, 152, 153,
        155, 156, 166, 211, 242, 332, 334, 451, 461, 462,
        463, 464, 516, 527, 596, 689, 692, 693, 697
Nikolaev, A. R., 468
Nikulin, V. V., 107, 351, 366, 453, 456
Ninaus, M., 210, 211, 222
Nirjon, Shahriar, 201
Nishida, S., 33
Nishikawa, N., 462
Nishimura, T., 33
Nishizaka, S., 237
Nissenbaum, 655
Nitzan, M.-B., 114
NKambou, 606
N'Kaoua, B., 4, 257, 331
Noirhomme, Q., 90, 259
Nolte, G., 351, 366, 453, 456
Nordin, S., 152, 155
Normann, R. A., 279, 702
Norris, D. G., 106
Northoff, G., 107
Novotny, E. J., 270, 271
Nowak, M. A., 127
Nugent, C., 462
Nunez, 704
Nunez, L., 299
Nunez, P. L., 16, 105
Nurmikko, A. V., 22
Nuttin, M., 29, 257
Nuwer, Marc., 508
Nuzhdin, Y. O., 76
Nyström, M., 468, 470

**O**

Obbink, 693
Obermaier, B., 33, 34t, 703
O'Brien, T. G., 564
O'Brien, T. J., 309, 312
Ochsner, K. N., 148, 149
O'Connell, R. G., 63
O'Doherty, J. E., 246, 704, 709, 710
O'Donovan, M., 117
Oeltermann, A., 299
Offenhauser, N., 20
Ogle, J. H., 228
Ohnhaus, E. E., 575
Oie, K. S., 82
Oja, E., 29
Ojakangas, C., 300
Ojeda, A., 13, 82, 167, 177, 327
Ojemann, G. A., 299
Ojemann, J., 4, 21, 270, 271, 299, 300, 301, 302, 303, 304,
        307, 308, 313, 334
Okabe, Y., 59
Okamoto, T., 116
Okanoya, K., 167
Okazaki, 626
Oken, B., 182

Okiyama, R., 107
Okorokova, 705, 706, 709
Okun, M., 299, 302, 306, 307, 308
Olausson, H., 260
Oldfield, R. C., 172
Oleson, K. B., 78
Oliveira, Aluizio, 198
Olivetti, 620
Olivetti, M., 256
Olivetti Belardinelli, M., 466
Olivi, A., 303
Oliviero, A., 306
Oller, E. D., 226
Olofsson, J. K., 152, 155
Olson, J. D., 270, 271
Olson, J. S., 127
Omori, M., 116
Onaral, B., 221
Onaran, I., 34
O'Neill, K., 313
Ono, T., 38t, 679
Onose, G., 38t
Oostenveld, R., 300, 327, 456, 624
Op de Beeck, M., 168
Open Sound Control (OSC), 181
Opisso, E., 4, 70, 90, 210, 461, 463, 464
Opris, J., 121
Opwis, K., 211
Orabona, F., 167
Ordikhani-Seyedlar, M., 116, 552, 554
Orhan, U., 489
Oriolo, G., 334
O'Rourke, B., 257
Orr, J. M., 75
Orsborn, A. L., 596
Ortner, R., 35t, 38t, 90, 95, 97, 258, 259, 329
Ossadtchi, Alexei, 116
Ostrem, J. L., 302, 306, 307, 308
Ota, N., 105
Ota, T., 38t, 105
Otake, M., 222
Otsuki, T., 116
Ottens, T., 305, 309, 310
Ottens, T. H., 334
Ouzounian, Gascia, 197
Ovarlez, J.-P., 381
Oweiss, K., 118
Owen, 658
Owen, J. P., 420
Ozaki, I., 552
Ozyurt, 663

**P**

Paganoni, S., 179
Paggiaro, A., 259
Pahwa, M., 314, 334
Pais-Vieira, 702, 712
Paiva, A., 211, 222
Pak, A. W., 125
Palaniappan, 465
Palaniappan, R., 33, 194
Pálfia, M., 382
Palko, K., 330

Pallas-Areny, R., 168
Palmer, C. I., 260
Palmowski, A., 586
Palomäki, T., 210
Palomares, M., 554
Paluch, K., 105
Pammer, V., 226
Pammer-Schindler, V., 211, 220, 221, 225, 226
Pan, 686, 702
Pan, J., 529
Pan, S. J., 61, 62
Panicker, R. C., 528, 529
Panicker, Rajesh C., 515
Panko, M., 283, 289, 292
Pannek, H., 300
Pantic, M., 149, 152, 154
Panych, L. P., 223
Paolucci, S., 38t, 95, 102, 105, 446, 451
Papadelis, C. L., 152
Pappas, C., 152
Para, M. P., 330
Paralescu, Sorin, 198
Paramesran, R., 33
Parasuraman, R., 72, 73, 78
Paré, Ambroise, Dr., 115
Parent, A., 115
Paret, 626
Paret, C., 211
Parini, S., 331
Parisi, L., 215, 227
Park, H., 223
Park, K., 39
Park, Y.-M., 462
Parkkonen, L., 327
Parks, A., 123
Parra, L. C., 70, 75, 171, 453, 468
Parvaz, M., 107
Parviz, B. A., 246
Parvizi, J., 299, 300
Pascal, F., 381
Pascarella, 704
Pasley, B. N., 305, 334
Pasqualotto, E., 334, 466, 564
Pastor, M. A., 373, 465, 507, 512
Pastrana, E., 117
Patki, S., 167, 168, 169, 171, 179
Patras, I., 152, 153, 154
Patrick, T. A., 314
Patton, J. L., 305, 334
Pauls, J., 299
Pauly, J. M., 223, 227
Paus, T., 108
Pavlov, S., 152, 153
Pawelzik, H., 334
Pawlitzki, J., 82
Pazzaglia, 706
Pca, Á., 33
Pearlmutter, B. A., 21, 329
Pearlson, G. D., 302
Peck, E. M., 4, 78
Peckham, P. H., 3, 72, 327
Peer A., 329
Pei, X., 299, 305, 334
Pelley, 663

Pellise, D., 270
Pels, E., 305, 309, 310, 334
Penaranda, B. N., 457
Penders, J., 166, 167, 168, 169, 171, 179
Penfield, 673, 709
Penfield, W., 60, 298
Peng, H.-L., 17
Peng, S.-H., 137
Penn, R., 4
Pennec, X., 383, 384
Penny, W. D., 33
Perdikis, S., 38
Perdoni, C., 451
Perego, P., 244, 331, 332, 479
Pereira, G., 211, 222
Perelmouter, J., 3, 13
Pérez, Miguel Angel Ortiz, 201, 299
Perez-Benitez, J. A., 37t
Perez-Benitez, J. L., 37t
Perez-Marcos, D., 243
Perge, J. A., 280, 293
Perrig, S., 270
Perrin, E. C., 105
Perrin, M., 596
Perrone-Bizzozero, N. I., 302
Perry, J., 116
Pesaran, B., 300, 303
Peters, J., 102, 103, 105, 255, 256
Peters, John F., 508
Peters, P. J. F., 219
Petersen, S. E., 550
Peterson, D., 31, 32
Petit, D., 244
Petkova, V. I., 244
Petr, D., 29
Petrantonakis, P., 152, 153, 154
Pettersson, L. M. E., 704
Petti, M., 38t, 95, 102, 105, 226, 243, 446, 451
Pfurtscheller, G., 3, 4, 12, 15, 17, 23, 24, 25, 27, 31, 32, 33,
        34t, 35t, 36, 37t, 38t, 54, 62, 70, 71, 89, 94, 101,
        106, 108, 133, 134, 151, 152, 154, 155, 171, 174,
        210, 211, 216, 218, 219, 224, 226, 227, 237, 238,
        239, 241, 242, 243, 259, 260, 299, 300, 304,
        327, 347, 349, 351, 362, 363, 366, 373, 408, 446,
        447, 451, 452, 453, 455, 462, 463, 465, 476, 514,
        515, 526, 527, 528, 531, 544, 554, 586, 596, 605,
        618, 623, 703, 705, 708
Pfurtscheller, J., 211
Phan, A.-H., 420
Philips, J., 29
Phillips, V. L., 568, 686, 691
Phua, K. S., 105, 408
Pi, Z., 410, 420
Piaggio, N., 107
Piccione, F., 101, 241, 703
Pichiorri, F., 38t, 39, 95, 102, 105, 226, 243, 334, 446, 451,
        589, 669
Picht, B., 167
Picton, T. W., 22, 105
Pikov, V., 117
Pilcher, W., 303
Pillen, S., 102, 106, 212, 219, 226
Pine, K., 115
Pineda, J. A., 102, 106, 211, 212, 219, 226, 239

Pineda, M., 102
Pino, 646
Pirker, J., 211
Pisansky, M. T., 38t, 214, 240, 334
Pisotta, I., 38t, 95, 102, 105, 226, 446, 451
Pistohl, 710
Pistohl, T., 300, 303
Pistor, 708
Pitsch, H., 329
Piyathaisere, D., 303
Pizer, S. M., 384
Placidi, 708
Plass-Oude Bos, D., 211, 588, 589
Platsko, 691
Platsko, V., 334
Plis, S. M., 37t
Plow, E. B., 108
Plum, F, 532
Poel, M., 13, 76, 152, 153, 154, 155, 156, 211, 242, 451,
        463, 689
Pogosyan, A., 107, 306
Pohl, P. S., 21
Pohlmeyer, E. A., 708
Pokorny, C., 259, 260, 261
Polak, M., 33, 101
Poldrack, Russell A., 662, 663
Poli, R., 687, 688, 689, 692, 694
Polich, J., 152, 155, 512, 554
Poline, Jean-Baptiste, 662
Pollick, F., 167
Polprasert, C., 489, 498
Pomeroy, V. M., 102, 105
Pons, J. L., 95, 117
Ponticelli, R., 167
Pope, K. J., 300
Popescu, F., 38t, 451
Popma, A., 181
Popp, J., 467
Pop Research Group, 32
Porteous, J. J., 152
Posner, M. I., 105, 550
Potes, C., 300, 305, 334
Potter-Baker, K., 108
Poulin-Charronnat, Bénédicte, 194
Power, S. D., 222
Powers, J., 14, 305
Powers, J. C., 565
Praamstra, P., 551
Prabhakaran, V., 105
Prada, R., 211, 222
Pradhapan, P., 169, 171, 174, 182
Prasad, G., 102, 103, 105, 464, 469, 552
Prataksita, N., 38
Prats-Sedano, M.A., 259
Preece, J., 75
Preissl, H., 334
Prelec, D., 74
Presacco, A., 279
Prewett, M. S., 254
Priftis, K., 90, 241
Principe, J. C., 171, 299
Principe, Jose, 3
Priori, A., 306
Pröll, M., 211, 220

Protzak, J., 76
Prsa, 711
Prückl, R., 258, 259, 329
Prueckl, R., 334
Prvulovic, D., 22
Pryor, H. L., 246
Pudenz, R. H., 303
Pun, T., 152, 200
Punsawad, Y., 257, 260, 538, 539, 554
Purdy, P., 17
Puthusserypady, S., 33, 554
Putze, F., 467, 468

## Q

Qi, Y., 242
Qian, K., 408
Qin, L., 60
Quandt, F., 300
Quatrano, L. A., 3
Quek, C., 410
Quigg, M., 270
Quitadamo, L. R., 90
Quyen, M. L. V., 155

## R

Rabbi, A., 465, 512, 516
Rachels, James, 661
Racine, E., 657
Rackham, H., 115
Raco, V., 35t, 36, 171
Raffel, C., 314
Raffone, A., 151
Räikkä, Juha, 657
Rajagovindan, R., 300
Rajangam, Sankaranarayani, 516
Rajdev, P., 280, 293
Rakotomamonjy, A., 32, 409
Ram, D., 329
Rama, P., 467
Ramage, D., 31
Ramanna, 508
Ramirez, R., 35t, 200
Ramos, A., 257
Ramoser, H., 3, 27, 62, 70, 347, 349, 363, 366, 446, 447,
    448f, 449f, 450t, 453, 476
Ramos-Murguialday, A., 95, 101, 102, 106, 120, 303, 314,
    408, 542, 669, 679
Rampini, P. M., 306
Ramsay, A., 38
Ramsey, L., 211, 464
Ramsey, N., 90, 300, 301, 303, 304, 305, 309, 310, 313,
    461, 463, 464
Ramsey, N. F., 334
Rana, M., 108
Rand, D. G., 127
Randolph, A. B., 599
Rao, B. D., 410, 420
Rao, J., 420
Rao, R., 35t, 36, 63, 299, 303, 304, 307, 313, 334
Rao, R. P. N., 457, 702, 712
Raouzaiou, A., 150
Rasmussen, R., 257

Rasmussen, T., 60, 298
Raspopovic, 710
Ratel, D., 22, 309, 311
Ray, 673
Ray, S., 299, 552
Ray, W., 237
Rayner, K., 467
Raz, A., 105, 210
Raz, G. G., 152
Rea, M., 95, 102, 106, 108
Reardon, S., 121
Reason, J., 75
Rebsamen, B., 532
Rechtsteiner, A., 28
Rees, 659
Regan, D., 373
Reichert, J. L., 102, 104, 106, 210, 215, 224, 226, 227, 228
Reid, 703
Reilly, R. B., 4, 37t, 217, 465
Reiner, M., 451
Reisenzein, R., 150
Reissland, J., 242
Reithler, J., 223
Remsik, A., 105
Renard, Y., 134, 239, 240, 242, 244, 331, 332, 449, 457,
    479
Rene, K. M., 105
Renner, G., 334
Reuderink, B., 4, 152, 153, 154, 155, 156, 242, 451, 579
Reuter, E. M., 554
Reva, N., 152, 153
Revathi, A., 118
Reynolds, M., 176
Rezeika. A., 135
Rheinberg, F., 575
Rhiu, Ilsun, 13, 122
Rhoton, C. J., 237
Riccio, 578, 588
Riccio, A., 4, 239, 256, 334, 564
Richards, C., 451
Richards, J., 176
Richmond, 657, 659
Rick, S., 74
Rickert, J., 21
Ridder, S., 211
Rieger, J., 305
Rieger, J. W., 313
Riehle, A., 171
Riikkila, K., 150
Rijkhoff, N. J. M., 116
Rincon-Gonzalez, L., 119
Risetti, M., 90
Ritaccio, A. L., 298, 299, 300, 301, 303, 305, 313, 334
Ritter, H., 35t, 468
Rivet, B., 35t, 686, 687, 688, 689, 690, 691, 697
Rizzolatti, G., 21, 226, 551
Rizzuto, D. S., 300
Roach, P., 150
Robben, A., 37t, 472
Roberts, S. J., 33
Robertson, I. H., 181
Robineau, F., 211
Robinson, C. J., 3
Robinson, C. W., 35t

Rocchi, G., 107
Rocha, L., 28
Rockstroh, B., 349
Roco, M.C., 114
Rodríguez, Angel, 198
Rodriguez, E., 155
Rodriguez, J., 35t, 90
Rodríguez Méndez, S. J., 175
Roesch, E., 150, 152, 155, 196, 200, 201
Rogala, J., 105
Rogenmoser, L., 152, 153
Rogers, J., 334
Rogers, L. J., 299
Rogers, Y., 75
Rogin, E., 38t, 240, 334
Rohm, M., 408, 588
Roland, J., 305, 313, 334
Rolandi, M., 125
Roman, S. A., 238
Romano, D., 463
Romo, 709
Romo, R., 300
Ron-Angevin, 606
Ron-Angevin, R., 213, 220, 227, 240
Ros, 626
Ros, T., 211, 224
Rosa, M., 306
Rose, M., 103, 107, 211, 240, 270
Rosenboom, David, 166, 167, 177, 193, 195
Rosenow, J., 334
Rosenow, J. M., 305
Rosenqvist, A., 152, 153
Rosenstiel, W., 35t, 73, 78, 134, 210, 243, 303, 305, 313, 314, 334
Rosler, D. M., 280, 293
Rossi, P., 302, 306, 307
Rossignol, S., 117
Rossini, P. M., 550, 552
Rossiter, 627
Rossiter, H. E., 106
Rost, T., 35t
Roth, C., 37t
Rothbart, M. K., 550
Rothenberger, A., 15, 25
Rothkrantz, L., 149
Rötting, M., 70, 71, 75, 255, 260
Roudsari, A. F., 125
Rousche, P. J., 279
Rouse, A., 303, 304, 305, 309, 313, 314
Roy, A., 543
Royer, A. S., 211, 240, 334
Royl, G., 20
Rubel, 655
Rubel, Alan, 126
Rubin, M., 127
Ruedebusch, V., 309, 312
Ruf, C., 347
Ruf, C. A., 35t, 239, 334, 408, 466
Ruffini, G., 4
Rumelhart, D. E., 32
Rupp, R., 4, 134, 152, 154, 155, 210, 211, 464
Rusconi, M., 362
Russel, G. S., 169
Russell, J. A., 148, 150

Russell, James, 200
Rusyniak, W., 303
Rutkowski, T., 420
Rutkowski, T. M., 35t, 152, 155, 167, 259, 420, 462, 535, 538
Ryan, D.B., 402
Ryapolova-Webb, E., 306
Ryapolova-Webb, E. S., 302, 307, 308
Ryberg, 657

**S**

Saab, J., 167
Saab, R., 259
Saeedi, S., 588, 589, 602
Saeki, M., 171
Saetang, J., 257, 260
Sagebaum, M., 221
Sagha, H., 464
Sahin, M., 117
Said, S., 394
Saiwaki, N., 33
Sajda, P., 70, 75, 171, 238, 242, 244, 245, 246, 453, 464, 468
Sakhavi, S., 456
Sakurada, T., 554
Salanova, V., 309, 311
Salari, N., 103, 107
Saleh, M., 4
Salinari, S., 479
Salinas, C. M., 334
Salinet, 670
Salinsky, M., 182
Salomon, P., 90, 461, 463, 464
Salovey, P., 150
Salt, J.D., 115
Salvaris, M., 32, 503
Salvendy, G., 568
Salzmann, M., 377
Samaha, H., 243
Samek, W., 60, 408, 430, 451
Sanchez, 625, 707
Sanchez, G., 4
Sanchez, J. C., 299, 596
Sanchez-Vives, M. V., 224, 238, 243
Sander, D., 150
Sander, T. H., 327
Sanders, David Adrian, 516
Sandin, D. J., 237
Sanei, S., 550, 552
Sankarasubramanian, V., 108
San Luciano, M., 307, 308
Sannelli, C., 210, 211, 347, 349, 451, 457, 464
Santana, E., 171
Santosh, P., 105
Santvoord, A. V., 179
Saproo, S., 238, 242, 245, 246, 464, 468
Sarcinelli-Filho, M., 15
Sarma, A., 479
Sarma, D., 152, 153, 154, 155, 270, 271
Sarmah, E., 292
Sarnacki, W. A., 101, 102, 104, 106, 107, 210, 211, 334, 462
Sartori, G., 215, 227
Sassaroli, A., 4

Satti, A., 457
Satti, A. R., 38t
Sattin, J. A., 105
Sauter-Starace, F., 22, 309, 311
Savotina, L. N., 152
Savvidou, S., 150, 156, 157
Sawey, M., 150, 156, 157
Saxena, T., 22
Sayres, C., 313
Sbattella, L., 38t
Sburlea, 676, 677
Scabini, D., 299, 307
Schäfer, C., 70
Schäfer, J., 361, 381, 385, 409
Schalk, G., 3, 4, 15, 17, 21, 23, 27, 33, 34, 39, 54, 72, 134,
    242, 244, 270, 297, 298, 299, 300, 301, 302,
    303, 304, 305, 307, 313, 330, 331, 332, 334, 362,
    446, 449, 455, 456, 457, 462, 465, 466, 479,
    494, 703, 708
Scharinger, J., 95
Scharnowski, F., 20
Scharre, D., 116
Schartz, G., 211
Scheeringa, R., 106
Schelldorfer, J., 62
Schellenberg, E. Glenn, 200
Scherer, K. R., 149, 150, 200
Scherer, R., 4, 15, 31, 35t, 36, 37t, 38t, 76, 94, 151, 152,
    154, 155, 171, 210, 211, 218, 219, 220, 221, 224,
    225, 226, 227, 237, 239, 240, 241, 243, 259,
    260, 299, 449, 451, 462, 512, 575, 588, 619
Scherffig, L., 242
Scherg, M., 22, 105
Schettini, F., 334, 479, 575, 588
Scheuermann, J., 330
Schiavone, G., 176, 177, 181
Schierholz, I., 4
Schiff, N. D., 90
Schimmack, U., 148, 149, 200
Schlögl, 597, 598, 601, 637
Schlögl, A., 28, 32, 211, 239, 244, 327, 361, 362, 408,
    589
Schlosberg, H., 150
Schmader, T., 211, 224
Schmalstieg, D., 37t, 241, 243
Schmansky, N., 280, 293
Schmidt, A., 75
Schmidt, K., 299
Schmidt, L. A., 28, 152, 181, 623
Schmidt, N. M., 70, 347, 464
Schmidt, R.N., 449
Schmidt, S., 462
Schmorrow, Dylan D., 516
Schnakers, C., 90
Schneider, 657
Schneider, A. L., 270
Schneider, G. H., 107
Schoenmakers, 657
Schoffelen, J.-M., 300, 327, 456
Scholkmann, F., 242, 243
Schölkopf, B., 36, 37t, 61, 102, 103, 105, 255, 256, 303,
    305, 313, 334, 434, 553
Schomer, D. L., 236
Schoner, B., 176

Schooler, J. W., 211, 224
Schouenborg, J., 704
Schrauwen, B., 389
Schreiner, C. E., 118
Schreuder, M., 35t, 151, 239, 260, 347, 588
Schröder, M., 61, 150, 156, 157, 362
Schubert, E., 150
Schuele, S. U., 305, 334
Schuettler, M., 21
Schuh, L. A., 299
Schuller, B., 156
Schultz, T., 305, 334, 467, 468
Schultze-Kraft, M., 362, 464, 689, 692, 697
Schulz, R., 300
Schulz, S. M., 334
Schulze-Bonhage, A., 21, 300, 303
Schumacher, J., 597
Schuner, J., 3
Schupp, H. T., 152, 155
Schwaiger, M., 21
Schwalger T., 121
Schwartz, 706
Schwartz, A. B., 4, 13, 270, 299, 303, 313, 330
Schwartz, N. E., 334
Schwarz, 704, 708
Schwarz, A., 38t, 220, 221, 225, 226
Schwarz, D. A., 550
Schweiger, D., 102, 104, 106, 210, 215, 224, 226, 227,
    228
Schweinberger, S. R., 24
Schweizer, R., 15
Scipione, A., 33
Scolari, M., 105
Scott, D., 116
Sebastiano, F., 167
Secundo, L., 299, 307
Sederberg, P. B., 300
Seeck, M., 270
Seed, A., 114
Seeland, A., 79
Seemann, G., 276
Segalowitz, S. J., 28
Seibert, S., 280
Seidl-Rathkopf, K.N., 105
Sejnowski, 662
Sejnowski, T. J., 17, 73, 182, 299
Sekihara, K., 420
Sellers, E. W., 15, 22, 34, 35t, 36, 210, 305, 334, 347,
    355, 362, 401, 402, 408, 409, 462, 513, 586,
    661, 703
Senekowitsch-Schmidtke, R., 21
Seo, Dongjin, 123, 124f
Sepulchre, R., 378
Sepulveda, F., 17, 19, 20, 32
Sepulveda, Francisco, 503
Sequeira, H., 152, 155
Sereno, M. I., 56, 59
Sereno, S., 467
Sergius, Marcus, 115
Serruya, 706
Serruya, M., 4, 117
Settgast, V., 239
Severens, M., 23, 35t, 36, 37t, 258, 259
Seymour, N. E., 238

Sforza, C., 179
Shackel, B., 564, 566
Shackman, A. J., 29
Shadden, B. B., 13, 14
Shades, K., 38t, 240, 334
Shah, B. B., 118
Shahid, S., 464, 552
Shami, N. S., 127, 566
Shamir, R. R., 306
Shanechi, 706, 707
Shannon, 645, 709
Shannon, R. V., 118
Shapiro, D., 211
Sharma, M., 300, 303, 305, 334
Sharma, N., 102, 105
Sharmah, U., 38t
Sharman, Ken, 196
Sharp, H., 75
Sharpe, S. M., 283
Shawe-Taylor, J., 465
Shaw-Taylor, J., 376
Sheffield, W. D., 309, 312
Shen, Guobin, 201
Shen, J., 210
Sheng, X., 257
Shenoy, 601
Shenoy, K. V., 126, 596
Shenoy, P., 35t, 36, 334, 457
Sheridan, T. B., 78
Sherrington, 705
Shetty, K., 75
Shewokis, P., 221
Shi, B. E., 468
Shi, C., 15
Shi, J., 125
Shi, T., 13
Shibasaki, H., 171
Shieh, C. K., 175
Shih, 653
Shih, J. J., 305, 334
Shih, J. Y., 118
Shih, N., 293
Shih, V., 238, 242, 246, 464, 468
Shimamoto, S., 302
Shimizu, K., 4, 259
Shin, D. I., 211, 213, 224, 225, 227
Shin, H.-C., 409
Shin, J., 15
Shin, Y., 457
Shindo, K., 38t, 105
Shishkin, S., 35t, 36
Shishkin, S. L., 76
Shlens, J., 28
Shneiderman, B., 564
Shoemaker, 645, 646, 647
Shokur, S., 246
Shouse, M.N., 102
Shriberg, E., 150
Shupe, L., 299
Shute, J., 302, 306, 307
Shyu, K.-K., 137
Siebert, S. A., 283, 289, 292
Sieracki, J. M., 300
Sijercic, Z., 3

Silbergeld, D. L., 299
Silk, T. J., 181
Sillanmäki, L., 152, 153
Silva Cunha, J. P., 167
Silverman, D. S., 239
Silvoni, S., 101, 171, 259
Simeral, 645
Simeral, J. D., 280, 293
Simic, V., 116
Simione, L., 256
Simmons, F. Blair, 117–118
Simon, J., 226
Simon, N., 239, 573
Simonoff, E., 105
Simpson, A. J., 491
Sinai, A., 299
Sinescu, C. J., 38t
Singer, 622
Singer, M. J., 224
Singer, W., 299, 300, 302
Singha, H., 33
Singla, R., 330
Sinha, R. K., 464
Sinkjaer, 678
Sitaram, R., 4, 101, 107, 108, 114, 151, 210, 236, 705
Siuly, S., 409
Sivanathan, A., 102, 106, 211, 212, 219, 226
Skidmore, E. R., 330
Slater, M., 4, 15, 35t, 216, 218, 224, 227, 236, 237, 238, 239, 241, 243
Slobounov, E., 237, 672, 673, 674
Slobounov, S. M., 237
Sloutsky, V. M., 35t
Slutzky, 708
Slutzky, M. W., 256, 305, 313, 334
Smallwood, J., 211, 224
Smart, R., 214, 224, 226, 227
Smith, D. J., 259
Smith, J. R., 123
Smith, M. C., 309, 311
Smith, Melissa M., 73, 120
Smith, R., 37t, 217, 465
Smyth, M. D., 4, 303, 304, 313, 334
Sneddon, I., 150
Snyder, D., 309, 312
Snyder, Joel S., 198
Snyder, L. H., 300
Soares, E., 102, 106
Sobell, Nina, 2
Soddu, A., 90
Sodini, C. G., 64
Soekadar, 653, 655, 659
Soekadar, S., 334
Soekadar, S. R., 70, 102, 105, 106, 108, 538, 539
Soleymani, M., 152, 154
Solis, J., 305, 334
Solis-Escalante, T., 4, 15, 38t, 94, 95, 151, 154, 155
Sollfrank, T., 226
Solomon, B., 152, 153
Solovey, E. T., 4, 242
Soltani, M., 299, 302, 307
Solzbacher, F., 330
Somersalo, E., 59
Soneji, D., 223

Song, 601, 708
Song, J., 105
Song, Y., 224
Sonuga-Barke, E.J., 105
Soraghan, C., 21, 329
Sorani, 663
Sørensen, J. A., 270
Sorensen, L., 313
Sorensen, L. B., 299
Sorger, B., 223
Soucaret, V., 36, 199
Soukoreff, 645
Sourina, O., 214
Souza, A. P., 33, 34t
*Spacecraft*, 195
Spanlang, B., 238
Sparing, R., 544
Spataro, R., 90, 97
Speier, 644
Spelmezan, D., 257
Spence, C. D., 70, 75, 453
Sprague, T. C., 549
Spronk, D., 181
Spueler, M., 303, 314
Spüler, M., 134, 243, 334, 463
Srikameswaran, A. V., 330
Srinivasan, 704
Srinivasan, R., 105, 299
Srivastava, K. H., 120
Staba, R. J., 21
Staiger-Sälzer, P., 4
Stambaugh, C. R., 70
Stanford, T. E., 535
Stangl, M., 210, 211
Stanic, U., 116
Stankovic, John A., 201
Stanslaski, S., 305, 309
Stanslaski, S. R., 305, 309
Stark, 658
Starr, P. A., 302, 306, 307, 308
Stawicki, P., 133, 134, 135, 136, 137, 138, 139, 140, 141,
        373, 465, 466, 472
Stearns, Stephen, 115
Steed, A., 214, 216, 218, 224, 226, 227, 236, 239, 241
Steffert, T., 214, 224, 226, 227
Steffert, Tony, 198
Stefitz, R., 211, 222
Stegeman, D.F., 107
Stehman, 638
Stein, B. E., 535
Stein, C., 361
Steiner, H., 550, 552, 555
Steiner, N. J., 105
Stenberg, C. C., 116
Stephani, Ulrich, 198
Stepp, C. E., 259
Steriade, M., 17, 73
Sterman, M.B., 106
Sterr, A., 4, 108
Stevens, B., 108
Stevens, C., 150
Stevens, R. H., 152, 153, 154, 195
Stevens, S., 150
Stevenson, J., 105

Stewart, D. R., 125
Steyrl, 619
Steyrl, D., 126
Steyvers, M., 451
Stieglitz, T., 21
Stikic, M., 152, 153, 154
Stinear, C.M., 451
Stirpe, P., 167
Stiver, S. I., 299, 307
Stocks, N. G., 33
Stoica, 694
Stokes, M. J., 33
Stolcke, A., 150
Stollfuss, J., 21
Stork, D. G., 31, 355
Strangman, G., 540
Straube, S., 79
Strehl, U., 25, 104, 211
Strick, P.L., 108
Strimmer, K., 361, 381, 385, 409
Stringaris, A., 105
Strohmeier, D., 327
Strojnik, P., 116
Strukov, D. B., 125
Studer, P., 25
Sturm, I., 211, 305, 464
Stypulkowski, P., 305, 309
Su, S., 554, 710
Su, Y., 242
Suárez, O.Y., 449
Subramanian, S., 257, 331
Subramaniyam, N. P., 276
Suchman, L. A., 75, 80, 82
Sugiyama, M., 384
Suk, H. I., 33, 34t, 420
Sulzer, J., 211
Suminski, 707
Summerfelt, A., 37t
Sun, H., 32
Sun, S., 451, 457, 601, 711
SuperCollider, 181
Susila, I. P., 331, 332, 479
Susila, P., 244
Sussillo, D., 428
Sutter, E. E., 402
Suttie, N., 102, 106, 211, 212, 219, 226
Sutton, 488
Sutton, J., 150
Sutton, S., 54
Suzuki, A., 59
Suzuki, T., 33
Svirin, E. P., 76
Swaine, Joel S., 200
Swami, A., 125
Swann, N. C., 307, 308
Swanson, D. P., 330
Sweller, J., 598, 599
Swetz, S., 330
Swinnen, S.P., 451
Sykacek, 601
Szczepanski, S., 299, 300
Szedmak, S., 376, 465
Szrama, N., 305, 314, 334
Szuromi, D., 331

**T**

Taberner, A. M., 33
Tabie, M., 79
Tabot, 704, 709
Taherian, S., 586
Tai, 705
Takahashi, A., 116
Takahashi, T., 373
Takano, K., 244
Takata, Y., 171
Talla, V., 123
Tallgren, P., 168
Tamburella, F., 95
Tameesh, M., 303
Tan, D., 4, 70, 155
Tan, Desney, 516, 596, 710
Tan, G., 211
Tan, L. F., 224
Tan, L.-H., 20
Tan, T., 156, 226
Tan, V., 152, 153, 154
Tanaka, T., 152, 155
Taner, M., 3
Tang, H. Y., 124f
Tang, K. Y., 105
Tangermann, M., 4, 35t, 61, 72, 210, 211, 221, 239, 255,
        260, 303, 305, 313, 347, 464
Taniguchi, M., 107
Tanikawa, T., 237
Tao, J., 156
Tarnita, C.E., 127
Tarrin, N., 35t
Tate, M. C., 305
Taub, E., 3, 300
Tavella, M., 38
Taylor, 707, 708
Taylor, D., 4, 237
Taylor, J. G., 150
Tecchio, F., 17, 19, 20
Tedesco, R., 38t
Tee, B.C.-K., 120
Teillet, 604
Teitelbaum, Richard, 195, 197, 199
Telaar, D., 305, 334
Temurtas, F., 33
Tenke, C. E., 27, 28
Tennison, 658
Tentler, A., 241
Teplan, M., 16, 17
Terada, 672, 673
Terasawa, H., 167
Terekhin, P., 108
Tesneli, A. Y., 33
Thabit, K., 27
Thaker, G. K., 37t
Thakor, N. V., 257, 300, 303
Thaut, M. H., 31, 32
Thayer, J. F., 149
Théberge, J., 211, 224
Thibault, R. T., 105, 210
Thomas, E., 32
Thomas, P., 566, 601, 638
Thompson, 621, 636, 637, 644, 647

Thompson, David E., 513
Thompson, J., 25
Thompson, William F., 200
Thomson, E., 462, 470
Thomson, K., 305, 313
Thonnard, M., 90
Thorbergsson, P. T., 704
Thorn, C., 299
Thornby, J., 211
Throckmorton, C. S., 402, 495
Thulasidas, M., 4
Thurlings, M. E., 35t, 242, 258, 259, 260, 535, 538
Thurlings, Marieke E., 512
Thurston, A. J., 115
Thut, G., 553
Tian, H.-C., 17
Tibarewala, D. N., 16, 21
Tibshirani, Lasso, 411
Tibshirani, R., 355, 411
Tierra-Criollo, C. J., 33, 34t
Tikhonov, A., 58
Tillery, S. H., 119
Timperi, A., 33
Timperley, H., 598
Tindale, 689
Tipping, M. E., 409, 410, 411, 414
Tkach, 707
Tocci, A., 334
Todd, D. A., 37t
Todorov, 706
Todorov, E., 116
Toharia, Pablo, 198
Toiviainen, P., 150
Tombini, M., 17, 19, 20
Tomioka, R., 29, 352, 353, 355, 360, 361, 362, 364, 366,
        377, 408, 410, 418, 453, 456, 601
Tonali, P., 306
Tonet, O., 17, 19, 20, 126
Tonin, L., 408, 550
Tonin, P., 241
Tootell, R. B., 59
Toppi, J., 38t, 90, 95, 102, 105, 226, 446, 451
Toro, C., 300
Torrellas, S., 237, 240
Torres, G., 303
Torres, R. R., 256
Tort, A. B., 299
Tourville, J. A., 283, 289, 292
Touyama, H., 4
Townsend, D. W., 21
Townsend, G., 35t, 334, 489, 493, 498, 586, 691
Townsend, J., 299
Trainor, 623
Trainor, L. J., 152
Tranel, D., 149
Travers, B., 280, 293
Treder, M. S., 35t, 70, 347, 350, 355, 360, 361, 362, 381,
        409, 464, 466, 489
Trejo, L. J., 237
Trimper, 657
Trinath, T., 299
Triponyuwasin, P., 39
Troen, T., 149
Trofimov, A. G., 76

Trösterer, S., 70, 71, 75
Truccolo, W., 280, 293
Trudeau, D. L., 102
Trujillo, N. J., 373
Tsanakalis, F., 704
Tsapatsoulis, N., 150
Tsoneva, T., 13
Tsuzuki, D., 18
Tu, W., 451
Tuch, A.N., 211
Tucker, D. M., 169
Tudor, Anca, 198
Tufte, E. R., 75
Tur, G., 150
Turolla, A., 101
Tyler, M., 105, 257
Tyler-Kabara, E. C., 4, 13, 270, 299, 303, 313, 330
Tyrrell, R.A., 228
Tzouvaras, V., 150

U

Uematsu, S., 300, 303
Ugawa, Y., 108
Uhl, 672
Uhlhaas, P. J., 19, 302
Ullestad, D., 305, 309
Ušc'umlic, M., 464, 468
Ushiba, J., 38t, 105, 107
Usoh, M., 227, 236
Uutela, K., 59

V

V. Kostic, 679
Väisänen, J., 276
Valbo, Å. B., 260
Valbuena, D., 135, 136, 138, 139, 465, 469, 476
Valdés-Sosa, P., 373
Valencia, M., 373, 465
Valera, E., 551
Valeriani, 689, 694
Väljamäe, Anastasiia, 198
Vallabhaneni, A., 15
Vallender, E. J., 114
Vamvakousis, Z., 35t, 200
van Aart, J., 219
Vanacker, G., 29, 257, 350
van Boxtel, G., 181
van de Laar, B., 76, 211, 242, 579, 692
Van Den Boom, M. A., 334
Van den Bosch, W. E., 672, 673
van den Broek, E., 152, 153
VandenEboom, M., 305, 309, 310, 313
van der Heiden, L., 347
Vanderheyden, L., 168
van der Waal, M., 35t, 36, 258, 259, 554
van der Werf, Y., 156
van de Steeg, C., 107
van de Ville, D., 211
Van de Weijer, J., 468, 470
Van Dijk, H., 300
Van Dokkum, L. E. H., 242
van Dongen-Boomsma, M., 181

van Drongelen, W., 59
Van Erp, J. B. F., 464, 692
Van Erp, Jan B., 13, 15, 22, 35t, 70, 72, 73, 76, 156, 196,
     254, 255, 256, 258, 259, 260, 261
van Gerven, M., 347, 512
Van Gompel, J. J., 314
Vanhala, J., 123
Vanhatalo, S., 21, 168
Vanhaudenhuyse, A., 90
Van Hoof, C., 168
Van Horn, 662
Van Hulle, M. M., 37t, 409, 472
Vanken, E., 116
van Koningsbruggen, 711
Vankov, A., 239
Van Langhenhove, A., 240
Van Leeuwen, C., 468
van Mourik, T., 106
van Nieuwenhuizen, C., 181
Van Os, T.W.D.P., 104
van Rijen, P., 303, 304, 305, 309, 310, 313, 334
van Roon, P., 105
Van Rotterdam, A., 56, 57
van Schouwenburg, M.R., 106
Vansteensel, M., 60, 303, 304, 305, 309, 310, 313, 334
Vansteensel, M. J., 588, 708
Vanstreels, K., 168
van't Ent, D., 61
van Veen, B. D., 59
van Vliet, M., 37t, 472
van Vugt, M., 299
van Wouwe, N., 152, 153
Varela, F. J., 155
Vargas, M. I., 270
Varghese, L. A., 259
Varkuti, 679
Varkuti, B., 210
Varlamov, A., 152, 153
Varnerin, N., 108
Varnet, L., 35t
Varsta, M., 3
Vassanelli, S., 125
Vatta, F., 27, 63
Vaughan, T. M., 3, 4, 12, 23, 24, 35t, 70, 72, 89, 104, 105,
     133, 210, 304, 334, 347, 355, 362, 373, 401, 408,
     409, 462, 586, 589, 590
Vavken, E., 116
Veit, R., 20, 108, 151, 210, 211, 236
Velasco, A. L., 116
Velasco, F., 116
Velasco, M., 116
Velasco-Alvarez, F., 240
Velichkovsky, B. M., 76
Velliste, M., 283, 292, 330, 702, 708
Venkatesh, V., 564
Venthur, B., 244, 332, 479
Ventura, M., 90
Verhoeven, T., 491, 498
Vernon, D., 627
Verschore, H., 389
Verschure, P., 226
Verschure, P. F. M. J., 243
Verschure, Paul, 200
Verstraeten, D., 389

Verwegen, A., 167, 168, 169
Veser, S., 259
Vesin, J., 31
Vesin, J. M., 409, 413
Vetter, R. J., 704
Vi, C., 257
Vialatte, F.-B., 373
Vicente, L. M., 33
Vidal, J. J., 687
Vidal, Jacques J., 2, 54, 70, 81
Vidaurre, C., 210, 211, 221, 327, 347, 349, 361, 408, 457,
        464, 512, 554, 586, 602
Viemerö, V., 152, 153
Viirre, E. III., 246
Vilimek, R., 463, 467, 469, 479
Villagran, C. T., 238
Villamira, M., 152, 153, 154
Villarejo, M. V., 149
Villringer, A., 20
Vilos, C., 125
Vinjamuri, R. K., 270, 303, 313, 330
Vitiello, N., 70
Viventi, 704
Viventi, J., 299, 300
Voipio, J., 168
Vollebregt, M. A., 552, 553
Volosyak, I., 15, 24, 133, 134, 135, 136, 137, 138, 139, 140,
        141, 373, 465, 466, 469, 470, 472, 476, 479
Volpato, C., 101, 259
Volta, Alessandro, 115
von Arnim, C., 151
von Bünau, P., 349
von Guericke, Otto, 115
Votsis, G., 150
Vourvopoulos, A., 606
Voytek, B., 299, 307
Vuckovic, A., 605
Vuèkovi, 688, 692
Vukelic, M., 243
Vukicevic, T., 150
Vullers, R., 166, 167, 168, 179
Vulliemoz, S., 270
Vuoskoski, J. K., 150
Vuoskoski, Jonna K., 200
Vygotsky, L.S., 606
Vyziotis, A., 102, 106

**W**

Wadeson, A., 13, 166
Wagner, J., 38t, 220, 225
Wagner, N., 228
Wahab, A., 152, 153
Wahl, M., 107
Wahnoun, R., 707
Wairagkar, M., 155, 156
Wald, P., 355
Waldert, S., 126
Walker, A. E., 303
Walker, I., 456, 703
Walker, J.E., 102, 103, 104, 108
Wall, M., 28
Wallace, M., 150
Wallstrom, G. L., 434

Walpulski, M., 152, 153, 154
Walter, A., 243, 303, 314
Walter, C., 73, 78
Walter, P., 118
Walter, W. G., 660, 671
Walterspacher, D., 327
Walton, L. M., 257, 332
Walton, L. M., 105
Walvoord, A. G., 254
Wan, F., 15, 37t, 138
Wander, J., 63, 270, 271
Wang, B., 15, 37t
Wang, C., 105, 408
Wang, Chi-Hong, 200
Wang, F., 13, 535, 543
Wang, H., 13, 532, 538, 539
Wang, J., 211, 215, 224
Wang, L., 127
Wang, M., 420
Wang, P., 29
Wang, Q., 214
Wang, T., 15
Wang, W., 4, 126, 270, 299, 303, 313, 330
Wang, X., 15, 37t, 134, 224, 408, 409, 410, 413, 414, 416,
        418, 420, 462, 463, 465, 708
Wang, Y., 4, 15, 24, 27, 29, 36, 82, 136, 168, 260, 349, 366,
        376, 377, 392, 393, 404, 405, 410, 418, 456, 458,
        464, 465, 476, 686, 688, 689, 692, 694
Wang, Y.-T., 136, 168, 175, 376, 377, 392
Wang, Z., 300
Wangler, S., 552, 554
Ward, L. M., 552
Ward, M. F., 299
Ward, M. P., 280, 293
Ward, N. S., 106
Ward, R. K., 30, 468
Ward, T., 167, 177, 242
Ward, T. E., 13, 15, 20, 21, 222, 329
Wårdell, K., 116
Ware, M. P., 470
Warp, R., 13, 167, 177
*The Warren*, 195
Warren, J. P., 119
Warwick, K., 155
Washizawa, Y., 420
Watchorn, A., 181
Waters, R. L., 116
Waytowich, N. R., 238, 242, 394, 464, 468
Weaver, 645
Weaver, J., 149, 152, 153, 154, 155, 156, 196, 199, 201, 202
Weaver, K., 270, 271
Weber, C., 105, 334
Weber, D. J., 4, 13, 126, 270, 299, 303, 313, 330
Weber, M. J., 123
Webster, J. G., 168
Wei, C.-S., 82
Weihing, J., 22
Weiland, J., 303
Weinand, 703
Weiskopf, N., 20, 236
Welford, 645
Welke, S., 70, 255, 260
Wendel, K., 276
Wenzel, M. A., 344, 464, 467

Werkhoven, P., 35t, 258, 259, 260
Wessberg, 702, 706, 707, 708
Wessberg, J., 70, 260
Wessig, C., 334
Westerfield, M., 299
Westerveld, M., 334
Wetherall, D., 123
Weyand, S., 578
Whang, M., 39
Wheeler, J. J., 314
Whitaker, K. W., 82
Whitfield, S., 227
Whitham, 617
Whitman, M., 167, 177
Whitmer, D., 463
Whittingstall, K., 299
Whrle, H., 79
Wibral, M., 22
Wichmann, T., 283, 292
Wickens, C. D., 73, 78
Widge, 711, 712
Widman, G., 303, 305, 313
Wieder, H., 21
Wieser, M. J., 24
Wilcox, T., 20
Wilding, K., 211, 226
Wiles, J. A., 148
Wilfried, M., 118
Wilhelm, B., 210
Wilke, 674
Wilke, C., 334
Wilkins, A., 373, 465
Williams, D., 149, 152, 153, 154, 155, 156, 194, 196, 199,
    200, 201, 202
Williams, J., 105, 257, 299, 300, 301, 303, 313, 331, 332
Williams, J. C., 332, 334
Williams, J. J., 314
Williams, O., 410
Williamson, J., 38
Willier, A., 176
Willis, H., 127
Willoughby, J. O., 300
Wills, R.F., 228
Wilschut, E.S., 256
Wilson, 465, 708, 709
Wilson, A. J., 332
Wilson, C. L., 21
Wilson, J., 4, 257, 300, 301, 303, 304, 313, 334
Wilson, John J., 194
Wilson, M. T., 300
Wilson, S., 13, 133
Wimmer, G. E., 74
Wingrave, C. A., 237
Winstein, C. J., 21
Winter, W.R., 105
Wipf, D. P., 420
Wise, S. P., 551
Wisneski, K. J., 334
Witkowski, M., 70
Witmer, B. G., 224
Witte, 626
Witte, H., 300
Witte, M., 210, 211
Wittenberg, E., 13, 25

Wodlinger, B., 4, 13, 270, 303, 313, 330
Woehrle, H., 598, 601, 602
Wöhrle, H., 79
Wojtowicz, J., 329
Wolf, M., 242, 243, 361, 381
Wolff, A., 107
Wolpaw, 661
Wolpaw, E. W., 4, 12, 25, 53, 70, 90, 101, 133, 237, 446
Wolpaw, J. R., 446, 449, 455, 456, 457, 462, 465, 466,
    476, 526, 550, 551, 554, 596, 598, 639, 686,
    691
Wolpaw, Jonathan, 2, 3, 4, 12, 15, 21, 22, 23, 24, 25, 27,
    32, 35t, 39, 53, 54, 70, 72, 89, 90, 101, 102, 104,
    105, 106, 107, 133, 134, 147, 210, 211, 237, 242,
    244, 270, 299, 300, 301, 303, 304, 305, 313,
    330, 331, 332, 334, 347, 349, 355, 362, 363, 373,
    401, 408, 409, 426
Wolpe, 657, 658
Wolpert, D. M., 706
Womelsdorf, T., 300
Won, D. O., 136
Wong, C. M., 138
Wong, K. M., 378
Wong-Lin, K., 469
Wongsawat, Y., 39, 257, 260, 554
Woo, J., 13, 34
Wood, G., 102, 104, 106, 210, 211, 215, 222, 224, 226, 227,
    228
Wood, R. B., 238
Woods, R., 20
Woodside., D. B., 116
Woolrich, M. W., 59
*World of Warcraft*, 209, 240
Worrell, G. A., 314
Worsley, 624
Wörz, S., 25
Wriessnegger, S., 171, 211
Wright, E. J., 280, 283, 289, 292
Wright, Z. A., 305, 334
Wrobel, A., 105
Wronkiewicz, Mark, 59, 61, 62, 63, 126
Wruck, E., 20
Wu, C., 420
Wu, D., 177, 434
Wu, J., 553
Wu, S., 14, 305
Wu, T., 32
Wu, Tien-Lin, 200
Wu, W., 347, 375, 376, 392, 393, 420, 465
Wu, Z., 137, 554
Wyler, A. R., 703

**X**

Xie, S. Q., 37t, 38, 134, 373, 375, 420
Xing, S., 37t, 38
Xu, B., 17
Xu, D., 465, 528
Xu, J., 167, 168, 169
Xu, M., 224
Xu, P., 409
Xu, R., 95, 671, 672, 676, 678
Xu, X., 136
Xu, Y., 409, 412

**Y**

Yamawaki, N., 334
Yameen, B., 125
Yan, N., 211, 215, 224
Yan, S., 456
Yan, Z., 347, 366, 403
Yang, B., 17, 32
Yang, C.-S., 17
Yang, G.-Z., 75
Yang, H., 408, 420
Yang, J. J., 125
Yang, L., 550
Yang, P., 409
Yang, Q., 61, 62, 211, 215, 224
Yang, Y., 20, 210
Yao, D. Z., 409
Yao, L., 37t, 38, 210, 257
Yao, S., 626
Yazacioglu, R. F., 167, 168, 169
Yazawa, S., 676
Yazdan-Shahmorad, A., 710
Yeon, P., 123
Yerra, R., 309, 312
Yger, F., 377, 378, 384
Yilmaz, O., 102, 106
Yin, E., 15, 259, 334, 463, 528, 535, 537
Yokochi, F., 107
Yong, X., 468
Yoo, D. J., 211
Yoo, J. H., 211
Yoo, P. B., 705
Yoo, S.-S., 151, 223
Yoon, H., 34
Yoshinobu, T., 331
You, C. K., 175
Young, B. M., 105, 669
Young, G. B., 270
Young, M. S., 73
Yu, B. M., 63
Yu, C., 175
Yu, S. B., 15
Yu, T., 38, 408, 420, 528, 531, 532, 534
Yu, Z., 409, 412, 420
Yuan, H., 60, 451, 639, 640, 647, 694
Yuchtman, M., 59
Yue, J., 38, 211, 215, 224
Yuen, T. G., 303
Yuksel, B. F., 78
Yun, M. H., 13

**Z**

Zaborowska, Katarzyna A., 200
Zacksenhouse, M., 706
Zaepffel, M., 171
Zaghloul, K. A., 103
Zander, T. O., 4, 13, 39, 70, 71, 72, 73, 75, 76, 80, 82, 94,
        147, 151, 154, 155, 167, 237, 238, 242, 255, 256,
        260, 463, 464, 467, 469, 479, 564, 614, 618, 658
Zanini, P., 394
Zanos, S., 299, 303, 304, 313, 334
Zao, J. K., 175

Zapirain, B. G., 149
Zarin, D. A., 550
Zarshenas, H., 133
Zavala, B., 306
Zawallich, L., 82
Zentner, M., 149, 150
Zen Wheels, 173, 175
Zeyl, T., 259
Zhang, Ben, 201
Zhang, C., 13, 347, 375, 376, 392, 393, 457, 465, 601
Zhang, D., 15, 37t, 38, 257, 260
Zhang, G., 210
Zhang, H., 4, 236, 366, 408, 418, 420, 453, 554, 708
Zhang, L., 213, 239, 420
Zhang, R., 541, 543
Zhang, Y., 134, 408, 409, 410, 413, 414, 416, 418, 420, 462,
        463, 465, 554, 704
Zhang, Z., 4, 27, 410, 420
Zhao, Feng, 201
Zhao, J., 331
Zhao, Q., 152, 155, 213, 239, 408, 409, 410, 413, 414, 416,
        420, 601
Zhao, R., 33, 34
Zhao, X., 210
Zhao, Z., 152
Zheng, C., 29
Zheng, H. Y., 553
Zheng, S. D., 15, 465
Zhigalov, A., 35t, 36
Zhong, C., 125
Zhong, S., 33, 34
Zhou, F., 237
Zhou, G., 134, 409, 410, 413, 414, 418, 420, 465
Zhou, L., 105
Zhou, S., 408
Zhou, Z., 15, 38, 259, 334, 463
Zhu, D., 15, 24, 136, 373, 465
Zhu, X., 37t, 38, 257
Zhuang, K. Z., 246
Ziarani, A. K., 37t
Ziat, M., 4
Zich, C., 4, 64, 626
Zickler, C., 4, 239, 334
Zickler, Claudia, 516, 517, 575, 578, 588
Ziefle, Martina, 512
Ziegler, S., 21
Ziemann, U., 114
Zimmerli, L., 226
Zioga, P., 167, 694
Zippo, A. G., 704
Zobova, L.N., 256
Zoccoli, E., 13
Zollinger, N., 152, 153
Zong, L., 211, 215, 224
Zopf, R., 15
Zorrilla, A. M., 149
Zotev, V., 626
Zrenner, C., 114
Zrenner E., 119f
Zrinzo, L., 306
Zuberer, A., 104, 105
Zubin, J., 54
Zygierewicz, J., 462, 472

# Subject Index

Page numbers followed by f and t indicate figures and tables, respectively.

## A

Abductor pollicis brevis (APB), 670
Accuracy, 470, 564, 589
  binary classification *vs.* task, 637–639
    binomial models, 638–639, 639f
    confusion matrix, 638
  predicted, 642–644
  projected, 643–644
Acquisition device, 568, 572t
Acquisition of signals (BCI experiments), design guidelines
  differential amplification, 616–617
  mental states, 618–619
  muscular activity interference with EEG activity, control of, 617–618, 617f
  sensor type, location, number selection, 615–616
Action potential process, 16
Activa PC+S devices, 306, 309, 310f
Activa RC+S system, 309
Active aBCIs, 155, 156
Active BCIs, 237, 255, 614; *see also specific entries*
  haptic feedback in, 256–257
Active multimind BCIs, 687
Active sensors, 168
Actuation techniques, 170
Acute intraoperative ECoG strips, implantation, 306
Adaptation; *see also* Adaptive BCI systems
  automated, 79–81
  closed-loop, 77–79
  model
    calibration-free decoding and, 437, 438f
    transfer learning, 437, 438f
  open-loop, 75–77
  principles of, 598
    human learning, 598–599
    machine learning, 598
  reasons for, 597
Adaptive automation, 78
Adaptive AutoRegressive (AAR) features, 601
Adaptive BCI systems
  framework, 599–600, 599f
    conductor, 600, 606–607
    feedback, 606
    instructions and stimuli, 606
    literature review on adaptive signal processing/ machine learning, 601–602
    machine output, 606
    system pipeline, 600–602, 600f
    task model, 603, 603f, 605
    user model, 603–604, 603f, 604t
  motivations and principles, 597–599
    human learning, 598–599
    machine learning, 598
    reasons for adaptation, 597–598
    signal variability, causes of, 597–598

  overview, 596–597
  perspectives and challenges, 607
Adaptive biofeedback, concept of, 195
Adaptive classifiers, 601–602
Adaptive decision methods, 602
Adaptive feature extraction, 601
Adaptive Gaussian Representation, 601
Adaptive logic network (ALN), 33
Adjacency problem, BCI paradigms design and, 509, 511
Affect, in aBCIs, 155–156
Affective BCIs (aBCIs), 147–158
  aBCMI, case study, 156–158
  affective states
    continuous affective state reporting tools, 150–151
    defined, 148
    detection, 151–155, 158
    discrete affective state reporting tools, 149–150
    overview, 148–149
    reporting, 149–151
  categories, 155, 158
  developing, guide for, 158–159
  intertrial and interuser variability, 158
  nonstationarity of affect, 158
  overview, 147–148
  purpose, 158
  use of affect in, 155–156, 158
Affective brain–computer music interface (aBCMI), 147, 155–157, 198
Affective computing, aBCIs, use, 156
Affective state control, BCMI, 199–201
Affective states
  defined, 148
  detection, 151–155
  mapping, 200
  overview, 148–149
  reporting, 149–151
    continuous methods, 150–151
    discrete methods, 149–150
Afferent/sensory NIs, 702, 709
Afferent volley, 679
Affine invariant Riemannian (AIR) distance, 384, 392, 429
Algorithms, MI BCI training session, 451–456, 452f
  classification, 454–455, 455f, 456
  discussions, 456
  feature extraction, 453–454, 454f, 456
  preprocessing, 451–453, 452f, 456
Alzheimer's disease, 116
Amplitude modulations, of brain rhythms, 351–353, 363
Amplitude threshold criterion, single-trial EEG analysis, 344–345
Amyotrophic lateral sclerosis (ALS), 254, 255, 305
Ankle dorsiflexion, 676
Anorexia nervosa, 116
Anthropomorphic robotic limbs, 120

Apical dendrite, 56
Application example
    brain and body sonification, juggling performance, 180–181
    competitive toy car racing using motor imagery BCI, 175–176
    monitoring, children during entertainment and learning, 186, 187f
Application level
    defined, 688
    multi-mind system at, 689
Application phase, ERP-based BCIs, 596
Application programming interfaces (APIs), 324
Applications, BCIs
    aBCIs, see Affective BCIs (aBCIs)
    artistic BCIs, practical BCI solutions, see Practical BCI solutions
    BCMI, see Brain–computer music interface (BCMI)
    CSP analysis, feature extraction, 366
    entertainment and multimedia, control of
        games, see Games
        mediating interaction in VR/AR, see Virtual and augmented reality (VR/AR)
    interaction technology, example, 34–39; see also Interaction technology
        ERD/ERS-based BCI application, 38–39
        P300-based BCIs, 34–36
        SSVEP-based BCIs, 36–38
    multi-mind BCIs, 690–695
        communication, 691
        control of external devices, 691–692
        music, 694–695
        target detection and decision making, 693–694
        tutorial, 695
        video games, 692–693
    neuroscience; see also Neuroscience
        classification accuracy, improving, 59–61
        transfer learning, 61–63
    passive BCIs, see Passive BCIs
    research, for VR/AR, 238
    SSVEP-based, see SSVEP-based BCI applications
    therapeutic, see Therapeutic applications
    TMS, 108
Application-specific integrated circuit (ASIC) board, 124f
*ARHGAP11A* gene, replication of, 114
*ARHGAP11B* gene, 114
Arousal
    decreasing/increasing, 157–158
    defined, 148
Artifacts, removing, 25–26, 158
Artificial General Intelligence (AGI), 125
Artificial neural network (ANN) classifiers, 32–33
    MLP, 32–33
    other architectures, 33
Artificial sensations, 709–710
Artificial somatosensory feedback, 117
Artistic BCIs
    BMCI, see Brain–computer music interface (BCMI)
    practical BCI solutions, see Practical BCI solutions
Asperger's syndrome, 200
Assistive Technology Device Predisposition Assessment device form (ATD-PA device form), 575

Associative BCIs, MRCP-based, 677–680
    overview, 677–678
    potential and challenges, 679–680
    type of neurofeedback, 678–679
Associative plasticity induced by BCI, 669–680
    MRCP and, see Movement-related cortical potentials (MRCPs)
    overview, 669–671
Asymmetry features, aBCI system, 151, 152, 152t
Asynchronous BCIs, 15, 29, 152, 154
Attention
    covert, 551
    mechanisms, 551
    neuroscience of, 550–551
    orientation of, 551
    overt, 551
    overview, 549–550
    premotor theory of, 551
    spatial, 551
Attention-based BCIs; see also Neurofeedback therapy
    emergence of, 551–552
    future directions, 554–555
    neural features for, 552
        event-related potentials, 553–554
        importance of selection, 552
        oscillations, 552–553
        steady-state visual evoked potentials, 554
Attention-deficit/hyperactivity disorder (ADHD), 550
    neurofeedback therapy, 550
    treatment, 102, 104, 105, 106, 550
Attention monitoring, 516
Attenuation, of MRCP, 674
Audio cues, personalized, 226
Audio-tactile P300 BCIs, 537–538, 537f
Audio-visual P300 BCIs, 535–537, 536f
Auditory evoked potential (AEP) approach, mindBEAGLE system, 91, 92f
Auditory senses, neuroprosthetics, 117–118
Auditory steady-state responses (ASSRs), 36
Auditory stimulation
    P300-based BCI, 34–36
    SSVEP-based BCIs, 36–38
Auditory stimuli, 571
Augmentation, cognitive, 516
Augmented reality (AR)
    BCIs and, 243–244
    mediating interaction, see Virtual and augmented reality (VR/AR)
Autism, 102, 106, 198, 224, 225
Automated adaptation, 79–81
    examples from literature, 80
    overview, 79–80
    reflection, 80–81
Automation
    adaptive, 78
    level of, 77–78
    purpose, 78
Autonomous navigation system, intelligent wheelchair based on, 541–542, 541f
Avatar
    video games, 692, 693
    VR/AR, 243
Averaged periodogram method, 272

**B**

Band-pass–filtered signals
    data matrices of, 363
    variance of, 363
Band-power–based features, aBCI system, 151, 152, 152t,
        153t–154t
Band power changes
    frequency, low- and high-, 273–274
    mu, beta, and high gamma, 272
Basal ganglia–cortical networks, 306
Bayesian DS algorithm, 490–491
Bayesian learning, for EEG analysis, 407–420
    discriminant analysis, 413–414
    discussion, 419–420
    experimental study, 415–419
        ERP data set, 415–417
        SMR data set, 418–419
    LDA and LSR, equivalence between, 410–411
    maximum likelihood and regularized least squares,
        411–413
    overview, 408–410
    SBL, 414–415, 416–417
Bayesian linear discriminant analysis (BLDA), 409, 410,
        414, 416–417
Bayesian logistic regression neural network (BLRNN), 33
Bayesian model, 526
BCILAB, 244–245, 327, 328f, 449
BCIs, *see* Brain–computer interfaces (BCIs)
BCI2000 system, 134, 242, 325, 329, 330–333, 398, 449,
        451, 456, 457, 494–495
Bereitschaftspotential (BP), 671, 672
Bernoulli distribution, logistic model prediction through,
        436
Beta band, 24–25
Beta distribution, logistic model prediction through, 436
Beta rhythm desynchronization, 107
Between-class (within-class) scatter, 31
Biases, avoidance of, 626–627
Bidirectional neural interfaces, 710–711; *see also* Neural
        interfaces (NIs)
Big data (BCI), privacy and, 662–664
Binary classification accuracy, *vs.* task accuracy, 637–639
    binomial models for accuracy, 638–639, 639f
    confusion matrix, 638
Binomial models, for accuracy, 638–639, 639f
BioComputing laboratory, 446, 451
Biofeedback, 2, 102, 103–105, 107–108
Biomimetic neuroprosthetics, 125
Biomuse, 195
Bionanoprotonics, 125
Biosemi ActiveTwo system, 446
BioSig, 327
Bipolar reference, 26, 27
Bladder dysfunction, treatment, 116
Blood oxygen level–dependent (BOLD) contrast, 20
Bluetooth, 169, 170, 175
Body schema, concept of, 706
Body-transfer illusion, 238
Bonferroni correction, 624
Boosting classification performance, 155
Botulinum toxin injections, 116
Boundary avoidance task (BAT), 246
Boundary element models (BEMs), 37

Braille, 118, 252
Brain, mapping noninvasive signals to, 56–59
Brain activity
    discriminative features of, 349–353
        amplitude modulations of brain rhythms, 351–353
        ERPs, modulations of, 350–351
        overview, 349, 350
    initial recording of, 74
    in multi-mind BCIs, 687, 688f
    pattern generation, 13
BrainAmp, 568, 573
Brain and body sonification, juggling performance,
        176–181
    application example, 180–181
    data analysis, 179
    experimental protocols, 177–179
    overview, 176–177
    preprocessing, 179
    results, 179–180
    study population, 177
BrainArena, 692
BrainBall, 693
Brain–computer interfaces (BCIs), 461–462, 550; *see also*
        Motor imagery (MI)–based brain–computer
        interface (BCI)
    active BCIs, 237, 255, 256
    adaptive systems, *see* Adaptive BCI systems
    application, 568, 573t
    applications, *see* Applications, BCIs
    associative plasticity induced by, *see* Associative
        plasticity induced by BCI
    attention-based, *see* Attention-based BCIs
    BCI system
        categories, 13, 14–15, 14f
        framework, 13, 14f
    categories, 462
    challenges, 526–527
    concept, 446, 526
    constraints, 463
    data acquisition, 526
    defined, 3–4, 12, 653–654
    design guidelines for experiments, *see* Design
        guidelines, BCI experiments
    evolution, *see* Evolution, BCIs
    exercise, 605
    eye gaze with, 466–469, 467f
    feature extraction, 526
    future perspectives, 464, 722–723
    haptics and, *see* Haptics, BCI and
    *hybrid, see hybrid* brain–computer interface (*h*BCI)
    mouse, MI-and-P300–based, 532–534, 533f
    multi-mind, *see* Multi-mind BCIs
    multiple systems, 463–464
    for music making, *see* Brain–computer music interface
        (BCMI)
    NIs, *see* Neural interfaces (NIs)
    paradigms; *see also* P300- and -SSVEP–based BCIs;
        SSVEP paradigms
        dependence of BCI applications, 513
        design-related challenges, 509–512
        efficiency and, 512–513
        hybrid SSVEP–P300 paradigm, 513–516, 514f,
            515f
        issues and challenges, 501–517

new applications evolvement, 516–517
overview, 502–503
role of, 502
spontaneous, 596
visual, 502–503
passive, *see* Passive BCIs
performance measurement, *see* Performance
  measurement
perspectives on, 721–723
preprocessing, 526
privacy and, *see* Privacy, and BCI
purpose of, 605
reactive BCIs, 238, 255, 256
rehabilitation, 516
research, UCD and, 590–591
research articles, 19
scope of, 4
signature, 568, 572t
software, *see* Software, BCI
SSVEP-based, 465–466
SSVEP BCI component, 472
strategy, 605
system architecture, 526, 526f
technology and historical events, 1
therapeutic applications, *see* Therapeutic applications
therapy, 550
transfer learning for, *see* Transfer learning
translation algorithms, 526
UCD in, *see* User-centered design (UCD)
usability dimension, 578f
usability evaluation for, *see* Usability evaluation
utility, 640–642
  for P300 speller, 641–642
visual paradigms, 502–503
for VR/AR, *see* Virtual and augmented reality
  (VR/AR)
Brain–computer music interface (BCMI), 193–202
affective, 147, 155–157, 198
BCI and music, overview, 194–196
challenges, 193
future, 201–202
generic, 195, 196f
historical approaches, 196–199
hybrid, 195
hybrid systems and affective state control, 199–201
overview, 193–194
BrainGate trial, 656, 659
BRAIN Initiative Public-Private Partnership Program, 309
BrainInterchange system, German, 310–311, 312f
Brain–machine interfaces, *see* Neural interfaces (NIs)
Brain painting (BP), 517, 588
task, 568, 569
BrainPong, 693
BRAIN project, 470
Brain rhythms, amplitude modulations of, 351–353, 363
Brain signal patterns, 13–14, 22–25
overview, 22, 23f, 24f
P300 ERPs, 22
SCPs, 25
SMRs, 24–25
SSEPs, 22–24
Brain signals, fusion of, 696–697
Brain–spine interface, 711
Brain switch, P300-and-SSVEP–based, 529–530, 530f

Brainwave patterns, categories of, 17
Broadband gamma activity, ECoG, 299–300
Butterworth filter, 272

**C**

C++, 327, 331, 332
Calibration
  CSP analysis, feature extraction, 366
  free decoding and model adaptation, 437, 438f
  single-trial EEG, 349, 350f
Calibration phase, ERP-based BCIs, 596
Canonical correlation
  analysis (CCA), 363, 366, 374, 375–377, 392–393, 403,
    404, 532
  classifying SSVEP signals, 374, 375–377
Cardiac pacemaker implantations, 293
Cartan mean, 382
Case study, aBCMI, 156–158
CAVE-based VR, 224, 239, 241
Centroids, defined, 353
Centromedian-parafascicular (Cm-Pf) complex, 306
Cerebral palsy, 225, 226
CertiViBE, 331
Challenges
  MRCP-based associative BCIs, 679–680
  multi-mind BCIs, 690
  neuroprosthetics, 122t
Chance level
  for classified data, BCI experiments, 620–622
  defined, 621
Chart, defined, 378
Checkerboard paradigm (CBP), 505, 505f–506f
Children
  monitoring vigilance, during entertainment and
    learning, 181–182
    application example, 186, 187f
    data analysis, 184
    experimental protocol, 182–184
    overview, 181–182
    preprocessing, 184
    results, 185
    study population, 182
Chronic pain, treatment, 116
Classical conditioning, neuroplasticity and, 101
Classification
  accuracy, improving, applying neuroscience, 59–61
  BCI systems, 13–15, 14f
  boosting, 155
  competitive toy car racing using motor imagery BCI, 174
  four-class P300 oddball, 401–402
  MI BCI training algorithms, 454–455, 455f, 456
  *n*-class SSVEP, 404–405
  problems, MTL in, 435–437
  Riemannian, feature space approach, 428–429
  Riemannian, for SSVEP-based BCI, *see* Riemannian
    classification, for SSVEP-based BCI
  single-trial EEG; *see also* Single-trial EEG analysis
    discriminative features of brain activity, signal and
      noise, 349–353
    LDA, remark on assumptions of, 359–361
    linear classification, 353–362
    multivariate approach to, 347–349, 350f
    other methods, 362

Classifier-based latency estimation (CBLE), 644
Classifier(s), 600
    adaptive, 601–602
    ANNs, 32–33
    for ECoG-based BCIs, 33–34
    for EEG-based BCIs, 33–34
    HMM, 33–34
    linear, 30–32
    MDM, 384–386
    selection, BCI experiments, 619–620
    single trials of EEG data into, 362
    training, 401
ClinicalTrials.gov, 309, 310
Closed-loop adaptation, 77–79
    examples from literature, 77–79
    overview, 77
    reflection, 79
Closed-loop DBS system, 306
Closed task, 568, 569, 570t
Cochlear implants, 118, 709
Codebook, PBP
    development of, 493–494
    error-correcting capacity, 491
    minimum Hamming distance, 491
    pseudo-code for design, 494
Coding theory, 489
Cognition, neuroprosthetics, 120–122
Cognitive augmentation, 516
Cognitive efforts, BCI, 15
Cognitive neural prosthesis, 702
Cognitive rehabilitation task, 568
Cohen's κ coefficient, 637, 638
Coherence spectrum, magnitude squared, 272,
    274–275
Collaborative BCIs, 686, 690, 692, 694
Collaborative music generation, 200
Collective brain, implementing, 688–689
Coma, 90–95, 97t
Commercial algorithms use, in BCI experiments, 622
Commercial high-level platforms, BCI software platforms
    using, 327–330
    LabVIEW, 329–330
    MATLAB®, 327–328
    SIMULINK, 329
Common average reference (CAR) methods, 26, 28
Common sparse spectral spatial pattern (CSSSP), 29
Common spatial patterns (CSP), 3, 349, 446, 455, 455f,
    456, 532, 534
    analysis, feature extraction, 363–366
    changes of, 96, 97f
    data-dependent spatial filtering, 28, 29–30, 60
    for feature extraction, 453–454, 454f
    feature extraction and classification, 174
    formalization, as two-step procedure, 366–367
    regularized CSP, 429–431, 439
    for SMR feature extraction, 418
Common spatio-spectral pattern (CSSP), 29
Communication
    assessment, 89–90, 90–95, 97t
    information, 170
    multi-mind BCIs, application, 691
Communication applications
    aBCIs, use, 156
    ECoG BCIs for, 304–304

ERD/ERS-based BCIs, 38
P300-based BCIs, 34–36
SSVEP-based BCIs, 36
Competitive BCIs, 686, 690
Competitive toy car racing using motor imagery BCI,
    171–176
    application example, 175–176
    cue-based measurement, 173, 175t
    data analysis, 174
    evaluation, 174
    experimental protocol, 172–173
    feature extraction and classification, 174
    overview, 171
    preprocessing, 174
    results, 174–175
    self-paced measurements, 173, 175t
    study population, 171–172
Competitive video game, 693
Complementary metal-oxide semiconductor (CMOS)
    circuits, 123
Complete LIS (CLIS) patients, 90–95, 97t
Complex devices, control of, 691
Components, 597
    long-term user, 598
    short-term user, 598
Computational biology, 33
Computer-oriented systems, BCMI, 197
Conditioning of units, examples of, 289–292
Conductive gel, 167–168
Conductor, adaptive BCI systems, 600
Confounds, minimizing, 617–618
Confusion matrix, 638
Consciousness, assessment, 89–90, 90–95, 97t
Considerations
    four-class P300 oddball, 402
    n-class SSVEP, 405
Contingent negative variation (CNV), 671–672
Continuous BCI, 644–646
    Fitts's law, 645–646
    Shannon's theory, 645
    Shannon–Welford model, 646
Continuous tools, affective state reporting, 150–151
Control; see also specific applications
    of entertainment and multimedia
        games, see Games
        mediating interaction in VR/AR, see Virtual and
            augmented reality (VR/AR)
    of external devices, 691–692
Control applications
    aBCIs, use, 156
    ECoG BCIs, 303–304
    ERD/ERS-based BCIs, 38–39
    P300-based BCIs, 36
    SSVEP-based BCIs, 36–38
    VR-BCIs for, 238–242
Control interface (CI), 637, 637f
Control task, 569
Convenient EEG electrodes, 167–168
Conventional music therapy, 201
Cooperative video game, 693
CorTec, 310–311, 312f
Cortical excitability and excitation, 302
Cortical excitation, 299
Cortically coupled computing, 468

Cortical microcircuits, 711
Cortical multielectrode implants, in monkeys, 710
Cortical plasticity, 678, 679
cortiQ, 334
Cost(s)
    BCI device, 722
    of MATLAB, 327
Counteracting, 361
Counterbalancing, 626–627
Covariance estimators, evaluation of, 390, 391f
Covariance matrices, 355, 356f, 357, 372–373
    assumptions of LDA, 360–361
    defined, 380
    determinant, 383
    distances and means, 382–384
    estimation of, 380–382
    LDA with shrinkage of, 361
    MDM, 384–386
    Riemannian geometry, 378–380
Covariate Shift minimization, 601
Covert attention, 551
Craniux, 329–330
Cross-correlation analysis, 286
Cross-validation (CV), 409, 620, 620n
Crowding effect, BCI paradigms design and, 509
CSP, *see* Common spatial patterns (CSP)
Cue-based measurement, 173, 175t
Cue-based MRCP, 672
Cues in reactive BCIs, haptic, 257–260
    ERP-based BCIs, 258–259
    other paradigms, 260
    overview, 257
    SSSEP-based BCIs, 258–259
Current matrix, defined, 385
Current source density (CSD), 299
Curse of dimensionality, 408
Curve direction criterion, 389, 390
Customization
    SSVEP-based BCI applications, *see* SSVEP-based BCI
        applications
    SSVEP parameters, 135–138
        number of classes, 136–137, 138t
        overview, 135
        stimulation frequencies, 136–137, 138t
        time windows, 137, 138, 139f, 139t, 140f
Cutaneous sensing, 254, 255f
Cybathlon 2016, 693
Cyborg-turtle, BCI-controlled, 244

**D**

Data, utilizing subdermal electrodes
    acquisition, 272
    preprocessing, 272
Data acquisition, 526
Data analysis
    brain and body sonification, juggling performance, 179
    competitive toy car racing using motor imagery BCI,
        174
    monitoring, in children during entertainment and
        learning, 184
Data collection
    four-class P300 oddball, 398
    $n$-class SSVEP, 403

Data-dependent spatial filtering, 28–30
    CSP, 29–30
    ICA, 28, 29
    PCA, 28
Data description
    ERP data set, 415–416
    SMR data set, 418
Data Fusion Module, 474
Data likelihood, defined, 432
Data preprocessing
    four-class P300 oddball, 398–399
    $n$-class SSVEP, 404
Data processing
    BCI experiments, design guidelines, 619
        chance level for classified data, 620–622
        classifier selection, 619–620
        commercial algorithms use, 622
        multiple comparisons correction, 623–624
        neurophysiological markers, relevance of, 622–623
        training data set separation from testing data set,
            620
    practical BCI solutions, 170
Data scarcity and predicted accuracy, discrete BCI,
        642–644
    classifier-based latency estimation, 644
    projected accuracy metric, 643–644
Data segmentation
    four-class P300 oddball, 399–400
    $n$-class SSVEP, 404–405
Data set
    ERP, Bayesian learning, 415–417
        data description, 415–416
        performance evaluation, 416
        results, 416–417
    SMR, Bayesian learning, 418–419
        data description, 418
        performance evaluation, 418
        results, 419
    SSVEP, experimental evaluation on, 390–393
        covariance estimators, evaluation of, 390, 391f
        description, 390
        offline classification of SSVEP, 392
        online classification of SSVEP, 392–393
Decisional privacy, 655t, 656
Decision making, multi-mind BCIs, 693–694
Decision methods, adaptive, 602
Decision module, single-user BCI, 688
Decoders, defined, 705
Decoding
    calibration-free, 437, 438f
    neural signals, 705–708
Deep brain stimulation (DBS), 116
    clinical value of, 306
    closed-loop DBS system, 306
    electrode, implantation, 305–306
    neural correlates of, 307
    open-loop DBS system, 306
Delta brainwaves, 17
Demographic information, 567, 568
Deoxygenated blood (deoxy-Hb), 20
Depression, 102
Design guidelines, BCI experiments, 613–629
    acquisition of signals
        differential amplification, 616–617

mental states, 618–619
    muscular activity interference with EEG activity,
        control of, 617–618, 617f
    sensor type, location, number selection, 615–616
data processing, 619
    chance level for classified data, 620–622
    classifier selection, 619–620
    commercial algorithms use, 622
    multiple comparisons correction, 623–624
    neurophysiological markers, relevance of, 622–623
    training data set separation from testing data set,
        620
key points, 628t–629t
overview, 613–614
user component
    biases, avoidance of, 626–627
    good control group, 625–626
    state of mind in new BCI experiment, 624–625
    statistical tests selection, 627, 628t, 629
Designs; see also Design guidelines
    GUI, 138, 139, 140–141
    neurotrophic electrode, 280, 281f–282f
    SSVEP-based BCI applications, see SSVEP-based BCI
        applications
    training protocol, 211
Detectability index, 491
Detection
    affective state, 151–155
    MRCP
        during gait, 676–677
        during motor tasks and imagery, 675–676
Diagonal loading, defined, 430
Differential amplification, 616
Dimensionality reduction in EEG, feature decomposition,
    437, 438–439
Direct current (DC) battery, 446
Directions for further research, ECoG, 312–314
Discrete BCI, 637–644
    BCI utility, 640–642
        for P300 speller, 641–642
    binary classification accuracy vs. task accuracy,
        637–639
        binomial models for accuracy, 638–639, 639f
        confusion matrix, 638
    data scarcity and predicted accuracy, 642–644
        classifier-based latency estimation, 644
        projected accuracy metric, 643–644
    information gain, 639–640
        information transfer rate (ITR), 639–640
        rate of information gain (RIG$_B$), 640
Discrete tools, affective state reporting, 149–150
Discriminant analysis
    Bayesian learning, 413–414
    LDA, see Linear discriminant analysis (LDA)
Discriminative features of brain activity, 349–353
    amplitude modulations of brain rhythms, 351–353
    ERPs, modulations of, 350–351
    overview, 349, 350
Disorder of consciousness (DOC), 537
    patients with, 89–90, 90–95, 97t
Distances, SPD matrices, 382–384
Divergences, SPD matrices, 382–384
Dorsal premotor cortex (PMd), 551
Double blindness, 626–627

Dry (dry-contact) electrodes, EEG systems with, 166, 167,
    168
Dwell time, 76, 466, 466n
Dynamic stopping (DS) algorithm, 490
    Bayesian, 490–491
Dystonia, 116, 305, 306f

E

ECM, see Extended confusion matrix (ECM)
EEG- and -EMG–based BCIs, 539
EEG- and -EOG–based BCIs, 539–540
EEG-based BCIs, 526
EEG features, adaptive BCI systems, 600
EEGlab MATLAB toolbox, 327, 451, 456
    "event" variable, 451–452
    "latency" variable, 451, 452
    "position" variable, 451, 452
    "type" variable, 451, 452
EEGs, see Electroencephalograms (EEGs)
EEG signal, key factors, 508, 509t
Effectiveness, 578, 589
Efferent NIs, 702, 705, 709
Efficiency (Eff.), 469, 470, 578, 589
    BCI paradigms and, 512–513
EFRPs, see Eye fixation-related potentials (EFRPs)
Eigenvalue decomposition (EVD), 357, 366–367
Eigenvalue problem, 31, 364–365
Elderly people, SSVEP-based BCI applications for, see
    SSVEP-based BCI applications
Electrical stimulation, transcranial, 711
Electrocorticography (ECoG), 15, 21–22, 33–34, 295–312,
    526
    bidirectional NI, implementation, 702, 703f
    current ECoG-based BCIs, 303–309
        for communication, 304–305
        for control, 303–304
        for neuromodulation, 305–308
    current implantable devices, 309–312
    ECoG-based sensory NI, 711
    electrodes, 276, 707
    epidural, 314
    in epileptic patients, 704
    implants, 710
    invasive approach, 703
    motor NIs, 708
    neural sources of, 704, 705f
    overview, 297–298
    potential advantages, 705
    questions and directions for further research, 312–314
    recordings, neural signals, 270
    signal acquisition, 298–299
    signal physiology, 299–303
    subdural, 314
Electrode(s)
    activation of, 616–617
    DBS, 305–306
    dry (dry-contact), 166, 167, 168
    ECoG, 21, 301, 707
    EEG, 17–19, 57, 165–166
    intracortical, 303
    micro-ECoG, 313, 314
    neurotrophic, validation of, see Neurotrophic
        electrode, validation of

silver/silver chloride (Ag/AgCl), 167, 168, 169
subcortically implanted, 306
subcutaneous, 271
subdermal, utilizing, *see* Subdermal electrodes, utilizing
subgaleal, 270
surface, 271
Electrode-tissue impedance (ETI) signals, with EEG, 168
Electroencephalograms (EEGs), 446, 461
 acquisition device, 472
 in *h*BCI, *see* hybrid brain–computer interface (*h*BCI)
 MI data recording, 446, 447f
 in rapid serial visual presentation, 468
 SSVEP, 465–466
Electroencephalography (EEG), 526, 597
 aBCIs for, 151–152, 153t–154t
 action potential, 16
 actuation/information communication, 170
 analysis, Bayesian learning for, *see* Bayesian learning, for EEG analysis
 for art and entertainment, 166–167
 BCI research articles, 19
 brain and body sonification, juggling performance, 177, 179, 180–181
 changes in, 104
 classifiers, 33–34
 concept, 2
 data, in BCMI, 197
 data processing, 170
 dimensionality reduction in, 437, 438–439
 dry (dry-contact) electrodes, 166, 167, 168
 electrodes, 17–19, 57
  convenient, 167–168
 ETI signals with, 168
 features, 2
 forward modeling process, 57–58, 64
 headsets, 169–170
 hyperscanning results, 687
 low frequency band of, 676
 monitoring, subdermal electrodes, *see* Subdermal electrodes
 musification, 198
 neurophysiological origin of, 16
 noninvasive method, 15, 16–19
 nonstationarities of, 408
 potential advantages, 705
 power spectrum, motion artifacts and, 179
 recordings, neural activity and, 57
 signal amplitude, 3
 for single-trial EEG analysis, *see* Single-trial EEG analysis
 SSVEPs in, 193, 194, 197, 198f, 199
 time window for, 137
 wearable and wireless system, 188
Electromyography (EMG), 617
 electrodes, placement, 270
 recordings
  hand and forearm muscles, 708
  spinal motoneurons and, 703
Electronic design, practical BCI solutions, 168–169
Electrooculography (EOG), 617
Eligibility criteria, usability evaluation, 565
Emotional reactivity, fMRI detection of, 107

Emotions, 72
 perceived and induced, 200
 state, improving, 201
Emotiv algorithm, 622
Emotiv EPOC, 568, 573
Endogenous NIs, 703
End-stage retinitis pigmentosa, 118
Engineering Village, 566
Enhanced motor imagery training, 102, 103
Ensemble activity, 9 years after implantation, 286–289
Entertainment
 aBCIs, use, 156
 control of
  games, *see* Games
  mediating interaction in VR/AR, *see* Virtual and augmented reality (VR/AR)
 EEG for, 166–167
 ERD/ERS-based BCI controls, 38–39
 monitoring vigilance in children during, 181–186
  application example, 186, 187f
  data analysis, 184
  experimental protocol, 182–184
  overview, 181–182
  preprocessing, 184
  results, 185
  study population, 182
 P300-based BCI controls, 36
 practical BCI solutions for, *see* Practical BCI solutions
 SSVEP-based BCI controls, 36–38
Environment, MI data recording in MI BCI training session, 447, 451
Environment characteristics, usability evaluation and, 567, 567t, 571–573, 571t
EOG/EMG artifacts, 617, 617f
EOG/EMG confounds, 618
Epidural ECoG, 314
Epilepsy, 106, 116, 305, 306f, 307, 312, 704
Epochs, defined, 347, 374
ERD/ERS, *see* Event-related desynchronization/synchronization (ERD/ERS)
ERP-based BCIs, 488–489, 573
 application phase, 596
 calibration phase, 596
 training phase, 596
ERPs, *see* Event-related responses (ERPs)
Error-correcting capacity, 491
Error-related negativity (ERN), 75, 76
Essential tremor (ET), 116, 306
Ethics, in BCI research, 653–664; *see also* Privacy, and BCI
Euclidean Riemannian distance, 392
European Space Agency, 126
Evaluation; *see also* Performance measurement
 competitive toy car racing using motor imagery BCI, 174
 experimental, on SSVEP data set, 390–393
  covariance estimators, evaluation of, 390, 391f
  description, 390
 role of, 589; *see also* Usability evaluation
Event-related desynchronization/synchronization (ERD/ERS), 15, 24–25, 38–39, 169, 297, 363, 526
 of somatosensory rhythm (SMR), 452–453, 452f
Event-related potentials (ERPs), 2, 487, 488, 526, 568, 596
 aBCI systems, feature, 151–152, 152t, 155
 active multi-mind BCIs, 687

AEP approach and, 91, 92f
attention-based BCIs and, 553–554
data set, Bayesian learning, 415–417
    data description, 415–416
    performance evaluation, 416
    results, 416–417
ECoG signals, 299
EP BCIs, *see* Evoked potential (EP) BCIs
ERP-based guilty knowledge tests, 74
guideline for transient activity, 362
modulations of, 350–351
morphology, by affective and cognitive processes, 73
non–phase-locked activity in, 360
P300, 14, 22, 34–36, 54, 134, 255, 408; *see also* Four-class P300 oddball
reactive BCIs, 255
tactile ERP-based reactive BCIs, 258–259
transient response, 373
Event-related responses (ERPs), 462
"Event" variable, EEGlab, 451–452
Evidence method, 413
Evoked potential (EP) BCIs, signal processing for, 397–405
    four-class P300 oddball, 398–402
      classification, 401–402
      classifier training, 401
      considerations, 402
      data collection, 398
      data preprocessing, 398–399
      data segmentation and feature extraction, 399–400
      overview, 398
    *n*-class SSVEP, 402–405
      considerations, 405
      data collection, 403
      data preprocessing, 404
      data segmentation and classification, 404–405
      overview, 402–403
    overview, 397–398
Evolution, BCIs, 1–6
    modern history, 4
    origins, 2
    overview, 1
    pioneers, 2–3
    research field, bloom of, 3–4
Evolutionary neurobiology, BCI and, 114–115
Excitability and excitation, cortical, 302
Exocortical cognition (ECC), 125
Exogenous NIs, 703
Experimental complexity, BCI software, 325
Experimental evaluation, on SSVEP data set, 390–393
    covariance estimators, evaluation of, 390, 391f
    description, 390
    offline classification of SSVEP, 392
    online classification of SSVEP, 392–393
Experimental paradigm, MI data recording in MI BCI training session, 447–448, 448f, 448t, 451
    design, 447–448, 448f
    procedure, 448t
    six types of noise data, 447
Experimental protocols
    brain and body sonification, juggling performance, 177–179
    competitive toy car racing using motor imagery BCI, 172–173

*h*BCI, 475–476
    monitoring, in children during entertainment and learning, 182–184
Experimental study, Bayesian learning, 415–419
    ERP data set, 415–417
      data description, 415–416
      performance evaluation, 416
      results, 416–417
    SMR data set, 418–419
      data description, 418
      performance evaluation, 418
      results, 419
Experimental validation, VR/AR, 246
Explicit input, 75
Exploration, VR-BCIs for, 238–242
Exponential mapping, defined, 379–380
Extended confusion matrix (ECM), 638
Extensible file format (XDF), 244
External devices, control of, 691–692
Eye blinking, 27
Eye fixation-related potentials (EFRPs), 467
    ET with, 468
Eye gaze technology
    cortically coupled computing, 468
    *h*BCI with, 466–469, 467f
    Midas Touch problem, 468, 470
    and SSVEP *h*BCI, 469
      architecture, 472–475, 473f, 474t
      ET component, 470, 471, 471f
      ET inclusion, 469–470
      experimental protocol, 475–476
      postprocessing, 476–477, 476f–478f
      SSVEP BCI component, 472
      visual interface application design, 470, 471f
Eye Tracker signal, 466
Eye tracking (ET), 464, 466; *see also* Eye gaze technology
    as complementary technology, 470
    devices, 135
    with EFRPs, 468
    with SSVEP, 468–469
    system, 305
    use of, 467–468, 467f
    using EyeTribe, 469
    zones, 470–471, 471f
EyeTribe, 469

**F**

Fast Fourier transform (FFT), 272
FastICA, 29
Fatigue, BCI paradigms design and, 511–512
Fault detection, 33
Fault tolerance, MLP, 32
Feature classification methods, 30–34
    ANNs, 32–33
      MLP, 32–33
      other architectures, 33
    HMM classifiers, 33–34
    linear classifiers, 30–32
      LDA, 31
      overview, 30
      SVM, 31–32
Feature decomposition, dimensionality reduction in EEG, 437, 438–439

Feature extraction, 13, 25–30, 526
  adaptive, 601
  competitive toy car racing using motor imagery BCI, 174
  defined, 353
  four-class P300 oddball, 399–400
  MI BCI training algorithm, 453–454, 454f, 456
  overview, 25
  removing noisy signals and artifacts, 25–26
  single-trial EEG analysis, 362–366; *see also* Single-trial EEG analysis
    CCA, 366
    CSP analysis, 363–366
    guideline for transient activity, ERP and LRP, 362
    oscillatory brain activity, guideline for, 362–363
    overview, 362
  spatial filtering methods, 26–30
    bipolar reference, 26, 27
    CAR, 26, 28
    CSP, 29–30
    data-dependent, 28–30
    ICA, 28, 29
    PCA, 28
    referencing methods, 26–28
    surface Laplacian reference, 26, 27
  SSVEP, 30
Feature extraction module, single-user BCI, 688
Feature space approaches, 427–431
  nonlinear representations, 428
  overview, 427
  regularized CSP, 429–431
  Riemannian classification, 428–429
Feature vector, defined, 347, 353
Federal Drug Administration, 295
Feedback (FB), 568, 571
  BCI/NF studies using games as, 211–212, 213t–223t
  designs, need for, 210–211
  game-like, potential value of using, 212, 224–227
    attract users' attention and reduce mind wandering, 224–225
    flow, immersion, and presence, 224
    increasing BCI/NF performance, 227
    intuitive feedback and interactions, 225–226
    mirror neuron system, activating, 226
    motivation and interest, 212, 224
    real-world behavior, transfer to, 226–227
  haptic, in active BCIs, 256–257
  machine output of adaptive BCI systems, 606
  types of, 606
  vibrotactile, 257
FEELTRACE tool, 150, 151f, 156, 157
Felt affect, 149
Fidelity, VR/AR, 236, 237
FieldTrip, 327
Filter bank canonical correlation analysis (FBCCA), 376, 392–393
Filter bank CSP (FBCSP), 418, 419
Finite impulse response neural network (FIRNN), 33
Fisher linear discriminant (FLD), 526
Fisher's linear discriminant analysis (FLDA), 408–409, 446, 454–455
  for feature extraction, 453–454, 454f
  SVM and, 456
Fitts's law, 645–646

FLDA, *see* Fisher's linear discriminant analysis (FLDA)
Flow, defined, 224
Fludeoxyglucose, 21
Food and Drug Administration (FDA), 299
Force, MRCP during sensorimotor behavior, 674
Formalization, of CSP as two-step procedure, 366–367
Forward modeling process, EEG, 57–58, 64
Four-class P300 oddball, 398–402
  classification, 401–402
  classifier training, 401
  considerations, 402
  data collection, 398
  data preprocessing, 398–399
  data segmentation and feature extraction, 399–400
  overview, 398
Fourier transform, 465–466
Frame-based stimulus approximation method, 136
Framework
  adaptive BCI systems, 599–600, 599f
    conductor, 600, 606–607
    feedback, 606
    instructions and stimuli, 606
    literature review on adaptive signal processing/machine learning, 601–602
    machine output, 606
    system pipeline, 600–602, 600f
    task model, 603, 603f, 605
    user model, 603–604, 603f, 604t
  usability, 566–569, 566f, 567t
Frechet mean, 382
Free-Floating Wireless Neural Interface Wireless Implantable Neural Recording (FF-WINeR), 123
Frequency band power changes, low- and high-, 273–274
Frequency bands, personalized, 184, 185
Frobenius distance, 429
Frobenius inner product, 382
Frontal–parietal theta–alpha asymmetry, in EEG activity, 73
Fugl–Meyer Assessment, 243
Fugl-Meyer Motor Assessment (FMMA) score, 542
Fully adaptive signal processing, 602
Functional complexity, BCI software, 325
Functional electrical stimulation (FES), 708
Functional electrical stimulator (FES), 95–96, 97
Functionality, 9 years of implantation, neurotrophic electrode, 289–292
Functional magnetic resonance imaging (fMRI), 54, 526, 657
  aBCIs for, 151
  BCMI and, 201–202
  detection of emotional reactivity, 107
  discriminative activity in separate cortical areas, 74
  NIs, 705
  overview, 15, 20
Functional mapping system, 334
Functional near-infrared spectroscopy (fNIRS), 620
  aBCIs, 151
  learning speed using, 78
  for neurorehabilitation, 242
  NIs, 705
  overview, 15, 20–21
Fusion, of brain signals, 696–697
Fuzzy ARTMAP neural network, 33

## G

Gait, MRCP detection during, 676–677
Games, 210–228
  BCI/NF studies using games as feedback, 211–212, 213t–223t
  drawbacks, lack of evaluation of effects, 227–228
  new feedback designs, need for, 210–211
  overview, 210
  P300-based BCI controls, 36
  potential value of using game-like FB, 212, 224–227
    attract users' attention and reduce mind wandering, 224–225
    flow, immersion, and presence, 224
    increasing BCI /NF performance, 227
    intuitive feedback and interactions, 225–226
    mirror neuron system, activating, 226
    motivation and interest, 212, 224
    real-world behavior, transfer to, 226–227
  SSVEP-based BCI controls, 38
Game task, 568
Gamma dynamic neural network (GDNN), 33
Gartner 2016 Hype Cycle, "Innovation Trigger" phase, 464
Gaussian distributions
  charactcristics, 355
  related transformations and, 356–359
Gaussian kernel, in BCI research, 32
Gaze-based HCI, 76
Gaze shifting period, 140
g.BCIsys, 327, 329
Generalizability, MLP, 32
Generic BCMI, 195, 196f
Geneva Emotional Music Scale (GEMS), 149, 150
Geodesic curve, defined, 378
Geodesics, defined, 384
Geometric mean, 382
GigaDB, 446
Glabrous skin, 254, 255f
g.MOBIlab, 568
GNU Affero General Public License, 331
GNU Octave software, 327
GO/NO-GO paradigm, 182
Good control group, for BCI experiments, 625–626
Graphical user interface (GUI), 528
  design of, 135, 138, 139, 140–141
  of hybrid BCI combining MI and P300 potentials, 532–533, 533f
  Tic-Tac-Toe, 226
Ground electrode, 17
gTec MobiLab Amp, 390
GTRACE tool, 150
GugerTec, 272
Guilty knowledge tests, ERP-based, 74
g.USBamp, 568, 573
Gwangju Institute of Science and Technology (GIST), 446, 447

## H

Hairy skin, 254, 255f
Hand movement, imagining, 305
Haptics, BCI and, 253–261
  cues in reactive BCIs, 257–260
    ERP-based BCIs, 258–259
    other paradigms, 260

    overview, 257
    SSSEP-based BCIs, 259–260
  cutaneous/tactile sensing, 254, 255f
  feedback in active BCIs, 256–257
  overview, 253–256
  potential, for HCI and BCI, 254, 255–256
  recommendations, 261
Hardware capacity, BCI paradigms design and, 512
Harmonic sum decision (HSD), 531
HCI, *see* Human–computer interaction (HCI)
Head-mounted displays (HMDs), 237, 239, 240, 241, 244
Headsets, EEG, 169–170
Hebbian plasticity, 105
Hebb's theorem, 670
Hex-o-Spell, 258
Hidden Markov model (HMM) classifiers, 33–34
Hilbert transform, 352, 466
Histograms, interspike interval, 283, 286, 287f
Historical approaches, BCMI, 196–199
History, multi-mind BCIs, 687–688
*Homo neanderthalensis*, 114
Human–computer interaction (HCI), 461, 564, 645
  BCI and, potential of haptics, 254, 255–256
  gaze-based HCI, 76
  open-loop adaptation, 75, 76
  response and machine errors, 70
Human cortex, long-term recordings, *see* Neurotrophic electrode, validation of
Human factors and ergonomics (HFE), 579
Human learning, 598–599
Human–machine interaction
  ERD/ERS-based BCI controls, 38–39
  P300-based BCI controls, 36
  SSVEP-based BCI controls, 36–38
Hybrid BCMI, 195, 199–201
*hybrid* brain–computer interface (*h*BCI), 94, 236, 240, 573, 686, 694; *see also* Multimodal BCIs
  advantages, 463
  architecture, 469–470
  based on multibrain patterns, 527, 527f, 528–535
    MI- and -P300–based BCIs, 532–535
    MI- and -SSVEP–based BCIs, 531–532
    P300- and -SSVEP–based BCIs, 528–530
  based on multiple signals, 527f, 528, 538–540, 538t
    EEG- and -EMG–based BCIs, 539
    EEG- and -EOG–based BCIs, 539–540
  classes of, 527–528, 527f; *see also specific classes*
  concepts for ET inclusion into, 469–470
  dataflow, 473f
  definitions, 463, 463f
  with eye gaze, 466–469, 467f
  eye gaze and SSVEP, 469
    architecture, 472–475, 473f, 474t
    ET component, 470, 471, 471f
    ET inclusion, 469–470
    experimental protocol, 475–476
    postprocessing, 476–477, 476f–478f
    SSVEP BCI component, 472
    visual interface application design, 470, 471f
  factors, 464
  on multiple intelligent techniques, 527f, 528, 541–543

intelligent wheelchair based on BCI and
        autonomous navigation system, 541–542, 541f
    rehabilitative system based on BCI and intelligent
        robot, 542–543
multisensory hybrid BCIs, 527, 527f, 535–538
    audio -tactile P300 BCIs, 537–538, 537f
    audio -visual P300 BCIs, 535–537, 536f
    overview, 463–464, 527
    signal processing, 527
    SSVEP, 465–466
    system components, 469–470, 478f, 527
    vs. BCI system, 527
Hybrid SSVEP–P300 paradigm, 513–516, 514f, 515f;
        see also P300 paradigms; SSVEP paradigms
Hyperkinetic disorder, TS, see Tourette syndrome (TS)
Hyperscanning technique, 686, 687
Hypertension, 116
Hypokinetic disorder, PD, see Parkinson's disease (PD)

I

ICA, see Independent component analysis (ICA)
IEEE Xplore, 566
Illiteracy phenomenon, BCI, 210, 228
Imagery, motor, MRCP during, 674–676
ImageryHands condition, 180
Imagination of tongue/hand movement, ECoG studies, 305
IMEC, 167, 168, 169, 170, 172, 180, 186
Immersion
    game-like environments, 224
    VR/AR, context of, 236, 239
Impedance
    measurements in humans, 281f–282f, 283
    tests of, 280
Implantable devices, ECoG, 309–312
Implantation
    acute intraoperative ECoG strips, 306
    DBS electrode, 305–306
    neurotrophic electrode
        cardiac pacemaker, 293
        discussion, 292–293
        four years after, 283–285
        functionality, 9 years of implantation, 289–292
        nine years after, 286–289
Implementation, BCI software, 325–335
    platforms using commercial high-level platforms,
        327–330
        LabVIEW, 329–330
        MATLAB®, 325, 326–327, 327–328
        overview, 325–327
        SIMULINK, 329
    self-contained BCI software platforms, 330–335
        BCI2000, 327, 331, 332–335
        OpenViBE, 331, 332f, 335f
Implementation, online and offline, SSVEP-based BCI,
        373–374
Implicit dialogue, 79
Implicit input, 75
Independent component analysis (ICA), 28, 29, 60, 465
Index finger flexion and extension, 673
Index of performance (IP), 645
Individual alpha peak frequencies (IAF), 182, 184, 188
Induced emotions, 200
Inducing, plasticity, 669–680

MRCP and, see Movement-related cortical potentials
        (MRCPs)
    overview, 669–671
Informational privacy, 655, 655t
Information communication, 170
Information gain, 639–640
    information transfer rate (ITR), 639–640
    rate of information gain (RIG_B), 640
Information security, defined, 126
Information transfer rate (ITR), 376–377, 457–458, 462,
        466, 506, 526, 564, 639–640, 690
InfoSec, 126
Inquiry method, 568, 574t
Insomnia, 102
Inspection method, 568, 574t, 579
Institutional Review Board, 270, 295
Instructions, machine output of adaptive BCI systems, 606
Integration, of modern neuroscience, see Neuroscience
Intelligent neuroprosthesis, 125
Intelligent robot, rehabilitative system based on BCI and,
        542–543
Intelligent Tutoring Systems (ITS), 606
Intelligent wheelchair based on BCI and autonomous
        navigation system, 541–542, 541f
Interactions, intuitive, 225–226
Interaction technology, 11–39
    example BCI applications, 34–39
        ERD/ERS-based BCI application, 38–39
        P300-based BCIs, 34–36
        SSVEP-based BCIs, 36–38
    feature classification methods, 30–34
        ANNs, 32–33
        HMM classifiers, 33–34
        LDA, 31
        linear classifiers, 30–32
        MLP, 32–33
        SVM, 31–32
    overview, 12–15, 14f
    signal acquisition methods, 15–25, 16f
        brain signal patterns for BCI operation, 22–25
        ECoG, 15, 21–22
        EEG, 15, 16–19
        fMRI, 15, 20
        fNIRS, 15, 20–21
        INR, 15, 22
        invasive methods, 15, 21–22
        MEG, 15, 19
        noninvasive methods, 15, 16–21
        P300 ERPs, 22
        PET, 15, 21
        SCPs, 25
        SMRs, 24–25
        SSEPs, 22–24
    signal quality and feature extraction methods,
        improving, 25–30
        overview, 25
        removing noisy signals and artifacts, 25–26
        spatial filtering methods, 26–30
        SSVEP, 30
Interactivity, defined, 71
Interest, NF/BCI performance and, 212, 224
Interfaces, between user and VR/AR, 246
Internal context, 589
Internal model theory, body schema, 706

International Organization for Standardization (ISO), 587
10/20 International system of electrode placement, EEG, 18
Interspike interval histograms, 283, 286, 287f
Interstimulus interval (ISI), 536
Intertrial and interuser variability, aBCIs, 158
Intracortical electrodes, 303
Intracortical microstimulation, 117
Intracortical neuronal recording (INR), 15, 22
Intracortical stimulation (ICMS), 709, 710
Intracranial EEG, 15, 21–22
Intractable major depression, 116
Intuitive feedback and interactions, game-like FB,
    225–226
Invasive neuroprosthetics, noninvasive *vs.*, 126
Invasive NIs, 703
Invasive recording methods, 15, 21–22
    ECoG, 15, 21–22
    INR, 15, 22
    overview, 21
Inverse problems, defined, 19, 57
Investigational device exemption (IDE), FDA, 306, 309
Ischemic stroke, 116
ISO 9241, 469
ISO 9241–210, 586, 587

**J**

Jaw clenching, 27
Jigsaw puzzle, 226
Juggling performance, brain and body sonification,
    176–181
    application example, 180–181
    data analysis, 179
    experimental protocols, 177–179
    overview, 176–177
    preprocessing, 179
    results, 179–180
    study population, 177

**K**

Kalman filter tuning model, 706
Karcher mean, 382
Kernel trick, defined, 32
Keywords, for search engines, 565
Kinesthesis, defined, 254
Kullback–Leibler divergence (KLD), 493

**L**

LabRecoder, 244
Labstreaming Layer (LSL), 244–245
LabVIEW (Laboratory Virtual Instrument Engineering
    Workbench), 326, 327, 329–330
Latency and jitter of processing, VR/AR, 245–246
"Latency" variable, EEGlab, 451, 452
Lateralized readiness potential (LRP), guideline for
    transient activity, 362
Learnability, MLP, 32
Learning
    Bayesian, for EEG analysis, *see* Bayesian learning, for
        EEG analysis
    to control BCI/NF applications, 211
    model space, *see* Model space learning

monitoring vigilance in children during, 181–186
    application example, 186, 187f
    data analysis, 184
    experimental protocol, 182–184
    overview, 181–182
    preprocessing, 184
    results, 185
    study population, 182
NF/BCI, 227
transfer, *see* Transfer learning
Learning vector quantization (LVQ) neural network, 33
Least-squares regression (LSR)
    framework, 409
    LDA and LSR, equivalence between, 410–411
    maximum likelihood and regularized least squares,
        411–413
Leyden jar, use, 115
Lie detector, 74
Light-emitting diodes (LEDs), 23, 76, 168
Limitations, VR/AR in context of BCI, 246
Linear classification, single-trial EEG analysis, 353–362
    Gaussian distributions and related transformations,
        356–359
    LDA, 355–356
        remark on assumptions of, 359–361
        with shrinkage of covariance matrix, 361
    LDA to NCC, whitening, and mahalanobis distance,
        relation of, 359
    motivation, NCC, 353–354
    other methods, 362
    overview, 353
Linear classifiers, 30–32
    LDA, 31
    overview, 30
    SVM, 31–32
Linear decoders, optimal, 706
Linear discriminant analysis (LDA)
    BLDA, 409, 410, 414, 416–417
    classification, 534, 601
    classifier, 174, 309
    continuous decoding method, 708
    CSP filtering and, 170, 175
    from EMGs, 708–709
    FDA, 408–409
    feature classification method, 31
    LDA and LSR, equivalence between, 410–411
    linear classification, 353, 355–356
    NCC, whitening, and mahalanobis distance, relation
        of, 359
    remark on assumptions of, 359–361
    RFDA, 409
    with shrinkage of covariance matrix, 361
    simple binary classifier on, 401
    SKLDA, 409
    SWLDA, 409, 416–417
Literature, examples from
    automated adaptation, 80
    closed-loop adaptation, 77–79
    mental state assessment, 72–74
    open-loop adaptation, 75–76
Literature review
    of adaptive methods
        related to task model, 605
        related to user model, 604, 604t

on adaptive signal processing/machine learning,
    601–602
    adaptive classifiers, 601–602
    adaptive decision methods, 602
    adaptive feature extraction, 601
    fully adaptive signal processing, 602
Local field potentials (LFPs), 22, 307
Locality preserving projection (LPP), 676
Local motor potentials (LMPs), 303, 314
Location, 568
    selection, BCI experiments, 615–616
Locked-in syndrome (LIS), 89, 90, 97t, 257
Logarithmic mapping, 377, 379–380
Log-Euclidean distance, 384
Log-Euclidean kernels, 377
Log-Euclidean Riemannian distance, 392
Logistic sigmoid function, defined, 436
Long-term potentiation (LTP)
    defined, 670
    LTP-like plasticity, 670
    properties, 677
Long-term recordings in human cortex, *see* Neurotrophic
    electrode, validation of
Long-term robustness, 526
Long term variability, 597
"Löschen," command, 139
Low-frequency oscillations, ECoG, 300–302

## M

Machine learning, 598, 619
    for BCIs, 3, 54, 61, 193
    in conditioning approach, 347, 350f
    literature review, 601–602
    optimization of spatial filters in, 349, 350f
    Riemannian geometry, 377
Machine output, adaptive BCI systems, 606
    feedback, 606
    instructions and stimuli, 606
Macular degeneration, 118, 119
Magnetic resonance imaging (MRI), 19, 61
Magnetic stimulation, transcranial, 711
Magnetoencephalography (MEG), 15, 19, 105, 151, 526
    NIs, 705
Magnitude squared coherence, 272, 274–275
Mahalanobis distance and LDA, relation, 359
Manifold, Riemannian, 378
Man–machine adaptability, 526
Mann–Whitney *U* tests, 184
Mapping
    affective state, 200
    exponential, defined, 379–380
    logarithmic, 377, 379–380
    music, 194, 195–196, 199
    noninvasive signals to brain, 56–59
Masses, practical BCI solutions for, 166–167
Massively multiplayer online (MMO), 240
Materials, subdermal electrodes, 270–272
Mathematical notation, transfer learning, 427
MATLAB, 451, 453, 477, 621; *see also* EEGlab MATLAB
    toolbox
MATLAB® (MATrix LABoratory), 179, 244–245, 325,
    326–327, 327–328, 399–400
Matrix spellers, 691

Maximum likelihood estimation, 411–413
Maximum likelihood estimator (MLE), 381
Mean distance to Riemannian mean (MDRM) method,
    429
Means, Riemannian geometry, 382–384
Measurement characteristics, usability evaluation and,
    567t, 569, 575–578, 576t–577t, 578f
Mechanoreceptors, in human skin, 254, 255f
Mediating interaction, in VR/AR, *see* Virtual and
    augmented reality (VR/AR)
Meditation, 71
Meissner corpuscles, 254, 255f
Memory, neuroprosthetics, 120–122
Mental Imagery–based BCI (MI-BCI), 615
Mental privacy, 656–660
Mental state assessment, 72–74
    examples from literature, 72–74
    overview, 72
    reflection, 74
Mental states, BCI experiments, 618–619
Mental task, 568
Merkel receptors, 254, 255f
Method characteristics, usability evaluation and, 567t,
    568, 574t, 575
Methods
    neurotrophic electrode, validation of, 280,
        281f–282f
    utilizing subdermal electrodes, 270–272
Methyl methacrylate glue, 280, 281f
MI, *see* Motor imagery (MI)
MI-and-P300–based BCI mouse, 532–534, 533f
MI- and -P300–based BCIs, 532–535
    MI-and-P300–based BCI mouse, 532–534, 533f
    MI-and-P300–based wheelchair control, 534–535
MI-and-P300–based wheelchair control, 534–535
MI- and -SSVEP–based BCIs, 531–532
    MI-and-SSVEP–based MI training, 531–532
    MI-and-SSVEP–based orthosis control, 531
MI-and-SSVEP–based MI training, 531–532
MI-and-SSVEP–based orthosis control, 531
MI BCI, *see* Motor imagery (MI)–based brain–computer
    interface (BCI)
Micro-ECoG, 313, 314
Microelectrodes, polymer-based, 704
Microns, 280
Microscale BCIs, 122–124
Midas Touch problem, 468, 470
MI data recording, in MI BCI training session,
    446–451
    device and software, 446, 447f, 449
    discussions, 449, 451
    EEG channel labeling, 446, 447f
    environment, 447, 451
    experimental paradigm, 447–448, 448f, 448t, 451
    MI instructions, 449, 449f, 451
    questionnaire, 449, 450t, 451
    subjects, 447, 449, 451
MI instructions, 449, 449f, 451
Mil, 280, 292
mindBEAGLE system, 90–94
Mindfulness, defined, 224
Mind state, in new BCI experiment, 624–625
Mind wandering, 224–225
Minimally conscious state (MCS), 90–95, 97t

Minimum distance to mean (MDM)
  classifier, 384–386
  online, 386, 388–390
  for SSVEP, 386, 387f
Minimum distance to Riemannian mean (MDRM), 377–378
Minimum energy combination (MEC), 472
Minimum Hamming distance, codebook, 491
Minimum-norm estimate (MNE) approach, 58, 59
Mirror neuron system, activating, 226
Mixed National Institute of Standards and Technology
    (MNIST), 54, 55
(M,l)-code, 490
Mobile usability framework, 567
Modality, 568
Model space learning, 431–440
  calibration-free decoding and model adaptation, 437,
    438f
  dimensionality reduction in EEG, feature
    decomposition, 437, 438–439
  MTL in classification problems, 435–437
  MTL in regression problems, 434–435
  multitask linear regression, 434–435
  overview, 431–433
Mode of operation, for BCI, 15
Modern history, 4
Modulations
  amplitude, of brain rhythms, 351–353, 363
  ERPs, 350–351
Monitoring, children during entertainment and learning,
    181–186
  application example, 186, 187f
  data analysis, 184
  experimental protocol, 182–184
  overview, 181–182
  preprocessing, 184
  results, 185
  study population, 182
Monkeys
  cortical multielectrode implants in, 710
  ICMS patterns, 709, 710
  quadrupedal locomotion in, 711
Mood disorders, 116
Morlet wavelet coefficients, 708
Motivation
  NCC, 353–354
  NF/BCI performance and, 212, 224
Motor-based BCIs, noninvasive alternative for
  subdermal electrodes as, utilizing, see Subdermal
    electrodes, utilizing
Motor control and movement, nuroprosthetics, 116–117
Motor imagery (MI), 462, 468, 469, 526, 588, 596
  MRCP during, 674–676
Motor Imagery (MI) approach, mindBEAGLE system, 94
Motor imagery–based BCIs, 3, 15
  competitive toy car racing using, 171–176
    application example, 175–176
    cue-based measurement, 173, 175t
    data analysis, 174
    evaluation, 174
    experimental protocol, 172–173
    feature extraction and classification, 174
    overview, 171
    preprocessing, 174
    results, 174–175

    self-paced measurements, 173, 175t
    study population, 171–172
  MI BCIs, 94
  SMR BCI, 102, 105
Motor imagery (MI)–based brain–computer interface
    (BCI), 445–458, 596
  concept, 446
  information transfer rate (ITR), 457–458
  overview, 445–446
  testing session
    adaptive approaches, 457
    co-adaptive approaches, 457
    discussion, 457–458
    online experiment, 456–457, 457f
  training session
    algorithms and offline analysis, 451–456
    classification, 454–455, 455f, 456
    discussions, 449, 451, 456
    environment, 447, 451
    experimental paradigm, 447–448, 448f, 448t, 451
    feature extraction, 453–454, 454f, 456
    MI data recording, 446–451
    MI instructions, 449, 449f, 451
    preprocessing, 451–453, 452f, 456
    questionnaire, 449, 450t, 451
    recording device and software, 446, 447f, 449
    subjects, 447, 449, 451
Motor neural interfaces, 708–709
Motor potential (MP), 671, 673
Motor rehabilitation, BCI for, 89–90, 95–97, 97t
Mouse model
  brain-to-brain communications, 712
  motor cortex using bidirectional NI, 711
Movement, MRCP during sensorimotor behavior
  speed/velocity, 673–674
  type, 673
Movement control, 568, 569
Movement disorders, 116
Movement-related cortical potentials (MRCPs), 669–680
  characteristics, 675
  components, 670
  detection
    during gait, 676–677
    during motor tasks and imagery, 675–676
    during motor imagery, 674–675
  MRCP-based associative BCIs, 677–680
    overview, 677–678
    potential and challenges, 679–680
    type of neurofeedback, 678–679
  overview, 669–673
  during sensorimotor behavior, 673–674
    force, 674
    speed/velocity of movement, 673–674
    type of movement, 673
  signal-to-noise ratio, 675
Movement time (MT), 645
Mu, beta, and high gamma band power changes, 272
Mu band ERD, 24–25
Multi-Attribute Task Battery, 73
Multibrain patterns, hybrid BCIs based on, 527, 527f,
    528–535
  MI- and -P300–based BCIs, 532–535
    MI-and-P300–based BCI mouse, 532–534, 533f
    MI-and-P300–based wheelchair control, 534–535

MI- and -SSVEP–based BCIs, 531–532
  MI-and-SSVEP–based MI training, 531–532
  MI-and-SSVEP–based orthosis control, 531
  P300- and -SSVEP–based BCIs, 528–530
    P300-and-SSVEP–based BCI spellers, 528–529
    P300-and-SSVEP–based brain switch, 529–530,
      530f
Multidimension/function control, 526
Multielectrode NIs, 704
Multilayer perceptron (MLP), 32–33
Multimedia, control of
  games, see Games
  mediating interaction in VR/AR, see Virtual and
    augmented reality (VR/AR)
Multi-mind BCIs, 685–697
  applications, 690–695
    communication, 691
    control of external devices, 691–692
    music, 694–695
    target detection and decision making, 693–694
    video games, 692–693
  challenges, 690
  collective brain, implementing, 688–689
  future directions, 697
  history, 687–688
  influence of participant similarity, forming groups,
    689–690
  minds, need, 689
  overview, 685–687
  P300-based BCIs for, 691
  single-trial, 691
  theoretical aspects, 687–690
  tutorial, 695–697
    application, 695
    fusion of brain signals, 696–697
    number of users, 695–696
    operation mode, 696
    real-time requirement, 696
Multimodal BCIs, 527; see also hybrid brain–computer
    interface (hBCI)
Multimodal brain orchestra, 695
Multimodal stimuli, 571
Multiple comparisons, correction of, 623–624
Multiple intelligent techniques, hybrid BCIs based on,
    527f, 528, 541–543
  intelligent wheelchair based on BCI and autonomous
    navigation system, 541–542, 541f
  rehabilitative system based on BCI and intelligent
    robot, 542–543
Multiple signals, hybrid BCIs based on, 527f, 528,
    538–540, 538t
  EEG- and -EMG–based BCIs, 539
  EEG- and -EOG–based BCIs, 539–540
Multisensory hybrid BCIs, 527, 527f, 535–538
  audio -tactile P300 BCIs, 537–538, 537f
  audio -visual P300 BCIs, 535–537, 536f
Multisensory stimulation, 260
Multitask learning (MTL), 439
  approach, flow of using, 433
  Bayesian framework for, 432
  in classification problems, 435–437
  defined, 432
  in regression problems, 434–435
Multitask linear regression, 434–435

Multitask logistic regression, 437
Multi-unit activity (MUA), 22
Multivariate approach, to classification of single-trial
    EEG, 347–349, 350f
Multivariate features, single-trial EEG analysis, 346–347
Mu power, 226
Mu rhythm, 300
Music
  application of multi-mind BCIs, 694–695
  BCI and, overview, 194–196
  making, BCI for, see Brain–computer music interface
    (BCMI)
  therapy, aBCMI, 147, 155–157
Musification, of brainwave data, 197–198
Mutually oriented systems, BCMI, 197
Myoelectric interface, 708

N

Nanobiotechnology, 125
NASA Task Load Index (NASA-TLX), 575, 578
National Center for Adaptive Neurotechnologies, 331, 332
National Instruments, 329
N-class SSVEP, 402–405
  considerations, 405
  data collection, 403
  data preprocessing, 404
  data segmentation and classification, 404–405
  overview, 402–403
Nearest centroid classifier (NCC)
  defined, 353
  LDA and, 355
  LDA to NCC, relation of, 359
  motivation, 353–354
Near-infrared spectroscopy (NIRS), 526
NEDE, 244–245
Network features, aBCI system, 151, 152t, 155
Neural activity, EEG recordings and, 57
Neural cliques, 122
Neural dust, 123–124
Neural engineering/neuroengineering, 116
Neural interfaces (NIs), 701–712
  artificial sensations, 709–710
  bidirectional, 710–711
  decoding neural signals, 705–708
  defined, 702
  futuristic ideas, 711–712
  motor, 708–709
  neural recordings, 704–705
  overview, 701–702
  types, 702–703
Neural oscillations, in EEG signals, 17
Neural prostheses, see Neural interfaces (NIs)
Neural recordings, 704–705
Neural rehabilitation, 516
Neural signals, decoding, 705–708
Neural tuning, 706
Neuralynx Inc., 283
Neurites, 280, 292
Neuroadaptive systems, 69–70, 82
  automated adaptation, 79–81
  closed-loop adaptation, 77–79
  open-loop adaptation, 75–77
Neurobiohybrids, 125

Neurochip, use, 107
Neuroergonomics, 72
Neurofeedback (NF), 550, 551
  BCI/NF performance, 209, 210–211
    attract users' attention and reduce mind wandering, 224–225
    flow, immersion, and presence, 224
    increasing, 227
    motivation and interest, 212, 224
    studies using games as feedback, 211–212, 213t–223t
  overview, 2, 3
  rehabilitation paradigms, 102, 103–105, 107–108
  type, associative BCIs, 678–679
Neurofeedback therapy, 550, 551–552; see also Attention-based BCIs
Neurological and neurologically related disorders, 116
Neuromarketing, 74
Neuromodulation
  closed-loop BCI systems for, 679
  ECoG BCIs for, 305–308
  inducing plasticity, 669
Neuropace RNS system, 309, 311f
Neurophysiological markers, relevance of, 622–623
Neuropil, 279, 280, 292
Neuroprosthetics, 113–126
  challenges, 122t
  current, 115–122
    memory, cognition, and volition, 120–122
    motor control and movement, 116–117
    neurological and neurologically related disorders, 116
    overview, 115–116
    sensory neuroprosthetics, 117–120
  evolutionary neurobiology and toolmaking, 114–115
  future, 124–125
    bionanoprotonics, 125
    intelligent, biomimetic, and neurobiohybrid, 125
    nanobiotechnology, 125
    synthetic biology, 125
  invasive vs. noninvasive, 126
  microscale BCIs, 122–124
  overview, 114
  security and standards, 126
Neurorehabilitation, 446
Neuroscience, modern, facilitating integration of, 53–63
  applications
    classification accuracy, improving, 59–61
    transfer learning, 61–63
  future directions, 63–64
  mapping noninvasive signals to brain, 56–59
  overview, 53–56
Neuroscience, of attention, 550–551
Neurosky algorithm, 622
Neurotherapy, 2, 102, 103–105, 107–108
Neurotrophic electrode, validation of, 279–293
  conflicts of interest, 295
  discussion, 292–293
  Federal Drug Administration, 295
  functional studies at year 9, 289–292
  implantation, four years after, 283–285
  implantation, nine years after, 286–289
  Institutional Review Board, 295
  methods, 280, 281f–282f
  overview, 279–280
  placements, 283

results, 280, 283
Neurovascular coupling, fMRI principle, 20
NeuroVista device, Australian, 309, 312f
New BCI applications, evolvement of, 516–517
NI-DAQ hardware, 329
NO-GO trials, 182, 184
Noise, discriminative feature of brain activity, 349–353
  amplitude modulations of brain rhythms, 351–353
  ERPs, modulations of, 350–351
  overview, 349, 350
Noisy signals and artifacts, removing, 25–26
Non–BCI-based human–machine interaction, UCD in, 586
Noninvasive alternative for motor-based BCIs
  subdermal electrodes as, utilizing, see Subdermal electrodes, utilizing
Noninvasive BCIs
  facilitating integration of modern neuroscience, see Neuroscience
  recording methods, 15, 16–21
    EEG, 15, 16–19
    fMRI, 15, 20
    fNIRS, 15, 20–21
    MEG, 15, 19
    overview, 16
    PET, 15, 21
  signals to brain, mapping, 56–59
Noninvasive neuroprosthetics, invasive vs., 126
Noninvasive NIs, 703
Nonlinearity, MLP, 32
Nonlinear representations, feature space approach, 428
Non-retinal prosthesis, 709
Nonstationarities, defined, 426
Notations, SSVEP signals, 374, 375f
Number
  selection, BCI experiments, 615–616
Nyquist–Shannon sampling theorem, 403

## O

Objective measures, 569
Occurrence criterion, 389
Ocular prosthetics, 115
Ocular senses, neuroprosthetics, 118–119
Oddball paradigm, 14, 22, 73, 93, 236, 350
Offline analysis, MI BCI training session, 452–453, 452f, 456
Offline BCIs, 690, 696
Offline classification, of SSVEP, 392
Offline estimation, of Riemannian centers of classes, 385
One-versus-the-rest (OVR) strategy, 31
Online and offline implementations, SSVEP-based BCI, 373–374
Online BCIs, 690, 696
Online classification of SSVEP, 392–393
Online experiments, 625
  MI BCI testing session, 456–457, 457f
Online MDM, 386, 388–390
On My Feet Again, 656
Opal Kelly FPGA board, 124f
OpenBCI, 329
OpenEEG, 329
Open-loop adaptation, 75–77
  defined, 75
    examples from literature, 75–76

overview, 75
reflection, 76–77
Open-loop DBS system, 306
Open Sound Control (OSC) protocol, 181
Open task, 568, 569–570, 570t
OpenViBE, 134, 242, 325, 329, 330f, 333f, 457
Operant conditioning, neuroplasticity and, 101
Operating BCIs, brain signal patterns for, 22–25
    overview, 22, 23f, 24f
    P300 ERPs, 22
    SCPs, 25
    SMRs, 24–25
    SSEPs, 22–24
Operation mode, multi-mind BCIs, 696
Operation strategy, BCI, 15
Opportunistic sensing, 246–247
Opportunity for privacy, BCI and, 660–662
Optimal linear decoders, 706
Optogenetics, 117
Orientation, of attention, 551
Origins, BCIs, 2
Orthosis, 95, 102, 103, 105, 106
Orthosis control, MI-and-SSVEP–based, 531
Oscillations, attention-related, 552–553
Oscillations, ECoG low-frequency, 300–302
Oscillatory brain activity, guideline for, 362–363
Overfitting problem, 349, 361, 411–412
Overt attention, 551
Oxyhemoglobin in blood (oxy-Hb), 20

**P**

Pacinian corpuscles, 254, 255f
Paired stimulation (PS), 95
P300- and -SSVEP–based BCIs, 528–530
    P300-and-SSVEP–based BCI spellers, 528–529
    P300-and-SSVEP–based brain switch, 529–530,
        530f
P300-and-SSVEP–based BCI spellers, 528–529
P300-and-SSVEP–based brain switch, 529–530, 530f
*Pan troglodytes* (chimpanzees), 114
PAR (Participatory Action Research), 590
Paradigms
    BCI, *see* Brain–computer interface (BCI), paradigms
    SSVEP, 134–135
Paralysis, 303
Parkinson's disease (PD), 116, 304, 305, 306f
Participant similarity, influence of, 689–690
Passive BCIs, 69–83, 236, 614; *see also specific entries*
    automated adaptation, 79–81
        examples from literature, 80
        overview, 79–80
        reflection, 80–81
    BCI class and paradigm, 255f
    brain patterns, 256
    closed-loop adaptation, 77–79
        examples from literature, 77–79
        overview, 77
        reflection, 79
    cognitive or emotional state, measurement, 256
    measure of user's neurological activity, 155
    mental state assessment, 72–74
        examples from literature, 72–74
        overview, 72

reflection, 74
open-loop adaptation, 75–77
    defined, 75
    examples from literature, 75–76
    overview, 75
    reflection, 76–77
overview, 70–71
Passive multi-mind BCIs, 687
Passive NIs, 703
P300-based BCI applications, 241
    example, 34–36
        communication applications, 34–36
        control applications, 36
P300-based BCIs, 691
PBP, *see* Performance-based paradigm (PBP)
PCA, *see* Principal component analysis (PCA)
Peak negative (PN) phase, of MRCP, 671, 677
Perceived affect, 149
Perceived emotions, 200
Performance, juggling
    by brain and body sonification, 176–181
        application example, 180–181
        data analysis, 179
        experimental protocols, 177–179
        overview, 176–177
        preprocessing, 179
        results, 179–180
        study population, 177
Performance-based paradigm (PBP)
    Bayesian DS algorithm, 490–491
    codebook development, 493–494
    discussion and future work, 498
    methods
        BCI implementation, 494–495
        P300 speller task, 495
    overview, 488–490, 488f
    parameters, 491–493, 492f
    results, 495–498, 496f–497f, 496t
Performance-based parameters, 491–493, 492f
Performance evaluation
    ERP data set, 416
    SMR data set, 418
Performance measurement, BCI system
    continuous BCI, 644–646
        Fitts's law, 645–646
        Shannon's theory, 645
        Shannon–Welford model, 646
    discrete BCI, 637–644
        BCI utility, 640–642
        binary classification accuracy *vs.* task accuracy,
            637–639
        binomial models for accuracy, 638–639, 639f
        classifier-based latency estimation, 644
        confusion matrix, 638
        data scarcity and predicted accuracy, 642–644
        information gain, 639–640
        information transfer rate (ITR), 639–640
        projected accuracy metric, 643–644
        rate of information gain, 640
        utility for P300 speller, 641–642
    general framework, 636–637, 637f
        control interface (CI), 637
        transducer (TR) level, 636–637
    overview, 636

Performance measures, 577t
Peripheral nerve stimulation, 710
P300 ERPs, 14, 22, 34–36, 54, 134, 255, 408; *see also*
    Four-class P300 oddball
Personalized audio cues, 226
Personalized frequency bands, 184, 185
Phase–amplitude coupling (PAC), 302
Physical privacy, 655–656, 655t
Physiology, ECoG signal, 299–303
Pilot-induced oscillations (PIOs), 246
Pioneers, BCIs, 2–3
Placements
    neurotrophic electrode, 283
    subdermal electrodes, 270–271
Plasticity, inducing, 669–680
    cortical, 678, 679
    MRCP and, *see* Movement-related cortical potentials
        (MRCPs)
    overview, 669–671
Platforms, BCI software
    self-contained, 330–335
        BCI2000, 327, 331, 332–335
        OpenViBE, 331, 332f, 335f
    using commercial high-level platforms, 327–330
        LabVIEW, 329–330
        MATLAB®, 327–328
        SIMULINK, 329
Polarization, after-hyperpolarization, 283
Polymer-based microelectrodes, 704
Population vector, defined, 706
"Position" variable, EEGlab, 451, 452
Positron annihilation, phenomenon, 21
Positron emission tomography (PET), 15, 21
Postprocessing, *h*BCI-based ET, 476–477, 476f–478f
Postsynaptic potentials (PSPs), 56
Potential of haptics, for HCI and BCI, 254, 255–256
Potential value, of using game-like FB, 212, 224–227
    attract users' attention and reduce mind wandering,
        224–225
    flow, immersion, and presence, 224
    increasing BCI /NF performance, 227
    intuitive feedback and interactions, 225–226
    mirror neuron system, activating, 226
    motivation and interest, 212, 224
    real-world behavior, transfer to, 226–227
P300 paradigms, 501, 503–506, 503f–506f, 526
    advantages, 462
    audio-tactile P300 BCIs, 537–538, 537f
    audio-visual P300 BCIs, 535–537, 536f
    dependence of BCI applications, 513
    design-related challenges, 509
        adjacency problem, 509, 511
        crowding effect, 509
        fatigue, 511–512
        hardware capacity, 512
        repetition blindness, 511
        user comfortability, 512
        user training, 512
    detection, 508, 509t, 510t–511t
    efficiency and, 512–513
    hybrid SSVEP–P300 paradigm, 513–516, 514f, 515f
    signal processing methods, 508, 510t
Practical BCI solutions, for entertainment and art
    performance, 166–188

brain and body sonification, juggling performance,
    176–181
    application example, 180–181
    data analysis, 179
    experimental protocols, 177–179
    overview, 176–177
    preprocessing, 179
    results, 179–180
    study population, 177
competitive toy car racing using motor imagery BCI,
    171–176
    application example, 175–176
    cue-based measurement, 173, 175t
    data analysis, 174
    evaluation, 174
    experimental protocol, 172–173
    feature extraction and classification, 174
    overview, 171
    preprocessing, 174
    results, 174–175
    self-paced measurements, 173, 175t
    study population, 171–172
discussion, 186, 187–188
for masses, 166–167
monitoring, in children during entertainment and
    learning, 181–186
    application example, 186, 187f
    data analysis, 184
    experimental protocol, 182–184
    overview, 181–182
    preprocessing, 184
    results, 185
    study population, 182
overview, 166–167
technology required for, 167–170
    active sensors, 168
    actuation/information communication, 170
    convenient EEG electrodes, 167–168
    data processing, 170
    EEG headsets, 169–170
    electronic design, 168–169
Predicted accuracy, 642–644
Preferred Reporting Items for Systematic reviews and
    Meta-Analyses (PRISMA), 565
Prefrontal cortex (PFC)
    activity during attentional tasks, 550–551
Premotor theory of attention, 551
Pre-movement potential (PMP), 671
Preprocessing, 526
    MI BCI training session, 451–453, 452f, 456
Preprocessing step
    brain and body sonification, juggling performance,
        179
    competitive toy car racing using motor imagery BCI,
        174
    monitoring, in children during entertainment and
        learning, 184
Presence
    game-like environments, 224
    VR/AR, context of, 236, 239
Primary current, defined, 56
Principal component analysis (PCA), 28, 465
PRISMA (Preferred Reporting Items for Systematic
    reviews and Meta-Analyses), 565

Privacy, and BCI
  and BCI big data, 662–664
  decisional, 655t, 656
  definitions, 654–656, 655t
  informational, 655
  mental privacy, 656–660
  opportunity for, 660–662
  overview, 653–654
  physical, 655–656
Probability estimating guarded neural classifier (PeGNC), 33
Projected accuracy metric, 643–644
Prosthetic hand
  touch and position sensors, 702
  touch feedback in, 257
Prosthetic leg with hinged joints, 115
P300 Speller, 2, 34–36, 462, 487, 488–489, 488f, 495, 614
  BCI session with, 495, 496–497, 497f
P300 speller, 637
  utility for, 641–642
Psychological therapy, 550
Psychostimulants, 550
Psychtoolbox, 398
PubMed, 134, 566
P300 waveform, 462
Pyramidal neurons, 56
Python, 326

## Q

Quadratic discriminant analysis (QDA), 355, 601–602
Quebec User Evaluation of Satisfaction with assistive Technology 2.0 (QUEST 2.0), 575
Questionnaire
  MI data recording in MI BCI training session, 449, 450t, 451
Questionnaire for Current Motivation (QCM), 575
Questions for further research, ECoG, 312–314

## R

Radial basis function (RBF)
  based SVMs, 32
  neural network, 33
Randomization, 626–627
Rapid serial visual presentation
  EEG analysis during, 468
Rapid serial visual presentation (RSVP), 506
Rate of information gain ($RIG_B$), 640
Reactive BCIs, 238, 255, 256, 614; *see also specific entries*
  haptic cues in, 257–260
    ERP-based BCIs, 258–259
    other paradigms, 260
    overview, 257
    SSSEP-based BCIs, 259–260
Readiness potential (RP), 671, 673
Real-time requirement, multi-mind BCIs, 696
Real-world behavior, transfer to, 226–227
Recommendations, haptics and BCI, 261
Recording methods, in BCIs, 15
  invasive, 15, 21–22
    ECoG, 15, 21–22

INR, 15, 22
  overview, 21
noninvasive, 15, 16–21
  EEG, 15, 16–19
  fMRI, 15, 20
  fNIRS, 15, 20–21
  MEG, 15, 19
  overview, 16
  PET, 15, 21
Recordings
  EEG, neural activity and, 57
  FF-WINeR, 123
  initial, of brain activity, 74
  INR, 15, 22
  long-term, in human cortex, validation of neurotrophic electrode, *see* Neurotrophic electrode, validation of
  neural, 704–705
  subdermal and surface electrodes
    low- and high-frequency band power changes, 273–274
    magnitude squared coherence, 272, 274–275
    mu, beta, and high gamma band power changes, 272
  subgaleal, neural signals, 270
recoveriX system, 95–97
Reference electrodes, 17
Referencing methods, 26–28
  bipolar reference, 26, 27
  CAR, 26, 28
  surface Laplacian, 26, 27
Reflection
  automated adaptation, 80–81
  closed-loop adaptation, 79
  mental state assessment, 74
  open-loop adaptation, 76–77
Refractory period, 283
Regional cerebral blood flow (rCBF), 20
Regional cerebral blood oxygenation (rCBO), 20
Region-based paradigm (RBP), 504, 504f, 506
regress() function, 401
Regression problems, MTL in, 434–435
Regularized CSP, feature space approach, 429–431, 439
Regularized Fisher's discriminant analysis (RFDA), 409
Regularized least squares, 411–413
Rehabilitation
  of brain disorders, 107
  ERD/ERS-based BCI controls, 38–39
  fNIRS-based BCI, 242–243
  motor, TMS, 108
  of motor function, 104
  paradigms, current BCI, 102–103
  process, nature, 107
  protocols, development, 106
  SSVEP-based BCI controls, 36–38
  stroke, 243
Rehabilitative system based on BCI and intelligent robot, 542–543
Relevance vector machine, 414
Repetition blindness, BCI paradigms design and, 511
Reporting, affective states, 149–151
  continuous methods, 150–151
  discrete methods, 149–150
Requirements, for software, 324

Research applications
  ECoG-based BCI, 312–314
  for VR/AR, 238
Research field, bloom of, 3–4
Research findings, overview of, 103–107
Responsive Neurostimulator (RNS) system, 309, 311f
Results
  brain and body sonification, juggling performance,
      179–180
  competitive toy car racing using motor imagery BCI,
      174–175
  ERP data set, 416–417
  monitoring, in children during entertainment and
      learning, 185
  neurotrophic electrode, validation of, 280, 283
  SMR data set, 419
  utilizing subdermal electrodes, 273–275
Retinal prosthesis, 709
Retinitis pigmentosa, 118, 119f
Review, of SSVEP-based BCI, 373–374
  online and offline implementations, 373–374
Rhythm, 198
Riemannian centers of classes, offline estimation of, 385
Riemannian classification, feature space approach, 428–429
Riemannian classification, for SSVEP-based BCI, 372–394
  data set, experimental evaluation on, 390–393
      covariance estimators, evaluation of, 390, 391f
      description, 390
      offline classification of SSVEP, 392
      online classification of SSVEP, 392–393
  online and offline implementations, 373–374
  overview, 372–373
  review of SSVEP-based BCI, 373–374
  Riemannian geometry, 378–390
      centers of classes, offline estimation of, 385
      covariance matrices, 378–380
      distances and means, 382–384
      estimation of covariance matrices, 380–382
      MDM classifier, 384–386
      MDM for SSVEP, 386, 387f
      online MDM, 386, 388–390
      overview, 378
  SSVEP signals, classifying, 374–378
      canonical correlation, 374, 375–377
      notations, 374, 375f
      Riemannian geometry, 377–378
Riemannian geometry, 378–390
  centers of classes, offline estimation of, 385
  classifying SSVEP signals, 377–378
  covariance matrices
      estimation of, 380–382
      geometry of, 378–380
  defined, 372
  distances and means, 382–384
  MDM classifier, 384–386
  MDM for SSVEP, 386, 387f
  online MDM, 386, 388–390
  overview, 378
Riemannian manifold, defined, 378
Riemannian Potato, 378
Risk alpha, 624
Robot(s)
  control, P300-based BCI, 36
  humanoid, 334

SSVEP-based collaborative BCIs, 692
  therapy, BCI-controlled, 106
Row–column matrix speller paradigm, 503
Row–column paradigm (RCP), 489, 503
RSVP-based BCI speller, 506
rtsBCI, 327
Ruffini endings/corpuscles, 254, 255f

**S**

Sample covariance matrix (SCM), defined, 381
Sample mean and covariance, defined, 355
Satisfaction, 578, 589
Scalp, convenient EEG electrodes, 167–168
Schimack and Grob three-dimensional model, 148,
      149
Scientific complexity, BCI software, 325
Scope of investigation, BCI software, 325, 326f
Scopus, 566
Second Sight Argus II System, 118
Security, neuroprosthetics, 126
Seizures, 293, 309
Selection control, 568
Selective attention, BCI, 15
Self-assessment manikin (SAM), 149–150
Self-contained BCI software platforms, 330–335
  BCI2000, 327, 331, 332–335
  OpenViBE, 331, 332f, 335f
Self-paced measurements, 173, 175t
Self-paced MRCP, 672
Sensitivity, in ECoG, 21
Sensorimotor behavior, MRCP during, 673–674
  force, 674
  speed/velocity of movement, 673–674
  type of movement, 673
Sensorimotor loop, closing, 102, 103, 105, 106
Sensorimotor rhythms (SMR), 568, 596
Sensorimotor rhythms (SMR)-based BCI
  for ADHD, 106
  beta rhythms, 107
  data set, Bayesian learning, 418–419
      data description, 418
      performance evaluation, 418
      results, 419
  desynchronization, 102
  feedback based on, 102
  modulations, 106–107, 235
  overview, 2–3, 15, 24–25, 54, 408
  sensor space features for, 60
  training, 102, 104, 106
  voluntary desynchronization, 106
  VR and, 137, 237–239
Sensors
  selection, BCI experiments, 615–616
Sensor space
  defined, 55
  source space vs., 55f, 56
Sensory neuroprosthetics, 117–120
  auditory, 117–118
  ocular, 118–119
  somatosensory system, 119–120
Separating hyperplane
  classification and, 353–354
  defined, 353

Sequential processing, 463
Serious games, defined, 211
Setups, VR/AR, 237–238
    BCI/VR, example architecture for, 244–245
Sham control, 626–627
Shannon's theory, 645
Shannon–Welford model, 646
Short term variability, 597
Shrinkage LDA (SKLDA), 409
Shrinkage parameter, 361
Signals
    noninvasive, to brain, 56–59
    SSVEP, classifying, 374–378
        canonical correlation, 374, 375–377
        notations, 374, 375f
        Riemannian geometry, 377–378
Signal, discriminative feature of brain activity, 349–353
    amplitude modulations of brain rhythms, 351–353
    ERPs, modulations of, 350–351
    overview, 349, 350
Signal, ECoG
    acquisition, 298–299
    physiology, 299–303
Signal acquisition and open source platform
    ECoG-based BCIs, see Electrocorticography (ECoG)
    neurotrophic electrode, validation of, see Neurotrophic
        electrode, validation of
    software, see Software, BCI
    subdermal electrodes, utilizing, see Subdermal
        electrodes, utilizing
Signal acquisition methods, 13, 15–25
    brain signal patterns for BCI operation, 22–25
        overview, 22, 23f, 24f
        P300 ERPs, 22
        SCPs, 25
        SMRs, 24–25
        SSEPs, 22–24
    invasive methods, 15, 21–22
        ECoG, 15, 21–22
        INR, 15, 22
        overview, 21
    noninvasive methods, 15, 16–21
        EEG, 15, 16–19
        fMRI, 15, 20
        fNIRS, 15, 20–21
        MEG, 15, 19
        overview, 16
        PET, 15, 21
Signal acquisition module, single-user BCI, 688
Signal processing, feature extraction, and classification
    Bayesian learning, for EEG analysis, see Bayesian
        learning, for EEG analysis
    EP BCIs, see Evoked potential (EP) BCIs
    Riemannian classification, for SSVEP-based BCI, see
        Riemannian classification, for SSVEP-based BCI
    for single-trial EEG analysis, see Single-trial EEG analysis
    transfer learning, for BCIs, see Transfer learning
Signal quality, improving, 25–30
    overview, 25
    removing noisy signals and artifacts, 25–26
    spatial filtering methods, 26–30
        bipolar reference, 26, 27
        CAR, 26, 28
        CSP, 29–30

        data-dependent, 28–30
        ICA, 28, 29
        PCA, 28
        referencing methods, 26–28
        surface Laplacian reference, 26, 27
Signals acquisition (BCI experiments), see Acquisition of
        signals (BCI experiments), design guidelines
Signal-to-noise ratio, of MRCPs, 675
Signal variability, 598
    causes of, 597–598
SigViewer, 244
Silver/silver chloride (Ag/AgCl) electrodes, 167, 168, 169
SIMULINK, 326, 327, 329
Simultaneous processing, 463
Single-character paradigm (SCP), 503–504, 504f
Single-trial EEG analysis, 343–367
    classification, multivariate approach to, 347–349, 350f
    discriminative features of brain activity, signal and
        noise, 349–353
        amplitude modulations of brain rhythms, 351–353
        ERPs, modulations of, 350–351
        overview, 349, 350
    feature extraction, 362–366
        CCA, 366
        CSP analysis, 363–366
        guideline for transient activity, ERP and LRP, 362
        oscillatory brain activity, guideline for, 362–363
        overview, 362
    formalization of CSP as two-step procedure, 366–367
    linear classification, 353–362
        Gaussian distributions and related transformations,
            356–359
        LDA, 355–356
        LDA, remark on assumptions of, 359–361
        LDA, with shrinkage of covariance matrix, 361
        LDA to NCC, whitening, and mahalanobis
            distance, relation of, 359
        motivation, NCC, 353–354
        other methods, 362
        overview, 353
    overview, 343–344
    uni- to multivariate features, 346–347
    univariate features and amplitude threshold criterion,
        344–345
Single unit activity (SUA), 22
Single-user BCIs, 692
Slater–Usoh–Steed questionnaire, 236
Sleep disorders, 106
Slow cortical potentials (SCPs), 3, 15, 25, 462
SMR, see Somatosensory rhythm (SMR)
Social Mirroring Game, 226
Socio-Cognitive Model of Technology, 591
Software, BCI, 323–335
    impact, 335
    implementation, 325–335
        BCI2000, 327, 331, 332–335
        LabVIEW, 329–330
        MATLAB®, 325, 326–327, 327–328
        OpenViBE, 331, 332f, 335f
        overview, 325–327
        platforms using commercial high-level platforms,
            327–330
        self-contained BCI software platforms, 330–335
        SIMULINK, 329

overview, 323–325
purpose, 323
requirements for, 324
scope of investigation, 325, 326f
technical demands, 324–325, 326f
Software and device
for MI data recording, 446, 447f, 449
Solutions, practical BCI, *see* Practical BCI solutions
Somatosensory rhythm (SMR)
event-related desynchronization/synchronization
(ERD/ERS) of, 452–453, 452f, 596
Somatosensory sensations, artificial, 709
Somatosensory system, neuroprosthetics, 119–120
Sonification
brain and body, juggling performance, 176–181
application example, 180–181
data analysis, 179
experimental protocols, 177–179
overview, 176–177
preprocessing, 179
results, 179–180
study population, 177
brainwave data, 197–198
Source estimation, 56, 57
Source imaging, 53, 56, 58, 59, 61
Source space
defined, 56
sensor space *vs.*, 55f, 56
*Space Invaders*, 693
Sparse Bayesian learning (SBL), 410, 414–415, 416–417,
418, 419
Spatial attention, 551
Spatial filtering, 526
algorithm, 3
defined, 347
Spatial filtering methods, 26–30
data-dependent, 28–30
CSP, 29–30
ICA, 28, 29
PCA, 28
referencing methods, 26–28
bipolar reference, 26, 27
CAR, 26, 28
surface Laplacian reference, 26, 27
Spatial filters, 349, 377
Spatial resolution, 616–617
of INR, 22
Spatio-spectral decomposition (SSD), 366
Speech recognition, 33
Speed/velocity of movement, 673–674
Spelling task, 568, 569
Spherical morphing procedure, 59
Spikes, 283, 284f–285f, 286, 286f–287f
Spontaneous BCIs paradigms, 596
SSVEP, *see* Steady-state visual evoked potential
(SSVEP)
SSVEP-based BCI applications
for elderly people, 133–141
GUI, design of, 138, 139, 140–141
number of classes, 136–137, 138t
overview, 133–134
paradigm, 134–135
parameters, customization of, 135–138
stimulation frequencies, 136–137, 138t

time windows, 137, 138, 139f, 139t, 140f
example, 36–38
communication, 36
control, 36–38
SSVEP-BCI ITR, 470
SSVEP paradigms, 501, 507–508, 507f
amplitudes with different frequencies, 507, 507f
dependence of BCI applications, 513
design-related challenges, 509
adjacency problem, 509, 511
crowding effect, 509
fatigue, 511–512
hardware capacity, 512
repetition blindness, 511
user comfortability, 512
user training, 512
detection, 508, 509t, 510t–511t
efficiency and, 512–513
hybrid SSVEP–P300 paradigm, 513–516, 514f, 515f
signal processing methods, 508, 510t
Stability, 526
Standards, neuroprosthetics, 126
State-dependent trial presentations, 103, 107
Statistical learning framework, model space learning, *see*
Model space learning
Statistical tests, selection of, 627, 628t, 629
Steady-state auditory evoked potentials (SSAEPs), 14–15,
23, 332
Steady-state evoked potentials (SSEPs), 14–15, 22–24,
236, 253, 255, 257–258
Steady-state response (SSR), 373
Steady-state somatosensory evoked potentials (SSSEPs),
15, 23, 255, 257–258
Steady-state visual evoked potentials (SSVEPs), 465–466,
501, 526, 568, 596
attention-based BCIs and, 554
BCI2000, 334
CCA method, 366
collaborative BCIs, 692
defined, 238
in EEG, 193, 194, 197, 198f, 199
ET with, 468–469
eye gaze and, 469
architecture, 472–475, 473f, 474t
ET component, 470, 471, 471f
ET inclusion, 469–470
experimental protocol, 475–476
postprocessing, 476–477, 476f–478f
SSVEP BCI component, 472
visual interface application design, 470, 471f
multi-mind BCI, 688
musical control, 193, 194, 197, 198f, 199f
*n*-class SSVEP, 402–405
considerations, 405
data collection, 403
data preprocessing, 404
data segmentation and classification, 404–405
overview, 402–403
overview, 3, 15, 23–24, 30, 54, 462–463
Riemannian classification, *see* Riemannian
classification, for SSVEP-based BCI
SSVEP-based BCI application, *see* SSVEP-based BCI
applications
VR/AR, 241

Stein kernel, 377
Stepwise linear discriminant analysis (SWLDA), 409,
    416–417
Stimulation frequencies, 136–137, 138t
Stimulator with surface electrodes, 116
Stimulus, 568, 571
    machine output of adaptive BCI systems, 606
    modality, 13–14, 15
Stimulus-responsive input measures, 197
Stroke patients
    associative BCI, 677
    BCI as rehabilitation tool, 242, 243
    BCI for, 89–90, 95–97, 97t
    BCI2000 for, 334
    detecting gait initiation from MRCPs, 676, 677
    epidural ECoG, 314
    ipsilateral ECoG activity, 303
    neurofeedback for, 102
Study population
    brain and body sonification, juggling performance, 177
    competitive toy car racing using motor imagery BCI,
        171–172
    monitoring vigilance in children during entertainment
        and learning, 182
Study selection, usability evaluation, 565–566, 565f
Subcortically implanted electrodes, 306
Subcutaneous electrodes, 271
Subdermal electrodes, utilizing, 270–275
    discussion, 275–276
    materials and methods, 270–272
        data acquisition, 272
        data preprocessing, 272
        magnitude squared coherence, 272
        mu, beta, and high gamma band power changes, 272
        placement, 270–271
        subjects, 270
        task, 271–272
    overview, 270
    results, 273–275
        low- and high-frequency band power changes,
            273–274
        magnitude squared coherence, 274–275
Subdural cavity, 123
Subdural ECoG, 314
Subgaleal recordings, neural signals, 270
Subjective measures, 569
Subjects, MI data recording in MI BCI training session,
    447, 449, 451
Substance use disorders, 102
Substitutive strategy, defined, 101
Sulcal/gyral regions, 59
SuperColider, 181
Superconducting quantum interference device (SQUID),
    19
Support vector machine (SVM), 31–32, 376, 416–417, 419,
    456, 526, 602
Suprachoroidal retinal implants, 118, 119f
Surface electrodes
    placement, 271
    recordings
        low- and high-frequency band power changes,
            273–274
        magnitude squared coherence, 272, 274–275
        mu, beta, and high gamma band power changes, 272

Surface Laplacian reference methods, 26, 27
Sustained Attention to Response Task (SART) protocol,
    182–184
Swelling effect, defined, 383
Symmetric and positive-definite (SPD) covariance
    matrices, 377, 379t, 382–384
Synchronous BCIs, 15, 29, 152, 154
Synthetic biology, neuroprosthetics, 125
System pipeline, adaptive BCI systems, 600–602, 600f
    classifier, 600
    decision, 600
    EEG features, 600
    literature review on adaptive signal processing/
        machine learning, 601–602
        adaptive classifiers, 601–602
        adaptive decision methods, 602
        adaptive feature extraction, 601
        fully adaptive signal processing, 602
System Usability Scale survey (SUS survey), 575

T

Tactile feedback, 257
Tactile sensing, 254, 255f
Tactile speller, 258
Tactile stimulation
    P300-based BCI, 34–36
    SSVEP-based BCIs, 36–38
Tangent space approximation, 429
Target detection, multi-mind BCIs, 693–694
Target-to-target interval (TTI), 489, 492–493
Task accuracy, vs. binary classification accuracy, 637–639
    binomial models for accuracy, 638–639, 639f
    confusion matrix, 638
Task characteristics, usability evaluation and, 567t,
    569–571, 570t
Task model, adaptive BCI systems, 603, 603f, 605
Technical demands, BCI software, 324–325, 326f
Technical validation, VR/AR, 245–246
Technologies
    for practical BCI solutions, 167–170
        active sensors, 168
        actuation/information communication, 170
        convenient EEG electrodes, 167–168
        data processing, 170
        EEG headsets, 169–170
        electronic design, 168–169
    therapeutic applications, 101–108
        current BCI rehabilitation paradigms, 102–103
        discussion, 107–108
        overview, 101–102
        research findings, overview of, 103–107
Technology characteristics, usability evaluation and, 567t,
    568, 572t–573t, 573–574
Telemetry unit, implantable, 310, 311, 312f
Temporal filtering, 347, 526
Temporalis, 117
Temporal resolution, of INR, 22
Tension, defined, 148
Testing data set, BCI experiments, 620
Testing method, 568, 574t
Testing session, MI BCI
    discussion, 457–458
    online experiment, 456–457, 457f

Tetraplegia, 303
Tetraplegic patient, 709
Tetris, 78
Thalamocortical networks, of disease, 306
Theoretical aspects, multi-mind BCIs, 687–690
    challenges, 690
    collective brain, implementing, 688–689
    history, 687–688
    influence of participant similarity, forming groups,
        689–690
    minds, need, 689
Therapeutic applications, BCIs
    aBCIs, 156
    of BCI technologies, *see* Technologies, therapeutic
        applications
    DOC, patients with, 89–90, 90–95, 97t
    motor rehabilitation, 89–90, 95–97, 97t
    neuroprosthetics, *see* Neuroprosthetics
    SSVEP-based BCI application, *see* SSVEP-based BCI
        applications
    stroke patients, 89–90, 95–97, 97t
Therapeutic intervention, VR-BCIs for, 242–243
Theta-contingent group, 107
Thought Translation Device (TTD), 3, 25
Three dimentions (3D), game-like feedback scenario,
    224–225, 227–228
Tic-Tac-Toe game, 226
Tikhonov regularization, 58
Tikhonov regularizer, 431
Time windows, 137, 138, 139f, 139t, 140f
Tines, 279–280, 293
Toolmaking, BCI and, 114–115
Touch
    defined, 254
    feedback in prosthetic hand, 257
Tourette syndrome (TS), 116, 304–305, 306f
Toy car racing using motor imagery BCI, 171–176
    application example, 175–176
    cue-based measurement, 173, 175t
    data analysis, 174
    evaluation, 174
    experimental protocol, 172–173
    feature extraction and classification, 174
    overview, 171
    preprocessing, 174
    results, 174–175
    self-paced measurements, 173, 175t
    study population, 171–172
TrainERPs, input argument, 401
Training
    BCI and NF, 211
    classifier, 401
    CSP-based classification, 366
    data set, BCI experiments, 620
    ECoG BCIs, 304
    EEG features for, 105–106
    enhanced motor imagery, 102, 103
    game-like NF, 224, 227
    goal, feedback and, 102
    NI session, 707
    paradigm, 102
    protocol, design of, 211
    recoveriX, 95–97
    SMR, 102, 104, 106

Training phase, ERP-based BCIs, 596
Training session, MI BCI
    algorithms and offline analysis, 451–456, 452f
        classification, 454–455, 455f, 456
        discussions, 456
        feature extraction, 453–454, 454f, 456
        preprocessing, 451–453, 452f, 456
    MI data recording, 446–451
        device and software, 446, 447f, 449
        discussions, 449, 451
        environment, 447, 451
        experimental paradigm, 447–448, 448f, 448t,
            451
        MI instructions, 449, 449f, 451
        questionnaire, 449, 450t, 451
        subjects, 447, 449, 451
Transcranial magnetic stimulation (TMS), use, 108
Transcranial magnetic stimulation/electrical stimulation,
    711
Transducer (TR) level, 636–637, 637f
Transductive transfer learning, 62
Transfer learning, for BCIs, 61–63, 425–440
    drawback for, 439
    feature space approaches, 427–431
        nonlinear representations, 428
        overview, 427
        regularized CSP, 429–431
        Riemannian classification, 428–429
    mathematical notation, 427
    model space learning, 431–440
        calibration-free decoding and model adaptation,
            437, 438f
        dimensionality reduction in EEG, feature
            decomposition, 437, 438–439
        MTL in classification problems, 435–437
        MTL in regression problems, 434–435
        multitask linear regression, 434–435
        overview, 431–433
    overview, 425–427
Transformations, related, Gaussian distributions and,
    356–359
Transient activity, guideline for, 362
Translation algorithms, 526
Translational research, goals, 722
Traumatic brain injury, 242
Treatment-resistant obsessive–compulsive disorder, 116
Trial presentations, 103, 107
Trophic factors, 280, 281f, 283, 293
Tutorial, multi-mind BCIs, 695–697
    application, 695
    fusion of brain signals, 696–697
    number of users, 695–696
    operation mode, 696
    real-time requirement, 696
Twitches, defined, 260
Two dimentions (2D), game-like feedback scenario, 224
Two-sided *t* test, 624
"Type" variable, EEGlab, 451, 452


U

UCD, *see* User-centered design (UCD)
Unisensory stimulation, 260
Unity 3D, 244–245

Univariate features, single-trial EEG analysis, 344–345, 346–347
Unresponsive wakeful state (UWS), 90–95, 97t
Unscented Kalman filter (UKF), 706, 710
Usability, 564
Usability evaluation, for BCIs, 563–579
  defined, 589
  overview, 564
  PRISMA flow diagram, 565–566, 565f
  recommendations, 579
  results
    environment characteristics, 571–573, 571t
    measurement characteristics, 575–578, 576t–577t, 578f
    method characteristics, 574t, 575
    task characteristics, 569–571, 570t
    technology characteristics, 572t–573t, 573–574
    user characteristics, 569, 569t, 570f
  review method, 565
    eligibility criteria, 565
    study selection, 565–566, 565f
    usability framework, 566–569, 566f, 567t
USC/DARPA trial, 121
USE Questionnaire, 575
"User activity," 567
User and VR/AR, interfaces between, 246
User-centered design (UCD), 579, 585–591
  BCI research and, 590–591
  defined, 587
  described, 586–588, 587f
  do-it-yourself UCD and evaluation, 591
  end-users, 586
  goal of, 586–587, 590
  implementation in BCI applications, 588
  in non–BCI-based human–machine interaction, 586
  overview, 586
  relevance of, 586
  role of evaluation, 589
  user involvement, 589–590
  user-oriented BCI applications, 589
User characteristics, usability evaluation and, 567–568, 567t, 569, 569t, 570f
User comfortability, BCI paradigms design and, 512
User component (BCI experiments), design guidelines
  biases, avoidance of, 626–627
  good control group, 625–626
  state of mind in new BCI experiment, 624–625
  statistical tests selection, 627, 628t, 629
User Datagram Protocol (UDP) packet, 474
User experiences (UX), 579
User involvement, UCD in BCI applications and, 589–590
User model, adaptive BCI systems, 603–604, 603f, 604t
User-oriented approaches, BCMI, 196–197
User-oriented BCI applications, UCD in, 589
Users
  number, multi-mind BCIs, 695–696
  training, BCI paradigms design and, 512
  variability, 598
Users' attention, attracting, 224–225
User's emotions
  modulating, 156
  understanding, 156
Utah array, 704, 710

**V**

Valance
  defined, 148
  increasing, 157, 158
Valance–arousal circumplex model, 148
Validation
  of example architecture, VR/AR, 245–246
    experimental, 246
    latency and jitter of processing, 245–246
    technical, 245–246
  neurotrophic electrodes, *see* Neurotrophic electrode, validation of
Variability, 597
  long term, 597
  short term, 597
  signal, causes of, 597–598
  user, 598
Variance, of band-pass–filtered signals, 363
Vibrotactile-2 (VTP2) approach, mindBEAGLE system, 91, 92f
Vibrotactile-3 (VTP3) approach, mindBEAGLE system, 91, 92, 93–94
Vibrotactile feedback, 257
Video games
  cooperative and competitive, 693
  multi-mind BCIs, application, 692–693
Vigilance
  monitoring, in children during entertainment and learning, 181–186
    application example, 186, 187f
    data analysis, 184
    experimental protocol, 182–184
    overview, 181–182
    preprocessing, 184
    results, 185
    study population, 182
Virtual and augmented reality (VR/AR), 236–247
  AR and BCIs, 243–244
  fidelity, immersion and presence, 236
  future developments, 246–247
    novel interfaces between user and, 246
    opportunistic sensing, 246–247
  general research applications for, 238
  limitations, 246
  measures of interest, 236
  overview, 236–238
  setups, 237–238
  validation of example architecture, 245–246
    experimental validation, 246
    latency and jitter of processing, 245–246
    technical, 245–246
  VR and BCIs, 238–243
    for control and exploration, 238–242
    setup, example architecture for, 244–245
    therapeutic intervention, 242–243
Virtual limbs, 226
Virtual reality (VR)
  BCIs and, 238–243; *see also* Virtual and augmented reality (VR/AR)
    for control and exploration, 238–242
    setup, example architecture for, 244–245
    therapeutic intervention, 242–243
  game-like FB, 210, 211, 224, 226, 227, 228

Visual Analog Scale (VAS), 575
Visual evoked potential (VEP), 465
Visual image classification, 516
Visual interface application design, *h*BCI, 470, 471
Visual paradigms, BCI, 502–503; *see also specific types*
Visual prosthesis, 709
Visual speller, 258
Visual stimulation
    P300-based BCI, 34–36
    SSVEP-based BCIs, 36–38
Visual stimulus, SSVEP-based BCI, 373
Viterbi algorithm, 33
Volition, 120–122
Voluntary desynchronization, in SMRs, 106

**W**

Wavelet common spatial pattern (WCSP), 29
Web of Science, 566
Welch method, 179, 184, 272
Welford's model, 646
Wernicke's area, 305
Wheelchair, 35t, 37t, 38t
    control, 36, 208, 237, 332
    control, P300-based BCI, 36
    intelligent, based on BCI and autonomous navigation
        system, 541–542, 541f
    virtual, 258
    in VR, 226–227
Wheelchair control, MI-and-P300–based, 534–535
Whitening and LDA, relation, 359
Wiener filters, 706
Wii Remote, 695
Wilcoxon signed-rank test, 495
WIMAGINE system, French, 309, 311f
Wireless multi-electrode arrays, 117
Wireless neuroprosthetics technology study, 117
Workload, measures of
    online operation, 77–78
    questionnaire, 72–73
World of Warcraft, 692

**Z**

Zen Wheels micro cars, 175
"zurück," command, 139

T - #0454 - 071024 - C816 - 254/178/38 - PB - 9780367375454 - Gloss Lamination